Commonly Used Symbols and Abbreviations

$(A-a)PO_2diff$	difference between partial pressure of oxygen in alveoli and arterial blood
$a-vO_2diff$	difference in oxygen content between arterial and venous blood
A	actin
ACh	acetylcholine
ACTH	adrenocorticotrophic hormone
ADH	antidiuretic hormone
ADL	activities of daily living
ADP	adenosine diphosphate
AI	adequate intake
AIDS	acquired immune deficiency syndrome
AMP	adenosine monophosphate
ANS	autonomic nervous system
AP	action potential
ATP	adenosine triphosphate
ATP-PC	phosphagen system
ATPS	atmostpheric temperature and pressure, saturated air
AV	atrioventricular
BCAA	branched chain amino acids
BF	body fat
BMC	bone mineral content
BMD	bone mineral density
BMI	body mass index
BMR	basal metabolic rate
BP	blood pressure
BTPS	body temperature and pressure, saturated air
BW	body weight
CAD	coronary artery disease
CHD	coronary heart disease
CHO	carbohydrate
CNS	central nervous system
CP	creatine phosphate
CR-10	category ratio scale of perceived exertion
D_B	density of the body
D_W	density of water
DBP	diastolic blood pressure
DOMS	delayed-onset muscle soreness
DRI	daily reference intake
DXA	dual-energy X-ray absorptiometry
E	epinephrine
ECG	electrocardiogram
EDV	end diastolic volume
EF	ejection fraction
EIAH	exercise-induced arterial hypoxemia
EMG	electromyogram
EPOC	excess postexercise oxygen consumption
ERT	estrogen replacement therapy
ESV	end systolic volume
ETAP	exercise-related transient abdominal pain
ETS	electron transport system
F_ECO_2	fraction of expired carbon dioxide
F_EN_2	fraction of expired nitrogen
F_EO_2	fraction of expired oxygen
F_G	fraction of a gas
F_ICO_2	fraction of inspired carbon dioxide
F_IN_2	fraction of inspired nitrogen
F_IO_2	fraction of inspired oxygen
f	frequency
FAD	flavin adenine dinucleotide
FEV	forced expiratory volume
FFA	free fatty acids
FFB	fat-free body mass
FFM	fat-free mass
FFW	fat-free weight
FG	fast twitch, glycolytic muscle fibers
FI	fatigue index
FOG	fast twitch, oxidative-glycolytic muscle fibers
FT	fast twitch muscle fibers
GAS	General Adaptation Syndrome
GH	growth hormone
GLUT-1	non-insulin regulated glucose transporter
GLUT-4	insulin regulated glucose transporter
GTO	Golgi tendon organ
Hb	hemoglobin
HbO_2	oxyhemoglobin
HDL-C	high-density lipoprotein
HIV	human immunosupression virus
HR	heart rate
HRmax	maximal heart rate
HRR	heart rate reserve
HT	height
ICD	isocitrate dehydrogenase
ICP	isovolumetric contraction period
IRP	isovolumetric relaxation period
LA	lactic acid/glycolytic system
LBM	lean body mass
LBP	low back pain
LDL-C	low-density lipoprotein
LSD	long, slow distance
LT	lactate threshold
M_A	mass of the body in the air
M_W	mass of the body underwater
M	myosin
MAOD	maximal accumulated oxygen deficit
MAP	mean arterial pressure
MCT1	extracellular and intracellular monocarboxylate lactate transporter
MCT4	extracellular monocarboxylate lactate transporter
MET	metabolic equivalent
MLSS	maximal lactate steady state

MP	mean power
MVC	maximal voluntary contraction
MVV	maximal voluntary ventilation
NAD	nicotinamide adenine dinucleotide
NE	norepinephrine
NK	natural killer
NKCA	natural killer cell activity
NMJ	neuromuscular junction
NMS	neuromuscular spindle
NT	neurotransmitter
OBLA	onset of blood lactate accumulation
OP	oxidative phosphorylation
OTS	overtraining syndrome
P_A	pressure in the alveoli
P_ACO_2	partial pressure of carbon dioxide in the alveoli
P_AO_2	partial pressure of oxygen in the alveoli
P_B	barometric pressure
P_G	partial pressure of a gas
P_i	inorganic phosphate
P	pressure
$PaCO_2$	partial pressure of carbon dioxide in arterial blood
PaO_2	partial pressure of oxygen in arterial blood
PC	phosphocreatine
PCO_2	partial pressure of carbon dioxide
PFK	phosphofructokinase
pH	hydrogen ion concentration
PN_2	partial pressure of nitrogen
PNF	proprioceptive neuromuscular facilitation
PNS	peripheral nervous system
PO_2	partial pressure of oxygen
PP	peak power
PRO	protein
PvO_2	partial pressure of oxygen in venous blood
$PvCO_2$	partial pressure of carbon dioxide in venous blood
$\dot{Q}$	cardiac output
R_a	rate of appearance
R_d	rate of disappearance
R	resistance
RBC	red blood cells
RDA	recommended daily allowance
RER	respiratory exchange ratio
RH	relative humidity
RHR	resting heart rate
RM	repetition maximum
RMR	resting metabolic rate
RMT	respiratory muscle training
ROM	range of motion
RPE	rating of perceived exertion
RPP	rate pressure product
RQ	respiratory quotient
RV	residual volume
$SaO_2\%$	percent saturation of arterial blood with oxygen
$SbO_2\%$	percent saturation of blood with oxygen
$SvO_2\%$	percent saturation of venous blood with oxygen
SBP	systolic blood pressure
SO	slow twitch, oxidative muscle fibers
SR	sarcoplasmic reticulum
SSC	stretch shortening cycle

ST	slow-twitch muscle fibers
STPD	standard temperature and pressure, dry air
SV	stroke volume
T	temperature
T_{amb}	ambient temperature
TC	total cholesterol
T_{co}	core temperature
TEF	thermic effect of feeding
TEM	thermic effect of a meal
TExHR	target exercise heart rate
$TExVO_2$	target exercise oxygen consumption
TG	triglycerides
TLC	total lung capacity
TPR	total peripheral resistance
T_{re}	rectal temperature
T_{sk}	skin temperature
T_{tym}	tympanic temperature
URTI	upper respiratory tract infection
$\dot{V}_A$	alveolar ventilation
$\dot{V}_D$	volume of dead space
$\dot{V}_E$	volume of expired air
$\dot{V}_G$	volume of a gas
V_I	volume of inspired air
V_T	tidal volume
$\dot{V}$	volume per unit of time
V	volume
VAT	visceral abdominal tissue
VC	vital capacity
VCO_2	volume of carbon dioxide produced
VEP	ventricular ejection period
VFP	ventricular filling period
VLDL	very low density lipoproteinn
$\dot{V}O_2$	volume of oxygen consumed
$\dot{V}O_2max$	maximal volume of oxygen consumed
$\dot{V}O_2peak$	peak volume of oxygen consumed
$\dot{V}O_2R$	oxygen consumption reserve
VT	ventilatory threshold
$v\dot{V}O_2max$	velocity at maximal oxygen consumption
W/H	waist-to-hip ratio
WBC	white blood cells
WT	weight

Icon Identification Guide

Short-term, light to moderate submaximal aerobic

Long-term, moderate to heavy submaximal aerobic

Incremental aerobic to maximum

Static

Dynamic resistance

Very short-term, high-intensity anaerobic exercise

Exercise Physiology

FOR HEALTH, FITNESS, AND PERFORMANCE

Fourth Edition

Sharon A. Plowman
Northern Illinois University

Denise L. Smith
Skidmore College

Wolters Kluwer | Lippincott Williams & Wilkins
Health

Philadelphia · Baltimore · New York · London
Buenos Aires · Hong Kong · Sydney · Tokyo

Acquisitions Editor: Emily Lupash
Product Manager: Linda G. Francis
Production Project Manager: Cynthia Rudy
Marketing Manager: Sarah Schuessler
Designer: Stephen Druding
Compositor: SPi Global

Fourth Edition

Library of Congress Cataloging-in-Publication Data
Plowman, Sharon A.
  Exercise physiology for health, fitness, and performance / Sharon A. Plowman, Denise L. Smith. — 4th ed.
       p. ; cm.
  Includes bibliographical references and index.
  ISBN 978-1-4511-7611-7
  I. Smith, Denise L. II. Title.
  [DNLM: 1. Exercise—physiology. WE 103]

612'.044—dc23

2012038286

DISCLAIMER
Care has been taken to confirm the accuracy of the information present and to describe generally accepted practices. However, the authors, editors, and publisher are not responsible for errors or omissions or for any consequences from application of the information in this book and make no warranty, expressed or implied, with respect to the currency, completeness, or accuracy of the contents of the publication. Application of this information in a particular situation remains the professional responsibility of the practitioner; the clinical treatments described and recommended may not be considered absolute and universal recommendations.

The authors, editors, and publisher have exerted every effort to ensure that drug selection and dosage set forth in this text are in accordance with the current recommendations and practice at the time of publication. However, in view of ongoing research, changes in government regulations, and the constant flow of information relating to drug therapy and drug reactions, the reader is urged to check the package insert for each drug for any change in indications and dosage and for added warnings and precautions. This is particularly important when the recommended agent is a new or infrequently employed drug.

Some drugs and medical devices presented in this publication have Food and Drug Administration (FDA) clearance for limited use in restricted research settings. It is the responsibility of the health care provider to ascertain the FDA status of each drug or device planned for use in their clinical practice.

To purchase additional copies of this book, call our customer service department at **(800) 638-3030** or fax orders to **(301) 223-2320**. International customers should call **(301) 223-2300**.

Visit Lippincott Williams & Wilkins on the Internet: http://www.lww.com. Lippincott Williams & Wilkins customer service representatives are available from 8:30 am to 6:00 pm, EST.

9 8 7 6 5 4 3 2 1

To our teachers and students,
past, present, and future:
sometimes one and the same.

About the Authors

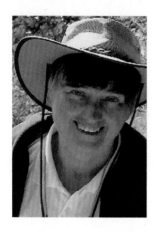

SHARON A. PLOWMAN earned her Ph.D. at the University of Illinois at Urbana–Champaign under the tutelage of Dr. T. K. Cureton Jr. She is a professor emeritus from the Department of Kinesiology and Physical Education at Northern Illinois University. Dr. Plowman taught for, 36 years, including classes in exercise physiology, stress testing, and exercise bioenergetics. She has published over 70 scientific and research articles in the field as well as numerous applied articles on physical fitness with emphasis on females and children in such journals as *ACSM's Health & Fitness Journal; Annals of Nutrition and Metabolism; Human Biology; Medicine & Science in Sports & Exercise; Pediatric Exercise Science;* and *Research Quarterly for Exercise and Sport.* She is a coauthor of the Dictionary of the Sport and Exercise Sciences (M. H. Anshel ed., 1991) and has published several chapters in other books.

Dr. Plowman is a Fellow Emeritus of the American College of Sports Medicine, and served on the Board of Trustees of that organization from 1980 to 1983. In 1992 she was elected an Active Fellow by the American Academy of Kinesiology and Physical Education. She serves on the Advisory Council for FITNESSGRAM®. The American Alliance for Health, Physical Education, Recreation and Dance (AAHPERD) recognized her with the Mabel Lee Award in 1976 and the Physical Fitness Council Award in 1994. Dr. Plowman received the Excellence in Teaching Award (at Northern Illinois University at the department level in 1974 and 1975 and at the university level in 1975) and the Distinguished Alumni Award from the Department of Kinesiology at the University of Illinois at Urbana–Champaign in 1996. In 2006 the President's Council on Physical Fitness and Sports presented her with their Honor Award in recognition of her contributions made to the advancement and promotion of the science of physical activity.

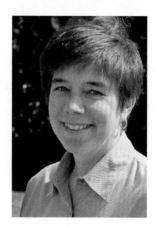

DENISE L. SMITH is a Professor of Exercise Science and recipient of the Class of 1961 Chair at Skidmore College. She also serves as the Director of the First Responder Health and Safety Research Laboratory. With a Ph.D. in kinesiology and specialization in exercise physiology from the University of Illinois at Urbana–Champaign, Dr. Smith has taught for over 20 years, including classes in anatomy and physiology, exercise physiology, clinical aspects of cardiovascular health, cardiorespiratory aspects of human performance, neuromuscular aspects of human performance, and research design. Her research is focused on the cardiovascular strain associated with heat stress, particularly as it relates to cardiac, vascular, and coagulatory function. She has published her research findings in such journals as *American Journal of Cardiology; Cardiology in Review; Medicine & Science in Sports & Exercise; Vascular Medicine; Ergonomics; European Journal of Applied Physiology; Journal of Applied Physiology;* and *Journal of Cardiopulmonary Rehabilitation.* She is also a coauthor of "Advanced Cardiovascular Exercise Physiology," an upper-level text that is part of the Advanced Exercise Physiology series.

Dr. Smith is a Fellow in the American College of Sports Medicine and has served as secretary for the Occupational Physiology Interest Group and as a member of the National Strategic Health Initiative Committee. She has served on the executive board and as an officer for the Mid-Atlantic Regional Chapter of ACSM. She is a member of the National Fire Protection Agency Technical Committee on Fire Service Occupational Safety and Health. She is also a Research Scientist at the University of Illinois Fire Service Institute at Urbana–Champaign.

Preface

The fourth edition of *Exercise Physiology for Health, Fitness, and Performance* builds upon and expands the strength of the first three editions. The purpose of the current edition, however, remains unchanged from that of the first three editions. That is, the goal is to present exercise physiology concepts in a clear and comprehensive way that will allow students to apply fundamental principles of exercise physiology in the widest variety of possible work situations. The primary audience is kinesiology, exercise science, health, coaching, and physical education majors and minors, including students in teaching preparation programs and students in exercise and sport science tracts where the goal is to prepare for careers in fitness, rehabilitation, athletic training, or allied health professions.

As with other textbooks in the field, a great deal of information is presented. Most of the information has been summarized and conceptualized based on extensive research findings. However, we have occasionally included specific research studies to illustrate certain points, believing that students need to develop an appreciation for research and the constancy of change that research precipitates. **Focus on Research** boxes, including some that are labeled as **Clinically Relevant**, are integrated into the text to help students understand how research informs our understanding of exercise physiology and how research findings can be applied in the field. Our definition of the designation "Clinically Relevant" is used in the broadest sense to refer to a variety of situations that students of exercise physiology might find themselves in during an internship situation or eventual employment. All Focus on Research boxes highlight important classic or recent basic and applied studies in exercise physiology, as well as relevant experimental design considerations.

All chapters are thoroughly referenced and a complete list of references is provided at the end of each chapter. These references should prove to be a useful resource for students to explore topics in more detail for laboratory reports or term projects. The extensive referencing also reinforces the point that our knowledge in exercise physiology is based on a foundation of rigorous research.

The body of knowledge in exercise physiology is extensive and growing every day. Each individual faculty member must determine what is essential for his or her students. To this end, we have tried to allow for choice and flexibility, particularly in the organization of the content of the book.

A Unique Integrative Approach

The intent of this textbook is to present the body of knowledge based on the traditions of exercise physiology but in a way that is not bound by those traditions. Instead of proceeding from a unit on basic science, through units of applied science, to a final unit of special populations or situations (which can lead to the false sense that scientific theories and applications can and should be separated), we have chosen a completely integrative approach to make the link between basic theories and applied concepts both strong and logical.

Flexible Organization

The text begins with an introductory chapter: The Warm-Up. This chapter is intended to prepare students for the chapters that follow. It explains the text's organization, provides an overview of exercise physiology, and establishes the basic terminology and concepts that will be covered in each unit. Paying close attention to this chapter will help the student when studying the ensuing chapters.

Four major units follow: Metabolic System, Cardiovascular-Respiratory System, Neuromuscular-Skeletal System, and Neuroendocrine Immune System. Although the units are presented in this order, each unit can stand alone and has been written in such a way that it may be taught before or after each of the other three with the assumption that Chapter 1 (The Warm-Up) will always precede whichever unit the faculty member decides to present first. Figure 1.1 depicts the circular integration of the units reinforcing the basic concepts that all of the systems of the body respond to exercise in an integrated way and that the order of presentation can logically begin with any unit. Unit openers and graphics throughout the text reinforce this concept.

Consistent Sequence of Presentation

To lay a solid pedagogical foundation, the chapters in each unit follow a consistent sequence of presentation: basic anatomy and physiology, the measurement and meaning of variables important to understanding exercise physiology, exercise responses, training principles and adaptations, and special applications, problems, and considerations.

Basic Sciences

It is assumed that the students using this text will have had a basic course in anatomy, physiology, chemistry, and math. However, sufficient information is presented in the basic chapters to provide a background for what follows if this is not the case. For those students with a broad background, the basic chapters can serve as a review; for those students who do not need this review, the basic chapters can be de-emphasized.

Measurement

Inclusion of the measurement sections serves two purposes—to identify how the variables most frequently used in exercise physiology are obtained and to contrast criterion or laboratory test results with field test results. Criterion or laboratory results are essential for accurate determination and understanding of the exercise responses and training adaptations, but field test results are often the only items available to professionals in school or health club settings.

Exercise Responses and Training Adaptations

The chapters or sections on exercise responses and training adaptations present the definitive and core information for exercise physiology. Exercise response chapters are organized by exercise modality and intensity. Specifically, physiological responses to the following six categories of exercise (based on the duration, intensity, and type of muscle contraction) are presented when sufficient data are available: (1) short-term, light to moderate submaximal aerobic exercise; (2) long term, moderate to heavy submaximal aerobic exercise; (3) incremental aerobic exercise to maximum; (4) static exercise; (5) dynamic resistance exercise; and (6) very short-term, high intensity anaerobic exercise. Training principles for the prescription of exercise training programs are presented for each physical fitness component: aerobic and anaerobic metabolism, body composition, cardiovascular endurance, muscular strength and endurance, and flexibility and balance. These principles are followed by the training adaptations that will result from a well-prescribed training program.

Special Applications

The special applications chapters always relate the unit topic to health-related fitness and then deal with such diverse topics as altitude and thermoregulation (Cardiovascular-Respiratory Unit); making weight and eating disorders (Metabolic Unit); muscle fatigue and soreness (Neuromuscular-Skeletal Unit); and Overreaching/Overtraining Syndrome (Neuroendocrine Immune Unit).

Focus on Application and **Focus on Application—Clinically Relevant** boxes emphasize how research and underlying exercise physiology principles are relevant to the practitioner.

Complete Integration of Age Groups and Sexes

A major departure from tradition in the organization of this text is the complete integration of information relevant to all age groups and both sexes. In the past, there was good reason to describe evidence and derive concepts based on information from male college students and elite male athletes. These were the samples of the population most involved in physical activity and sport, and they were the groups most frequently studied. As more women, children, and older adults began participating in sport and fitness programs, information became available on these groups. Chapters on females, children/adolescents, and the elderly were often added to the back of an exercise physiology text as supplemental material. However, most physical education, kinesiology, and exercise science professionals will be dealing with both male and female children and adolescents in school settings, average middle-aged adults in health clubs or fitness centers, and older adults in special programs. Very few will be dealing strictly with college-aged students, and fewer still will work with elite athletes. This does not mean that information based on young adult males has been excluded or even de-emphasized. However, it does mean that it is time to move coverage of the groups that make up most of the population from the back of the book and integrate information about males and females at various ages throughout the text. That being said, these sections are typically stand-alone, allowing the faculty member to give the individual students freedom to select a population they are primarily interested in.

Pedagogical Considerations

This text incorporates multiple pedagogical techniques to support student learning. These techniques include a list of learning objectives at the beginning of each chapter as well as a chapter summary, review questions, and references at the end of each chapter. Another pedagogical aid is the use of a running glossary. Terms are highlighted in definition boxes as they are introduced and are highlighted and defined in the text where they first appear to emphasize the context in which they are used. A glossary is included in the back matter of the book for easy reference. Additional important technical terms with which students should be familiar are italicized in the text to emphasize their importance. Because so many are used, a complete list of commonly used symbols and abbreviations with their meanings is printed on the front endpapers of the text for quick and easy reference. Each chapter contains a multitude of tables, charts, diagrams, and photographs to underscore the pedagogy, to aid in the Organization of material, and to enhance the visual appeal of the text.

Unique Color-Coding

A unique aspect of the graphs is color-coding, which allows for quick recognition of the condition represented. Because it is so critical to recognize the differences among exercise responses to different types of exercise, we use a specific background color for each category of exercise. Further, we differentiate the responses to an acute bout of exercise from training adaptations that occur as a result of a consistent training program with a specific background color. For exercise response patterns, each of the six exercise categories has its own shaded representative color and accompanying icon. A key to these colors and icons is included in Table 1.2.

Active Learning

Throughout the text, **Check Your Comprehension** boxes engage the student in active learning beyond just reading. In some instances, the boxes require students to work through problems that address their understanding of the material. In other instances, students are asked to interpret a set of circumstances or deduce an answer based on previously presented information. Scattered throughout the text and occasionally used in Check Your Comprehension boxes are equations and problems used to calculate specific variables in exercise physiology. Examples using all equations are included in discrete sections in the text. Individual faculty members can determine how best to use or not use these portions of the text to best fit their individual situations and student needs. Each chapter ends with a set of essay review questions.

Appendices

Appendix A provides information on the metric system, units, symbols, and conversion both with and between the metric and English systems. Appendix B offers supplementary material, consisting of three parts that deal with aspects of oxygen consumption calculation. Appendix C provides Answers to the Check Your Comprehension boxes that appear throughout the text.

Online Resources

A comprehensive set of ancillary materials designed to facilitate classroom preparation and ease the transition into a new text is available to students and instructors using *Exercise Physiology for Health, Fitness, and Performance, Fourth Edition.*

For Students

- E-book
- Crossword puzzles using key terms and definitions. Answers are accessible.
- Quiz Bank, including multiple choice and drop and drag questions to assist in studying the material or for self-testing. Answers are accessible.
- Worksheets that include true/false questions (with space for correcting false statements), fill-in tables, figure labeling, matching, and calculation to assist in studying or for self-testing. Worksheet answers are also available to students.
- Laboratory manual
- Online animations

For Faculty

- E-book
- Image bank of all figures in the text
- PowerPoint lecture outlines
- Brownstone test generator
- Answers to in-text chapter review questions

User's Guide

This User's Guide explains the key features found in the fourth edition of *Exercise Physiology for Health, Fitness, and Performance.*

Get the most out of your learning and study time so you can master exercise physiology principles and move on to career success!

Commonly Used Symbols and Abbreviations

You can find this useful resource just inside the front cover of the text.

Commonly Used Symbols and Abbreviations

Commonly Used Symbols and Abbreviations

(A-a)PO₂diff	difference between partial pressure of oxygen in alveoli and arterial blood	F_EN₂	fraction of expired nitrogen
a-vO₂diff	difference in oxygen content between arterial and venous blood	F_EO₂	fraction of expired oxygen
		F_G	fraction of a gas
A	actin	F_ICO₂	fraction of inspired carbon dioxide
ACh	acetylcholine	F_IN₂	fraction of inspired nitrogen
ACTH	adrenocorticotrophic hormone	F_IO₂	fraction of inspired oxygen
ADH	antidiuretic hormone	f	frequency
ADL	activities of daily living	FAD	flavin adenine dinucleotide
ADP	adenosine diphosphate	FEV	forced expiratory volume
AIDS	acquired immune deficiency syndrome	FFA	free fatty acids
AMP	adenosine monophosphate	FFB	fat-free body mass
ANS	autonomic nervous system	FFM	fat-free mass
AP	action potential	FFW	fat-free weight
ATP	adenosine triphosphate	FG	fast, glycolytic muscle fibers
ATP-PC	phosphagen system	FI	fatigue index
ATPS	atmospheric temperature and pressure, saturated air	FOG	fast, oxidative-glycolytic muscle fibers
		FT	fast-twitch muscle fibers
AV	atrioventricular	GAS	General Adaptation Syndrome
BCAA	branched chain amino acids	GH	growth hormone
BF	body fat	GLUT-1	non-insulin regulated glucose transporter
BMC	bone mineral content	GLUT-4	insulin regulated glucose transporter
BMD	bone mineral density	GTO	Golgi tendon organ
BMI	body mass index	Hb	hemoglobin
		HbO₂	oxyhemoglobin

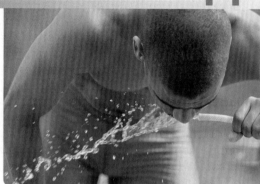

Thermoregulation 14

OBJECTIVES

After studying the chapter, you should be able to:

> Identify environmental factors that affect thermoregulation and be able to use indices of heat stress and windchill to assess the risks associated with exercise under various conditions.

> Describe thermal balance and discuss factors that contribute to heat gain and heat loss.

> Define the mechanisms by which heat is lost from the body, and describe how they differ under exercise conditions.

> Describe the body's regulatory system for temperature control in terms of the sensory input, neural integration, and effector responses to increase or decrease heat loss.

> Identify the factors that influence heat exchange between an individual and the environment.

> Describe the challenges to the cardiovascular system during exercise in a hot environment and in a cold environment.

> Describe the goals for fluid ingestion before, during, and after exercise.

> Differentiate among the types of heat illness in terms of severity and symptoms.

> Identify ways in which an exercise leader can prevent heat and cold injuries and illness.

Chapter Objectives

These are the learning objectives that you need to meet after reading the chapter.

Data Graphs

Each chapter contains a multitude of graphs, tables, charts, and diagrams that clarify and enhance points made in the text.

FIGURE 21.11 Epinephrine and Norepinephrine Responses to Various Categories of Exercise.
Sources: Galbo, H.: *Hormonal and Metabolic Adaptation to Exercise.* New York, NY: Thieme-Stratton (1983); Kraemer, W.J.: Endocrine responses to resistance exercise. *Medicine and Science in Sports and Exercise.* 20(5):S152–S157 (1988).

Epinephrine — A: Short-term, light to moderate submaximal aerobic exercise; C: Long-term, moderate to heavy submaximal aerobic exercise; E: Incremental aerobic exercise to maximum; G: Static exercise (40%MVC; 1 leg); I: Dynamic resistance exercise (10 RM)

Norepinephrine — B, D, F, H, J

Icons and Color Coding

Color tints and bold icons within figures and figure legends help you quickly distinguish the exercise response to six different categories of exercise.

Exercise Category	Color	Icon
Short-term, light to moderate submaximal aerobic		
Long-term, moderate to heavy submaximal aerobic		
Incremental aerobic to maximum		
Static		
Dynamic resistance		
Very short-term, high-intensity anaerobic		

Focus on Research Boxes

Classic, illustrative, and cutting-edge research studies are presented to help you develop an appreciation for how research affects changing practices in the field.

Clinically Relevant Boxes

Specially identified boxes highlight clinical information, situations, or case studies that you may experience during an internship or future employment.

Focus on Application Boxes

These features apply basic concepts, principles, or research findings to relevant practical situations, concerns, or recommendations.

Body System Responses to Exercise

Consistently formatted diagrams clearly show how each body system responds to exercise in an integrated fashion and how those responses are interdependent.

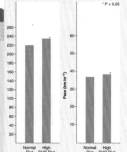

CHAPTER 6 ● Nutrition for Fitness and Athletics 175

FOCUS ON RESEARCH: *Clinically Relevant*

The Impact of Increased Glycogen Storage on Exercise Performance

In this study, well-trained male endurance cyclists completed two exercise trials separated by at least 4 days. Each trial consisted first of 2 hours of cycling at approximately 73% VO₂max. Every 20 minutes, an all-out 60-second sprint

than after the normal diet. This enabled the cyclists to maintain a significantly higher power output and a faster overall pace during the time trial. Interestingly, muscle glycogen levels after the time trial were similar between groups

trial. Furthermore, although the term glycogen depletion is often used, glycogen concentrations do not actually reach zero at exhaustion.
Source: Rauch, H. G. L., A. St. Clair Gibson, E. V. Lambert, & T. D. Noakes: A signaling role for muscle glycogen in the regulation of pace during prolonged exercise. *British Journal of Sports Medicine.* 39:34–38 (2005).

334 Cardiovascular-Respiratory System Unit

FOCUS ON APPLICATION: *Clinically Relevant*

Are All Elevations in Heart Rate Equal?

Heart rate (HR) can be elevated by a variety of factors mediated by the neural and hormonal systems (see Figures 11.16 and 11.17). One of these factors is movement (exercise), but others include emotion and environmental temperatures. Does an individual derive the same benefit from HR elevation caused by emotion or heat as from HR elevation caused by exercise? That is, is it possible to improve one's cardiovascular function while sitting in a sauna or hot tub or when frightened, angry, or anxious?

A regular, sustained elevation in HR is recognized as an important factor for improving cardiovascular fitness (techniques of exercise prescription

changes occur in energy expenditure; hence there is no training stimulus.

The importance of an increase in oxygen consumption has been demonstrated by individuals on medications such as beta blockers, which markedly suppress HR at rest and during exercise, and by those with constant heart-rate pacemakers. Both of these

groups routinely show improvements in exercise capacity and fitness as a result of exercise programs, despite the fact that the exercise-induced increase in HR is dampened. Although HR can be elevated by other factors, you do not derive the health-related benefits unless the elevated HR is accompanied by physical activity.

Source: Franklin and Munnings (1998).

hormonal levels (Sedlock, 2008). Overall, ...ed in this section, there were "respond-...ved) and "nonresponders" (who did not ... fat loading and carbohydrate loading. ... ust be reemphasized that each athlete ... what benefits himself or herself most. ...y not enough evidence to support carbo-...n either children or older adults (Nemet ...9; Tarnopolsky, 2008).

...hydrate loading is intended for endurance ...ilders often follow a version of the modi-...e-loading technique (Kroculick, 1988). ...fference is a restriction of water and ... body builders during the high-carbohy-...hase. This water restriction has nothing ...y requirements during competition; it is ...f that water will be sucked from beneath

370 Cardiovascular-Respiratory System Unit

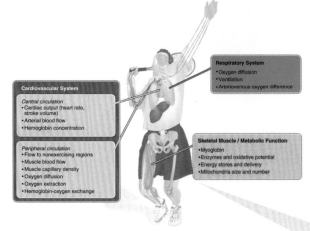

Cardiovascular System

Central circulation
- Cardiac output (heart rate, stroke volume)
- Arterial blood flow
- Hemoglobin concentration

Peripheral circulation
- Flow to nonexercising regions
- Muscle blood flow
- Muscle capillary density
- Oxygen diffusion
- Oxygen extraction
- Hemoglobin-oxygen exchange

Respiratory System
- Oxygen diffusion
- Ventilation
- Arteriovenous oxygen difference

Skeletal Muscle / Metabolic Function
- Myoglobin
- Enzymes and oxidative potential
- Energy stores and delivery
- Mitochondria size and number

FIGURE 12.9 Possible Limitations to Maximal Oxygen Consumption.
Source: Modified from Rowell (1993).

During the *isovolumetric relaxation period (IRP)* both the ... nd the semilunar valves are closed (**Figure 11.5D**). ..., ventricular volume is again unchanged (isovolu-...ic), but pressure is low because the ventricles are ...ed.

...ll these events occur within a single cardiac cycle, ...h repeats with every beat of the heart. **Figure 11.6** ...narizes the cardiac cycle graphically, showing con-...nt information about the electrocardiogram; the ...ure in the left atrium, the left ventricle, and aorta; ...eft ventricular volume; the heart phase; the period

Possibly, the factors limiting VO₂max vary with the fitness level of the individual. According to this hypothesis, in an untrained individual the respiratory capacity for gas exchange exceeds the cardiovascular system's capacity to deliver oxygen. A training program results in little change in the respiratory capacity but large changes in the cardiovascular capacity. Thus, in some highly trained individuals who have exercise-induced arterial hypoxemia (Chapter 10), the increased cardiovascular capacity may exceed the respiratory capacity (Dempsey, 1986; Legrand et al., 2005; Powers et al., 1989). In this case the respiratory system becomes the factor limiting VO₂max. One final point to remember, although it is interesting to probe the question, "what limits VO₂max?" we must resist the temptation to allow the search for an answer to obscure the fact that a close interaction exists among the various systems ensuring a continuous supply of oxygen to the working tissue during exercise (Mitchell and Saltin, 2003).

The reduction in plasma volume during submaximal exercise also occurs in incremental exercise to maximum. Because the magnitude of the reduction depends on the intensity of exercise, the reduction is greatest at maximal exercise. A decrease of 10–20% can be seen during incremental exercise to maximum (Wade and Freund, 1990).

Considerable changes in cardiac output occur during maximal incremental exercise. Figure 12.10 illustrates the distribution of cardiac output at rest and at maximal aerobic exercise. Maximum cardiac output in this example is 25 L·min⁻¹. Again, the most striking change is the tremendous amount of cardiac output that is directed to the working muscles (88%). At maximal exercise, skin blood flow is reduced to direct the necessary blood to the muscles. Renal and splanchnic blood flows also decrease considerably. Blood flow to the brain and cardiac muscle is maintained.

Table 12.1 summarizes the cardiovascular responses to exercise.

Age of Females (yr)

10–15	20–30	50–60
85	76	82
40	75	62

Check Your Comprehension Boxes

These engaging mini-quizzes challenge you to work through problems, interpret circumstances, or deduce answers to reinforce your learning as you move through each chapter.

---

by the NCAA. Several high school associations allow bioelectrical impedance analysis (BIA) as well, although BIA has been shown to have a high prediction error in wrestlers and research indicates that skinfolds and BIA body composition values cannot be used interchangeably (Clark et al., 2002, 2005).

The Lohman skinfold equation is as follows:

body density $(g \cdot cc^{-1}) = 1.0982 - [[0.000815 \times$ sum of triceps + subscapular + abdominal skinfolds (mm)] + [0.0000084 × sum of triceps + subscapular + abdominal skinfolds squared (mm)]]

$D_B = 1.0982 - (0.000815$ sum of skinfolds $+ 0.0000084$ sum of skinfolds^2)(American College of Sports Medicine, 1983)

EXAMPLE

If a 17-year-old wrestler weighs 165 lb and his sum of skinfolds for the selected sites is 46 mm, the calculation would be

$$D_B = 1.0982 - [0.000815(46) = 0.0000084(2116)]$$
$$= 1.0429 g \cdot cc^{-1}$$

The D_B value is then substituted into the age-appropriate formula presented in Table 7.1 in Chapter 7 for a male adolescent to determine %BF. For a 17-year-old this is

$$\%BF = \left[\frac{5.03}{D_B} - 4.59\right] \times 100 = 23.31$$

Equations 7.4, 7.5, and 7.6 are then used to determine the wrestler's most appropriate competitive weight. Using Equation 7.4,

$$FFW = 165 lb \times \left[\frac{100\% - 23.3\%}{100}\right] = 126.6 lb$$

Using Equation 7.5,

$$WT_2 = \left[\frac{100 \times 126.6}{100\% - 16.3\%}\right] = 151.3 lb$$

Note: 16% is used here as the desirable %BF, not 5%, which is the lowest recommended %BF for a wrestler of this age. The 16.3% complies with the recommendation that weight loss not exceed 7% of body weight.

To get down to 5% BF, this wrestler would need to lose 18.3% of his body weight, and that is too much. Using Equation 7.6,

$$151.3 lb - 165 lb = -13.7 lb$$

To achieve his recommended body weight, this wrestler needs to lose 13.7 lb.

Complete the problem in the Check Your Comprehension 2 box.

Specific guidelines for making weight have not been established for other sports, but the principles discussed here can and should be applied.

CHECK YOUR COMPREHENSION 2

Calculate the weight at which the following 14-year-old wrestler should compete.

   Name: Zachary   Triceps skinfold: 8 mm
   Weight: 138 lb   Subscapular skinfold: 9 mm
                  Abdominal skinfold: 12 mm

How much weight does Zachary need to gain or lose to achieve this weight?
Check your answer in Appendix C.

Several studies have [...] new regulations. A 1[...] (Oppliger et al., 200[...] during the season was [...] weekly weight loss wa[...] that the then-new NC[...] loss behaviors, appr[...] mately 28% used sau[...] vapor-barrier suits at [...] ever, compared to col[...] behavior was less extr[...] et al., 2006) of 811 c[...] national championshi[...] showed that weight [...] son to postseason co[...] certified minimum w[...] 9.2 kg versus 67.9 ± [...] ment between the pr[...] actual end-of-season [...] weigh-in was found [...] small (~1.7% of bod[...] at the tournaments w[...] from the preseason [...] above the minimum [...] that the NCAA weig[...] to be effective in re[...] behaviors (although [...] they achieved weight[...] equity.

This is an examp[...] between science and [...] pants, but it needs to [...] of wrestling and mo[...] weight-category sport[...]

Example Boxes

These highlighted equations enable you to visualize working out problems and calculate specific variables in exercise physiology.

Clear and Accurate Artwork

Detailed anatomic illustrations and practice-related photos place key concepts in context.

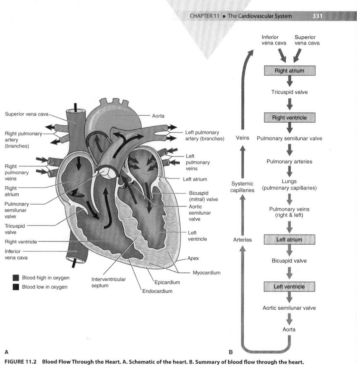

FIGURE 11.2   Blood Flow Through the Heart. A. Schematic of the heart. B. Summary of blood flow through the heart.

linked by **intercalated discs (Figure 11.3)**. The intercalated discs contain specialized intracellular junctions (gap junctions) that allow the electrical activity in one cell to pass to the next. Thus, the individual cells of the myocardium function collectively: when one cell is stimulated electrically, the stimulation spreads from cell to cell over the entire area. This electrical coupling allows the myocardium to function as a single coordinated unit, or a functional **syncytium**. Each of the two functional syncytia, the atrial and ventricular, contracts as a unit.

The Heart as Excitable Tissue

Cardiac muscle cells are excitable cells that are polarized (have an electrical charge with the inside being negative relative to the outside of the cell) in the resting state and

Intercalated Discs The junction between adjacent cardiac muscle cells that forms a mechanical and electrical connection between cells.

Syncytium A group of cells of the myocardium that function collectively as a unit during depolarization.

Definition Boxes

Important terms are boldfaced in the text where they first appear to emphasize the context in which they are used. Definitions are provided in a callout box to create an on-the-spot glossary.

Chapter Review Questions

Essay-style questions help you build your critical-thinking, problem-solving, and decision-making skills.

Chapter Summaries

Concise copy points review the chapter's core content.

Online Animations and Other Resources

Icons throughout the text direct readers to useful resources that are available online.

References and Suggested Readings

Key published articles are identified for further in-depth exploration and can be used as a source of additional information for laboratory reports and class papers.

---

512 Neuromuscular-Skeletal System Unit

SUMMARY

1. The skeletal system serves a number of important functions, including support, protection, movement, mineral storage, and hematopoiesis (blood cell formation).

...lesterol uptake at the cellular or tissue level. HDL definitely carries cholesterol away from the sites of deposit to the liver, where the cholesterol can be broken down and eliminated in the bile.

6. Arteriosclerosis is characterized by a thickening of the arterial wall, inflammation, loss of elastic connective tissue, and hardening of the vessel wall.

7. Atherosclerosis is a pathological process that results in the buildup of plaque (composed of connective tissue, smooth muscle cells, cellular debris, and cholesterol) inside the vessel. The buildup of plaque obstructs blood flow and increases the risk of thrombosis. Depending on the amount of obstruction, the result can be pain, a heart attack, or a stroke.

5. High-density lipoproteins (HDL) may block cholesterol uptake at the cellular or tissue level. HDL definitely carries cholesterol away from the sites of deposit to the liver, where the cholesterol can be broken down and eliminated in the bile.

6. Arteriosclerosis is characterized by a thickening of the arterial wall, inflammation, loss of elastic connective tissue, and hardening of the vessel wall.

7. Atherosclerosis is a pathological process that results in the buildup of plaque (composed of connective tissue, smooth muscle cells, cellular debris, and cholesterol) inside the vessel. The buildup of plaque obstructs blood flow and increases the risk of thrombosis. Depending on the amount of obstruction, the result can be pain, a heart attack, or a stroke.

8. Active individuals generally have lipid profiles that indicate a reduced risk for coronary heart disease (CHD).

9. The atherosclerotic process is accelerated in individuals who smoke cigarettes. Smoking injures the arterial wall lining, increases the levels of circulating TC, and decreases the amount of HDL-C. Smoking also causes blood platelets to adhere to each other, speeds up the rate of internal blood clotting, and makes the clots tougher to dissolve.

10. Individuals who are at high risk for developing hyper-...

REVIEW QUESTIONS

1. Compare and contrast cortical and trabecular bone.
2. Diagram the stages of bone remodeling, citing the specific role of the different types of bone cells.
3. What is the relationship between the hormonal control... their relationship with cardiovascular disease.
4. Identify contributing and nontraditional risk factors, and discuss their relationship with cardiovascular disease.
5. Discuss metabolic syndrome.
6. What is the impact of exercise training on each CHD risk factor?
7. What is the importance of identifying cardiovascular disease risk factors in children?

For further review and additional study tools, visit the website at http://thePoint.lww.com/Plowman4e

3. Identify the major modifiable risk factors, and discuss their relationship with cardiovascular disease.
4. Identify contributing and nontraditional risk factors, and discuss their relationship with cardiovascular disease.
5. Discuss metabolic syndrome.
6. What is the impact of exercise training on each CHD risk factor?
7. What is the importance of identifying cardiovascular disease risk factors in children?

For further review and additional study tools, visit the website at http://thePoint.lww.com/Plowman4e

REFERENCES

Alcazar, O., R. C. Ho, & L. J. Goodyear: Physical activity, fitness, and diabetes mellitus. In Bouchard, C., S. N. Blair, & W. L. Haskell (eds.): *Physical Activity and Health.* Champaign, IL: Human Kinetics, 191–204 (2006).
Alpert, B. S. & J. H. Wilmore: Physical activity and blood pressure in adolescents. *Pediatric Exercise Science.* 6(4):361–380 (1994).
American College of Sports Medicine: Position stand: Exercise and hypertension. *Medicine & Science in Sports & Exercise.*...

ADDITIONAL LEARNING AND TEACHING RESOURCES

Learning goes beyond the pages of this textbook! Interactive materials are available to students and faculty via thePoint companion Website.

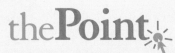

http://thePoint.lww.com/Plowman4e

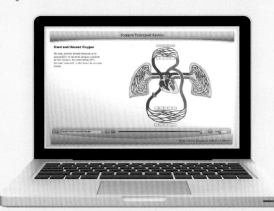

Dynamic 3-D animation clips bring key concepts to life.

Log on to thePoint with your personal access code to access all of these valuable tools:

Student Resource Center

- **Full Text Online**
- **Crossword Puzzles: Key Terms and Definitions**
- **Quiz Bank Questions**
  Multiple Choice
  Drop & Drag
- **Worksheets**
  True/false (with space for corrections)
  Tables to fill in
  Matching
  Calculations

- **Laboratory Manual**
- **Reference List of American College of Sports Medicine Position Stands**
- **Answers to Crossword Puzzles, Quiz Bank Questions and all Worksheets**

Faculty Resource Center

- **E-book**
- **Image bank of all figures in text**
- **PowerPoint lecture outlines**
- **Brownstone test generator**
- **Answers to in-text chapter review questions.**

Acknowledgments

The completion of this textbook required the help of many people. A complete list of individuals is impossible, but four groups to whom we are indebted must be recognized for their meritorious assistance. The first group is our families and friends who saw less of us than either we or they desired due to the constant time demands. Their support, patience, and understanding were much appreciated. The second group contains our many professional colleagues, known and unknown, who critically reviewed the manuscript at several stages and provided valuable suggestions for revisions along with a steady supply of encouragement. This kept us going. The third group is our students, who provided much of the initial motivation for undertaking the task. Some went far beyond that by using the text in manuscript form and providing valuable feedback that helped shape the text. The final group is the editors and staff at Lippincott Williams & Wilkins, particularly our Aquisition Editor, Emily Lupash, and our Product Manager, Linda Francis, whose faith in the project and commitment to excellence in its production are responsible for the finished product you now see. We thank you all.

Sharon A. Plowman
Denise L. Smith

Contents

The Warm-Up

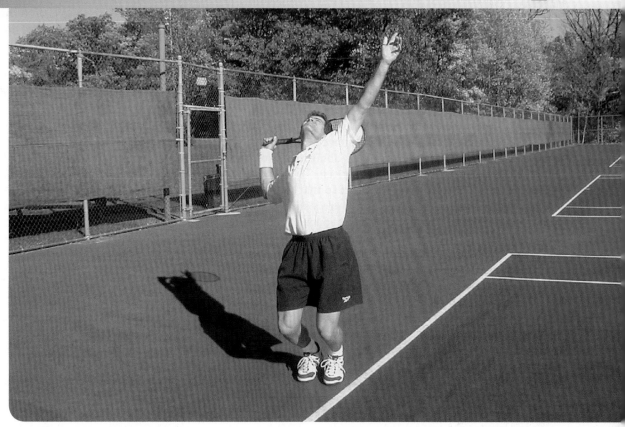

OBJECTIVES

After studying the chapter, you should be able to:

> Describe what exercise physiology is and discuss why you need to study it.

> Identify the organizational structure of this text.

> Differentiate between exercise responses and training adaptations.

> List and explain the six categories of exercise whose responses are discussed throughout this book.

> List and explain the factors involved in interpreting an exercise response.

> Describe the graphic patterns that physiological variables may exhibit in response to different categories of exercise and as a result of training adaptations.

> List and explain the training principles.

> Describe the differences and similarities between health-related and sport-specific physical fitness.

> Define and explain periodization.

> Define detraining.

> Relate exercise and exercise training to Selye's theory of stress.

Introduction

In the 1966 science fiction movie *Fantastic Voyage* (CBS/Fox), a military medical team is miniaturized in a nuclear-powered submarine and injected through a hypodermic needle into the carotid artery. Anticipating an easy float into the brain, where they plan to remove a blood clot by laser beam, they are both awed by what they see and imperiled by what befalls them. They see erythrocytes turning from an iridescent blue to vivid red as oxygen bubbles replace carbon dioxide; nerve impulses appear as bright flashes of light; and when their sub loses air pressure, all they need to do is tap into an alveolus. Not all of their encounters are so benign, however. They are sucked into a whirlpool caused by an abnormal fistula between the carotid artery and jugular vein. They have to get the outside team to stop the heart so that they will not be crushed by its contraction. They are jostled about by the conduction of sound waves in the inner ear. They are attacked by antibodies. And finally, their submarine is destroyed by a white blood cell—they are, after all, foreign bodies to the natural defense system. Of course, in the end, the "good guys" on the team escape through a tear duct, and all is well.

Although the journey you are about to take through the human body will not be quite so literal, it will be just as incredible and fascinating, for it goes beyond the basics of anatomy and physiology into the realm of the moving human. The body is capable of great feats, whose limits and full benefits in terms of exercise and sport are still unknown.

Consider these events and changes, all of which have probably taken place within the life span of your grandparents.

- President Dwight D. Eisenhower suffered a heart attack on September 23, 1955. At that time, the normal medical treatment was 6 weeks of bed rest and a lifetime of curtailed activity (Hellerstein, 1979). Eisenhower's rehabilitation, including a return to golf, was, if not revolutionary, certainly progressive. Today, cardiac patients are mobilized within days and frequently train for and safely run marathons.
- The 4-minute mile was considered an unbreakable limit until May 6, 1954, when Roger Bannister ran the mile in 3:59.4. Hundreds of runners (including some high school boys) have since accomplished that feat. The men's world record for the mile, which was set in 1999, is 3:43.13. The women's mile record, of 4:12.56 set in 1996, is approaching the old 4-minute "barrier."

> **Exercise Physiology** A basic and an applied science that describes, explains, and uses the body's response to exercise and adaptation to exercise training to maximize human physical potential.

- The 800-m run was banned from the Olympics from 1928 to 1964 for women because females were considered to be "too weak and delicate" to run such a "long" distance. In the 1950s when the 800-m run was reintroduced for women in Europe, ambulances were stationed at the finish line, motors running, to carry off the casualties (Ullyot, 1976). In 1963, the women's world marathon record (then not an Olympic sport for women) was 3:37.07, a time now commonly achieved by females not considered to be elite athletes. The women's world best (set in 2003) was 2:15.25, an improvement of 1:21.42 (37.5%).
- In 1954, Kraus and Hirschland published a report indicating that American children were less fit than European children (Kraus and Hirschland, 1954). These results started the physical fitness movement. At that time, being fit was defined as being able to pass the Kraus-Weber test of minimal muscular fitness, which consisted of one each of the following: bent-leg sit-up; straight-leg sit-up; standing toe touch; double-leg lift, prone; double-leg lift, supine; and trunk extension, prone. Today (as is discussed in detail later in this chapter), physical fitness is more broadly defined in terms of both physiology and specificity (health-related and sport-related), and its importance for individuals of all ages is widely recognized.

These changes and a multitude of others that we readily accept as normal have come about as a combined result of formal medical and scientific research and informal experimentation by individuals with the curiosity and courage to try new things.

What Is Exercise Physiology and Why Study It?

The events and changes described above exemplify concerns in the broad area of exercise physiology, that is, athletic performance, physical fitness, health, and rehabilitation. **Exercise physiology** can be defined as both a basic and an applied science that describes, explains, and uses the body's response to exercise and adaptation to exercise training to maximize human physical potential.

No single course or textbook, of course, can provide all the information a prospective professional will need. However, knowledge of exercise physiology and an appreciation for practice based on research findings help set professionals in the field apart from mere practitioners. It is one thing to be able to lead yoga routines. It is another to be able to design routines based on predictable short- and long-term responses of given class members, to evaluate those responses, and then to modify the sessions as needed. To become respected professionals in fields related to exercise science and physical education, students need to learn exercise physiology in order to:

1. Understand how the basic physiological functioning of the human body is modified by various types of exercise as well as the mechanisms causing these changes. Unless one knows what responses are normal, one cannot recognize an abnormal response or adjust to it.
2. Understand how the basic physiological functioning of the human body is modified by various training programs and the mechanisms responsible for these changes. Adaptations will be specific to the training program used.
3. Provide quality fitness programming and physical education programs in schools that stimulate children and adolescents both physically and intellectually. To become lifelong exercisers, individuals need to understand how physical activity can benefit them, why they take physical fitness tests, and what to do with fitness test results.
4. Apply the results of scientific research to maximize health, rehabilitation, and/or athletic performance in a variety of subpopulations.
5. Respond accurately to questions and advertising claims, as well as recognize myths and misconceptions regarding exercise. Good advice should be based on scientific evidence.

Overview of the Text

Just as the fitness participant, athlete (**Figure 1.1**), or even musician warms up before working out, competing, or performing, this chapter is intended to provide you, the learner, with an essential warm-up for the rest of the text. That is, it provides the basic information that will prepare you to successfully understand what follows in the text and accomplish the goals stated above. To do this, the textbook is first divided into four units: metabolic system, cardiovascular-respiratory system, neuromuscular-skeletal system, and neuroendocrine-immune system. To facilitate learning, each unit follows a consistent format:

1. Basic information
   a. Anatomical structures
   b. Physiological function
   c. Laboratory techniques and variables typically measured
2. Exercise responses
3. Training
   a. Application of the training principles
   b. Adaptations to training
4. Special applications, problems, and considerations

Each unit first deals with basic anatomical structures and physiological functions necessary to understand the material that follows. Then each unit describes the acute

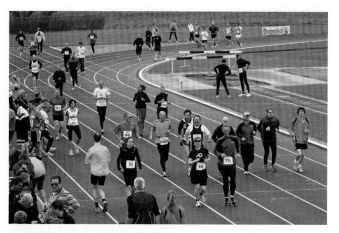

FIGURE 1.1 Warming up in Preparation for Performance.

responses to exercise. Following are specific applications of the training principles and discussion of the typical adaptations that occur when the training principles are applied correctly. Finally, each unit ends with one or more special application topics, such as thermal concerns, weight control/body composition, and osteoporosis. This integrated approach demonstrates the relevance of applying basic information.

More exercise physiology research has been done on college-age males and elite male athletes than on any other portion of the population. Nonetheless, wherever possible, we provide information about both sexes as well as children and adolescents at one end of the age spectrum and older adults at the other, throughout the unit.

Each unit is independent of the other three, although the body obviously functions as a whole. Your course, therefore, may sequence these units of study in a different order other than just going from Chapter 1 to Chapter 22. After this first chapter, your instructor may start with any unit and then move in any order through the other two. This concept is represented by the circle in (**Figure 1.2**).

Figure 1.2 also illustrates two other important points: (1) all of the systems respond to exercise in an integrated fashion, and (2) the responses of the systems are interdependent. The metabolic system produces cellular energy in the form of adenosine triphosphate (ATP). ATP is used for muscular contraction. For the cells (including muscle cells) to produce ATP, they must be supplied with oxygen and fuel (foodstuffs). The respiratory system brings oxygen into the body via the lungs, and the cardiovascular system distributes oxygen and nutrients to the cells of the body via the blood pumped by the heart through the blood vessels. During exercise, all these functions must increase. The neuroendocrine-immune system regulates and integrates both resting and exercise body functions.

Each unit is divided into multiple chapters depending on the amount and depth of the material. Each chapter begins with a list of learning objectives that present an

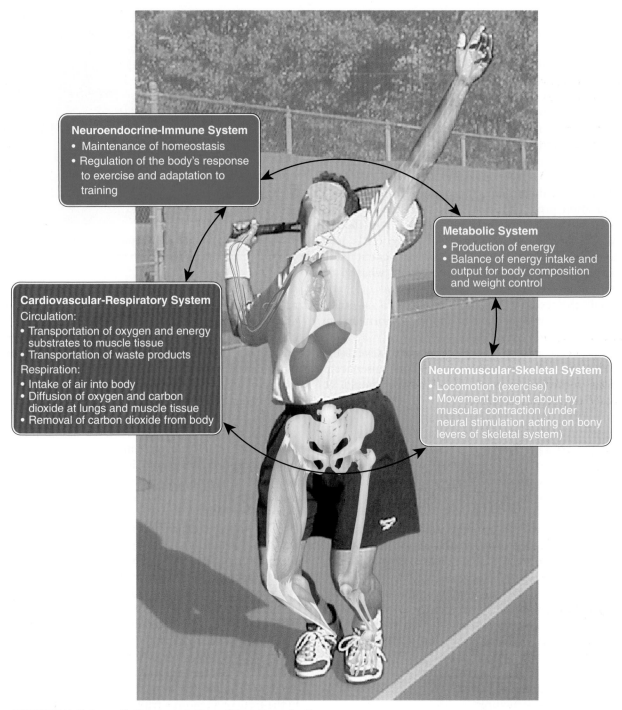

FIGURE 1.2 Schematic Representation of Text Organization.

overall picture of chapter content and help you understand what you should learn. Definitions are highlighted and boxed as they are introduced. Each chapter ends with a summary and review questions. Appearing throughout the text are Focus on Research and Focus on Application boxes, which present four types of research studies:

1. Analytical—an evaluation of available information in a review

2. Descriptive—a presentation of some variable (such as heart rate or blood lactate) or population (such as children or highly trained endurance athletes)

3. Experimental—a design in which treatments have been manipulated to determine their effects on selected variables

4. Quasi-experimental—designs such as used in epidemiology that study the frequency, distribution, and risk of disease among population subgroups in real-world settings

Focus on Research boxes present classic, illustrative, or cutting-edge research findings. Focus on Application boxes show how research may be used in practical contexts. Some of each type of focus box have been designated as Clinically Relevant.

Clinically Relevant boxes present information, situations, or case studies related to clinical experiences students of exercise physiology often have. These include selected topics in athletic training, cardiac or other rehabilitation, coaching, personal training, physical therapy, and/or teaching. An additional feature is the Check Your Comprehension box. The Check Your Comprehension boxes are problems for you to complete. Occasionally the Check Your Comprehension boxes will be clinically relevant. Answers to these problems are presented in Appendix C. When appropriate, calculations are worked out in examples. The appendices and endpapers provide supplemental information. For example, Appendix A contains a listing of the basic physical quantities, units of measurement, and conversions within the Système International d'Unités (SI or metric system of measurement commonly used in scientific work) and between the metric and English measurement systems. In the front of the book, you will find a list of the symbols and abbreviations used throughout the book, along with their full names. You may need to refer to these appendices/endpapers frequently if these symbols and measurement units are new to you.

Exercise physiology is a dynamic area of study with many practical implications. Over the next few months, you will gain an appreciation for the tremendous range in which the human body can function. At the same time, you will become better prepared as a professional to carry out your responsibilities in your particular chosen field. Along the way, you will probably also learn things about yourself. Enjoy the voyage.

The Exercise Response

Let's begin with some definitions and concepts required for understanding all the units to come. **Exercise** is a single acute bout of bodily exertion or muscular activity that requires an expenditure of energy above resting level and that in most, but not all, cases results in voluntary movement. Exercise sessions are typically planned and structured to improve or maintain one or more components of physical fitness. The term *physical activity*, in contrast, generally connotes movement in which the goal (often to sustain daily living or recreation) is different from that of exercise, but which also requires the expenditure of energy and often provides health benefits. For example, walking to school or work is physical activity, while walking around a track at a predetermined heart rate is exercise. Exercise is sometimes considered a subset of physical activity with a more specific focus (Caspersen et al., 1985). From a physiological standpoint, both involve the process of muscle

action/energy expenditure and bring about changes (acute and chronic). Therefore, the terms exercise and physical activity are often used interchangeably in this textbook. Where the amount of exercise can actually be measured, the terms workload or work rate may be used as well.

Homeostasis is the state of dynamic equilibrium (balance) of the body's internal environment. Exercise disrupts homeostasis, causing changes that represent the body's response to exercise. An **exercise response** is the pattern of change in physiological variables during a single acute bout of physical exertion. A physiological *variable* is any measurable bodily function that changes or *varies* under different circumstances. For example, heart rate is a variable with which you are undoubtedly already familiar. You probably also know that heart rate increases during exercise. However, to state simply that heart rate increases during exercise does not describe the full pattern of the response. For example, the heart rate response to a 400-m sprint is different from the heart rate response to a 50-mi bike ride. To fully understand the response of heart rate or any other variable, we need more information about the exercise itself. Three factors are considered when determining the acute response to exercise:

1. The exercise modality
2. The exercise intensity
3. The exercise duration

Exercise Modality

Exercise modality (or **mode**) means the type of activity or the particular sport. For example, rowing has a very different effect on the cardiovascular-respiratory system than does football. Modalities are often classified by the type of energy demand (aerobic or anaerobic), the major muscle action (continuous and rhythmical, dynamic resistance, or static), or a combination of the energy system and muscle action. Walking, cycling, and swimming are examples of continuous, rhythmical aerobic activities; jumping, sprinting, and weight lifting are anaerobic and/or dynamic resistance activities. To determine the effects

Exercise A single acute bout of bodily exertion or muscular activity that requires an expenditure of energy above resting level and that in most, but not all, cases results in voluntary movement.

Homeostasis The state of dynamic equilibrium (balance) of the internal environment of the body.

Exercise Response The pattern of homeostatic disruption or change in physiological variables during a single acute bout of physical exertion.

Exercise Modality or Mode The type of activity or sport; usually classified by energy demand or type of muscle action.

TABLE 1.1   Absolute and Relative Submaximal Workloads

	Absolute Workload		Relative Workload	
	Maximal Lift	**No. of Times 80 lb Can Be Lifted**	**75% of Maximal Lift**	**No. of Times 75% Can Be Lifted**
Gerry	160	12	120	10
Pat	100	6	75	10
Terry	80	1	60	10

of exercise on a particular variable, you must first know what type of exercise is being performed.

Exercise Intensity

Exercise intensity is most easily described as maximal or submaximal. **Maximal (max) exercise** is straightforward; it simply refers to the highest intensity, greatest load, or longest duration an individual is capable of doing. Motivation plays a large part in the achievement of maximal levels of exercise. Most maximal values are reached at the endpoint of an *incremental exercise test to maximum*; that is, the exercise task begins at a level the individual is comfortable with and gradually increases until he or she can do no more. The values of the physiological variables measured at this time are labeled as "max"; for example, maximum heart rate is symbolized as HRmax.

Submaximal exercise may be described in one of two ways. The first involves a *set load*, which is a load that is known or is assumed to be below an individual's maximum. This load may be established by some physiological variable, such as working at a specific heart rate (perhaps 150 b·min^{-1}); at a specific work rate (e.g., 600 kgm·min^{-1} on a cycle ergometer); or for a given distance (perhaps a 1-mi run). Such a load is called an **absolute workload**. If an absolute workload is used, and the individuals being tested vary in fitness, then some individuals will be challenged more than others. Generally, those who are more fit in terms of the component being tested will be less challenged and so will score better than those who are less fit and more challenged. For example, suppose the exercise task is to lift 80 lb in a bench press as many times as possible, as in the YMCA bench press endurance test. As illustrated in **Table 1.1**, if the individuals tested were able to lift a maximum of 160, 100, and 80 lb once, respectively, it would be anticipated that the first individual could do more repetitions of the 80-lb lift than anyone else. Similarly, the second individual would be expected to do more repetitions than the third, and the third individual would be expected to do only one repetition. In this case the load is not submaximal for all the individuals, because Terry can lift the weight only one time (making it a maximal lift for Terry). Nonetheless, the use of an absolute load allows for the ranking of individuals based on the results of a single exercise test and is therefore often used in physical fitness screenings or tests.

The second way to describe submaximal exercise is as a percentage of an individual's maximum. A load may be set at a percentage of the person's maximal heart rate, maximal ability to use oxygen, or maximal workload. This value is called a **relative workload** because it is prorated or relative to each individual. All individuals are therefore expected to be equally challenged by the same percentage of their maximal task. This should allow the same amount of time or number of repetitions to be completed by most, if not all, individuals. For example, for the individuals described in **Table 1.1**, suppose that the task now is to lift 75% of each one's maximal load as many times as possible. The individuals will be lifting 120, 75, and 60 lb, respectively. If all three are equally motivated, they should all be able to perform the same total number of repetitions. Relative workloads are occasionally used in physical fitness testing. They are more frequently used to describe exercises that are light, moderate, or heavy in intensity or to prescribe exercise guidelines.

There is no universal agreement about what exactly constitutes light, moderate, or heavy intensity. In general, this book uses the following classifications:

1. Low or light: ≤54% of maximum
2. Moderate: 55–69% of maximum
3. Hard or heavy: 70–89% of maximum
4. Very hard or very heavy: 90–99% of maximum
5. Maximal: 100% of maximum
6. Supramaximal: >100% of maximum

Maximal (max) Exercise The highest intensity, greatest load, or longest duration exercise of which an individual is capable.

Absolute Submaximal Workload A set exercise load performed at any intensity from just above resting to just below maximum.

Relative Submaximal Workload A workload above resting but below maximum that is prorated to each individual; typically set as some percentage of maximum.

Maximal Voluntary Contraction (MVC) The maximal force that the muscle can exert.

1-RM The maximal weight that an individual can lift once during a dynamic resistance exercise.

Maximum is defined variously in terms of workload or work rate, heart rate, oxygen consumption, weight lifted for a specific number of repetitions, or force exerted in a voluntary contraction. Specific studies may use percentages and definitions of maximum that vary slightly.

Exercise Duration

Exercise duration is simply a description of the length of time the muscular action continues. Duration may be as short as 1–3 seconds for an explosive action, such as a jump, or as long as 12 hours for a full triathlon (3.2-km [2-mi] swim, 160-km [100-mi] bicycle ride, and 42.2-km [26.2-mi] run). In general, the shorter the duration, the higher the intensity that can be used. Conversely, the longer the duration, the lower the intensity that can be sustained. Thus, the amount of homeostatic disruption depends on both the duration and intensity of the exercise.

Exercise Categories

This textbook combines the descriptors of exercise modality, intensity, and duration into six primary categories of exercise. Where sufficient information is available, the exercise response patterns for each are described and discussed:

1. *Short-term, light to moderate submaximal aerobic exercise.* Exercises of this type are rhythmical and continuous in nature and utilize aerobic energy. They are performed at a constant workload for 10–15 minutes at approximately 30–69% of maximal work capacity.
2. *Long-term, moderate to heavy submaximal aerobic exercise.* Exercises in this category also utilize rhythmical and continuous muscle action. Although predominantly aerobic, anaerobic energy utilization may be involved. The duration is generally between 30 minutes and 4 hours at constant workload intensities ranging from 55 to 89% of maximum.
3. *Incremental aerobic exercise to maximum.* Incremental exercises start at light loads and continue by a predetermined sequence of progressively increasing workloads to an intensity that the exerciser cannot sustain or increase further. This point becomes the maximum (100%). The early stages are generally light and aerobic, but as the exercise bout continues, anaerobic energy involvement becomes significant. Each workload/work rate is called a stage, and each stage may last from 1 to 10 minutes, although 3 minutes is most common. Incremental exercise bouts typically last between 5 and 20 minutes for the total duration.
4. *Static exercise.* Static exercises involve muscle contractions that produce an increase in muscle tension and energy expenditure but do not result in meaningful movement. Static contractions are measured as some percentage of the muscle's **maximal voluntary contraction (MVC)**, the maximal force that the muscle can exert. The intent is for the workload to remain constant, but fatigue sometimes makes that impossible. The duration is inversely related to the percentage of maximal voluntary contraction (%MVC) that is being held, but generally ranges from 2 to 10 minutes.
5. *Dynamic resistance exercise.* These exercises utilize muscle contractions that exert sufficient force to overcome the presented resistance, so that movement occurs, as in weight lifting. Energy is supplied by both aerobic and anaerobic processes, but anaerobic is dominant. The workload is constant and is based on some percentage of the maximal weight the individual can lift (**1-RM**) or a resistance that can be lifted for a specified number of times. The number of repetitions, not time, is the measure of duration.
6. *Very-short-term, high-intensity anaerobic exercise.* Activities of this type last from a few seconds to approximately 3 minutes. They depend on high-power anaerobic energy and are often supramaximal.

Complete the Check Your Comprehension 1 box.

CHECK YOUR COMPREHENSION 1

Describe each of the following activities using the terms of the six exercise response categories.

1. A male cheerleader holds a female cheerleader overhead.

2. A body builder poses.

3. A new mother pushes her baby in a stroller in the park for 20 minutes.

4. A freshman in high school takes the FITNESSGRAM® PACER (Progressive Aerobic Cardiovascular Endurance Run) test in physical education class.

5. An adult male completes a minitriathlon in 2:35.

6. A basketball player executes a fast break ending with a slam dunk.

7. A volleyball player performs two sets of six squats.

8. A cyclist completes a 25-mi time trial in 50:30.6

9. An exercise physiology student completes a graded exercise test on a cycle ergometer with 3-minute stages and + 50 kgm·min⁻¹ per stage to determine $\dot{V}O_2$max.

10. A barrel racer warms up her horse for 15 minutes prior to competition.

11. A middle-aged individual performs 18 repetitions in the YMCA bench press endurance test.

12. A college athlete participates in a 400-m track race.

Check your answers in Appendix C.

Exercise Response Patterns

Throughout the textbook, the exercise response patterns for the six categories of exercise are described verbally and depicted graphically. For ease of recognition, consistent background colors and icons represent each category of exercise (**Table 1.2**). **Figure 1.3** presents six of the most frequent graphic patterns resulting from a constant workload/work rate, that is, all of the exercise categories except incremental exercise to maximum and very-short-term, high-intensity anaerobic exercise. Frequent incremental exercise patterns are depicted in **Figure 1.4**. The verbal descriptors used throughout the book are included on these graphs and in the following paragraphs. Note that the y-axis can be any variable that is measured with its appropriate unit of measurement. Examples are heart rate (b·min^{-1}), blood pressure (mmHg), and oxygen consumption (mL·kg·min^{-1}). Only specific graphic patterns are applicable to any given variable. These combinations of pattern and variable are described in the exercise response sections in each unit. Although not indicated in the figure, curvilinear changes can also be described as exponential—either positive or negative. For each exercise response, the baseline, or starting point against which the changes are compared, is the variable's resting value. Your goal here is to become familiar with the graphic patterns and the terminology used to describe each.

The patterns showing an initial increase or decrease with a plateau at steady state (**Figure 1.3A and B**) are the most common responses to short-term, light to moderate submaximal aerobic exercise. Patterns that include a drift seen as the gradual curvilinear increase or decrease from a plateau despite no change in the external workload (**Figure 1.3C and D**), typically result from

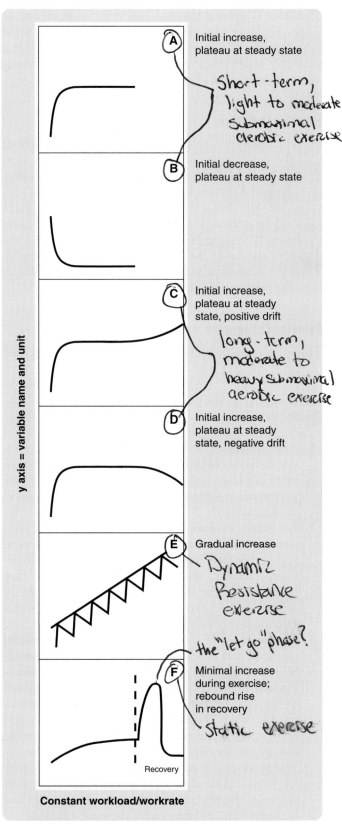

FIGURE 1.3 Graphic Patterns and Verbal Descriptors for Constant Workload/Work Rate Exercise Responses.

TABLE 1.2	Color and Icon Interpretation for Exercise Response Patterns		
Exercise Category		**Color**	**Icon**
Short-term, light to moderate submaximal aerobic			
Long-term, moderate to heavy submaximal aerobic			
Incremental aerobic to maximum			
Static			
Dynamic resistance			
Very short-term, high-intensity anaerobic			

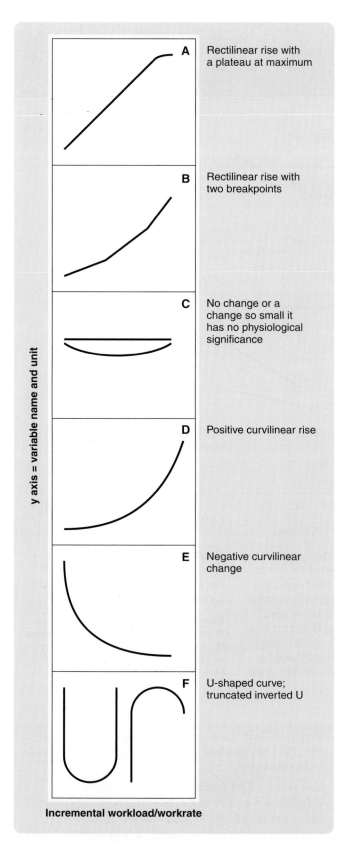

A Rectilinear rise with a plateau at maximum

B Rectilinear rise with two breakpoints

C No change or a change so small it has no physiological significance

D Positive curvilinear rise

E Negative curvilinear change

F U-shaped curve; truncated inverted U

y axis = variable name and unit

Incremental workload/workrate

FIGURE 1.4 Graphic Patterns and Verbal Descriptors for Incremental Workload/Work Rate Exercise Responses.

long-term, moderate to heavy submaximal aerobic exercise. Another form of gradual increase despite no change in the external workload (**Figure 1.3E**), is frequently seen during dynamic resistance exercise as a saw tooth pattern resulting from the sequential lifting and lowering of the weight. Finally, some categories of exercise may show a smooth, gradual increase (the straight rising line of **Figure 1.3E**). Minimal change during exercise with a rebound rise in recovery is almost exclusively a static exercise response (**Figure 1.3F**).

As the title of **Figure 1.4** indicates, all of these patterns of response routinely result from incremental exercise to maximum. Panel **1.4F** shows two versions of the U-shaped pattern. You may see either a complete or truncated (shortened) U, either upright or inverted. No specific patterns are shown for very-short-term, high-intensity anaerobic exercise, because these tend to be either abrupt rectilinear or curvilinear increases or decreases.

Exercise Response Interpretation

When interpreting the response of variables to any of the exercise categories, keep four factors in mind:

1. Characteristics of the exerciser
2. Appropriateness of the selected exercise
3. Accuracy of the selected exercise
4. Environmental and experimental conditions

Characteristics of the Exerciser

Certain characteristics of the exerciser can affect the magnitude of the exercise response. The basic pattern of the response is similar, but the magnitude of the response may vary with the individual's sex, age (child/adolescent, adult, older adult), and/or physiological status, such as health and training level. Where possible, these differences will be pointed out. See the Focus on Research Box for an example.

Appropriateness of the Selected Exercise

The exercise test used should match the physiological system or physical fitness component one is evaluating. For example, you cannot determine cardiovascular endurance using dynamic resistance exercise. However, if the goal is to determine how selected cardiovascular variables respond to dynamic resistance exercise, then, obviously, that is the type of exercise that must be used.

The modality used within the exercise category should also match the intended outcome. For example, if the goal is to demonstrate changes in cardiovascular-respiratory fitness for individuals training on a stationary cycle, then an incremental aerobic exercise to maximum test should be conducted on a cycle ergometer, not a treadmill or other piece of equipment.

The Effects of Age, Sex, and Physical Training on the Response to Exercise

Exercise professionals and exercise participants have long been interested in how personal characteristics influence the body's response to exercise. In this study, the authors investigated the effects of age, sex, and physical training on cardiovascular responses to exercise. They separated 110 healthy subjects into eight groups based on three variables: age (young [mid 20s] or old [mid 60s]), sex (male or female), and physical training (trained or untrained). The table below identifies the eight groups based on these three subject characteristics.

	Males	**Females**
Young	Trained (TR)	Trained (TR)
	Untrained (UT)	Untrained (UT)
Old	Trained (TR)	Trained (TR)
	Untrained (UT)	Untrained (UT)

Results of this study are shown in the figure at the right, which depicts for each group the systolic blood pressure responses to incremental treadmill tests to maximum. These data reveal:

1. Systolic blood pressure response to incremental exercise to maximum was significantly greater in older persons than in younger persons. This is true for males and females regardless of training status.

2. Maximal systolic blood pressure was significantly lower in trained females than in untrained females.

Although the authors investigated many variables, we describe only systolic

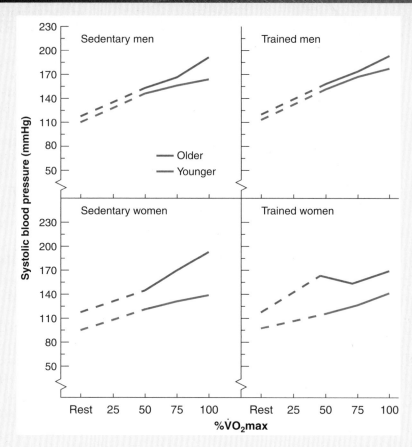

blood pressure because the purpose here is only to demonstrate how characteristics of the exerciser affect exercise response. Throughout this book, exercise response is discussed in terms of age, sex, and physical training. This study is an excellent example of how these characteristics influence the exercise response of a given variable. Exercise professionals

should understand such relationships in order to recognize normal and abnormal responses to exercise and respond accordingly.

Source: Ogawa, T., R. J. Spina, W. H. Martin, W. M. Kohrt, K. B. Schectman, & J. O. Holloszy: Effects of aging, sex, and physical training on cardiovascular responses to exercise. *Circulation*. 86:494–503 (1992).

Accuracy of the Selected Exercise

The most accurate tests are called **criterion tests**. They represent a standard against which other tests are evaluated. Most criterion tests are **laboratory tests**—precise, direct measurements of physiological function that usually involve monitoring, collection, and analysis of expired air, blood, or electrical signals. Typically, these require expensive equipment and trained technicians. Not all laboratory tests, however, are criterion tests.

Field tests can be conducted almost anywhere, such as a school gymnasium, playing field, or health club. Field tests are often performance-based and estimate the values

Criterion Test The most accurate tests for any given variable; the measurement standard against which other tests are judged.

Laboratory Test Precise, direct measurement of physiological functions for the assessment of exercise responses or training adaptations; usually involves monitoring, collection, and analysis of expired air, blood, or electrical signals.

Field Test A performance-based test that can be conducted anywhere and that estimates the values measured by the criterion test.

measured by the criterion test. The mile run is a field test used to assess cardiovascular-respiratory fitness, which is more directly and accurately measured by the criterion test of maximal oxygen consumption ($\dot{V}O_2$max). Both laboratory and field tests are discussed in this text.

Environmental and Experimental Conditions

Many physiological variables are affected by environmental conditions, most notably temperature, relative humidity (RH), and barometric pressure. Normal responses typically occur at neutral conditions (~20–29°C [68–84°F]; 50% RH; and 630–760 mm Hg, respectively). Likewise, when a response to exercise is described, it is assumed that the exerciser had adequate sleep, was not ill, had not recently eaten or exercised, and was not taking any prescription or nonprescription drugs or supplements that could affect the results. If any of these assumed conditions is not met, the expected exercise response might not occur.

Training

Training is a consistent or chronic progression of exercise sessions designed to improve physiological function for better health or sport performance. The two main goals for exercise training are (1) health-related physical fitness and (2) sport-specific physical fitness (sometimes called athletic fitness).

Health-Related Versus Sport-Specific Physical Fitness

In this textbook the phrase **health-related physical fitness** refers to that portion of physical fitness directed toward the prevention of or rehabilitation from disease, the development of a high level of functional capacity

---

Training A consistent or chronic progression of exercise sessions designed to improve physiological function for better health or sport performance.

Health-Related Physical Fitness That portion of physical fitness directed toward the prevention of or rehabilitation from disease, the development of a high level of functional capacity for the necessary and discretionary tasks of life, and the maintenance or enhancement of physiological functions in biological systems that are not involved in performance but are influenced by habitual activity.

Hypokinetic Diseases Diseases caused by and /or associated with lack of physical activity.

Sport-specific Physical Fitness That portion of physical fitness directed toward optimizing athletic performance.

---

for the necessary and discretionary tasks of life, and the maintenance or enhancement of physiological functions in biological systems that are not involved in performance but are influenced by habitual activity. The individual's goal may be to participate minimally in an activity to achieve some health benefit before disease occurs. The goal may be to participate in a substantial amount of exercise to improve or maintain a high level of physical fitness. Or a disabled individual's goal may be to participate in an activity to recover and/or attain the maximal function possible. All goals should include avoiding injury during the process.

Three components of health-related physical fitness are generally recognized: cardiovascular-respiratory endurance (aerobic power), body composition, and muscular fitness (strength, muscular endurance, and flexibility) (American College of Sports Medicine, 2010; Canadian Society for Exercise Physiology, 2004; The Cooper Institute, 2010). **Figure 1.5** (inner circle) shows that these components form the core of physical fitness. The relationships between each of these fitness components and **hypokinetic disease** are described in appropriate later units. Hypokinetic diseases are diseases caused by and/or associated with a lack of physical activity. Health-related physical fitness is important for everyone.

Sport-specific physical fitness has a more narrow focus; it is that portion of physical fitness directed toward optimizing athletic performance. **Figure 1.5** shows that sport-specific (athletic) fitness (outer circle) expands from the core of health-related physical fitness. Higher levels of cardiovascular-respiratory endurance and anaerobic power and capacity are generally needed for successful performance. Body composition values may be more specific than health levels in order to optimize performance. The muscular fitness attributes of power, balance, and flexibility are frequently more specific in certain athletic performances than for health.

To determine the importance of each component of fitness and develop a sport-related fitness program, you first analyze the specific sport's physiological demands. Then the athlete is evaluated in terms of those requirements. These elements allow for a specifically designed, individualized program. This program should:

- Work specific musculature while achieving a balance between agonist and antagonistic muscle groups
- Incorporate all motor fitness attributes that are needed
- Use the muscles in the biomechanical patterns of the sport
- Match the cardiovascular and metabolic energy requirements of the sport
- Attend realistically to body composition issues

The demands of the sport will not change to accommodate the athlete. The athlete must be the one to meet the demands of the sport to be successful.

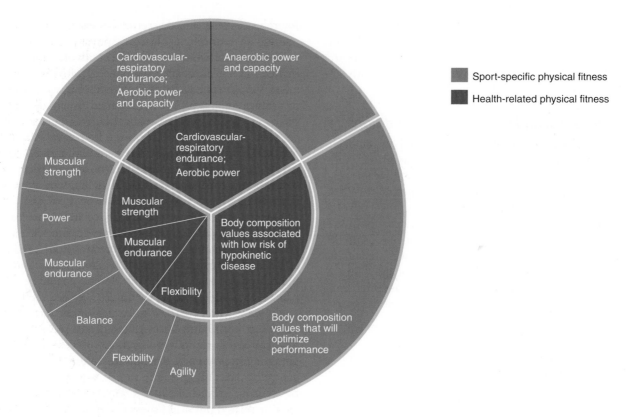

FIGURE 1.5 Physical Fitness.
Physical fitness consists of health-related physical fitness (inner circle) and sport-specific physical fitness (outer circle). Health-related physical fitness is composed of components representing cardiovascular-respiratory endurance, metabolism, and muscular fitness (strength, muscular endurance, and flexibility). Sport-specific physical fitness builds on health-related physical fitness and adds motor attributes (such as agility, balance, and power) and anaerobic power and capacity, as needed.

Putting all of these elements together, **physical fitness** may be defined as a physiological state of well-being that provides the foundation for the tasks of daily living, a degree of protection against hypokinetic disease, and a basis for participation in sport (American Alliance for Health, 1988). It is a product, the result of the process of doing physical activity/exercise.

Dose-Response Relationships

Major questions in exercise physiology revolve around "how much exercise/activity is enough?" and "what is the relationship between specific amounts of exercise/activity or physical fitness levels and the benefits achieved?" To the exercise scientist, these are what are called dose-response relationship questions. A **dose-response relationship** describes how a change in one variable is associated with a corresponding change in another variable. In this context, the training dose refers to the characteristics of the training program, that is, the type, intensity, frequency, duration, and/or volume of the exercise program or physical activity undertaken by the individual or group. The response means the changes that occur when a specific volume or dose of exercise/physical activity is performed.

Thus, for physical activity and health, dose-response describes the health-related changes obtained for the particular level of physical activity performed. Likewise, for physical fitness and health, the dose-response describes the health-related changes that occur with experimentally documented changes or levels of fitness (Haskell, 2007). These experimentally derived relationships can be graphed and are often called curves. Although it is clear, for example, that exercise/physical activity reduces the risk of many diseases and improves cardiovascular function, it is far less clear what the minimal dose of physical activity may be to acquire risk reduction or how much additional activity/fitness is needed to confer additional benefits. The shape of the dose-response curve may vary (large benefit for minimal increase, small benefit for large

Physical Fitness A physiological state of well-being that provides the foundation for the tasks of daily living, a degree of protection against hypokinetic disease, and a basis for participation in sport.

Dose-response relationship A description of how a change in one variable is associated with a corresponding change in another variable.

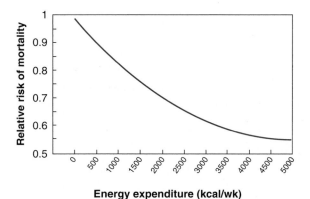

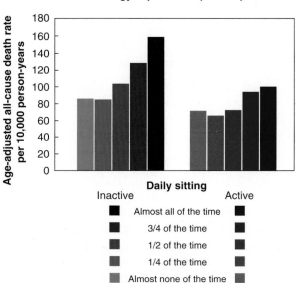

FIGURE 1.6 Data Showing Dose-Response Relationships. Panel A shows the relative risk for all-cause mortality and its relationship to baseline physical activity energy expenditure in elderly males and females with coronary artery disease. Panel B shows age-adjusted all-cause mortality and its relationship in both male and females to daily sitting amount.

Sources: (A) Janssen, I. & C. J. Jolliffe: Influence of physical activity on mortality in elderly with coronary artery disease. *Medicine & Science in Sports & Exercise.* 38(3):418–423 (2006). (B) Modified from Katzmarzyk, P.T., T.S. Church, C.L. Craig, & C. Bouchard. *Medicine & Science in Sports & Exercise.* 41(5): 998–1005 (2009).

increase, etc.) depending upon the health benefit or physiological variable being measured, and the population that is being studied.

Two examples of dose-response curves are presented in **Figure 1.6**. Panel **A** is an actual curve and depicts an inverse or negative dose-response relationship. That is, the higher the weekly energy expenditure, the lower the relative risk of mortality. Panel **B** is an example where the curve is implied by the relative heights of the bars in the graph. In contrast to Panel **A**, this dose-response relationship is a direct or positive one. That is, the higher the amount of daily sitting time, the higher the pro-rated all-cause death rate. Note that the mortality rate varies between those who are active and those who are inactive. However, although lower even within the active group (defined as participating in at least 30 min of moderate intensity exercise 5 d·wk⁻¹) there is a strong association between sitting and risk of mortality.

Considerable research is currently being done to discern the shapes of the dose-response curves in order to clarify exercise/physical activity recommendations for various benefits and populations. Until more dose-response information is available, we can only cite variations for the upper and lower recommendations in order to acknowledge that these guidelines do not represent a threshold below which no benefits are achieved. There is undoubtedly a point of diminishing return, where more exercise is not necessarily better. Conversely, it is also absolutely clear that some activity is always better than no activity. Somewhere between the minimal and maximal doses of exercise/physical activity may be an optimal dose. Such a dose would provide the greatest health benefit for the least amount of time and effort and the least risk of injury (American College of Sports Medicine, 2010; Haskell, 2007). Similarly both athletes and coaches would like to know dose-response and optimal levels of training or fitness to maximize performance. Ideally, one dose would also be optimal for all possible desirable health/performance outcomes and all populations. This is highly unlikely, but unknown at this point. As a result a variety of public health statements on the amount of exercise/physical activity/fitness necessary for obtaining health-related benefits are available. These are discussed in this text, as well as considerations for sport performance in the context of the application of the training principles.

Training Principles

Although there is much we do not know about training, and new training techniques appear often, eight fundamental guidelines are well established and should form the basis for the development of any training program. These **training principles** are defined and briefly discussed in the following sections, but the specific details for applying each principle, as well as the anticipated results or adaptations, are discussed in appropriate later units.

1. *Specificity.* This principle is sometimes called the SAID principle, which stands for "specific adaptations to imposed demands"; that is, what you do is what you get.

Training Principles Fundamental guidelines that form the basis for the development of an exercise training program.

When you develop an exercise training program, you first determine the goal. Fitness programs for children and adolescents, for example, differ from those for older adults. Training programs for non-athletes differ from training programs for athletes. Athletic training programs vary by sport, by event, or even by position within the same sport.

Second, you analyze the physiological requirements for meeting the goal. What physiological system is being stressed: the cardiovascular-respiratory, the metabolic, or the neuromuscular-skeletal? What is the major energy system involved? What motor fitness attributes (agility, balance, flexibility, strength, power, muscular endurance) need to be developed? The more closely the training program matches these factors, the greater its chance for success.

2. *Overload*. Overload is a demand placed on the body greater than that to which it is accustomed. To determine the overload, first evaluate the individual's critical physiological variables (specificity). Then consider three factors: frequency—the number of training sessions daily or weekly; intensity—the level of work, energy expenditure, or physiological response in relation to the maximum; and duration—the amount of time spent training per session or per day. **Training volume** is the quantity or amount of overload (frequency times duration for anaerobic or aerobic continuous exercise or number of sets times number of repetitions for resistance exercise), whereas training intensity represents the quality of overload.

3. *Rest/Recovery/Adaptation*. Adaptation is the change in physiological function that occurs in response to training. Adaptation occurs during periods of rest, when the body recovers from the acute homeostatic disruptions and/or residual fatigue and, as a result, may compensate to above-baseline levels of physiological functioning. This is sometimes called *supercompensation* (Bompa, 1999; Freeman, 1996). It is therefore critical for exercisers to receive sufficient rest between training sessions, after periods of increased training overload, and both before and after competitions. Adaptation allows the individual to either do more work or to do the same work with a smaller disruption of baseline values. Keeping records and retesting individuals are generally necessary to determine the degree of adaptation.

4. *Progression*. Progression is the change in overload in response to adaptation. The best progression occurs in a series of incremental steps (called *steploading*), in which every third or fourth change is actually a slight decrease in training load (Bompa, 1999; Freeman, 1996). This step-down allows for recovery, which leads to adaptation. Each step should be small, controlled and flexible. A continuous unbroken increase in training load should be avoided. Complete the Check Your Comprehension 2 box.

CHECK YOUR COMPREHENSION 2

Below are three patterns of overload progression in the general conditioning phase of an athlete's training. Select the one that is best, and justify your answer.

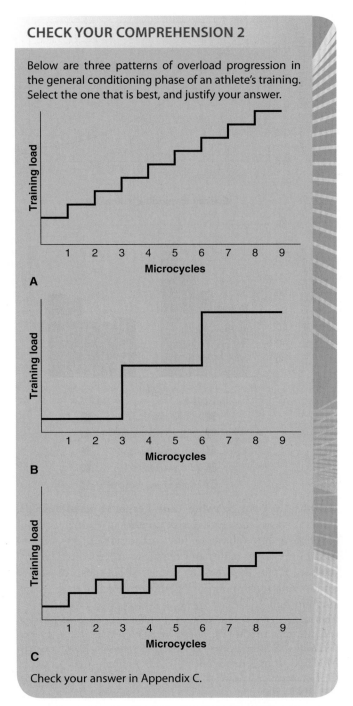

A

B

C

Check your answer in Appendix C.

5. *Retrogression/Plateau/Reversibility*. Progress is rarely linear, predictable, or consistent. When an individual's adaptation or performance levels off, a plateau has been reached. If it decreases, retrogression has occurred. A plateau should be interpreted relative to the training regimen. Too much time spent doing the same type of

Training Volume The quantity of training overload calculated as frequency times duration for anaerobic or aerobic continuous exercise or number of sets times number of repetitions for resistance exercise).

workout using the same equipment in the same environment can lead to a plateau. Either too little or too much competition can lead to a plateau. Plateaus are a normal consequence of a maintenance overload, and may also occur normally, even during a well-designed, well-implemented steploading progression. Variety and rest may help the person move beyond a plateau. However, if a plateau continues for some time or if other signs and symptoms appear, then the plateau may be an early warning signal of overreaching or overtraining (Chapter 22). Retrogression may signal overreaching or overtraining. Reversibility is the reversal of achieved physiological adaptations that occurs after training stops (detraining).

6. *Maintenance.* Maintenance is sustaining an achieved adaptation with the most efficient use of time and effort. At this point, the individual has reached an acceptable level of physical fitness or training. The amount of time and effort required to maintain this adaptation depends on the physiological systems involved. For example, more time and effort are needed to maintain adaptations in the cardiovascular system than in the neuromuscular system. In general, intensity is the key to maintenance. That is, as long as exercise intensity is maintained, frequency and duration of exercise may decrease without losing positive adaptations.

7. *Individualization.* Individuals require personalized exercise prescriptions based on their fitness levels and goals. Individuals also adapt differently to the same training program. The same training overload may improve physiological performance in one individual, maintain physiological and performance levels in a second individual, and result in maladaptation and performance decreases in a third. Such differences often result from lifestyle factors, particularly nutritional and sleep habits, stress levels, and substance use (such as tobacco or alcohol). Age, sex, genetics, disease, and the training modality also all affect individual exercise prescriptions and adaptations.

8. *Warm-Up/Cooldown.* A warm-up prepares the body for activity by elevating the body temperature. Conversely, a cooldown allows for a gradual return to normal body temperature. The best type of warm-up is specific to the activity that will follow and individualized to avoid fatigue.

Another important element beyond the physiological training principles is motivation. Except at a military boot camp, it is very difficult to force anyone to train. Therefore, any training program should also be fun. Intersperse games,

> **Periodization** Plan for training based on a manipulation of the fitness components with the intent of peaking the athlete for the competitive season or varying health-related fitness training in cycles of harder or easier training.

CHECK YOUR COMPREHENSION 3

Mark, a 30-year-old teacher, was disappointed when he ran the local 10-km (6.2 mi) Corn Harvest race in 49:04, which was within seconds of his previous year's time under similar weather conditions. To prepare for the race, he had been training for the previous 6 months. His training consisted of walking for 30 minutes on the Stairmaster at level 10, 2 days per week; running 3 mi in 25–30 minutes on another 2 days; and swimming or bicycling for 45–60 minutes on a 5th day. He did his runs and cycling with Kristi, a 25-year-old fellow teacher, and let her set the pace. She did not run the race.

Considering all eight training principles, identify three principles that apply here and that Mark may not have followed very well. For each one, make a suggestion as to how he might better apply it to prepare more successfully for the upcoming Turkey Trot 10-km race in 3 months.

variations, and special events with the training, and strive to make normal training sessions as enjoyable as possible.

Complete the Check Your Comprehension 3 box now.

Periodization

A training program should be implemented in a pattern that is most beneficial for adaptations. This pattern is called the training cycle or periodization. **Periodization** is a plan for training based on a manipulation of the sport's fitness components and the training principles. The objective is to peak the athlete's performance for the competitive season or some part of it while managing fatigue and avoiding overtraining (Plisk and Stone, 2003). In general, periodized training progresses from high-volume, low-intensity training to high-intensity, low-volume training for both endurance and resistance weight training as the program progresses (Plisk and Stone, 2003). There are a variety of ways of organizing periodization schedules. See the Focus on Application box for an example of a study that tested two variations of periodization in previously untrained female college students. An individual training for health-related physical fitness should also use periodization to build in cycles of harder or easier training, or to emphasize one component or another, to prevent monotony.

Figure 1.7 is an example of how periodization might be arranged for an athlete, in this case a basketball player whose season lasts approximately 4.5 months. This is intended as an example only, because periodization depends on the individual's situation and abilities. The time frame in our example is for 1 year—presented as 52 weeks (outer circle)—and is divided into four phases or cycles (Bompa, 1999; Freeman, 1996; Kearney, 1996):

1. The general preparation phase (sometimes labeled off-season)
2. The specific preparation phase (also known as preseason)

FOCUS ON APPLICATION

Linear versus Undulating Periodization

Two of the basic periodization models for resistance training are the linear (also know as traditional or stepwise) model and the undulating (also known as the nontraditional, nonlinear or mixed methods) model. Linear periodization starts with the typical high-volume/low-intensity training and progresses through an emphasis on hypertrophic adaptation (strength-endurance) to basic strength and finally to strength and power thus gradually reversing the emphasis to high-intensity/low-volume training. In undulating training, however, volume and intensity vary on a weekly or daily basis.

Kok et al. (2009) compared these two methods in twenty college students when total workload and average training intensity were matched by the end of the training. All participants received four familiarization sessions prior to testing and 3 weeks of pretraining conditioning before baseline testing. The actual training routines are presented in the accompanying table. Note that in the linear training group (LP) the exercise prescription is by phase and varies only in terms of the % of 1-RM (percentage of the maximal amount of weight the individual could lift one time) for each set, whereas for the undulating training group (UP) both the number of repetitions per set and the % 1-RM vary by day.

Results of the training adaptations for the 1-RM bench press (kg) and 1-RM Squat (kg) are presented in the accompanying figure. Both groups improved significantly in these two lifts at T2 (week 6), T3 (week 9), and T4 (week 12) tests when compared to the baseline testing at T1 (week 3). Squat jump height and bench press throw, indicators of power, (not shown) improved similarly. It was concluded that both programs improved strength and power equally and therefore, either technique may be used.

Source: Kok et al. (2009).

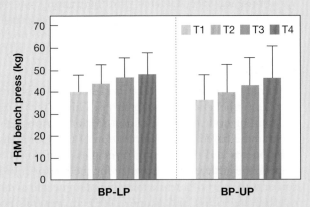
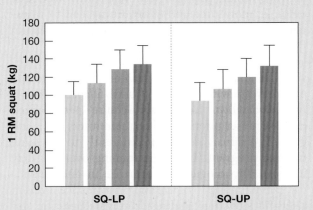

Pretraining Conditioning: Weeks 1-3			T1: Division of Subjects into Groups	Training Phase I: Weeks 4-6			Training Phase II: Weeks 7-9			Training Phase III: Weeks 10-12		
All subjects perform the same training			LP	Week 1 (H)	Week 2 (H)	Week 3 (H)	Week 1 (S)	Week 2 (S)	Week 3 (S)	Week 1 (P)	Week 2 (P)	Week 3 (P)
				$\frac{75}{10}$ 3	$\frac{77}{10}$ 3	$\frac{80}{10}$ 3	$\frac{85}{6}$ 3	$\frac{90}{6}$ 3	$\frac{90}{6}$ 4	$\frac{30}{8}$ 3	$\frac{40}{8}$ 3	$\frac{40}{8}$ 4
				10RM × 3	10RM × 3	10RM × 3	6RM × 3	6RM × 3	6RM × 3	$\frac{30}{8}$ 3	$\frac{40}{8}$ 3	$\frac{40}{8}$ 3
Week 1	Week 2	Week 3	UP	Day 1 (H)	Day 2 (S)	Day 3 (P)	Day 1 (H)	Day 2 (S)	Day 3 (P)	Day 1 (H)	Day 2 (S)	Day 3 (P)
$\frac{70}{10}$ 2	$\frac{70}{10}$ 3	$\frac{70}{12}$ 3		$\frac{75}{10}$ 3	$\frac{85}{6}$ 3	$\frac{30}{8}$ 3	$\frac{77}{10}$ 3	$\frac{90}{6}$ 3	$\frac{40}{8}$ 3	$\frac{80}{10}$ 3	$\frac{90}{6}$ 4	$\frac{40}{8}$ 4
15RM × 2	12RM × 3	10RM × 3		10RM × 3	6RM × 3	$\frac{30}{8}$ 3	10RM × 3	6RM × 3	$\frac{40}{8}$ 3	10RM × 3	6RM × 3	$\frac{40}{8}$ 3

$\left[\frac{70}{10}\ 2 \right]$ denotes $\left[\frac{\text{% of 1RM}}{\text{repetitions}}\ \text{number of sets} \right]$ for the bench press and squat exercises, and all power exercises.

(15RM × 2) denotes the number of maximum repetitions to be performed for the required number of sets for all other exercises (except abdominal and back exercises).

(H), hypertrophy training; (P), power training; (S), maximal strength training.

---

3. The competitive (or in-season) phase
4. The transition (active rest) phase

Overload is rated on a scale of 0 (complete rest) to 10 (maximal) and is shown in the boxes on the inner circle. These values are relative to the individual athlete and do not represent any given absolute training load.

General Preparation Phase

The general preparation (off-season) phase should be preceded by a sport-specific fitness evaluation to guide both the general and specific preparation training program. Another evaluation might be conducted before the season if desired, or evaluations might be conducted systematically throughout the year to determine how the individual is responding to training and to make any necessary adjustments. All evaluation testing should be done at the end of a regeneration cycle so that fatigue is not a confounding factor. As the name implies, the general preparation phase (off-season) is a time of general preparation when health-related physical fitness components are emphasized to develop cardiovascular-respiratory endurance (an aerobic base), flexibility, and muscular strength and endurance. Any needed changes in body composition should be addressed during this phase (Kibler and Chandler, 1994). An aerobic base is important for all athletes, even those whose event is primarily anaerobic. A high aerobic capacity allows the individual to work at a higher intensity before accumulating large quantities of lactic acid. A high aerobic capacity also allows the individual to recover faster, which is important in itself and allows for a potentially greater total volume of work during interval sessions (Bompa, 1999).

The general preparation phases may occupy most of the year for a fitness participant. During this phase, overload progresses by steps in both intensity and volume (frequency times duration/sets times repetitions), with volume typically being relatively more important than intensity (Bompa, 1999).

Specific Preparation Phase

During the specific preparation phase (preseason phase), the athlete shifts to specific preparation for the fitness and physiological components needed to succeed in the intended sport. The training program is very heavy and generally occupies at least 6–8 weeks before the first competition or longer (in the example it is 12 weeks) before league competition. About midway through the specific preparatory phase, intensity may surpass volume in importance. Alternately, this shift to more emphasis on intensity than volume may not occur until the following competitive phase. This varies according to the physiological demands of particular sports and the relative length of the two phases. Sport technical skill training typically increases as the specific preparation phase progresses (Kibler and Chandler, 1994; Plisk and Stone, 2003).

Competitive Phase

Once the athlete begins the competition phase, the emphasis first shifts to maintaining the sport-specific fitness developed during the preseason. Although both volume and intensity may be maintained or intensity may even increase, heavy work should immediately follow a competition instead of directly preceding one. During the late season, when the most important competitions are usually held (such as conference championships or bowl games), the athlete should do only a minimum of training or taper gradually so that he or she is rested without being detrained. An analysis of 27 tapering studies revealed that the optimal taper for maximizing performance consists of 2 weeks during which training volume

is exponentially reduced by 41–60% without any modification of either training intensity or frequency (Bosquet et al., 2007).

Transition Phase

The transition phase begins immediately after the last competition of the year. The athlete should take a couple days of complete rest and then participate in active rest using noncompetitive physical activities outside the primary sport. This type of activity is often called cross-training. In this transition phase, neither training volume nor intensity should exceed low levels (Kibler and Chandler, 1994).

Macrocycles

Each periodization phase is typically divided into several types of *macrocycles* that may each vary in length from 2 to 6 weeks (Fry et al., 1992; Kibler and Chandler, 1994). It should be noted that some systems use the term macrocycle to indicate the total yearly plan and the term mesocycle to indicate phases that last 2–6 weeks (Plisk and Stone, 2003). In this text, we will use the definitions as indicated. Each type of cycle aims for an optimal mixture of work and rest. Macrocycles have five basic goals or patterns, described in the following sections. Different types of macrocycles may be used in a single phase of training.

1. *Developmental macrocycle.* **Figure 1.7A** illustrates a developmental macrocycle typically used in the preparatory stages. It is designed to improve either general or specific fitness attributes, such as strength, progressively. Overloading is achieved by a stepwise progression from low to medium to high by gradually increasing the load for three cycles (e.g., weeks 9, 10, and 11), followed in week 12 by a regeneration cycle back to the level of the second load or first increase, week 9). This level then becomes the base for the next loading cycle. This is what is meant by steploading.

2. *Shock macrocycle.* Shock macrocycles, such as the one illustrated in **Figure 1.7B**, are used primarily during the two preparatory phases and are designed to increase training demands suddenly. They should always be followed by an unloading regeneration cycle consisting of a drastically reduced training load.

3. *Competitive macrocycle.* Competitive macrocycles are based on maintaining physiological fitness while optimizing performance for competitions. Obviously, competitive macrocycles occur during the competitive phase.

4. *Tapering or unloading regeneration macrocycle.* Tapering or unloading regeneration macrocycles involve systematic decreases in overload to facilitate a physiological fitness peak or supercompensation (Bompa, 1999). As noted, unloading regeneration cycles are used both as breaks between other cycles and as the basis of the active transition phase (Bompa, 1999; Freeman, 1996; Kibler and Chandler, 1994).

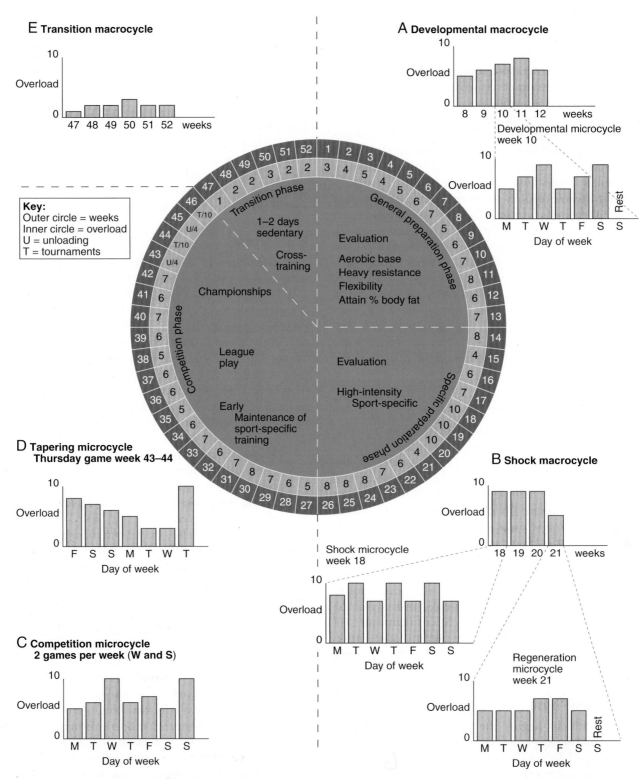

FIGURE 1.7 Periodization Phases and Overload.
The annual training plan consists of four phases: the general preparatory phase (which concentrates on developing the health-related physical fitness components), the specific preparatory phase (which emphasizes development of the sport-specific physical fitness components), the competitive phase (which emphasizes maintenance of all the physical fitness components), and the transition phase (which allows rest and recovery from the season but emphasizes cross-training to avoid complete detraining). Overload is rated on a scale of 0 (complete rest) to 10 (maximal) and is shown in the tan boxes on the inner circle. Three of the five types of macrocycles are illustrated [A (developmental), B (shock), and E (transition)] in the phases where they typically are used. Four of the five types of microcycles are also shown [A (developmental), B (shock), C (competitive), B and D (regeneration/tapering)] where they are typically used.

5. *Transition macrocycles.* Transition or regression macrocycles (**Figure 1.7E**) occur during the transition phase and involve very little overload. Tapering (regeneration) and transition phrases are intended to remove fatigue, emphasize relaxation, and prevent overreaching/overtraining. Some reversal (regression) of conditioning is expected. These phases are just as valuable for the fitness participant as the athlete.

Microcycles

Macrocycles are further divided into *microcycles*, each lasting 1 week (Fry et al., 1992; Kibler and Chandler, 1994) (**Figure 1.7A–D**). Similar to macrocycles, microcycles can be developmental, shock, competitive or maintenance, tapering or unloading regeneration, or transition or regression. Different types of microcycles may also be used in a single phase or macrocycle. For example, **Figure 1.7B** illustrates a shock macrocycle that contains both shock microcycles and a regeneration (unloading) microcycle. Likewise, **Figure 1.7 C** and **D** depict a tapering microcycle and a competitive microcycle in the competition phase. Microcycles are further subdivided into specific daily workouts or lesson plans designed by the coach for the athlete. Depending on the athlete's maturity and experience and the level of competition, a training day may entail one, two, or three workouts (Bompa, 1999).

Where possible throughout this text, periodization will be considered in the application of the training principles.

Training Adaptations

Training (**Figure 1.8**) brings about physical and physiological changes typically labeled adaptations. **Training adaptations** are physiological changes or adjustments resulting from an exercise training program that promote optimal functioning. Whereas exercise responses (those physiological changes that occur during a single exercise bout) use resting values as the baseline, training adaptations are evaluated against the same condition prior to training. That is, posttraining values for the variable of interest (on the y-axis) at rest are compared to pretraining values of that variable at rest. Posttraining values in the variable of interest during submaximal exercise are compared to pretraining values under the same submaximal exercise conditions. Similarly, posttraining maximal values of the variable of interest can be compared to pretraining maximal values. Time or exercise intensity, as always, is on the x-axis for the line graphs. Training adaptations may be presented as exercise response patterns using a line graph where T = trained state and UT = untrained state (**Figure 1.9 A–C**) or simply as specific values using a bar graph where T1 (Time 1) indicates the pretraining value and T2 (Time 2) indicates the post training value (**Figure 1.9D**).

Training results in adaptations that are an increase, a decrease, or unchanged in relation to the untrained state. For example, in **Figure 1.9A**, there is no difference in the values of this variable between the trained and untrained individuals either at rest or during submaximal exercise. However, the trained group increased at maximum over the untrained. In **Figure 1.9B**, training resulted in an increase at rest, during submaximal exercise, and at maximum. **Figure 1.9C** and **D** present the same adaptations in both a line graph and a bar graph to show how each might look. Both graphs indicate that training resulted in a decrease at rest and submaximal work, but no change at maximum.

Training adaptations at rest show more variation than either submaximal or maximal changes. In general, if the exercise test is an absolute submaximal test, the physiological responses will probably be decreased after training. For example, heart rate at a work rate of 600 kgm·min^{-1} might be 135 b·min^{-1} for an individual before training, but 128 b·min^{-1} after training. If the exercise test is a relative submaximal test, the physiological responses will probably show no change after training. That is, if an individual were to cycle at 75% $\dot{V}O_2$max both before and after training, it would be assumed that the $\dot{V}O_2$max, and therefore the amount of external work done at 75%, had increased because of the training. However, both the before and after training heart rate could be 142 b·min^{-1}. If the comparison is made at maximal effort, most physiological responses will increase, such as the $\dot{V}O_2$max in the preceding absolute example. These results do not hold for all variables but are general patterns.

The predominant way of looking at training adaptations (as opposed to during exercise responses) is that not only do they result from the chronic application of exercise but also they themselves represent *chronic changes*. Such adaptations become greater with harder training, are thought to exist as long as the training continues, and gradually return to baseline values when training stops (detraining). In reality, however, not all training adaptations follow this standard pattern. Some benefits occur only immediately after

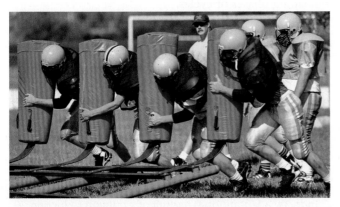

FIGURE 1.8 Training to Improve Physiological Function and Skill for Improved Performance.

Training Adaptations Physiological changes or adjustments resulting from an exercise training program that promote optimal functioning.

levels. The acute response of blood pressure to continuous aerobic endurance exercise is an increase in systolic blood pressure but little or no change in diastolic blood pressure. In the recovery period after exercise, systolic blood pressure decreases. In normal individuals, the decrease is back to the exerciser's normal resting value in a matter of minutes. In individuals with high blood pressure, this postexercise decrease can result in values below their abnormally high resting level for up to 3 hours after exercise. After 3 hours, the high resting values return. In some cases the last-bout effect can be augmented. That is, assuming the individual participates in a training program of sufficient frequency, intensity, and duration for a period of one to several weeks, the positive change occurring after each exercise bout may be increased. In the example just referred to, the decrease in systolic blood pressure might be 2 mmHg initially, but after several weeks the post exercise blood pressure decrease might be 6 mmHg for several hours. However, the adjustments that can occur are finite. Once the level of the *augmented last-bout effect* is reached, no further increase in training will bring about additional benefit (Haskell, 1994). This may be the reason why frequency and consistency are so important in overload for adaptation.

Overall, then, the adaptations that result from training can occur on three levels: (1) a chronic change, (2) a last-bout effect, and (3) an augmented last-bout effect. The majority of the training adaptations are dealt with in this book as if they are chronic changes unless otherwise specified.

Detraining

As noted in the retrogression/plateau/reversibility training principle, training adaptations are reversible. This is called detraining. **Detraining** is the partial or complete loss of training-induced adaptations as a result of a training reduction or cessation. Detraining may occur due to a lack of compliance with an exercise training program, injury, illness, or a planned periodization transition phase. Detraining should not occur during the tapering/unloading phases or cycles.

The magnitude of the reversal of physiological adaptations depends on the training status of the individual when the training is decreased or ceased, the degree of reduction in the training (minimal to complete), which element of training overload is impacted most (frequency, intensity, or duration), and how long the training is reduced or suspended.

Just as all physiological variables do not adapt at the same rate (days versus months), so all physiological

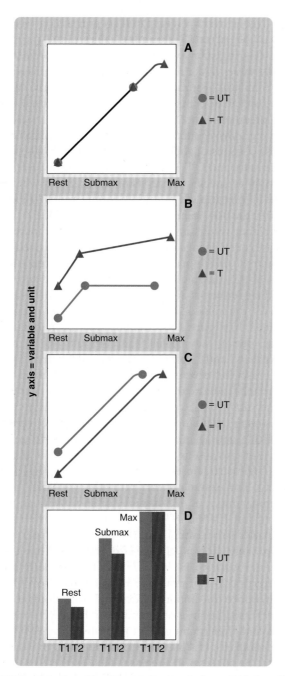

FIGURE 1.9 Graphic Patterns Depicting Training Adaptations.
Training adaptations are evaluated by comparing variables of interest before and after the training program during the same condition; that is, at rest, during submaximal exercise, or at maximal exercise. Before and after are either depicted by separate lines for untrained (UT) or trained (T) individuals or by the designations T1 and T2 indicating the first test and second test separated by the training program. Compared with the untrained state, training may cause no change, an increase, or a decrease in the measured variable.

the exercise session. These effects are called *last-bout effects* and should not be confused with the exercise response. For example, a last-bout effect can occur with blood pressure

Detraining The partial or complete loss of training-induced adaptations as a result of a training reduction or cessation.

variables do not reverse at the same rate. Unfortunately, less information is available about detraining than training. The timeline for the loss/reversal of adaptation for all variables and in all populations is unknown. Compounding this issue, it is often difficult to distinguish among changes resulting from illness, normal aging, and detraining. What is known will be discussed in this text within each unit, following the training adaptation sections.

Exercise and Training as Stressors

Exercise and training are often considered only in a positive manner, but both acute exercise and chronic training are stressors.

Selye's Theory of Stress

A stressor is any activity, event, or impingement that causes stress. **Stress** is defined most simply as a disruption in body homeostasis and all attempts by the body to regain homeostasis. Selye defines stress more precisely as "the state manifested by a specific syndrome that consists of all the nonspecifically induced changes within a biological system." The biological system here is the human body. The specific syndrome is the general adaptation syndrome (GAS), a step-by-step description of the bodily reactions to a stressor. It consists of three major stages (Selye, 1956):

1. The Alarm-Reaction: shock and countershock
2. The Stage of Resistance
3. The Stage of Exhaustion

In the *Alarm-Reaction stage*, the body responds to a stressor with a disruption of homeostasis (shock). It immediately attempts to regain homeostasis (countershock). If the body can adjust, the response is mild and advantageous to the organism; the *Stage of Resistance* or adaptation ensues. If the stress becomes chronic or the acquired adaptation is lost, the body enters the *Stage of Exhaustion*. At this point, the nonspecifically induced changes, which are apparent during the Alarm-Reaction but disappear during the Stage of Resistance, become paramount. These changes are labeled the triad of symptoms and include enlargement of the adrenal glands, shrinkage of thymus and lymphatic tissue, and bleeding ulcers of the digestive tract. Specifically induced changes directly related to the stressor may also occur; for example, if the stressor is cold (shock), the body may shiver to produce heat (countershock). Ultimate exhaustion is death (Selye, 1956).

> **Stress** The state manifested by the specific syndrome that consists of all the nonspecifically induced changes within a biological system; a disruption in body homeostasis and all attempts by the body to regain homeostasis.

Selye's Theory of Stress Applied to Exercise and Training

In the context of Selye's theory of stress, the pattern of responses exhibited by physiological variables during a single bout of exercise results directly from the disruption of homeostasis. This is the shock phase of the Alarm-Reaction stage. For many physiological processes (respiration, circulation, energy production, and so forth), the initial response is an elevation in function. The degree of elevation and constancy of this elevation depends on the intensity and duration of the exercise. Appropriate changes in physiological function begin in the countershock phase of the Alarm-Reaction and stabilize in the Stage of Resistance if the same exercise intensity is maintained for at least 1–3 minutes. The Stage of Exhaustion that results from a single bout of exercise, even incremental exercise to maximum, is typically some degree of fatigue or reduced capacity to respond to stimulation, accompanied by a feeling of tiredness. This fatigue is temporary and readily reversed with proper rest and nutrition.

Training programs are made up of a series of acute bouts of exercise organized in such a way as to provide an overload that puts the body into the Alarm-Reaction stage followed by recovery processes that not only restore homeostasis but also encourage supercompensation or adaptation (Kenttä and Hassmén, 1998; Kuipers, 1998; O'Toole, 1998). This can be manifested by altered homeostatic levels at rest, dampened homeostatic disruptions to absolute submaximal exercise loads, and/or enhanced maximal performances or physiological responses. When these adaptations occur, the body has achieved a Stage of Resistance. **Table 1.3** shows how the training principles previously introduced operate in the three stages of Selye's general adaptation syndrome.

The goal of a training program is to alternate the exerciser between Stages I and II and to avoid time in Stage III where recovery is not possible in a reasonable time. This process primarily proceeds by the cyclical interaction (shown by the arrows in **Table 1.3**) between adaptation (changes that occur in response to an overload) and progression (change in overload in response to adaptation). Each progression of the overload should allow for adaptation. However, this is not always accomplished.

Training Adaptation and Maladaptation

The results of exercise training can be positive or negative depending on how the stressors are applied. Training is related to fitness goals and athletic performance on a continuum that is best described as an inverted U (**Figure 1.10**) (Fry et al., 1991; Kuipers, 1998; Rowbottom et al., 1998). At one end of the continuum are individuals who are undertrained and whose fitness level and performance abilities are determined by genetics, disease, and

TABLE 1.3   Selye's Theory of Stress Applied to Exercise Physiology

Stage	Exercise Response	Training Principle	Training Adaptation/Maladaptation
I. Alarm-Reaction	Neuroendocrine system stimulated	Warm-up/Cooldown	
a. Shock	a. Homeostasis disrupted	Overload	Dampened response to equal
b. Countershock	b. Begin to attain elevated steady state	Progression*	acute exercise stimulus
II. State of Resistance	Elevated homeostatic steady state maintained if exercise intensity is unchanged	Adaptation Maintenance Specificity (SAID) Individualization	Enhanced function/physical fitness/health; increased maximal exercise depending on imposed demand and individual neuroendocrine physiology
		Reversibility	Adaptation is reversible with detraining
			Overreaching†
III. Stage of Exhaustion	Fatigue, a temporary state, reversed by proper rest and nutrition	Retrogression/ plateau reversibility	Overreaching Overtraining syndrome Maladaptation changes in neuroendocrine systems

*The cycle of adaptation and progression occurs repeatedly during a training program.
†If overreaching is planned and recovery is sufficient, positive adaptation results; if overreaching is accompanied by insufficient recovery and additional overload, overtraining will result.

nonexercise lifestyle choices. Individuals whose training programs lack sufficient volume, intensity, or progression for either improvement or maintenance of fitness or performance are also undertrained. The goal of optimal periodized training is the attainment of peak fitness and/or performance. However, if the training overload is too much or improperly applied, then *maladaptation* may occur.

The first step toward maladaptation may be *overreaching (OR)*, a short-term decrement in performance capacity that is easily recovered from and generally lasts only a few days to 2 weeks. Overreaching may result from planned shock microcycles, as described in the periodization section,

or result inadvertently from too much stress and too little planned recovery (Fry et al., 1991; Fry and Kraemer, 1997; Kuipers, 1998). If overreaching is planned and recovery is sufficient, positive adaptation and improved performance, sometimes called *supercompensation*, result. If, however, overreaching is left unchecked or the individual or coach interprets the decrement in performance as an indication that more work must be done, overreaching may develop into overtraining. Overtraining, more properly called the **overtraining syndrome (OTS)** (or staleness), is a state of chronic decrement in performance and ability to train, in which restoration may take several weeks, months, or even years (Armstrong and vanHeest, 1997; Fry et al., 1991; Fry and Kraemer, 1997; Kreider et al., 1998). The neuroendocrine-immune basis of all stress responses, and the maladaptations of overreaching and the overtraining syndrome, are discussed in the neuroendocrine-immune unit of this text.

The stress theory enhances our understanding of exercise, exercise training, and physical fitness. As emphasized previously, both exercise and exercise training are stressors. Thus, from the standpoint of stress theory, physical fitness may be defined as achieved adaptation to the stress imposed by muscular exercise. It results as an adaptation from a properly applied training program,

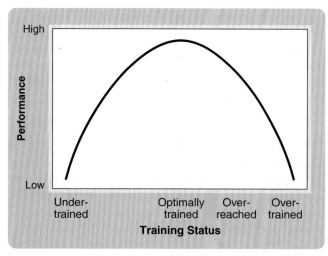

FIGURE 1.10 Training Status and Performance.

Overtraining Syndrome (OTS) A state of chronic decrement in performance and ability to train, in which restoration may take several weeks, months, or even years.

is usually exhibited in response to an acute exercise task, and implies avoidance of the OTS.

Strictly speaking, according to stress theory, supercompensation occurs because of a cause-effect relationship between fatigue and fitness. Recent periodization literature emphasizes the opposing effects of fitness and fatigue and is guided by the attempt to maximize the fitness responses to training stimuli while minimizing fatigue. Because fatigue is a natural consequence of training stress and because adaptations are manifested during recovery periods, fatigue management tactics become extremely important (Brown and Greenwood, 2005; Plisk and Stone, 2003).

SUMMARY

1. This chapter presents the general organization of the text and provides background information that will help you interpret and understand the information presented in later chapters.
2. This chapter differentiates between exercise responses to a single acute bout of exercise and training adaptations to a program of regular exercise.
3. The response to exercise, which is always a disruption in homeostasis, depends on the exercise modality, intensity, and duration. Interpretation of exercise responses must consider characteristics of the exerciser (age, sex, training status), appropriateness of the exercise test used (match between the intended physiological system and outcome), accuracy of the selected exercise (criterion or field test), and environmental and experimental conditions (temperature, relative humidity, barometric pressure, and subject preparation).
4. The baselines against which the exercise-caused disruptions of homeostasis are compared are normal resting values of the measured variables.
5. Health-related physical fitness is composed of components representing cardiovascular-respiratory endurance, metabolism, and muscular fitness (strength, muscular endurance, and flexibility).
6. Sport-specific physical fitness builds on health-related physical fitness and adds motor fitness attributes (such as agility, balance, and power) and anaerobic power and capacity, as needed.
7. Dose-response relationships describe how a change in one variable (such as exercise training, physical activity, or physical fitness level) is associated with a corresponding change in another variable (for example, training adaptations, health risk factors, or mortality).
8. Eight general training principles provide guidance for establishing and applying training programs: specificity, overload, rest/recovery/adaptation, progression, retrogression/plateau/reversibility, maintenance, individualization, and warm-up/cooldown.
9. Periodization provides a timeline for the planning of training programs that progresses through four phases or cycles: the general preparatory phase (off-season), the specific preparatory phase (preseason), the competitive phase (in-season), and the transition phase (active rest).
10. To prescribe a training program:
    a. analyze the physiological demands of the physical fitness program, rehabilitation, or sport goal;
    b. evaluate the individual relative to the established physiological demands; and
    c. apply the training principles relative to the established physiological demands in periodization cycles that allow for a steploading pattern of varying levels of exercise and rest or recovery.
11. Exercise training brings about adaptations in physiological function. Training adaptations are compared to corresponding pretraining conditions (the baseline).
12. Training adaptations may occur on at least three levels: a last-bout effect, an augmented last-bout effect, or a chronic change.
13. Detraining is the reversal of training adaptations caused by a decrease or cessation of exercise training. It depends upon the training status of the individual, the degree of reduction in the exercise training, which overload component is impacted most, and the length of time training is interrupted. The timeline for detraining is different for different physiological variables.
14. In the context of Selye's theory of stress, exercise is a stressor that causes a disruption of the body's homeostasis. During an acute bout of exercise, the body may progress from the Alarm-Reaction stage to the Stages of Resistance and (occasionally) Exhaustion. Training programs should be designed to provide an overload that allows adaptation and gradual progression, but avoids nonrecoverable time in the Stage of Exhaustion and the Overtraining Syndrome.

REVIEW QUESTIONS

1. Define exercise physiology, exercise, and exercise training.
2. Define and differentiate between exercise response and training adaptation.
3. Graph the most frequent responses physiological variables might exhibit in response to a constant workload/work rate exercise. Verbally describe these responses.
4. Graph the most frequent responses physiological variables might exhibit in response to an incremental exercise to maximum. Verbally describe these responses.
5. Differentiate between an absolute and relative submaximal workload/work rate exercise, and give an example other than weight lifting.
6. Fully describe an exercise situation, including all elements needed to accurately evaluate the exercise response.

7. Compare the components of health-related physical fitness with those of sport-specific physical fitness.
8. Define dose-response relationship. Give an example relevant to exercise physiology.
9. List and explain the training principles.
10. Explain the phases and cycles of a periodization training program.
11. Differentiate among the three levels of training adaptation, and state which level of adaptation is most common.
12. Relate detraining to the training principle of retrogression/plateau/reversibility. What factors does the degree of detraining depend on?
13. Explain the relationship of Selye's theory of stress to exercise, training, and physical fitness.

For further review and study, you can find lab exercises, worksheets, a quiz bank, and crossword puzzles at http://thePoint.lww.com/Plowman4e. ✳ ◉

REFERENCES

American Alliance for Health, Physical Education, Recreation and Dance: *Physical Best: A Physical Fitness Education and Assessment Program*. Reston, VA: Author (1988).

American College of Sports Medicine: *ACSM's Guidelines for Exercise Testing and Prescription* (8th ed.). Philadelphia, PA: Lippincott Williams & Wilkins (2010).

Armstrong, L. E. & J. L. vanHeest: The unknown mechanism of the overtraining syndrome: Clues from depression and psychoneuroimmunology. *SportsMedicine*. 32(3):185–209 (2002).

Bompa, T. O.: *Periodization: Theory and Methodology of Training*. Champaign, IL: Human Kinetics (1999).

Bosquet, L., J. Montpettit, D. Arvisais, & I. Mujika. Effects if tapering on performance: A meta-analysis. *Medicine & Science in Sports & Exercise*. 39(8):1358–1365 (2007).

Brown, L. E. & M. Greenwood: Periodization essentials and innovations in resistance training protocols. *Strength and Conditioning Journal*. 24(4):80–84 (2005).

Canadian Society for Exercise Physiology: *Canadian Physical Activity, Fitness & Lifestyle Approach: CSEP-Health & Fitness Program's Health-Related Appraisal and Counselling Strategy* (3rd ed). Ottawa, ON: Author (2004).

Caspersen, C. J., K. E. Powell & G.M. Christenson: Physical activity, exercise and physical fitness. *Public Health Reports*. 100:125–131 (1985).

Freeman, W. H.: *Peak When It Counts: Periodization for American Track & Field* (3rd ed.). Mountain View, CA: Tafnews Press (1996).

Fry, A. C., & W. J. Kraemer: Resistance exercise overtraining and overreaching: Neuroendocrine responses. *Sports Medicine*. 23:106–129 (1997).

Fry, R. W., A. R. Morton, & D. Keast: Overtraining in athletes: An update. *Sports Medicine*. 12(1):32–65 (1991).

Fry, R. W., A. R. Morton, & D. Keast: Periodisation and the prevention of overtraining. *Canadian Journal of Sports Science*. 17(3):241–248 (1992).

Haskell, W. L.: Dose-response issues in physical activity, fitness, and health. In: Bouchard, C., S. N. Blair, & W. L. Haskell: *Physical Activity and Health*. Champaign, IL: Human Kinetics (2007).

Haskell, W. L.: Health consequences of physical activity: Understanding and challenges regarding dose response. *Medicine and Science in Sports and Exercise*. 26(6):649–660 (1994).

Hellerstein, H. K.: Cardiac rehabilitation: A retrospective view. In M. L. Pollock & D. H. Schmidt (eds.), *Heart Disease and Rehabilitation*. Boston, MA: Houghton Mifflin, 511–514 (1979).

Janssen, I. & C. J. Jolliffe: Influence of physical activity on mortality in elderly with coronary artery disease. *Medicine & Science in Sports & Exercise*. 38(3):418–423 (2006).

Katzmarzyk, P. T., T. S. Church, C. L. Craig, & C. Bouchard. *Medicine & Science in Sports & Exercise*. 41(5): 998–1005 (2009).

Kearney, J. T.: Training the Olympic athlete. *Scientific American*. 274(6):52–63 (1996).

Kenttä, G., & P. Hassmén: Overtraining and recovery: A conceptual model. *Sports Medicine*. 26:1–16 (1998).

Kibler, W. B., & T. J. Chandler: Sport-specific conditioning. *American Journal of Sports Medicine*. 22(3):424–432 (1994).

Kraus, H., & R. Hirschland: Minimum muscular fitness tests in school. *Research Quarterly*. 25:178–188 (1954).

Kok, L. -Y., P. W. Hamer, & D. J. Bishop: Enhancing muscular qualities in untrained women: Linear versus undulating periodization. *Medicine & Science in Sports & Exercise*. 41(9): 1797–1807 (2009).

Kreider, R. B., A. C. Fry, & M. L. O'Toole: Overtraining in sport: Terms, definitions, and prevalence. In Kreider, R. B., A. C. Fry, & M. L. O'Toole (eds.): *Overtraining in Sport*. Champaign, IL: Human Kinetics, vii-is, (1998).

Kuipers, H.: Training and overtraining: An introduction. *Medicine & Science in Sports & Exercise*. 30(7):1137–1139 (1998).

O'Toole, M. L.: Overreaching and overtraining in endurance athletes. In Kreider, R. B., A. C. Fry, & M. L. O'Toole (eds.), *Overtraining in Sport*. Champaign, IL: Human Kinetics, 3–17 (1998).

Ogawa, T., R. J. Spina, W. H. Martin, W. M. Kohrt, K. B. Schectman, & J. O. Holloszy: Effects of aging, sex, and physical training on cardiovascular responses to exercise. *Circulation*. 86:494–503 (1992).

Plisk, S. S., & M. H. Stone: Periodization strategies. *Strength and Conditioning Journal*. 25(6):19–37 (2003).

Rowbottom, D. G., D. Keast, & A. R. Morton: Monitoring and preventing of overreaching and overtraining in endurance athletes. In Kreider, R. B., A. C. Fry, & M. L. O'Toole (eds.), *Overtraining in Sport*. Champaign, IL: Human Kinetics, 47–66 (1998).

Selye, H.: *The Stress of Life*. New York, NY: McGraw-Hill (1956).

The Cooper Institute: *FITNESSGRAM/ACTIVITYGRAM® Test Administration Manual*. (updated 4th ed.) Meredith, M. D. & G. J. Welk (eds.). Champaign, IL: Human Kinetics (2010).

Ullyot, J.: *Women's Running*. Mountain View, CA: World Publications (1976).

Metabolic System Unit

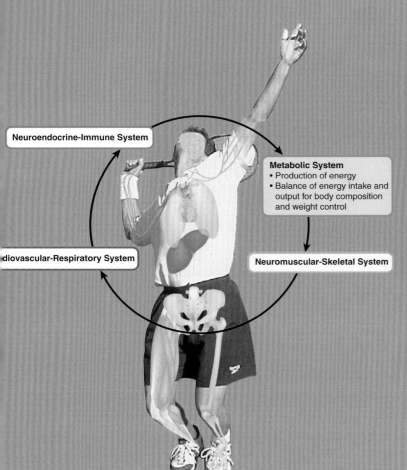

Neuroendocrine-Immune System

Cardiovascular-Respiratory System

Metabolic System
- Production of energy
- Balance of energy intake and output for body composition and weight control

Neuromuscular-Skeletal System

etabolism refers to the sum of all chemical processes that occur within the body. For the study of exercise physiology, the most important metabolic process is how muscle cells convert foodstuffs with or without oxygen to chemical energy (in the form of adenosine triphosphate) for physical activity. Without the production of adenosine triphosphate through metabolic processes, there could be no movement by the neuromuscular system; indeed, there could be no life. Because most energy production requires the presence of oxygen, metabolism largely depends on the functioning of the cardiorespiratory system.

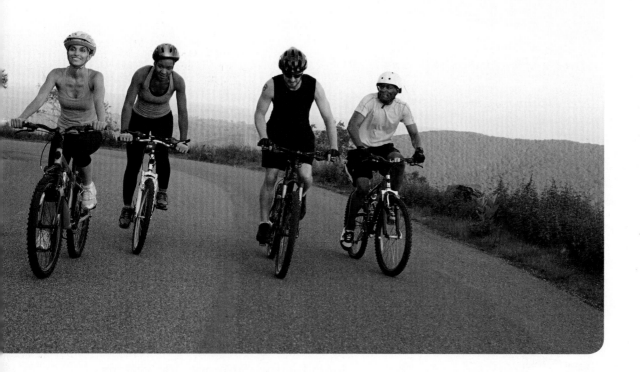

2 Energy Production

OBJECTIVES

After studying the chapter, you should be able to:

❭ Describe the role of adenosine triphosphate (ATP).

❭ Summarize the processes of cellular respiration for the production of ATP from carbohydrate, fat, and protein fuel substrates.

❭ Calculate the theoretical and actual number of ATP produced from glucose or glycogen, fatty acid, and amino acid precursors.

❭ Describe the goals of metabolic regulation during exercise.

❭ Explain how the production of energy is regulated by intracellular and extracellular factors.

❭ Compare the relative use of carbohydrate, fat, and protein fuel substrates based on the intensity and duration of exercise.

Introduction

Most individuals eat at least three meals a day. Eating is necessary to provide the energy that is essential for all cellular—and thus bodily—activity. To provide this energy, food must be transformed into chemical energy.

The total of all energy transformations that occur in the body is called **metabolism**. When energy is used to build tissues—as when amino acids are combined to form proteins that make up muscle—the process is called *anabolism*. When energy is produced from the breakdown of foodstuffs and stored so that it is available to do work, the process is called *catabolism*.

It is catabolism that is of primary importance in exercise metabolism. Energy is needed to support muscle activity, whether a little or a lot of muscle mass is involved or the exercise is light or heavy, submaximal or maximal. In providing this needed energy, the human body is subject to the *First Law of Thermodynamics*, which states that energy is neither created nor destroyed, but only changed in form. Figure 2.1 depicts this law and the changes in form representing catabolism. Potential chemical energy—or fuel—is ingested as food. Carbohydrates, fats, and protein can all be used as fuels, although they are not used equally by the body in that capacity. The chemical energy produced from the food fuel is stored as **adenosine triphosphate (ATP)**. The ATP then transfers its energy to energy-requiring physiological functions, such as muscle contraction during exercise, in which some energy performs the work and some is converted into heat. Thus, ATP is stored chemical energy that links the energy-yielding and the energy-requiring functions within all cells. The aim of this chapter is to fully explain ATP and how it is produced from carbohydrate, fat, and protein food sources.

Adenosine Triphosphate (ATP)

Structurally, ATP is composed of a carbon-nitrogen base called adenine, a 5-carbon sugar called ribose, and three phosphates, symbolized by P_i (inorganic phosphate). Each phosphate group is linked by a chemical bond. When one phosphate is removed, the remaining compound is

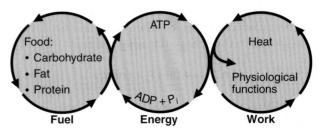

FIGURE 2.1 Generalized Scheme of Catabolic Energy Transformation in the Human Body.
Energy is the capacity to do work. Energy exists in six forms: chemical, mechanical, heat, light, electrical, and nuclear. Movement of the human body (work) represents mechanical energy that is supported by the chemical energy derived from food fuels. See animation, Catabolism, at http://thepoint.lww.com/plowman4e

adenosine diphosphate (ADP). When two phosphates are removed, the remaining compound is adenosine monophosphate (AMP).

The ATP energy reaction is reversible. When ATP is synthesized from ADP and P_i, energy is required. The addition of P_i is known as **phosphorylation**.

$$ADP + P_i + energy \rightarrow ATP$$

When ATP is broken down, energy is released. **Hydrolysis** is a chemical process in which a substance is split into simpler compounds by the addition of water. ATP is split by hydrolysis.

$$ATP \rightarrow ADP + P_i + energy\ for\ work + heat$$

The energy-requiring and energy-releasing reactions involving ATP are **coupled reactions**. Coupled reactions are linked chemical processes in which a change in one substance is accompanied by a change in another; that is, one of these reactions does not occur without the other. As the chemical agent that links the energy-yielding and energy-requiring functions in the cell, ATP is also a universal agent. It is the immediate source of energy for virtually all reactions requiring energy in all cells.

ATP is often referred to as cellular energy. Actually, ATP is a high-energy molecule. The term high energy means that the probability is high that when a phosphate is removed, energy will be transferred (Brooks et al., 2004). To better understand how the breakdown of ATP releases energy, consider the analogy of a spring-loaded dart gun. The dart can be considered analogous to P_i. It takes energy to "spring-load" the dart; this energy corresponds to the energy involved in the energy-requiring reaction:

$$ADP + P_i + energy \rightarrow ATP$$

Metabolism The total of all energy transformations that occur in the body.

Adenosine Triphosphate (ATP) Stored chemical energy that links the energy-yielding and energy-requiring functions within all cells.

Phosphorylation The addition of a phosphate (P_i).

Hydrolysis A chemical process in which a substance is split into simpler compounds by the addition of water.

Coupled Reactions Linked chemical processes in which a change in one substance is accompanied by a change in another.

Once the dart is loaded, the compressed spring has potential energy, which is released when the gun is fired. Firing corresponds to the energy-releasing reaction:

$$ATP \rightarrow ADP + P_i + energy$$

The ATP content of skeletal muscle at rest is about $6\,mmol \cdot kg^{-1}$. If not replenished, this amount could supply energy for only about 3 seconds of maximal contraction. The total amount of ATP stored in the body at any given time is approximately 0.1 kg, which is enough energy for only a few minutes of physiological function. However, ATP is constantly being hydrolyzed and resynthesized. The average adult produces and breaks down (turns over) approximately 40 kg (88 lb) of ATP daily, and an athlete may turn over 70 kg (154 lb) a day. The rate of hydrolysis of ATP during maximal exercise may be as high as $0.5\,kg \cdot min^{-1}$ (Mougois, 2006).

ATP can be resynthesized from ADP in three ways:

1. By interaction of ADP with CP (creatine phosphate, which is sometimes designated as PC, or phosphocreatine)
2. By anaerobic respiration in the cell cytoplasm
3. By aerobic respiration in the cell mitochondria

Phosphocreatine is another high-energy compound stored in muscles. It transfers its phosphate—and, thus, its potential energy—to ADP to form ATP, leaving creatine:

$$ADP + PC \rightarrow C + ATP$$

Resting muscle contains more CP ($\sim$20 mmol$\cdot$kg^{-1}) and C ($\sim$12 mmol$\cdot$kg^{-1}) than ATP. The maximal rate of ATP resynthesis from CP is approximately 2.6 mmol$\cdot$kg$\cdot$sec^{-1} and occurs within 1–2 seconds of the onset of maximal contraction. CP stores are used to regenerate ATP and in a working muscle will be depleted in 15–30 seconds. The rest of this chapter will concentrate on the more substantial production of ATP by the second and third techniques listed, namely, anaerobic and aerobic cellular respiration.

Cellular Respiration

The process by which cells transfer energy from food to ATP in a stepwise series of reactions is called **cellular respiration**. This term is used because, to produce energy, the cells rely heavily on the oxygen that the respiratory system provides. In addition, the by-product of energy production, carbon dioxide, is exhaled through the respiratory system. Cellular respiration can be either anaerobic or aerobic. **Anaerobic** respiration means it occurs in the absence of oxygen, does not require oxygen, or does not use oxygen. **Aerobic** means it occurs in the presence of oxygen, requires oxygen, or uses oxygen. Brain cells cannot produce energy anaerobically, and cardiac muscle cells have only a minimal capacity for anaerobic energy production. Skeletal muscle cells, however, can produce energy aerobically and/or anaerobically as the situation demands.

Figure 2.2 outlines the products and processes of cellular respiration, which are discussed in detail in the following sections. Following are some basic points about these processes:

1. All three major food nutrients, fats (FAT), carbohydrates (CHO), and proteins (PRO), can serve as fuel or **substrates**—the substances acted upon by enzymes—for the production of ATP.
2. The most important immediate forms of the substrates utilized are glucose (GLU), free fatty acids (FFA), and amino acids (AA). Both FFA and glycerol are derived from the breakdown of triglycerides. Some cells can use glycerol directly in glycolysis, but muscle cells cannot.
3. Acetyl coenzyme A (acetyl CoA) is the central converting substance (usually called the universal or *common intermediate*) in the metabolism of FAT, CHO, and PRO. Although the process of glycolysis provides a small amount of ATP as well as acetyl CoA, both beta-oxidation and oxidative deamination or transamination are simply preparatory steps by which FFA and AA are converted to acetyl CoA. That is, beta-oxidation and oxidative deamination or transamination are simply processes for converting FFA and AA, respectively, to a common substrate that allows the metabolic pathway to continue. The end result is that the primary metabolic pathways of the Krebs cycle, electron transport system (ETS), and oxidative phosphorylation (OP) are the same regardless of the type of food precursor. This is certainly more efficient than having totally different pathways for each food nutrient.
4. Each of the energy-producing processes or stages (glycolysis, formation of Acetyl CoA, Krebs cycle, ETS/OP) consists of a series of steps. Each step represents a small chemical change to a substrate resulting in a slightly different product in a precise, unvarying sequence with a designed first and last step. This is known as a **metabolic pathway**. That is, a metabolic pathway is a sequence of enzyme-mediated chemical reactions resulting in a specific product. Each stage may be made up of one or more metabolic pathways. These sequences of steps are important for the body because they allow energy to be released gradually. If all of the energy contained in food nutrients were released at one time, it would be predominantly released as heat and would destroy tissue.

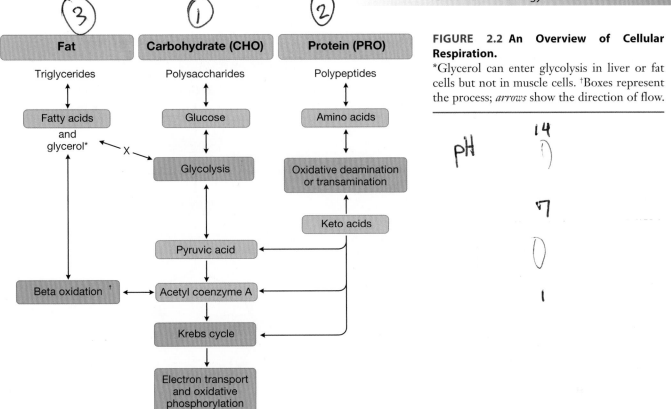

FIGURE 2.2 An Overview of Cellular Respiration.
*Glycerol can enter glycolysis in liver or fat cells but not in muscle cells. †Boxes represent the process; *arrows* show the direction of flow.

It is easy to be intimidated by or uninterested in so many steps, each with its own chemical structure, enzyme, and long, complicated name. There is a logic to these steps, however. It is on this logic and understanding (rather than the chemical structures) that the following discussion concentrates.

Carbohydrate Metabolism

The discussion of ATP production begins with carbohydrate metabolism for several reasons. First, many of the energy requirements of the human body are met by carbohydrate metabolism. Second, carbohydrate is the only food nutrient that can be used to produce energy anaerobically. Energy for both rest and exercise

is provided primarily by aerobic metabolism. However, exercise often requires anaerobic energy production, and then carbohydrate is essential. Third, carbohydrate is the preferred fuel of the body because carbohydrate requires less oxygen in order to be metabolized than fat. Finally, once you understand carbohydrate metabolism, it is relatively simple to understand how fats and proteins are metabolized.

Carbohydrates are composed of carbon (C), oxygen (O), and hydrogen (H). The complete metabolism of carbohydrate requires oxygen, which is supplied by the respiratory system and is transported by the circulatory systems to the muscle cells. The metabolism of carbohydrate also produces carbon dioxide (CO_2), which is removed via the circulatory and respiratory systems, and water.

The form of carbohydrate that is exclusively metabolized is glucose, a 6-carbon sugar arranged in a hexagonal formation and symbolized as $C_6H_{12}O_6$. Thus, all carbohydrates must be broken down into glucose in order to continue through the metabolic pathways. In its most simplistic form, the oxidation of glucose can be represented by the equation

$$C_6H_{12}O_6 + 6O_2 \rightarrow 6H_2O + 6CO_2$$

or

$$glucose + oxygen \rightarrow water + carbon\ dioxide$$

Cellular Respiration The process by which cells transfer energy from food to ATP in a stepwise series of reactions. It relies heavily on the use of oxygen.

Anaerobic In the absence of, not requiring, nor utilizing, oxygen.

Aerobic In the presence of, requiring, or utilizing, oxygen.

Substrate Fuel substance acted on by an enzyme.

Metabolic Pathway A sequence of enzyme-mediated chemical reactions resulting in a specified product.

In the skeletal muscle, cell oxidation is tightly coupled with phosphorylation to produce energy in the form of ATP. Therefore, the equation becomes

$$C_6H_{12}O_6 + O_2 + (ADP + P_i) \rightarrow CO_2 + ATP + H_2O$$

or

glucose + oxygen + (adenosine diphosphate + inorganic phosphate) → carbon dioxide + adenosine triphosphate + water

When excess glucose is available to the cell, it can be stored as **glycogen**, which is a chain of glucose molecules chemically linked together, or it can be converted to and stored as fat. The formation of glycogen from glucose is called *glycogenesis*. Glycogen is stored predominantly in the liver and muscle cells, as shown in the electron micrograph in **Figure 2.3**. When additional glucose is needed, stored glycogen is broken down (hydrolyzed) to provide glucose, through a process called **glycogenolysis**. Because glycogen must first be broken down into glucose, the production of energy from glucose or glycogen is identical after that initial step. The complete breakdown of glucose and glycogen follows the four-stage process outlined in **Figure 2.4** and detailed in later figures.

Stage I: Glycolysis Overview

Glycolysis is important in part because it prepares glucose to enter the next stage of metabolism (see **Figure 2.4**) by converting glucose to pyruvate. Also very important is the fact that ATP is produced directly during glycolysis. This process is the only way ATP is produced in the absence of oxygen (anaerobically).

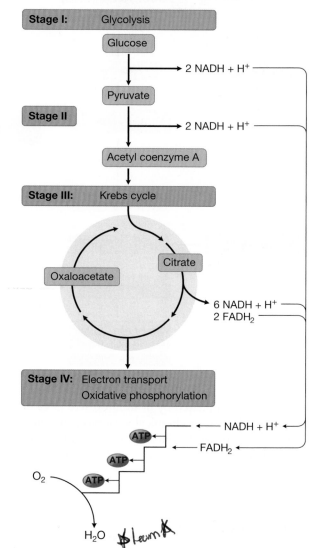

Embden-Meyerhof Pathway

FIGURE 2.4 The Four Stages of Carbohydrate Cellular Respiration.

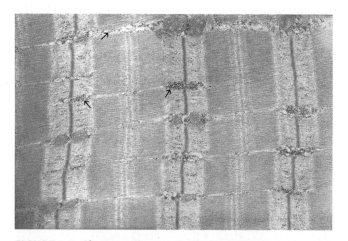

FIGURE 2.3 Glycogen Storage in Skeletal Muscle.
In this electron micrograph of skeletal muscle (EM: 25,000×), stored glycogen is visible as the small round black dots.
Source: Photo courtesy of Lori Bross, Northern Illinois University Electron Microscope Laboratory.

Glycolysis literally means the breakdown or dissolution of sugar. It is the energy pathway responsible for the initial catabolism of glucose in a 10- or 11-step process. Glycolysis begins with either glucose or glycogen and ends with the production of either pyruvate (pyruvic acid) by aerobic glycolysis or lactate (lactic acid) by anaerobic glycolysis (Frisell, 1982; Lehninger, 1971; Marieb and Hoehn, 2010; Mougois, 2006; Newsholme and Leech, 1983). (Note that names ending in *-ate* technically indicate the salts of their respective acids; that is lactate is the salt of lactic acid. However, the salt and acid forms are often used interchangeably in descriptions of the metabolic pathways.)

Each step is catalyzed by a specific enzyme. An **enzyme** is a protein that accelerates the speed of a chemical reaction without itself being changed by the reaction. It does

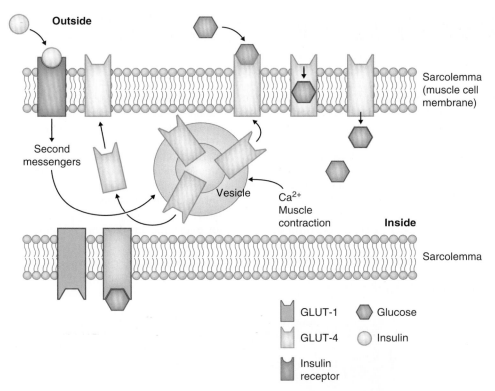

FIGURE 2.5 Glucose Transport into Muscle Cells.

In the resting muscle, when blood glucose levels are relatively stable, glucose enters by the non-insulin-regulated GLUT-1 transporters. Following a meal, insulin interacts with its receptors, and second messengers stimulate GLUT-4 to translocate from their storage vesicles to the sarcolemma and glucose is transported into the cell. During exercise and early recovery, muscle contraction involves Ca^{2+} release that stimulates the translocation of GLUT-4.

not cause a reaction that would not otherwise occur; it simply speeds up one that would occur anyway. Metabolic enzymes are easy to identify because their names usually end in the suffix *-ase*. Generally, their names are also related to the substrate or type of reaction (or both) they are catalyzing. For those reactions that are reversible, a specific single enzyme will catalyze the reaction in both directions.

The activity of enzymes is affected by the concentrations of the substrate acted upon and of the enzyme itself, temperature, pH, and the presence or absence of other ions, poisons, or medications. The following discussions describe how enzymes act in a normal physiological environment. Only a few selected enzymes that are especially important or function in regulatory or rate-limiting roles

Glycogen Stored form of carbohydrate composed of chains of glucose molecules chemically linked together.

Glycogenolysis The process by which stored glycogen is broken down (hydrolyzed) to provide glucose.

Glycolysis The energy pathway responsible for the initial catabolism of glucose in a 10- or 11-step process that begins with glucose or glycogen and ends with the production of pyruvate (aerobic glycolysis) or lactate (anaerobic glycolysis).

Enzyme A protein that accelerates the speed of a chemical reaction without itself being changed by the reaction.

are described here. *Regulatory or rate-limiting enzymes* are the enzymes that are critical in controlling the rate and direction of energy production along a metabolic pathway—just as a traffic light regulates the flow of vehicles along a road.

As a metabolic pathway, glycolysis begins with the absorption of glucose into the bloodstream from the small intestine or with the release of glucose into the bloodstream from the liver. Either step supplies the fuel. Glucose is then transported into the muscle cell. Transport occurs across the cell membrane via facilitated diffusion, utilizing a protein carrier and occurring down a concentration gradient. The carriers are called *glucose transporter carrier proteins, or GLUT*, and are differentiated by numbers, from 1 to 12 with a 13th labeled as HMIT (Wilson-O'Brien et al., 2010; Zhoa and Keating, 2007). Transport is a passive process that does not require the expenditure of energy.

The predominant transports of glucose in human skeletal and cardiac muscle and adipose cells are GLUT-1 (non–insulin-regulated) and GLUT-4 (insulin-regulated) transporters (**Figure 2.5**). GLUT-1 transporters are located in the sarcolemma or cell membrane. In resting muscles when blood glucose levels are relatively stable, most glucose enters by GLUT-1 transport. When glucose and insulin levels are high, such as after a meal, or when insulin levels are low, such as during exercise, most glucose enters by GLUT-4 transport. The GLUT-4 transporters are thus activated both by insulin, through a second messenger system, and by muscle contraction. Calcium (Ca^{2+})

FOCUS ON APPLICATION: *Clinically Relevant*

Diabetes

As described in the text and shown in Figure 2.5, for glucose to enter muscle cells and be used as fuel, insulin and GLUT-4 translocation or muscle contraction and GLUT-4 translocation is required. Malfunction of this process can result in diabetes mellitus.

Type 1 diabetes is an autoimmune disease that involves the destruction of the beta cells (β-cells) in the pancreas that normally secrete insulin. This leads to a deficiency of insulin, glucose intolerance (the inability to use carbohydrate effectively), and increased blood glucose levels (hyperglycemia).

Type 2 diabetes is characterized by a progression of steps indicating impaired regulation of glucose metabolism. The initial step is insulin resistance (the inability to achieve normal rates of glucose uptake in response to insulin). Insulin resistance is indicated by glucose intolerance, sometimes called impaired fasting glucose (IFG). IFG may be diagnosed in an individual more than 10 years before the disease fully develops. In response to insulin resistance, the β-cells increase insulin secretion (hyperinsulinemia), which may compensate for the insulin resistance for a while. However, at some point, the β-cells will fail and hyperglycemia occurs.

This signals that the clinical development of the disease, but not the consequences, is complete.

Research evidence indicates that the initial step of insulin resistance is due to dysfunction in the GLUT-4 translocator process. That is, insulin resistance results from a reduced ability to stimulate GLUT-4 cells to migrate to the cell surface. Precisely what in the insulin-signaling pathway is defective is unknown. The number of both GLUT-1 and GLUT-4 transporters is similar in those with and without Type 2 diabetes.

Although there is a genetic component to Type 2 diabetes, obesity and physical inactivity are strongly related to the expression of this predisposition. Conversely, exercise training increases GLUT-4 function in skeletal muscle that, in turn, improves insulin action on glucose metabolism and can be important in the prevention of, or delay in, the development of Type 2 diabetes

Sources: Alcazar et al. (2007); Dengel and Reynolds (2004).

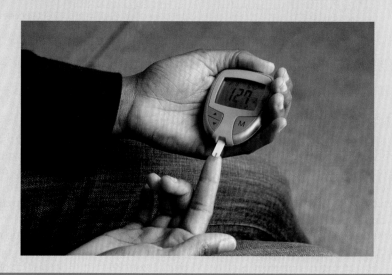

is probably one of the second messengers (Brooks et al., 2004; MacLean et al., 2000; Wilson-O'Brien et al., 2010; Zhoa and Keating, 2007). Within skeletal muscle, the number of GLUT-4 transporters is highest in fast-twitch oxidative glycolytic (FOG, Type IIA) fibers, followed by slow-twitch oxidative (SO, Type I) fibers, and is lowest in fast-twitch glycolytic (FG, Type IIX fibers (Sato et al., 1996).

GLUT-4 transporters exist intracellularly in small sacs or vesicles within the cytoplasm. When activated, they literally move to the cell surface (translocate) and serve as portals through which glucose enters the cell. The maximal rate of muscle glucose transport is determined both by the total number of GLUT-4 molecules and the proportion that are translocated to the cell membrane (Houston, 1995; Sato et al., 1996). The dual stimulation of GLUT-4 translocation by insulin and contraction is important because insulin secretion is suppressed during exercise. Thus, during exercise, the predominant activator of GLUT-4 transporters is the muscle contraction itself. When total work performed is equal, GLUT-4 increases are similar despite differences in exercise intensity and duration (Kraniou et al., 2006). The effect of muscle contraction persists into the early recovery period to help rebuild depleted glycogen stores (Houston, 1995).

Glycolysis takes place in the cytoplasm of the cell. The enzymes that catalyze each step float free in the cytoplasm. The substances acted upon by the enzymes and the resultant products are transferred by diffusion, which is the tendency of molecules to move from a region of high concentration to one of low concentration. All of the intermediates (everything but glucose and the pyruvate or lactate) are phosphorylated compounds—that is, they contain phosphates. All of the phosphate intermediates, ADP, and ATP are unable to pass through the cell membrane. The cell membrane, however, is freely permeable to glucose and lactate.

FIGURE 2.6 Stage I: Glycolysis.

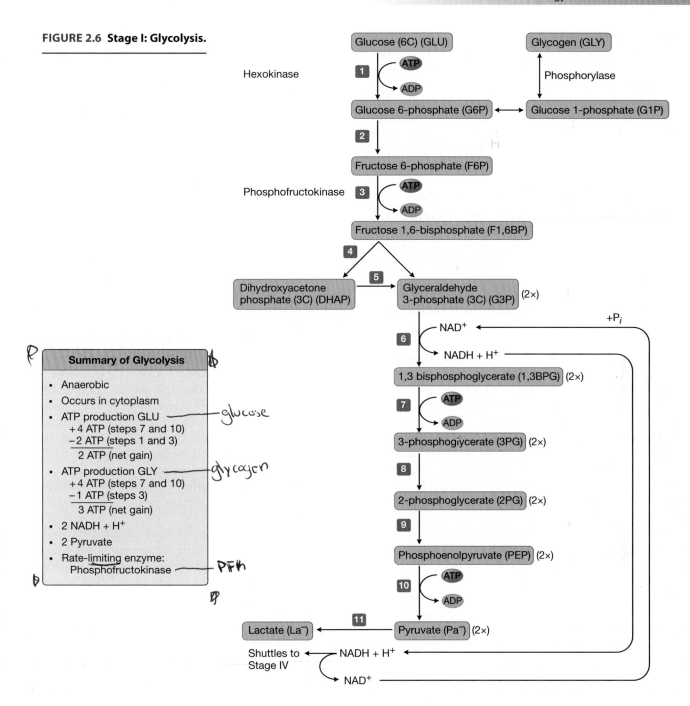

Glycolysis, as depicted in **Figure 2.6**, involves both the utilization and production of ATP. One ATP molecule is used in the first step if the initial fuel is glucose, but not if the initial fuel is glycogen. One ATP is used in step 3 regardless of whether the initial fuel is glucose or glycogen. Thus, 1 ATP is used for activation if the initial fuel is glycogen, but 2 ATP are used if the

initial fuel is glucose. ATP is produced from ADP + P_i at steps 7 and 10 by a process known as substrate-level phosphorylation. **Substrate-level phosphorylation** is the transfer of P_i directly from the phosphorylated intermediates or substrates to ADP without any oxidation occurring. A net total of 3 ATP are gained if glycogen is the initial fuel, but only 2 ATP are gained if glucose is the initial fuel.

Exactly how glycolysis is accomplished is explained in the following step-by-step analysis. First, however, one should understand the processes of oxidation and reduction and the role of nicotinamide adenine dinucleotide (NAD) and flavin adenine dinucleotide (FAD).

Substrate-Level Phosphorylation The transfer of P_i directly from a phosphorylated intermediate or substrates to ADP without any oxidation occurring.

OXIDATION-REDUCTION There are three kinds of **oxidation**: a gain of oxygen (hence the name), a loss of hydrogen, or the direct loss of electrons by an atom or substance.

The process whereby an atom or substance gains electrons is called **reduction**. The electron's negative charge reduces the molecule's overall charge. A good way to remember that electrons are gained through reduction, not oxidation, is to associate the "e" in reduction with the "e" in electron: reduction = +e⁻. Reduction can also mean a loss of oxygen or a gain of hydrogen by an atom or a substance. Electron donors are known as reducing agents, and electron acceptors as oxidizing agents. The major electron donors are organic fuels, such as glucose. Oxygen is the final electron acceptor or oxidizing agent in cellular respiration.

When one substance is oxidized, another is simultaneously reduced. The substance that is oxidized also loses energy; the substance that is reduced also gains energy.

Oxidation in the form of hydrogen removal occurs in several of the intermediary steps in cellular respiration. When hydrogen atoms are removed, they must be transported elsewhere. The two most important hydrogen carriers in cellular respiration are **nicotinamide adenine dinucleotide (NAD)** and **flavin adenine dinucleotide (FAD)**. Both NAD and FAD can accept two electrons and two protons from two hydrogen atoms. Each does so in a slightly different manner, however. FAD (the oxidized form is FAD_{ox}) actually binds both protons and is written as $FADH_2$ (or FAD reduced, written FAD_{red}). NAD actually exists as NAD^+ (or NAD oxidized, written NAD_{ox}); when bonded to hydrogen, it is written as $NADH + H^+$ (or NAD reduced, written as NAD_{red}). The symbols NAD^+ and FAD will be used to indicate the oxidized form in this text, and $NADH + H^+$ and $FADH_2$ will be used to indicate the reduced form of these carriers, so that it is clear where the hydrogen atoms are. NAD^+ is by far the more important hydrogen carrier in human metabolism.

A helpful analogy of the roles of FAD and NAD is a taxicab. The purpose of NAD and FAD is to transport (serve as taxis for) the hydrogen. NAD and FAD must pick up hydrogen passengers (be reduced) and they must drop them off (be oxidized) at another point without either the carrier (taxi) or the hydrogen (passengers) being permanently changed.

THE STEPS OF STAGE I Refer to **Figure 2.6** as each step is explained in the text (Frisell, 1982; Lehninger, 1971; Marieb and Hoehn, 2010; Mougios, 2006; Newsholme and Leech, 1983; Salway, 1994).

Step 1. The glucose molecule, which has 6 carbons indicated by the (6C), is phosphorylated (has a phosphate attached) through the transfer of one phosphate group from ATP to the location of the sixth carbon on the glucose hexagon, producing glucose-6-phosphate. Hexokinase is the enzyme that catalyzes this process. This phosphorylation effectively traps the glucose in that particular cell, because the electrical charge of the phosphate group prohibits glucose from crossing the membrane, and the enzyme that can break this phosphate bond is not present in muscle cells.

The same is true for the glycogen in the cells; that is, it is trapped in the muscle where it is stored. On the other hand, the liver has enzymes to break down glycogen and release glucose into the bloodstream.

These facts are important because during high-intensity, long-term exercise, glycogen stored in specific muscles must be used there. Furthermore, glycogen that is stored in muscles but not used in an activity (e.g., the upper body during a running event) cannot be transported from the inactive muscles to the active ones. Therefore, high levels of glycogen need to be stored in the muscles that will be used.

Step 2. The atoms that make up the glucose-6-phosphate are simply rearranged to form fructose-6-phosphate.

Step 3. Another molecule of ATP is broken down and the phosphate added at the first carbon. This addition places a phosphate group at each end of the molecule and results in the product fructose-1,6-bisphosphate. The prefixes *di-* and *bis-* both mean "two," but *di-* indicates two groups attached to the same spot and *bis-* at different positions. Two phosphates are now part of the molecule. This step is catalyzed by the enzyme phosphofructokinase (PFK), which is the rate-limiting enzyme in glycolysis.

Step 4. This is the step from which glycolysis, meaning sugar breaking or splitting, gets its name, for here the 6-carbon sugar is split into two 3-carbon sugars indicated by the (3C). The two sugars are identical in terms of their component atoms but have different names (dihydroxyacetone phosphate, or DHAP, and glyceraldehyde-3-phosphate, or G3P) because the component atoms are arranged differently.

Step 5. The atoms of dihydroxyacetone phosphate are rearranged to form glyceraldehyde 3-phosphate, with the phosphate group at the third carbon. From this point on, each step occurs twice (indicated by 2X in **Figure 2.6**), once for each of the three carbon subunits.

Step 6. Two reactions that are coupled occur in this step. In the first, a pair of hydrogen atoms is transferred from the G3P to the hydrogen carrier NAD^+, reducing this to $NADH + H^+$. The fate of this $NADH + H^+$ will be dealt with later. This reaction releases enough energy to perform the second reaction, which adds a phosphate from the P_i always present in the cytoplasm to the first carbon, so that the product becomes 1,3-bisphosphoglycerate.

Step 7. ATP is finally produced from ADP in this step when the phosphate from the first carbon is transferred to ADP, storing energy. Since this step is also doubled, 2 ATP molecules are formed.

Step 8. This is simply another rearrangement step where the phosphate is moved from the number 3 to the number 2 carbon.

Step 9. A water molecule is removed, which weakens the bond between the remaining phosphate group and the rest of the atoms.

Step 10. The remaining phosphate is transferred from phosphoenolpyruvate (PEP) to ADP, forming ATP and pyruvate. The enzyme that catalyzes this step is pyruvate kinase. Again, since the reaction happens twice, 2 ATP molecules are produced.

Step 11. If the hydrogen atoms carried by NADH + H$^+$ are unable to enter the electron transport chain (as described in Stage IV), they are transferred instead to pyruvate (pyruvic acid), forming lactate (lactic acid), which regenerates the NAD$^+$. The enzyme catalyzing this reaction is lactic dehydrogenase.

The formula for pyruvate is $C_3H_3O_3$ whereas the formula for lactate is $C_3H_5O_3$. The formula for pyruvic acid is $C_3H_4O_3$ and the formula for lactic acid is $C_3H_6O_3$. Both the number of carbon atoms and the number of oxygen atoms are the same; however, there are four fewer hydrogen atoms in two molecules of pyruvate/pyruvic acid than lactate/lactic acid. These are the hydrogen atoms that are carried by the NAD$^+$ from step 6 and used to produce the lactate ($2C_3H_5O_3$)/lactic acid ($2C_3H_6O_3$) from pyruvate/pyruvic acid. If lactate/lactic acid is not formed, the hydrogen atoms from step 6 may be carried further down the metabolic chain. Currently, there is some unresolved controversy as to whether skeletal muscle actually produces lactate or lactic acid. What has just been presented represents the accepted classic view and the interchangeable use of the salt and acid forms in the metabolic pathways and discussions will be maintained throughout this textbook (Brooks, 2010; Marcinek et al., 2010; Robergs et al., 2004).

When the end product of glycolysis is pyruvate/pyruvic acid, the process is called *aerobic glycolysis* (or *slow glycolysis*). When the end product of glycolysis is lactate/lactic acid, the process is called *anaerobic glycolysis* (or *fast glycolysis*). Glucose predominates as the fuel for slow glycolysis, and glycogen predominates as the fuel for fast glycolysis.

MITOCHONDRIA Mitochondria (the plural form of the singular mitochondrion) are subcellular organelles that are often called the powerhouses of the cell. The formation of acetyl CoA, Krebs cycle, electron transport, and oxidative phosphorylation all take place in the mitochondria.

Figure 2.7 presents a diagram and an electron micrograph of a mitochondrion: a three-dimensional, discretely encapsulated, bean-shaped structure. In actual living tissue mitochondria exist in many different shapes—and, indeed, they constantly change shapes.

As shown in **Figure 2.7**, mitochondria have seven distinct components. The first component is the outer membrane (labeled 1 in the figure). As is usual, this membrane serves as a barrier; however, it contains many channels

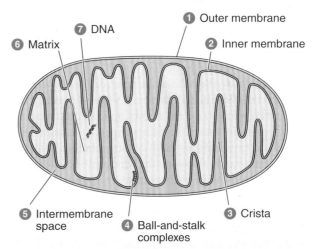

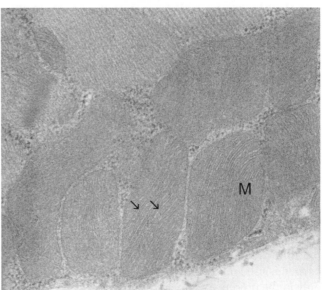

FIGURE 2.7 Mitochondrion.
The electron micrograph is of skeletal muscle mitochondria (EM: 40,000×).
Source: Electron micrograph provided by Lori Bross, Northern Illinois University Electron Microscope Laboratory.

Oxidation A gain of oxygen, a loss of hydrogen, or the direct loss of electrons by an atom or substance.

Reduction A loss of oxygen, a gain of electrons, or a gain of hydrogen by an atom or substance.

Nicotinamide Adenine Dinucleotide (NAD) A hydrogen carrier in cellular respiration.

Flavin Adenine Dinucleotide (FAD) A hydrogen carrier in cellular respiration.

Mitochondria Cell organelles in which the formation of acetyl CoA, Krebs cycle, electron transport, and oxidative phosphorylation take place.

through which solutes can pass and so is permeable to many ions and molecules. The second component (2) is an inner membrane. The inner mitochondrial membrane is impermeable to most ions and molecules unless each has a specific carrier. It is, however, permeable to water and oxygen. The inner membrane is parallel to the outer membrane in spots, but it also consists of a series of folds or convolutions called crista (3) (the plural is cristae). Extending through and protruding from the inner membrane are a series of protein-enzyme complexes called ball-and-stalk complexes (4) that look like a golf ball on a tee. Although the inner membrane has transport functions, the crista portion and especially the ball-and-stalk apparatus are specialized as the locations where ATP synthesis actually takes place.

The area between the two membranes is known simply as the intermembrane space (5). The center portion of the mitochondria is known as the matrix (6). The matrix is filled with a gel-like substance composed of water and proteins. Metabolic enzymes and DNA (7) for organelle replication are stored here.

The fact that mitochondria contain their own DNA means that they are self-replicating. When a need for more ATP arises, mitochondria simply split in half and then grow to their former size. This property, discussed later, has specific implications for how an individual adapts to exercise training. It also explains why some cells have only a few mitochondria but others have thousands. Red blood cells are unique in that they contain no mitochondria.

Mitochondria tend to be located where they are needed. Within muscle cells they lie directly beneath the cell membrane (called sarcolemmal or subsarcolemmal mitochondria) and among the contractile elements (called interfibrillar mitochondria).

Stage II: Formation of Acetyl Coenzyme A

Stage II (**Figure 2.8**) is a very short metabolic pathway consisting solely of the conversion of pyruvate to acetyl CoA (Frisell, 1982; Lehninger, 1971; Marieb and Hoehn, 2010; Newsholme and Leech, 1983). No ATP is either used or produced directly. However, a pair of hydrogen atoms (because all reactions still happen twice) are removed and picked up by NAD$^+$ to be transferred to the electron transport chain.

The conversion of pyruvate to acetyl CoA takes place within the mitochondrial matrix (**Figure 2.7**). This conversion requires that the pyruvate be transported across the mitochondrial membranes via a specific carrier. No oxygen is used directly in this stage, but these steps occur only in the presence of oxygen. As usual, enzymes catalyze each reaction.

THE STEPS OF STAGE II Refer to the diagram in **Figure 2.8** for the two steps of Stage II (Frisell, 1982; Lehninger, 1971; Marieb and Hoehn, 2010; Mougois, 2006; Newsholme and Leech, 1983; Salway, 1994).

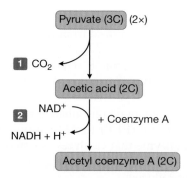

Summary of the Formation of Acetyl CoA

- Does not directly utilize O_2 but must be aerobic
- Occurs in mitochondrial matrix
- No ATP produced
- 2 NADH + H$^+$
- 2 CO_2
- 2 Acetyl CoA

FIGURE 2.8 Stage II: The Formation of Acetyl Coenzyme A.

Step 1. Pyruvate is converted to acetic acid. In the process, one molecule of CO_2 is removed. This CO_2, as well as the CO_2 that will be formed in Stage III, diffuses into the bloodstream and is ultimately exhaled via the lungs.

Step 2. Acetic acid is combined with coenzyme A to form acetyl Coenzyme A (acetyl CoA). A **coenzyme** is a nonprotein substance derived from a vitamin that activates an enzyme. The conversion of pyruvate to acetyl CoA commits the pyruvate to Stages III and IV since there is no biochemical means of reconverting acetyl CoA back to pyruvate.

Stage III: Krebs Cycle

The **Krebs cycle** is a cycle because it begins and ends with the same substance, called oxaloacetate (or oxaloacetic acid, abbreviated as OAA). The cycle is an eight-step process (see **Figure 2.9**) that actually comprises two metabolic pathways: one pathway for steps 1–3 and the second pathway for steps 4–8.

No ATP is used in the Krebs cycle, and only one step (5) results in the substrate-level phosphorylation production of ATP. However, four steps (3, 4, 6, and 8) result in the removal of hydrogen atoms, which are picked up by either NAD$^+$ or FAD. This result is critically important, because these are the hydrogen atoms that will provide the electrons for the electron transport system. Carbon dioxide is produced at steps 3 and 4. As with every step since the 6-carbon glucose molecule was split into two 3-carbon units in Stage I (step 4, **Figure 2.6**), every reaction and product is doubled.

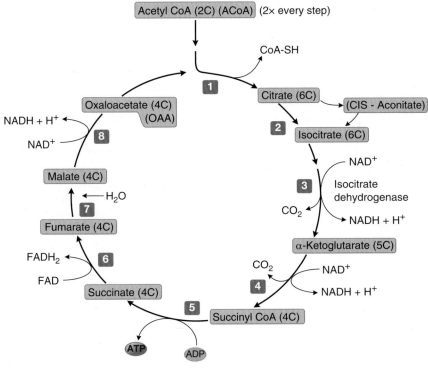

FIGURE 2.9 Stage III: The Krebs Cycle.

All of the enzymes and hence all of the reactions for the Krebs cycle occur within the mitochondrial matrix, with one exception. The enzyme succinate dehydrogenase that catalyzes step 6 is located in the inner mitochondrial membrane.

The intermediate molecules as well as the preliminary molecules, pyruvic acid and acetyl CoA, are keto acids. Although no oxygen is used directly, this stage requires the presence of oxygen.

THE STEPS OF STAGE III The steps for the Krebs cycle (Frisell, 1982; Lehninger, 1971; Marieb and Hoehn, 2010; Mougois, 2006; Newsholme and Leech, 1983; Salway, 1994) are presented in **Figure 2.9**, which you should refer to while reading the discussion.

Step 1. The 2-carbon acetyl CoA combines with the 4-carbon molecule oxaloacetate (OAA) to form citrate or citric acid. This cycle is thus also known as the citric

acid cycle. In the reaction, the coenzyme A (CoA-SH) is removed from acetyl CoA and is free to convert more pyruvate to acetyl CoA or to be used later in the cycle.

Step 2. The atoms of citric acid (citrate) are rearranged to become isocitrate. This rearrangement sometimes involves an intermediary substrate, cis-aconitate, being produced between citrate and isocitrate (shown in parenthesis is **Figure 2.9**). However, this step is not obligatory, and a single enzyme, aconitase, catalyzes both reactions (Newsholme and Leech, 1983).

Step 3. Two reactions occur. In the first, hydrogen atoms are removed and accepted by the carrier NAD^+, forming $NADH + H^+$. In the second reaction, a CO_2 is removed, leaving the 5-carbon α-ketoglutarate.

Step 4. Step 4 is basically a repetition of step 3 in that a pair of hydrogen atoms are removed and picked up by NAD^+ and a CO_2 is also removed. In addition, the remaining structure is attached to coenzyme A (CoA-SH). The resultant succinyl CoA has four carbons, which will remain intact throughout the rest of the cycle.

Step 5. In this step coenzyme A is displaced by a phosphate group, which in turn is transferred to a substance called guanosine diphosphate (GDP), resulting in guanosine triphosphate (GTP). GTP is equivalent to ATP in terms of energy and is labeled and counted as ATP in this book. This is the only step in the Krebs cycle that produces and stores energy directly. As in glycolysis, this ATP is produced by substrate-level phosphorylation.

Coenzyme A nonprotein substance derived from a vitamin that activates an enzyme.

Krebs Cycle A series of eight chemical reactions that begins and ends with the same substance; energy is liberated for direct substrate phosphorylation of ATP from ADP and P_i carbon dioxide is formed and hydrogen atoms removed and carried by NAD and FAD to the electron transport system; does not directly utilize oxygen but requires its presence.

Step 6. More hydrogen atoms are removed, but this time the carrier substance is FAD, forming $FADH_2$.

Step 7. Water is added, converting fumarate to malate.

Step 8. A pair of hydrogen atoms is removed and accepted by NAD^+. The remaining atoms once more make up oxaloacetate, and the cycle is ready to begin again.

The ATP produced in Stages I and III can be used immediately to provide energy for the cell. The CO_2 produced in Stage II diffuses into the bloodstream, is transported to the lungs, and is exhaled. Now we will describe what happens to all of the hydrogen atoms that are carried as $NADH + H^+$ and $FADH_2$.

Stage IV: Electron Transport and Oxidative Phosphorylation

The **electron transport system (ETS)** or respiratory chain is the final metabolic pathway in the production of ATP. It proceeds as a series of chemical reactions in the mitochondria that transfer electrons from the hydrogen atom carriers NAD and FAD to oxygen. Water is formed as a by-product, and the electrochemical energy released by the hydrogen ions is coupled to the formation of ATP from ADP and P_i (Frisell, 1982; Lehninger, 1971; Marieb and Hoehn, 2010; Mougois, 2006; Newsholme and Leech, 1983). The chain itself consists of a series

of electron (e^-) carriers and proton pumps embedded in the inner membrane of the mitochondria. Most carriers are proteins or proteins combined with metal ions (such as iron, Fe) that attract e^-. The major carriers are indicated in **Figure 2.10**. Four of these carriers are stationary: Complexes I, II, III, and IV. Three (I, III, and IV) are embedded into the inner membrane of the mitochondria, while Complex II is attached to the inner membrane on the matrix side. Cytochromes b and c_1 are part of Complex III, and cytochromes a and a_3 are part of Complex IV. Coenzyme Q and cytochrome c are mobile and diffuse through the inner membrane carrying electrons. Coenzyme Q moves from Complexes I and II to Complex III, and cytochrome c moves from Complex III to IV.

The H^+ and e^- come from the breakdown of the hydrogen atoms released in Stages I, II, and III and transported to the electron transport chain by NAD^+ and FAD:

$$2H = 2H^+ + 2e^-$$

The H^+ are deposited first into the mitochondrial matrix and then move via the proton pumps into the intermembrane space. The e^- are shuttled along from one electron acceptor to the next (see **Figure 2.10**). The e^- move along in a series of oxidation-reduction reactions, because each successive carrier in the sequence has a greater affinity

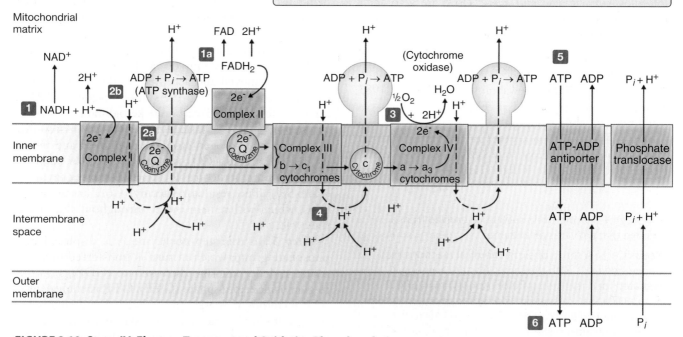

Summary of Electron Transport (ETS) and Oxidative Phosphorylation (OP)

- Directly utilizes O_2 as the final electron acceptor
- Occurs in inner mitochondrial membrane
- Includes 3 steps for ATP production for each $NADH + H^+$ and 2 for each $FADH_2$
- $2H^+ + 2e^- + \frac{1}{2}O_2 \rightarrow H_2O$
- Rate-limiting enzyme: Cytochrome oxidase

FIGURE 2.10 Stage IV: Electron Transport and Oxidative Phosphorylation.

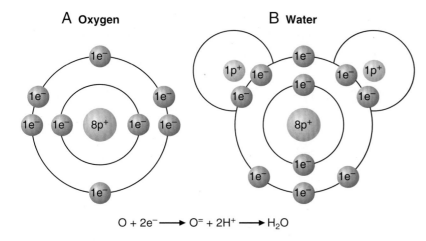

$$O + 2e^- \longrightarrow O^= + 2H^+ \longrightarrow H_2O$$

FIGURE 2.11 Oxygen as the Final Electron Acceptor.
A. The outer shell of oxygen has room for eight electrons but contains only six. Thus it can accept two electrons at the end of electron transport. **B.** When oxygen accepts these two electrons, it then has a double negative charge (O^{2-}). Two hydrogen ions (H^+) are thus attracted, and water (H_2O) is formed.

(force of chemical attraction) for them than the preceding one. Oxygen has the greatest affinity of all for e^- and acts as the final e^- acceptor. The additional electrons on the oxygen give it a negative charge and attract the positively charged H^+, thus forming water (**Figure 2.11**). Other H^+ move back from the intermembrane space to the matrix through the ball-and-stalk apparatus. This movement of the H^+ activates ATP synthetase, which phosphorylates ADP to ATP.

Thus, the formation of ATP from ADP and P_i is coupled to the movement of H^+ and e^- through and along the electron transport chain. The movement of those ions releases energy that is harnessed when ADP is phosphorylated to ATP. Because phosphate is added (phosphorylation) and the NADH + H^+ and $FADH_2$ are oxidized (electrons removed), the term **oxidative phosphorylation (OP)** is used to denote this formation of ATP. Oxidative phosphorylation is the process in which NADH + H^+ and $FADH_2$ are oxidized in the electron transport system and the energy released is used to synthesize ATP from ADP and P_i. Remember that the process of producing ATP directly in glycolysis and the Krebs cycle was called substrate-level phosphorylation because the P_i was transferred directly from phosphorylated intermediates to ADP without any oxidation occurring.

Electron Transport System (ETS) The final metabolic pathway, which proceeds as a series of chemical reactions in the mitochondria that transfer electrons from the hydrogen atom carriers NAD and FAD to oxygen; water is formed as a by-product; the electrochemical energy released by the hydrogen ions is coupled to the formation of ATP from ADP and P_i.

Oxidative Phosphorylation (OP) The process in which NADH + H^+ and $FADH_2$ are oxidized in the electron transport system and the energy released is used to synthesize ATP from ADP and P_i.

THE STEPS OF STAGE IV Again, the series of steps (Frisell, 1982; Lehninger, 1971; Marieb and Hoehn, 2010; Mougois, 2006; Newsholme and Leech, 1983) presented in **Figure 2.10** are necessary so that the energy is preserved rather than released all at once and lost as heat, which would destroy tissue.

Step 1. NADH + H^+ arrives at Complex I, transfers the electrons (e^-) to the complex, and deposits the protons (H^+) into the mitochondrial matrix.

Step 1a. This step is really a variation and not a sequential step. If the original hydrogen carrier was FAD instead of NAD^+, the transfer of electrons and protons occurs at Complex II instead of Complex I.

Step 2a. The electrons shuttle down the cytochromes, alternately causing the cytochromes to gain (become reduced) and lose (become oxidized) the electrons.

Step 2b. In this process, electrons also move across the width of the inner membrane driving the proton pumps that shuttle H^+ from the matrix to the inner membrane space.

Step 3. Oxygen accepts the electrons. This increase in negative charge attracts hydrogen ions and causes the formation of water. **Figure 2.11** depicts this step graphically.

Step 4. The H^+ that have been transported into the intermembrane space create an electrochemical gradient. Since the drive is to equalize that gradient, the H^+ leak back into the mitochondrial matrix through the ball-and-stalk complexes that are the enzyme ATP synthase. The movement of H^+ creates an electrical current, and this electrical energy, along with the enzyme action, is somehow used to synthesize ATP from ADP + P_i, both of which are present in the matrix. This occurs three times if the carrier is NADH + H^+ and twice if the carrier is $FADH_2$.

Step 5. ATP moves into the intermembrane space through the ATP-ADP antiporter protein. For every ATP molecule exported, an ADP molecule is imported. P_i is moved into the mitochondrial matrix via the phosphate translocase protein along with one H^+.

Step 6. In the final step, the ATP moves out of the mitochondria in exchange for the inward movement of ADP needed for the continual production of energy.

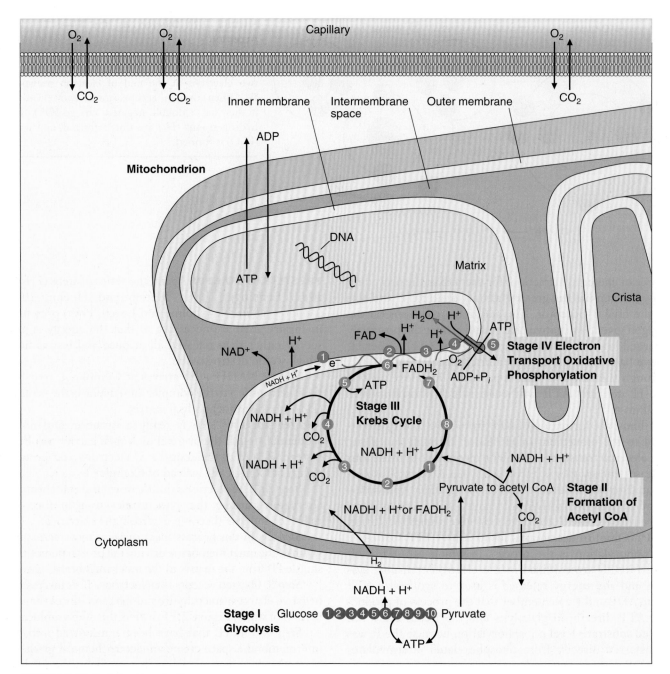

FIGURE 2.12 Cellular Respiration.

Figure 2.12 summarizes the process of cellular respiration just described and shows the interrelationships in a cell. As you study the figure, refer to the individual stage explanations as needed.

ATP Production from Carbohydrate

The number of ATP produced directly by substrate-level phosphorylation and the number of hydrogen atoms being carried by NAD+ and FAD were described above for each stage. These numbers are summarized in **Table 2.1**. From this summary, we can compute the total yield of ATP from one molecule of glucose or glycogen.

Stage I (glycolysis) yields a gross production of 4 ATP but uses 2 ATP, yielding a net gain of 2 ATP from direct substrate-level phosphorylation, if the substrate is glucose. If the substrate is glycogen, only 1 ATP is used and the net gain is 3 ATP.

Two molecules of NADH + H+ are also produced. These hydrogen atoms are transported from the cytoplasm, where glycolysis has taken place, into the mitochondria, if the level of pyruvate is not too high and if

TABLE 2.1   ATP Production from Carbohydrate

Metabolic Process Stage	ATP				Hydrogen Atoms and Carrier	
	Heart Muscle		Skeletal Muscle		Heart Muscle	Skeletal Muscle
I. Glycolysis	+4	+4	+4	+4	2 NADH + H$^+$	2 NADH + H$^{+\ddagger}$ → 2 FADH$_2$
Glucose	$\dfrac{-2}{2}$	$\dfrac{-1^*}{}$	$\dfrac{-2}{2}$	$\dfrac{-1^*}{}$		
Glycogen*		3		3		
II. Pyruvate → acetyl CoA	0	0	0	0	2 NADH + H$^+$	2 NADH + H$^+$
III. Krebs cycle	2	2	2	2	6 NADH + H$^+$ 2 FADH$_2$	6 NADH + H$^+$ 2 FADH$_2$
IV. ETS/OP: Hydrogen atoms from						
Stage I	(6)†5	(6)5	(4)‡3	(4)‡3		
Stage II	(6)5	(6)5	(6)5	(6)5		
Stage III	(22)18	(22)18	(22)18	(22)18		
Total						
Glucose	(38)32		(36)30			
Glycogen		(39)33		(37)31		

*If glycogen, not glucose, is fuel.

†Numbers in parentheses indicate theoretical ATP production values; numbers without parentheses indicate actual values.

‡Owing to shuttle differences in crossing into mitochondrial membrane, these hydrogen atoms are actually carried by FAD in the mitochondria, reducing the ATP production.

there is enough oxygen to accept the electrons at the end of the ETS. However, the inner mitochondrial membrane is impermeable to NADH + H$^+$, meaning that the membrane does not allow it to pass through. Therefore, a shuttle system must be employed.

Actually, two shuttle systems appear to operate—one in cardiac muscle and the other in skeletal muscle. The cardiac muscle shuttle system is called the *malate-aspartate shuttle*. It operates by the NADH + H$^+$ in the cytoplasm giving up the hydrogens to malate, which carries them across the inner mitochondrial membrane. Here, mitochondrial NAD$^+$ picks up the H$^+$ and enters the ETS (Newsholme and Leech, 1983).

The skeletal muscle shuttle system is called the *glycerol-phosphate shuttle*. It operates by the NADH + H$^+$ in the cytoplasm giving up the hydrogens to glycerol phosphate, which carries them into the inner mitochondrial membrane. Here, FAD picks up the H$^+$ and enters the ETS. This shuttle predominates in skeletal muscle (Frisell, 1982; Lehninger, 1971; Marieb and Hoehn, 2010; Mougios, 2006; Newsholme and Leech, 1983), although there is some evidence that the malate-aspartate shuttle may operate in Type I slow-twich oxidative skeletal muscle (Houston, 1995).

Because of these different shuttle systems, in heart muscle the ATP yield from the glycolytic hydrogens is higher than in skeletal muscle. In heart muscle the shuttle releases H$^+$ to NADH$^+$, whereas in skeletal muscle the shuttle releases H$^+$ to FAD. As detailed in step 4 above, the amount of ATP produced in ETS/OP depends on where the carrier enters the ETS, with NADH + H$^+$ resulting in more ATP produced than FADH$_2$. No differences between cardiac and skeletal muscle exist in the ATP production count for any of the remaining stages.

The counts for ATP produced during the oxidative phosphorylation are a little different from those in substrate-level phosphorylation. Theoretically and historically, because the H$^+$ moves through ATP synthase ball-and-stalk apparatus in three locations if deposited by NADH + H$^+$ and two locations if deposited by FADH$_2$, it was assumed that 3 ATP molecules were produced for each NADH + H$^+$ and 2 ATP molecules were produced for each FADH$_2$. The actual number may be less. Biochemists are currently uncertain (Mougois, 2006) because the numbers of H$^+$ moving are not necessarily constant, but may depend on the energy state of the cell. The best available estimate is that it takes 3 H$^+$ moving through ATP synthase to form 1 ATP. However, this actually involves 4 H$^+$ to compensate for the 1 H$^+$ that enters the mitochondrial matrix with P$_i$ through the phosphate translocase (**Figure 2.10**). Thus the movement of 4 H$^+$ results in 1 ATP. The number of H$^+$ expelled by the three complexes (I, III, and IV) is thought to be 4 at complex I, 2 at complex III, and 4 at complex IV for a total of 10 H$^+$ per NADH + H$^+$. Dividing 10 H$^+$ by 4 H$^+$ for each ATP = 2.5 ATP per NADH + H$^+$. FADH$_2$ bypasses complex I. Therefore, the total is only 2 H$^+$ at complex III and 4 H$^+$ at complex IV for a total of 6 H$^+$. Dividing 6 H$^+$ by 4 H$^+$ per ATP = 1.5 ATP per FADH$_2$.

Stage II (the conversion of pyruvate to acetyl CoA) yields no substrate-level ATP, but it does produce 2 NADH + H⁺. Since these molecules are already in the mitochondria, they directly enter the ETS. Theoretically, this would result in the production of 6 ATP (2 NADH + H⁺ × 3) but actually the yield is 5 ATP (2 NADH + H⁺ × 2.5).

Stage III (the Krebs cycle) produces 2 ATP directly by substrate-level phosphorylation, NADH + H⁺ at three steps, and FADH₂ at one step. Thus, (3 NADH + H⁺ × 3 = 9 ATP theoretically, but 3 NADH + H⁺ × 2.5 = 7.5 by actual count) + (1 FADH₂ × 2 = 2 ATP theoretically, but 1 FADH₂ × 1.5 ATP actually). Since each step occurs twice for each 6-carbon glucose molecule, this yield must be doubled: 9 ATP + 2 ATP = 11 ATP × 2 = 22 ATP theoretically, but only 7.5 ATP + 1.5 ATP = 9 ATP × 2 = 18 ATP actually.

If we add all of these (with the higher theoretical values indicated in the parentheses) results for skeletal muscle when glucose is the fuel, we get:

2 ATP	(substrate – level phosphorylation, glycolysis)
(4) 3 ATP	(2 NADH + H⁺ → 2 FADH₂, glycolysis)
(6) 5 ATP	(2 NADH + H⁺, Stage II)
2 ATP	(substrate – level phosphorylation, Krebs cycle)
(22) 18 ATP	(2 FADH₂ + 6 NADH + H⁺, Krebs cycle ETS/OP) for a total of
(36) 30 ATP	for the aerobic oxidation of one molecule of glucose by skeletal muscle.

Complete the Check your Comprehension 1.

CHECK YOUR COMPREHENSION 1

Determine the theoretical and actual count of total ATP produced when the aerobic oxidation takes place in heart muscle and the initial fuel is glucose. Check your answer against the value given in Table 2.1. Next, do the same computations assuming that glycogen, not glucose, is the energy substrate. Again, check your answer against the value given in Table 2.1.

Fat Metabolism

Although the body may prefer to use carbohydrate as fuel from the standpoint of oxygen cost, the importance of fat as an energy source should not be underestimated. Fat is found in many common foods. Fat, in the form of triglyceride (sometimes known as triacylglycerol), is the major storage form of energy in humans. Some triglyceride is stored within muscle cells (**Figure 2.13**), but the vast majority is deposited in adipose cells (**Figure 2.14**), which comprise at least 10–15% of the body weight of average young males and 20–25% of the body weight of average young females (Malina and

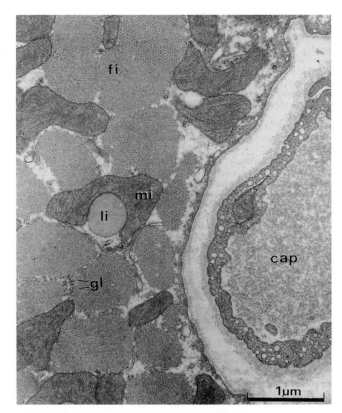

FIGURE 2.13 Electron Micrograph of Cross-Sectional Muscle Area (EM:28,500×). A lipid droplet is labeled as "li."
Source: Vogt, M., A. Puntschart, H. Howald, B. Mueller, C. Mannhart, L. Gfeller-Tuescher, P. Mullis, & H. Hoppeler: Effects of dietary fat on muscle substrates, metabolism, and performance in athletes. *Medicine & Science in Sports & Exercise.* 35(6):952–960, 2003.

Bouchard, 1991). Roughly half of this adipocyte storage occurs subcutaneously (under the skin). The remaining stores surround the major organs of the abdominothoracic cavity as support and protection. Triglycerides are turned over constantly in the body. Because body fat is turned over completely about every 3–4 weeks, no one is literally still carrying their "baby fat" (Marieb and Hoehn, 2010).

Fat is an excellent storage fuel for several reasons. First, fat is an energy-dense fuel yielding 9.13 kcal·gm⁻¹; both carbohydrate and protein yield slightly less than 4 kcal·gm⁻¹. The difference is due to the chemical structure of the substrates—specifically, the amount of oxidizable carbon and hydrogen. It is easy to appreciate the difference by looking at the chemical composition of the free fatty acid palmitate, which is $C_{16}H_{32}O_2$. This fatty acid has almost three times as much C and H, but only a third as much O as glucose ($C_6H_{12}O_6$). Remember that it is H atoms that donate the electrons (e⁻) and protons (H⁺) used during electron transport and oxidative phosphorylation.

Second, carbohydrate, in the form of glycogen, is stored in the muscles with a large amount of water: 2.7 g

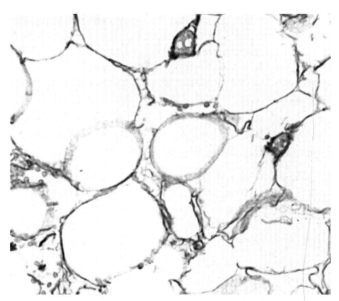

FIGURE 2.14 Triglyceride Stored in Adipose Tissue.
Source: Mills, S.E. *Histology for pathologists*, 3rd edition. Philadelphia: Lippincott Williams & Wilkins (2007).

of water per gram of dried glycogen. Triglyceride is stored dry. Thus, the energy content of fat is not diluted, and hard as it may be to believe, body bulk is less than would otherwise be necessary. If humans had to store the comparable amount of energy as carbohydrates, we would be at least twice as big (Newsholme and Leech, 1983)!

Third, glycogen stores are relatively small in comparison to fat stores. A person can deplete stored glycogen in as little as 2 hours of heavy exercise or 1 day of bed rest, whereas fat supplies can last for weeks, even with moderate activity. Although many North Americans are concerned about having too much body fat, this storage capacity is undoubtedly important for survival of the species when food is not readily available.

The triglycerides stored in adipose tissue must first be broken down into glycerol and free fatty acids before they can be used as fuel (see earlier **Figure 2.2**). One glycerol and three fatty acids make up a triglyceride. Seven fatty acids predominate in the body, but since three fatty acids combine with a glycerol to make up a triglyceride, 343 (7 × 7 × 7) different combinations are possible (Péronnet et al., 1987). Some common fatty acids include oleic acid, palmitic acid, stearic acid, linoleic acid, and palmitoleic acid.

Fatty acids may be saturated, unsaturated, or polyunsaturated. A saturated fatty acid has a chemical bonding arrangement that allows it to hold as many hydrogen

Beta-oxidation A cyclic series of steps that breaks off successive pairs of carbon atoms from FFA, which are then used to form acetyl CoA.

atoms as possible. Thus, the term "saturated" means "saturated with hydrogen." Unsaturated fatty acids have a chemical bonding arrangement with a reduced-hydrogen binding potential and therefore are unsaturated with respect to hydrogen atoms. Polyunsaturated means several bonds are without hydrogen.

The breakdown of triglycerides into glycerol and fatty acids is catalyzed by the enzyme hormone-sensitive lipase. The glycerol is soluble in blood, but the free fatty acids (FFAs) are not. Glycerol can enter glycolysis in the cytoplasm (as 3-phosphoglycerate, the product of step 7 in **Figure 2.6**), but it is not typically utilized by muscle cells in this way (Newsholme and Leech, 1983; Péronnet et al., 1987). The direct role of glycerol as a fuel in the muscle cells during exercise is so minor that it need not be considered. However, glycerol can be converted to glucose by the liver.

FFA must be transported in the blood bound to albumin. Specific receptor sites on the muscle cell membrane take up the FFA into the cell. The FFA must then be translocated or transported from the cytoplasm into the mitochondria. Once in the mitochondrial matrix, the FFA undergoes the process of beta-oxidation (**Figure 2.15**).

Beta-Oxidation

Beta-oxidation is a cyclic series of steps that breaks off successive pairs of carbon atoms from FFA, which are then used to form acetyl CoA. Remember that acetyl CoA is the common intermediate by which all foodstuffs enter the Krebs cycle and ETS/OP stage. The number of cycles depends upon the number of carbon atoms; most fatty acids have 14–24 carbons.

When there is an adequate supply of oxaloacetate to combine with, the fat-derived acetyl CoA enters the Krebs cycle and proceeds through electron transport and oxidative phosphorylation. **Figure 2.15** diagrams the steps of beta-oxidation, which are explained next.

As with glycolysis, ATP is used for activation; but unlike glycolysis, beta-oxidation produces no ATP directly by substrate-level phosphorylation.

THE STEPS OF BETA-OXIDATION *Step 1*. The fatty acid molecule is activated by the breakdown of 1 ATP to AMP, releasing the energy equivalent of 2 ATP if broken down as it is normally to ADP. Concurrently, coenzyme A is added.

Step 2. FAD is reduced to $FADH_2$. The $FADH_2$ enters the electron transport chain and produces 1.5 ATP (actual count).

Step 3. A molecule of water is added, and NAD^+ is reduced to NADH + H$^+$. The NADH + H$^+$ will enter the electron transport chain and produce 2.5 ATP (actual count). Steps 2 and 3, with the removal of the hydrogen atoms, account for the oxidation portion of the name for this process.

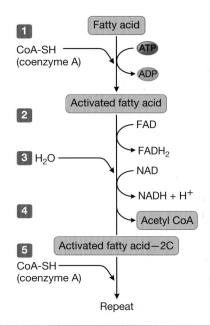

FIGURE 2.15 Beta-Oxidation.

Step 4. The bond between the alpha (α) carbon (C_2) and the beta (β) carbon (C_3) is broken, resulting in the removal of two carbon atoms (C_1 and C_2), which are then used to form acetyl coenzyme A. The cleavage of carbons at the site of the beta carbon explains why the process is called beta-oxidation.

Step 5. Steps 1–4 are repeated for each pair of carbons except the last, since the last unit formed is acetyl CoA itself. Therefore, the number of cycles that must be completed to oxidize the fat can be computed using the formula $n/2 - 1$ where n is the number of carbons. The acetyl CoA can enter the Krebs cycle and electron transport system (see earlier **Figures 2.2, 2.9,** and **2.10**).

ATP Production from Fatty Acids

The number of ATP produced from the breakdown of fat depends on which fatty acid is utilized. The following example shows a calculation of ATP production by

actual count for palmitate. As with carbohydrate, the actual number of ATP molecules produced is lower than the theoretical number would be.

Calculate the number of ATP actually produced from the breakdown of palmitate (palmitic acid). The steps in the calculation follow:

1. Palmitate is a 16-carbon fatty acid. Therefore, as noted in the previous step 5, it cycles through beta-oxidation $n/2-1 = 16/2 - 1 = 7$ times.
2. Each cycle produces 1 $FADH_2$ and 1 NADH + H^+, as follows:

$FADH_2$ $\rightarrow$ FAD $\quad$ 1.5 ATP
NADH + H^+ $\rightarrow$ NAD^+ $\quad$ +2.5 ATP
$\qquad\qquad\qquad\qquad$ 4.0 ATP

This reaction happens 7 times: $7 \times 4 = 28$ ATP.

3. Each cycle (7) plus the last step (1) produces acetyl CoA, for a total of 8. Each acetyl CoA yields 1 ATP, 3 NADH + H^+, and 1 $FADH_2$ in the Krebs cycle. The 3 NADH + H^+ will produce 7.5 ATP, and the $FADH_2$ will produce 1.5 ATP in the electron transport system. Thus, 10 ATP are produced for each acetyl CoA, for a total of 8 acetyl CoA × 10 ATP = 80 ATP.
4. Add the results of steps 2 and 3: 80 ATP + 28 ATP = 108 ATP produced.
5. 1 ATP was utilized in step 1 of beta-oxidation to activate the fatty acid. Furthermore, this ATP was broken down to AMP, not ADP; thus the equivalent of 2 ATP was used.
6. Subtracting the ATP used from the total ATP produced, we get 108 ATP–2 ATP = 106 net ATP from palmitate.

Recall that three acids plus one glycerol make up a triglyceride. These calculations apply to a single specific fatty acid. Complete the Check your Comprehension 2.

CHECK YOUR COMPREHENSION 2

To check your understanding of the ATP yield from fatty acids, calculate the theoretical and actual count for ATP produced from an 18-carbon fatty acid, such as stearate. Check your answer in Appendix C.

Ketone Bodies and Ketosis

As mentioned earlier, in order for the acetyl CoA produced by beta-oxidation to enter the Krebs cycle, a sufficient amount of oxaloacetate is necessary. When carbohydrate supplies are sufficient, this is no problem, and fat is said to burn in the flame of carbohydrate. However, when carbohydrates are inadequate (perhaps as a result of fasting, prolonged exercise, or diabetes mellitus), oxaloacetate is converted to glucose. The production of glucose from noncarbohydrate sources under these conditions is necessary because some tissue, such as the brain and nervous system, rely predominantly on glucose for fuel (Marieb and Hoehn, 2010).

When oxaloacetate is converted to glucose and is therefore not available to combine with acetyl CoA to form citrate, the liver converts the acetyl CoA derived from the fatty acids into metabolites called *ketones* or *ketone bodies*. Despite the similarity in the names, do not confuse ketones with keto acids (pyruvic acid and the Krebs cycle intermediates) (**Figure 2.9**). There are three forms of ketones: acetoacetic acid, beta-hydroxybutyric acid, and acetone. All are strong acids. Acetone gives the breath a very characteristic fruity smell.

Ketone bodies themselves can be used as fuel by muscles, nerves, and the brain. If the ketones are not used but instead, accumulate, a condition called *ketosis* occurs. The high acidity of ketosis can disrupt normal physiological functioning, especially acid-base balance. Ketosis is more likely to result from an inadequate diet (as in anorexia nervosa) or diabetes than from prolonged exercise, since the muscles will use the ketones as fuel. During exercise, aerobically trained individuals can utilize ketones more effectively than untrained individuals.

Protein Metabolism

Proteins are present in many food sources. Proteins are large molecules consisting of varying combinations of amino acids linked together. Approximately 20 amino acids occur naturally (Kapit et al., 1987). Because there are so many ways these amino acids can combine, the number of possible proteins is almost infinite. Like carbohydrates and fats, amino acids contain atoms of carbon, oxygen, and hydrogen. In addition, they may include sulfur, phosphorus, and iron. All amino acids have in common an amino group containing nitrogen (NH_2).

Proteins are extremely important in the structure and function of the body. Among other things they are components of hemoglobin, contractile elements of the muscle, hormones, fibrin for clotting, tendons, ligaments, and portions of all cell membranes. Because proteins are so important in the body, the constituent amino acids are used predominantly as building blocks, not as a source of energy.

However, amino acids can be, and in certain instances are, used as a fuel source. When amino acids are used as a fuel source, muscles appear to preferentially, but not exclusively, utilize the group of amino acids known as branched-chain amino acids (BCAA), leucine, isoleucine, and valine. In this situation, as with carbohydrate and fat metabolism, the final common pathways of the Krebs cycle, electron transport, and oxidative phosphorylation are utilized. The site of entry into the metabolic pathways varies, as shown in **Figure 2.2**, with the amino acid.

Six amino acids can enter metabolism at the level of pyruvic acid, 8 at acetyl CoA, 4 at alpha-ketoglutarate, 4 at succinate, 2 at fumarate, and 2 at oxaloacetate. All of these intermediates except acetyl CoA are, in turn, converted to pyruvate before being used to produce energy. The acetyl CoA is used directly in the Krebs cycle and electron transport, as previously described.

Transamination and Oxidative Deamination

Before amino acids can be used as a fuel and enter the pathways at any place, the nitrogen-containing amino group (the NH_2) must be removed. It is removed by the process of transamination and sometimes by oxidative deamination (Frisell, 1982; Lehninger, 1971; Marieb and Hoehn, 2010; Mougios, 2006; Newsholme & Leech, 1983). These processes are summarized in **Table 2.2**.

All but two amino acids appear to be able to undergo **transamination**. Transamination involves the transfer of the NH_2 amino group from an amino acid to a keto acid. Remember that keto acids include pyruvic acid, acetyl CoA, and the Krebs cycle intermediates. This process occurs in both the cytoplasm and the mitochondria, predominantly in muscle and liver cells. Transamination results in the formation of a new amino acid and a different keto acid. The most frequent keto acid acceptor of NH_2 is α-ketoglutarate, with glutamate being the amino acid formed (Marieb and Hoehn, 2010; Mougios, 2006).

Two fates for glutamate are shown in **Table 2.2**. In the first, glutamate is transaminated to alanine, another amino acid. Alanine, in turn, can be converted to glucose in a process called gluconeogenesis (Frisell, 1982; Marieb and Hoehn, 2010). **Gluconeogenesis** is the creation of glucose in the liver from noncarbohydrate sources, particularly glycerol, lactate or pyruvate, and alanine.

In the second process, glutamate undergoes oxidative deamination. In oxidative deamination, the oxidized form of NAD is reduced, and the amino group (NH_2) is removed and becomes NH_3. NH_3 is ammonia, which in high concentrations in the body is extremely toxic. The dominant pathway for NH_3 removal is by conversion to urea in the liver (via the urea cycle) and excretion in urine by the kidneys. Oxidative deamination is used much less frequently than transamination.

Transamination The transfer of the NH_2 amino group from an amino acid to a keto acid.

Gluconeogenesis The creation of glucose in the liver from noncarbohydrate sources, particularly glycerol, lactate or pyruvate, and alanine.

TABLE 2.2   Transamination and Oxidative Deamination

Transamination	Oxidative Deamination
Generalized	**Generalized**
Amino acid (1) + keto acid (1) ⇌ amino acid (2) + keto acid (2) The NH$_2$ group from amino acid (1) is transferred to keto acid (1), forming a different amino acid (2) and a different keto acid (2)	Amino acid ⇌ keto acid + NH$_3$ The NH$_2$ group is removed from an amino acid, forming a keto acid and ammonia
Most common	**Most common**
Any 1 of 12 different amino acids + α-ketoglutarate ⇌ glutamate + keto acid	Glutamate+H$_2$O + NAD$^+$ ⇌ NH$_3$ + α-ketoglutarate + NADH + H$^+$
Specific example	**Fate of products**
Glutamate + pyruvate ⇌ alanine + α-ketoglutarate	1. NADH + H$^+$ enters the electron transport system. 2. α-ketoglutarate is a Krebs cycle intermediate. 3. NH$_3$ (ammonia) is removed in urine. The urea cycle is $2NH_3 + CO_2 \rightarrow NH_2CONH_2$ (urea) + H$_2$O

ATP Production from Amino Acids

Because the amino acid derivatives are ultimately utilized as pyruvate or acetyl CoA, the ATP production count from the amino acids is the same as for glucose from that point on, except that it is not doubled (Péronnet et al., 1987). Refer to **Figure 2.6** to remind yourself why the double count occurs with glucose and to **Figure 2.2** to see amino acids entering the pathways denoted next. All of these computations are for ATP produced by actual, not theoretical, count.

Pyruvate → acetyl CoA = 1 NADH + H$^+$		2.5 ATP
Krebs cycle		1 ATP
ETS/OP	3 NADH + H$^+$	7.5 ATP
	1 FADH$_2$	1.5 ATP
		12.5 ATP

This is the first time we have seen a total indicating a fraction of ATP. Interpret this as an average, not literally. ATP molecules do not exist in halves.

Acetyl CoA would produce 10 ATP, because the NADH + H$^+$ production from pyruvate to acetyl CoA would be the only step missing.

The Regulation of Cellular Respiration and ATP Production

Intracellular Regulation

Intracellularly, the production of ATP—and, hence, the flow of substrates through the various metabolic pathways—is regulated predominantly by feedback mechanisms. Again, each step in each metabolic pathway is catalyzed by a specific enzyme. At least one of these enzymes in each pathway can be acted on directly by other chemicals in the cell and, as a result, increases or decreases its activity. Such an enzyme is called a *rate-limiting enzyme*, and the other factors that influence it are called modulators. When the rate-limiting enzyme is inhibited, every step in the metabolic pathway beyond that point is also inhibited. When the rate-limiting enzyme is stimulated, every step in the metabolic pathway beyond that point is also stimulated.

The primary rate-limiting enzyme in glycolysis is phosphofructokinase (PFK), the enzyme that catalyzes step 3. PFK is stimulated, and subsequently the rate of glycolysis increased, by modulators such as ADP, AMP, P$_i$, and a rise in pH. ADP, AMP, and P$_i$ modulators are the result of the breakdown of ATP. This is an example of a positive-feedback system in which the by-product of the utilization of a substance stimulates a greater production of that original substance. Conversely, PFK is inhibited, and subsequently the rate of glycolysis decreased, by the modulators ATP, CP, citrate (a Krebs cycle intermediate), FFA, and a drop in pH. Each of these modulators signals that sufficient substances exist to supply ATP. This is an example of a negative-feedback system in which the formation of a product or other similarly acting product inhibits further production of the product (Newsholme and Leech, 1983).

The primary rate-limiting enzyme in the Krebs cycle is isocitrate dehydrogenase (ICD), which catalyzes step 3. ICD is stimulated by ADP, P$_i$, and calcium (positive feedback), and is inhibited by ATP (negative feedback) (Newsholme and Leech, 1983).

Cytochrome oxidase—which catalyzes the transfer of electrons to molecular oxygen, resulting in the formation of water—is the rate-limiting enzyme for the electron transport system. It is stimulated by ADP and P$_i$ (positive feedback) and is inhibited by ATP (negative feedback) (Newsholme and Leech, 1983).

A pattern in the modulators is readily evident, with ATP, ADP, and P$_i$ being universally important. When

ATP is present in sufficient amounts to satisfy the needs of the cell and to provide some reserve in storage, there is no need to increase its production. Thus, key enzymes in the metabolic pathways are inhibited. However, when muscle activity begins and ATP is broken down into ADP and P_i, these by-products stimulate all the metabolic pathways to produce more ATP so that the muscle contractions can continue.

Extracellular Regulation

During exercise, metabolic processes must provide ATP for energy and maintain blood glucose levels at near-resting values for the proper functioning of the entire organism. This is because the brain and nervous tissue must have glucose as a fuel. One of the ways of maintaining glucose levels is by the process of gluconeogenesis.

Gluconeogenesis

As defined earlier, gluconeogenesis is the creation (-genesis) of new (-neo) glucose (gluco-) in the liver from noncarbohydrate sources. The primary fuel sources for gluconeogenesis are glycerol, lactate or pyruvate, and alanine. Glycerol is released into the bloodstream when triglycerides are broken down (**Figure 2.16A**).

Pyruvate is the end product of glycolysis. The majority of the pyruvate is converted to acetyl CoA and enters the Krebs cycle and electron transport system. However, a small portion diffuses out of the muscle cell and into the bloodstream (Péronnet et al., 1987). Still another portion of the pyruvate is converted to lactate, which also diffuses into the bloodstream. About 10 times as much lactate as pyruvate diffuses out of the muscle cells (**Figure 2.16B**).

Alanine is formed by transamination when the amino group from one amino acid (preferentially, the BCAA or an amino acid derived from glutamate) is transferred to pyruvate (**Figure 2.16C**). Note that in the liver alanine is first reconverted to pyruvate (freeing the NH_3 to enter the urea cycle and be excreted) before being converted to glucose.

In all cases, the conversion to glucose takes place in the liver. For each gram of glucose produced, 1.02 g of glycerol, 1.43 g of pyruvate, 1.23 g of lactate, or 1.45 g of alanine is utilized (Péronnet et al., 1987).

The glycerol-glucose cycle has no special name, but the pyruvate/lactate-glucose cycle is known as the *Cori cycle*, and the alanine-glucose cycle is called the *Felig cycle*. The Cori and Felig cycles help maintain normal blood glucose levels so that the brain, nerves, and kidneys as well as the muscles may draw from this supply.

Neurohormonal Coordination

The regulation of blood glucose levels, including gluconeogenesis, is governed jointly by the autonomic nervous

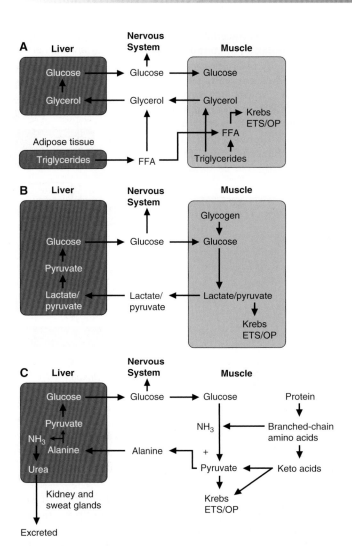

FIGURE 2.16 Gluconeogenesis.
A. Glycerol-glucose cycle. **B.** Cori cycle. **C.** Felig cycle.

system (particularly the sympathetic division) and the endocrine system, which function in a coordinated fashion. **Figure 2.17** shows this integration of the two control systems for the regulation of energy production in response to exercise. Chapter 21 provides a comprehensive explanation of the functioning of the neurohormonal system.

When exercise begins, signals from the working muscles and motor centers in the central nervous system bring about a neurohormonal response mediated through the hypothalamus. The hypothalamus stimulates both the anterior pituitary and the sympathetic nervous system. The neurotransmitter norepinephrine is released directly from sympathetic nerve endings, and the hormones epinephrine and norepinephrine are released from the adrenal medulla. Epinephrine and norepinephrine both act directly on fuel sites and stimulate the anterior pituitary and pancreas. As a result of the dual stimulation of the anterior pituitary, hormones are released—namely, growth hormone, cortisol, and thyroxine. The release

FIGURE 2.17 Extracellular Neurohormonal Regulation of Metabolism.
TRH is thyroid-releasing hormone; ACTH is adrenocorticotrophic hormone; GHRH is growth hormone–releasing hormone; CRH is corticotrophin-releasing hormone; TSH is thyroid-stimulating hormone. ↓, decrease; ↑, increase.
Sources: Bunt (1986); Marieb and Hoehn (2010); Van de Graaff and Fox (1989).

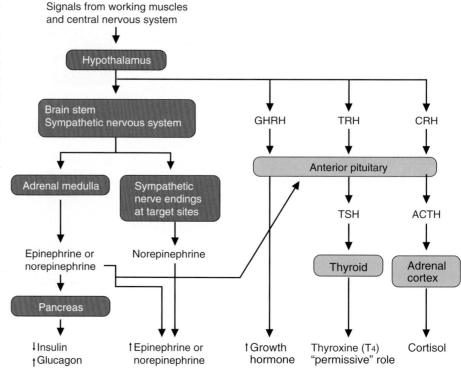

of insulin is inhibited from the pancreas, but glucagon release is stimulated (Bunt, 1986; Galbo, 1983). In general, there are three results (see also **Table 2.3**):

1. An increase in the mobilization and utilization of free fatty acid stores from extramuscular (adipose tissue) and intramuscular stores
2. An increase in the breakdown of extramuscular (liver) and intramuscular stores of glycogen and the formation of glucose from noncarbohydrate sources (gluconeogenesis) in the liver

3. A decrease in the uptake of glucose into the non-working cells

A two-tier system of hormonal involvement appears to operate on the basis of either a fast or slow time of response. The catecholamines (epinephrine and norepinephrine) and glucagon react to an increase in muscular activity in a matter of seconds to minutes. Both assist in all three metabolic functions listed above, although not equally. Epinephrine's influence on fat metabolism is far greater than its effect on glucose metabolism (Guyton and Hall, 2011).

TABLE 2.3	Hormonal Regulation of Metabolism during Exercise			
Effect		**Hormone**		
	Glucagon	**Epinephrine and Norepinephrine**	**Growth Hormone***	**Cortisol**
Glucose uptake and utilization	↓†		↓†	↓†
Glycogen breakdown (glycogenolysis)	↑	↑	↑	↑
Glycogen formation (glycogenesis)	↓	↓	↑	↑
Gluconeogenesis	↑	↑	↑	↑
FFA storage (lipogenesis)	↓		↓	↓
FFA mobilization	↑	↑	↑	↑
Amino acid transport and uptake			↑	↑
Protein breakdown				↑
*Heavy exercise.				
†Nonactive cells.				
↑, Increases; ↓, Decreases.				

FOCUS ON APPLICATION

Metabolic Pathways: The Vitamin Connection

Many individuals mistakenly believe that vitamins are a source of energy for the body. Although this is not true, vitamins do participate in many of the chemical reactions described in this chapter that convert the potential energy of food sources into ATP. Your body cannot produce energy without vitamins. In general, the ingestion of a well-balanced diet (the fuel source) provides the needed vitamins. Conversely, the ingestion of excessive amounts of vitamins does not increase the activity of the enzymes for which the vitamins act as coenzymes. Listed in the table are the six vitamins that are particularly important for energy metabolism, their actions, and selected dietary sources. Check to see that you are getting all of these in your diet.

Source: vanderBeek (1985)

Vitamin	Function in Metabolism	Selected Dietary Sources
B_1 (thiamine)	Coenzyme involved in the conversion of pyruvate to acetyl CoA during carbohydrate metabolism	Lean meats, eggs, whole grains, leafy green vegetables, legumes
B_2 (riboflavin)	Basis of coenzyme FAD which serves as hydrogen acceptor in the mitochondria	Milk, eggs, lean meat, green vegetables
Niacin (nicotinamide)	Basis of coenzyme NAD which is the primary hydrogen carrier in both the cytoplasm and mitochondria	Lean meat, fish, legumes, whole grains, peanuts
B_6 (pyridoxine)	Functions as coenzyme in amino acid transamination reactions; required coenzyme for glycogenolysis action of the enzyme phosphorylase	Meat, poultry, fish, white and sweet potatoes, tomatoes, spinach
Pantothenic acid	Functions as coenzyme A in the formation of acetyl CoA from pyruvate	Meat, legumes, whole grains, eggs
Biotin	Essential as coenzyme for a number of enzymes in the Krebs cycle and gluconeogenesis	Eggs, legumes, nuts

The actions of the catecholamines and glucagon are backed up by growth hormone and cortisol, respectively. The response of growth hormone and cortisol may take hours to become maximal. Thus, these latter two hormones are probably most important for carbohydrate conservation during long-duration activity. This explains why growth hormone and cortisol can bring about glycogen synthesis, while glucagon and the catecholamines cannot (Guyton and Hall, 2011).

Insulin secretion is suppressed during exercise. This decrease in insulin and the increase in glucagon, growth hormone, and cortisol cause a decrease in the glucose uptake into cells other than the working muscles. The available glucose is thus spared for the working muscles and the nervous system.

During exercise, the working muscles become highly permeable to glucose despite the lack of insulin. As previously noted, the muscle contraction itself stimulates GLUT-4 translocation to the cell surface for the movement of glucose into the working muscle (Houston, 1995; Sato et al., 1996). The contractile process also helps to break down the intramuscular stores of glycogen and triglycerides (Galbo, 1983; Guyton and Hall, 2011).

The increases in protein breakdown and in amino acid transport caused by growth hormone and cortisol are important in providing protein precursors for gluconeogenesis. The fact that these hormones are slow responders also explains why protein is not used in significant amounts except in long-duration activity.

Because the mobilization of free fatty acids involves the breakdown of triglycerides, glycerol is also released and made available for gluconeogenesis. Note that an accumulation of the other gluconeogenic precursor, lactate, inhibits free fatty acid release from adipose tissue. Therefore, gluconeogenesis serves a dual purpose in helping to provide glucose and reducing the levels of lactate so that it does not interfere as much with fat utilization.

Thyroxine itself has a number of metabolic functions. However, its role in exercise metabolism appears to be one of potentiation or permissiveness. That is, it helps to create an environment in which the other metabolic hormones can function more effectively, rather than having any major effect itself.

The level of response and reaction to all of these hormones depends on the following:

1. The type, duration, and intensity of the exercise; relative intensity appears to be more important than the absolute workload.
2. The nutritional status, health, training status, and fiber-type composition of the exerciser.
3. The size of the fuel depots, the state of the hormone receptors, and the capacity of the involved enzymes (Galbo, 1983).

Fuel Utilization at Rest and during Exercise

Preceding sections explain how each of the major fuel sources—fats, carbohydrates, and proteins—are converted to ATP energy for the human body. At rest, it has been estimated that fats contribute 41–67%, carbohydrates 33–42%, and proteins from just a trace to 17% of the total daily energy requirements of the human body (Lemon and Nagel, 1981).

During exercise, various forms of each fuel are utilized to supply working muscles with the additional ATP energy needed to sustain movement. To understand which energy sources are used during exercise, it is first necessary to know approximately how much of each energy substrate is available. **Table 2.4** shows the tissue fuel stores in an average adult male who weighs 65 kg, has 8.45 kg (13%) body fat, and 30 kg of muscle. Protein stores are omitted because the major tissue storage of protein is in the muscles, and complete degradation (breakdown) of muscle to sustain energy metabolism is neither realistic nor desirable under normal circumstances.

Several important points should be noted in **Table 2.4**. First, triglycerides provide the greatest source of potential energy (77,150 kcal is enough energy to sustain life for ~47 days!). Second, comparatively, very little carbohydrate is actually stored. In fact, the human body's stores of carbohydrate are only enough to support life for 1 1/4 days, if all three sources (muscle glycogen, liver glycogen, and circulating glucose) are added together. Thus, carbohydrate replenishment on a regular basis is essential. Third, exercise has a major impact on how long each fuel can supply energy.

Table 2.4 assumes that each fuel is acting independently, which in fact never happens. **Tables 2.5** and **2.6** provide more realistic views of what actually happens during exercise. **Table 2.5** depicts the relative utilization of each substrate source based on the type, intensity, and duration of the activity. Very short-duration, very high-intensity dynamic activity and static contractions are special cases that rely predominantly on energy substrates stored in the muscle fibers—that is, ATP-PC and glycogen (which can quickly be broken down into ATP to provide energy).

The other exercises listed in **Table 2.5** are assumed to be predominantly dynamic and to a large extent aerobic (utilizing oxygen). In general, the lower the intensity, the more important fat is as a fuel; the higher the intensity, the more important carbohydrates are as fuel. Duration has a similar effect: the shorter the duration, the more important carbohydrates are as a fuel, with fat being utilized more and more as the duration lengthens. Fats come into play over the long term because the glycogen stores can and will be depleted. Indeed, long-duration activities often exhibit a three-part sequence in which muscle glycogen, bloodborne glucose (including glucose that has been broken down from liver glycogen and glucose that has been created by gluconeogenesis), and fatty acids successively predominate as the major fuel source. Protein may account for 5–15% of the total energy supply in activities lasting more than an hour (Felig and Wharen, 1975; Lemon and Nagel, 1981; Pernow and Saltin, 1971).

TABLE 2.4 Tissue Fuel Stores in Average Adult Males (Body Weight = 65 kg, Percent Body Fat = 13)						
Tissue Fuel	**Total Energy***			**Estimated Period Fuel Would Supply Energy**[†]		
	g	**kJ**	**Kcal**	**Basal**[‡] **(d)**	**Walk**[‡] **(d)**	**Run**[‡] **(min)**
Triglycerides[§] (fatty acids)	8450	322,789	77,150	47.46	11.25	5223
Liver glycogen[‖]	80	1275	305	0.19	0.05	20.7
Muscle glycogen (28.25 kg muscle[#])	425	7384**	1743**	1.07	0.25	118
Circulating glucose (blood + extracellular)	20	319	76	0.05	0.01	5.2

*Conversion factors utilized: glucose, 3.81 kcal·g⁻¹; fatty acid, 9.13 kcal·g⁻¹; kcal × 4.184 = kJ (Burszstein et al., 1989; Péronnet et al., 1987).

[†]Calculations assume that each fuel is the only fuel utilized. In reality, the fuels are utilized with mixtures that depend on the type, intensity, and duration of the activity and the training, fiber-type proportions, and nutritional status of the exerciser.

[‡]Kilocalorie cost of exercise: basal 0.174 kcal·kg⁻¹·10 min⁻¹ walking at 3.5 mi·hr⁻¹ = 0.733 kcal·kg⁻¹·10 min⁻¹; running at 8.7 mi·hr⁻¹ (6:54 mile) =2.273 kcal·10 min⁻¹ (Consolazio et al., 1963).

[§]65 kg body weight × 0.13 (fraction of body fat) = 8.45 kg fat.

[‖]Liver equals approximately 2.5% body weight. Normal glycogen content is 50 g·kg⁻¹; extracellular glucose includes the portion in liver available to circulation (Péronnet et al., 1987).

[#]Weight of the muscle is approximately equal to half the lean body mass.

**Muscle fatty acid values would equal this value because 1 kg of muscle contains approximately 13.5 g fatty acid and 1.5 g glycerol. The triglyceride value includes the muscle store (Péronnet et al., 1987).

Sources: Based on Kapit, W., R. I. Macey, & E. Meisami: *The Physiology Coloring Book* (2nd edition). San Franciso, CA: Addison Wesley Longman (2000); Newsholme, E. A. & A. R. Leech: *Biochemistry for the Medical Sciences.* New York: John Wiley (1983).

Sex Differences in Substrate Utilization

The data presented in Tables 2.5 and 2.6 show variations not only in the reliance on carbohydrate, fat, and protein substrates based on exercise intensity, but also among the various components of carbohydrate used as a fuel (glucose, and muscle and liver glycogen). Data from this study by Friedlander et al. demonstrate that there might also be meaningful variations among fuel substrates between the sexes. Substrate utilization in young adult males and females was determined at rest and at 45% $\dot{V}O_2$peak and 65% $\dot{V}O_2$peak exercise intensities on a cycle ergometer. Although only those comparisons marked with an asterisk (*) in the accompanying graphs attained statistical significance, the overall pattern seen in panel (A) is that carbohydrates provided a higher percentage of the total

energy supply for males than for females. Conversely, the pattern in panel (B) shows that the females used relatively more glucose than other carbohydrate sources (presumably glycogen and lactate) than the males. Both of these trends were true at rest before (UT) and after (TR) training, at the two submaximal power outputs pretraining (45% UT and 65% UT), at the same absolute power output pretraining and posttraining (65% UT and 65% TR), and at the new relative power output posttraining (65% TR).

The mechanism that explains these differences is unknown. However, the authors speculate that hormonal differences may have been the cause. Factors that may influence these differences include the amount of circulating epinephrine (although these values did not

differ between the males and females in this study), receptor availability and affinity for epinephrine (which was not tested), or the interaction of other circulating hormones, especially estrogen and progesterone (higher, of course, in the females) with epinephrine. It is also possible, because many of the differences were significant only after training, that the sympathetic nervous system in males and females may adapt differently to exercise training.

Source: Friedlander, A. L., G. A. Casazza, M. A. Horning, M. J. Huie, M. F. Piacentini, J. K. Trimmer, & G. A. Brooks: Training-induced alterations of carbohydrate metabolism in women: Women respond differently from men. *Journal of Applied Physiology.* 85(3):1175–1186 (1998).

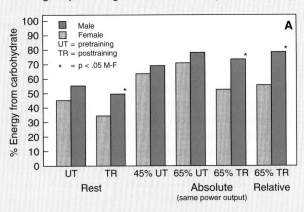

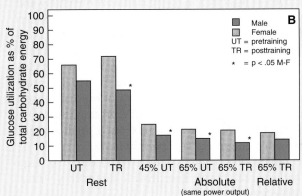

TABLE 2.5	Relative Degree of Fuel Utilization in Muscle for Various Types of Exercise					
Fuel	**Rest**	**Exercise Condition**				
		Very high-intensity, very short-duration (<3 min), and static contractions	**High-intensity (80–85% max), short-duration (<40 min)**	**High-intensity (70–80% max), moderate-duration (40–150 min)**	**Moderate-intensity (60–70% max), long-duration (>150 min)**	**Low-intensity (<50% max), long-duration (>150 min)**
Muscle glycogen	Negligible	High	High	High	Moderate	Low
Liver glycogen/ blood glucose	Moderate	Negligible	High	High	Moderate	Moderate
Free fatty acid (FFA)	Moderate	Negligible	Low	Moderate	High	High
Amino acid	Low	Negligible	Negligible	Low	Low	Low

Sources: Based on Felig, P. & J. Wahren: Fuel homeostasis in exercise. *The New England Journal of Medicine.* 293(4):1078–1084 (1975); Pernow, B. & B. Saltin (eds.): *Muscle Metabolism During Exercise.* New York: Plenum (1971).

TABLE 2.6	Fuel Utilization by 70-kg Male Runner at Different Distances and Levels of Performance			
	10 km (6.2 mi)		**42.2 km (26.2 mi)**	
	Fast	**Slow**	**Fast**	**Slow**
Performance (hr:min:sec)	0:30:00	1:00:00	2:21:00	5:12:00
Circulating glucose (g)	9.7	13.4	120.5	217.8
Muscle glycogen (g)	149.0	134.0	403.0	69.0
Liver glycogen (g)	20.1	10.9	73.7	103.9
Fatty acids (g)	7.0	12.0	104.0	229.0
Branched-chain amino acids (g) (BCAA)	0.7	0.9	15.7	48.5

Source: Péronnet, F., G. Thibault, M. Ledoux, & G. Brisson: *Performance in Endurance Events: Energy Balance, Nutrition, and Temperature Regulation in Distance Running.* London, ON: Spodym (1987).

Table 2.6 provides an estimation of how fuel utilization varies by race distance (10 km [6.2 mi] and 42.2 km [26.2 mi], or marathon distance) and performance (a "fast" and a "slow" time for each distance). Compare the muscle glycogen utilization in the fast and the slow conditions. At the short distance (10 km) there is not much difference, but during the marathon almost six times as much muscle glycogen is used by the faster runner. Conversely, the greatest amount of fat is utilized by the slow marathoner. Circulating glucose use is much higher in marathoners because the longer duration and lower intensity permit the liver to generate (by gluconeogenesis) and release glucose into the bloodstream. The 10-km runner has sufficient muscle glycogen stores and does not need to rely on external glucose production. Very little protein (BCAA) is used by either of the 10-km runners, but a small amount provides some energy for the marathoners.

A complex interaction exists between exercise energy needs and the fuel sources that provide this energy within the human organism.

SUMMARY

1. The process by which ATP is formed from food is called cellular respiration.
2. Carbohydrate metabolism consists of four stages that convert glucose or glycogen into carbon dioxide, water, and ATP energy.
3. Stage I of carbohydrate metabolism is known as glycolysis. Glycolysis consists of a series of 10 or 11 steps; it occurs in the cytoplasm of cells and is anaerobic. It begins with glucose or glycogen and ends with pyruvate (pyruvic acid) or lactate (lactic acid). In the process, a net gain of 2 ATP molecules is achieved by substrate-level phosphorylation if the fuel was glucose and 3 ATP if the fuel was glycogen. A pair of NADH + H$^+$ also results.
4. Stage II of carbohydrate metabolism has no identifying name, but it results in the formation of acetyl coenzyme A from pyruvate. These two steps occur in the mitochondrial matrix; although no oxygen is used directly, the process must be aerobic. No ATP is produced, but two pairs of hydrogen atoms are released and picked up by NAD$^+$, forming NADH + H$^+$.
5. Stage III of carbohydrate metabolism is the Krebs cycle. This stage consists of eight steps and also occurs in the mitochondrial matrix; again, no oxygen is used directly, but it also must be aerobic. Two ATP are produced by substrate-level phosphorylation and pairs of hydrogen atoms are removed at four separate steps. In three cases, the hydrogen ions are picked up by NAD$^+$ and in the fourth by FAD.
6. Stage IV of carbohydrate metabolism is known as electron transport and oxidative phosphorylation. Electron transport takes place in the inner mitochondrial membrane and consists of relaying electrons from the hydrogen atoms from one protein carrier to another and transporting the hydrogen ions into the intermembrane space. In the process, an electrical current is created. This electrical energy is then used to synthesize ATP from ADP by the addition of a phosphate as the H$^+$ move through the ball-and-stalk apparatus into the mitochondrial matrix. For each hydrogen carried to the ETS by NAD+, 2.5 ATP molecules are formed. For each hydrogen carried by FAD to the electron transport chain, 1.5 ATP are formed, lower than the previously thought theoretical values of 3 and 2, respectively.
7. A total of 30 ATP molecules are produced if the fuel substrate is glucose and the muscle is skeletal. A total of 31 ATP are produced if the fuel substrate is glycogen and the muscle is skeletal. A total of 32 ATP are produced if the fuel substrate is glucose and the muscle is cardiac. A total of 33 ATP are produced if the fuel substrate is glycogen and the muscle is cardiac. Theoretically, these values would be 36, 37, 38, and 39, respectively.
8. Triglycerides stored in adipose cells or stored intramuscularly are the major storage form of energy in humans. Triglycerides are composed of fatty acids and glycerol. Muscle cells can only use fatty acids as a fuel.

9. Fatty acid can only be utilized as a fuel source aerobically within the mitochondria. Fatty acids must undergo the process of beta-oxidation—which involves the removal of hydrogen atoms (oxidation) and the removal of pairs of carbons (at the beta carbon location) to form acetyl coenzyme A—before entering the Krebs cycle and electron transport.

10. The ATP produced from each fatty acid depends upon the number of carbon pairs.

11. When glucose supplies are inadequate and oxaloacetate must be converted to glucose, the acetyl coenzyme A derived from fatty acids is converted into three forms of ketones: acetoacetic acid, beta-hydroxybutyric acid, and acetone.

12. Amino acids are used primarily in anabolic processes in human cells, building proteins such as hemoglobin and the contractile elements of muscle. However, amino acids—and especially the branched-chain amino acids (valine, leucine, and isoleucine)—can be used as a fuel source and may contribute as much as 5–15% of the energy supply in long-term, dynamic-endurance activity.

13. All amino acids contain an amino group (NH_2). Before an amino acid can be used as a fuel, this amino group must be removed. Removal of the amino group is accomplished by two processes: oxidative deamination or transamination (most common). Entry into the Krebs cycle and electron transport then occurs at several locations, but ultimately all of the intermediates except acetyl CoA are converted to pyruvate before being used to produce energy.

14. Twelve-and-a-half ATP are derived from each of the amino acid derivatives utilized as pyruvate, and 10 ATP are produced from each derivative utilized as acetyl CoA, less than the historical theoretical values of 15 and 12, respectively.

15. ATP energy production has both intracellular and extracellular regulation. Intracellular regulation operates primarily by the feedback stimulation (by ADP, AMP, P_i, and a rise in pH) or inhibition (by ATP, CP, citrate, and a drop in pH) of the rate-limiting enzyme. Extracellular regulation is achieved by the coordinated action of the sympathetic nervous system (via norepinephrine) and the hormonal system (norepinephrine, epinephrine, glucagon, growth hormone, and cortisol).

16. The goal of metabolism during exercise is threefold:
    a. To increase the mobilization and utilization of free fatty acid from adipose tissue and intramuscular stores.
    b. To decrease the uptake of glucose into nonworking muscle cells while at the same time providing glucose for nerve and brain cells.
    c. To increase the breakdown of liver and muscle stores of glycogen and create glucose from noncarbohydrate sources in the liver.

17. The creation of glucose from noncarbohydrate sources is called gluconeogenesis. The primary fuel sources for gluconeogenesis are glycerol, lactate or pyruvate, and alanine.

18. Fatty acids comprise the largest fuel supply. Other fuels, in descending order, are total muscle glycogen, liver glycogen, and circulating glucose.

19. Which energy substrate is utilized and in what amounts depends upon the complex interaction of the type, duration, and intensity of exercise; the proportion of muscle fiber types involved; and the training status, long-term nutritional state, and short-term dietary status of the exerciser.

20. In general, very short-duration, high-intensity dynamic activity and static contractions are special cases that rely predominantly on the ATP-PC and glycogen stored in the muscle fibers.

21. In dynamic aerobic activity the higher the intensity, the more important carbohydrates (glucose and glycogen) are as a fuel; the lower the intensity, the more important fats are as a fuel. Likewise, the shorter the duration, the more important carbohydrates are as a fuel; the longer the duration, the more that fat is utilized. In activities lasting more than an hour, protein makes a small but important contribution to the energy supply.

REVIEW QUESTIONS

1. Distinguish between anabolism and catabolism. Is cellular respiration anabolic or catabolic?
2. Name and briefly summarize the four steps of carbohydrate metabolism.
3. Explain how a theoretical count of 36 ATP is achieved by cellular respiration if the fuel substrate is glucose in skeletal muscle. Why is the theoretical count for ATP production from carbohydrate sometimes 37, 38, or 39 instead of 36? Why is the count often 30, 31, 32, and 33 instead of the 36–39 values?
4. Why is beta-oxidation necessary before fat can be used as an energy substrate? Describe what occurs during beta-oxidation.
5. State how the calculation is completed to determine the number of ATP produced from fatty acids. Complete an example using a fat having 24 carbons.
6. Name and describe the process that amino acids must undergo before being used as a fuel substrate. Why is this process necessary?
7. Identify the locations in the metabolic pathways where amino acids may enter. How does the ATP count differ between these locations?
8. Why is acetyl CoA called the universal common intermediate?
9. Why might the breath of someone suffering from anorexia nervosa smell sweet?
10. Describe the role of enzymes in the metabolic pathways. Identify the rate-limiting enzymes in Stages

I, III, and IV of carbohydrate metabolism. How are enzymes regulated?

11. What are the goals of metabolic regulation during exercise? How are these goals achieved by the interaction of the sympathetic nervous system and the hormonal system?

12. Compare the relative availability and use of carbohydrate, fat, and protein fuel substrates on the basis of the intensity and duration of exercise.

For further review and study, you can find lab exercises, worksheets, a quiz bank, and crossword puzzles at http://thePoint. lww.com/Plowman4e. ✷ ▶

REFERENCES

Alcazar, O., R. C. Ho, & L. J. Goodyear: Physical activity, fitness, and diabetes mellitus. In Bouchard, C., S. N. Blair, & W. L. Haskell (eds.): *Physical Activity and Health*. Champaign, IL: Human Kinetics, 191–204, (2007).

Brooks, G. A.: What does glycolysis make and why is it important? *Journal of Applied Physiology*. 108:1450–1451 (2010).

Brooks, G. A., T. D. Fahey, & K. M. Baldwin: *Exercise Physiology: Human Bioenergetics and Its Applications* (4th edition). Boston, MA: McGraw-Hill (2004).

Bunt, J. C.: Hormonal alterations due to exercise. *Sports Medicine*. 3(5):331–345 (1986).

Bursztein, S., D. H. Elwyn, J. Askanazi, & J. M. Kinney: *Energy Metabolism, Indirect Calorimetry and Nutrition*. Baltimore, MD: Williams & Wilkins (1989).

Consolazio, C. F., R. E. Johnson, & L. J. Pecora: *Physiological Measurements of Metabolic Functions in Man*. New York, NY: McGraw-Hill (1963).

Dengel, D. R. & T.H. Reynolds: Diabetes. In LeMura, L. M., & S. P. von Duvillard (eds.): *Clinical Exercise Physiology*. Philadelphia, PA: Lippincott Williams & Wilkins (2004).

Felig, P. & J. Wahren: Fuel homeostasis in exercise. *New England Journal of Medicine*. 293(4):1078–1084 (1975).

Friedlander, A. L., G. A. Casazza, M. A. Horning, M. J. Huie, M. F. Piacentini, J. K. Trimmer, & G. A. Brooks: Training-induced alterations of carbohydrate metabolism in women: Women respond differently from men. *Journal of Applied Physiology*. 85(3):1175–1186 (1998).

Frisell, W. R.: *Human Biochemistry*. New York, NY: Macmillan (1982).

Galbo, H.: *Hormonal and Metabolic Adaptation to Exercise*. New York, NY: Thieme-Stratton, (1983).

Guyton, A. C. & J. E. Hall: *Textbook of Medical Physiology* (12th edition). Philadelphia, PA: Saunders (2011).

Houston, M. E.: *Biochemistry Primer for Exercise Science*. Champaign, IL: Human Kinetics (1995).

Kapit, W., R. I. Macey, & E. Meisami: *The Physiology Coloring Book*. New York, NY: Harper & Row (1987).

Kraniou, G. N., D. Cameron-Smith, & M. Hargreaves: Acute exercise and GLUT4 expression in human skeletal muscle: influence of exercise intensity. *Journal of Applied Physiology*. 101:934–937 (2006).

Lehninger, A. L.: *Bioenergetics* (2nd edition). Menlo Park, CA: Benjamin (1971).

Lemon, P. W. R. & F. J. Nagel: Effects of exercise on protein and amino acid metabolism. *Medicine and Science in Sports and Exercise*. 13(3):141–149 (1981).

MacLean, P. S., D. Zheng, & G. L. Dohm: Muscle glucose transporter (GLUT 4) gene expression during exercise. *Exercise and Sport Sciences Reviews*. 28(4):148–152 (2000).

Malina, R. M. & C. Bouchard.: *Growth, Maturation and Physical Activity*. Champaign, IL: Human Kinetics (1991).

Marcinek, D.J., M. J. Kushmerick, & K. E. Conley: Lactic acidosis in vivo: Testing the link between lactate generation and H+ accumulation in ischemic mouse muscle. *Journal of Applied Physiology*. 108:1479–1486 (2010).

Marieb, E. N. & K. Hoehn: *Human Anatomy and Physiology* (8th edition). San Francisco, CA: Benjamin Cummings (2010).

Mougios, V.: *Exercise Biochemistry*. Champaign, IL: Human Kinetics (2006).

Newsholme, E. A. & A. R. Leech: *Biochemistry for the Medical Sciences*. New York, NY: John Wiley (1983).

Pernow, B. & B. Saltin (eds.): *Muscle Metabolism During Exercise*. New York, NY: Plenum (1971).

Péronnet, F., G. Thibault, M. Ledoux, & G. Brisson: *Performance in Endurance Events: Energy Balance, Nutrition, and Temperature Regulation in Distance Running*. London, Ontario, Canada: Spodym (1987).

Robergs, R. A., F. Ghiasvand, & D. Parker: Biochemistry of exercise-induced metabolic acidosis. *American Journal of Physiology-Regulatory Integrative and Comparative Physiology*. 287: R502–R516 (2004).

Salway, J. G.: *Metabolism at a Glance*. Oxford, England: Blackwell Science (1994).

Sato, Y., Y. Oshida, I. Ohsawa, N. Nakai, N. Ohsaki, K. Yamanouchi, J. Sato, Y. Shimomura, & H. Ohno: The role of glucose transport in the regulation of glucose transport by muscle. In R. J. Maughm & S. M. Shirreffs (eds.): *Biochemistry of Exercise IX*. Champaign, IL: Human Kinetics (1996).

vanderBeek, E. J.: Vitamins and endurance training: Food for thought for running, or faddish claims? *Sports Medicine* 2:175–197 (1985).

Wilson-O'Brien, A. L., N. Patron, & S. Rogers: Evolutionary ancestry and novel functions of the mammalian glucose transporter (GLUT) family. *BMC Evolutionary Biology*. 10:152–163 (2010).

Zhao, F.-Q. & A. F. Keating: Functional properties and genomics of glucose transporters. *Current Genomics*. 8:113–128 (2007).

Anaerobic Metabolism during Exercise

3

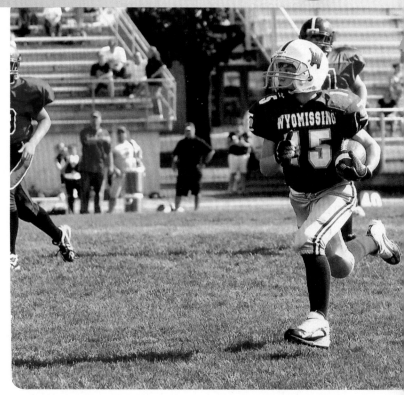

OBJECTIVES

After studying the chapter, you should be able to:

> Describe the energy continuum as it relates to varying durations of maximal maintainable exercise.

> Provide examples of sports or events within sports in which the ATP-PC, lactic, or oxygen system predominates.

> List the major variables that are typically measured to describe the anaerobic response to exercise and, where appropriate, the actual exercise test itself.

> Explain the physiological reasons why lactate may accumulate in the muscles and blood.

> Distinguish among the ATP-PC, lactic, and oxygen systems in terms of power and capacity.

> Identify oxygen deficit and excess postexercise oxygen consumption and explain the causes of each.

> Describe the changes in ATP and PC that occur during constant-load, heavy exercise lasting 3 minutes or less.

> Describe the changes in lactate accumulation that occur during short-term, high-intensity, anaerobic exercise lasting 3 minutes or less; short-term, light to moderate, and moderate to heavy submaximal aerobic exercise; long-term moderate to heavy submaximal

aerobic exercise; incremental exercise to maximum; and dynamic resistance exercise.

> Differentiate among the terms anaerobic threshold, ventilatory threshold, and lactate threshold and explain why anaerobic threshold is a misnomer.

> Discuss why the accumulation of lactate is a physiological and performance problem.

> Explain the fate of lactate during exercise and recovery.

> Compare anaerobic metabolic capacities during exercise for males versus females; children and adolescents versus young and middle-aged adults; and the elderly versus young and middle-aged adults and cite possible reasons for these differences.

Introduction

Chapter 2 explained how ATP, the ultimate energy source for all human work, is produced by the metabolic pathways. The emphasis there was on the energy substrate (carbohydrate, fat, or protein) utilized as fuel. This chapter and the next look at ATP production and utilization on the basis of the need for oxygen. Anaerobic metabolism does not require oxygen to produce ATP, whereas aerobic metabolism does. Critical to understanding anaerobic and aerobic exercise metabolism is the fact that these processes are not mutually exclusive; that is, anaerobic metabolism and aerobic metabolism are not either/or situations in terms of how ATP is provided. Both systems can and usually do work concurrently. When describing muscular exercise, the terms aerobic or anaerobic refer to the system predominating at the time.

The Energy Continuum

Figure 3.1 reviews the three sources of ATP production introduced in Chapter 2. **Figure 3.1A** describes *alactic anaerobic metabolism*, sometimes called the *phosphagen* or *ATP-PC system*. Once produced, ATP is stored in the muscle. This amount is relatively small and can provide energy for only 2–3 seconds of maximal effort (Mougios, 2006). However, another high-energy compound, phosphocreatine (PC), also known as creatine phosphate (CP), can be used to resynthesize ATP from ADP almost instantaneously. The amount of PC stored in muscle is about three times that of ATP (Gollnick and King, 1969). Muscles differ in the amount of stored PC by fiber type. Muscle fiber types are fully described in Chapter 17, but briefly, fibers that produce energy predominantly by anaerobic glycolysis are called glycolytic; those that produce energy predominantly aerobically are called oxidative. In terms of contraction speed, muscle fibers are either fast twitch or slow twitch. When contractile and metabolic characteristics are combined, three fiber types are generally described: fast-twitch glycolytic (FG also known as Type IIX), fast-twitch oxidative glycolytic (FOG also known as Type IIA), and slow-twitch oxidative (SO). Fast-twitch fibers have proportionally more PC than ATP compared to slow-twitch exidative fibers. Any time the energy demand is increased—whether the activity is simply turning a page of this book, coming out of the blocks for a sprint, or starting out on a long bicycle ride—at least part of the immediate need for energy is supplied by these stored forms (ATP, PC), which must ultimately be replenished. These sources are also used preferentially in high-intensity, very short-duration activity. Most resynthesis of ATP from PC takes place in the first 10 seconds of maximal muscle contraction; little, if any, occurs after 20 seconds of maximal activity (Gastin, 2001). This ATP-PC system neither uses oxygen nor produces lactic acid and is thus said to be *alactic anaerobic*.

Figure 3.1B represents *anaerobic glycolysis*, also called the *lactic acid (LA) system*. When the demand for ATP exceeds the capacity of the phosphagen system and the aerobic system (at the initiation of any activity or during high-intensity, short-duration exercise), *fast* (anaerobic) glycolysis is used to produce ATP. This is rather like calling in the reserves, for glycolysis can provide the supplemental energy quickly. The rate of ATP production from glycolysis reaches its maximum about 5 seconds after initiation of contraction and is maintained at this rate for several seconds (Gastin, 2001). This system predominates in activities such as a 1500-m speed skating event. Other sport activities with a heavy reliance on the LA system include middle distances (e.g., track 200 to 800 m, swimming 100 m, slalom, and downhill skiing); gymnastic floor exercise; parallel bars; a round of boxing; and a period of wrestling. The ability to perform the events with speed and power is the benefit. The cost is that the production of lactic acid often exceeds clearance, and lactate accumulates. Because this system does not use oxygen but does result in the production of lactic acid, it is said to be *lactic anaerobic*.

Figure 3.1C shows *aerobic oxidation*, also termed the *O_2 system*. The generation of ATP from *slow* (aerobic) glycolysis, the Krebs cycle, and electron transport–oxidative phosphorylation is constantly in operation at some level. In resting conditions, this system provides basically all of the energy needed. When activity begins or occurs at moderate levels of intensity, oxidation increases quickly and proceeds at a rate that supplies the needed ATP. If the workload is continuously increased, aerobic oxidation proceeds at a correspondingly higher rate until its maximal limit is reached. The highest amount of oxygen the body can consume during heavy dynamic exercise for the aerobic production of ATP is called maximal oxygen uptake, or $\dot{V}O_2$max Because $\dot{V}O_2$max is primarily an index of cardiorespiratory power, and as such is used as a measure of cardiovascular-respiratory fitness, it is discussed in depth in that unit. However, because $\dot{V}O_2$max reflects the

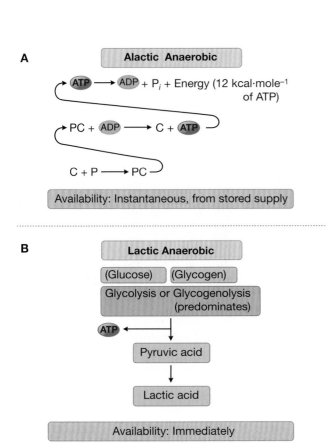

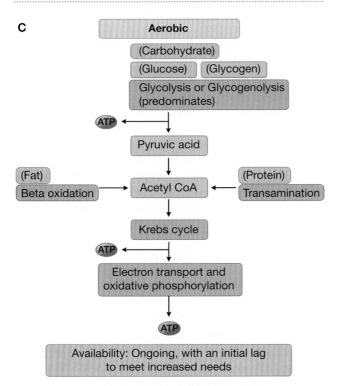

FIGURE 3.1   Anaerobic and Aerobic Sources of ATP.

$\dot{V}O_2$max). Anaerobic metabolic processes are important at the onset of all aerobic exercise, contribute significantly at submaximal levels, and increase their contribution as the exercise intensity gets progressively higher. Depending on an individual's fitness level, lactic anaerobic metabolism begins to make a significant contribution to dynamic activity at approximately 40–60% $\dot{V}O_2$max. However, even then the ability to use oxygen is most important. Historically the contribution of aerobic metabolism to intense exercise has probably been underestimated and the contribution of anaerobic metabolism overestimated because of the difficulty in measuring the anaerobic metabolism accurately. By between 1 and 2 minutes of maximal exercise, the relative contributions of ATP production from the aerobic and anaerobic energy systems are approximately equal (Gastin, 2001). Because the aerobic system involves the use of oxygen and proceeds completely to oxidative phosphorylation, it is said to be *aerobic* or *oxidative*. Sport activities that rely predominantly on the O_2 system include long-distance events, such as the 5000 and 10,000 m in track; marathons; swimming 1500 m; cross-country running, skiing, and orienteering; field hockey, soccer, and lacrosse; and race walking.

These three sources of ATP—the phosphagen system (ATP-PC), the glycolytic system (LA), and the oxidative system (O_2)—contribute to maximal exercise of different durations in a pattern called the *time-energy system continuum*. This continuum assumes that the individual is working at a maximal maintainable intensity for a continuous duration. This means that it is assumed that an individual can go all out for 5 minutes or less or can work at 100% $\dot{V}O_2$max for 10 minutes, at 95% $\dot{V}O_2$max for 30 minutes, at 85% $\dot{V}O_2$max for 60 minutes, and at 80% $\dot{V}O_2$max for 120 minutes. Of course, there are individual differences, but these assumptions are reasonable in general.

Figure 3.2 differentiates the anaerobic systems into the ATP-PC and LA as well as indicates that the O_2 system participates quickly in all-out maximal exercise lasting

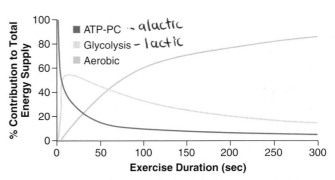

FIGURE 3.2   Relative Contributions of the ATP-PC, LA, and O_2 Energy Systems to Maximal Exercise.
Source: Gastin, P. B.: Energy system interaction and relative contribution during maximal exercise. *Sports Medicine*. 31(10):725–741 (2001). Reprinted by permission.

amount of oxygen available for the aerobic production of ATP, it is also an important metabolic measure. Both aerobic and anaerobic exercises are often described in terms of a given percentage of $\dot{V}O_2$max (either < or >100%

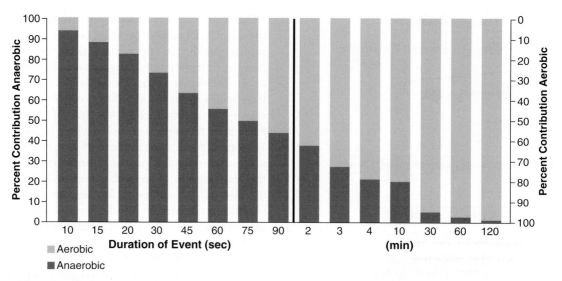

FIGURE 3.3   Time-Energy System Continuum.
Approximate relative contributions of aerobic and anaerobic energy production at maximal maintainable intensity for varying durations.
Note: The graphs assume 100% $\dot{V}O_2$max at 10 minutes; 95% $\dot{V}O_2$max at 30 minutes; 85% $\dot{V}O_2$max at 60 minutes; and 80% $\dot{V}O_2$max at 120 minutes. ATP-PC ≤ 10 s.

300 seconds (5 minutes) or less (Gastin, 2001). Note that both anaerobic systems respond immediately but neither can sustain the high level of ATP production needed. The LA system contributes more than the ATP-PC by approximately 10 seconds. Conversely, the aerobic energy system (O_2) is incapable of meeting the immediate energy demands but contributes to a meaningful degree quickly.

Figure 3.3 shows the best estimates available of the relative contributions of the combined anaerobic (ATP-PC plus LA) systems and the aerobic energy system to the total energy requirement for exercise durations up to 120 minutes. Again, initially the anaerobic systems predominate, but by 30 seconds almost 27% of the ATP is being supplied by oxidative phosphorylation. The point at which the aerobic and anaerobic contribution becomes approximately equal is 75 seconds (**Figure 3.2**). From then on, the aerobic system dominates.

Four basic patterns can be discerned from this continuum. Understanding these patterns is helpful when developing training programs.

1. All three energy systems (ATP-PC, LA, O_2) are involved in providing energy for all durations of exercise.
2. The ATP-PC system predominates in activities lasting 10 seconds or less. Since the ATP-PC system is involved primarily at the onset of longer activities, it becomes a smaller portion of the total energy supply as duration gets longer.
3. Anaerobic metabolism (ATP-PC and LA) predominates in supplying energy for exercises lasting between 1 and 2 minutes. The equal contribution point for anaerobic and aerobic energy contribution to maxi-

mal exercise is probably close to 75 seconds. However, even exercises lasting as long as 10 minutes use at least 15% anaerobic sources. Within the anaerobic component the longer the duration, the greater the relative importance of the lactic acid system in comparison to the phosphagen system.
4. By 2 minutes of exercise, the O_2 system clearly dominates. The longer the duration, the more important it becomes.

The rest of this chapter concentrates on the anaerobic contribution to energy metabolism. Chapter 4 then focuses on the aerobic contribution to energy metabolism, although again it must be emphasized that the two systems work together, with one or the other predominating primarily on the duration and intensity of the activity.

Anaerobic Energy Production

Alactic Anaerobic PC Production

As previously described, alactic anaerobic production of ATP involves the use of phosphocretine PC, which is simply creatine bound to inorganic phosphate. An adult human has a creatine level of approximately 120–140 mmol·kg^{-1} of dry muscle, although there is considerable individual variation from a low of 90–100 mmol·kg^{-1} to a high of about 150–160 mmol·kg^{-1}. Each day approximately 2 g of creatine are degraded in a nonreversible reaction to creatinine. This creatinine is ultimately excreted by the kidneys in urine. The loss is counterbalanced under normal dietary conditions by the ingestion of about 1 g of creatine from meat, poultry, and/or fish and the synthesis of another gram in the liver from the amino acids arginine, glycine, and methionine. Close to 95% of the creatine in the body is stored in skeletal muscle. Thirty to forty percent is stored as free creatine and the rest as phosphocreating.

Figure 3.4 shows the breakdown of ATP and PC during heavy exercise. It also shows the restoration of ATP from energy substrate sources and the restoration of PC from the regenerated ATP. The process continues until the resting levels of both PC and ATP are regained. Specifically, when ATP is hydrolyzed by the contractile proteins in muscle (1) (large inner circle), the resulting ADP is rephosphorylated in the cytoplasm by the PC available there (2) (small inner circle). In turn, the now free creatine is rephosphorylated at the inner mitochondrial membrane from the breakdown of ATP produced at that site (3) (large outside oval). The remnant (4) ADP is then free, in turn, to be phosphorylated again by oxidative phosphorylation using energy substrates. In addition to providing ATP rapidly, this mechanism, called the creatine phosphate shuttle, is one way in which electron transport and oxidative phosphorylation are regulated (Brooks et al., 1999).

See the Focus on Application box on the use of creatine as an ergogenic aid.

Lactic Acid/Lactate Levels

Lactic acid is produced in muscle cells when the $NADH + H^+$ formed in glycolysis (step 6; see **Figure 2.6** in Chapter 2)

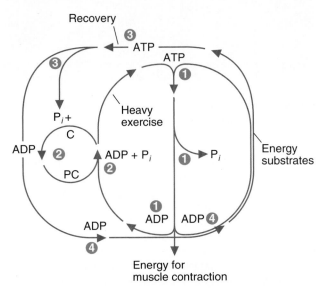

FIGURE 3.4   Use and Regeneration of ATP-PC.
1. $ATP \rightarrow ADP + P_i$ + energy for muscle contraction (*large inner circle*). 2. During heavy exercise the ADP is regenerated to ATP by the breakdown of PC ($PC + ADP \rightarrow C + ATP$) (*small inner circle*). 3. Only in recovery will the nearly depleted PC stores be restored from the breakdown of ATP resulting from aerobic metabolic production (*large outside oval*). 4. $ADP \rightarrow ATP$ from energy substrates.

is oxidized to NAD^+ by a transfer of the hydrogen ions to pyruvic acid ($C_3H_4O_3$), which in turn is reduced to lactic acid ($C_3H_6O_3$) (Brooks, 1985; Newsholme and Leech, 1983). In muscle tissue, lactic acid is produced in amounts that are in equilibrium with pyruvic acid under normal resting conditions. As stated in Chapter 2 there is some unresolved controversy as to whether skeletal muscle actually produces lactate or lactic acid although lactic acid, not lactate, represents the accepted classic view (Brooks, 2010; Marcinek et al., 2010; Robergs et al., 2004). Even if lactic acid of is the substance actually produced, at physiological pH 99% of the lactic acid is dissociated immediately to H^+ and La^- (lactate) (Brooks, 1985; Gladden, 2004). In addition, lactic acid is always produced by red blood cells, portions of the kidneys, and certain tissues within the eye. Both resting and exercise blood lactate values depend on the balance between lactic acid/lactate *production* (*appearance*) and *removal* (*disappearance* or *clearance*). This balance of appearance and disappearance is called *turnover*. When production exceeds removal, lactate is said to accumulate. The issues, then, especially during exercise, focus on what conditions result in lactic acid/lactate production and what processes lead to lactate removal. When blood lactate levels are measured they reflect the balance of lactate production and removal. The major contributors to lactate production and removal are summarized in **Figure 3.5**.

Lactic Acid/Lactate Production

In general, the relative rates of glycolytic activity (Stage I of carbohydrate metabolism) and oxidative activity (Stages II, III, and IV) determine the production of lactic acid/lactate. Specifically, five factors play important roles: muscle contraction, enzyme activity, muscle fiber type, sympathetic nervous system activation, and insufficient oxygen (anaerobiosis, the onset of anaerobic metabolism).

1. Muscle contraction. During exercise, muscle activity obviously increases. Muscle contraction involves the release of calcium (Ca^{2+}) from the sarcoplasmic reticulum. In addition to its role in the coupling process of actin and myosin, calcium also causes glycogenolysis by activating the enzyme glycogen phosphorylase. Glycogen is processed by fast glycolysis and results in the production of lactic acid/lactate regardless of whether oxygen levels are sufficient or not (Brooks et al., 1999; Fox, 1973).

2. Enzyme activity. The conversion of pyruvate and $NADH + H^+$ to lactate and NAD^+ is catalyzed by specific isozymes of the enzyme lactic dehydrogenase (LDH), whereas the conversion of pyruvate to acetyl CoA (Stage II) prior to entry into the Krebs cycle is catalyzed by the enzyme pyruvate dehydrogenase (PDH). LDH has the highest rate of functioning of any of the glycolytic enzymes and is much more active

Creatine as an Ergogenic Aid

Creatine (C) [primarily in the form of creatine monohydrate (CM)] continues to enjoy unprecedented popularity as an ergogenic aid. It has been established that oral creatine supplementation can increase muscle creatine (C) content by approximately 10–40%, depending on an individual's starting muscular concentration. There is an upper limit for storage, so if an individual is already at that point (~160 mmol·kg^{-1} of dry muscle) supplementation will not further increase storage. Excess ingested creatine is excreted in the urine (American College of Sports Medicine [ACSM], 2000; Buford et al., 2007). This can explain why one individual might respond to creatine monohydrate supplementation and another might be a "nonresponder." Training status may impact C uptake during a loading phase because intramuscular levels may already be elevated (Bemben and Lamont, 2005).

Metabolically, there are three primary mechanisms to explain how increased levels of creatine in muscle could impact anaerobic energy production: (1) increased C means increased levels of PC for increased rephosphorylation of ADP to ATP; (2) stimulation of phosphofructokinase (PFK), the rate-limiting enzyme of glycolysis, occurs when PC levels decline as PC is used for the increased rephosphorylation of ATP (Bemben and Lamont, 2005); (3) increased muscle glycogen (Rawson and Persky, 2007). Molecular adaptation, that is, an increased gene expression of growth factors, and reduced muscle damage also occur (Poortmans et al., 2010). These adaptations allow an individual to train harder and recover faster (Buford et al., 2007). A number of studies have also indicated that creatine supplementation, along with heavy resistance training, enhances the normal training adaptation (American College of Sports Medicine, 2000). Creatine does not increase skeletal muscle protein synthesis (Poortmans et al., 2010).

There are studies that have shown no improvement with creatine supplementation (Misic and Kelley, 2002) and others that have shown significant improvement (Branch, 2003). On the whole, of the several hundred peer-reviewed published research studies nearly 70% have reported a significant improvement in exercise capacity (American College of Sports Medicine, 2000; Buford et al., 2007; Jäger et al., 2011). The effectiveness of creatine depends in large part on the exercise category. The greatest improvement in performance seems to occur in the later bouts of a repetitive series of exercises in which the high power output lasts only a matter of seconds separated by rest periods of 20–60 seconds (American College of Sports Medicine, 2000). A 2005 analysis by Bemben and Lamont concurred that the use of CM is effective for short-term high-intensity activities, especially when the activity involves repeated bouts. They also concluded, however, that whether or not peak force appeared to benefit from CM supplementation depended on the type of muscle contraction. Dynamic isotonic peak force measures seem to benefit, isokinetic results are mixed, and there is little benefit for isometric measures. Typical improvement ranges from approximately 2% in increased lean body mass, approximately 11% in muscle strength, and approximately 8% in high-intensity exercise performance. No studies have reported an impairment of

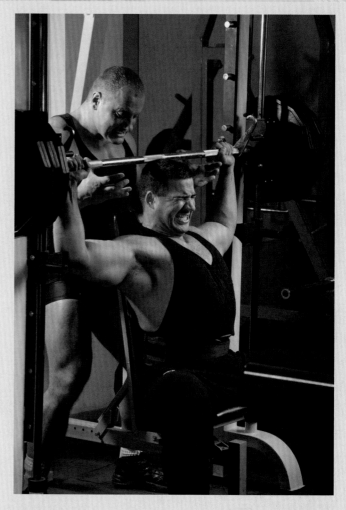

Athletes using heavy resistance training appear to benefit the most from CM supplementation.

exercise performance. The International Society of Sports Nutrition position stand—Creatine Supplementation and Exercise (2007, p. 1)—concluded that "creatine monohydrate is the most effective ergogenic nutritional supplement currently available to athletes in terms of increasing high-intensity exercise capacity and lean body mass during training." The addition of carbohydrate or carbohydrate and protein combined to creatine appears to increase muscular retention of creatine; however, the effect on performance currently does not appear to be any greater than using CM alone. (Buford

FOCUS ON APPLICATION

Creatine as an Ergogenic Aid *(Continued)*

et al., 2007). There is no evidence that any of the newer forms of creatine are more effective and/or safer than CM whether ingested alone or in combination with other ingredients (Jäger et al., 2011).

As with any supplement, concerns have been expressed regarding the safety of creatine ingestion. Although there have been numerous anecdotal reports of gastrointestinal disturbances (nausea, vomiting, diarrhea), liver and kidney dysfunction, cardiovascular/thermal impairment, and muscular damage (cramps, strains), credible reviews have concluded that, with the notable exception of individuals with medically documented preexisting kidney problems (that were aggravated with creatine supplementation and resolved when the supplementation was stopped), there is no scientific evidence that the short- or long-term use of CM has any detrimental effects on otherwise healthy individuals (Buford et al., 2007; Jäger et al., 2011). In addition, recent evidence suggests that creatine neither hinders the body's ability to dissipate heat nor negatively affects body fluid balance (Lopez et al., 2009). Creatine may actually enhance performance in hot/humid conditions by maintaining hematocrit, aiding thermoregulation, reducing exercising heart rate and sweat rate, and maintaining plasma volume (Dalbo et al., 2008). The evidence of safety is strong at intakes up to 5 g·d^{-1} for chronic supplementation (Shao and Hathcock, 2006). This does not mean that there are no precautions. The following are advised (American College of Sports Medicine, 2000; Bemben and Lamont, 2005; Poortmans and Francaux, 2000; Poortmans et al., 2010):

1. Individuals with preexisting kidney dysfunction or those at high risk for kidney disease (e.g., diabetics and individuals with a family history of kidney disease) should either avoid creatine supplementation or undergo regular medical monitoring. Regular checkups are recommended for everyone taking creatine because any individual may react adversely to any substance, and excess creatine is a burden that must be eliminated by the kidneys.

2. Individuals wishing to maintain or decrease body weight while participating in strenuous exercise should avoid creatine supplementation.

3. Adequate fluid and electrolytes should always be ingested.

4. Pregnant or lactating females should not supplement with creatine.

5. The ingestion of creatine during exercise should be avoided.

There appears to be no systematic sex or age difference in the results of C supplementation (Bemben and Lamont, 2005). While fewer studies have been conducted using children or adolescent participants, and these have primarily been therapeutic interventions, none have shown CM to have adverse effects in this population. Thus the International Society of Sports Nutrition (2007) recommends the following guidelines for the use of CM by adolescents:

1. The athlete should be postpubertal and involved in competitive training of the type of activity that would benefit from CM supplementation.

2. The athlete should be eating a well-balanced, performance-enhancing diet.

3. The athlete and his or her parents should understand the truth concerning the effects of CM supplementation.

4. The athlete's parents should have approved the supplementation.

5. CM supplementation should be supervised by the parents, trainers, coaches, and/or physician.

6. Quality supplements should be used.

7. The athlete should not exceed recommended dosages.

The quickest method of increasing muscle C stores appears to be by ingesting approximately 0.3 g·kg·d^{-1} of CM for at least 3 days followed by 3–5 g·d^{-1} to maintain the elevated stores.

CM products are readily available as a dietary supplement and are regulated by the U.S. Food and Drug Administration as a dietary ingredient. The legal and regulatory status of other forms is somewhat ambiguous. CM is approved as a natural health product in Canada by the Natural Health Products Directorate (Jäger et al., 2011). Creatine supplementation is not currently banned by any athletic organization although the National Collegiate Athletic Association (NCAA) does not allow institutions to provide CM supplements for athletes. The International Olympic Committee (IOC) ruled that there was no need to ban creatine since it is naturally found in food and there is no valid test to determine supplementation (Buford et al., 2007). These rulings, of course, can change at any time so the wise athlete will check before supplementing.

Sources: American College of Sports Medicine Roundtable (2000), Bemben and Lamont (2005), Branch (2003), Buford et al. (2007), Dalbo et al. (2008), Jäger et al. (2011), Lopez et al. (2009), Misic and Kelley (2002), Poortmans and Francaux (2000), Rawson and Persky (2007), Shao and Hathcock (2006).

than the enzymes that provide alternate pathways for pyruvate metabolism, including PDH and the rate-limiting enzymes in the Krebs cycle. Any increase in pyruvate and NADH + H$^+$ further increases the activity of LDH and results in the production of lactic acid/lactate (Spriet et al., 2000). Therefore, lactic acid production is an inevitable consequence of glycolysis (Brooks, 1986; Gaesser and Brooks, 1975; Spriet et al.,

2000). The more pyruvate provided, the more lactate produced. The shifting of the hydrogen atoms from NADH + H$^+$ to pyruvate-forming lactate serves to maintain the redox potential of the cell. The redox, or oxidation-reduction, potential is the ratio of NADH + H$^+$ to NAD$^+$. There is a finite amount of NAD$^+$ available in the cytoplasm to accept hydrogen atoms in step 6 and keep glycolysis going. To maintain this supply,

FIGURE 3.5 The Balance between Lactate Production and Clearance.
Lactate accumulation in the blood is the result of the balance between lactate production and lactate clearance. Normal resting blood values are usually ≤ 2.0 mmol·L⁻¹.

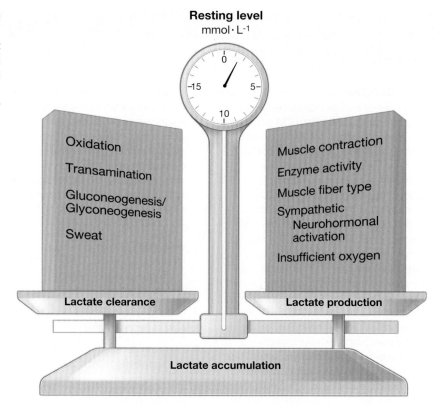

NADH + H⁺ must either transfer the hydrogen atoms into the mitochondria to the electron transport chain or give them up to pyruvate.

3. Muscle fiber type. During high-intensity, short-duration activities, fast-twitch glycolytic (FG) muscle fibers are preferentially recruited. These fast-contracting glycolytic fibers produce lactic acid/lactate when they contract, regardless of whether oxygen is present in sufficient amounts or not. This response appears to be a function of the specific lactic dehydrogenase isozyme and the low mitochondrial density found in these fibers. Different lactic dehydrogenase isozymes are found in different fibers (Green, 1986). Lactic dehydrogenase isozymes 4 and 5 predominate in fast-twitch fibers and facilitate the conversion of pyruvate to lactate. Conversely, LDH isozymes 1 and 2 predominate in cardiac, slow-twitch oxidative, and fast-twitch mitochondria and catalyze the conversion of lactate to pyruvate (Houston, 1995).

4. Sympathetic neurohormonal activation. During heavy exercise, activity of the sympathetic nervous system stimulates the release of epinephrine and glucagon and suppression of insulin (see **Figure 2.17** in Chapter 2). The result is the breakdown of glycogen, leading ultimately to high levels of glucose-6-phosphate (G6P). (Refresh your memory by referring to **Figure 2.6**, if necessary, to locate G6P in glycolysis.) High levels of G6P increase the rate of glycolysis and thus the production of pyruvic acid (Brooks, 1986). As previously described, any increase in pyruvate and NADH + H⁺

ultimately results in an increase in lactic acid/lactate. In addition, late in prolonged endurance activity, epinephrine-mediated glycogen breakdown may bring about the release of lactate from resting muscle when an increased lactate release is no longer occurring in contracting muscles (Stallknecht et al., 1998).

5. Insufficient oxygen (anaerobiosis, onset of anaerobic metabolism). Finally, during high-intensity, short-duration or near-maximal exercise or during static contractions when blood flow is impeded (Stallknecht et al., 1998), the delivery of oxygen to the mitochondria—and thus the availability of oxygen as the final electron acceptor at the end of the respiratory chain—can become deficient. In these circumstances, glycolysis proceeds at a rate that produces larger quantities of NADH + H⁺ than the mitochondria have oxygen to accept. Again, "something" has to be done with the hydrogen atoms so that the NAD⁺ can be regenerated. That "something" is the transfer of the hydrogen atoms to pyruvic acid and the formation of lactic acid, which dissociates quickly to lactate.

Thus, although lactic acid is associated with high-intensity, short-duration exercise, this is not the only exercise condition that results in the production of lactic acid/lactate. Furthermore, although a lack of oxygen can contribute to the production of lactic acid, the presence of lactic acid/lactate does not absolutely indicate a lack of oxygen. The presence of lactate simply reflects the use of the anaerobic glycolytic pathway for ATP production and the balance between glycolytic and mitochondrial activity. Furthermore, rather than lactic acid being a "waste product," lactate provides a means of coordinating carbohydrate metabolism in diverse tissues (Brooks et al., 1999). The formation, distribution, and utilization of lactate is a way for glycogen reserves to be mobilized and used within either the working muscle cell or other cells. In the process, blood glucose is spared for use by other tissues (Brooks, 2002; Gladden, 2004). The use or reconversion of lactate, or both, comprise lactate clearance.

Lactate Clearance

As stated earlier, blood lactate levels reflect the balance between lactic acid/lactate production (appearance) and clearance (removal). Lactate clearance (**Figure 3.5**) occurs primarily by three processes: oxidation (50–75%), gluconeogenesis/glyconeogenesis (10–25%), and transamination (5–10%). All three processes can involve the movement of lactate, either within or between cells.

As stated previously, although produced as lactic acid, at physiological pH more than 99% quickly dissociates into lactate (La^-) anions and protons (H^+) (Gladden, 2004). Lactate moves readily between cytoplasm and mitochondria, muscle and blood, blood and muscle, active and inactive muscle, glycolytic and oxidative muscle, blood and heart, blood and liver, and blood and skin (Brooks, 2000). Lactate moves between lactate-producing and lactate-consuming sites through intracellular and extracellular lactate shuttles (Brooks, 2002). Transport across cellular and mitochondrial membranes occurs by facilitated exchange down concentration and hydrogen ion (pH) gradients using lactate transport proteins known as monocarboxylate transporters (MCTs) (Brooks, 2000; Gladden, 2004).

As of 2006, 14 monocarboxylate transporters had been reported in the literature (Bonen et al., 2006). MCT1 is abundant in oxidative skeletal and cardiac muscle fibers and mitochondrial membranes. MCT4 is most prevalent in the cell membranes of glycolytic skeletal fibers (Bonen, 2000).

The *intracellular lactate shuttle* (**Figure 3.6A**) involves the movement of lactate by MCT1 transporters between the cytoplasm, where it is produced, and the mitochondria. Once inside the mitochondria, lactate is oxidized to pyruvate under the influence of the isozyme LDH1 and NAD^+ is reduced to $NADH + H^+$. Although originally it seemed that this occurred inside the mitochondrial matrix, recent evidence points to the intermembrane space adjacent to the inner mitochondrial membrane as the location. The pyruvate proceeds through Stages II, III, and IV of aerobic metabolism, while the $NADH + H^+$ goes directly to Stage IV. This is a relatively new and somewhat controversial concept that indicates that muscle cells can both produce and consume lactate at the same time (Brooks, 2000; Gladden, 2004, 2008a; Hashimoto and Brooks, 2008; Rasmussen, 2002; Sahlin, 2002).

Extracellular lactate shuttles act to move lactate between tissues (**Figure 3.6B**). Muscle cell membrane lactate proteins

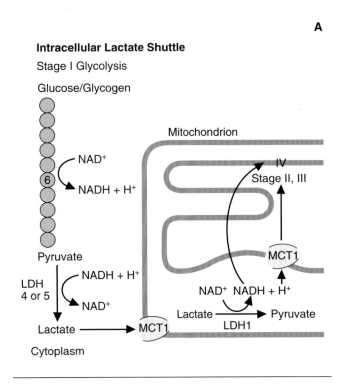

A

Intracellular Lactate Shuttle

Stage I Glycolysis

Glucose/Glycogen

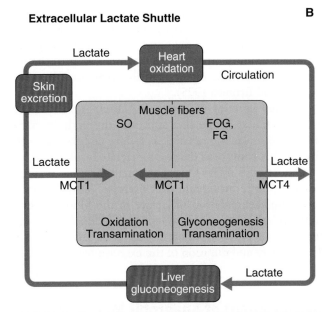

B

Extracellular Lactate Shuttle

FIGURE 3.6 Intracellular and Extracellular Lactate Shuttles.
A. The intracellular lactate shuttle transports lactate from the cytoplasm into the mitochondria by MCT1 transporters, where it is reconverted to pyruvate and proceeds through Stages II, III, and IV of metabolism. **B.** The extracellular lactate shuttle moves lactate directly between lactic acid-producing fast-twitch glycolytic fibers (FOG and FG) and lactate-consuming slow-twitch oxidative fibers. It also transports lactate through the circulation to the liver, skin, and heart, where it is cleared by oxidation, transamination, gluconeogenesis, or excretion. Most lactate remaining in fast-twitch glycolytic fibers is reconverted to glycogen by glyconeogenesis.

(MCT1 and MCT4) move the lactate both out of and into tissues. Intermuscularly, most lactate moves out of active fast-twitch glycolytic skeletal muscle cells (both fast-twitch oxidative glycolytic [FOG] and fast-twitch glycolytic [FG]) and into active slow-twitch oxidative (SO) skeletal muscle cells. This can occur either by a direct shuttle between the skeletal muscle cells or through the circulation. Once lactate is in the bloodstream, it can also circulate to cardiac cells. During heavy exercise, lactate becomes the preferred fuel of the heart. In this manner glycogenolysis in one cell can supply fuel for another cell. In each of these cases the ultimate fate of the lactate is oxidation to ATP, CO_2, and H_2O by aerobic metabolism (Brooks, 1986, 2000; Chatham, 2002).

Lactate circulating in the bloodstream can also be transported to the liver where, as described in Chapter 2, it is reconverted into glucose by the process of gluconeogenesis. Indeed, the liver appears to preferentially make glycogen from lactate rather than glucose. In human glycolytic muscle fibers (both fast-twitch oxidative glycolytic and fast-twitch glycolytic), some of the lactate produced during high-intensity exercise is retained, and in the postexercise recovery period it is reconverted to glycogen in that muscle cell. This process is called glyconeogenesis (Brooks et al., 1999; Donovan and Pagliassotti, 2000; Gladden, 2000).

Both oxidative and glycolytic fibers can also clear lactate by transamination. Transamination forms keto acids (Krebs cycle intermediates) and amino acids. The predominant amino acid produced is alanine. In turn, alanine can undergo gluconeogenesis in the liver (Brooks, 1986; Gaesser and Brooks, 1975).

A small amount of lactate in the circulation moves from the blood to the skin and exits the body in sweat. Finally, some lactate remains as lactate circulating in the blood. This comprises the resting lactate level.

Oxidation is by far the predominant process of lactate clearance both during and after exercise. As stated previously, the accumulation of lactate in the blood depends on the relative rate of appearance (production) and disappearance (clearance), which in turn is directly related to the intensity and duration of the exercise being done.

Measurement of Anaerobic Metabolism

Laboratory Procedures

Unfortunately, there is no generally accepted means by which to directly measure the contribution of anaerobic energy to exercise. Two general approaches are used, however, to describe the anaerobic exercise response. One approach describes changes in the chemical substances either used in alactic anaerobic metabolism (specifically, ATP and PC levels) or produced as a result of lactic anaerobic metabolism (lactate). The second approach quantifies the amount of work performed or the power generated during short-duration, high-intensity activity.

The assumption is that such activity could not be done without anaerobic energy; therefore, measuring such work or power indirectly measures anaerobic energy utilization and provides an indication of anaerobic capacity.

ATP-PC and Lactate

Muscle ATP, PC, and lactate can be measured by chemical analysis of muscle biopsy specimens. Lactate is the most frequently measured variable, in part because it can also be measured from blood samples. The blood sample may be obtained by venipuncture or finger prick, both of which are less invasive than a muscle biopsy. Another reason for the popularity of lactate analysis is the availability of user-friendly, fast, accurate, and relatively inexpensive analyzers. **Figure 3.7** shows an analyzer that requires a minimal blood sample (a 25-mL capillary tube obtained by a finger prick); it is portable and takes less than 5 minutes for each sample analysis.

Remember that at normal pH levels, lactic acid almost completely dissociates into hydrogen ions (H^+) and lactate ($C_3H_5O_3^-$, designated as La^-). Thus, technically, lactic acid may or may not be what is formed, but lactate is what

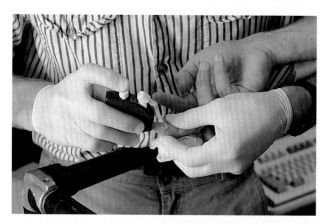

A

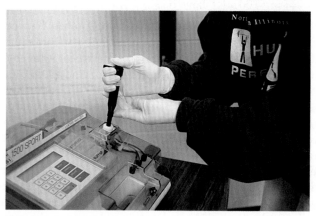

B

FIGURE 3.7 Lactate Analysis.
A small sample of blood is obtained by a finger prick **(A)** and injected into a lactate analyzer **(B)** for determination of lactate concentration [La^-].

TABLE 3.1 Estimated Maximal Power and Capacity in Untrained Males

Energy system	Power		Time	Capacity	
	kcal·min⁻¹	kJ·min⁻¹	hr:min:sec	kcal	kJ
ATP-PC (phosphagen)	72	300	:09–:10	11	45
LA (anaerobic glycolysis)	36	150	1:19.8	48	200
O₂ (aerobic glycolysis + Krebs cycle +ETS-OP; fuel = CHO)	7.2–19.1	30–80	2:21:00*	359–1268	1500–5300

*When all fuels are considered, the time is unlimited.
Sources: Bouchard et al. (1982, 1991).

is measured in the bloodstream. Despite this distinction, the terms lactic acid and lactate are often used synonymously (Brooks, 1985; Gladden, 2004).

Lactate is a small molecule that moves easily from the muscles to the blood and most other fluid compartments. However, much of the lactate that is produced does not get into the bloodstream. It takes time for the portion that does get into the bloodstream to reach equilibrium between muscle and blood. This equilibrium and the achievement of peak blood values may take as long as 5–10 minutes. Until equilibrium occurs, muscle lactate values will be higher than blood lactate values. This also means that the highest blood lactate values are typically seen after several minutes of recovery, not during high-intensity work (Gollnick and Hermansen, 1973).

Lactate levels are reported using a variety of units. The two most common are millimoles per liter (mmol·L⁻¹, sometimes designated as mM) or milligrams per 100 mL of blood (mg 100·mL⁻¹, sometimes designated as mg% or mgd·L⁻¹). One mmol·L⁻¹ is equal to 9 mg·100 mL⁻¹. Resting levels of lactate of 1–2 mmol·L⁻¹ or 9–18 mg·100 mL⁻¹ are typical. A value of 8 mmol·L⁻¹ or 72 mg·100 mL⁻¹ is usually taken to indicate that an individual has worked maximally (Åstrand et al., 2003). Peak values as high as 32 mmol·L⁻¹ or 288 mg·100 mL⁻¹ have been reported.

Tests of Anaerobic Power and Capacity

Energy system capacity is the total amount of energy that can be produced by an energy system. **Energy system power** is the maximal amount of energy that can be produced per unit of time. **Table 3.1** clearly shows that the phosphagen (ATP-PC) system is predominantly a power system with very little capacity. The lactic anaerobic glycolytic system has almost equal power and capacity, just slightly favoring capacity. The information on the aerobic (O₂) system is included here just to show how truly high in power and low in capacity the anaerobic systems are.

Energy System Capacity The total amount of energy that can be produced by an energy system.

Energy System Power The maximal amount of energy that can be produced per unit of time.

Although the ATP-PC system can put out energy at the rate of 72 kcal·min⁻¹, it can sustain that value when working maximally only for 9–10 seconds, for a total output of only 11 kcal (72 kcal·min⁻¹/60 sec·min⁻¹ = 1.2 kcal·sec⁻¹; 11 total kcal/1.2 kcal·sec⁻¹ = 9.17 seconds). The LA system has a lower power (36 kcal·min⁻¹) but can sustain it for almost 1 minute and 20 seconds (48 kcal/36 kcal·min⁻¹ = 1.33 minutes =1:19.8). By comparison, if the O₂ system worked at a power output of 9 kcal·min⁻¹, exercise could be sustained for more than 2 hours (1268 kcal/9 kcal·min⁻¹ = 141 minutes = 2:21) just using carbohydrate fuel sources. In fact, when all fuel supplies are included within a healthy, well-fed body, the capacity of the aerobic system is, for all intents and purposes, unlimited.

For measuring the anaerobic systems, an ideal test could distinctly evaluate alactic anaerobic power, alactic anaerobic capacity, lactic anaerobic power, and lactic anaerobic capacity. Because no such test exists, attempts have been made to get this information indirectly by measuring (1) the total mechanical power generated during high-intensity, short-duration work; (2) the amount of mechanical work done in a specific period of time; or (3) the time required to perform a given amount of presumably anaerobic work (Green, 1995). Two such tests are commonly used in laboratory settings: the Wingate Anaerobic Test (WAT) and the Maragaria-Kalamen Stair Climb (Bouchard et al., 1982).

THE WINGATE ANAEROBIC TEST The Wingate Anaerobic Test depicted in **Figure 3.8** is probably the most well-known of several bicycle ergometer tests used to measure anaerobic power and capacity. The test is an all-out ride for 30 seconds against a resistance based on body weight. Both arm and leg versions are available, although the leg test is most frequently used and will be the only version discussed here. Resistance values of 0.075 kg·kg⁻¹ body weight for children, 0.086 kg·kg⁻¹ body weight for adult females, and 0.095 kg·kg⁻¹ body weight for adult males appear to be optimal. Athletes may need values as high as 0.10 kg·kg⁻¹ of body weight, but the most common value used (as in the example that follows) is 0.075 kg·kg⁻¹ body weight (Vandewalle et al., 1987). The revolutions (rev) of the flywheel are counted per second during the test, and from the available information three variables are determined.

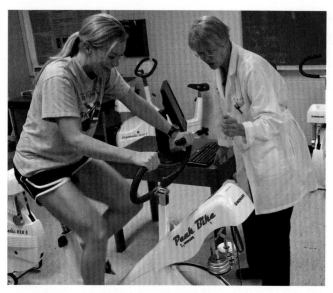

FIGURE 3.8   Wingate Anaerobic Test.
This subject is performing the Wingate Anaerobic Test. Once she is pedaling as fast as she can, the tester releases the weight, providing a resistance based on the subject's body weight. The subject then continues to pedal as quickly as possible for 30 seconds. Data from sensors attached to the flywheel are relayed to the computer for calculation of peak power, mean power, and fatigue index.

Computer-generated results from a typical test are given in **Table 3.2**. The subject was a 129-lb female physical education major, but not an athlete. Calculations for the resistance used (4.4 kg) are shown in **Table 3.2**. The data can be used to calculate three variables: peak power, mean power, and fatigue index. **Peak power (PP)** is the maximal power (force times distance divided by time) exerted during very short- (5 seconds or less) duration work. **Mean power (MP)** is the average power (force times distance divided by time) exerted during short (typically 30 seconds) duration work. The **fatigue index (FI)** is the percentage of peak power (PP) drop-off during high-intensity, short-duration work. Each of these variables requires the use of different time periods in the calculations.

The first variable computed is peak power (PP), the maximum power exerted during the highest 5-second period. This usually occurs early in the activity and, in the example given, is the time between 2 and 6 seconds when 10.25 rev were completed. Peak power can be expressed in absolute terms as kgm·5 sec^{-1} or prorated to a full minute as kgm·min^{-1} or watts (W). Peak power can also be expressed relative to body weight as kgm·5 sec^{-1}·kg^{-1}, kgm·min^{-1}·kg^{-1}, or W·kg^{-1}. The formula for peak power is

3.1   peak power (kgm · 5 sec^{-1}) = maximal revolutions in 5 seconds × distance that the flywheel travels per revolution (m) × force settiing (kg)

or

PP = rev (max) in 5 seconds × D · rev^{-1} × F

Thus for this example the calculation is

PP = 10.25 rev × 6 m·rev^{-1} × 4.4 kg = 270.6 kgm·5 sec^{-1}

Prorated to a full minute, PP is

PP = 270.6 kgm · 5 sec^{-1} × 12
(60 sec · min^{-1} ÷ 5 seconds = 12)
= 3247.2 kgm · min^{-1}

Relative to body weight PP is

PP = 3247.2 kgm · min^{-1} ÷ 58.5kg
= 55.50 kgm · min^{-1} · kg^{-1}

When converted to watts (1 W = 6.12 kgm·min^{-1}), the relative value is

PP = 55.5 kgm · min^{-1} ÷ 6.12 kgm · min^{-1} · W^{-1}
= 9.07 W · kg^{-1}

Peak power was originally thought to reflect only alactic processes—alactic anaerobic capacity, in particular. However, subsequent research has shown that muscle lactate levels rise to high values as early as 10 seconds into such high-intensity work. This indicates that glycolytic processes are occurring almost immediately along with ATP-CP breakdown. Therefore, peak power cannot be interpreted as being only alactic (Bar-Or, 1987).

The second variable calculated is mean power, which can also be expressed in both absolute and relative units. Mean power is the average power sustained throughout the 30-second ride. The formula for mean power is

3.2   mean power (kg · 30 sec^{-1}) = total number of revolutions in 30 seconds × distance that the flywheel travels per revolution (m) × force settiing (kg)

or

MP = rev (total) in 30 seconds × D · rev^{-1} × F

Thus for this example the calculation is

MP = 45.25 rev × 6 m · rev^{-1} × 4.4 kg
= 1194.6 kgm · 30 seconds

Prorated to a full minute, MP is

MP = 1194.6 kgm × 2 (60 sec · min^{-1} ÷ 30 seconds = 2)
= 2389.2 kgm · min^{-1}

Related to body weight MP is

MP = 2389.2 kgm · min^{-1} ÷ 58.5 kg
= 40.84 kgm · min^{-1} · kg^{-1}

When converted to watts MP is

MP = 40.84 kgm · min^{-1} · kg^{-1} ÷ 6.12 kgm · min^{-1} · W^{-1}
= 6.67 W · kg^{-1}

TABLE 3.2 Results for the Wingate Leg Test

Weight is 129 lb = 58.50 kg; resistance for legs is 58.50 kg × 0.075 kg·kg^{-1} body weight = 4.4 kg.

Inclusive Time (sec)	5-sec Total Revolutions	kgm·min^{-1}·kg^{-1}	W·kg^{-1}
1–5	10.00	54.15	8.85
2–6	10.25	55.50	9.07
3–7	9.75	52.80	8.63
4–8	9.50	51.44	8.41
5–9	9.25	50.09	8.18
6–10	9.00	48.74	7.96
7–11	8.25	44.67	7.30
8–12	8.00	43.32	7.08
9–13	7.75	41.97	6.86
10–14	7.50	40.61	6.64
11–15	7.50	40.61	6.64
12–16	7.50	40.61	6.64
13–17	7.25	39.26	6.41
14–18	7.25	39.26	6.41
15–19	7.00	37.91	6.19
16–20	7.00	37.91	6.19
17–21	6.75	36.55	5.97
18–22	6.75	36.55	5.97
19–23	6.50	35.20	5.75
20–24	6.50	35.20	5.75
21–25	6.25	33.84	5.53
22–26	6.25	33.84	5.53
23–27	6.00	32.49	5.31
24–28	6.00	32.49	5.31
25–29	5.75	31.14	5.09
26–30	5.50	29.78	4.87

Total pedal revolutions = 45.25.

Highest 5-sec absolute peak power = 3247.20 kgm·min^{-1}.

Highest 5-sec relative peak power = 55.50 kgm·min^{-1}·kg^{-1} = 9.07 W·kg^{-1}.

Mean absolute power = 2389.20 kgm·min^{-1}.

Mean relative power = 40.84 kgm·min^{-1}·kg^{-1} = 6.67 W·kg^{-1}.

Fatigue index = 100 − (lowest 5 sec divided by highest 5 sec) × 100 = 46.34%.

Mean power is sometimes said to represent lactic anaerobic capacity, although this has not been substantiated (Bar-Or, 1987). And, as previously shown in **Figure 3.3**, by 30 seconds, approximately 27% of the energy is being supplied by aerobic processes.

Peak Power (PP) The maximum power (force times distance divided by time) exerted during very short-duration (5 seconds or less) work.

Mean Power (MP) The average power (force times distance divided by time) exerted during short-duration (typically 30 seconds) work.

Fatigue Index (FI) Percentage of peak power drop-off during high-intensity, short-duration work.

The third variable that can be computed is the fatigue index (FI)or the percentage of peak power drop-off during high-intensity, short-duration work. It is calculated using the highest 5-second power (PP) and the lowest 5-second power (LP). Little is known about the relationship of the fatigue index to anaerobic fitness (Bar-Or, 1987).

Although the WAT is not a purely anaerobic test (a meaningful aerobic component has been measured), it is predominantly anaerobic. It compares well (with correlations generally above 0.75) with other tests of anaerobic

3.3 fatigue index (%) = 1− [(lowest power kgm · 5 sec^{-1}) ÷ (peak power kgm · 5 sec^{-1})] × 100

or

FI = [1−(LP ÷ PP)] × 100

In our example the highest 5-second power is 270.6 kgm. Using the peak power formula of Equation 3.1 but with the lowest 5-second total, we get

$$LP = 5.50 \text{ rev} \times 6 \text{ m} \cdot \text{rev}^{-1} \times 4.4 \text{ kg}$$
$$= 145.2 \text{ kg} \cdot 5 \text{ sec}^{-1}$$

$$[1-(145.2 \text{ kg} \cdot 5 \text{ sec}^{-1} \div 270.6 \text{ kg} \cdot 5 \text{ sec}^{-1})]$$
$$\times 100 = 46.34\%$$

power and capacity and is widely used (Bar-Or, 1987; Patton and Duggan, 1987).

THE MARGARIA-KALAMEN STAIR CLIMB To perform the Margaria-Kalamen test, an individual runs for 6 m on the level and then climbs a staircase, taking three steps at a time. Power in kgm·sec⁻¹ is calculated from the weight of the subject, the vertical height between the third and ninth steps, and the time between the third and ninth steps (Bouchard et al., 1982; Vandewalle et al., 1987). The use of electronic switch mats or photoelectric cells is essential for accuracy. This test is considered to be a test of alactic anaerobic power because of the short time involved—usually less than 5 seconds for the entire test and close to 1 second for the measured time between the third and ninth steps.

Field Tests

No field tests are available to estimate the ATP-PC used or the lactate produced during exercise. However, performance in high-intensity, short-duration activity can give an indication of anaerobic power and capacity. Two types of activities are commonly used: vertical jump tests and sprints (sometimes done as shuttles) or middle-distance runs.

In vertical jump tests, several different protocols are used, including variations in the starting posture, the use or nonuse of arms, and what body part displacement is measured. The one commonality is the end value measured: the height jumped. When the jump is performed on a force platform, actual power values can be calculated, and the test is considered a laboratory test. When the jump is performed as a field test on a normal surface, an estimate of work (force × distance), not power, is calculated. The height of the vertical jump and peak power as determined from force plate data has been shown to be highly correlated ($r = 0.92$). For these reasons, vertical jump height is seen as an acceptable indicator of anaerobic alactic power (Payne et al., 2000; Vandewalle et al., 1987).

For sprints, shuttle, or middle-distance runs, the involvement of the various energy systems is related to the time of the all-out activity, as shown in **Figure 3.3**. Therefore, runs whose distance can be covered in a distinct time range (depending somewhat on age, sex, and training status) can be used as field tests of anaerobic metabolism (Cheetham et al., 1986; Thomas et al., 2002). For example, dashes of 40, 50, or 60 yd or m will take approximately 4–15 seconds and can be used as an indication of alactic anaerobic power and/or capacity. Longer runs, probably between 200 and 800 m (or 220 and 880 yd) and lasting 40–120 seconds, can be used as an indication of lactic anaerobic power and capacity. Faster speeds covering a given distance would indicate increased anaerobic power and/or capacity.

The Anaerobic Exercise Response

Oxygen Deficit and Excess Postexercise Oxygen Consumption

When exercise begins, regardless of how light or heavy it is, there is an immediate need for additional energy. Thus, the most obvious exercise response is an increase in metabolism. All three energy systems are involved in this response, their relative contributions being proportional to the intensity and duration of the activity.

Figure 3.9 shows two scenarios for going from rest to different intensities of exercise. In **Figure 3.9A** the activity is a moderate submaximal bout. The oxygen requirement for this exercise is 1.4 L·min⁻¹. The individual has a $\dot{V}O_2$max of 2.5 L·min⁻¹. Therefore, this individual is working at 56% $\dot{V}O_2$max. The area under the smoothed curve during both exercise and recovery represents oxygen used. Notice, however, that there is an initial lag during which the oxygen supplied and utilized is below the oxygen requirement for providing energy. This difference between the oxygen required during exercise and the oxygen supplied and utilized is called the **oxygen deficit**. Because of this discrepancy between supply and demand, anaerobic sources must be involved in providing energy at the onset of all activity.

The O_2 deficit has traditionally been explained as the inability of the circulatory and respiratory systems to deliver oxygen quickly enough to meet the increased energy demands. Evidence now indicates, however, that the O_2 deficit is probably due to limited cellular utilization of O_2 as a result of metabolic adjustments in both the anaerobic and aerobic systems. The relatively slow response time of aerobic ATP production is determined by the faster speed of response of the ATP-PC system and by the content of mitochondria in the muscle. The fact that the ATP-PC system responds rapidly does not indicate any intrinsic delay or inertia of activation for either the LA or O_2 systems. All three pathways respond simultaneously in an integrated fashion. The metabolic response is regulated by a series of feedback control systems that are sensitive to the release of Ca^{2+} from muscle contraction and the breakdown of ATP (Grassi, 2005;

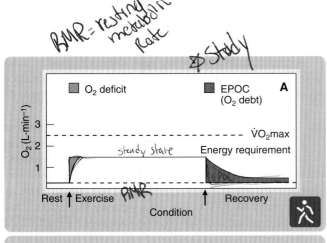

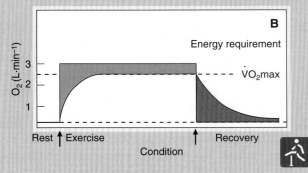

FIGURE 3.9 Oxygen Deficit and Excess Postexercise Oxygen Consumption (EPOC) during Submaximal Exercise and Supramaximal Exercise.
A. During light to moderate submaximal exercise, both the oxygen deficit, indicated by the convex curve at the start of exercise, and the excess post exercise oxygen comsumption, indicated by the concave curve during the recovery time period, are small. **B.** During heavy or supramaximal exercise both the O_2 deficit and the EPOC are large. Under both conditions energy is supplied during the O_2 deficit period by using stored ATP-PC, anaerobic glycolysis, and oxygen stores in capillary blood and bound to myoglobin. The heavier the exercise the more the reliance on anaerobic glycolysis. The EPOC is a result of the restoration of ATP-PC, removal of lactate, restoration of O_2 stores, elevated cardiovascular and respiratory function, elevated hormonal levels, and especially, the elevated body temperature.

Hughson et al., 2001; Meyer and Wiseman, 2006; Sahlin et al., 1988). The metabolic systems simply respond at different speeds. Therefore, during the transition from rest to work, energy is supplied by

1. O_2 transport and utilization;
2. Utilization of O_2 stores in capillary blood and bound to myoglobin;

Oxygen Deficit The difference between the oxygen required during exercise and the oxygen supplied and utilized. Occurs at the onset of all activity.

Supramaximal Exercise An exercise bout in which the energy requirement is greater than what can be supplied aerobically at $\dot{V}O_2$max.

3. The splitting of stored ATP-PC; and
4. Anaerobic glycolysis, with the concomitant production of lactic acid.

Eventually, if the exercise intensity is low enough (as in the example in **Figure 3.9A**), the aerobic system will predominate and the oxygen supply will equal the oxygen demand. This condition is called steady-state, steady-rate, or steady-level exercise.

Figure 3.9B shows a smoothed plot of O_2 consumption at rest and during and after an exercise bout in which the energy requirement is greater than $\dot{V}O_2$max, sometimes called **supramaximal exercise**. The initial lag period between O_2 supply and demand is once again evident, and as in the first example, the added energy is provided by stored ATP-PC, anaerobic glycolysis, and stored O_2. However, in this case, when the O_2 consumption plateaus or levels off, it is at $\dot{V}O_2$max, and more energy is still needed if exercise is to continue.

This plateau is not considered to be a steady state because the energy demands are not totally being met aerobically. Supplemental energy is provided by anaerobic glycolysis. The exact energy demand in this situation is difficult to determine precisely because, as stated before, lactic acid levels do not reflect production alone. However, without the anaerobic energy contribution, this activity could not continue. The maximal ability to tolerate lactic acid accumulation will determine to a large extent how long the activity can continue.

A practical application of oxygen deficit theory is a measurement called *maximal accumulated oxygen deficit (MAOD)*. MAOD is the difference between the estimated accumulated oxygen demand (based on an extrapolation from 4 to 10 bouts of at least 4 minutes each of submaximal exercise and a maximal test to determine power output-oxygen uptake relationships) and the accumulated oxygen uptake measured during exhausting supramaximal exercise of 110–125% $\dot{V}O_2$max (Bortolotti et al., 2010; Medbo et al., 1988; Noordhof et al., 2010). MAOD relates highly to the WAT, and is interpreted as a direct measure of anaerobic capacity (Weber and Schneider, 2001). Not surprisingly, sprinters and middle-distance runners have been shown to have higher MAOD values than endurance-distance runners (Scott et al., 1991).

During recovery from exercise represented by the concave curves after exercise in **Figure 3.9A**, B, oxygen consumption drops quickly (a fast component lasting 2–3 minutes) and then tapers off (a slow component lasting 3–60 minutes). The magnitude and duration of this elevated postexercise oxygen consumption depends on the duration, intensity, and modality of the preceding exercise. After light submaximal work (**Figure 3.9A**), recovery takes place quickly; after heavy exercise (**Figure 3.9B**) recovery takes much longer. Note that although the oxygen consumption is expressed as $L \cdot min^{-1}$ in this figure, it can also be prorated by body weight and expressed as $mL \cdot kg \cdot min^{-1}$.

Historically, this period of elevated metabolism after exercise has been called the O_2 debt, based on the assumption being that the "extra" O_2 consumed during the "debt" period was used to "pay back" the deficit incurred in the early part of exercise (Bahr, 1992; Stainsby and Barclay, 1970). More recently, the terms *O_2 recovery* or **excess postexercise oxygen consumption (EPOC)** have come into favor. EPOC is defined as the oxygen consumption during recovery that is above normal resting values.

The relationship between the size of the EPOC and the intensity of aerobic exercise is curvilinear, whereas the relationship between the size of the EPOC and the duration of aerobic exercise in more linear. The relationship between EPOC and resistance exercise is less well defined, but intensity seems important here as well (Børsheim and Bahr, 2003) However, a recent study (Scott et al., 2011) found that for a single set of resistance training to fatigue the recovery energy expenditure was similar in both strength and muscular endurance protocols; moreover, recovery energy expenditure had little to no relationship with aerobic and anaerobic exercise energy expenditure or work.

CHECK YOUR COMPREHENSION

You are working as a fitness trainer at a wellness center. Yeen Kuen is a new client who wants to work out three days a week combining aerobic and resistance exercise. Yeen Kuen does not need to lose weight but wants to tone muscles and improve endurance. Using the data presented below from a study by Drummond et al. (2005), make a recommendation as to whether this client should do the resistance workout first or the aerobic workout first. Explain your reasoning.

Check your answer in Appendix C.

Physiological Responses to Sequential Activity

Sequence	Activity	HR (b·min⁻¹) during	V̇O₂ (mL·kg·min⁻¹) during	V̇O₂ (mL·kg·min⁻¹) EPOC (10 min)
RE-RU	Treadmill (25 min) 3 sets/ 10 reps	$172 \pm 4.0^*$ 140 ± 9.0	$40.0 \pm 1.3^*$	$5.14 \pm 0.2^*$
RU-RE	Treadmill (25 min) 3 sets/ 10 reps	161 ± 4.0 144 ± 5.0	38.0 ± 1.3	5.7 ± 0.1

RE = Resistance exercise, 7 lifts at 70% 1-RM; RU = Treadmill running at 70% V̇O₂max; *$P < 0.05$ compared to RU-RE.

A critical question is what causes this elevated metabolism in recovery. Although EPOC cannot be completely explained at this time, seven factors have been suggested.

1. Restoration of ATP-PC stores: About 10% of the EPOC is utilized to rephosphorylate creatine and ADP to PC and ATP, respectively, thus restoring these substances to resting levels (Bahr, 1992; Gaesser and Brooks, 1975). Approximately 50% of the ATP-PC is restored in 30 seconds (Margaria et al., 1933). This time is called the half-life restoration of ATP-PC. Full recovery requires 2–8 minutes (Fox, 1973; Harvis et al, 1976; Hultman, 1967).

2. Restoration of O_2 stores: Although the amount of O_2 stored in the blood (bound to hemoglobin) and muscle (bound to myoglobin) is not large, it does need to be replenished when exercise stops. Replenishment probably occurs completely within 2–3 minutes (Bahr, 1992; Stainsby and Barclay, 1970).

3. Elevated cardiovascular-respiratory function: Both the respiratory system and the cardiovascular system remain elevated postexercise; that is, neither the breathing rate and depth nor heart rate recover instantaneously. Although this enables the extra amounts of oxygen to be processed, the actual energy cost of these cardiovascular-respiratory processes probably accounts for only 1–2% of the excess oxygen (Bahr, 1992; Stainsby and Barclay, 1970).

4. Elevated hormonal levels: During exercise the circulating levels of the catecholamines (epinephrine and norepinephrine), thyroxine, and cortisol are all increased (see **Figure 2.17** and **Table 2.3** in Chapter 2). In addition to their fuel mobilization and utilization effects, these hormones increase Na^+–K^+ pump activity in muscles and nerves by changing cell membrane permeability to Na^+ and K^+. As an active transport process, the Na^+–K^+ pump requires ATP. The increased need for ATP means an increased need for O_2. Until the hormones are cleared from the bloodstream, the additional O_2 and ATP use is a significant contributor to the EPOC (Bahr, 1992; Gaesser and Brooks, 1975).

5. Elevated body temperature: When ATP is broken down to supply the energy for chemical, electrical, or mechanical work, heat is produced as a by-product. During exercise, heat production may exceed heat dissipation, causing a rise in body core temperature. For each degree Celsius that body temperature rises, the metabolic rate increases approximately 13–15% (Kapit et al., 2000). Thus, in recovery, although high levels of energy are no longer needed to support the exercise, the influence of the elevated temperature remains, because cooling takes some time to occur. This temperature effect is by far the most important reason for EPOC, accounting for as much as 60–70% of the slow component after exercise at 50–80% V̇O₂max (Bahr, 1992; Gaesser and Brooks, 1975).

6. Lactate removal: The lactate that has accumulated must be removed. Historically, it was thought that the majority of this lactate was converted to glycogen and that this conversion was the primary cause of the slow component of EPOC. As previously described, the fate of lactic acid is now seen as more complex, and its contribution as a causative factor for EPOC is minimal (Gaesser and Brooks, 1975; Stainsby and Barclay, 1970).

7. Energy substrate shift: During recovery the primary fuel utilized shifts from carbohydrate to fat. Fat requires more oxygen to process than does CHO and thus may be important in prolonging the slow component of EPOC (Børsheim and Bahr, 2003).

ATP-PC Changes

Figure 3.10 indicates what happens to ATP and PC levels in muscle during constant-load, supramaximal exercise (105–110% $\dot{V}O_2$max) lasting 3 minutes or less. As shown in the figure, the ATP level in the muscle decreases only slightly. In fact, the maximum ATP depletion observed in skeletal muscle after heavy exercise is only about 30–40% in both males and females. Thus, even after exhaustive work, 60–70% of the resting amount of ATP is still present (Cheetham et al., 1986; Gollnick and King, 1969).

Conversely, the level of PC changes dramatically and it is nearly depleted. The greatest depletion of PC occurs in the initial 20 seconds of exercise, with the result that ATP is maintained almost at resting levels during that time span. From 20 to 180 seconds, the decline in PC and ATP is both gradual and parallel (Gollnick and Hermansen, 1973). Obviously, the ATP level is maintained at the expense of the PC. However, some ATP is also being provided from glycolysis, as indicated by the rise in lactate in both muscle and blood, and an additional amount by oxidation.

Lactate Changes

Lactate levels in response to exercise depend primarily on the intensity of the exercise. Acute exercise does not result in any meaningful enhancement of lactate transporters. Instead, transmembrane lactate and hydrogen ion gradients increase. Lactate transport is faster in oxidative fibers than in glycolytic ones. The fast transport of lactate by oxidative fibers may reflect lactate's role as an energy substrate, while the slower transport in glycolytic fibers may contribute to a greater retention of lactate during recovery for reconversion into glycogen (Gladden, 2000).

Short-Term, High-Intensity Anaerobic Exercise

Figure 3.10 includes both muscle and blood lactate responses to high-intensity, short-duration (3 minutes or less), supramaximal exercise. As the figure shows, muscle lactate levels rise immediately with the onset of such hard work (105–110% $\dot{V}O_2$max) and continue to rise throughout the length of the task. Blood lactate values show a similar pattern, if the lag for diffusion time is taken into account. This lactate response (a rapid and consistent accumulation) is representative of what occurs when the exercise bout is greater than 90% $\dot{V}O_2$max (Gollnick and Hermansen, 1973).

Short- and Long-Term, Light to Moderate Submaximal Aerobic Exercise

Figure 3.11 depicts what occurs in both short-term and long-term low-intensity submaximal aerobic activity. During the first 3 minutes of such steady-state work the lactate (La⁻) level rises (Figure 3.11A). This increase reflects the lactate accumulated during the oxygen deficit (Gollnick and Hermansen, 1973). When a similar workload is continued for 60 minutes, the lactate level remains unchanged after the initial rise (Figure 3.11B). The reason for this result lies in the balance between lactate production (the rate of lactate appearance) and lactate clearance (the rate of lactate disappearance).

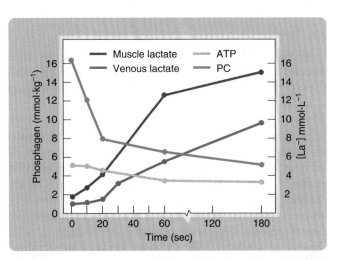

FIGURE 3.10 Time Course for the Depletion of PC and ATP and the Accumulation of Lactate in Muscle and Veins.
Muscle levels of ATP are maintained relatively constant during high-intensity, short-duration exercise at the expense of PC. Muscle lactate levels rise sooner and higher than venous levels owing to the diffusion time lag and dilution.
Source: Modified from Gollnick, P. D. & L. Hermansen: Biochemical adaptation to exercise: Anaerobic metabolism. In Wilmore, J. H. (ed.): *Exercise and Sport Sciences Reviews*. New York: Academic Press (1973). Reprinted by permission of Williams & Wilkins.

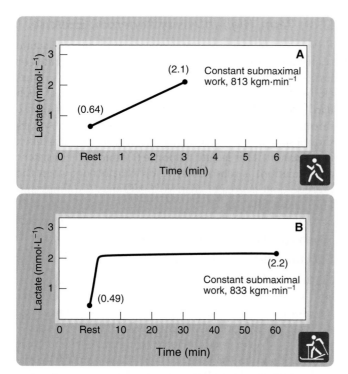

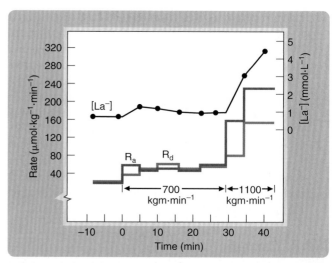

FIGURE 3.11 Lactate Accumulation during Short- and Long-Term Dynamic Aerobic Constant Submaximal Work.
After an initial rise in accumulation during the oxygen deficit period **(A)**, lactate levels off and remains relatively constant during long-duration submaximal aerobic work **(B)**.
Source: Based on data from Freund et al. (1990).

FIGURE 3.12 The Impact of the Rates of Lactate Appearance and Disappearance on Lactate Accumulation during Light and Heavy Submaximal Aerobic Exercise.
During light (700 kgm·min⁻¹ submaximal aerobic exercise, the rate of lactate disappearance (R_d) (left y-axis) lags behind the rate of lactate appearance (R_a) (left y-axis) to a small extent, but then catches up so that the 30-minute lactate concentration [La⁻] value (right y-axis) approximates rest. During heavy submaximal exercise (minutes 30–45) the R_d lags behind R_a and [La⁻] increases.
Source: Brooks, G. A. Anaerobic threshold: Review of the concept and directions for further research. *Medicine and Science in Sports and Exercise*. 17(1):22–31 (1985). Reprinted by permission.

Figure 3.12 shows the results from a study that directly measured the rate of lactate appearance (R_a) and the rate of lactate disappearance (R_d) by radioactive tracers as well as the blood levels of lactate concentration ([La⁻]) (Brooks, 1985). In the transition from rest to steady-state submaximal exercise, the rate of both lactate appearance and lactate disappearance increased. During the next 30 minutes of exercise, the turnover rate was higher than at rest. The result was an initial increase in [La⁻], which declined after 5 minutes of activity to almost resting levels by 30 minutes. When the workload was increased, the rate of clearance (R_d) was no longer able to keep up with the rate of production (R_a), and the lactate concentration in the blood [La⁻] increased sharply.

Figure 3.13 shows how lactate level varies with competitive distance (and thus duration) in highly trained male runners. At the shorter distances the predominant energy source is anaerobic, and the anticipated high lactate values occur. As the distance increases and more energy is supplied aerobically, the intensity that can be maintained decreases. As a result, lactate also decreases, doing so in a negative exponential curvilinear pattern. By approximately 30 km (18 mi) the lactate levels are almost the same as at rest.

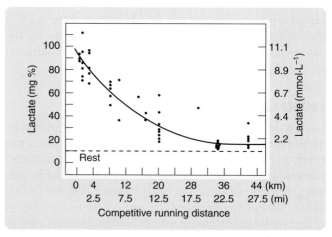

FIGURE 3.13 Lactate Accumulation Resulting from Increasing Distances of Competitive Running Races.
Blood lactate accumulation shows an inverse curvilinear relationship with distance in running races.
Source: Costill, D. L.: Metabolic responses during distance running. *Journal of Applied Physiology*. 28(3):251–255 (1970). Modified and reprinted by permission of the American Physiological Society.

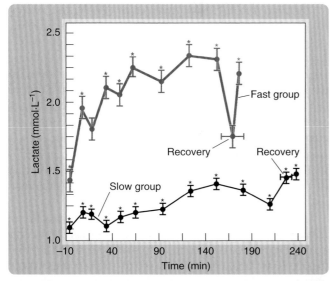

FIGURE 3.14   Blood Lactate Accumulation during the Marathon.

Blood lactate accumulation during a fast marathon (2 hours and 45 minutes or less) was greater than the accumulation during a slow marathon (3 hours and 45 minutes or less). The lactate levels for the slow marathoners never exceeded normal resting levels, and the lactate levels for the fast marathoners barely exceeded normal resting levels.

Source: O'Brien, M. J., C. A. Viguie, R. S. Mazzeo, & G. A. Brooks: Carbohydrate dependence during marathon running. *Medicine and Science in Sports Exercise.* 25(9):1009–1017 (1993). Reprinted by permission.

Long-Term, Moderate to Heavy Submaximal Aerobic Exercise

The importance of the intensity of exercise, even at the marathon distance, is illustrated in **Figure 3.14**. Two groups of runners were matched according to their $\dot{V}O_2$max. One group ran a simulated marathon on the treadmill at 73.3% $\dot{V}O_2$max (in 2 hours 45 minutes or less); the other group ran the same distance but at 64.5% $\dot{V}O_2$max (in 3 hours 45 minutes or slightly less). Within the slow group, blood lactate values remained relatively stable and at a level considered to be within normal resting amounts. The blood lactate levels in the fast group were statistically significantly higher throughout the marathon than those of the slow group. As absolutes, however, both sets of values were low, with the slow group being within a normal resting range and the fast

group slightly above normal resting levels (O'Brien et al., 1993).

In general, during light to moderate work (i.e., <50–60% of $\dot{V}O_2$max), the blood lactate level is likely to rise slightly at first. Then it either remains the same or decreases slightly, even if the exercise lasts 30–60 minutes.

At moderate to heavy intensities between 50% and 85% $\dot{V}O_2$max (depending on the individual's genetic characteristics and training status), lactate levels rise rapidly during the first 5–10 minutes of exercise. If the workload continues for more than 10 minutes, the lactate level may continue to rise, may stabilize, or may decline, depending on the individual and other conditions.

One of these "other conditions" may be the exercise intensity in relation to the individual's maximal lactate steady state. **Maximal lactate steady state (MLSS)** is the highest workload that can be maintained over time without a continual rise in blood lactate; it indicates an exercise intensity above which lactate production exceeds clearance. MLSS is assessed by a series of workloads performed on different days. Each succeeding workload gets progressively harder until the blood lactate accumulation increases more or less steadily throughout the test or increases more than $1\,mmol·L^{-1}$ after the initial rise and establishment of a plateau in the early minutes. Thus, in a 30-minute test, changes in the first 10 minutes are ignored and only the last 20 minutes used to determine if the change is less than or greater than $1\,mmol·L^{-1}$. When the blood lactate concentration meets this criterion, the previous workload that exhibited a plateau in lactate throughout the duration (after the initial rise) is labeled as the MLSS workload. Often the MLSS workload is compared to the individual's maximal workload and expressed as a percentage known as MLSS intensity. Performances at the MLSS intensity result in a steady state for lactate; performances below this intensity show declining lactate values, and performances above this level exhibit progressively increasing lactate values. Extensive endurance performance cannot be completed above the MLSS, but portions of the event certainly may be (Beneke et al., 2000; Billat et al., 2003).

Incremental Aerobic Exercise to Maximum

Figure 3.15 depicts physiological responses during incremental exercise to maximum. Heart rate and oxygen consumption (**Figure 3.15A, B**) increase in a rectilinear pattern to meet the increasing demands for energy, but both ventilation and blood lactate (**Figure 3.15C, D**) show very little initial change and then increases more sharply. As depicted, this pattern is often described as a rectilinear rise with two breakpoints or thresholds. Alternately, by smoothing these points, the pattern can be described as positively accelerating exponential curves.

Since the early 1970s much attention has been paid to a concept that has been labeled variously as the *anaerobic*

Maximal Lactate Steady State (MLSS) The highest workload that can be maintained over time without a continual rise in blood lactate; it indicates an exercise intensity above which lactate production exceeds clearance.

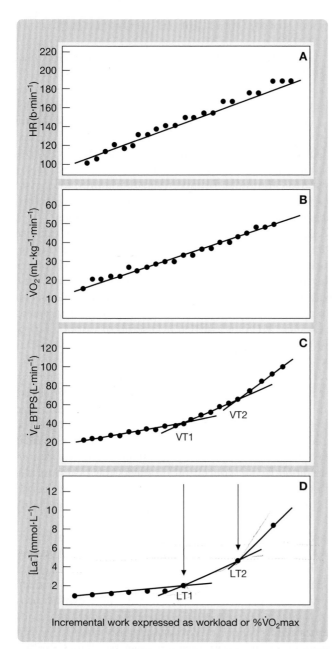

FIGURE 3.15 Ventilatory and Lactate Thresholds during Incremental Work to Maximum.
Both heart rate **(A)** and O₂ consumption **(B)** increase in direct rectilinear patterns during an incremental work task whether the work is expressed in terms of absolute workload or percentage of $\dot{V}O_2$max. In contrast, both ventilation **(C)** and lactate **(D)** appear to exhibit two distinct breakpoints as they rise. The circumstance of VT1 occurring at the same time as LT1 and VT2 occurring at the same time as LT2 is coincidental.

As espoused by Wasserman et al. (1973), the *anaerobic threshold* is defined as the exercise intensity, usually described as a percentage of $\dot{V}O_2$max or absolute workload, above which blood lactate levels rise and minute ventilation increases disproportionately in relation to oxygen consumption. The onset of anaerobic metabolism (or anaerobiosis), which is assumed to lead to the lactate accumulation, is attributed to the failure of the cardiovascular system to supply the oxygen required to the muscle tissue. The disproportionate rise in ventilation is attributed to excess carbon dioxide resulting from the buffering of the lactic acid (Jones and Ehrsam, 1982; Wasserman and McIlroy, 1964).

Theoretically, these interactions can occur as follows: lactic acid is a strong acid, and as noted earlier in this chapter, it readily dissociates into hydrogen ions (H⁺) and lactate lactic acid. Because excess hydrogen ions would change the pH (or acid-base balance) of the muscles and blood, the body attempts to bind these hydrogen ions to a chemical buffer. For example, sodium bicarbonate (a weak base) may be used as a buffer in the reaction:

$$NaHCO_3 + HLa \leftrightarrow NaLa + H_2CO_3$$
sodium bicarbonate + lactic acid ↔ sodium lactate + carbonic acid

Carbonic acid is a much weaker acid than LA and can be further dissociated into water and carbon dioxide:
$$H_2CO_3 \leftrightarrow H_2O + CO_2$$

Carbon dioxide is a potent stimulant for respiration and can easily be removed from the body through respiration, thereby assisting in the maintenance of pH (Pitts, 1974). The carbon dioxide thus formed is said to be *nonmetabolic carbon dioxide*, since it does not result from the immediate breakdown of an energy substrate (carbohydrate, fat, or protein).

Figure 3.15 clearly shows distinct breaks from linearity in respiration (**Figure 3.15C**) despite a continuous rectilinear rise in heart rate (**Figure 3.15A**) and oxygen consumption (**Figure 3.15B**) during incremental work to maximum. These breakpoints (**Figure 3.15C**) have been labeled VT1 (the first ventilatory threshold) and VT2 (the second ventilatory threshold). They were originally thought to result from corresponding lactate thresholds (labeled in **Figure 3.15D** as LT1 and LT2 for the first and second lactate threshold) as a result of the buffering of lactic acid. The original work by Wasserman and others postulated only one anaerobic threshold (which would have been VT1 in **Figure 3.16C**), but later work identified at least two thresholds, which were given various names (Carey et al., 2010; Jacobs, 1986; Reinhard et al., 1979; Skinner and McLellan, 1980). The designations VT1 and VT2 and LT1 and LT2 are used here for simplicity and because no causal mechanism is implied.

threshold, the *ventilatory threshold(s)*, or the **lactate threshold(s)**. The original concept of an anaerobic threshold is based on the lactate response to incremental exercise, as depicted in **Figure 3.15D**, and the relationship of the lactate response to minute ventilation (the volume of air breathed each minute, **Figure 3.15C**).

The idea that the point of lactate accumulation can be determined noninvasively by respiratory values typically measured during laboratory exercise testing of oxygen consumption is appealing, since few people enjoy having a catheter inserted or multiple blood samples taken. However, the terminology, determination, and mechanistic explanations are not without controversy (Walsh and Banister, 1988). Four concerns have been raised, as described below.

The primary concern is that the presence of lactate does not automatically mean that the oxygen supply is inadequate (Gladden, 2004; Hughes et al., 1982). This fact was discussed in detail earlier in this chapter. Lactate accumulation occurs not at the time of increased production but when the turnover rate (or balance between production and removal) cannot keep up and appearance exceeds clearance.

Figure 3.16A shows this concept graphically for incremental exercise. That is, as the exercise and oxygen consumption increase, the rate of lactate appearance (R_a) in the muscle does also (**Figure 3.16B**). At low-intensity exercise, the rate of lactate disappearance (R_d) does not differ much from R_a. However, as the intensity increases, the gap between R_a and R_d grows progressively wider. The result is the blood lactate concentration [La$^-$] depicted in **Figure 3.16A**. Thus, it is incorrect to consider the appearance of elevated levels of lactic acid in the blood an anaerobic threshold.

A second concern is exactly how to interpret the lactate response to incremental work. Look closely at the lactate pattern in **Figure 3.15** and recall that this pattern can be described as either a rectilinear rise with two breakpoints, or thresholds (Skinner and McLellan, 1980) or as an exponential curve (Hughson et al., 1987). Experimental evidence and mathematical models (Hughson et al., 1987) support the curvilinear interpretation. Nevertheless, the term *lactate threshold* continues to be used to indicate marked increases in the accumulation of lactate. The ventilatory thresholds are always considered to be true breakpoints.

A third concern involves carbon dioxide. Carbon dioxide is involved in the control of respiration (see Chapter 9). An excess of hydrogen ions from a source such as lactic acid can cause an increased amount of carbon dioxide through the bicarbonate buffering system described earlier. However, the presence of lactic acid is not the only mechanism that can account for the increased carbon dioxide or the concomitant increase in minute ventilation (Inbar and Bar-Or, 1986). Evidence is particularly strong in McArdle's syndrome patients. McArdle's syndrome patients are deficient in the enzyme glycogen

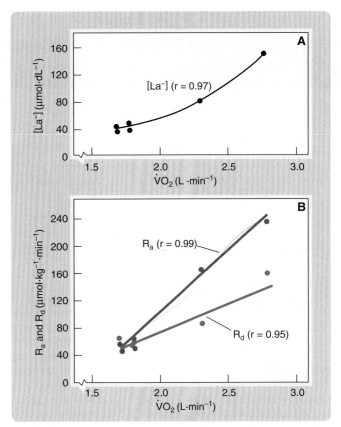

FIGURE 3.16 The Rate of Appearance (R_a), the Rate of Disappearance (R_d), and the Resultant Accumulation of Lactate as a Consequence of Incremental Exercise.
The measured change in lactate concentration [La$^-$] (**A**) is a result of a growing imbalance between the rate of appearance (R_a) and the rate of disappearance (R_d) (**B**) as exercise intensity increases.
Source: Brooks, G. A.: Anaerobic threshold: Review of the concept and directions for future research. *Medicine and Science in Sports and Exercise*. 17(1):22–31 (1985). Reprinted by permission.

phosphorylase, which is necessary for breaking down glycogen, which can ultimately be converted to lactic acid. Thus, no matter how hard these patients exercise, their lactic acid values remain negligible. On the other hand, their minute ventilation values have the same distinctive breakpoints shown by anyone not deficient in glycogen phosphorylase (Hagberg et al., 1982). Recent evidence by Péronnet and Aguilaniu (2006) has shown that the decrease in bicarbonate concentration is not the mirror image of the increase in lactate concentration. These researchers believe that the disproportionate increase in $\dot{V}CO_2$ is due to hyperventilation and low plasma pH—not that the hyperventilation is due to the increased CO_2.

A fourth concern is that the lactate thresholds and the ventilatory thresholds do not change to the same extent in the same individuals as a result of training, glycogen depletion, caffeine ingestion, and/or varying pedaling

Lactate Thresholds Points on the linear-curvilinear continuum of lactate accumulation that appear to indicate sharp rises, often labeled as the first (LT1) and second (LT2) lactate threshold.

FOCUS ON RESEARCH

The Impact of Dehydration on the Lactate Threshold

Seven collegiate female rowers participated in two incremental exercise bouts to maximum on a cycle ergometer. One trial (hydrated state) was preceded the night before by a 45-minute submaximal ride at a heart rate of 130–150 b·min^{-1} during which the participants were allowed unlimited access to fluid. The other trial (dehydrated state) consisted of the same submaximal exercise, but the participants performed in a full sweat suit and were denied fluid until after the incremental test the next morning. See the table for results.

Despite only a mild dehydration—associated with a net drop of 1.5% in body weight—a statistically significant ($P < 0.05$) shift did occur in the lactate threshold, defined as the first lactate threshold (LT1), to a lower percentage of peak oxygen consumption. This was accompanied by a significant decrease in

Variable	Hydrated Trial	Dehydrated Trial
Body weight loss (kg)	0.8 ± 0.2	1.8 ±0.2*
Performance time (min)	17.3 ± 0.7	16.3 ±0.7*
Power output at max (W)	250.0 ± 7.7	235.7 ± 9.21*
$\dot{V}O_2$ (L·min^{-1})	3.1 ±0.2	3.0 ± 0.1
HRmax (b·min^{-1})	181.± 62.9	180.6 ±2.4
Lactate max (mmol·L^{-1})	4.65 ± 0.27	5.36 ± 0.83
Lactate threshold LT1 (%$\dot{V}O_2$ peak)	72.2 ± 1.1	65.5 ± 1.8*

*$P < 0.05$.

work performance in terms of both power output and time to exhaustion. However, similar values were attained for maximal heart rate, oxygen consumption, and lactate. Thus, it appears that dehydration (or the failure to rehydrate adequately after exercise) alters the relative contributions of aerobic and anaerobic metabolism to an external workload and

negatively affects performance. Guidelines for hydration are presented in Chapters 6 and 14. The effects of dehydration on cardiovascular responses to exercise are detailed in Chapter 14.

Source: Moquin, A. & R. S. Mazzeo: Effect of mild dehydration on the lactate threshold in women. Medicine & Science in Sports & Exercise 32(2):396–402 (2000).

rates (Hughes et al., 1982; Poole and Gaesser, 1985). If they were causally linked, they should change together.

Current theory, therefore, concludes that although lactic acid increases and ventilatory breaks or thresholds often occur simultaneously, these responses are due to coincidence, not cause and effect (Brooks, 1985; Walsh and Banister, 1988). Exactly what these various thresholds mean is still unknown.

Despite a lack of complete understanding of the lactate threshold, the amount of work an athlete can do before accumulating large amounts of lactate has a definite bearing on performance. Distance running performance, for example, depends to a large extent on some combination of $\dot{V}O_2$max, the oxygen cost of running at a given submaximal speed (called economy), and the ability to run at a high percentage of $\dot{V}O_2$max without a large accumulation of lactate (Costill et al., 1973; Farrell et al., 1979; Kinderman et al., 1979). An indication of the running speed that represents the optimal percentage of $\dot{V}O_2$max can be achieved by determining the lactate thresholds. The first lactate threshold (LT1) generally occurs between 40 and 60% of $\dot{V}O_2$max the second lactate threshold (LT2) is generally over 80% of $\dot{V}O_2$max and possibly as high as 95% of $\dot{V}O_2$max. LT1 is sometimes equated with a lactate concentration of 2 mmol·L^{-1}, and LT2 with a lactate concentration of 4 mmol·L^{-1}. This 4 mmol·L^{-1} level, also called the *onset of blood lactate accumulation (OBLA)*, is frequently used to

decide both training loads and racing strategies (Hermansen et al., 1975; Jacobs, 1986). Running at a pace that results in a continual accumulation of lactate is generally associated with a detrimental effect on endurance time that is often attributed to changes brought about by the lactate.

Dynamic Resistance Exercise

Lactate responses to dynamic resistance exercise vary greatly because of the many different possible combinations of exercises, repetitions, sets, and rest periods, In addition, samples are generally not taken repeatedly during the workout; instead, the most frequently reported values are only postexercise. In general, postexercise lactate values have been shown to range from approximately 4 to 21 mmol·L^{-1}. The higher values result from high-volume, moderate-load, short rest period sequences and circuit-type exercise bouts (Bangsbo et al., 1994; Burleson et al., 1998; Keul et al., 1978; Reynolds et al., 1997; Tesch, 1992). Concentric contractions elicit higher lactate responses than eccentric contractions (Durand et al., 2003). Resistance programs designed to increase strength primarily through hypertrophy (increased muscle size) produce greater lactate responses than those designed to increase strength primarily through neural adaptation or dynamic power programs (Crewther et al., 2006).

Table 3.3 summarizes the anaerobic metabolic exercise responses discussed in this section.

TABLE 3.3   Lactic Anaerobic Exercise Response

Short-Term, Light to Moderate, Submaximal Aerobic Exercise	Short-Term, Moderate to Heavy, Submaximal Aerobic Exercise	Long-Term, Moderate to Heavy, Submaximal Aerobic Exercise	Short-Term, High-Intensity, Anaerobic Exercise	Incremental Exercise to Maximum	Dynamic Resistance Exercise
$\leq 2\,mmol\cdot L^{-1}$	~ 4–$6\,mmol\cdot L^{-1}$	Depends on relationship to MLSS	Large increase; interval may go to $32\,mmol\cdot L^{-1}$	Positive exponential curve; LT1 $\sim 2\,mmol\cdot L^{-1}$, LT2 $\sim 4\,mmol\cdot L^{-1}$; max $\geq 8\,mmol\cdot L^{-1}$	4–$21\,mmol\cdot L^{-1}$; greatest with high volume and circuit type

Why Is Lactic Acid Accumulation a Problem?

It is the hydrogen ions (H^+) that dissociate from lactic acid, rather than undissociated lactic acid or lactate (La^-), that present the primary problems to the body. This distinction is important, because at normal pH levels, 99% of the lactic acid is dissociated immediately to H^+ and La^- ($C_3H_5O_3^-$) (Brooks, 1985; Gladden, 2004). As long as the amount of free H^+ does not exceed the ability of the chemical and physiological mechanisms to buffer them and maintain the pH at a relatively stable level, there are few problems. Most problems arise when the amount of lactic acid—and thus H^+—exceeds the body's immediate buffering capacity and the pH decreases (Gladden, 2004). The blood has become more acidic. At that point pain is perceived and performance suffers. The mechanisms of these results are as follows.

Pain

Anyone who has raced or run the 400-m distance all out understands the pain associated with lactic acid production. The 400-m run takes between approximately 45 seconds and 3 minutes (depending on the ability of the runner) and relies heavily on the ATP-PC and LA systems to supply the needed energy. The resultant hydrogen ions accumulate and stimulate pain nerve endings in the muscle (Guyton and Hall, 2011).

Performance Decrement

The decrement in performance associated with lactic acid results from fatigue that is both metabolic and muscular in origin.

METABOLIC FATIGUE Metabolic fatigue results from a reduced production of ATP linked to enzyme changes, changes in membrane transport mechanisms, and changes in substrate availability.

Enzymes—in particular, the rate-limiting enzymes in the metabolic pathways—can be inactivated by high hydrogen ion concentrations (low pH). The hydrogen ion attaches to these enzyme molecules and in so doing changes their size and shape and thus their ability to function. phosphofructokinase (PFK) is thought to be particularly sensitive, although oxidative enzymes can also be affected (Hultman and Sahlin, 1980).

At the same time, changes occur in membrane transport mechanisms (either to the carriers in the membrane or to the permeability channels). These changes affect the movement of molecules across the cell membrane and between the cytoplasm and organelles such as the mitochondria (Hultman and Sahlin, 1980).

Energy substrate availability can be inhibited by a high concentration of hydrogen ions. Glycogen breakdown is slowed by the inactivation of the enzyme glycogen phosphorylase. Fatty acid utilization is decreased because lactic acid inhibits mobilization. Thus, a double-jeopardy situation occurs. With fatty acid availability low, a greater reliance is placed on carbohydrate sources at the time when glycogen breakdown is inhibited. At the same time, phosphocreatine breakdown is accelerated, leading to a faster depletion of substrate for ATP regeneration (Åstrand et al, 2003; Davis, 1985; Hultman and Sahlin, 1980).

Thus, both the inactivation of enzymes and the decrement in substrate availability will lead to a reduction in the production of ATP and, ultimately, a decrement in performance.

MUSCULAR FATIGUE Muscular fatigue is evidenced by reduced force and velocity of muscle contraction. The contraction of skeletal muscle and the influence of lactic acid on muscular fatigue are detailed in Chapters 17 and 18, respectively. Suffice it to say here that the lactic acid hypothesis of muscular fatigue is based primarily on two major effects of a lowered pH on muscle contraction. The first is an inhibition of actomyosin ATPase, the enzyme responsible for the breakdown of ATP to provide the immediate energy for muscle contraction. The second is an interference of H^+ with the actions and uptake of calcium (Ca^{2+}) that is necessary for the excitation-contraction coupling and relaxation of the protein cross-bridges within the muscle fiber. High levels of lactate ions (La^-) may also interfere with cross-bridging (Gladden, 2004; Hogan et al., 1995). These actions result in a decrease in both the force a muscle can exert and the velocity of muscle contraction. Recent studies question these traditionally accepted roles of lactic acid in muscular fatigue, even to the point of considering changes brought about by lactate and acidosis during exercise to be beneficial. That is, it is unclear whether lactate is a causative or a preventive agent of muscle fatigue (Gladden, 2008b; Robergs et al., 2004). While the controversy remains, what is certain is that although lactate/H^+ may contribute to fatigue, lactic acid is not the sole cause of muscular fatigue (Bangsbo, 2006; Cairns, 2006; Lamb, 2006).

Time Frame For Lactate Removal Postexercise

Lactate is removed from the bloodstream relatively rapidly following exercise (Gollnick et al., 1986). However, removal does not occur at a constant rate. If it did, then higher levels of lactate would take proportionately longer to dissipate than lower levels. By analogy, if you do one push-up in 2 seconds and you couldn't change that rate or speed, then 10 push-ups would take twice as long to do as 5 push-ups (20 versus 10 seconds). On the other hand, if you could change the rate, you might do 10 in the same time as you did 5 (in 10 seconds). Many chemical reactions have this ability to change the rate or speed at which they occur. The rate is proportional to the amount of substrate and product present. The more substrate available and the less product, the faster the reaction proceeds, and vice versa. This characteristic is called the *mass action effect*. Lactate appears to be one of those substrates whose utilization and conversion is linked with the amount of substrate present (Bonen et al., 1979).

Thus, despite wide differences among individuals (which may be related to muscle fiber type), in a resting recovery situation approximately half of the lactate is removed in about 15–25 minutes regardless of the starting level. This time is called the *half-life of lactate*. Near-resting levels are achieved in about 30–60 minutes, regardless of the starting level. Thus, the initial postexercise concentration of lactate is the first factor that influences the rate of removal. The higher the concentration, the faster is the rate of removal (Bonen et al., 1979; Hermansen and Stensvold, 1972; Hogan et al., 1995).

Figure 3.17 shows typical resting recovery curves from cycling and running studies. Note that in each case the value close to 50% (shown in parentheses) of the initial postexercise lactate levels occurs between 15 and 25 minutes of recovery.

The second factor that determines the rate of lactate removal is whether the individual follows a rest (passive) recovery or an exercise (active) recovery regimen. Third, with exercise recovery, the intensity of the exercise (expressed as a percentage of $\dot{V}O_2max$) makes a difference. Fourth, the modality of the exercise used in the recovery phase may influence the optimal percentage of $\dot{V}O_2max$ at which removal occurs. And finally, whether the recovery exercise is continuous or intermittent seems to make a difference.

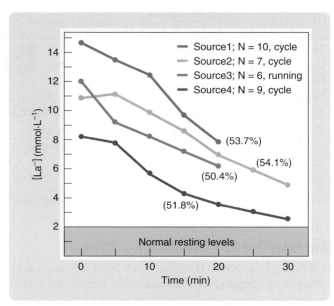

FIGURE 3.17   The Time Course of Lactate Removal during Resting Recovery from Exercise.
During resting recovery from exercise, lactate exhibits a half-life of 15–25 minutes.
Based on data from Bonen et al. (1979), Belcastro and Bonen (1975), Bonen and Belcastro (1976), McGrail et al. (1978).

Evidence suggests that lactate removal occurs more quickly when an individual exercises during recovery than when he or she sits quietly (Bangsbo et al., 1994). **Figure 3.18** shows the results of a study conducted by Bonen and Belcastro (1976). Six trained runners completed a mile run on three different occasions. In randomized order they then performed three different 20-minute recoveries: (1) seated rest, (2) continuous jogging at a self-selected pace, and (3) self-selected active recovery. During self-selected active recovery, the subjects did calisthenics, walked, jogged, and rested for variable portions of the total time.

As shown in **Figure 3.18**, after 5 minutes there is no appreciable difference in the level of lactate among the different recovery protocols. However, over the next 15 minutes, the rate of lactate removal was significantly faster for the jogging recovery than for either the self-selected active recovery or the rest recovery. The self-selected activity (what athletes typically do at a track meet), although not as good as continuous jogging (in part because it was intermittent), was still significantly better than resting recovery.

After 20 minutes of jogging recovery, the lactate that remained was within the normal resting levels of 1–2 mmol·L^{-1}. The self-selected active recovery had removed 70% of the lactate, but the resting recovery had only removed 50% of the lactate. Thus, full recovery was, and generally is, delayed with seated rest. Because athletes who run distances from 400 to 1500 m (or the English equivalents of 440 yd to 1 mi) often double at track meets, such a

The higher the concentration the faster is the rate of removal

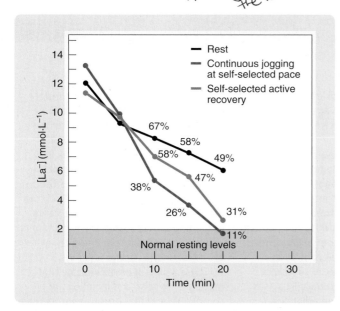

FIGURE 3.18 Lactate Removal in Active versus Passive Recovery.
Lactate removal is faster under active than passive conditions, although the magnitude of the benefit of active recovery depends on the type and intensity of the activity. In this study, continuous jogging at 61.4% $\dot{V}O_2$max was more effective than a mixture of walking, jogging, and calisthenics.
Source: Bonen and Belcastro (1976).

delay could impair their performances in the second event. Based on these results, athletes competing or training at distances that are likely to cause large accumulations of lactate should cool down with an active continuous recovery.

Why does activity increase the rate of lactate removal? The rate of lactate removal by the liver appears to be the same whether an individual is resting or exercising. However, during exercise, blood flow is increased, as is the oxidation of lactate by skeletal and cardiac muscles (Bangsbo et al., 1994; Belcastro and Bonen, 1975; Gollnick and Hermansen, 1973; Hogan et al., 1995; McGrail et al., 1978). These changes appear to be primarily responsible for the beneficial effects of an active recovery.

At what intensity should an active recovery be performed? Studies have found an inverted U-shaped response (Belcastro and Bonen, 1975; Hogan et al., 1995). That is, up to a point, a higher intensity of exercise (as measured by percentage of $\dot{V}O_2$max) during recovery is better. But after that point, as the intensity continues to rise, the removal rate decreases. The optimal rate for recovery from cycle ergometry is between 29% and 45% of $\dot{V}O_2$max. Data from track and treadmill exercises show the same type of inverted U-shaped curve response, but in the 55–70% $\dot{V}O_2$max range (Belcastro and Bonen, 1975; Hogan et al., 1995). This difference in optimal intensity may be a function of the modality (there is a higher static component for the cycle ergometer than for running) or of the training status of the subjects tested.

The actual value of these optimal percentages should not be surprising. The LT1 has been shown to occur between 40% and 60% of $\dot{V}O_2$max and may be higher in trained individuals. Thus, it appears that the optimal intensity for recovery would be just below an individual's lactate threshold, where lactate production is minimal but clearance is maximized. Direct measurement of lactate clearance when recovery intensity was set according to % LT1 has confirmed this (Menzies et al., 2010). The rate of blood lactate clearance exhibited a dose-response relationship during active recovery. Active recovery intensities at 80–100% of LT were more effective than exercise intensities at 60%, 40%, or 0% LT. Although there was a wide variation, in general, study participants self-selected a recovery intensity very close to the 80% LT value, so self-regulation may be possible for many individuals.

One word of caution: Although active recovery is best for lactate removal, it can delay glycogen resynthesis by further depleting glycogen stores (Choi et al., 1994). This has more relevance for an individual attempting to recover from a hard interval-training session than for someone just completing a middle-distance race and preparing for another. Glycogen depletion is likely to be more severe in the former case, and removing lactate quickly is a more immediate concern in the latter case. For athletes recovering from an interval training session or competing in heats on successive days, the best procedure may be to combine an initial dynamic active recovery (just to the point of regaining a near-resting heart rate) with stretching and then engage in a passive recovery during which carbohydrates are consumed.

Male Versus Female Anaerobic Exercise Characteristics

The anaerobic characteristics of females are generally lower than those of males in the young and middle-aged adult years. Much of the difference is undoubtedly related to the smaller overall muscle mass of the average female compared with that of the average male (Wells, 1991).

The Availability and Utilization of ATP-PC

Neither the local resting stores of ATP per kilogram of muscle nor the utilization of ATP-PC during exercise varies between the sexes (Brooks, 1986; Gollnick et al., 1986). However, in terms of total energy available from these phosphagen sources, males will have more than females because of muscle mass differences.

The Accumulation of Lactate

Resting levels of lactate are the same for males and females. Lactate thresholds, when expressed as a percentage of

FOCUS ON APPLICATION

Exercise, Lactic Acid, and Lactation

The impact of the accumulation of lactic acid/lactate following exercise on infants' acceptance of postexercise breast milk is an area of special interest. Some of the lactate present in the blood diffuses into breast milk.

In 1991, Wallace and Rabin reported that the concentration of lactic acid in breast milk following maximal treadmill exercise increased from $0.79 \, mmol \cdot L^{-1}$ pre-exercise to $1.62 \, mmol \cdot L^{-1}$ postexercise and remained elevated for at least 30 minutes. This milk [HLa] was approximately 25% of the postexercise blood concentration. Infants' acceptance of the postexercise milk was not tested in this study, but the investigators speculated that because these levels were high enough to change the taste of the breast milk, this could be a problem. Infants have fully developed taste buds at birth and can detect sour tastes such as that produced by lactic acid.

A follow-up study (Wallace et al., 1992) again revealed elevated postmaximal-exercise milk [HLa] ($2.84 \, mmol \cdot L^{-1}$ at 10 minutes and $2.97 \, mmol \cdot L^{-1}$ at 30 minutes). Infants were fed 2 mL of the pre- and two postexercise milk samples in a randomized fashion through a medicine dropper. Mothers' ratings of their infants' acceptance of the milk were significantly lower for both postexercise samples than the pre-exercise sample.

Reasoning that nursing mothers typically would not be doing maximal exercise, Quinn and Carey (1999) compared three exercise intensities on three separate days (maximal, at LT1, and 20% below LT1 abbreviated as LT1-20) to a resting control trial. Mothers were divided into two groups based on controlled carbohydrate intakes of 63% or 52% of total caloric intake. Breast milk [HLa] was significantly increased immediately after maximal exercise (1.27 and $1.52 \, mmol \cdot L^{-1}$) and LT1 exercise (0.19 and $0.25 \, mmol \cdot L^{-1}$), but not after the LT1-20 exercise (0.11 and $0.12 \, mmol \cdot L^{-1}$). Only the level following maximal exercise remained elevated 30 minutes after exercise.

More recently, Wright et al. (2002) tested the impact of maximal- and moderate-(LT1-20) intensity exercise compared to a resting control session on acceptance of postexercise breast milk by infants in a well-designed, controlled experiment. As in the prior research, breast milk [HLa] was significantly elevated over the control condition after maximal exercise (0.21 versus $0.09 \, mmol \cdot L^{-1}$) but not after the moderate-intensity exercise. Infants were offered the posttesting milk in a bottle. The mother and three lactation consultants (via videotape) rated the infants' acceptance of the milk. Both the mothers and the lactation consultants judged no differences in the infants' milk acceptance. Infants consumed an average of 104 mL of milk at the feedings.

These results seem to indicate that moderate exercise and lactation are compatible and that nursing mothers can enjoy the benefits of both for themselves and for their infants. Indeed, a 1994 study (Dewey et al., 1994) demonstrated fitness benefits for lactating women participating in a moderate submaximal aerobic exercise program (60–70%HRR progressing from 20 to 45 $min \cdot d^{-1}$, 5 $d \cdot wk^{-1}$ for 12 weeks). Although not a primary interest in this study, these researchers reported that none of these mothers mentioned any difficulties with nursing after exercise.

Sources: Dewey et al. (1994); Quinn and Carey (1999); Wallace and Rabin (1991); Wright et al. (2002).

$\dot{V}O_2max$, are also the same for both sexes, although the absolute workload at which the lactate thresholds occur is higher for males than females. Thus, at any given absolute workload that is still submaximal but above LT1 or LT2, females have a higher lactate value than males. Consequently, the workload is more stressful for females and requires a greater anaerobic contribution. However, at a given relative workload or percentage of $\dot{V}O_2max$ above the lactate thresholds, lactate concentrations are equal for both sexes (Wells, 1991).

Lactate values at maximal exercise from ages 16 through 50 are higher by approximately $0.5–2.0 \, mmol \cdot L^{-1}$ for males than for females (see **Figure 3.19**). Once again, females are generally doing less in terms of an absolute workload than males at maximum.

Mechanical Power and Capacity

As previously mentioned, on average males produce higher absolute work output than females. Data available from the Wingate Anaerobic Test show that values for peak power for women are approximately 65% of values for men if expressed in watts, improve to 83% if expressed in watts per kilogram of body weight, and come close to being equal at 94% when expressed in watts per kilogram of lean body mass. The corresponding comparisons for mean power are 68%, 87%, and 98%, respectively. The peak power of women (in watts per kilogram of body weight) is very similar to the mean power of men. The fatigue index does not show a significant sex difference, indicating that both sexes tire at the same rate (Makrides et al., 1985). It has been shown that females provide a relatively higher portion of the energy for the WAT aerobically than males. This may mean that the total power output during a WAT actually underestimates the sex difference in anaerobic capacity between males and females (Hill and Smith, 1993).

The maximal accumulated oxygen deficit (MAOD) expressed relative to the active muscle mass for cycling is significantly higher in males than females (Weber and Schneider, 2000).

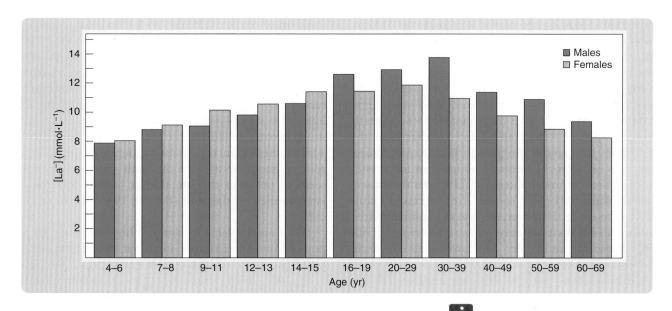

FIGURE 3.19   Lactate Values after Maximal Exercise as a Function of Age and Sex.
Sources: Compiled from computed mean values data for 4- to 20-year-old subjects: Cumming et al. (1985), Saris et al. (1985), Åstrand et al. (1963), and Eriksson (1972). Computed mean values data for 20- to 60-year-old subjects: Bouhuys et al. (1966), Sidney and Shephard (1977), Åstrand (1960), Robinson (1938), and Åstrand (1952).

Anaerobic Exercise Characteristics of Children

The anaerobic characteristics of children are not as well developed as those of adults. Furthermore, children tend not to exhibit metabolic specialization as adults do. For example, one would not expect Usain Bolt (the 2009 world record holder in the 100-m dash, with a time of 9.58) to do well at the marathon distance, nor Paula Radcliffe (who set the women's marathon world best at 2:15:25 in 2003) to be successful at the sprint distances. Yet watch children at play (**Figure 3.20**) and, more often than not, the fastest at short distances or strength-type events also do well at long distances or in aerobic-type games such as soccer. Although more research is needed to explain the anaerobic differences between children and adults, some patterns are apparent (Bar-Or, 1983; Rowland, 2005).

The Availability and Utilization of ATP-PC

Local resting stores of ATP per kilogram of wet muscle weight appear to be the same for children and adults (Boisseau and Delamarche, 2000; Rowland, 2005). Levels of resting PC per kilogram of wet muscle weight have been reported as slightly lower in children (Bar-Or, 1983; Shephard, 1982) or no different from adult levels (Eriksson, 1972; Shephard, 1982). There is agreement that the rate of utilization of these reserves during exercise does not differ. However, because children are smaller than adults, the total amount of energy that can

be generated from this source is lower. Children have been shown to have faster intramuscular PC restoration and recovery half-times after exercise than adults (Falk and Dotan, 2006). From a practical standpoint, the capacity for youngsters to perform at high intensity in exercises of 10–15 seconds in duration is not impaired compared with adults (Boisseau and Delamarche, 2000).

The Accumulation of Lactate

On the average, blood lactate values obtained during submaximal exercise and after maximal exercise are lower in children than in adults (Boisseau and Delamarche, 2000; Rowland, 1990, 2005; Shephard, 1982; Van Praagh, 2007).

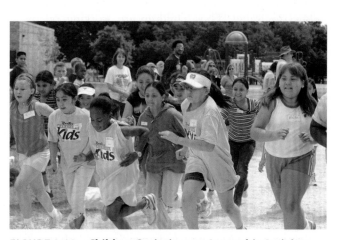

FIGURE 3.20   Children Sprinting, an Anaerobic Activity.

Furthermore, peak lactate values after maximal exercise exhibit a relatively positive rectilinear increase with age until adulthood. This increase can be as much as 50% for boys between the ages of 6 and 14 years and slightly less for girls (Rowland, 2005). **Figure 3.19** depicts children's values. It also shows that there is no meaningful sex difference in children in the accumulation of lactate, although the girls' values are slightly higher than the boys' values throughout the growth period. Anatomical differences between children and adults allow for a faster transition time for metabolites (La^-, H^+) from the muscle to blood; thus [La^-] peaks sooner after exercise in children than in adults. However, the rate of elimination (the time for half-life disappearance of La^-) is the same in children, adolescents, and adults. The lower lactate levels in children and adolescents is also reflected in higher pH levels during intense exercise although there is no difference in resting muscle pH between children and adults. Children appear to recover from physical exertion more quickly than adults, in large part because their lower maximal power output means they have less to recover from. However, the early peak of lactate is also a major advantage over adults in recovery. As a consequence, children and adolescents may require shorter rest periods between high-intensity bouts of activity (Boisseau and Delamarche, 2000; Falk and Dotan, 2006).

The Lactate Threshold(s)

The phenomenon of ventilatory breakpoints and lactate accumulation is seen in children as well as in adults, but they typically occur at a higher % $\dot{V}O_2$max than for adults (Gaisl and Buchberger, 1979; Klentrou et al., 2006; Rowland, 2005). Because children do not utilize anaerobic metabolism as early in work as adults do, the work level of children at the fixed lactate levels of $4\,mmol\cdot L^{-1}$ is relatively higher than that of adults (Kanaley and Boileau, 1988; Reybrouck, 1989). Williams et al. (1990) report a value of almost 92% of $\dot{V}O_2$max for $4\,mmol\cdot L^{-1}$ of lactate in 11- to 13-year-old boys and girls. Values for adults tend to be about 15% below this value. Thus, children are working relatively harder (at a higher %$\dot{V}O_2$max) than adults at the same lactate level. Consequently, the assessment of exercise capacity and the monitoring of training by a 4-$mmol\cdot L^{-1}$ value is inappropriate in prepubertal children. MLSS ($mmol\cdot L^{-1}$) is independent of age and sex between children and adults despite the fact that the MLSS workload is significantly higher in adults than in children (Beneke et al., 2009).

Mechanical Power and Capacity

Peak power and peak power per kilogram of body weight have consistently been shown to be lower in prepubertal boys and girls than in adolescents or young adults when evaluated by the Margaria-Kalamen Stair Climb test. The results are similar to those for the Wingate Anaerobic Test, although information is lacking about females for

the Wingate Anaerobic Test except for isolated ages (10–13 years) (Armstrong et al., 1997, 2000; Chia et al., 1999) (**Figure 3.21**). In boys, peak power and mean power increase consistently from age 10 yr to young adulthood. This is true both in absolute terms (watts) and when corrected for body weight (watts per kilogram). The absolute differences between children and adults, however, are much greater (children can achieve only about 30% of adult values) than the relative differences (children can achieve about 60–85% of the adult values). Peak values seem to occur in the late thirties for the legs and the late twenties for the arms (Bar-Or, 1988; Hughson et al., 1987).

Data are available to compare boys and girls on peak power from a variation of an all-out cycle ergometer test called the force-velocity test (Martin et al., 2004; Santos et al., 2002, 2003). The results of the most comprehensive study in terms of age range are shown in **Figure 3.22**. These results indicate that from ages 7 to 16 yr girls increased peak power by 273% and then plateaued between ages 16 and 17 yr. Boys' peak power increased by 375% between ages 7 and 17 yr. Sex differences were not apparent in peak power until age 14 yr (Martin et al., 2004).

Fatigue resistance to high-intensity intermittent exercise (maximal knee flexion and extension) shows a gradual decline from childhood through adolescence to young adulthood in males. In females, fatigue resistance declines from childhood to adolescence but plateaus from there to young adulthood (Dipla et al., 2009).

Mechanisms

Several theories, described in the following sections, have been postulated to explain children's inability to function at a high level anaerobically in activities lasting 15 seconds to 2 minutes and/or requiring large power outputs. These theories are based on two assumptions: that the children tested did indeed put forth a maximal effort and that there is a physiological cause for the observed differences.

The Muscle Enzyme Theory

Eriksson (1972) and others have shown that phosphofructo kinase (PFK) activity in 11- to 13-year-old boys is 2.5–3 times lower than in trained or sedentary adult men. Since PFK is a rate-limiting enzyme of glycolysis, this lowered activity may indicate a decreased ability to produce lactic acid. In addition, the availability and the utilization of glycogen as a substrate, as well as the activity of lactic dehydrogenase (LDH), are both lower in children than in adults. Studies have shown that the glycogen content of children's muscles is approximately 50–60% that of adults (Boisseau and Delamarche, 2000). Anaerobic enzymes evolve with pubertal maturation, however, and by 12–14 years of age LDH activity has reached adult levels (Berg et al., 1986). Therefore, it appears that prepubertal youngsters do have lower glycolytic enzyme activity than fully mature individuals (Boisseau and Delamarche, 2000; Rowland, 2005).

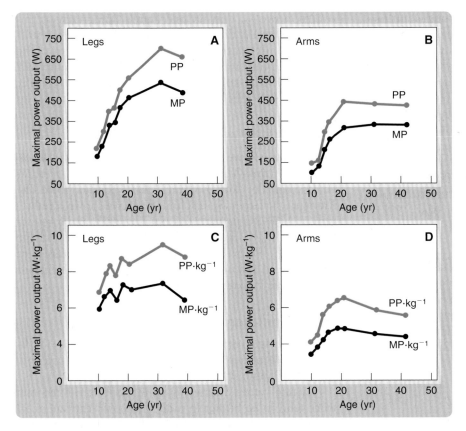

FIGURE 3.21   The Effect of Age on Anaerobic Performance.
Cross-sectional data on 306 males who performed both an arm and a leg Wingate Anaerobic Test. The pattern of increase in values from childhood to young adulthood is similar for leg (**A, C**) and arm (**B, D**) cycling whether the unit of measurement is absolute (**A, B**) or relative (**C, D**). *Source*: Inbar & Bar-Or. Anaerobic characteristics in male children and adolescents. *Medicine and Science in Sports and Exercise*. 18(3):264–269 (1986). Reprinted by permission.

In general, the oxidative enzymes show higher activity in young children than in older individuals (Berg, 1986; Williams et al., 1990). This result, along with higher mitochondrial density and intracellular lipids, means that lipid utilization is greater in children. Thus, it may be that children have a finer balance between aerobic and anaerobic metabolism than adults. Additional evidence for this observation comes from the fact that children show a lower oxygen deficit and reach a steady state faster than adults (Åstrand, 1952; Boisseau and Delamarche, 2000; Reybrouck, 1989; Rowland, 2005; Shephard, 1982).

Muscle Characteristics Theory

Several muscle characteristics have been suggested as explanations for the lower glycolytic anaerobic function in children and adolescents than adults. These include muscle fiber differentiation, muscle fiber recruitment, contractile properties, muscle fiber size, muscle size, and muscle mass (Boisseau and Delamarche, 2000; Falk and Dotan, 2006; Van Praagh, 2000, 2007).

The development of muscle fiber-type distribution continues from birth to approximately 6 years of age, when the individual achieves his or her profile of slow-twitch and fast-twitch fibers. However, the relative proportion of fast-twitch oxidative glycolytic (FOG) and fast-twitch glycolytic (FG) fibers continues to change through late adolescence. Typically FOG fibers predominate more than FG fibers during childhood and adolescence. Boys develop greater FG cross-sectional area than girls as they mature. The contractile properties of FG fibers favor force and power expression. Children may be limited in their ability to recruit FG fibers.

Muscle fiber size, measured as diameter, and muscle size, measured as cross-sectional area, both increase

FIGURE 3.22   Peak Power by Age in Boys and Girls.
Force-velocity test results indicate that both boys and girls increase the production of PP from 7 to approximately 17 years of age. Sex differences are not apparent until age 14, when boys' PP production increased more than girls'. Based on data from Martin et al. (2004).

rectilinearly with age from birth to young adulthood. Muscle force changes closely parallel changes in cross-sectional area, and these power changes during growth favor boys over girls after puberty. However, when normalized for muscle cross-sectional area, age and sex differences in muscle force disappear.

Finally, total muscle mass is directly related to the ability to generate force/power. As the child grows, obviously so does his or her total muscle mass. However, even normalized for muscle mass, force production is lower in children and adolescents than adults (Van Praagh, 2000). Body composition changes (more total muscle mass, less fat for boys) favor males in force production (Armstrong et al., 1997).

Sexual Maturation Theory

Limited evidence suggests that the increase in glycolytic capacity (and thus the production of lactate) in children is related to the hormonal changes that bring about sexual maturation. In particular, testosterone is thought to have a role, but research evidence has not been definitive (Boisseau and Delamarche, 2000; Rowland, 2005; Williams et al., 1990).

Neurohormonal Regulation Theory

It has been shown that sympathoadrenal system activity is significantly lower in children than in adults at maximal exercise (Boisseau and Delamarche, 2000). Epinephrine is a potent stimulator of muscle glycolysis. Another result of sympathetic stimulation during exercise is hepatic vasoconstriction. The liver plays a major role in the clearance of lactate. If blood flow to the liver is reduced, less lactate is cleared. Thus, because the child maintains a higher liver blood flow, more lactate can be cleared. This implies that children are not deficient in the production of lactate but are, instead, better able to remove or reconvert it than adults (Berg and Keul, 1988; Mácek and Vávra, 1985; Rowland, 1990, 2005).

Which of these theories—muscle enzyme, muscle characteristics, sexual maturation, neurohormonal regulation—or which combination of them is correct remains to be shown.

Anaerobic Exercise Characteristics of Older Adults

Detailed evidence of the anaerobic characteristics of the elderly is scarce, undoubtedly in part because of caution by researchers and in part because of the uncertain motivation of subjects facing high-intensity exercise. The available data indicate that anaerobic variables show a common aging pattern; that is, there is a peak in the second or third decade and then a gradual decline into the sixth decade. One must always remember when interpreting aging

results, however, that no one knows how much of this reduction results directly from aging, how much results from detraining accompanying the reduced activity of the elderly, and how much results from disease. Despite this, older adults can still participate successfully in basically anaerobic activities (**Figure 3.23**).

The Availability and Utilization of ATP-PC

Local resting stores of ATP-PC are reduced and levels of creatine and ADP are elevated in muscles of older adults (Kanaley and Boileau, 1988). Results from the Margaria-Kalamen Stair Climb test have shown a reduction in ATP-PC power of as much as 45% and a reduction in ATP-PC capacity of 32% from youth to old age (Shephard, 1982). This means that ATP-PC stores are both reduced and unable to be used as quickly. The result is a decrease in alactic anaerobic power.

The Accumulation of Lactate

On the average, resting levels of blood lactate are remarkably consistent across the entire age span, varying only from 1 to 2 mmol·L^{-1}.

Lactate values during the same absolute submaximal work tend to be higher in individuals over the age of 50 (I. Åstrand, 1960; P.-O. Åstrand, 1952, 1956; Robinson, 1938). However, this generalization is confounded by the fact that at any given absolute load of work, the older individual is working at a higher percentage of his or

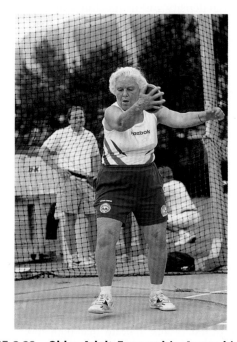

FIGURE 3.23   Older Adult Engaged in Anaerobic Activity. Anaerobic metabolic processes function less effectively in the elderly than in younger adults, but participation in anaerobic sports such as throwing the discus can still be enjoyed.

her maximal aerobic power, which would be expected to involve more anaerobic metabolism (Sidney and Shephard, 1977). When younger and older individuals work at the same relative workload (%V̇O₂max), lactate concentrations are lower in older people than in the young, probably because the elderly are using less muscle mass to do less work (Kohrt et al., 1993).

Maximal lactate levels as a result of incremental dynamic exercise to maximum reach a peak between 16 and 39 years of age and then show a gradual decline (see **Figure 3.19**). Both males and females exhibit the same pattern, although the absolute values of females are considerably lower than those of males.

Direct measurement of ATP produced from anaerobic glycolysis indicates that older males have an overall lower production than younger males (Lanza et al., 2005) during 60 seconds maximal static contraction. Because this reflects a lower utilization of the glycolytic pathway, exercise lactate values should be lower.

Physiological factors appear to contribute to the decline in anaerobic ATP production and maximal lactate values with age (Shephard, 1982; Smith and Serfass, 1981). First, activity of the enzyme lactate dehydrogenase (which catalyzes the conversion of pyruvic acid to lactic acid) decreases in all muscle fiber types. This decrease effectively slows glycolysis. The reduction in glycolysis may also be related to reduced amounts of glycogen stored in the skeletal muscles of the elderly.

Second, the elderly possess a smaller ratio of muscle mass to blood volume, a smaller ratio of capillary to muscle fiber, and a concomitant slower diffusion of lactic acid out of active muscle fibers and into the bloodstream (Shephard, 1982). Thus, it may not be that the elderly have a large deficiency in anaerobic capacity at the cellular level; rather, it may simply be that measurements from blood samples are underestimations. Of course, a combination of the first and second factors may also be operating.

Lactate Threshold(s)

Although individuals continue to exhibit at least one lactate threshold as they age, the point at which this is evident, expressed as %V̇O₂max, appears to shift to a higher value in both sexes. In a study of 111 male and 57 female runners from 40 to 70 years of age, the lactate threshold increased from approximately 65% to 75% across the decades. In addition, there is some controversy about the ability of the LT to predict endurance performance in this age group (Wiswell et al., 2000).

Mechanical Power and Capacity

The average peak power value obtained on the Margaria-Kalamen Stair Climb test (**Figure 3.24A**) declines precipitously from 20 to 70 years of age (Bouchard et al., 1982). There are no published results for the Wintage Anaerobic

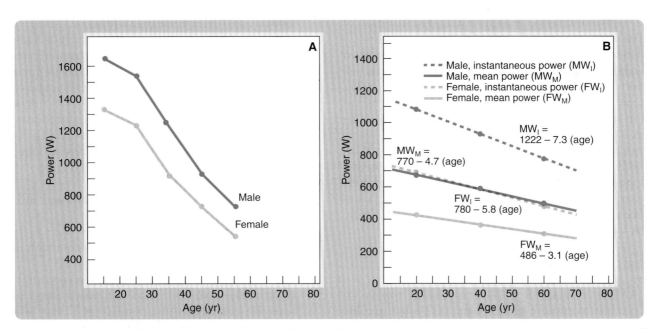

FIGURE 3.24 Mechanical Power Changes with Age in Males and Females.
A. Average peak power ratings determined from the Margaria-Kalamen Stair Climb are higher for males than females across the age span from adolescence to middle adulthood. Males and females show steady and parallel declines in peak power during the adult years. **B.** Instantaneous peak power and mean power measured during a 30-second cycle ergometer test are higher for males (MW$_I$ and MW$_M$, respectively) than for females (FW$_I$ and FW$_M$, respectively) across the age span from late adolescence to older adulthood. Female instantaneous peak power (FW$_I$) is equal to male mean power (MW$_M$). Instantaneous peak power and mean power show rectilinear and parallel declines with age in males and females. Each line was calculated from the experimentally determined equation associated with that line on the graph.
Sources: **A.** Data from Bouchard et al. (1982). **B.** Data from Makrides et al. (1985).

Test for individuals over the age of 40 and for females except in the 18- to 28-year range (Maud and Shultz, 1989). However, Makrides et al. (1985) presented data on 50 male and 50 female subjects from 15 to 70 on a test similar to the WAT (**Figure 3.24B**). In this case peak power represented an instantaneous value rather than a 5-second value. Mean power was still the average of 30 seconds of pedaling but at a controlled rate of 60 rev·min^{-1}. The results in this study showed a decline of approximately 6% for each decade of age for sedentary individuals of both sexes. However, the absolute values for the females were consistently lower than those for the males. Indeed, in the Makrides study the peak power of the females coincided with the mean power of the males. For both sexes, lean thigh volume was closely related to peak power and mean power, but this did not account for all the variation in the values or in the decline with age. A more recent study (Kostka et al., 2009) has shown a decline in maximal anaerobic power per kg of body weight of approximately 10.3% per decade from 20 to 88 years in males.

An analysis of weight lifting (e.g., snatch, clean, and jerk) and power lifting (e.g., dead lift, squat, bench press) records for males and females from 40 to 70 years showed declines in anaerobic muscle performance. The decline was greatest (and curvilinear) in the weight-lifting tasks that required explosive coordinated movements and high-balance skills. The decline in weight lifting was higher in females (~–70%) than males (~–50%). The overall decline in the power lifts was rectilinear and similar in males (~–40%) and females (~–50%). Upper and lower body muscular power demonstrated similar rates of decline with aging (Anton et al., 2004).

Undoubtedly, muscle mass is lost with age. Between the ages of 30 and 70, almost 25% of muscle mass is lost in both males and females (Rogers and Evans, 1993). Obviously, the loss of muscle mass leads to a concomitant loss in force and power production. In addition, as individuals age, the percentage of fast-twitch muscle fibers, particularly fast-twitch glycolytic fibers, decreases. With this shift there is a decline in potential glycolytic function and force production. Finally, neural activation and integration decline with age. Thus, moves requiring high levels of coordination may present a greater risk (Anton et al., 2004; Larsson et al., 2001).

SUMMARY

1. Anaerobic metabolism does not require oxygen to produce adenosine triphosphate (ATP), but aerobic metabolism does.

2. Anaerobic and aerobic metabolism work together to provide ATP and thus energy for exercise. Depending on the duration and intensity of the activity, one or the other predominates.

3. The adenosine triphosphate-phosphocreatine (ATP-PC) system predominates in high-intensity exercise that lasts 30 seconds or less. The LA system predominates in high-intensity exercise lasting 30–75 seconds. The aerobic system predominates in exercise lasting from approximately 2 minutes to hours. This sequence is called the time-energy system continuum.

4. There is no generally accepted way to directly measure the anaerobic energy contribution to exercise. One indirect approach is to describe the changes in ATP, PC, and lactate levels. Another is to quantify the amount of work performed or power generated during short-duration, high-intensity activity.

5. Lactic acid/lactate production depends on the use of glycogen as fuel, the formation of pyruvate, and the necessity of preserving the redox potential of the cell. It involves:
   a. muscle contraction that in turn depends on calcium release and results in glycogenolysis;
   b. the high activity of the enzyme lactate dehydrogenase compared with other glycolytic and oxidative enzymes;
   c. recruitment of fast-twitch glycolytic (FG, Type IIA and FOG, Type IIX) muscle fibers;
   d. activation of the sympathetic nervous system, which ultimately results in glycogenolysis; and
   e. insufficient oxygen, which results in anaerobiosis or the onset of anaerobic metabolism.

6. Lactic acid/lactate clearance utilizes both an intracellular and extracellular shuttle system. MCT1 and MCT4 transporters move lactate by facilitated exchange down concentration and pH gradients.

7. Lactate accumulation results when production (appearance) exceeds clearance (disappearance).

8. The onset of all exercise is characterized by a discrepancy between oxygen demand and oxygen utilization known as the oxygen deficit. This deficit is due not to the cardiovascular-respiratory system's inability to deliver oxygen but to the varying speeds of response of the two anaerobic and aerobic systems to the contraction of muscle and the breakdown of ATP.

9. During the transition from rest to exercise—the O_2 deficit period—energy is supplied by:
   a. oxygen transport and utilization
   b. the use of oxygen stores in venous blood and on myoglobin
   c. the splitting of stored ATP-PC
   d. anaerobic glycolysis with the concomitant production of lactic acid

10. During recovery from exercise, oxygen consumption remains elevated, a phenomenon called excess postexercise oxygen consumption (EPOC). The following factors appear to occur during recovery.
    a. Restoration of ATP-PC stores
    b. Restoration of oxygen stores
    c. Elevated cardiorespiratory function
    d. Elevated hormonal levels
    e. Elevated body temperature
    f. Lactate removal
    g. Energy substrate shift from CHO to fat

11. During exercise, the balance between aerobic and anaerobic metabolism depends on the intensity of the activity in relation to the individual's maximal ability to produce energy using oxygen ($\dot{V}O_2$max).

12. During high-intensity, short-duration (3 minutes or less) anaerobic exercise, ATP levels decrease 30–40%, PC levels decrease 60–70%, and lactate accumulation can increase well over 1000%.

13. The lactate response (increase, decrease, no change after an initial rise) to long-term moderate to heavy submaximal exercise depends to a large extent on the intensity of the exercise in relation to the maximal lactate steady state (MLSS) intensity.

14. During incremental work to maximum, lactate accumulates slowly until approximately 40–60% $\dot{V}O_2$max when the continual accumulation is exponentially curvilinear. The term lactate threshold (LT) is commonly used (although not absolutely accurately) to describe the point where large increases in lactate accumulation occur.

15. LT1 is typically found between 40% and 60% $\dot{V}O_2$max, and LT2 is found between 80% and 95% $\dot{V}O_2$max. An absolute value of $4\,mmol\cdot L^{-1}$ is termed the onset of blood lactate accumulation (OBLA) and is often used as a training and racing guideline for adults.

16. The relationship between the lactate thresholds and ventilatory thresholds appears to be primarily coincidental.

17. The term anaerobic threshold is a misnomer and should not be used because the presence of lactate does not automatically mean that the oxygen supply is inadequate.

18. Performance decrements are related to high concentrations of H^+ because of:
    a. pain
    b. reduced production of ATP through inactivation of enzymes or changes in membrane transport
    c. inhibition of energy substrate availability because glycogen breakdown is slowed or because fatty acid mobilization is slowed
    d. reduced force and velocity of muscle contraction

19. Lactate removal from the bloodstream after exercise follows the law of mass action: The more lactate present, the faster the rate of removal. The half-life of lactate is approximately 15–25 minutes, with full removal achieved between 30 and 60 minutes.

20. The time required for lactate removal can be decreased by doing an active recovery at an intensity of approximately 30–45% $\dot{V}O_2$max for cycling and 55–70% $\dot{V}O_2$max for running—at or slightly below the first lactate threshold.

21. The anaerobic capacities of children are not well-developed compared to adults. The lower amount of ATP-PC available is related to children's small body size.

22. Peak lactate values after incremental exercise to maximum are lower in children than adults and vary directly with age throughout the growth years. There is no meaningful male-female difference in the ability to accumulate lactate during childhood.

23. Mechanical power and capacity are lower for children and adolescents than for adults, whether expressed in absolute terms or corrected for body weight.

24. During the adult years males accumulate higher levels of blood lactate as a result of maximal work than females, and males exhibit higher mechanical power and capacity even when they are adjusted for body weight.

25. Anaerobic metabolic processes decline from young and middle-aged adults to older adults. The decline includes lower resting levels of ATP-PC.

26. Peak lactate values after incremental exercise to maximum decline after approximately 40 years of age. Females exhibit considerably lower peak values than males.

27. The mechanical power and capacity of the elderly decline steadily. The decline is greater in females than in males.

REVIEW QUESTIONS

1. Describe the energy continuum. For each of the following sports or events, determine the percentage contribution from the anaerobic and aerobic systems.
   a. 100-m dash
   b. 800-m run
   c. soccer (not goalie)
   d. triathlon
   e. volleyball spike
   f. 100-m swim
   g. mile run
   h. stealing a base
   i. wrestling period

2. List the major variables typically measured to describe the anaerobic response to exercise. Where possible, provide an example of an exercise test that can measure the variable.

3. Explain the five physiological reasons for the production of lactic acid. What determines whether or not lactate accumulates in the blood? How is lactate cleared?

4. Rank the ATP-PC, LA, and O_2 systems from highest to lowest in terms of (a) power and (b) capacity. What is the difference between power and capacity?

5. Diagram the oxygen deficit and excess postexercise oxygen consumption for an activity that requires 110% $\dot{V}O_2$max in an individual whose $\dot{V}O_2$max equals $4\,L\cdot min^{-1}$ and whose resting oxygen is $0.25\,L\cdot min^{-1}$. Explain how energy is provided during the oxygen deficit time period and why oxygen remains elevated during recovery.

6. Diagram and explain the changes that take place in ATP, PC, and [La$^-$] during constant-load, heavy exercise lasting 3 minutes or less.

7. Explain the concept of maximal lactate steady state and why MLSS is important in endurance performance.

8. Diagram the lactate response to incremental work to maximum. The ventilatory and lactate thresholds often occur at approximately the same time. Debate whether this is a result of cause and effect or coincidence. Can either the lactate thresholds or the ventilatory thresholds be accurately described as anaerobic thresholds? Why or why not?

9. What are the physiological effects of lactic acid production and lactate accumulation according to the lactate acidosis hypothesis of muscular fatigue?

10. What is the best way to clear lactate quickly during recovery?

11. What are the effects of sex and age on anaerobic metabolism during exercise?

For further review and additional study tools, visit the website at http://thePoint.lww.com/Plowman4e ✳ ◉

REFERENCES

American College of Sports Medicine Roundtable: The physiological and health effects of oral creatine supplementation. *Medicine & Science in Sports & Exercise.* 32(3):706–717 (2000).

Anton, M. M., W. W. Spirduso, & H. Tanaka: Age-related declines in anaerobic muscular performance: Weightlifting and power lifting. *Medicine & Science in Sports & Exercise.* 36:143–147 (2004).

Armstrong, N., J. R. Welsman, & B. J. Kirby: Performance on the Wingate Anaerobic Test and maturation. *Pediatric Exercise Science.* 9:253–261 (1997).

Armstrong, N., J. R. Welsman, C. A. Williams, & B. J. Kirby: Longitudinal changes in young people's short-term power output. *Medicine & Science in Sports & Exercise.* 32:1140–1145 (2000).

Åstrand, I.: Aerobic work capacity in men and women with special reference to age. *Acta Physiologica Scandinavica (Suppl.).* 169:1–92 (1960).

Åstrand, P.-O.: *Experimental Studies of Physical Working Capacity in Relation to Sex and Age.* Copenhagen: Munksgaard (1952).

Åstrand, P.-O.: Human physical fitness with special reference to sex and age. *Physiological Reviews.* 36(3):307–335 (1956).

Åstrand, P.-O., L. Engstrom, B. O. Eriksson, P. Karlberg, I. Nylander, B. Saltin, & C. Thoren: Girl swimmers: With special reference to respiratory and circulatory adaption and gynecological and psychiatric aspects. *Acta Paediatrica (Suppl.).* 147:1–73 (1963).

Åstrand, P.-O., K. Rodahl, H. A. Dahl, & S. B. Strømme: *Textbook of Work Physiology: Physiological Bases of Exercise* (4th edition). Champaign, IL: Human Kinetics (2003).

Bahr, R.: Excess postexercise oxygen consumption—Magnitude, mechanisms and practical implications. *Acta Physiologica Scandinavica (Suppl.).* 605:9–70 (1992).

Bangsbo, J.: Counterpoint: Lactic acid accumulation is a disadvantage during muscle activity. *Journal of Applied Physiology.* 100:1412–1413 (2006).

Bangsbo, J., T. Graham, L. Johansen, & B. Saltin: Muscle lactate metabolism in recovery from intense exhaustive exercise: Impact of light exercise. *Journal of Applied Physiology.* 77(4):1890–1895 (1994).

Bar-Or, O.: *Pediatric Sports Medicine for the Practitioner: From Physiological Principles to Clinical Applications.* New York, NY: Springer-Verlag, 1–65 (1983).

Bar-Or, O.: The prepubescent female. In M. M. Shangold & G. Mirkin (eds.): *Women and Exercise: Physiology and Sports Medicine.* Philadelphia, PA: Davis, 109–119 (1988).

Bar-Or, O.: The Wingate Anaerobic Test: An update on methodology, reliability and validity. *Sports Medicine.* 4:381–394 (1987).

Belcastro, A. N. & A. Bonen: Lactic acid removal rates during controlled and uncontrolled recovery exercise. *Journal of Applied Physiology.* 39(6):932–936 (1975).

Bemben, M. G. & H. S. Lamont: Creatine supplementation and exercise performance: Recent findings. *Sports Medicine.* 35:107–125 (2005).

Beneke, R., H. Heck, H. Hebestreit, & R. M. Leithäuser: Predicting maximal lactate steady state in children and adults. *Pediatric Exercise Science.* 21:493–505 (2009).

Beneke, R., M. Hutler, & R. M. Leithauser: Maximal lactate-steady-state independent of performance. *Medicine & Science in Sports & Exercise.* 32(6):1135–1139 (2000).

Berg, A. & J. Keul: Biochemical changes during exercise in children. In R. M. Malina (ed.): *Young Athletes: Biological, Psychological, and Educational Perspectives.* Champaign, IL: Human Kinetics (1988).

Berg, A., S. S. Kim, & J. Keul: Skeletal muscle enzyme activities in healthy young subjects. *International Journal of Sports Medicine.* 7:236–239 (1986).

Billat, V. L., P. Sirvent, G. Py, J. P. Koralsztein, & J. Mercier: The concept of maximal lactate steady state: A bridge between biochemistry, physiology and sport science. *Sports Medicine.* 33(6):407–426 (2003).

Boisseau, N. & P. Delamarche: Metabolic and hormonal responses to exercise in children and adolescents. *Sports Medicine.* 30(6):405–422 (2000).

Bonen, A.: Lactate transporters (MCT proteins) in heart and skeletal muscles. *Medicine & Science in Sports & Exercise.* 32(4):778–789 (2000).

Bonen, A. & A. N. Belcastro: Comparison of self-selected recovery methods on lactic acid removal rates. *Medicine and Science in Sports.* 8(3):176–178 (1976).

Bonen, A., C. J. Campbell, R. L. Kirby, & A. N. Belcastro: A multiple regression model for blood lactate removal in man. *Pflügers Archives.* 380:205–210 (1979).

Bonen, A, M. Heynen, & H. Hatta: Distribution of monocarboxylate transporters MCT1-MCT8 in rat tissues and human skeletal muscle. *Applied Physiology, Nutrition, and Metabolism.* 31(1):31–39 (2006).

Børsheim, E. & R. Bahr: Effect of exercise intensity, duration and mode on post-exercise oxygen consumption. *Sports Medicine.* 33(14):1037–1060 (2003).

Bortolotti, H., L. R. Altimari, F. Y. Nakamura, E. B. Fontes, A. H. Okano, M. P. T. Chacon-Mikahil, A. C. Moraes, & E. S. Cyrino: Determination of the maximal accumulated oxygen deficit: Effects of the submaximal tests duration for prediction of oxygen demand. *Revista Brasileira de Medicina do esporte.* 16(6):445–449 (2010).

Bouchard, C., A. W. Taylor, & S. Dulac: Testing maximal anaerobic power and capacity. In MacDougall, J. D., H. W. Wenger, & H. J. Green (eds.): *Physiological Testing of the High-Performance Athlete* (2nd edition). Champaign, IL: Human Kinetics, 175–221 (1991).

Bouchard, C., A. W. Taylor, J. A. Simoneau, & S. Dulac: Testing anaerobic power and capacity. In J. D. MacDougall, H. A. Wenger, & H. J. Green (eds.): *Physiological Testing of the Elite Athlete*. Hamilton, ON: Canadian Association of Sport Sciences Mutual Press Limited, 61–73 (1982).

Bouhuys, A., J. Pool, R. A. Binkhorst, & P. van Leeuwen: Metabolic acidosis of exercise in healthy males. *Journal of Applied Physiology*. 21(3):1040–1046 (1966).

Branch, J. D.: Effect of creatine supplementation on body composition and performance: A meta-analysis. *International Journal of Sport Nutrition and Exercise Metabolism*. 13:198–226 (2003).

Brooks, G. A.: Anaerobic threshold: Review of the concept and directions for future research. *Medicine and Science in Sports and Exercise*. 17(1):22–31 (1985).

Brooks, G. A.: Intra- and extra-cellular lactate shuttles. *Medicine & Science in Sports & Exercise*. 32(4):790–700 (2000).

Brooks, G. A.: Lactate shuttles in nature. *Biochemical Society Transactions*. 30:258–264 (2002).

Brooks, G. A.: The lactate shuttle during exercise and recovery. *Medicine and Science in Sports and Exercise*. 18(3):360–368 (1986).

Brooks, G. A.: What does glycolysis make and why is it important? *Journal of Applied Physiology*. 108:1450–1451 (2010).

Brooks, G. A., T. D. Fahey, T. P. White, & K. M. Baldwin: *Exercise Physiology: Human Bioenergetics and Its Applications* (3rd edition). Mountain View, CA: Mayfield (1999).

Buford, T. W., R. B. Kreider, J. R. Stout, M. Greenwood, B. Campbell, M. Spano, T. Ziegenfuss, H. Lopez, J. Landis, & J. Antonio: International Society of Sports Nutrition position stand: Creatine supplementation and exercise. *Journal of the International Society of Sports Nutrition*. 4(6):1–8 (2007).

Burleson, M. A., Jr., H. S. O'Bryant, M. H. Stone, M. A. Collins, & T. Triplett-McBride: Effect of weight training exercise and treadmill exercise on post-exercise oxygen consumption. *Medicine & Science in Sports & Exercise*. 30(4):518–522 (1998).

Cairns, S. P.: Lactic acid and exercise performance: Culprit or friend? *Sports Medicine*. 36(4):279–291 (2006).

Carey, D. G., G. J. Pliego, & J. L. Rohwer: The ventilatory response to incremental exercise: Is it one or two breakpoints? *Journal of Strength and Conditioning Research*. 24(10):2840–2845 (2010).

Chatham, J. C.: Lactate—the forgotten fuel! *Journal of Physiology*. 542(2):333 (2002).

Cheetham, M. E., L. H. Boobis, S. Brooks, & C. Williams: Human muscle metabolism during sprint running. *Journal of Applied Physiology*. 61(1):54–60 (1986).

Chia, M. Y. H., N. Armstrong, M. B. A. De Ste Crois, & J. R. Welsman: Longitudinal changes in Wingate Anaerobic Test determined peak and mean power in 10 to 12 year olds. *Pediatric Exercise Science*. 11:272 (1999).

Choi, D., K. J. Cole, B. H. Goodpaster, W. J. Fink, & D. L. Costill: Effect of passive and active recovery on the resynthesis of muscle glycogen. *Medicine and Science in Sports and Exercise*. 26(8):992–996 (1994).

Costill, D. L.: Metabolic responses during distance running. *Journal of Applied Physiology*. 28(3):251–255 (1970).

Costill, D. L., H. Thomason, & E. Roberts: Fractional utilization of the aerobic capacity during distance running. *Medicine and Science in Sports*. 5(4):248–252 (1973).

Crewther, B., J. Cronin, & J. Keogh: Possible stimuli for strength and power adaptation: Acute metabolic responses. *Sports Medicine*. 36(1):65–78 (2006).

Cumming, G. R., L. Hastman, & J. McCort: Treadmill endurance times, blood lactate, and exercise blood pressures in normal children. In Binkhorst, R. A., H. C. G. Kemper, & W. H. M. Saris (eds.): *Children and Exercise XI*. Champaign, IL: Human Kinetics, 140–150 (1985).

Dalbo, V. J., M. D. Roberts, J. R. Stout, & C. M. Kerksick: Putting to rest the myth of creatine supplementation leading to muscle cramps and dehydration. *British Journal of Sports Medicine*. 42(7):567–573 (2008).

Davis, J. A.: Response to Brooks' manuscript. *Medicine and Science in Sports and Exercise*. 17(1):32–34 (1985).

Dewey, K. G., C. A. Lovelady, L. A. Nommsen-Rivers, M. A. McCrory, & B. Lonnerdal: A randomized study of the effects of aerobic exercise by lactating women on breast-milk volume and composition. *New England Journal of Medicine*. 330(7):449–453 (1994).

Dipla, K., T. Tsirini, A. Zafeiridis, V. Manou, A. Dalamitros, E. Kellis, & S. Kellis: Fatigue resistance during high-intensity intermittent exercise from childhood to adulthood in males and females. *European Journal of Applied Physiology*. 106(5):645–653 (2009).

Donovan, C. M. & M. J. Pagliassotti: Quantitative assessment of pathways for lactate disposal in skeletal muscle fiber types. *Medicine & Science in Sports & Exercise*. 32(4):772–777 (2000).

Drummond, J. K., P. R. Vehrs, G. B. Schaalje, & A. C. Parcell: Aerobic and resistance exercise sequence affects excess postexercise oxygen consumption. *Journal of Strength and Conditioning Research*. 19(2):332–337 (2005).

Durand, R. J., V. D. Castracane, D. B. Hollander, J. L. Tryniecki, M. M. Bamman, S. O'Neal, E. P. Hebert, & R. R. Kramer: Hormonal responses from concentric and eccentric muscle contractions. *Medicine & Science in Sports & Exercise*. 35(6):937–943 (2003).

Eriksson, B. O.: Physical training, oxygen supply and muscle metabolism in 11–13 year old boys. *Acta Physiologica Scandinavica (Suppl.)*. 384:1–48 (1972).

Falk, B. & R. Dotan: Child-adult differences in the recovery from high-intensity exercise. *Exercise and Sport Science Reviews*. 34(3):107–112 (2006).

Farrell, P. A., J. H. Wilmore, E. F. Coyle, J. E. Billing, & D. L. Costill: Plasma lactate accumulation and distance running performance. *Medicine and Science in Sports and Exercise*. 11:338–344 (1979).

Fox, E. L.: Measurement of the maximal lactic (phosphagen) capacity in man. *Medicine and Science in Sports (abstract)*. 5:66 (1973).

Freund, H., S. Oyono-Enguéllé, A. Heitz, C. Ott, J. Marbach, M. Gartner, & A. Pape: Comparative lactate kinetics after short and prolonged submaximal exercise. *International Journal of Sports Medicine*. 11(4):284–288 (1990).

Gaesser, G. A. & G. A. Brooks: Muscular efficiency during steady-rate exercise: Effects of speed and work rate. *Journal of Applied Physiology*. 38(6):1132–1139 (1975).

Gaisl, G. & J. Buchberger: Determination of the aerobic and anaerobic thresholds of 10–11 year old boys using blood-gas analysis. In K. Berg & B. O. Eriksson (eds.): *Children and Exercise IX*. Baltimore, MD: University Park Press, International Series of Sport Sciences, 93–98 (1979).

Gastin, P. B.: Energy system interaction and relative contribution during maximal exercise. *Sports Medicine*. 31(10):725–741 (2001).

Gladden, L. B.: A "lactic" perspective on metabolism. *Medicine & Science in Sports & Exercise*. 40(3):477–485 (2008a).

Gladden, L. B.: 200th anniversary of lactate research in muscle. *Exercise and Sport Sciences Reviews*. 36(3):109–115 (2008b).

Gladden, L. B.: Lactate metabolism: a new paradigm for the third millennium. *Journal of Physiology*. 558:5–30 (2004).

Gladden, L. B.: Muscle as a consumer of lactate. *Medicine & Science in Sports & Exercise*. 32(4):764–771 (2000).

Gollnick, P. D., W. M. Bayly, & D. R. Hodgson: Exercise intensity, training, diet, and lactate concentration in muscle and blood. *Medicine and Science in Sports and Exercise*. 18(3):334–340 (1986).

Gollnick, P. D. & L. Hermansen: Biochemical adaptations to exercise: Anaerobic metabolism. In J. H. Wilmore (ed.): *Exercise and Sport Sciences Reviews*. New York, NY: Academic Press (1973).

Gollnick, P. D. & D. W. King: Energy release in the muscle cell. *Medicine and Science in Sports*. 1(1):23–31 (1969).

Grassi, B.: Delayed metabolic activation of oxidative phosphorylation in skeletal muscle at exercise onset. *Medicine & Science in Sports & Exercise*. 37(9):1567–1573 (2005).

Green, H. J.: Muscle power: Fiber type recruitment, metabolism and fatigue. In Jones, N. L., M. McCartney, & A. J. McComas (eds.): *Human Muscle Power*. Champaign, IL: Human Kinetics (1986).

Green, S.: Measurement of anaerobic work capacities in humans. *Sports Medicine*. 19(1):32–42 (1995).

Guyton, A. C. & J. E. Hall: *Textbook of Medical Physiology* (12th edition). Philadelphia, PA: Saunders (2011).

Hagberg, J. M., E. F. Coyle, J. E. Carroll, J. M. Miller, W. H. Martin, & M. H. Brooke: Exercise hyperventilation in patients with McArdle's disease. *Journal of Applied Physiology*. 52:991–994 (1982).

Hashimoto, T. & G. A. Brooks: Mitochondrial lactate oxidation complex and an adaptive role for lactate production. *Medicine & Science in Sports & Exercise*. 40(3):486–494 (2008).

Hermansen, L., S. Maehlum, E. D. R. Pruett, O. Vaage, H. Waldum, & T. Wessel-Aas: Lactate removal at rest and during exercise. In Howald, H. & J. R. Poortmans (eds.): *Metabolic Adaptation to Prolonged Exercise*. Basel: Birkhäuser, 101–105 (1975).

Hermansen, L. & I. Stensvold: Production and removal of lactate during exercise in man. *Acta Physiologica Scandinavica*. 86:191–201 (1972).

Hill, D. W. & J. C. Smith: Gender difference in anaerobic capacity: Role of aerobic contribution. *British Journal of Sports Medicine*. 27(1):45–48 (1993).

Hogan, M. C., L. B. Gladden, S. S. Kurdak, & D. C. Poole: Increased [lactate] in working dog muscle reduces tension development independent of pH. *Medicine and Science in Sports and Exercise*. 27(3):371–377 (1995).

Houston, M. E.: *Biochemistry Primer for Exercise Science*. Champaign, IL: Human Kinetics (1995).

Hughes, E. F., S.C. Turner, & G. A. Brooks: Effect of glycogen depletion and pedaling speed an anaerobic threshold. *Journal of Applied Physiology*. 52 (6):1598–1607(1982).

Hughson, R. L., M. E. Tschakovsky, & M. E. Houston: Regulation of oxygen consumption at the onset of exercise. *Exercise and Sport Science Review*. 29(3):129–133 (2001).

Hughson, R. L., K. H. Weisiger, & G. D. Swanson: Blood lactate concentration increases as a continuous function in progressive exercise. *Journal of Applied Physiology*. 62(5):1975–1981 (1987).

Hultman, E. & K. Sahlin: Acid-base balance during exercise. In Hutton, R. S. & D. I. Miller (eds.): *Exercise and Sport Sciences Reviews*. 8:41–128 (1980).

Inbar, O. & O. Bar-Or: Anaerobic characteristics in male children and adolescents. *Medicine and Science in Sports and Exercise*. 18(3):264–269 (1986).

Jacobs, I.: Blood lactate: Implications for training and sports performance. *Sports Medicine*. 3:10–25 (1986).

Jäger, R., M. Purpura, A. Shao, T. Inoue, & R. B. Kreider: Analysis of the efficacy, safety, and regulatory status of novel forms of creatine. *Amino Acids*. 40:1369–1383 (2011).

Jones, N. L. & R. E. Ehrsam: The anaerobic threshold. In Terjung, R. L. (ed.): *Exercise and Sport Sciences Reviews*. 10:49–83 (1982).

Kanaley, J. A. & R. A. Boileau: The onset of the anaerobic threshold at three stages of physical maturity. *Journal of Sports Medicine and Physical Fitness*. 28(4):367–374 (1988).

Kapit, W., R. I. Macey, & E. Meisami: *The Physiology Coloring Book* (2nd edition). San Francisco: Addison Wesley Longman (2000).

Keul, J., G. Haralambie, M. Bruder, & H.-J. Gottstein: The effect of weight lifting exercise on heart rate and metabolism in experienced weight lifters. *Medicine and Science in Sports*. 10(1):13–15 (1978).

Kinderman, W., G. Simon, & J. Keul: The significance of the aerobic-anaerobic transition for the determination of workload intensities during endurance training. *European Journal of Applied Physiology*. 42:25–34 (1979).

Klentrou, P., M. L. Nishio, & M. Plyley: Ventilatory breakpoints in boys and men. *Pediatric Exercise Science*. 18:216–225 (2006).

Kohrt, W. M., R. J. Spina, A. A. Ehsani, P. E. Cryer, & J. O. Holloszy: Effects of age, adiposity, and fitness level on plasma catecholamine responses to standing and exercise. *Journal of Applied Physiology*. 75(4):1828–1835 (1993).

Kostka, T., W. Drygras, A. Jegier, & D. Zaniewicz: Aerobic and anaerobic power in relation to age and physical activity in 354 men aged 20-88 years. *International Journal of Sports Medicine*. 30(3):225–230 (2009).

Lanza, I. R., D. E. Befroy, & J. A. Kent-Brown: Age-related changes in ATP-producing pathways in human skeletal muscle in vivo. *Journal of Applied Physiology*. 99(5):1769–1744 (2005).

Lamb, G. D.: Point: Lactic acid accumulation is an advantage during muscle activity. *Journal of Applied Physiology*. 100:1410–1412 (2006).

Larsson, L., F. Yu, P. Hook, B. Ramamurthy, J. O. Marx, & P. Pircher: Effects of aging on regulation of muscle contraction at the motor unit, muscle cell, and molecular levels. *International Journal of Sport Nutrition and Exercise Metabolism*. 11(Suppl.):S28–S43 (2001).

Lopez, R. M., D. J. Casa, B. P. McDermott, M. S. Ganio, L. E. Armstrong, & C. M. Maresh: Does creatine supplementation hinder exercise heat tolerance or hydration status? A systematic review with meta-analysis. *Journal of Athletic Training*. 44(2):215–223 (2009).

Mácek, M. & J. Vávra: Anaerobic threshold in children. In Binkhorst, R. A., H. C. G. Kemper, & W. H. M. Saris (eds.): *Children and Exercise XI*. Champaign, IL: Human Kinetics Publishers, 110–113 (1985).

Makrides, L., G. J. F. Heigenhauser, N. McCartney, & N. L. Jones: Maximal short term exercise capacity in healthy subjects aged 15–70 years. *Clinical Science*. 69:197–205 (1985).

Marcinek, D. J., M. J. Kushmerick & K. E. Conley: Lactic acidosis in vivo: Testing the link between lactate generation and H^+ accumulation in ischemic mouse muscle. *Journal of Applied Physiology*. 108:1479–1486 (2010).

Margaria, R., M. T. Edwards, & D. B. Dill: The possible mechanisms of contracting and paying the oxygen debt and the role of lactic acid in muscular contraction. *American Journal of Physiology*. 106:689–715 (1933).

Martin, R. J. F., E. Dore, J. Twisk, E. van Praagh, C. A. Hautier, & M. Bedu: Longitudinal changes of maximal short-term peak power in girls and boys during growth. *Medicine & Science in Sports & Exercise*. 36:498–503 (2004).

Maud, P. J. & B. B. Shultz: Norms for the Wingate Anaerobic Test with comparison to another similar test. *Research Quarterly for Exercise and Sport*. 60(2):144–151 (1989).

McGrail, J. C., A. Bonen, & A. N. Belcastro: Dependence of lactate removal on muscle metabolism in man. *European Journal of Applied Physiology*. 39:87–97 (1978).

Medbo, J. I., A. C. Mohn, I. Tabata, R. Bahr, O. Vaage, & O. M. Sejersted: Anaerobic capacity determined by maximal accumulated O_2 deficit. *Journal of Applied Physiology*. 64:50–60 (1988).

Menzies, P., C. Menzies, L. McIntyre, P. Paterson, J. Wilson, & O. J. Kemi: Blood lactate clearance during active recovery after an intense running bout depends on the intensity of the active recovery. *Journal of Sports Sciences*. 28(9):975–982 (2010).

Meyer, R. A. & R. W. Wiseman: The metabolic systems; Control of ATP synthesis in skeletal muscle. In: Tipton, C. M. (ed): *ACSM's Advanced Exercise Physiology*. Philadelphia, PA: Lippincott Williams & Wilkins, 370–384 (2006).

Misic, M. M. & G. A. Kelley: The impact of creatine supplementation on anaerobic performance: A meta-analysis. *American Journal of Medicine & Sports*. 4:116–124, 2002.

Mougios, V.: *Exercise Biochemistry*. Champaign, IL: Human Kinetics (2006).

Moquin, A. & R. S. Mazzeo: Effect of mild dehydration on the lactate threshold in women. *Medicine & Science in Sports & Exercise*. 32(2):396–402 (2000).

Newsholme, E. A. & A. R. Leech: *Biochemistry for the Medical Sciences*. New York, NY: Wiley (1983).

Noordhof, D. A., J. J. de Koning, & C. Foster: The maximal accumulated oxygen deficit method: A valid and reliable measure of anaerobic capacity? *Sports Medicine*. 40(4):285–302 (2010).

O'Brien, M. J., C. A. Viguie, R. S. Mazzeo, & G. A. Brooks: Carbohydrate dependence during marathon running. *Medicine and Science in Sports and Exercise*. 25(9):1009–1017 (1993).

Patton, J. F., & A. Duggan: An evaluation of tests of anaerobic power. *Aviation and Space Environmental Medicine*. 58:237–242 (1987).

Payne, N., N. Gledhill, P. T. Katmarzyk, V. K. Jamnik, & P. J. Keir: Canadian musculoskeletal fitness norms. *Canadian Journal of Applied Physiology*. 25(6):430–442 (2000).

Péronnet, F. & B. Aguilaniu: Lactic acid buffering, nonmetabolic CO_2 and exercise hyperventilation: A critical reappraisal. *Respiratory Physiology and Neurobiology*. 150(1):4–18 (2006).

Pitts, R. F.: *Physiology of the Kidney and Body Fluids* (3rd edition). Chicago: Year Book Medical (1974).

Poole, D. C. & G. A. Gaesser: Response of ventilatory and lactate threshold to continuous and interval training. *Journal of Applied Physiology*. 58(4):1115–1121 (1985).

Poortmans, J. R. & M. Francaux: Adverse effects of creatine supplementation: Fact or fiction? *SportsMedicine*. 30(3):155–170 (2000).

Poortmans, J. R., E. S. Rawson, L. M. Burke, S. J. Stear, & L. M. Castell: A-Z of nutritional supplements: Dietary supplements, sports nutrition foods and ergogenic aids for health and performance Part 11. *British Journal of Sports Medicine*. 44:765–766 (2010).

Quinn, T. J. & G. B. Carey: Does exercise intensity or diet influence lactic acid accumulation in breast milk? *Medicine & Science in Sports & Exercise*. 31(1):105–110 (1999).

Rasmussen, H. N., G. Van Hall, & U. F. Rasmussen: Lactate dehydrogenase is not a mitochondrial enzyme in human and mouse vastus lateralis muscle. *Journal of Physiology*. 541:575–580 (2002).

Rawson, E. S. & A. M. Persky: Mechanisms of muscular adaptations to creatine supplementation. *International SportMed Journal*. 8(2):43–53 (2007).

Reinhard, V., P. H. Muller, & R. M. Schmulling: Determination of anaerobic threshold by the ventilation equivalent in normal individuals. *Respiration*. 38:36–42 (1979).

Reybrouck, T. M.: The use of the anaerobic threshold in pediatric exercise testing. In Bar-Or, O. (ed.): *Advances in Pediatric Sport Sciences*. Champaign, IL: Human Kinetics Publishers, 131–150 (1989).

Reynolds, T. H., IV, P. A. Frye, & G. A. Sforzo: Resistance training and the blood lactate response to resistance exercise in women. *Journal of Strength and Conditioning Research*. 11(2):77–81 (1997).

Robergs, R. A., F. Ghiasvand, & D. Parker: Biochemistry of exercise-induced metabolic acidosis. *American Journal of Physiology-Regulatory Integrative and Comparative Physiology*. 287:R502–R516 (2004).

Robinson, S.: Experimental studies of physical fitness in relation to age. *Arbeitsphysiologie*. 10:251–323 (1938).

Rogers, M. A. & W. J. Evans: Changes in skeletal muscle with aging: Effects of exercise training. In: Holloszy, J. O. (ed): *Exercise and Sport Sciences Reviews* (vol. 21). Baltimore, MD: Lippincott Williams & Wilkins, 65–101 (1993).

Rowland, T. W.: *Children's Exercise Physiology* (2nd edition). Champaign, IL: Human Kinetics (2005).

Rowland, T. W.: *Exercise and Children's Health*. Champaign, IL: Human Kinetics Publishers (1990).

Sahlin, K., J. M. Ren, & S. Broberg: Oxygen deficit at the onset of submaximal exercise is not due to a delayed oxygen transport. *Acta Physiologica Scandinavica*. 134:175–180 (1988).

Sahlin, K., M. Fernström M. Svenssan & M. Tankanogi: No evidence of an intracellular shuttle in rat skeletal muscle. *Journal of Physiology*. 541:569 (2002).

Santos, A. M. C., N. Armstrong, M. B. A., P. Sharpe, & J. R. Welsman: Optimal peak power in relation to age, body size, gender, and thigh volume. *Pediatric Exercise Science*. 15:406–418 (2003).

Santos, A. M. C., J. R. Welsman, M. B. A. De Ste Crois, & N. Armstrong: Age-and sex-related differences in optimal peak power. *Pediatric Exercise Science*. 14:202–212 (2002).

Saris, W. H. M., A. M. Noordeloos, B. E. M. Ringnalda, M. A. Van't Hof, & R. A. Binkhorst: Reference values for aerobic power of healthy 4 to 18 year old Dutch children: Preliminary results. In Binkhorst, R. A., H. C. G. Kemper, & W. H. M. Saris (eds.): *Children and Exercise XI*. Champaign, IL: Human Kinetics Publishers, 151–160 (1985).

Scott, C. B., B. H. Leighton, K. J. Ahearn, & J. J. McManus: Aerobic, anaerobic, and excess postexercise oxygen consumption energy expenditure of muscular endurance and strength: 1-set of bench press to muscular fatigue. *Journal of Strength and Conditioning*. 25(4): 903–908 (2011).

Scott, C. B., F. B. Roby, T. G. Lohman, & J. C. Bunt: The maximally accumulated oxygen deficit as an indicator of anaerobic capacity. *Medicine and Science in Sports and Exercise*. 23(5):618–624 (1991).

Shao, A. & J. N. Hathcock: Risk assessment for creatine monohydrate. *Regulatory Toxicology and Pharmacology*. 45:242–251 (2006).

Shephard, R. J.: *Physical Activity and Growth*. Chicago: Year Book Medical (1982).

Sidney, K. H. & R. J. Shephard: Maximum and submaximum exercise tests in men and women in the seventh, eighth, and ninth decade of life. *Journal of Applied Physiology: Respiratory, Environmental and Exercise Physiology*. 43(2):280–287 (1977).

Skinner, J. S. & T. H. McLellan: The transition from aerobic to anaerobic metabolism. *Research Quarterly for Exercise and Sport*. 51(1):234–248 (1980).

Smith, E. L; R. C. Serfass (eds.): *Exercise and Aging: The Scientific Basis*. Hillside, N.J.: Enslow Publishers (1981).

Spriet, L. L., R. A. Howlett, & G. J. F. Heigenhauser: An enzymatic approach to lactate production in human skeletal muscle during exercise. *Medicine & Science in Sports & Exercise*. 32(4):756–763 (2000).

Stainsby, W. N. & J. K. Barclay: Exercise metabolism: O2 deficit, steady level O2 uptake and O2 uptake for recovery. *Medicine and Science in Sports*. 2(4):177–181 (1970).

Stallknecht, B., J. Vissing, & J. Galbo: Lactate production and clearance in exercise: Effects of training. A mini review. *Scandinavian Journal of Sports Medicine*. 8:127–131 (1998).

Tesch, P. A.: Short- and long-term histochemical and biochemical adaptations in muscle. In Komi, P. V. (ed.): *Strength and Power in Sports*. Oxford, England: Blackwell Scientific, 239–248 (1992).

Thomas, C., S. A. Plowman, & M. A. Looney: Reliability and Validity of the Anaerobic Speed Test and the Field Anaerobic Shuttle Test for measuring anaerobic work capacity in soccer players. *Measurement in Physical Education and Exercise Science*. 6(3):187–205 (2002).

Vandewalle, H., G. Pérès, & H. Monod: Standard anaerobic exercise tests. *Sports Medicine*. 4:268–289 (1987).

Van Praagh, E.: Development of anaerobic function during childhood and adolescence. *Pediatric Exercise Science*. 12:150-173 (2000).

Van Praagh, E.: Anaerobic fitness tests; what are we measuring? *Medicine and Sport Science*. 50:26–45 (2007).

Wallace, J. P., G. Inbar, & K. Ernsthausen: Infant acceptance of postexercise breast milk. *Pediatrics*. 89(6):1245–1247 (1992).

Wallace, J. P. & J. Rabin: The concentration of lactic acid in breast milk following maximal exercise. *International Journal of Sports Medicine*. 12(3):328–331 (1991).

Walsh, M. L. & E. W. Banister: Possible mechanisms of the anaerobic threshold: A review. *Sports Medicine*. 5:269–302 (1988).

Wasserman, K. & M. B. McIlroy: Detecting the threshold of anaerobic metabolism in cardiac patients during exercise. *American Journal of Cardiology*. 14:844–852 (1964).

Wasserman, K., B. J. Whipp, S. N. Koyal, & W. L. Beaver: Anaerobic threshold and respiratory gas exchange during exercise. *Journal of Applied Physiology*. 35:236–243 (1973).

Weber, C. L. & D. A. Schneider: Maximal accumulated oxygen deficit expressed relative to the active muscle mass for cycling in untrained male and female subjects. *European Journal of Applied Physiology* 82(4):255–261 (2000).

Weber, C. L. & D. A. Schneider: Reliability of MAOD measured at 110% and 120% of peak oxygen uptake for cycling. *Medicine & Science in Sports & Exercise*. 33(6):1056–1059 (2001).

Wells, C. L.: *Women, Sport and Performance: A Physiological Perspective* (2nd edition). Champaign, IL: Human Kinetics Publishers (1991).

Williams, J. R., N. Armstrong, & B. J. Kirby: The 4mM blood lactate level as an index of exercise performance in 11–13 year old children. *Journal of Sport Sciences*. 8:139–147 (1990).

Wiswell, R. A., S. V. Jaque, J. J. Marcell, S. A. Hawkins, K. M. Tarpenning, N.Constantino, & D. M. Hyslop: Maximal aerobic power, lactate threshold, and running performance in master athletes. *Medicine & Science in Sports & Exercise*. 32:1165–1170 (2000).

Wright, K. S., T. J. Quinn, & G. B. Carey: Infant acceptance of breast milk after maternal exercise. *Pediatrics*. 109(4):585–589 (2002).

Aerobic Metabolism during Exercise

4

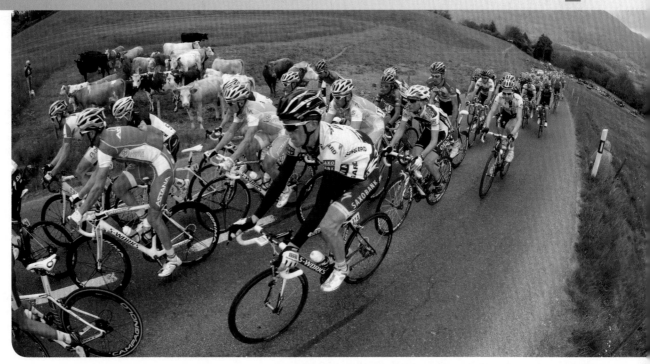

OBJECTIVES

After studying the chapter, you should be able to:

❯ List and explain the major variables used to describe the aerobic metabolic response to exercise.

❯ Explain the laboratory and field assessment techniques used to obtain information on aerobic metabolism during exercise.

❯ Compare and contrast oxygen consumption during aerobic (a) short-term, light- to moderate-intensity exercise; (b) long-term, moderate to heavy submaximal exercise; (c) incremental aerobic exercise to maximum; (d) static and dynamic resistance exercise; and (e) very short-term, high-intensity anaerobic exercise.

❯ Describe how the oxygen cost of breathing changes during exercise.

❯ Calculate the respiratory exchange ratio and interpret what it means in terms of energy substrate utilization.

❯ Calculate the metabolic cost of activity in both kilocalories and metabolic equivalents, and explain how each can be applied.

❯ Differentiate among gross efficiency, net efficiency, and delta efficiency; differentiate between the efficiency and the economy of movement.

❯ List the ways in which an exercising individual can optimize his/her efficiency in walking/running or cycling events.

❯ Compare the walking and running economy of children and older adults with young or middle-aged adults, and discuss possible reasons for the differences.

❯ Explain why efficiency and economy are important for exercise performance.

Introduction

Chapter 3 concentrated on anaerobic exercise responses: situations in which energy is provided predominantly by stored ATP-PC or by the production of ATP through anaerobic glycolysis. Chapter 3 also described anaerobic participation in exercises of lower intensity, longer duration, and incremental exercise to maximum. This chapter focuses on the aerobic responses to the different intensities, durations, and types of exercise. Keep in mind throughout this chapter that aerobic metabolism predominates in activity lasting approximately 2 minutes or longer but that the onset of all activity involves some amount of anaerobic metabolism during the oxygen deficit period. Excess postexercise oxygen consumption (EPOC) occurs following submaximal as well as maximal exercise and is evident following aerobic as well as dynamic resistance exercise.

Laboratory Measurement of Aerobic Metabolism

The primary goal of measuring aerobic metabolism is to quantify how much energy is needed to complete a given activity. This goal can be approached in two ways. To understand these approaches, consider two known aspects of aerobic metabolism. First, aerobic metabolism requires oxygen; and second, it produces heat as a by-product. Therefore, aerobic metabolism can be assessed by measuring oxygen consumption or heat production. Oxygen consumption is measured by indirect open-circuit spirometry, and heat production is measured by calorimetry, as summarized in **Figure 4.1**.

Calorimetry

The term *calorimetry* is derived from the word *calorie*, the basic unit of heat energy. **Calorimetry** is the measurement of heat energy liberated or absorbed in metabolic processes. *Direct calorimetry* actually measures heat production. This measurement requires the use of specially constructed chambers in which the heat produced by a subject increases the temperature of the air or water surrounding the walls and is thereby measured.

Accurate exercise data are difficult to obtain because exercise equipment, even if it fits into the usually small space required, can also emit heat. In addition, the body may store heat (as evidenced by a rise in body temperature) and/or sweat (which must be accounted for). Despite these drawbacks, the direct measurement of heat is the most precise use of the term *calorimetry*.

Spirometry

Spirometry is an indirect calorimetry method for estimating heat production in which expired air is measured and analyzed for the amount of oxygen consumed and

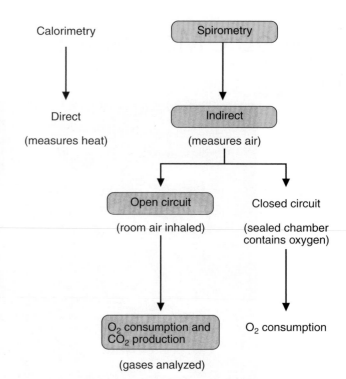

FIGURE 4.1 Measurement of Aerobic Metabolism.
Aerobic metabolism can be measured by direct calorimetry or indirect spirometry. In exercise physiology, open-circuit indirect spirometry/open-circuit indirect calorimetry, in which expired gases are analyzed for O_2 consumed and CO_2 produced, is typically used.
Note: Boxes indicate processes typically used in exercise physiology.

carbon dioxide produced. It is also the direct measurement of air breathed. This method is based on the fact that oxygen consumption at rest or during submaximal exercise is directly proportional to the aerobic production of ATP and, when expressed as calories, is equal to the heat produced by the body as measured by direct calorimetry. However, since heat is not measured directly, spirometry is an *indirect* measure.

In a *closed system*, the subject breathes from a sealed container filled with gas of a designated composition (often 99.9% O_2). Expired CO_2 is usually absorbed by a chemical such as soda lime. The rate of utilization of the available O_2 is then determined. This system has a large error and is rarely used. It is mentioned here so that the terminology of an open circuit can be understood.

In *open-circuit spirometry*, the subject inhales room or outdoor air from his or her surroundings and exhales into the same surroundings. The oxygen content of the inhaled air is normally 20.93%; the carbon dioxide does not need to be absorbed but is simply exhaled into the surrounding atmosphere. A sample of the expired air is analyzed for oxygen and carbon dioxide content.

Putting these factors together results in the descriptor *open-circuit indirect spirometry*. The term *open-circuit indirect calorimetry* should technically be reserved for use when calories are calculated from oxygen consumption, but, in fact, that term is often used interchangeably with open-circuit indirect spirometry, and we will do so in this text.

Measuring oxygen consumption by open-circuit indirect spirometry is a valid way to assess aerobic metabolism during resting and steady-state submaximal exercise, conditions when the relationship between oxygen consumption and ATP production remains linear. However, in situations also involving anaerobic energy production, the actual energy cost of the exercise will be underestimated, because the linear relationship no longer exists and there is no way to account for the anaerobic portion.

Open-circuit indirect spirometry can be used to measure oxygen consumption during any physical activity. However, the size, sensitivity, and lack of portability of the equipment have, until recently, limited its use to modalities that can be performed in a laboratory or a special swimming pool setup. By far, the most popular exercise-testing modalities in the laboratory are the motor-driven treadmill and the cycle ergometer. Measurements can be performed with the subject at rest, during submaximal exercise, or at maximal levels of exertion. The following sections describe in detail how these measurements are done and the aerobic responses to varying patterns of exercise.

Aerobic Exercise Responses

Figure 4.2 shows an individual attached to an analysis system for open-circuit indirect spirometry. The individual uses a breathing valve, which permits air to flow in only one direction at a time—in from room air and out toward the sampling chamber. The nose clip ensures that the individual breathes only through the mouth.

Oxygen Consumption and Carbon Dioxide Production

Figure 4.3 shows schematic configurations of an open-circuit system in which the volume of either inspired air (Figure 4.3A) or expired air (Figure 4.3B) is measured

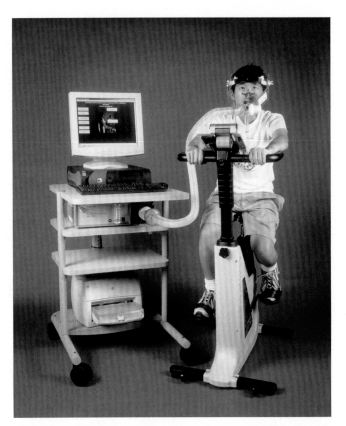

FIGURE 4.2 Subject Undergoing Assessment of Aerobic Metabolism during Exercise. See animation, Oxygen Consumption, at http://thePoint.lww.com/Plowman4e.

Calorimetry The measurement of heat energy liberated or absorbed in metabolic processes.

Spirometry An indirect calorimetry method for estimating heat production, in which expired air is analyzed for the amount of oxygen consumed and carbon dioxide produced.

Oxygen Consumption ($\dot{V}O_2$) The amount or volume of oxygen taken up, transported, and used at the cellular level.

Carbon Dioxide Produced ($\dot{V}CO_2$) The amount or volume of carbon dioxide generated during metabolism.

---

and the expired air is analyzed for the percentage of oxygen and carbon dioxide. Although oxygen consumption is the variable of primary interest, given its direct relationship with ATP, determining the amount of carbon dioxide produced is also important because that measure enables a determination about fuel utilization and caloric expenditure.

Oxygen consumption ($\dot{V}O_2$) is technically the *amount* of oxygen taken up, transported, and used at the cellular level. It equals the amount of oxygen inspired minus the amount of oxygen expired. However, as the symbol $\dot{V}O_2$ indicates, it is commonly labeled as the *volume* of oxygen consumed. Similarly, **carbon dioxide produced ($\dot{V}CO_2$)** is technically the amount of carbon dioxide generated during metabolism, primarily from aerobic cellular respiration. It equals the amount of carbon dioxide expired minus the amount of carbon dioxide inspired. As with $\dot{V}O_2$, $\dot{V}CO_2$ is commonly described as the volume of carbon dioxide produced.

The *amount* of a gas equals the volume of air (either inhaled or exhaled) times the percentage of the gas. Therefore, to determine these amounts, the volume of air either inhaled or exhaled is measured, as are the percentages of oxygen and carbon dioxide in the exhaled air. The percentages of oxygen and carbon dioxide in inhaled air are known to be 20.93% and 0.03%, respectively.

FIGURE 4.3 Open-Circuit Indirect Spirometry with Online Computer Analysis.

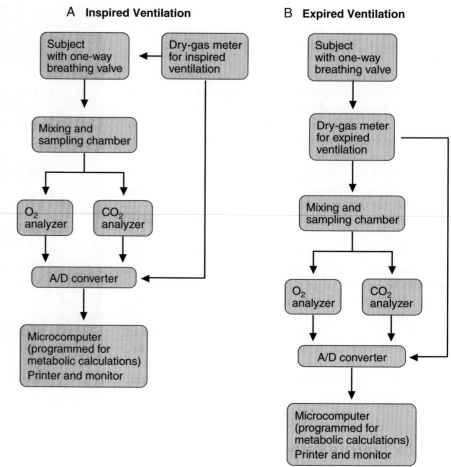

A Inspired Ventilation

Subject with one-way breathing valve ← Dry-gas meter for inspired ventilation

Subject with one-way breathing valve → Mixing and sampling chamber → O$_2$ analyzer / CO$_2$ analyzer → A/D converter → Microcomputer (programmed for metabolic calculations) Printer and monitor

B Expired Ventilation

Subject with one-way breathing valve → Dry-gas meter for expired ventilation → Mixing and sampling chamber → O$_2$ analyzer / CO$_2$ analyzer → A/D converter → Microcomputer (programmed for metabolic calculations) Printer and monitor

These mathematical relationships can be formulated as follows:

4.1 oxygen consumption (L·min^{-1}) = (volume of air inspired [L·min^{-1}] × percentage of oxygen in inspired air) − (volume of air expired [L·min^{-1}] × percentage of oxygen in expired air)

or

$$\dot{V}O_2 \text{ cons} = (\dot{V}_I \times \%O_2 \text{ insp}) - (\dot{V}_E \times \%O_2 \text{ expir})$$

4.2 carbon dioxide produced (L·min^{-1}) = (volume of air expired [L·min^{-1}] × percentage of carbon dioxide in expired air) × (volume of air inspired × percentage of carbon dioxide in inspired air)

or

$$\dot{V}CO_2 \text{ prod} = (\dot{V}_E \times \%CO_2 \text{ expir}) - (\dot{V}_I \times \%CO_2 \text{ insp})$$

The volume of air inhaled is usually not exactly equal to the volume of air exhaled. However, knowing either the value of air inhaled or exhaled and the gas percentages allows us to calculate the other air volume. These calculations are fully described in Appendix B.

Most laboratories use computer software to solve Equations 4.1 and 4.2. **Table 4.1** gives the results of such a computer program for a metabolic test. The first 3 minutes represent resting values. The values for the next 8 minutes were obtained during treadmill walking at 3.5 mi·hr^{-1} (94 m·min^{-1}, or 5.6 km·hr^{-1}) at 7% grade. Ignore for the time being minutes 33 through 37 as well as the missing minutes. Locate in **Figure 4.3** the pieces equipment referred to in the following discussion. The dot above the volume symbol ($\dot{V}$) indicates per unit of time, which is usually 1 minute.

The volume of air inspired ($\dot{V}_I$) or expired ($\dot{V}_E$) is measured by a pneumoscan or flowmeter (labeled as the dry gas meter in **Figure 4.3**). Typically, all ventilation values are reported as expired values that have been adjusted to standard temperature (0°C), standard pressure (760 mmHg), and dry (without water vapor) conditions, known as STPD. The process and rationale for standardizing ventilatory volumes are discussed fully in Chapter 9. Standardization permits comparisons between data collected under different conditions. Two things should be noted about the $\dot{V}_E$ STPD values. First, the values for exercise (Ex) are higher than those at rest (R) ($\overline{X}R = 7.93$ L·min^{-1}, $\overline{X}Ex = 25.41$).

TABLE 4.1   Aerobic Metabolic Responses at Rest and During Submaximal Exercise

Sex = Female Ambient Temperature = 18°C
Age = 22 yr Barometric Pressure = 752 mmHg
Weight = 53.4 kg Relative Humidity = 5%

Time (min)	$\dot{V}_E$ STPD ($L \cdot min^{-1}$)	O_2%	CO_2%	$\dot{V}O_2$ ($L \cdot min^{-1}$)	$\dot{V}CO_2$ ($L \cdot min^{-1}$)	$\dot{V}O_2$ ($mL \cdot kg^{-1} \cdot min^{-1}$)	RER	HR ($b \cdot min^{-1}$)
Rest (Standing)								
1	7.57	17.11	3.26	0.30	0.23	5.61	0.81	75
2	7.58	17.21	3.20	0.29	0.23	5.43	0.82	75
3	8.64	16.95	3.37	0.34	0.28	6.55	0.80	75
$\bar{X}$	7.93	17.09	3.28	0.31	0.25	5.86	0.81	75
3.5 $mi \cdot hr^{-1}$ Walking (Steady State); 7% Grade								
1	21.96	15.85	4.34	1.14	0.93	21.53	0.81	120
2	24.20	15.85	4.60	1.25	1.10	23.59	0.87	136
3	23.46	15.73	4.76	1.25	1.10	23.40	0.88	136
4	26.07	16.02	4.66	1.29	1.20	24.15	0.93	136
5	25.71	15.95	4.73	1.29	1.20	24.34	0.92	136
6	27.53	16.03	4.68	1.35	1.27	25.46	0.93	136
7	25.71	15.91	4.79	1.29	1.22	4.34	0.93	136
8	28.64	16.06	4.68	1.39	1.33	26.21	0.94	136
$\bar{X}$	25.41	15.93	4.66	1.28	1.17	24.13	0.90	136
3.5 $mi \cdot hr^{-1}$ Walking (Oxygen Drift); 7% Grade								
33	28.64	16.26	4.56	1.33	1.29	25.09	0.96	140
34	31.21	16.33	4.55	1.43	1.41	26.96	0.98	144
35	31.21	16.32	4.54	1.43	1.39	26.96	0.97	144
36	30.84	16.16	4.67	1.47	1.43	27.71	0.96	146
37	32.31	16.19	4.68	1.52	1.50	28.65	0.97	150

This individual had a $\dot{V}O_2$max of 47.64 $mL \cdot kg^{-1} \cdot min^{-1}$, or 2.54 $L \cdot min^{-1}$.

Second, within each condition, the values are very stable.

The air the subject exhales is sampled from a mixing chamber and analyzed by electronic gas analyzers that have been previously calibrated by gases of known composition. Data about the percentage of expired oxygen (O_2% in **Table 4.1**) and carbon dioxide (CO_2% in **Table 4.1**) are relayed from the gas analyzers along with ventilation values through an analog-to-digital (A/D) converter to the computer. Remember that room air is composed of 20.93% O_2, 0.03% CO_2, 79.04% N_2, and other trace elements such as argon and krypton. N_2 is considered to be inert in human metabolism. However, as we have seen in the metabolic pathways, O_2 is consumed and CO_2 is produced when ATP is generated aerobically. Therefore, in general, the exhaled O_2% will be lower than the value in ambient air, ranging around 15–16% during moderate exercise. Exhaled CO_2 values will be greater than that in room air, increasing to somewhere around 4–6% during moderate exercise. Note these values in **Table 4.1**. During rest, not much oxygen is used, so the percentage exhaled is relatively high ($\bar{X}R = 17.09\%$). The accompanying CO_2% is, as would be expected, relatively low ($\bar{X}R = 3.28\%$). During exercise, more O_2 is used to produce energy, so there is a lower percentage of O_2 exhaled ($\bar{X}E = 15.93\%$). The use of more O_2 to produce more energy also results in the production of more CO_2 ($\bar{X}Ex = 4.66\%$).

The computer software uses metabolic formulas to correct ventilation for temperature (room temperature if $\dot{V}_I$ is measured); expired air temperature (if $\dot{V}_E$ is measured), relative humidity (if $\dot{V}_I$ is measured), and barometric pressure. Then using the expired percentage values of O_2 and CO_2, it calculates values for the volume of O_2 consumed ($\dot{V}O_2$ $L \cdot min^{-1}$ and $\dot{V}O_2$ in $mL \cdot kg^{-1} \cdot min^{-1}$), CO_2 produced ($\dot{V}CO_2$ in $L \cdot min^{-1}$), and the ratio of the volume of CO_2 produced divided by the volume of O_2 consumed, known as the respiratory exchange ratio (RER).

Sometimes this relationship is designated simply as R, but this text will consistently use RER. The $\dot{V}O_2$ and $\dot{V}CO_2$ values are actual volumes of the gases that are used and produced by the body, respectively. The $L \cdot min^{-1}$ unit represents the absolute amount of gas on a per-minute basis. The $mL \cdot kg^{-1} \cdot min^{-1}$ unit takes into account body size (body weight [BW] is given at the top of the table) and is therefore considered a relative value; it describes how many milliliters of gas are consumed (or produced) for each kilogram of BW each minute.

The absolute unit (L·min^{-1}) is highly influenced by body size, with large individuals showing the highest values. Therefore, it is most useful when comparing an individual to himself or herself under different conditions, such as before and after a training program, to determine whether a change in fitness has occurred. Use of the absolute unit is particularly important if the individual has lost weight, because the mL·kg^{-1}·min^{-1} relative value goes up as weight goes down regardless of whether or not actual fitness has improved. The mL·kg^{-1}·min^{-1} value thus, to an extent, equates individuals by factoring out the influence of body size. It is therefore typically used for comparisons between individuals.

Another unit used to express O_2 consumed and CO_2 produced on a relative basis is mL·kg FFB^{-1}·min^{-1} or mL·kg LBM^{-1}·min^{-1}, where FFB stands for fat-free body and LBM stands for lean body mass. To calculate these units, the individual's percentage of body fat must be known and used to determine what portion of the total BW is fat free or lean. This unit is often used in comparisons between the sexes. However, it is not a very practical measure because no one has yet figured how to avoid carrying one's fat during exercise.

At rest, the subject in the example in **Table 4.1** is using about 0.31 L·min^{-1}, or 310 mL·min^{-1}, of oxygen and producing about 0.25 L·min^{-1} of carbon dioxide. During exercise, she is using 1.28 L·min^{-1} of oxygen and producing 1.17 L·min^{-1} of carbon dioxide.

Short-Term, Light- to Moderate-Intensity Submaximal Exercise

Look at minutes 1–8 in **Table 4.1**. During this light exercise, there is very little minute-to-minute variation in any of the variables after the first minute of adjustment. A comparison of the individual's mean oxygen cost of these 8 minutes (24.13 mL·kg^{-1}·min^{-1}) with her $\dot{V}O_2$max (47.64 mL·kg^{-1}·min^{-1}) shows that she is working at approximately 50% $\dot{V}O_2$max. When the exercise performed is at less than 70% $\dot{V}O_2$max and the duration is 5–10 minutes, the oxygen consumption should level off and remain relatively constant for the duration of the work after the initial rise (**Figure 4.4A**). This condition is known as *steady-state* or *steady-rate* exercise. The time to achieve steady state varies from 1 to 3 minutes in youths and young adults at low and moderate levels of intensity, but it increases with higher intensity exercise (Morgan et al., 1989b). The time to achieve steady state is longer in older adults.

Long-Term, Moderate to Heavy Submaximal Exercise

Now look carefully at minutes 33 through 37 in **Table 4.1**. Pay particular attention to the $\dot{V}O_2$ L·min^{-1} and mL·kg^{-1}·min^{-1} values. Despite the fact that the workload has not changed, a gradual increase occurs in these variables. When exercise is performed at a level greater

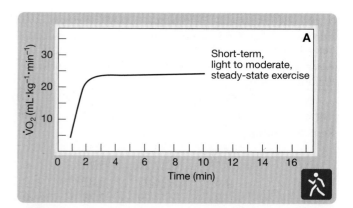

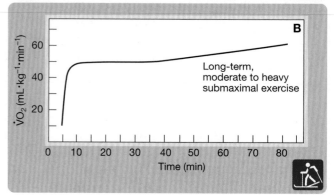

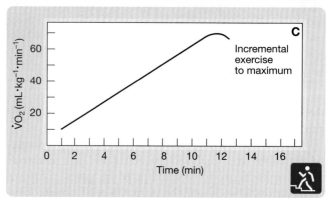

FIGURE 4.4 Oxygen Consumption Responses to Various Exercises.
A. Short-term, light to moderate, submaximal aerobic exercise. **B.** Long-term, moderate to heavy, submaximal dynamic aerobic exercise. **C.** Incremental aerobic exercise to maximum.

than 70% $\dot{V}O_2$max; or when exercise is performed at a lower percentage of $\dot{V}O_2$max, as in this case, but for a long duration; or if the conditions are hot and humid, a phenomenon known as **oxygen drift** occurs. In oxygen drift, the oxygen consumption increases despite the fact that the oxygen requirement of the activity has not changed. A schematic representation of oxygen drift is presented in **Figure 4.4B**.

The oxygen consumption increases (drifts upward) because of rising blood levels of catecholamine hormones (epinephrine and norepinephrine), lactate accumulation (if the % $\dot{V}O_2$ is high enough), shifting substrate utilization

TABLE 4.2 Aerobic Metabolic Responses during an Incremental Treadmill Test (Modified Balke Protocol)

Sex = Male   Ambient temperature = 23°C
Age = 22 yr   Barometric pressure = 739 mmHg
Weight = 66 kg   Relative humidity = 13%

Time (min)	$\dot{V}_E$ STPD	$O_2\%$	$CO_2\%$	$\dot{V}O_2$ (L·min^{-1})	$\dot{V}O_2$ (mL·kg^{-1}·min^{-1})	$\dot{V}CO_2$ (L·min^{-1})	RER	HR (b·min^{-1})
2	25.21	16.47	4.45	1.12	16.96	1.10	0.99	82
3	27.31	16.36	4.54	1.25	18.93	1.22	0.98	84
4	29.06	16.30	4.62	1.33	20.30	1.30	0.98	100
5	29.75	16.18	4.71	1.41	21.36	1.39	0.98	98
6	33.62	16.09	4.84	1.62	24.54	1.60	0.99	108
7	30.17	16.08	4.99	1.45	21.96	1.49	1.03	105
8	34.37	15.99	5.03	1.68	25.45	1.72	1.01	120
9	37.92	16.09	5.03	1.81	27.42	1.89	1.04	117
10	37.17	16.07	4.96	1.79	27.12	1.83	1.02	115
11	38.84	15.89	5.00	1.95	29.69	1.93	0.98	123
12	39.56	15.82	5.10	2.01	30.60	2.00	0.99	122
13	39.84	15.57	5.23	2.15	32.57	2.07	0.96	124
14	43.37	15.51	5.30	2.36	35.75	2.28	0.96	132
15	46.64	15.62	5.41	2.45	37.27	2.50	1.01	144
16	47.37	15.68	5.42	2.45	37.27	2.54	1.03	138
17	50.87	15.85	5.21	2.55	38.78	2.62	1.02	143
18	51.53	15.52	5.48	2.78	42.12	2.80	1.01	146
19	55.12	15.73	5.38	2.83	42.87	2.95	1.03	155
20	56.84	15.74	5.32	2.91	44.24	3.00	1.02	158
21	58.54	15.63	5.38	3.08	46.81	3.12	1.01	162
22	59.95	15.58	5.43	3.19	48.33	3.23	1.01	167
23	68.06	15.59	5.47	3.61	54.69	3.70	1.02	180
24	78.06	15.69	5.55	4.01	60.90	4.30	1.07	181
25	85.18	15.70	5.62	4.36	66.21	4.75	1.08	188
26	94.94	15.78	5.75	4.68	71.06	5.39	1.14	192
27	112.96	16.29	5.51	4.98	75.45	6.18	1.24	196
28	139.04	16.97	4.94	5.11	77.52	6.83	1.34	200

(to greater carbohydrate), increased cost of ventilation, and increased body temperature. Thus, although any given level of exercise typically requires a specific amount of oxygen, this amount has some individual and circumstantial variation (Daniels, 1985).

Incremental Aerobic Exercise to Maximum

Table 4.2 provides the results of a computer program for an incremental treadmill test to maximum. In this

> **Oxygen Drift** A situation that occurs in submaximal activity of long duration, or above 70% $\dot{V}O_2$max, or in hot and humid conditions where the oxygen consumption increases, despite the fact that the oxygen requirement of the activity has not changed.

case, the subject was a very fit male senior exercise science major who regularly and successfully competed in long-distance running, cycling, and duathlon events. In an incremental exercise test such as this, the participant is asked to continue to the point of *volitional fatigue*, that is, until he is too tired to go on any longer. Throughout the test, the speed and/or grade is systematically raised so that the exercise becomes progressively harder. The protocol used in this particular test is called the modified Balke. For this test, the speed was kept constant at 3.5 mi hr^{-1} (94 m·min^{-1}). The grade was 0% for the first minute and 2% for the second minute, increasing 1% per minute thereafter. At the treadmill limit of 25% grade, speed was then increased 13.4 m·min^{-1} each minute. Because the increments are small, the individual should be able to adjust to the load change in just 1 minute for most of the submaximal portion. Typically, the goal is for a maximal test to last 12–15 minutes. Because of his very high fitness, this individual was able to continue for 28 minutes.

Because the work is different, the ventilation, $\dot{V}O_2$, and $\dot{V}CO_2$ responses are also different from those of the submaximal steady-state exercise in **Table 4.1**. In the incremental task, ventilation ($\dot{V}_E$), $\dot{V}O_2$, and $\dot{V}CO_2$ values all increase as a result of the increasing demands for and production of energy. For this particular individual, the volume of expired air ($\dot{V}_E$ STPD) rose from 25.21 $L\cdot min^{-1}$ at minute 2 to 139.04 $L\cdot min^{-1}$ at minute 28. This demonstrates the reserve capacity in the ventilatory system. Oxygen consumption increased from slightly over 1 $L\cdot min^{-1}$ (or almost 17 $mL\cdot kg^{-1}\cdot min^{-1}$) to just over 5 $L\cdot min^{-1}$ at maximum. At this point, the individual was producing as much ATP as he could aerobically.

The highest amount of oxygen an individual can take in, transport, and utilize to produce ATP aerobically while breathing air during heavy exercise is called **maximal oxygen consumption ($\dot{V}O_2$max)**. The exercise tester has to decide whether any given test truly is a maximal effort before labeling the highest $\dot{V}O_2$ value as maximal. Several physiological criteria can be used to determine whether the test is a maximal test: (a) a lactate value greater than 8 $mmol\cdot L^{-1}$ (Åstrand, 1956; Åstrand and Rodahl, 1977); (b) a heart rate ±12 $b\cdot min^{-1}$ of predicted maximal heart rate (220 minus age) (Durstine and Pate, 1988); (c) a respiratory exchange ratio (RER) (which is described fully later in this chapter) of 1.0 or 1.1, primarily depending on the age of the subject (Holly, 1988; MacDougall et al., 1982); and (d) a plateau in oxygen consumption. The classic definition of a plateau is a rise of 2.1 $mL\cdot kg^{-1}\cdot min^{-1}$ or less, or a rise of 0.15 $L\cdot min^{-1}$ or less, in oxygen consumption ($\dot{V}O_2$) with an increase in workload that represents a change in grade of 2.5% while running at 7 $mi\cdot hr^{-1}$ (11.2 $km\cdot hr^{-1}$) with 3-minute stages (Taylor et al., 1955). Use of this criterion for all protocols, however, has been questioned (Howley et al., 1995). One alternative is to define a plateau as an increase of less than half the expected theoretical rise based on the change in speed, grade, or speed and grade (Plowman and Liu, 1999). The expected increase can be calculated using the American College of Sports Medicine [ACSM] (2010) equations provided in Appendix B. In this case, the expected difference in oxygen consumption between the last 2 minutes (27 and 28) is 5.8 $mL\cdot kg^{-1}\cdot min^{-1}$. Occasionally, a rating of perceived exertion (RPE) equal to or greater than 17 is used as a psychophysiological criterion (Howley et al., 1995). Complete the Check Your Comprehension 1 to apply these criteria.

CHECK YOUR COMPREHENSION 1

Did the individual in **Table 4.2** meet the HR and $\dot{V}O_2$ criteria for a true maximal test?
Check your answer in Appendix C.

The rectilinear increase in $\dot{V}O_2$ can be generalized to all healthy individuals, both male and female, young and old, and those who are high and low in fitness. This pattern is schematically represented in **Figure 4.4C**. However, the plateau is not always evident in children and the elderly. In these cases, the term *peak oxygen consumption* ($\dot{V}O_2$peak) to describe the highest value attained is more accurate than the term maximal oxygen consumption ($\dot{V}O_2$max).

As a result of the increasing ATP production, the amount of CO_2 produced also increases. Note in **Table 4.2** that the amount of CO_2 produced ($\dot{V}CO_2$) is generally not equal to the amount of O_2 consumed ($\dot{V}O_2$). Note also that despite the incremental nature of this test, the O_2% and CO_2% do not vary much. There is a slight decline in O_2% and a parallel rise in CO_2% after the first 10 minutes and then relatively steady values until the last 2 minutes, when the O_2% goes back up and the CO_2% goes back down just a little. Frequently, as a subject nears maximal exertion, the O_2% may rise to 17% and the CO_2% may drop to 3%. These small percentage changes, especially when they occur in the last couple of minutes, are compensated for by the increasingly larger volumes of air being ventilated.

Static and Dynamic Resistance Exercise

Physiological responses to static exercise are generally described in relation to the percentage of maximal voluntary contraction (MVC) at which they take place. Depending on the muscle group used, static contractions below 15–25% MVC do not fully occlude blood flow, such that oxygen can still be delivered to working muscles. At such loads, however, little extra energy above the resting level is required, and oxygen consumption increases minimally, perhaps as little as 50 $mL\cdot min^{-1}$, but for as long as half an hour (Asmussen, 1981; Shepard et al., 1981).

The higher the percentage of MVC of the static contraction, the greater the intramuscular pressure is, the more likely it is that the blood flow will be completely arrested or occluded, and the shorter the time that the contraction can be maintained. If occlusion of blood flow is not complete, oxygen consumption increases. This increased oxygen consumption is higher than the amount at lower percentages of MVC but still far below the rise in values that occurs during the aerobic endurance exercises previously described.

In addition to a lower oxygen consumption, there is one other major difference between static and dynamic-endurance exercise. At the cessation of static exercise, when blood flow is fully restored, a sudden increase in oxygen consumption occurs (**Figure 4.5**) before the slow, gradual decline of the typical EPOC curve begins (Asmussen, 1981; Shepard et al., 1981).

The primary source of energy for dynamic resistance activity such as weight lifting or wrestling is anaerobic

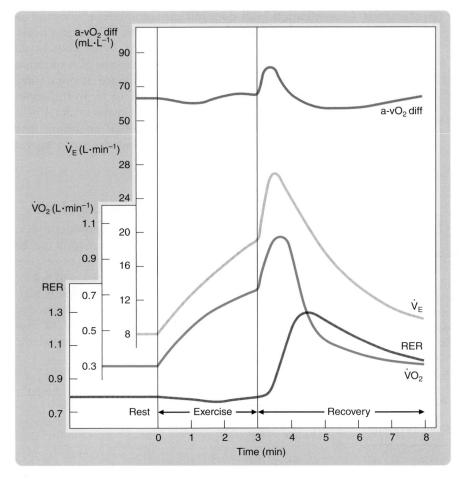

FIGURE 4.5 Respiratory and Metabolic Responses to Heavy Static Exercise. Heavy static exercise causes small respiratory (a-vO$_2$diff and $\dot{V}_E$) and metabolic ($\dot{V}O_2$ and RER) responses during the actual contraction. However, each of these variables shows an increased rebound effect immediately upon cessation of the exercise before slowly returning to preexercise values.
Source: Asmussen, E.: Similarities and dissimilarities between static and dynamic exercise. *Circulation Research (Suppl.).* 48 (6):I-3–I-10 (1981). Copyright 1981 by the American Heart Association. Reprinted by permission.

(Fleck and Kraemer, 1987; Fox and Mathews, 1974). In part, anaerobic energy is used because dynamic resistance exercise has a static component. In part, anaerobic energy is used due to the high intensity and short duration of the exercise. Despite the predominance of anaerobic energy sources, dynamic resistance activity has an aerobic component as well. The more the repetitions and the longer the duration of the sets in a weight-lifting workout, the greater is the aerobic contribution. Actual values are not available for different routines because such activities are intended for anaerobic, not aerobic, benefits. However, an example of the oxygen contribution to five sets of 6–12 repetitions per set of supine leg press exercise can be seen in **Figure 4.6** (Tesch et al., 1990). In this group of untrained males, a gradual rise in oxygen consumption occurs over the first three sets, at which point the oxygen consumption basically stabilizes for the remaining two sets. The oxygen cost represents approxi-

mately 33–47% of the average maximal oxygen consumption for these subjects. Thus, the aerobic contribution during weight-lifting exercise can be expected to be somewhat less than the oxygen costs of most aerobic endurance activities but higher than the cost of purely static exercise (Tesch et al., 1990).

Very Short-Term, High-Intensity Anaerobic Exercise

As stated in Chapter 3, historically the contribution of aerobic metabolism to short, intense exercise has probably been underestimated because of the difficulty of obtaining accurate measurements. However, data are available to show that even the most widely used anaerobic test, the 30-second Wingate Anaerobic Test, has an aerobic energy contribution of almost 25–30% (Bar-Or, 1987; Gastin, 2001).

The Oxygen Cost of Breathing

Part of the oxygen used both at rest and during exercise goes to support the respiratory muscles. This value does not remain constant but varies with the intensity of activity. During rest, the respiratory system uses about 1–2%

Maximal Oxygen Consumption ($\dot{V}O_2$max) The highest amount of oxygen an individual can take in, transport and utilize to produce ATP aerobically while breathing air during heavy exercise.

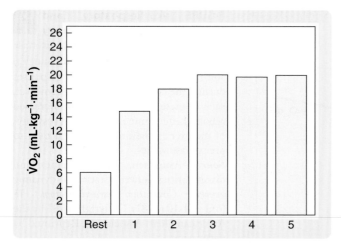

FIGURE 4.6 Aerobic Contribution to Dynamic Resistance Exercise.

Oxygen consumption was measured before and during five sets of 6–12 repetitions of supine leg presses. The values represent the combined results of two groups: one performed only the concentric (lifting) phase and the other performed both the concentric and eccentric (lowering) phases. The addition of the eccentric phase represented such a low additional energy cost above just the concentric energy expenditure that it was not separated out.

Source: Based on Tesch, P. A., P. Buchanan, & G. A. Dudley: An approach to counteracting long-term microgravity-induced muscle atrophy. *The Physiologist*. 33(Suppl. 1):S77–S79 (1990).

of the total body oxygen consumption, or 2.5 mL·min^{-1} of oxygen. The oxygen cost of ventilation is higher in children than in middle-aged or older adults (Bar-Or, 1983; Pardy et al., 1984).

During light to moderate submaximal dynamic aerobic exercise, where $\dot{V}_E$ is less than 60 L·min^{-1}, the respiratory oxygen cost changes to about 25–100 mL·min^{-1}. At heavy submaximal exercise, when $\dot{V}_E$ is between 60 and 120 L·min^{-1}, respiratory oxygen use may rise to 50–400 mL·min^{-1}. During incremental exercise to maximum, the initial $\dot{V}_E$ during the lower exercise stages shows a very gradual curvilinear rise, reflecting the submaximal changes described previously. At workloads above those requiring a $\dot{V}_E$ greater than 120 L·min^{-1}, a dramatic exponential curve occurs. In this curve, by the time a $\dot{V}_E$ of 180 L·min^{-1} is achieved in a very fit individual, 1000–1300 mL·min^{-1} of oxygen is used simply to support respiration (Pardy et al., 1984).

Theoretically, there may be a maximal level of ventilation above which any further increase in oxygen consumption would be used entirely by the ventilatory musculature, thus limiting maximal exercise (Bye et al., 1983; Otis, 1954; Pardy et al., 1984; Vella et al., 2006). At what precise point this critical level of ventilation occurs is unknown. However, even if a critical

ventilation level does not exist, respiration does utilize a significant portion, 3–18%, of the $\dot{V}O_2$ during heavy exercise (Bye et al., 1983; Shephard, 1966; Vella et al., 2006). Smoking increases the oxygen cost of respiration during exercise. However, an abstinence of even 1 day can substantially reduce this effect of cigarette smoking (Rode and Shephard, 1971; Shepard et al., 1981). In old age, the higher oxygen cost of breathing may be a significant factor in limiting exercise performance (Shepard et al., 1981).

Respiratory Quotient/Respiratory Exchange Ratio

When the $\dot{V}O_2$ consumed and $\dot{V}CO_2$ produced during exercise are known, much useful information can be derived. One such derived variable—**RER, or respiratory exchange ratio**—is given in both **Tables 4.1 and 4.2**.

The RER reflects on a total body level what is happening at the cellular level. The ratio of the amount of carbon dioxide (CO_2) produced to the amount of oxygen consumed (O_2) at the cellular level is termed the **respiratory quotient (RQ)**. The formula is

4.3   respiratory quotient = carbon dioxide produced (molecules) ÷ oxygen consumed (molecules)

or

$$RQ = \frac{CO_2}{O_2}$$

This formula may also be computed using L·g^{-1} in place of molecules.

The values of carbon dioxide produced and oxygen consumed are known for the oxidation of carbohydrate, fat, and protein, both on a cellular level and in absolute amounts (L·g^{-1}). The latter values are presented in **Table 4.3**. The amount of oxygen consumed and the amount of carbon dioxide produced vary among the major fuel sources because of the differences in their chemical composition. The following examples compute the cellular level RQ for each major fuel source both per mole of a specific substrate (the carbohydrate, glucose, $C_6H_{12}O_6$; the fat, palmitic acid, $C_{16}H_{32}O_2$; and the protein, albumin, $C_{72}H_{112}N_2O_{22}S$) and per gram of carbohydrate (glucose), fat (fatty acid), total protein, and branched-chain amino acids. In each case, the oxygen used (left side of the equation) and carbon dioxide produced (right side of the equation) are inserted into Equation 4.3 to determine the RQ. The values of 1.0 for carbohydrate, 0.7 for fat, and 0.81 for protein calculated in the example are the classic accepted values for RQ.

Because these values for RQ have been derived from the cellular oxidation of specific foodstuffs, knowing the RQ allows one to estimate the fuels utilized in

TABLE 4.3   Energy Production from Carbohydrate, Fat, and Protein

	Carbohydrate		Protein		Fat
Primary utilization in exercise	High-intensity, short-duration exercise		Ultradistance exercise and glucose precursor		Low-intensity, long-duration exercise and glucose precursor
Form in which utilized by muscles	Glucose	Glycogen	*	Branched-chain amino acids	Fatty acids
Oxygen needed to utilize per gram ($L \cdot g^{-1}$)	0.75 L·g^{-1}	0.83 L·g^{-1}	0.965 L·g^{-1}	1.24 L·g^{-1}	2.02 L·g^{-1}
Energy produced per gram ($kcal \cdot g^{-1}$)	3.75 kcal·g^{-1} 15.68 kJ·g^{-1}	4.17 kcal·g^{-1} 17.43 kJ·g^{-1}	4.3 kcal·g^{-1} 17.97 kJ·g^{-1}	3.76 kcal·g^{-1} 18.09 kJ·g^{-1}	9.3 kcal·g^{-1} 38.87 kJ·g^{-1}
Energy produced per liter of oxygen[†] ($kcal \cdot L^{-1} O_2$)	$5.03 \text{ kcal·L}^{-1} O_2$ $21.03 \text{ kJ·L}^{-1} O_2$	$5.03 \text{ kcal·L}^{-1} O_2$ $21.03 \text{ kJ·L}^{-1} O_2$	$4.46 \text{ kcal·L}^{-1} O_2$ $18.64 \text{ kJ·L}^{-1} O_2$	$3.03 \text{ kcal·L}^{-1} O_2$ $12.67 \text{ kJ·L}^{-1} O_2$	$4.61 \text{ kcal·L}^{-1} O_2$ $19.27 \text{ kJ·L}^{-1} O_2$
Carbon dioxide produced ($L \cdot g^{-1}$)	0.75 L·g^{-1}	0.83 L·g^{-1}	0.781 L·g^{-1}	0.92 L·g^{-1}	1.43 L·g^{-1}

*Values for protein are given. However, the BCAA values are more realistic for muscle activity per 1 g PRO = 1.17 g AA (Morgan et al., 1989b; Péronnet et al., 1987).

[†]Energy produced per liter of oxygen equals the caloric equivalent.

EXAMPLE

For carbohydrates:
Glucose (per mole)

$$C_6H_{12}O_6 + 6O_2 \rightarrow 6CO_2 + 6H_2O + \text{energy}$$

$$RQ = \frac{6CO_2}{6O_2} = 1.0$$

Glucose (per gram, from Table 4.3)

$$1g \text{ glucose} + 0.75 \text{ L O}_2 \rightarrow 0.75 \text{ L CO}_2 + H_2O + 3.75 \text{ kcal}$$

$$RQ = \frac{0.75 \text{ L CO}_2}{0.75 \text{ L O}_2} = 1.0$$

For fat:
Palmitic acid (per mole)

$$C_{16}H_{32}O_2 + 23O_2 \rightarrow 16CO_2 + 15H_2O + \text{energy}$$

$$RQ = \frac{16CO_2}{23O_2} = 0.7$$

Fatty acids (per gram, from Table 4.3)

$$1g \text{ fatty acid} + 2.02 \text{ L O}_2 \rightarrow 1.43 \text{ L CO}_2 + H_2O + 9.3 \text{ kcal}$$

$$RQ = \frac{1.43 \text{ L CO}_2}{2.02 \text{ L O}_2} = 0.71$$

EXAMPLE *(Continued)*

For protein:
Albumin (per mole)

$$C_{72}H_{112}N_2O_{22}S + 77O_2 \rightarrow 63CO_2 + 38H_2O + SO_3 + 9CO(NH_2)(\text{urea})$$

$$RQ = \frac{63CO_2}{77O_2} = 0.82$$

Protein (per gram, from Table 4.3)

$$1g \text{ protein} + 0.965 \text{ L O}_2 \rightarrow 0.781 \text{ L CO}_2 + H_2O + 4.3 \text{ kcal}$$

$$RQ = \frac{0.781 \text{ L CO}_2}{0.965 \text{ L O}_2} = 0.81$$

Note that if the branched-chain amino acids are used, the RQ would be lower:

$$1g \text{ BCAA} + 1.24 \text{ L O}_2 \rightarrow 0.92 \text{ L CO}_2 + H_2O + 3.76 \text{ kcal}$$

$$RQ = \frac{0.92 \text{ L CO}_2}{1.24 \text{ L O}_2} = 0.74$$

Respiratory Exchange Ratio (RER) Ratio of the volume of CO_2 produced divided by the volume of O_2 consumed in the body as a whole.

Respiratory Quotient (RQ) Ratio of the amount of carbon dioxide produced divided by the amount of oxygen consumed at cellular level.

different activities. However, because individuals seldom use only one fuel, these "classic values" are rarely seen. Nonetheless, in a resting individual, an RQ of 0.93 indicates a high reliance on carbohydrate, and an RQ of 0.75 indicates a high reliance on fat. An RQ of 0.82 indicates either a fasting individual burning protein (usually from muscle mass, as in a starvation situation) or, more likely, an individual using a normal mixed diet of all three fuels. Remember that protein is not normally used as a major fuel source, especially at rest.

Although these interpretations are acceptable for resting individuals, there are several difficulties interpreting the RQ during exercise. In the first place, the O_2 and CO_2 values measured in open-circuit indirect spirometry are ventilatory measures that indicate total body gas exchange and not just working muscle. Second, hyperventilation from any cause will result in an excess of CO_2 being exhaled, thus falsely elevating the ratio. This often occurs in stress situations such as in anticipation of an exercise test or in early recovery from maximal work. Third, if exercise is of a high enough intensity to involve anaerobic metabolism, causing an increase in acidity (a decrease in pH) and a concomitant rise in nonmetabolic CO_2 release, RQ no longer represents just fuel utilization. Values during exercise, especially as an individual approaches maximal effort, usually exceed 1.0. In this case, it is assumed that the fuel source is carbohydrate and the excess CO_2 is a result of anaerobic metabolism. Conversely, after an initial increase during recovery, CO_2 is retained, causing low values (Newsholme and Leech, 1983). For these reasons, the term RER is more accurate than RQ to describe the ratio of $\dot{V}CO_2$ produced to $\dot{V}O_2$ consumed when determined by open-circuit spirometry.

The involvement of anaerobic metabolism that results in RER values greater than 1.0 allows for use of RER as a criterion to determine whether an exercise test is truly maximal. The criterion for a true maximal test is an RER greater than 1.1 or at least 1.0, with the lower value predominating for children/adolescents and older adults (Holly, 1988; MacDougall et al., 1982).

Although RER is a more accurate description than RQ, RER values still do not distinguish between different forms of a fuel, such as glucose or glycogen, fatty acids, or ketone bodies. Also, when only ventilatory CO_2 and O_2 are measured, there is no indication of protein utilization. To measure protein utilization, the amount of nitrogen excreted (in urine and sweat) must be measured. This task is at best cumbersome and at worst almost impossible to perform in exercise situations (Bursztein et al., 1989; Consolazio et al., 1963). Thus, the RER that is measured by the $\dot{V}CO_2$ $L \cdot min^{-1} \div \dot{V}O_2$ $L \cdot min^{-1}$ during exercise is a *nonprotein RER*. Again, because protein is not thought to be utilized as fuel until long-duration activity is in progress, this simplification is not deemed to materially affect the relative percentage of carbohydrate and fat utilization in most situations.

Table 4.4 presents the relative percentages of calories used from carbohydrate and fat for all RER values between 0.7 and 1.0 (Carpenter, 1921). Referring to **Table 4.1**, we see that, during rest, the individual had an RER of 0.81. From **Table 4.4**, this value indicates that 35.4% of her fuel was carbohydrate and 64.6% fat. During her 8 minutes of steady-state work, the RER averaged 0.90, indicating a major shift in fuel supply, with 66% of the fuel being carbohydrate and 34% fat.

TABLE 4.4   Percentage of Calories from Carbohydrate (CHO) and Fat and the Caloric Equivalents for Nonprotein RER Values for Each Liter of Oxygen Used

RER	CHO%	Fat%	Caloric Equivalent ($kcal \cdot L^{-1}$ O_2)	RER	CHO%	Fat%	Caloric Equivalent ($kcal \cdot L^{-1}$ O_2)
0.70	0.0	100.0	4.686	0.86	52.4	47.6	4.875
0.71	1.4	98.6	4.690	0.87	55.8	44.2	4.887
0.72	4.8	95.2	4.702	0.88	59.2	40.8	4.899
0.73	8.2	91.8	4.714	0.89	62.6	37.4	4.911
0.74	11.6	88.4	4.727	0.90	66.0	34.0	4.924
0.75	15.0	85.0	4.739	0.91	69.4	30.6	4.936
0.76	18.4	81.6	4.751	0.92	72.8	27.2	4.949
0.77	21.8	78.2	4.764	0.93	76.2	23.8	4.961
0.78	25.2	74.8	4.776	0.94	79.6	20.4	4.973
0.79	28.6	71.4	4.788	0.95	83.0	17.0	4.985
0.80	32.0	68.0	4.801	0.96	86.4	13.6	4.998
0.81	35.4	64.6	4.813	0.97	89.8	10.2	5.010
0.82	38.8	61.2	4.825	0.98	93.2	6.8	5.022
0.83	42.2	57.8	4.838	0.99	96.6	3.4	5.035
0.84	45.6	54.4	4.850	1.00	100.0	0.0	5.047
0.85	49.0	51.0	4.862				

Source: Modified from Carpenter, T. M.: *Tables, Factors, and Formulas for Computing Respiratory Exchange and Biological Transformations of Energy* (4th edition). Washington, DC: Carnegie Institution of Washington, Publication 303C (1921).

TABLE 4.5 Aerobic Exercise Response

		O₂ Consumption	RER/Energy Substrate
Short-term, light to moderate submaximal exercise		Initial rise; plateau at appropriate steady state	0.85 to 0.90/mixed fat and CHO to predominantly CHO
Short-term, moderate to heavy submaximal exercise		Initial rise; plateau at appropriate steady state	0.85 to 0.90 to 1.0+/mixed fat and CHO to CHO
Long-term, moderate to heavy submaximal exercise		Initial rise; plateau at steady state; positive drift	0.85 to 0.90 to 1.0+ to 0.90 to 0.85/ mixed fat and CHO to CHO; if duration is long enough, RER will decrease as CHO supplies are depleted
Very short-term, high-intensity, anaerobic exercise		Small increase; provides ~30% or less of energy cost	0.90 to 1.0+/predominantly CHO to all CHO
Incremental exercise to maximum		Rectilinear rise; plateau at maximum	0.85 to ≥1.0/mixed fat and CHO to glycogen
Static exercise		Small gradual rise during exercise; rebound rise in recovery	0.80 to 1.1+/mixed fat and CHO during exercise with rebound rise in recovery/ glycogen
Dynamic resistance exercise		Small gradual rise during exercise; the lighter the load and the higher the reps, the greater the contribution	0.90 to 1.0+/glycogen

During the last 5-minute interval (minutes 33–37 in **Table 4.1**), an even greater reliance on carbohydrate occurs with approximately 90% of the energy used being supplied by carbohydrate sources. If submaximal exercise were to continue for another 2 hours or more, the RER values would drop back down, indicating a depletion of available carbohydrate fuel stores. How low the RER values would go depends on the amount of carbohydrate originally stored as well as the intensity and duration of the activity. For this reason, athletes often try to carbohydrate load before endurance events so that carbohydrate stores are initially high and will last longer. Carbohydrate loading is fully discussed in Chapter 6. **Table 4.5** summarizes the oxygen consumption and RER/energy substrate responses to various categories of exercise. Check your knowledge by completing the Check Your Comprehension 2.

Estimation of Caloric Expenditure

Table 4.3 not only shows the oxygen consumed and carbon dioxide produced when each of the energy substrates is utilized but also indicates the potential energy in terms of kilocalories per gram (kcal·g⁻¹) or kilocalories per liter of oxygen (kcal·L⁻¹ O₂) for each substrate. The kcal·L⁻¹ O₂ figures show that carbohydrates are most efficient in the use of oxygen to provide energy, followed by fat, and

Caloric Equivalent The number of kilocalories produced per liter of oxygen consumed.

CHECK YOUR COMPREHENSION 2

Using **Table 4.2**, determine the approximate percentages of carbohydrate and fat used at minutes 2, 14, and 28. Check your answer in Appendix C to see whether you are correct. The early minute RER values are higher than expected for the workload, probably from hyperventilation in anticipation of the maximal effort to come in the exercise test. The last three RER values listed in Table 4.2 are greater than 1.1 and indicate the involvement of anaerobic metabolism.

finally by protein—although the substrates do not really vary a great deal.

The potential energy for carbohydrate and for protein depends on whether the form is glucose (3.75 kcal·g⁻¹) or glycogen (4.17 kcal·g⁻¹) or all amino acids (4.3 kcal·g⁻¹) or just the branched-chain amino acids (3.76 kcal·g⁻¹). When food is ingested, these distinctions cannot be made; the net average energy values are rounded to the whole numbers of 4 kcal·g⁻¹ for carbohydrate and protein and 9 kcal·g⁻¹ for fat. These values are called *Atwater factors* and are used to represent the energy potential of food. From the known values of $\dot{V}O_2$ L·min⁻¹ and RER, it is possible to compute the kilocalorie (or kilojoule) energy expenditure.

Table 4.4 includes the **caloric equivalent**—the number of kilocalories produced per liter of oxygen consumed—for all values of RER between 0.7 and 1.0. The caloric equivalent varies from 4.686 kcal·L⁻¹ O₂ at an

RER of 0.7 to 5.047 kcal·L^{-1} O$_2$ at an RER of 1.0. If the amount of oxygen consumed and the caloric equivalent are known, the caloric cost of an activity can be computed.

To compute the kcal·min^{-1} cost, first find the caloric equivalent for the RER in **Table 4.4**. The rest of the computation is simply a matter of multiplying the oxygen cost by the caloric equivalent. The formula is

4.4   caloric cost of an activity (kcal·min^{-1}) = oxygen consumed (L·min^{-1}) × caloric equivalent (kcal·L^{-1} O$_2$)

EXAMPLE

Assume that an individual had an RER of 0.91 during exercise that used 2.15 L O$_2$·min^{-1}. The caloric equivalent for an RER of 0.91 is 4.936 kcal·L^{-1} O$_2$, so the calculation becomes

$$2.15 \text{ L O}_2 \cdot \text{min}^{-1} \times 4.936 \text{ kcal} \cdot \text{L}^{-1}\text{O}_2 = 10.61 \text{ kcal} \cdot \text{min}^{-1}$$

This **caloric cost** is the energy expenditure of the activity. It may be expressed in calories or joules per minute (kcal·min^{-1} or kJ·min^{-1}), relative to BW (kcal·kg^{-1}·min^{-1} or kJ·kg^{-1}·min^{-1}), or as total calories if the calories per minute is multiplied by the total number of minutes of participation.

If you know the oxygen consumed during any activity but do not know the RER, you can estimate the caloric value of that activity by multiplying by 5.0 kcal·L^{-1} O$_2$. The 5.0 kcal·L^{-1} O$_2$ value is very close to the average caloric equivalent and is easy to remember. Since 1 kcal = 4.18 kJ, to convert kcal·min^{-1} to kJ·min^{-1}, multiply by 4.18. For the same example as above, this is

$$10.61 \text{ kcal} \cdot \text{min}^{-1} \times 4.18 \text{ kJ} \cdot \text{kcal}^{-1} = 44.36 \text{ kJ} \cdot \text{min}^{-1}$$

Remember that this caloric cost is an estimate of the aerobic portion only. If we attempt to calculate the caloric cost of all 28 minutes of the incremental task, the result will be an underestimation because the anaerobic energy expenditure cannot be calculated. Furthermore, these values include what an individual would expend if he or she were resting quietly. *Gross energy expenditure* is the term used when resting energy expenditure is included. If resting energy expenditure is subtracted from gross energy expenditure, the *net energy expenditure*—the energy expended to do the exercise itself—is the result. Knowing the caloric costs of activities is helpful when prescribing exercise.
Complete the Check Your Comprehensions 3 and 4 and check your answers in Appendix C.

CHECK YOUR COMPREHENSION 3

Determine the caloric cost (in kilocalories and kilojoules) for minute 14 of **Table 4.2**. Check your answer in Appendix C.

CHECK YOUR COMPREHENSION 4

A reasonable and beneficial level of exercise for fat loss is 300 kcal per session (Åstrand, 1952). The oxygen cost of riding a bicycle ergometer at 2 Kp (600 kg·min^{-1}, or 100 W) at 60 rev·min^{-1} is 1200 mL O$_2$·min^{-1} above resting metabolism. At this rate, how long must an individual ride to burn an excess of 300 kcal? Ignore the cost involved in a warm-up or cooldown. Check your answer in Appendix C.

The Metabolic Equivalent

Although most people think of energy cost in terms of kilocalories (kcal), exercise physiologists and physicians often use metabolic equivalent (MET) values. MET is an acronym derived from the term *Metabolic EquivalenT*. One MET represents the average, seated, resting energy cost of an adult and is set at 3.5 mL·kg^{-1}·min^{-1} of oxygen, or 1 kcal·kg^{-1}·hr^{-1}.

In reality, resting metabolic rates vary among individuals. If an individual's resting, seated energy expenditure is known, that value can be used instead of the 3.5 mL·kg^{-1}·min^{-1} average. In practice, however, variations from the average value are not considered substantial enough to invalidate its use. Multiples of the 1-MET resting baseline represent the **MET** level or multiples of the resting rate of oxygen consumption of any given activity. Thus, an activity performed at the level of 5 METs would require five times as much energy as is expended at rest (5 × 3.5 mL·kg^{-1}·min^{-1} = 17.5 mL·kg^{-1}·min^{-1}).

To calculate MET levels from measures of oxygen consumption, divide the amount of oxygen utilized (in mL·kg^{-1}·min^{-1}) by 3.5. For example, if an individual expends 29 mL·kg^{-1}·min^{-1} of O$_2$ on a task, the MET level is 29 mL·kg^{-1}·min^{-1} ÷ 3.5 mL·kg^{-1}·min^{-1} = 8.3 METs.

To convert from MET to kcal·min^{-1}, it is necessary to know the individual's BW and use the relationship 1 kcal·kg^{-1}·hr^{-1} = 1 MET. For example, if the 8.3-MET activity is done by a female of average weight (68 kg), the calculation is

$$8.3 \text{ METs} = \frac{(8.3 \text{ kcal} \times 68 \text{ kg})}{60 \text{ min} \cdot \text{hr}^{-1}} = 9.4 \text{ kcal} \cdot \text{min}^{-1}$$

Alternately, the formula

kcal·min^{-1} =

$$\left[\frac{\text{METs} \times 3.5 \text{ mL} \cdot \text{kg} \cdot \text{min}^{-1} \times \text{body weight in kg}}{1000 \text{ mL} \cdot \text{L}^{-1}} \right] \times 5 \text{ kcal} \cdot \text{L}^{-1}$$

simplified as (METs × 3.5 mL·kg·min^{-1} × body weight in kg) ÷200 kcal·mL^{-1}; where 200 kcal·mL^{-1} is 1000 mL·L^{-1} ÷ 5 kcal·L^{-1}, (Swain, 2010) may be used.

Caloric Cost and Exercise Machines

After studying exercise physiology for hours, to take a break, you go to the campus recreation center to exercise. Your goal is to burn 300 kcal, so you hop on your favorite exercise equipment, punch in your BW, select manual protocol, and begin. When the console reads 300 kcal, you stop—proud of having attained your goal. But did you really?

The answer to that question depends on a number of factors. The console number for kcal is derived mathematically from a prediction equation that typically takes into account BW and one or more measures of workload, such as stride rate, stride length, belt speed, elevation, and resistance or power output, depending on whether the equipment is a stair-stepping machine, treadmill, elliptical strider, rowing machine, or cycle ergometer. Research studies have generally shown that under identical conditions, calorie cost estimations are very consistent (reliable). However, the same cannot be said for the accuracy (validity) of the caloric cost values. For example, Swain et al. (1999) found that an elliptical motion machine significantly overestimated caloric cost (from 39 to 79%), with the larger overestimations occurring at the higher exercise intensities. In another study on an elliptical striding machine, Heselton et al. (2000) found that although the mean caloric cost values at two of three workloads were not significantly different, the estimated values were systematically overestimated at levels above 300 kcal for a 30-min workout, and the percentage of individuals whose measured caloric cost fell within 30 kcal of their estimated caloric cost was only 60%, averaged over two trials. A third study using an elliptical strider by Mier and Feito (2006) measured overestimations averaging 20–30% in caloric expenditure regardless of whether the participants used their legs only or arms and legs combined. Similar overestimations have been found for stair-stepping machines (Riddle and Orringer, 1990; Ryan et al., 1998), and several studies have reported that holding on to the point where part of the BW is supported results in a significant overestimation of caloric expenditure for both stair-steppers and the treadmill (Åstrand, 1984; Butts et al., 1993; Howley et al., 1992). The manufacturers of these machines try to provide accurate information to the exerciser, but errors are part of predictions, and the mathematical program cannot adjust if you "cheat" by holding on. Therefore, the answer to the question of whether you actually burned 300 kcal is "probably not." Console values for caloric expenditure should be interpreted as approximations rather than absolutes, and that approximation is probably high.

Sources: Åstrand (1984), Butts et al. (1993), Heselton et al. (2000), Howley et al. (1992), Mier and Feito (2006), Riddle and Orringer (1990), Ryan et al. (1998), Swain et al. (1999).

The example then becomes

$$\left[\frac{8.3 \text{ METs} \times 3.5 \text{ mL} \cdot \text{kg} \cdot \text{min}^{-1} \times 68 \text{ kg}}{1000 \text{ mL} \cdot \text{L}^{-1}} \right] \times 5 \text{ kcal} \cdot \text{L}^{-1}$$

$$= 9.88 \text{ kcal} \cdot \text{min}^{-1}$$

Table 4.6 presents a classification of absolute intensity ranges for physical activity in METs across fitness levels, where fitness level is defined as $\dot{V}O_2max$ and is reported in METs. (Remember $\dot{V}O_2max$ mL·kg·min^{-1} ÷ 3.5 mL·kg·min^{-1} = maximal METs.) For example, an individual with a fitness level of 8 METs should select activities between 3.8 and 5.1 METs to exercise at a moderate level. Table 4.7 presents a classification of metabolic intensities in MET values for selected physical activities. This allows an individual to find activities for any of the intensity levels for exercise found in Table 4.6. For example, on average, water skiing (6 METs) would be appropriate as a moderate activity for an individual whose $\dot{V}O_2max$ is 10 or 12 METs, but not for those with lower MET max levels. Walking at 3.0 mi·hr^{-1} (3.5 METs) would be an appropriate activity for an individual whose $\dot{V}O_2max$ is 6 or 8 METs. Table 4.8 classifies work intensities as a rough guide for determining how long work can be sustained at each intensity. Individuals often work at different intensities in a laboratory setting than in the natural setting, so some variation in actual MET values is to be expected (Withers et al., 2006). Combining the information from this table and Table 4.6, for example, shows that most indoor household chores would be considered very light to light work intensity and, theoretically, could be sustained indefinitely. Conversely, working as a Navy Seal or frogman is maximal work even for individuals with a maximal MET fitness level of 12 and can be expected to be sustained for only 1–2 hours occasionally. (Note: 12 METs = 42 mL·kg·min^{-1} $\dot{V}O_2max$) Generically, sedentary behaviors are considered to be MET values less than 1.5; light-intensity activities 1.6–2.9; moderate-intensity 3–5.9; and vigorous ≥6 (Ainsworth et al., 2011). Happily

Caloric Cost Energy expenditure of an activity performed for a specified period of time. It may be expressed as total calories (kcal), calories or kilojoules per minute (kcal·min^{-1} or kJ·min^{-1}), or relative to body weight (kcal·kg^{-1}·min^{-1} or kJ·kg^{-1}·min^{-1}).

MET A unit that represents the MET in multiples of the resting rate of oxygen consumption of any given activity.

TABLE 4.6   Classification of Physical Activity Intensity: Absolute Intensity Ranges Based on METS by Fitness Level

		Fitness Level			
		12 MET $\dot{V}O_2$max	10 MET $\dot{V}O_2$max	8 MET $\dot{V}O_2$max	6 MET $\dot{V}O_2$max
Intensity	Very light	<3.2	<2.8	<2.4	<2.0
	Light	3.2–5.3	2.8–4.5	2.4–3.7	2.0–3.0
	Moderate	5.4–7.5	4.6–6.3	3.8–5.1	3.1–4.0
	Hard (vigorous)	7.6–10.2	6.4–8.6	5.2–6.9	4.1–5.2
	Very hard	≥10.3	≥8.7	≥7.0	≥5.3
	Maximal	12	10	8	6

Source: American College of Sports Medicine: *ACSM's Guidelines for Exercise Testing and Prescription* (8th edition). Baltimore, MD: Lippincott Williams & Wilkins (2010).

TABLE 4.7   MET Values for Selected Physical Activities and Sports: Adults

Activity	MET Level	Activity	MET Level	Activity	MET Level
Archery	4.3	Frisbee		Soccer	
Badminton		General	3.0	General	7.0
Social	5.5	Ultimate	8.0	Competitive	10.0
Competitive	7.0	Golf		Snow shoeing	5.3
Baseball/softball	5.0	Power cart	3.5	Squash	12.0
Basketball		Walking, carrying clubs	4.3	Swimming	
General	6.0	Gymnastics	3.8	Freestyle (slow)	5.8
Competitive	8.0	Handball	12.0	Freestyle (fast)	9.8
Officiating	7.0	Hockey		Backstroke	9.5
Shooting	4.5	Field	7.8	Breaststroke	9.5
Wheelchair	7.8	Ice	8.0	Butterfly	13.8
Bicycling		Horseback riding		Treading water	3.5
<10 mi·hr^{-1}	4.0	Walking	3.8	Tennis	
10–11.9 mi·hr^{-1}	6.5	Trotting	5.8	Doubles	6.0
12–13.9 mi·hr^{-1}	8.0	Canter/gallop	7.3	Singles	8.0
14–15.9 mi·hr^{-1}	10.0	Kickball	7.0	Video games	
16–19 mi·hr^{-1}	12.0	Lacrosse	8.0	Wii Fit balance and Yoga	2.3
BMX/mountain	8.5	Rope jumping	11.3	Wii Fit aerobic & resistance	3.8
Stationary		100–120 skips.min^{-1}		Exergames; dance, dance	7.2
50 W	3.5	Rowing and paddling		revolution, vigorous	
100 W	6.8	Ergometer		Volleyball	
150 W	8.8	50 W	3.5	General	3.0
200 W	11.0	100 W	7.0	Competitive	6.0
Bowling	3.8	150 W	8.5	Beach	8.0
Calisthenics		Canoe	5.8	Walking (level)	
Light, moderate	3.5	Moderate		2.0 mi·hr^{-1}	2.8
Circuit	4.3	Kayak	5.0	2.5 mi·hr^{-1}	3.0
Stretching	2.3	Running		3.0 mi·hr^{-1}	3.5
Dance		12 min·mi^{-1}	8.3	3.5 mi·hr^{-1}	4.3
Aerobic		10 min·mi^{-1}	9.8	4.0 mi·hr^{-1}	5.0
6–8-in. step	7.5	9 min·mi^{-1}	10.5	Using crutches	5.0
10–12-in. step	9.5	8 min·mi^{-1}	11.5	Pushing child	4.0
Ballroom		7 min·mi^{-1}	12.3	Water aerobics	5.3
Slow	3.0	6 min·mi^{-1}	14.5	Weight lifting	
Fast	5.5	Skateboarding	5.0	Light, moderate	3.5
Fencing	6.0	Skating		Heavy	6.0
		Ice	7.0	Wrestling	6.0
		Rollerblading	7.5	Yoga (Hatha)	2.5
		9 mi.hr^{-1}			

TABLE 4.7   MET Values for Selected Physical Activities and Sports: Adults *(Continued)*

Activity	MET Level	Activity	MET Level	Activity	MET Level
Football		Skiing		Track and field	
Touch	8.0	Cross-country		Shot, discus	4.0
Competitive	8.0	2.5 mi·hr^{-1}	6.8	Jumps	6.0
		4.0–4.9 mi·hr^{-1}	9.0	Hurdles	10.0
		5.0–7.9 mi·hr^{-1}	12.5		
		Downhill			
		Moderate	5.3		
		Water	6.0		

Note: 1 MET = 1 kcal·kg·hr^{-1}; 1 kcal·kg·hr^{-1}/60 min·hr^{-1} = kcal·kg·min^{-1}.

Source: Modified from Ainsworth, B. E., W. L. Haskell, S. D. Herrmann, et al: 2011 Compendium of physical activities: A second update of codes and MET values. *Medicine & Science in Sports & Exercise*. 43(8):1575–1581 (2011); http://sites.google.com/site/compendiumofphysicalactivities.

TABLE 4.8   Work Classifications (A) and MET Levels for Selected Occupational and Home Activities (B)

A. Classification	Time Work Can be Sustained
Very light to light	Indefinitely
Moderate	8 hr daily
Hard	8 hr daily for a few weeks only
Very hard	4 hr 2–3 times per week for a few weeks consecutively
Maximal	1–2 hr occasionally
Exhausting	Few minutes, rarely

B. Activities	MET Level
Carrying small children	3.0
Carpentry	4.3
Cleaning house	3.8
Construction	4.0
Cooking	2.0
Driving tractor	2.8
Food shopping	2.3
Electrical work/plumbing	3.3
Ironing	1.8
Fighting fires	9.0
Making bed-changing linens	3.3
Massaging	4.0
Masonry	4.3
Mowing lawn (walk)	5.0
(ride)	2.5
Moving boxes	7.5
Navy Seal/frogman	12.0
Playing trumpet	1.8
Painting	4.5
Playing drums	3.8
Racking leaves	3.8
Police directing traffic	2.5
Shoveling snow	5.3
Sitting in class	1.8
Snow blowing (walk)	2.5
Sitting studying	1.3
Washing dishes	2.5
Sitting talking (on/off phone)	1.5

Sources: Modified from Ainsworth, B. E., W. L. Haskell, S. D. Herrmann, et al: 2011 Compendium of physical activities: A second update of codes and MET values. *Medicine & Science in Sports & Exercise*. 43(8):1575–1581 (2011); http://sites.google.com/site/compendiumofphysicalactivities; Wells, J. G., B. Balke, & D. D. Van Fossan: Lactic acid accumulation during work. A suggested standardization of work classification. *Journal of Applied Physiology*. 10(1):51–55 (1957).

we can see that sitting in class, taking notes, participating in discussions, and studying are relatively light metabolic work that can be sustained indefinitely.

Active video games are a new addition to the compendium selected for **Table 4.7** because of their increasing popularity for individuals of all ages and in some physical education classes. Wii Fit values have been broadly categorized together into light effort (balance and yoga) 2.3 METs and moderate effort (aerobic and resistance) 3.8 METs. A more specific breakdown the MET values of 68 Wii activities has been determined by Miyachi et al. (2010). Forty-six activities were classified as light (<3 MET) and 22 as moderate (>6 MET); no Wii activities were classified as vigorous.

Note that the compendium of MET values is intended for use with adults. There is a lack of comparable information for children and adolescents. Ridley and Olds (2008) attempted to synthesize information available for these younger individuals by comparing techniques in the literature for estimating energy expenditure in children. The results provided evidence that using the adult MET levels was the best technique for estimating energy expenditure in children and adolescents when directly measured energy expenditure values are not available. However, resting metabolic rates vary in children from adults according to age, sex, and size but are higher, which would mean that in general MET levels are overestimated for youngsters. Thus, it would be best if adult METs could be prorated by a child-specific resting metabolic rate, either measured or estimated, but this is generally not practical.

Field Estimates of Energy Expenditure during Exercise

Metabolic Calculations Based on Mechanical Work or Standard Energy Use

In situations where an accurate assessment of mechanical work is possible, energy expenditure, expressed as oxygen consumption ($mL \cdot min^{-1}$, $mL \cdot kg^{-1} \cdot min^{-1}$, or METs), can be estimated through a series of calculations. The equations used are based on known oxygen costs for steady-state horizontal walking (0.1 $mL \cdot kg^{-1} \cdot min^{-1}$ for each $m \cdot min^{-1}$), horizontal running (0.2 $mL \cdot kg^{-1} \cdot min^{-1}$ for each $m \cdot min^{-1}$), vertical rise (1.8 $mL \cdot kg^{-1} \cdot min^{-1}$ for each $m \cdot min^{-1}$ of walking or 0.9 $mL \cdot kg^{-1} \cdot min^{-1}$ for each $m \cdot min^{-1}$ of running), leg ergometer work against resistance (2 $mL \cdot kgm^{-1}$), and arm ergometer work against resistance (3 $mL \cdot kgm^{-1}$) for adults (American College of Sports Medicine, 2010). These values do not include the resting metabolic rate of 1 MET or 3.5 $mL \cdot kg^{-1} \cdot min^{-1}$ of oxygen.

EXAMPLE

For an individual walking on a track at a 20 $min \cdot mi^{-1}$ pace (3 $mi \cdot hr^{-1}$), which is a velocity of 80.4 $m \cdot min^{-1}$ (3 $mi \cdot hr^{-1}$ × 26.8 $m \cdot min^{-1} \cdot mi \cdot hr^{-1}$), the calculation is as follows:

$$\begin{aligned} \text{Walking} \\ \text{oxygen} \\ \text{consumption} \end{aligned} = 80.4 \text{ m} \cdot \text{min}^{-1} \times \left(\frac{0.1 \text{ mL} \cdot \text{kg}^{-1} \cdot \text{min}^{-1}}{\text{m} \cdot \text{min}^{-1}} \right)$$
$$+ 3.5 \text{ mL} \cdot \text{kg}^{-1} \cdot \text{min}^{-1}$$
$$= 11.54 \text{ mL} \cdot \text{kg}^{-1} \cdot \text{min}^{-1}$$

This value can easily be converted to METs as previously described by dividing by 3.5 $mL \cdot kg^{-1} \cdot min^{-1}$. At the 20 $min \cdot mi^{-1}$ pace, this is 3.3 METs. **Table 4.7** shows this is close to the actual measured value of 3.5 MET value for walking at 3 $mi \cdot hr^{-1}$.

In addition to this equation for horizontal walking, other available equations are presented in Appendix B for uphill walking, horizontal and uphill running, bench stepping, leg cycle ergometry, and arm cycle ergometry (American College of Sports Medicine, 2010). These equations are useful for exercise prescription purposes in a college, health club, or clinical setting where it is not possible to directly measure energy expenditure. Physicians often prescribe exercise by MET level, assuming that the exercise leader will be able to determine the proper pace for walking or running, resistance on a cycle ergometer, or height and rate for step aerobics. The equations enable the exercise leader to do just that. Remember that the resultant values are just estimates for any given individual in any specific setting, however. Therefore, workloads should be fine-tuned using heart rate or RPE responses as described in Chapter 13.

CHECK YOUR COMPREHENSION 5

How many METs is the subject in **Table 4.2** exercising at in minute 14?
The answer is in Appendix C.

Motion Sensors and Accelerometers

Attempts have been made to determine the energy cost in the field by measuring movement, assuming that more movement means greater calories expended. A familiar type of motion sensor is the pedometer (**Figure 4.7**). Set to the individual's stride length, a pedometer records the distance traveled by foot. Crouter et al. (2003) studied the accuracy of eight pedometers that also displayed

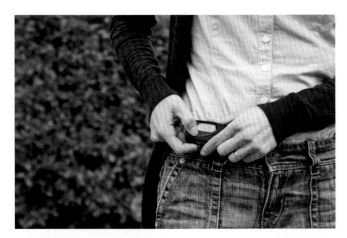

FIGURE 4.7 A Pedometer.
This woman is wearing a pedometer that measures step number and estimates distance and energy expenditure.

kilocalories. It was unclear whether the pedometers were displaying net or gross kilocalories. If net kcal, the general trend was an overestimation of energy expended at every treadmill speed from 54 to 107 m·min^{-1} (2–4 mi·hr^{-1}). If gross kcal, the accuracy of seven of the eight pedometers was within ±30% at all speeds. The authors concluded that pedometers are most accurate for measuring steps, less accurate for measuring distance, and even less accurate for assessing energy expenditure. These results were primarily supported in a 2011 study (Nielson et al., 2011) when steps counts were found to be accurate at 100, 110, and 120 steps·min^{-1} but not 80 or 90 steps·min^{-1}, and energy expenditure was significantly underestimated at 80 steps·min^{-1} but overestimated at all other stride frequencies.

Accelerometers are portable devices worn on the body that measure movement in terms of acceleration. Speed is a change in position relative to time. *Acceleration* is the change in speed relative to time. The unit of measurement is typically gravitational acceleration units (g; 1 g = 9.8 m·sec^{-2}). Depending on the level of electronic sophistication, accelerometers detect acceleration(s) in one to three planes or axes (anteroposterior, mediolateral, and/or vertical). The raw outputs of accelerometers are known as counts. These counts are processed by linear or nonlinear regression equation software to determine the estimated energy expenditure. Some newer technology uses multisensors applied to several body segments (e.g., arm, waist, and ankle) and/or combines accelerometry with physiological sensors (e.g., for heart rate, skin temperature, or body temperature) in a single device (Chen and Basset, 2005; Corder et al., 2007). As with pedometers, accelerometers often are not accurate indicators of energy expenditure/metabolic equivalents (Park et al., 2011).

Technology in pedometers and accelerometers continues to evolve in an attempt to get the best estimation of energy expenditure. An ear-worn activity recognition sensor may be the next generation cutting edge technology for use in the field to determine energy expenditure (Atallah et al., 2011).

Activity Recalls and Questionnaires

In terms of technology, the least complex system for estimating energy expenditure is a self- or observer activity report in which either all activities or just exercise sessions are recorded (Laporte et al., 1985). The caloric cost of a particular activity or exercise session depends on the activity performed, its intensity and duration, and the individual's BW. The caloric cost can be calculated from a chart such as the ones presented in **Tables 4.7** and **4.8** by converting METs to kcal·kg·min^{-1}. 1 MET = 1 kcal·kg·hr^{-1}; 1 kcal·kg·hr^{-1} ÷ 60 min·hr^{-1} = kcal·kg^{-1}·min^{-1}. The following formula is used:

> **4.5** total caloric cost of the activity (kcal) = caloric cost per kilogram of body weight per minute (kcal · kg^{-1} · min^{-1}) × body weight (kg) × exercise time (min)

EXAMPLE

If a 65-year-old, 84-kg female walks 3 mi in 1:15, how many kilocalories does she expend?

To use **Table 4.6**, first convert 3 mi in 1 hour and 15 minutes to mi per hour.

Table 4.6 shows that 2.5 mi·hr^{-1} at 3.0 METs is the closest approximation. Thus, an individual walking at 2.5 mi·hr^{-1} expends 0.05 kcal·kg^{-1}·min^{-1} (3.0 kcal·kg·hr^{-1} ÷ 60 min·hr^{-1} = 0.05 kcal·kg^{-1}·min^{-1}). Substituting into this formula:

$$0.05 \ \text{kcal} \cdot \text{kg}^{-1} \cdot \text{min}^{-1} \times 84 \ \text{kg} \times 75 \ \text{min} = 315 \ \text{kcal}$$

Therefore, this individual expends 315 kcal in her walk, which is a good fitness workout.

For an assessment of total daily energy expenditure or even weekly average expenditure, the process becomes more tedious and, as a result, is probably less exact. Even the most willing individuals have only so much time to write down everything they do; if activity is recorded after the fact, some activities will be forgotten. It is also possible that when asked to recall their activity and provide a record of that activity, some people may overestimate their energy expenditure. Nevertheless, keeping a diary both of approximate energy expended and ingested can provide valuable information for individuals.

Efficiency and Economy

Efficiency

Walk into an appliance store to buy a furnace, hot water heater, washer, dryer, air conditioner, or refrigerator and each of the choices will have a label proclaiming its efficiency rating. Brand X uses only so much electricity (for just pennies a day!) to heat 40 gallons of water, wash a load of clothes, and so on.

Down the street, the car dealer is shouting the praises of the latest midsized economy car or hybrid; it has plenty of leg room, holds five adults comfortably, and gets 35–50 mi·gallon^{-1} of gas. In each case, the concept is the same. We want to get the most output (in heating, cooling, or miles) for the least input and energy expense (electrical power, gas, or money). The same holds true for physical labor or exercise output: We want to get the most output (work) for the least input (ATP, kilocalories, or fuel used). One exception to this is probably the individual wishing to lose weight.

The human body follows the *First Law of Thermodynamics*, also called the *Law of Conservation of Energy*. Simply put, this law states that energy can neither be created nor destroyed but can only be changed in form. When an individual exercises or performs other external work, the actual work achieved represents only a portion of the total energy utilized. The rest of the energy appears as heat, which must be dissipated or body temperature will rise. The percentage of energy input that results in useful external work is called the **mechanical efficiency**, or simply the efficiency of that task.

Efficiency can be calculated in at least three ways. The simplest calculation of efficiency is as *gross efficiency*.

4.6
$$\text{gross efficiency} = \frac{\text{work output}}{\text{energy expended}} \times 100$$

EXAMPLE

Calculate the gross efficiency for a 22-year-old female whose BW is 65.5 kg. She has ridden a Monark cycle ergometer (flywheel distance = 6 m) at 50 rev·min^{-1} with a load of 2.5 kp for 15 minutes.

The external output is calculated as work equals force times distance (W = F × D).

$$W = 2.5 \text{ kp} \times (50 \text{ rev·min}^{-1} \times 6 \text{ m}) \times 15 \text{ min}$$
$$= 11{,}250 \text{ kg}$$

It takes 426.8 kg of work to equal 1 kcal. Therefore,

$$11{,}250 \text{ kg} \div 426.8 \text{ kcal·kgm}^{-1} = 26.36 \text{ kcal}$$
$$\text{of work output.}$$

EXAMPLE *(Continued)*

The amount of energy expended is calculated using Equation 4.4 and multiplying by the total time of the exercise. The average oxygen consumption for the ride was 1.73 L·min^{-1} and the RER was 0.91. At an RER of 0.91, the caloric equivalent (**Table 4.4**) is 4.936 kcal·L^{-1} O$_2$. Substituting into Equation 4.4, we get

$$1.73 \text{ L O}_2 \cdot \text{min}^{-1} \times 4.936 \text{ kcal·L}^{-1}\text{O}_2$$
$$= 29.95 \text{ kcal·min}^{-1} \times 15 \text{ min}$$
$$= 128.09 \text{ kcal of energy expended.}$$

Equation 4.6 can now be used to determine gross efficiency:

$$\text{gross efficiency} = \frac{26.36 \text{ kcal}}{128.09 \text{ kcal}} \times 100 = 20.58\%$$

A slightly more complex method uses net efficiency. In *net efficiency*, the energy expended is corrected for resting metabolic rate.

4.7
$$\text{Net efficiency} = \frac{\text{work output}}{\substack{\text{energy expended-resting} \\ \text{metabolic rate for the} \\ \text{same time period}}} \times 100$$

EXAMPLE

Calculate net efficiency using the same example as for gross efficiency; this means that the individual's resting metabolic rate (measured to be 1.11 kcal·min^{-1} or 16.6 kcal for the 15 min) must be subtracted from the total energy expenditure of 128.09 kcal before computing for efficiency. Thus, substituting in Equation 4.7, we get

$$\text{net efficiency} = \frac{26.36 \text{ kcal}}{128.09 \text{ kcal} - 16.6 \text{ kcal}} \times 100 = 23.64\%$$

The third technique for calculating efficiency requires the use of at least two workloads and is based on the difference between the two loads. It is called *delta efficiency*.

4.8
$$\text{Delta efficiency} = \frac{\substack{\text{difference in work output} \\ \text{between two loads}}}{\substack{\text{difference in energy} \\ \text{expenditure between} \\ \text{the same two loads}}} \times 100$$

EXAMPLE

Calculate the delta efficiency for the 22-year-old female in the last two examples whose BW is 65.5 kg. This time she has performed two exercise stages on a treadmill, the first at 0% grade and the second at 10% grade. The speed was a constant 94 m·min^{-1} (3.5 mi·hr^{-1}). The difference in work output is therefore primarily determined by the difference in percent grade—in this case, a 10% difference. Treadmill delta efficiency calculations are usually done on a per-minute basis. Therefore, instead of calculating the change in work (W = F × D) as in the first two examples, the change (Δ) in work rate or power (P), which is work divided by time, is used (Adams et al., 1972; Gaesser and Brooks, 1975):

$$\Delta P kg \cdot min^{-1} = BW (kg) \times speed (m \cdot min^{-1})$$
$$\times (\% \ slope/100)$$

Substituting, we get

$$\Delta P = 65.5 \ kg \times 94 \ m \cdot min^{-1} \times (10/100)$$
$$= 615.7 \ kg \cdot min^{-1}$$

Using the conversion of 426.8 kg of work is equal to 1 kcal, we then divide 615.7 kg·min^{-1} by 426.8 kg for a difference in work output of 1.44 kcal·min^{-1}.

As before, energy expenditure is calculated using Equation 4.4. The average oxygen consumption at 0% grade is 0.91 L·min^{-1} with an RER of 0.73. The caloric equivalent (**Table 4.4**) of the 0.73 RER is 4.714 kcal·L^{-1} O$_2$. Substituting into Equation 4.4, this becomes

$$0.91 \ LO_2 \cdot min^{-1} \times 4.714 \ kcal \cdot L^{-1} O_2 = 4.29 \ kcal \cdot min^{-1}$$

The average oxygen consumption at 10% grade was 1.75 L^{-1} O$_2$, and the RER was 0.86. The caloric equivalent of an RER of 0.86 is 4.875 kcal·L^{-1} O$_2$. Substituting these values into Equation 4.4 leads to

$$1.75 \ LO_2 \cdot min^{-1} \times 4.875 \ kcal \cdot L^{-1} O_2 = 8.53 \ kcal \cdot min^{-1}$$

To obtain the difference in energy expended at the two workloads, simply subtract:

$$8.53 \ kcal \cdot min^{-1} - 4.29 \ kcal \cdot min^{-1} = 4.24 \ kcal \cdot min^{-1}$$

Equation 4.8 can now be used to solve for delta efficiency:

$$delta \ efficiency = \frac{1.44 \ kcal \cdot min^{-1}}{4.25 \ kcal \cdot min^{-1}} \times 100 = 33.9\%$$

Mechanical Efficiency The percentage of energy input that appears as useful external work.

When used for the same exercise modality, these different methods of calculating efficiency yield very different results. For example, Gaesser and Brooks (1975) calculated gross efficiencies of 7.5–20.4%, net efficiencies of 9.8–24.1%, and delta efficiencies of 24.4–34% on the bicycle ergometer under the same controlled experimental conditions. Despite these differences, all these techniques are valuable because each technique is best suited for particular uses.

Gross efficiency is most useful for calculating values for specific workloads, speeds, or the like. For example, it answers the question: What is the efficiency of cycling into a 15 mi·hr^{-1} (24 km·hr^{-1}) head wind, and how might that change with body position? Gross efficiency is also important for applications in nutritional studies where gross energy expenditure is a concern for adequate replenishment, such as during the Tour de France, when replacement is essential if a cyclist is to continue hard riding day after day. Gross efficiency is also the measure reported most frequently, making it valuable for comparison purposes (Donovan and Brooks, 1977).

Net efficiency is a better indication of the efficiency of work per se because it eliminates resting levels of energy that are not used to perform the work. Nonetheless, it is not a realistic value because an individual performing any external work is still expending resting energy.

Delta efficiency is the most accurate means for determining the effect of speed or work rate on efficiency. It indicates the relative energy cost of performing an additional increment of work. Delta efficiency is also the technique of choice for calculating efficiency on a treadmill. Its use is necessary because technically no work (calculated as force × distance) is done when the treadmill is horizontal (0% grade), despite the fact that energy is used. The reciprocal arm and leg movements cancel each other out, and there is no gain in vertical distance. If the treadmill is elevated so that an individual is walking or running up a grade, then work can be calculated.

All efficiency calculations assume a submaximal steady-state or steady-rate condition and require that both work output and energy expenditure be expressed in the same units, typically kilocalories. The calculations may be done for the total time, as in the 15-minute bicycle ergometer ride used in the example for gross efficiency, or per unit of time, as in the per-minute calculations for the treadmill of delta efficiency. However, time can be a factor, since efficiency is generally high when a large amount of work is performed in a short period of time and low when a small amount of work is performed over a long period of time (Stegeman, 1981).

Because the same amount of physical work in any given exercise modality can cause different metabolic effects in individuals, the energy cost (V̇O$_2$ consumption) of the activity is the deciding factor in determining efficiency (Stegeman, 1981). **Figure 4.8** shows this basic relationship. As the energy cost (V̇O$_2$ mL·kg^{-1}·min^{-1} on the left y-axis) increases, efficiency (% efficiency on the right

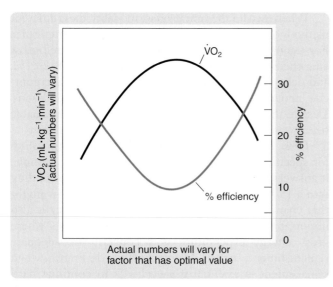

FIGURE 4.8 Optimizing Efficiency.
Note: Optimization means minimizing energy expenditure and maximizing work output. A variety of factors such as stride length, seat height, or pedaling frequency could be plotted on the *x*-axis.
Source: Cavanagh, P. R., & R. Kram: Mechanical and muscular factors affecting the efficiency of human movement. *Medicine and Science in Sports and Exercise.* 17(3):326–331 (1985).

y-axis) decreases, and vice versa. Some of the factors that have been investigated to try and optimize efficiency for physical activities are described in the following section. Each of these could be plotted on the *x*-axis in **Figure 4.8**.

Practical Application of Efficiency Information

Certain factors have been shown to change efficiency and thus can be manipulated by an individual to optimize efficiency and improve performance. For example, the optimal seat height on a bicycle at any given power output has been found to be approximately 109% of leg length. Optimal pedaling frequency at any given power output has been shown to be between 40 and 60 rev·min^{-1} for trained and untrained individuals, despite the fact that trained cyclists self-select a rate closer to 90 rev·min^{-1}. The reason for this difference is still unknown (Kohler and Boutellier, 2005). The higher revolutions per minute used by trained cyclists may optimize muscular forces and lower limb stresses but not metabolic efficiency (Widrick et al., 1992). Maximal power might not be reached at a pedaling rate near the most efficient one. It may be that the optimal pedaling rate is not fixed but depends on race duration (Kohler and Boutellier, 2005). In addition, at high values of mechanical power, the relationship between mechanical efficiency and pedaling frequency is relatively flat, so little efficiency is lost with the higher pedaling frequencies (Lazzer et al., 2011). When the revolutions per minute are kept constant on a cycle ergometer, efficiency

tends to increase from low to high workloads (Cavanagh and Kram, 1985; Hagberg et al., 1981; Stegeman, 1981).

The optimal speed for walking efficiency, when distance is held constant, is between 60 and 100 m·min^{-1} (about 2.25 and 3.75 mi·hr^{-1}, or 16–27 min·mi^{-1}). The optimal grade for efficiency, when speed is held constant, is approximately 5% downhill (25%). The optimal stride length for efficiency, when speed is held constant, varies considerably among individuals. Most runners, however, intuitively select a stride length that is very close to optimal for themselves. Therefore, coaches who attempt to alter stride length may be harming efficiency.

Exercise efficiency values are most frequently reported in the 20–25% range. These values may be slightly higher (20–45%) if they are calculated as delta efficiencies and slightly lower (5–20%) if the activity involves air or wind resistance. Overcoming air resistance requires additional energy at all speeds of running and velocities of wind (including no wind). Therefore, in a running or cycling race, participants often draft off of (or tuck in behind) the front competitor. The first athlete must work harder than the athlete tucked behind, who does less work, hoping to save sufficient energy to put on a surge at the end of the race and pass the more fatigued front competitor or designated teammates as in an event such as the Tour de France. It has been shown (Broker et al., 1999) that during a team pursuit cycling race, performed at approximately 37 mi·hr^{-1} (60 km·hr^{-1}) the average mechanical power was equal to 607 W in the lead position, 430 W (–29.2%) in the second position, and 389 W (–36%) in third and fourth position.

The extra energy cost due to air resistance is proportional to the velocity at which the runner is moving raised to the second power, or m·sec^2. Assuming there is no head wind, this amounts to approximately 2% extra energy expenditure for the marathon distance, 4–8% for middle-distance events, and 8–16% for sprints at world-class speeds. Although these percentages may not sound like much, they can be the equivalent of 5 minutes for a marathoner. At high levels of competition, this is a tremendous amount of time and would make a considerable difference in the results (Åstrand, 1952; Davies, 1980; Donovan and Brooks, 1977; Gaesser and Brooks, 1975; Pendergast et al., 1977; Pugh, 1970). Although running against a head wind can require additional energy, and thus decrease efficiency, the reverse is not true. A tailwind never assists the runner by decreasing the energy cost proportionally.

The mechanical efficiency of cycling, whether calculated as net efficiency or delta efficiency, is similar in prepubertal children, postpubertal adolescents, and adults (Klausen et al., 1985; Rowland, 1990). It may be slightly reduced in older adults such that a lower pedaling frequency is more efficient for older cyclists than younger ones (Sacchetti et al., 2010). These similarities are true whether the calculations are based on relative (%$\dot{V}O_2$max) or on absolute (kgm·min^{-1} or W) work rates. The similarities also hold for males and females although, if anything,

FOCUS ON RESEARCH

The Impact of Body Posture on Cycling Efficiency

Eight junior, national, and professional male competitive cyclists performed two sets of trials after determination of their peak power output (PPO). The first set of trials consisted of three Wingate anaerobic 30-second leg tests: one seated on a Monark ergometer, one seated on his personal bike on an ascending road, and one standing on his personal bike on an ascending road. The second set of trials consisted of five sessions of 6-minute duration at 75% PPO: two seated-level cycling; two seated-uphill cycling (5.3% grade); and one standing-uphill cycling.

The data for the 30-second cycling sprints revealed that power output was lowest (603 ± 81 W) when seated on the Monark ergometer, slightly higher when seated on personal bikes (635 ± 123 W), but highest in the standing position (803 ± 103 W)—a difference of 20–30%, respectively, over the two seated power outputs. These results clearly show an advantage in short-term power output in short sprints for the standing position.

Data from the second set of trials are presented in the table below.

Remember that the power output was held constant at 75% PPO. Despite this constancy, both velocity and cadence were significantly lower in both uphill conditions. However, neither gross efficiency nor economy changed by either terrain (level or uphill) or body position (seated or standing).

The researchers concluded that there is an advantage for the cyclist to stand during short high-intensity hill climbs but to remain seated in longer steady-state climbs. However, which combination of speed and hill gradient favors climbing in the standing position remains to be determined.

Source: Millet, G. P., C. Tronche, N. Fuster, & R. Candau: Level ground and uphill cycling efficiency in seated and standing positions. *Medicine & Science in Sports & Exercise.* 34(10):1645–1652 (2002).

Condition	Power (W)	Velocity (km·hr^{-1})	Cadence (rev·min^{-1})	Gross Efficiency (%)	Economy (kJ·L^{-1})
Seated level	279.6 ± 34.7	35.8 ± 1.7	90.5 ± 6.5	22.4 ± 0.8	4.7 ± 0.2
Seated uphill	286.6 ± 35.3	18.3 ± 1.3*	58.9 ± 4.1*	22.2 ± 1.3	4.8 ± 0.3
Standing uphill	292.1 ± 34.6	17.9 ± 1.2*	58.5 ± 4.1*	22.5 ± 1.9	4.7 ± 0.5

*P < 0.001 for differences with the seated-level condition.

females may be more efficient than males at the same cycling power outputs (Bal et al., 1953; Girandola et al., 1981; Hopker et al., 2010; Sidney and Shephard, 1977; Taylor et al., 1950). Because of the relative constancy of efficiency, cycling is a good family activity.

Economy of Walking and Running

As discussed earlier, the calculation of efficiency is a ratio of work output to energy expenditure input. However, measuring external work output may be impossible in many activities such as horizontal walking and running on the treadmill. Consequently, the energy expended to move mass or oxygen cost is often used alone for walking and running as a measure of economy, not efficiency.

Economy is the oxygen cost of any activity, but particularly walking or running at varying speeds. The relationship between oxygen cost and economy is inverse. That is, the more oxygen utilized in an activity, the lower the economy of that activity. This is similar to the concept that the more gas used to go any given distance at any given speed, the less economical the car.

The most basic generalization about economy is that, over a wide range of velocities of walking or running, the energy cost (in mL·kg^{-1}·min^{-1} of O_2) is rectilinearly related to the speed (in m·min^{-1}). That is, higher speeds are less economical. This generalization is true at least at 0% grade on a treadmill when the speed can be accomplished at a submaximal steady-state level (Costill, 1986). **Figure 4.9** shows this fundamental relationship. The black lines were computed from the equations recommended by the American College of Sports Medicine (2010). These equations, in turn, are based on a compilation of research. Note that the relationship between speed and oxygen consumption is not a continuous straight line encompassing both walking (**Figure 4.9A**) and running (**Figure 4.9B**). For walking speeds between approximately 50 and 100 m·min^{-1}, each m·min^{-1} adds 0.1 mL·kg^{-1}·min^{-1} above resting to the cost of the walk; for running speeds above 134 m·min^{-1}, the increment is 0.2 mL·kg^{-1}·min^{-1}. Speeds between 100 and 134 m·min^{-1} are awkward for most people because they are too fast to walk but too slow to run. Additionally, outdoor running over ground is probably more demanding in terms of oxygen cost than indoor running on the treadmill at any given velocity, although overground inclined running equals the oxygen cost of treadmill-grade running (Daniels, 1985; Morgan et al., 1989b).

For any given individual, running economy appears to be relatively stable if environmental, equipment, and testing factors (such as body temperature, air resistance, footwear, time of day, and training status) are controlled (Morgan et al., 1989b). Day-to-day variations from 1.6 to 11% have been reported in the literature for well-trained and elite male runners. On the other hand, differences

Economy The oxygen cost of any activity, but particularly walking or running at varying speeds.

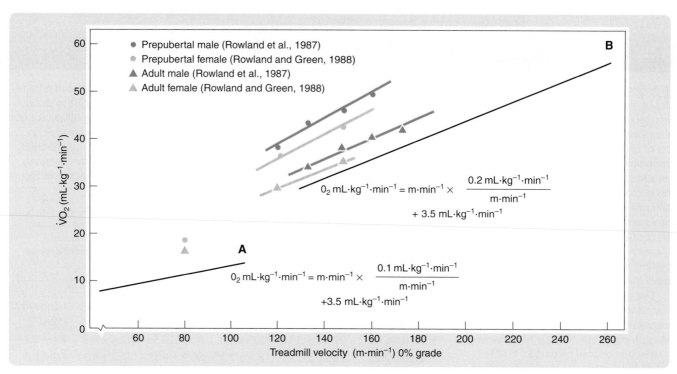

FIGURE 4.9 The Economy of Walking and Running for Children versus Adults.
The oxygen cost (expressed as V̇O₂ mL·kg⁻¹ min⁻¹) of walking **(A)** and running **(B)** increases rectilinearly as velocity increases. However, the slopes of the two lines are different, and the lines are not continuous from slow walking to fast running. Prepubertal males and prepubertal females are less economical than adult males and females as indicated by the higher oxygen cost at each and every velocity.
Sources: American College of Sports Medicine: *ACSM's Guidelines for Exercise Testing and Prescription* (8th edition). Baltimore, MD: Lippincott Williams & Wilkins (2010); Rowland, T. W., J. A. Auchinachie, T. J. Keenan, & G. M. Green: Physiologic responses to treadmill running in adult and prepubertal males. *International Journal of Sports Medicine.* 8(4):292–297 (1987); Rowland, T. W., & G. M. Green: Physiological responses to treadmill exercise in females: Adult-child differences. *Medicine and Science in Sports and Exercise.* 20(5):474–478 (1988).

among individuals in terms of running economy are often extensive, ranging from 20 to 30%, in subjects of equal training and performance status. The reason for these observations has not been determined (Conley and Krahenbuhl, 1980; Daniels, 1985; McCann and Higginson, 2008).

Male-Female Differences in Economy

The influence of sex on variations among individuals in economy is unclear. Different studies report that males expend more energy (**Figure 4.9**, green lines), less energy, or the same amount of energy in walking and running as do females (**Figure 4.9**, gold lines) when values are expressed relative to body mass (per kilogram of body weight). What is clear is that even if the oxygen cost is equal at any given speed, females, who typically have a lower V̇O₂max, will be working at a higher %V̇O₂max than males (Åstrand, 1956; Bhambhani and Singh, 1985; Bransford and Howley, 1977; Bunc and Heller, 1989; Cunningham, 1990; Daniels, 1985; Morgan et al., 1989b). This fact has implications for the pace at which long-distance events can be run.

Studies on sex differences in economy in children and adolescents are more or less equally divided between those showing no sex differences and those showing girls with a higher economy (lower V̇O₂ cost). No study has indicated that boys have a higher economy than girls (Rowland, 2005).

Economy in Children and Adolescents

Age has a clear-cut effect on economy in youths. Ample evidence shows that children and adolescents are less economical than adults when running/walking over a wide range of speeds, when economy is expressed as V̇O₂ mL·kg·min⁻¹ (Asmussen, 1981; Daniels, 1985; Girandola et al., 1981; Larish et al., 1987; Morgan et al., 1989b; Robinson et al., 1976; Rowland, 2005; Rowland and Green, 1988; Rowland et al., 1987, 1988; Van de Walle et al., 2010).

Figure 4.9A, B shows the results of two studies conducted in the same laboratory in which male prepubertal children (9–13 years) were compared with adult males (23–33 years) (Rowland et al., 1987) and female prepubertal children (8–12 years) were compared with adult females (22–35 years) (Rowland et al., 1988) and how the

FOCUS ON RESEARCH: *Clinically Relevant*
Wheelchair Propulsion Economy

Twelve able-bodied male participants (without prior preferences for frequency or strategy for wheelchair propulsion) completed four 5-minute exercise bouts at 32 W (52% $\dot{V}O_2$peak) in a randomized design on a basketball wheelchair ergometer. The purpose was to examine physiological responses to two selected push frequencies (40 push·min^{-1} and 70 push·min^{-1}) completed using either a synchronous (SYN) push strategy (both arms working simultaneously) or asynchronous (ASY) strategy (arms working alternately).

Results indicated that the SYN 40 condition was 9% more economical than the ASY 70, 12% more economical than the SYN 70 ($P < 0.01$), and 13% more economical than ASY 40 ($P < 0.01$). Heart rate values showed that the SYN 40 condition was significantly less stressful than all other conditions, and lactate concentrations were lower in both 40-push conditions as opposed to 70-push conditions. It was concluded that low push frequency combined with SYN arm motion provides the most economical form of wheelchair propulsion.

Source: Goosey-Tolfrey, V. L., & J. H. Kirk: Effect of push frequency and strategy variations on economy and perceived exertion during wheelchair propulsion. *European Journal of Applied Physiology.* 90:154–158 (2003).

four groups compared to the theoretical computed oxygen consumption values. In both sexes, the energy cost at all speeds of running was higher for children than adults relative to body mass. Males were not tested for walking, but in females, at 80 m·min^{-1}, there was no apparent walking economy difference with age. The differences at the running speeds held true whether expressed as an absolute load (m·min^{-1}) or relative load. The adult values were much closer to the calculated values than the children's, indicating that the equations should not be used for children.

Figures 4.10A and **4.10B** show that children and adolescents differ in economy of running not only from adults but also from each other by sex and age (Åstrand, 1952). Indeed, there is a progressive decline in oxygen cost (progressive increase in economy) from the youngest (4–6 years) to the oldest (16–17 years) age groups in both boys and girls. A compilation of studies shows the decline in oxygen cost to be about 2% per year from 8 to 18 years when the same work is performed (Morgan et al., 1989b). Similar data are available for both boys and girls walking at 80–100 m·min^{-1} at increasing grades. These changes are evident from cross-sectional studies in which different individuals are tested at each age and in longitudinal studies of the same individuals at different ages (Bar-Or, 1983; Costill, 1986; Daniels et al., 1978). The available data indicate that the oxygen cost of walking/running at any given speed decreases on average by 1.0 mL·kg·min^{-1} per year (Rowland, 2005).

There has been much speculation about the cause of this low economy in children. Five factors known to be affected by growth may offer at least a partial explanation.

1. *High basal metabolic rate.* Basal metabolic rate (BMR) is the minimum level of energy required to sustain the body's vital functions in a waking state, as measured by oxygen consumption. BMR is highest in young children and progressively declines to adulthood, where it stabilizes until it again declines in old age (Rowland, 1990) (see **Figure 4.11** and **Figure 8.4** in Chapter 8). Thus, gross exercise oxygen consumption values may be higher in children than in adults because resting metabolic rates are higher. Bar-Or (1983) has pointed out that this difference in resting metabolism is only 1–2 mL·kg^{-1}·min^{-1} and, although this value represents a 25–35% greater BMR in children than in adults, it alone is unlikely to account for all of the difference in submaximal exercise values. Indeed, when Åstrand (1952) used net oxygen values instead of gross (by subtracting the BMR), the difference between the age groups was reduced but not eliminated. Thus, the use of net, not gross, values is better when interpreting oxygen consumption of walking/running for children and adolescents (Van de Walle et al., 2010).

2. *Large surface area/mass ratio.* Throughout the animal kingdom, smaller animals (such as mice, squirrels, rabbits, or the young of any species) have higher resting metabolic rates per unit of body mass than larger animals (dogs, horses, elephants, or the adults of any species). However, when the unit of comparison is not body mass (per kilogram) but body surface area (per square meter), metabolic rates are similar. This is called the *surface law.* The surface law appears to be important for the maintenance of normal core temperatures, as body heat loss is directly related to surface area: The larger the surface area, the greater the heat loss. Smaller individuals, as is typically true of the young, have greater surface areas per unit of mass than larger individuals. Therefore, a higher resting metabolic rate is necessary to maintain body temperature in a smaller (younger) person. This phenomenon may be the reason for the elevated BMR in the young (Rowland, 1990; Rowland and Green, 1988; Rowland et al., 1987). When Rowland and colleagues (1988, 1987, 2005) changed the unit of comparison from mL·kg^{-1}·min^{-1} to mL·m^2·min^{-1}, the differences between the prepubertal and adult subjects of both sexes were no longer significant and were almost eliminated.

3. *Immature running mechanics.* Watching a young child and an adult run together reveals obvious differences

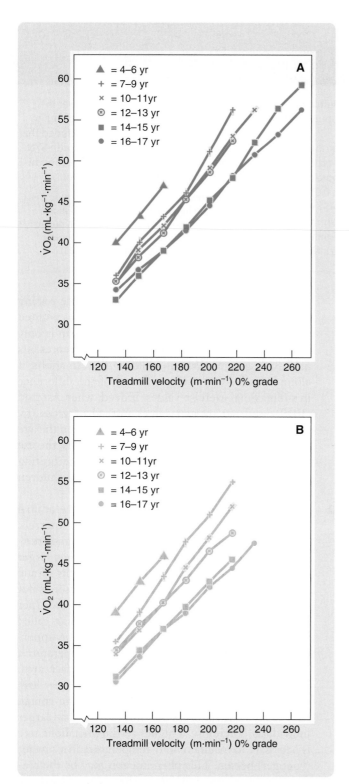

FIGURE 4.10 Running Economy of Children and Adolescents.
Running economy improves as both male **(A)** and female **(B)** children age. This can be seen by the almost parallel and successively lower V̇O₂ mL·kg⁻¹·min⁻¹ values across the tested velocities of running.
Source: Åstrand, P.-O.: *Experimental Studies of Physical Working Capacity in Relation to Sex and Age.* Copenhagen: Munksgaard (1952). Modified and printed by permission.

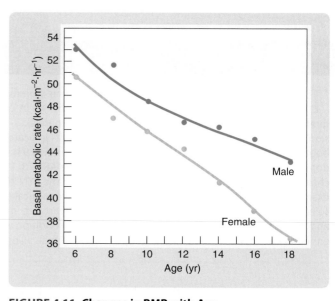

FIGURE 4.11 Changes in BMR with Age.
Source: From Rowland, T. W.: *Exercise and Children's Health.* Champaign, IL: Human Kinetics (1990). Data from Knoebel, L. K.: Energy metabolism. In Selkurt, E. E. (ed.): *Physiology.* Bostan: Little, Brown, 564–579, (1963). Reprinted with permission.

in motor skill (Rowland, 1990; Rowland et al., 1987). Young children seem to take numerous small, choppy steps involving lots of extraneous movements. At the same speed as an adult, the child has a higher stride frequency; a shorter stride length; a greater vertical displacement; increased ankle, knee, and hip extension at takeoff; increased cocontraction of antagonistic muscles; a longer nonsupport phase; and a shorter placement of the support foot in front of the center of gravity. The variable that seems to have the most direct effect on the oxygen cost of running is stride frequency. Each stride requires energy to accelerate and decelerate the body's mass. Per stride, the oxygen cost is the same in children and adults. Similarly, when speed is adjusted for body size using a leg length per second (LL·sec⁻¹) unit, children and adults are equally economical (Maliszewski and Freedson, 1996). However, at any given pace, the child has a greater frequency of strides simply because he or she is anatomically smaller. Thus, more oxygen is utilized (indicating lower economy) to provide the greater energy need (Rowland et al., 1987, 2005).

Remember that each individual intuitively selects the most economical combination of stride frequency and length for running. Therefore, one should not attempt to "make" children more economical by training them to lengthen their strides. Stride frequency decreases and stride length increases naturally as the child grows.

4. *Less efficient ventilation.* The volume of air breathed in to consume 1 L of oxygen is called the *ventilatory*

equivalent (*VE*). Children have a higher VE than adults. The processing of this additional air requires an added expenditure of energy. This increased metabolic cost of respiration may account for part of the increased oxygen cost at submaximal work in children, although not all research evidence agrees (Allor et al., 2000; Rowland, 1990; Rowland and Green, 1988; Rowland et al., 1987, 1988).

5. *Lower anaerobic capacity.* As discussed in the preceding chapter, children are less able to generate ATP anaerobically than adults. The measurement of economy by oxygen consumption evaluates only the aerobic energy contribution. It is possible that at higher, but still submaximal, workloads, adults provide more of the required energy anaerobically and thus exhibit artificially low oxygen cost values (Rowland, 1990; Rowland et al., 1987). Evidence from RER values supports this contention. Children typically show lower RERs during submaximal exercise than adults. Direct measurement of free fatty acid and glycerol levels shows, however, that the lower RERs are not the result of an increased utilization of fat as a fuel as might be expected. Instead, the lower RERs are thought to result from lower amounts of nonmetabolic "excess CO_2," that is, the CO_2 generated from the buffering of lactic acid.

Economy in Older Adults

Economy in older adults appears to be higher than that in children, approximately equal to adolescents, and lower than young adults (McCann and Adams, 2002). The difference from young adults in oxygen cost has been observed to be anywhere from 8 to 31% (Malatesta et al., 2003: Martin et al., 1992; McCann and Adams, 2002; Mian et al., 2006; Ortega and Farley, 2007).

As with children, the cause of the increased oxygen cost (lower economy) at any given speed of walking is unknown, although, unlike with children, there does not appear to be a size component (McCann and Adams, 2002). Mechanistic ideas about the difference include the following:

1. *Recruitment of additional motor units.* Aging brings a decline in the force-generating capacity of muscle. This may require the recruitment of additional motor units, including a higher proportion of less economical fast-twitch muscle fibers. More motor units require more oxygen to produce ATP (Martin et al., 1992).

2. *Gait instability.* Increased gait instability (based on stride time) and a greater energy expenditure needed to maintain balance during such instability have both been suggested as causes for the greater oxygen cost of walking in older adults. However, although Malatesta et al. (2003) found both greater stride time variability in 65-year-old and 80-year-old individuals and lower economy compared with 25-year-old individuals, these two variables were not significantly correlated. They concluded that the metabolic cost of the static contraction involved in maintaining balance was negligible.

3. *Antagonistic cocontraction.* Cocontraction or coactivation means that there is contraction or activation of antagonist muscles during agonist action. Excessive coactivation causes joint stiffening, limits range of movement, and may partly explain the elevated oxygen cost of walking in older adults. Again, more muscles require more oxygen for the production of ATP (Malatesta et al., 2003; Mian et al., 2006).

Practical Application of Economy Information

Economy and efficiency probably matter little in high-intensity, short-term activities such as maximal weight lifts and sprints or in skilled movements such as golf. However, economy is extremely important in endurance events. Among those factors critical for success in endurance performances are a high $\dot{V}O_2max$, the ability to work at a high $\%\dot{V}O_2max$ aerobically (sometimes measured as a high $\%\dot{V}O_2max$ at LT1 [first lactate threshold]), and a high economy measured as a low submaximal oxygen cost at high velocities (Almarwaey et al., 2003; Conley and Krahenbuhl, 1980; Costill, 1986; Costill et al., 1973; Cunningham, 1990; Morgan et al., 1989a,b; Saunders et al., 2004). What may matter most to competitive runners is a combination of economy and $\dot{V}O_2max$ known as velocity at $\dot{V}O_2max$ ($v\dot{V}O_2max$).

Although a high $\dot{V}O_2max$ is considered to be a prerequisite for success in distance or endurance events, it generally does not determine performance when participants are relatively homogeneous in that trait. For example, Costill (1986) presents data from two runners (Ted Corbitt and Jim McDonagh) who had similar $\dot{V}O_2max$ values (64 and 65 mL·kg^{-1}·min^{-1}). Over a period of 2 years, they competed against each other in 15 major races, and the same runner (McDonagh) won each and every time! Obviously, the physiological explanation did not lie in $\dot{V}O_2max$.

The importance of the ability to sustain a high $\%\dot{V}O_2max$ aerobically for long periods of time is exemplified by the success of such runners as Grete Waitz, Frank Shorter, and Derek Clayton (Costill, 1986). These world-class runners were estimated to use 85–90% $\dot{V}O_2max$ when they competed in marathons, whereas less successful marathoners average about 75–80% $\dot{V}O_2max$. Typically, such a high percentage (85–90%) can be maintained only for the shorter (10 mi or less) distance. By continuing at that rate over twice as long as normal, these individuals gained a competitive edge. A 2010 study (McLaughlin et al.) showed that when there was little variability in the $\%\dot{V}O_2max$ at LT1 during a 16-km race it ($\%\dot{V}O_2max$ at LT1) did not explain distance running ability similar to the situation that when

$\dot{V}O_2$max was homogeneous it ($\dot{V}O_2$max) did not explain endurance performance. However, the velocity (m·min⁻¹) at LT1 was highly correlated with the 16-km run time.

The importance of a high running economy is seen in several situations. If two runners of widely varying $\dot{V}O_2$max (runner A = 65 mL·kg⁻¹·min⁻¹; runner B = 50 mL·kg⁻¹·min⁻¹) but similar economy attempt to train together, say at an 8-minute pace ($\dot{V}O_2$max cost = 40 mL·kg⁻¹·min⁻¹), runner B would be working much harder (80% $\dot{V}O_2$max) than runner A (62% $\dot{V}O_2$max). This variation in effort often occurs when females (average lower $\dot{V}O_2$max, equal economy) run with males.

Differences in economy have a similar effect on performance. If, for example, runner A and runner B had the same $\dot{V}O_2$max (65 mL·kg⁻¹·min⁻¹) but widely varying economies at an 8-minute pace (runner A = 55 mL·kg⁻¹·min⁻¹; runner B = 40 mL·kg⁻¹·min⁻¹), then runner A would be working much harder (85% $\dot{V}O_2$max) than runner B (62% $\dot{V}O_2$max). This is the likely reason why McDonagh (above) continually beat Corbitt in their races. At all velocities faster than 8 min·mi⁻¹, Corbitt used significantly more oxygen than McDonagh (Costill, 1986). Corbitt could have won only by making up the difference by running at a higher %$\dot{V}O_2$max.

A similar situation occurs when a child (on average, equal in $\dot{V}O_2$max [in mL·kg·min⁻¹] to an adult but lower in economy) runs with an adult as seen in **Figure 4.12**. At any given speed, the child (unless there is a great disparity in his or her favor for $\dot{V}O_2$max) will be working harder than the adult. Although it is important for parents and teachers to encourage children to be active and for adults to do activities with children, the fact that the child will be working proportionally harder at any given running pace must be taken into account. The parent or teacher should match the child's pace or encourage just a slightly faster pace—not try to make the child keep up with what the adult finds comfortable. As a consequence, the adult will have to do his or her hard training without the child along, but the child will enjoy the experience much more. Since there appears to be no to little difference in efficiency in cycling as a function of sex or age as long as the wheel sizes are equal (allowing the same revolutions per minute), cycling may be a better family activity than running. Work through the Check Your Comprehension 6 box. Check your answer in Appendix C.

CHECK YOUR COMPREHENSION 6

The Fitt family plans to run the Cornfest 10-km (6.2 mi) race together. Dr Phyllis Fitt, the mother, is an exercise physiologist and recently tested all family members in her lab. Given the following information, what is the fastest time they can run with a reasonable chance of everyone finishing in good shape together?

	Daughter	Son	Mother	Father	Grand-mother
Age (yr)	12	8	37	45	57
$\dot{V}O_2$ max (mL·kg⁻¹·min⁻¹)	48	50	50	52	40
$\dot{V}O_2$ (mL·kg⁻¹·min⁻¹)					
10 min·mi⁻¹	37	39	30	32	33
9 min·mi⁻¹	40	43	32	34	36
8 min·mi⁻¹	45	48	38	41	40
7 min·mi⁻¹	48	50	43	46	

Hint: Competitive runners typically average 80–90% $\dot{V}O_2$max during distance races of 5–10 mi; fun runners might be expected to be at the lower end of this value.

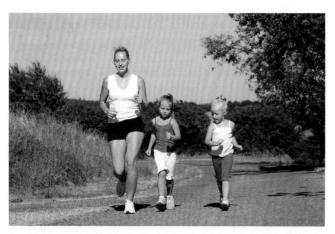

FIGURE 4.12 Children and Adults Exercising Together.
Because of the differences in running economy when children/adolescents and adults run together, the youngest individual should set the pace.

As stated previously, what may matter most to competitive runners is the combination of economy and $\dot{V}O_2$max known as velocity at $\dot{V}O_2$max (v$\dot{V}O_2$max). **Velocity at $\dot{V}O_2$max** is the speed at which an individual can run when working at his or her maximal oxygen consumption based on both submaximal running economy and $\dot{V}O_2$. **Table 4.9** and **Figure 4.13** show how this value is calculated and what it means. To calculate v$\dot{V}O_2$max, $\dot{V}O_2$ values (y-axis) are plotted at several submaximal speeds (x-axis) for each individual, and a regression line—a line that best fits the $\dot{V}O_2$ values—is established. The line is extended to reach the individual's measured $\dot{V}O_2$max. The speed (or velocity) at which the $\dot{V}O_2$max occurs is then determined by dropping a perpendicular line from the $\dot{V}O_2$max point to the x-axis. This velocity is taken as the velocity at $\dot{V}O_2$max (v$\dot{V}O_2$max). As the figure shows, it is possible to achieve the same v$\dot{V}O_2$max with a high economy (low energy cost at submaximal speeds) and a low $\dot{V}O_2$max (subject A) or with a low economy (high energy cost at submaximal speeds) and a high $\dot{V}O_2$max (subject B). Individuals such as these two with a similar

	VO₂ mL·kg⁻¹·min⁻¹ at Indicated Speed (m·min⁻¹)					vVO₂max (mL·kg⁻¹·min⁻¹)	vVO₂max (m·min⁻¹)	10-km Run Time	%vVO₂max for 10 km
Subject	196	215	230	248	268				
A	38.03	40.58	44.30	45.10	—	54.68	304.56	38:21	83.2
B	—	46.13	48.28	50.54	54.88	60.88	306.50	38:09	83.1

TABLE 4.9   Information for Predicted Velocity at VO₂max for Subjects A and B (Figure 4.13)

Source: Based on Bird, J.: The contribution of selected physiological variables to 10 km run time in trained, heterogeneous adult male runners. Unpublished master's thesis, Northern Illinois University, DeKalb, IL, 31 (1991).

vVO₂max would be expected to have similar performances in endurance running events (Bird, 1991; Morgan et al., 1989a). All other factors (such as %VO₂max) being relatively equal, an individual with a high vVO₂max would be expected to perform better than an individual with a low vVO₂max (Almarwaey et al., 2003; Kilding et al., 2006; McLaughlin et al., 2010; Sirotic and Coutts, 2007). The highest speed attained at the end of a graded exercise test with horizontal running can be used to predict performance, especially in a marathon, because it appears to reflect the physiological variables involved in vVO₂max (McLaughlin et al., 2010).

The low economy of children may help explain another phenomenon. Typically, endurance performance as measured by treadmill time to fatigue, 12-minute-run distance, mile-run time, and so on, improves in children with age despite a constant VO₂max (**Figure 4.14**). Furthermore, although young athletes generally have VO₂max values higher than those of nonathletes, when training programs are used, endurance performance often improves exclusively—or at least more than does VO₂max. Improvements in submaximal running economy (through improved skill in the short term) and age improvements in qualitative changes in oxygen delivery (not indicated by VO₂max) and/or the improvement of anaerobic strength and speed components in the long term may possibly account for the enhanced endurance performances regardless of what occurs with VO₂max. Indeed, submaximal running

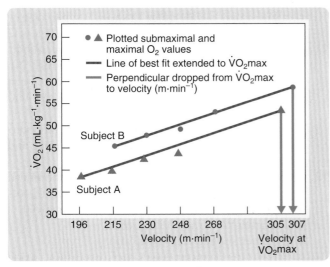

FIGURE 4.13 Predicted Velocity at VO₂max.
Source: Based on Bird, J.: The contribution of selected physiological variables to 10 kilometer run time in trained, heterogeneous adult male runners. Unpublished master's thesis, Northern Illinois University, DeKalb, IL, 31, (1991).

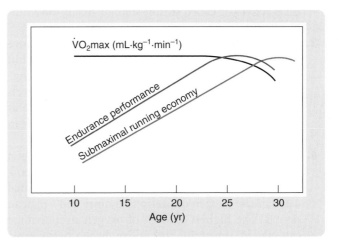

FIGURE 4.14 The Relationship between Maximal Oxygen Consumption, Endurance Performance, and Submaximal Running Economy from Childhood to Early Adulthood.
As children age, endurance performance typically improves often despite no improvement in VO₂max mL·kg⁻¹·min⁻¹. One possible explanation is the parallel improvement in submaximal running economy. In early adulthood, all three measures begin to decline.
Source: From Rowland, T. W.: *Exercise and Children's Health.* Champaign, IL: Human Kinetics (2004). Reprinted with permission.

Velocity at VO₂max The speed at which an individual can run when working at his or her maximal oxygen consumption, based on both submaximal running economy and VO₂max.

economy has been found to be statistically related to and to account for much of the variance in endurance performance in children and adolescents in most (but not all) studies. Since $\dot{V}O_2$max remains relatively stable and the O_2 cost of any given speed decreases, the child is working at a progressively lower %$\dot{V}O_2$max; as he or she ages. The individual is therefore expected to perform (endure) at the same speed for a longer period of time, cover more ground in the same time span, and/or increase the speed at which any given distance is covered (Bar-Or, 1983; Burkett et al., 1985; Daniels and Oldridge, 1971; Daniels et al., 1978; Krahenbuhl et al., 1989; Mayers and Gutin, 1979; McCormack et al., 1991; Rowland, 1990; Rowland et al., 1988).

Finally, for all the reasons discussed above, one cannot use adult prediction equations based on $\dot{V}O_2$/speed relationships to predict $\dot{V}O_2$max in children.

SUMMARY

1. Aerobic metabolism can be measured directly by calorimetry (the measurement of heat production) or indirectly by spirometry (the measurement of air breathed and the analysis of oxygen and carbon dioxide gases). Typically, open-circuit indirect spirometry/open-circuit indirect calorimetry is used.

2. During aerobic exercise, the amount of oxygen consumed and carbon dioxide produced increases. In a short-term submaximal activity, the metabolic costs level off where the energy requirements are met. This activity is called steady-state or steady-rate submaximal exercise.

3. If a submaximal exercise lasts for a long time, is above approximately 70% $\dot{V}O_2$max, or takes place under hot and humid conditions, oxygen drift occurs. The oxygen consumption drifts upward owing to rising levels of catecholamines, lactate, and body temperature as well as an increasing cost of ventilation and a shift in substrate utilization.

4. During incremental exercise to maximum, oxygen consumption rises in a rectilinear pattern proportional to the workload increments until the individual can increase oxygen utilization no more and a plateau occurs. The highest amount of oxygen an individual can take in, transport, and utilize during heavy exercise is called maximal oxygen consumption $\dot{V}O_2$max.

5. Very short, high-intensity anaerobic exercise and static and dynamic resistance activity are predominantly anaerobic activities. The oxygen contribution to the energy cost rarely exceeds one fourth to one half of the total energy cost but is a meaningful amount.

6. On the cellular level, the ratio of carbon dioxide produced to oxygen consumed is termed the respiratory quotient; as analyzed from expired air, it is termed the respiratory exchange ratio. Nonprotein RER is used most frequently in determining energy substrate utilization, with 0.7 being interpreted as fat, 1.0 as carbohydrate, and 0.85 as an approximate 50–50 mixture of both.

7. During exercise, the higher the intensity, the higher the RER value. During long-duration submaximal exercise, RER may decrease as the carbohydrate stores are depleted. During incremental exercise to maximum, RER may increase above 1.0, reflecting carbon dioxide increases from nonmetabolic sources. RERs for high-intensity static exercise and dynamic resistance exercise are between 0.8 and 1.0+, reflecting a mixed fuel supply during the static activity followed by hyperventilation and a reliance on glycogen during the dynamic resistance activity.

8. Given the amount of oxygen consumed, the RER during the same time span, and the caloric equivalent, caloric expenditure (kcal·min^{-1}) and metabolic equivalents (METs) can be calculated.

9. Energy expenditure can be estimated in field settings using a series of metabolic formulas, motion sensors/accelerometers, or activity recall questionnaires and previously established caloric cost charts.

10. Mechanical efficiency (gross, net, or delta) is some ratio of work output to energy expended. Economy is simply a measure of energy expended (oxygen consumed); it is used when measuring work output is difficult. Energy cost and economy are inversely related. Because the energy cost of walking and running is rectilinear over a wide range of speed, oxygen cost or MET values can be estimated when speed is known.

11. Variation in running economy is high between individuals but is low within the same individual. No clear-cut distinction in running economy has been shown between females and males. Children and adolescents are less economical than adults when running over a wide range of speeds. Older individuals are less economical when walking than young and middle-aged adults.

12. The exact reason why children are less economical than adults is unknown, but one or more of the following characteristics of children may be involved:
    a. A higher basal metabolic rate
    b. A larger surface area/mass ratio
    c. Immature running mechanics, especially stride frequency
    d. Less efficient ventilation
    e. Lower anaerobic capacity

13. The exact reason why older adults are less economical than younger adults is unknown, but the following factors have been considered possibilities:
    a. Recruitment of additional motor units
    b. Gait instability
    c. Antagonistic cocontraction

14. A high economy (low oxygen cost) at any given velocity of running is beneficial to performance, especially when combined with a high $\dot{V}O_2$max and

the ability to work consistently at a high percentage of $\dot{V}O_2$max aerobically (high % $\dot{V}O_2$max at LT1). The higher the velocity at $\dot{V}O_2$max and the greater the percentage of v$\dot{V}O_2$max an individual can maintain, the better his or her performance will be. Improvements in running economy may explain why, as they grow and/or train, children typically improve in endurance run performance (such as the mile run) but do not show any significant improvement in $\dot{V}O_2$max.

REVIEW QUESTIONS

1. List and define the variables used to describe aerobic metabolic responses to exercise. Describe how each is obtained from laboratory or field tests.
2. Diagram the oxygen consumption response during (a) short-term, light- to moderate-intensity submaximal aerobic exercise; (b) long-term, moderate to heavy submaximal aerobic exercise; (c) incremental aerobic exercise to maximum; (d) static exercise; and (e) dynamic resistance exercise.
3. Describe the relationship between the oxygen cost of breathing and the exercise intensity.
4. Explain the respiratory quotient and the respiratory exchange ratio. Relate them to the determination of energy substrate utilization, theoretically and numerically according to exercise intensity, duration, and type.
5. Explain the similarities and differences between describing activity by kilocalories and describing activity by MET levels. How can both be practically applied?
6. Differentiate, in terms of definition, calculation, and application, among gross efficiency, net efficiency, and delta efficiency. How can cyclists maximize efficiency?
7. Compare running economy by sex and age. Discuss possible reasons for any observed differences. Give three situations where observed differences could have significant practical meaning.
8. Show how efficiency or economy can affect exercise performance.

For further review and additional study tools, visit the website at http://thePoint.lww.com/Plowman4e ✳ ◉

REFERENCES

Adams, W. C., M. M. McHenry, & E. M. Bernauer: Multistage treadmill walking performance and associated cardiorespiratory responses of middle-aged men. *Clinical Science.* 42: 355–370 (1972).

Allor, K. M., J. M. Pivarnik, L. J. Sam, & C. D. Perkins: Treadmill economy in girls and women matched for height and weight. *Journal of Applied Physiology.* 89:512–516 (2000).

Almarwaey, O. A., A. H. Jones, & K. Tolfrey: Physiological correlates with endurance running performance in trained adolescents. *Medicine & Science in Sports & Exercise.* 35(3):480–487 (2003).

American College of Sports Medicine: *ACSM's Guidelines for Exercise Testing and Prescription* (8th edition). Baltimore, MD: Lippincott Williams & Wilkins (2010).

Ainsworth, B. E., W. L. Haskell, S. D. Herrmann, et al: 2011 Compendium of physical activities: A second update of codes and MET values. *Medicine & Science in Sports & Exercise.* 43(8):1575–1581 (2011); http://sites.google.com/site/compendiumofphysicalactivities.

Asmussen, E: Similarities and dissimilarities between static and dynamic exercise. *Circulation Research (Suppl. I).* 48(6):I-3–I-10 (1981).

Åstrand, P. O.: *Experimental Studies of Physical Working Capacity in Relation to Sex and Age.* Copenhagen: Munksgaard (1952).

Åstrand, P. O.: Human physical fitness with special reference to sex and age. *Physiological Reviews.* 36(3):307–335 (1956).

Åstrand, P -O.: Principles of ergometry and their implications in sport practice. *International Journal of Sports Medicine.* 5:102–105 (1984).

Åstrand, P. O. & K. Rodahl: *Textbook of Work Physiology: Physiological Bases of Exercise.* New York, NY: McGraw-Hill (1977).

Atallah, L., J. J. H. Leong, B. Lo, & G. Z. Yang: Energy expenditure prediction using a miniaturized ear-worn sensor. *Medicine & Science in Sports & Exercise.* 43(7):1369–1377 (2011).

Bal, M. E., E. M. Thompson, E. M. McIntosh, C. M. Taylor, & C. MacLeod: Mechanical efficiency in cycling of girls six to fourteen years of age. *Journal of Applied Physiology.* 6:185–188 (1953).

Bar-Or, O.: *Pediatric Sports Medicine for the Practitioner: From Physiological Principles to Clinical Applications.* New York, NY: Springer-Verlag, 1–65 (1983).

Bar-Or, O.: The Wingate Anaerobic Test: An update on methodology, reliability and validity. *Sports Medicine.* 4:381–394 (1987).

Bhambhani, Y., & M. Singh: Metabolic and cinematographic analysis of walking and running in men and women. *Medicine and Science in Sports and Exercise.* 17(1):131–137 (1985).

Bird, J.: The contribution of selected physiological variables to 10 kilometer run time in trained, heterogeneous adult male runners. Unpublished master's thesis, Northern Illinois University, DeKalb, IL, 31 (1991).

Bransford, D. R., & E. T. Howley: Oxygen costs of running in trained and untrained men and women. *Medicine and Science in Sports.* 9(1):41–44 (1977).

Broker, J. P., C. R. Kyle, & E. R. Burke: Racing cycling power requirements in the 4000-m individual and team pursuits. *Medicine & Science in Sports & Exercise.* 31(11):1677–1685 (1999).

Bunc, V., & J. Heller: Energy cost of running in similarly trained men and women. *European Journal of Applied Physiology.* 59:178–183 (1989).

Burkett, L. N., B. Fernhall, & S. C. Walter: Physiological effects of distance run training on teenage females. *Research Quarterly for Exercise and Sport.* 56(3):215–220 (1985).

Burszstein, S., D. H. Elwyn, J. Askanazi, & J. M. Kinney: *Energy Metabolism, Indirect Calorimetry and Nutrition*. Baltimore, MD: Lippincott Williams & Wilkins (1989).

Butts, N. K., C. Dodge, & M. McAlpine: Effect of stepping rate on energy costs during StairMaster exercise. *Medicine and Science in Sports and Exercise*. 25(3):378–382 (1993).

Bye, P. T. P., G. A. Farkas, & C. Roussos: Respiratory factors limiting exercise. *Annual Review of Physiology*. 45:439–451 (1983).

Carpenter, T. M.: *Tables, Factors, and Formulas for Computing Respiratory Exchange and Biological Transformations of Energy* (4th ed). Washington, DC: Carnegie Institution of Washington, Publication 303C (1921).

Cavanagh, P. R., & R. Kram: Mechanical and muscular factors affecting the efficiency of human movement. *Medicine and Science in Sports and Exercise*. 17(3):326–331 (1985).

Chen, K. Y., & D. R. Bassett, Jr.: The technology of accelerometry- based activity monitors: Current and future. *Medicine & Science in Sports & Exercise*. 37(11):S490–S500 (2005).

Conley, D. L., & G. S. Krahenbuhl: Running economy and distance running performance of highly trained athletes. *Medicine and Science in Sports and Exercise*. 12(5):357–360 (1980).

Consolazio, C. F., R. E. Johnson, & L. J. Pecora: *Physiological Measurements of Metabolic Functions in Man*. New York, NY: McGraw-Hill (1963).

Corder, K., S. Brage, & U. Ekelund: Accelerometers and pedometers: Methodology and clinical application. *Current Opinion in Clinical Nutrition and Metabolic Care*. 10(5):597–603 (2007).

Costill, D. L.: *Inside Running: Basics of Sport Physiology*. Indianapolis, IN: Benchmark Press (1986).

Costill, D. L., H. Thomason, & E. Roberts: Fractional utilization of the aerobic capacity during distance running. *Medicine and Science in Sports*. 5(4):248–252 (1973).

Crouter, S. E., P. L. Schneider, M. Karabulut, & D. R. Basset, Jr.: Validity of 10 electronic pedometers for measuring steps, distance and energy cost. *Medicine and Science in Sports*. 35(8):1455–1460 (2003).

Cunningham, L. N.: Relationship of running economy, ventilatory threshold, and maximal oxygen consumption to running performance in high school females. *Research Quarterly for Exercise and Sport*. 61(4):369–374 (1990).

Daniels, J. T.: A physiologist's view of running economy. *Medicine and Science in Sports and Exercise*. 17(3):332–338 (1985).

Daniels, J., & N. Oldridge: Changes in oxygen consumption of young boys during growth and running training. *Medicine and Science in Sports*. 3(4):161–165 (1971).

Daniels, J., N. Oldridge, F. Nagle, & B. White: Differences and changes in VO2 among young runners 10 to 18 years of age. *Medicine and Science in Sports and Exercise*. 10(3):200–203 (1978).

Davies, C. T. M.: Effects of wind assistance and resistance on the forward motion of a runner. *Journal of Applied Physiology: Respiratory, Environmental and Exercise Physiology*. 48(4):702–709 (1980).

Donovan, C. M., & G. A. Brooks: I. Muscular efficiency during steady-rate exercise. II. Effects of walking speed and work rate. *Journal of Applied Physiology: Respiratory, Environmental and Exercise Physiology*. 43(3):431–439 (1977).

Durstine, J. L., & R. R. Pate: Cardiorespiratory responses to acute exercise. In Blair, S. N., P. Palmer, R. R. Pate, L. K. Smith, & C. B. Taylor (eds.): *Resource Manual for Guidelines for Exercise Testing and Prescription*. Philadelphia, PA: Lea & Febiger, 38–54 (1988).

Fleck, S. J., & W. J. Kraemer: *Designing Resistance Training Programs*. Champaign, IL: Human Kinetics (1987).

Fox, E. L., & D. K. Mathews: *Interval Training: Conditioning for Sports and General Fitness*. Philadelphia, PA: W. B. Saunders (1974).

Gaesser, G. A., & G. A. Brooks: Muscular efficiency during steady-rate exercise: Effects of speed and work rate. *Journal of Applied Physiology*. 38(6):1132–1139 (1975).

Gastin, P. B.: Energy system interaction and relative contribution during maximal exercise. *Sports Medicine*. 31(10):725–741 (2001).

Girandola, R. N., R. A. Wiswell, F. Frisch, & K. Wood: Metabolic differences during exercise in pre- and post-pubescent girls. *Medicine and Science in Sports and Exercise* (abstract). 13(2):110 (1981).

Goosey-Tolfrey, V. L., & J. H. Kirk: Effect of push frequency and strategy variations on economy and perceived exertion during wheelchair propulsion. *European Journal of Applied Physiology*. 90:154–158 (2003).

Hagberg, J. M., J. P. Mullin, M. D. Giese, & E. Spitznagel: Effect of pedaling rate on submaximal exercise responses of competitive cyclists. *Journal of Applied Physiology: Respiratory, Environmental and Exercise Physiology*. 51(2):447–451 (1981).

Heselton, R., S. A. Plowman, N. S. Hannibal, L. Schuler, K. Jensen, & K. Harkness: The reliability and validity of the caloric expenditure values from an elliptical striding system. *Medicine & Science in Sports & Exercise (Abstract)*. 32(5):S301 (2000).

Holly, R. G.: Measurement of the maximal rate of oxygen uptake. In Blair, S. N., P. Palmer, R. R. Pate, L. K. Smith, & C. B. Taylor (eds.): *Resource Manual for Guidelines for Exercise Testing and Prescription*. Philadelphia, PA: Lea & Febiger, 171–177 (1988).

Hopker, J., S. Jobson, H. Carter, & L. Passfield: Cycling efficiency in trained male and female competitive cyclists. *Journal of Sports Science and Medicine*. 9(2):332–337 (2010).

Howley, E. T., D. R. Bassett, Jr., & H. G. Welch: Criteria for maximal oxygen uptake: Review and commentary. *Medicine and Science in Sports and Exercise*. 27(9):1292–1301 (1995).

Howley, E. T., D. L. Colacino, & T. C. Swensen: Factors affecting the oxygen cost of stepping on an electronic stepping ergometer. *Medicine and Science in Sports and Exercise*. 24(9):1055–1058 (1992).

Kilding, A. E., E. M. Winter, & M. Fysh: Moderate-domain pulmonary oxygen uptake kinetics and endurance running performance. *Journal of Sport Science*. 24(9):1013–1022 (2006).

Klausen, K., B. Rasmussen, L. K. Glensgaard, & O. V. Jensen: Work efficiency of children during submaximal bicycle exercise. In Binkhorst, R. A., H. C. G. Kemper, & M. Saris (eds.): *Children and Exercise XI*. Champaign, IL: Human Kinetics, 210–217 (1985).

Kohler, G. & U. Boutellier: The generalized force-velocity relationship explains why the preferred pedaling rate of cyclists exceeds the most efficient one. *European Journal of Applied Physiology*. 94(1–2):188–195 (2005).

Krahenbuhl, G. S., D. W. Morgan, & R. P. Pangrazi: Longitudinal changes in distance-running performance of young males. *International Journal of Sports Medicine*. 10(2):92–96 (1989).

Laporte, R. E., H. J. Montoye, & C. J. Caspersen: Assessment of physical activity in epidemiologic research: Problems and prospects. *Public Health Reports*. 100(2):131–146 (1985).

Larish, D. D., P. E. Martin, & M. Mungiole: Characteristic patterns of gait in the healthy old. *Annals of the New York Academy of Sciences*. 515:18–32 (1987).

Lazzer, S., L. Plaino, & G. Antonutto: The energetic of cycling on earth, moon and mars. *European Journal of Applied Physiology*. 111:357–366 (2011)

MacDougall, J. D., H. A. Wenger, & H. J. Green (eds.): *Physiological Testing of the Elite Athlete* (first edition). Hamilton, Ontario Canadian Association of Sport Sciences: Mutual Press Limited (1982).

McCann, D. J., & W. C. Adams: A dimensional paradigm for identifying the size-independent cost of walking. *Medicine & Science in Sports & Exercise*. 34(6):1009–1017 (2002).

McCann, D. J., & B. K. Higginson: Training to maximize economy of motion in running gast. *Current Sports Medicine Reports*. 7(3):158–162 (2008).

Malatesta, D., D. Simar, Y. Dauvilliers, R. Candau, F. Borrani, C. Préfaut, & C. Caillaud: Energy cost of walking and gait instability in healthy 65- and 80-yr-olds. *Journal of Applied Physiology*. 95:2248–2256 (2003).

Maliszewski, A. F., & P. S. Freedson: Is running economy different between adults and children? *Pediatric Exercise Science*. 8(4):351–360 (1996).

Martin, P. E., D. E. Rothstein, & D. D. Larish: Effects of age and physical activity status on the speed-aerobic demand relationship of walking. *Journal of Applied Physiology*. 73:200–206 (1992).

Mayers, N., & B. Gutin: Physiological characteristics of elite prepubertal cross-country runners. *Medicine and Science in Sports*. 11(2):172–176 (1979).

McCormack, W. P., K. J. Cureton, T. A. Bullock, & P. G. Weyand: Metabolic determinants of 1-mile run/walk performance in children. *Medicine and Science in Sports and Exercise*. 23(5):611–617 (1991).

McLaughlin, J. E., E. T. Howley, D. R. Basset, Jr., D. L. Thompson, & E. C. Fitzhugh: Test of the classic model for predicting endurance running performance. *Medicine & Science in Sports & Exercise*. 42(5):991–997 (2010).

Mian, O. S., J. M. Thom, L. P. Ardigò, M. V. Narici, & A. E. Minetti: Metabolic cost, mechanical work, and efficiency during walking in young and older men. *Acta Physiology*. 186(2):127–139 (2006).

Mier, C. M., & Y. Feito: Metabolic cost of stride rate, resistance, and combined use of arms and legs on the elliptical trainer. *Research Quarterly for Exercise and Sport*. 77(4):507–513 (2006).

Millet, G. P., C. Tronche, N. Fuster, & R. Candau: Level ground and uphill cycling efficiency in seated and standing positions. *Medicine & Science in Sports & Exercise*. 34(10):1645–1652 (2002).

Miyachi, M. K., K. Yamamoto, K. Ohkawara, & S. Tanaka: METS in adults while playing active video games: A metabolic chamber study. *Medicine & Science in Sports & Exercise*. 42(6):1149–1153 (2010).

Morgan, D., F. Baldini, P. Martin, & W. Kohrt: Ten km performance and predicted velocity of $\dot{V}O_2$max among well-trained male runners. *Medicine and Science in Sports and Exercise*. 21:78–83 (1989a).

Morgan, D. W., P. E. Martin, & G. S. Krahenbuhl: Factors affecting running economy. *Sports Medicine*. 7:310–330 (1989b).

Newsholme, E. A., & A. R. Leech: *Biochemistry for the Medical Sciences*. New York, NY: Wiley (1983).

Nielson, R., P. R. Vehrs, G. W. Fellingham, R. Hager, & K. A. Prusak: Step counts and energy expenditure as estimated by pedometry during treadmill walking at different stride frequencies. *Journal of Physical Activity & Health*. 8(7):1004–1013 (2011).

Otis, A. B: The work of breathing. *Physiological Reviews*. 34:449–458 (1954).

Ortega, J. D. & C. T. Farley: Individual limb work does not explain the greater metabolic cost of walking in elderly adults. *Journal of Applied Physiology*. 102:2266–2273 (2007).

Pardy, R. L., S. N. A. Hussain, & P. T. Macklem: The ventilatory pump in exercise. *Clinics in Chest Medicine*. 5(1):35–49 (1984).

Park, J., K. Ishikawa-Takata, S. Tanaka, Y. Mekata, & I. Tabata: Effects of walking speed and step frequency on estimation of physical activity using accelerometers. *Journal of Physiological Anthropology*. 30(3):119–127 (2011).

Pendergast, D. R., P. E. de Prampero, A. B. Craig, D. R. Wilson, & D. W. Rennie: Quantitative analysis of the front crawl in men and women. *Journal of Applied Physiology: Respiratory, Environmental and Exercise Physiology*. 43(3):475–479 (1977).

Péronnet, F., G. Thibault, M. Ledoux, & G. Brisson: *Performance in Endurance Events: Energy Balance, Nutrition, and Temperature Regulation in Distance Running*. London, ON: Spodym (1987).

Plowman, S. A., & N. Y. S. Liu: Norm-referenced and criterion-referenced validity of the one-mile run and PACER in college age individuals. *Measurement in Physical Education and Exercise Science*. 3(2):63–84 (1999).

Pugh, L. G. C. E.: Oxygen intake in track and treadmill running with observations on the effect of air resistance. *Journal of Physiology*. 207:823–835 (1970).

Riddle, S. J., & C. E. Orringer: Measurement of oxygen consumption and cardiovascular response during exercise on the StairMaster 4000PT versus the treadmill. *Medicine and Science in Sports and Exercise (Abstract)*. 22(2):S65 (1990).

Ridley, K., & T.S. Olds: Assigning energy costs to activities in children: A review and synthesis. *Medicine & Science in Sports & Exercise*. 40(8):1439–1446 (2008).

Robinson, S., D. B. Dill, R. D. Robinson, S. P. Tzankoff, & J. A. Wagner: Physiological aging of champion runners. *Journal of Applied Physiology*. 41(1):46–51 (1976).

Rode, A., & R. J. Shephard: The influence of cigarette smoking upon the oxygen cost of breathing in near-maximal exercise. *Medicine and Science in Sports*. 3(2):51–55 (1971).

Rowland, T. W.: *Exercise and Children's Health*. Champaign, IL: Human Kinetics (1990).

Rowland, T. W.: *Children's Exercise Physiology*. Champaign, IL: Human Kinetics (2005).

Rowland, T. W., & G. M. Green: Physiological responses to treadmill exercise in females: Adult-child differences. *Medicine and Science in Sports and Exercise*. 20(5):474–478 (1988).

Rowland, T. W., J. A. Auchinachie, T. J. Keenan, & G. M. Green: Physiologic responses to treadmill running in adult and prepubertal males. *International Journal of Sports Medicine*. 8(4):292–297 (1987).

Rowland, T. W., J. A. Auchinachie, T. J. Keenan, & G. M. Green: Submaximal aerobic running economy and treadmill performance in prepubertal boys. *International Journal of Sports Medicine*. 9(3):201–204 (1988).

Ryan, N. D., J. R. Morrow, Jr., & J. M. Pivarnik: Reliability and validity characteristics of cardiorespiratory responses on the StairMaster 4000PT®. *Measurement in Physical Education and Exercise Science*. 2(2):115–126 (1998).

Sacchetti, M., M. Lenti, A. S. Di Palumbo, & G. DeVito: Different effect of cadence on cycling efficiency between young and older cyclists. *Medicine & Science in Sports & Exercise*. 42(11):2128–2133 (2010).

Saunders, P. U., D. B. Pyne, R. D. Telford, & J. A. Hawley: Factors affecting running economy in trained distance runners. *Sports Medicine*. 34(7):465–485 (2004).

Shepard, J. T., C. G. Blomquist, A. R. Lind, J. H. Mitchell, & B. Saltin: Static (isometric) exercise: Retrospection and introspection. *Circulation Research (Suppl. I)*. 48(6):I179–I188 (1981).

Shephard, R. J.: The oxygen cost of breathing during vigorous exercise. *Quarterly Journal of Experimental Physiology*. 51:336–350 (1966).

Sidney, K. H., & R. J. Shepard: Maximum and submaximum exercise tests in men and women in the seventh, eighth, and ninth decade of life. *Journal of Applied Physiology: Respiratory, Environmental and Exercise Physiology*. 43(2):280–287 (1977).

Sirotic, A. C., & A. J. Coutts: Physiological and performance test correlates of prolonged, high-intensity, intermittent running performance in moderately trained women team sport athletes. *Journal of Strength and Conditioning Research*. 21(1):138–144 (2007).

Stegeman, J.: *Exercise Physiology: Physiological Bases of Work and Sport*. Chicago, IL: Year Book Medical Publishers (1981).

Swain, D. P.: Cardiorespiratory exercise prescription. In: J. K. Ehrman (ed.): *ACSM's Resource Manual for Guidelines for Exercise Testing and Prescription*. 6th ed. Baltimore, MD: Lippincott Williams and Wilkins, 448–462 (2010).

Swain, D. P., N. McClain, K. Davidson, A. Moseley, & N. Reed: Energy expenditure during elliptical motion exercise and comparison to treadmill walking. *Medicine & Science in Sports & Exercise Abstract*. 31(5):S153 (1999).

Taylor, C. M., M. E. Bal, M. W. Lamb, & G. MacLeod: Mechanical efficiency in cycling of boys seven to fifteen years of age. *Journal of Applied Physiology*. 2:563–570 (1950).

Taylor, H. L., E. Buskirk, & A. Henschel: Maximal oxygen intake as an objective measure of cardiorespiratory performance. *Journal of Applied Physiology*. 8:73–80 (1955).

Tesch, P. A., P. Buchanan, & G. A. Dudley: An approach to counteracting long-term microgravity-induced muscle atrophy. *The Physiologist*. 33(Suppl. 1): S77–S79 (1990).

Vella, C. A., D. Marks, & R. A. Roberts: Oxygen cost of ventilation during incremental exercise to VO_2max. *Respirology*. 11:175–181 (2006).

Wells, J. G., B. Balke, & D. D. Van Fossan: Lactic acid accumulation during work: A suggested standardization of work classification. *Journal of Applied Physiology*. 10(1):51–55 (1957).

Widrick, J. J., P. S. Freedson, & J. Hamill: Effect of internal work on the calculation of optimal pedaling rates. *Medicine and Science in Sports and Exercise*. 24(3):376–382 (1992).

Withers, R. T., A. G. Brooks, S. M. Gunn, J. L. Plummer, C. J. Gore, & J. Cormack: Self-selected exercise intensity during household/garden activities and walking in 55 to 65-year-old females. *European Journal of Applied Physiology*. 97(4):494–504 (2006).

Metabolic Training Principles and Adaptations

5

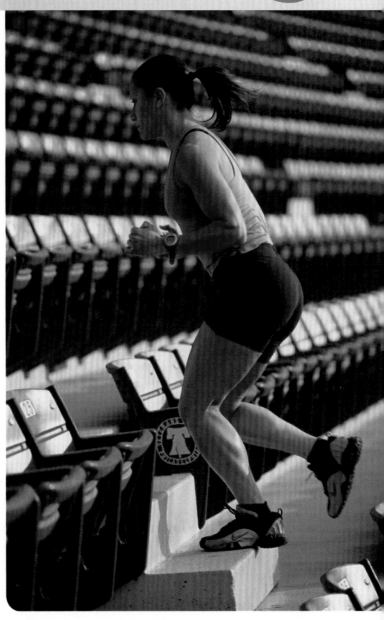

OBJECTIVES

After studying the chapter, you should be able to:

> Name and apply the training principles for metabolic enhancement.

> Describe and explain the metabolic adaptations that normally occur as a result of a well-designed and carefully followed training program.

> Discuss the influence of age and sex on the metabolic training adaptations.

> Discuss the detraining response that occurs in the metabolic system.

Introduction

To provide a training program that meets an individual's metabolic goals, the training principles must be systematically applied. How these principles are applied will determine the extent to which the body uses the aerobic and/or anaerobic systems of energy production. Which energy systems are emphasized will, in turn, determine the training adaptations that occur. Individualized training programs designed to bring about metabolic adaptations may be used to enhance performance in aerobic endurance or anaerobic events or health-related fitness.

Application of the Training Principles for Metabolic Enhancement

The training principles were described generically in Chapter 1. Each training principle can be applied specifically in relation to the metabolic production of energy to support exercise.

Specificity

In order to be specific and match the demands of the event, a training program must begin with determining the goal. For example, a 50-year-old male who is enrolled in a fitness program and wants to break 60 minutes in a local 10-km race will have a very different training program from a 16-year-old high school student competing in the 400- and 800-m distances.

With the goal established, the relative contributions of the major energy systems can be estimated using a graph such as the one shown in **Figure 3.3**. For the 50-year-old male described above, approximately 98% of the energy for his 60-minute, 10-km run is derived from the O_2 system, with the remaining 2% from the adenosine triphosphate-phosphocreatine (ATP-PC) and lactic acid (LA) systems. These percentages vary little even if an individual's time is considerably slower or even somewhat faster than 60 minutes. Thus, this individual's training regimen should emphasize the O_2 system.

For the high school middle-distance runner, it is a different story. Planning her training program requires knowing her typical times at those distances. In general, she would be expected to be in the 1:00–3:00-minute range for both distances. (The American National 2011 record for a high school female is 0:50.69 for the 400-m run [set in 2002] and 2:00.07 for the 800-m run [set in 1982].) Events in this range rely on approximately 60% anaerobic and 40% aerobic metabolism, with a heavier reliance on the ATP-PC and LA anaerobic systems as performance speed increases. Because a faster time is the goal, her training should emphasize the anaerobic systems without neglecting the O_2 system.

In general, only by stressing the primary energy system or systems used in the activity can improvement be expected. The one exception to this rule appears to be the development of at least a minimal level of cardiorespiratory fitness, often termed an *aerobic base* for all sports. An aerobic base does not need to be obtained through long distance running for all athletes. Other programs such as interval work may be more appropriate for sports that are basically anaerobic such as football (Kraemer and Gómez, 2001). Such a base should be achieved in the general preparatory phase (off-season) (see **Figure 1.7**). This base prepares the athletes for more intense and specific training for anaerobic sports and aids in recovery from anaerobic work. The most specific training for metabolic improvement should occur in the specific preparatory phase (preseason) (see **Figure 1.7**).

For those sports in which performance is not measured in time (such as basketball, football, softball, tennis, and volleyball), the sport's separate components must be analyzed to determine which energy system supports it. For example, the average football play lasts 4–7 seconds and the total action in a 60-minute game (although perhaps spread over 3 hours) may be only 12 minutes. Thus, football training must emphasize the ATP-PC system (the 4–7-second range), not the O_2 system (the 60-minute time). In all cases, drills or circuits should be devised to stress the energy systems most important for a specific sport or positions within a sport.

Specificity also applies to the major muscle groups and exercise modality involved. Most biochemical training adaptations occur only in the muscles that have been trained repeatedly in the way in which they will be used. Thus, a would-be triathlete who emphasizes bicycling and running in his or her program but spends little time on swimming should be more successful (in terms of individual potential) competing in duathlons instead.

Overload

Overload of the metabolic systems is typically achieved in one of two ways: first, by manipulating time and distance and, second, by monitoring lactate levels and adjusting work intensity accordingly. Maximal oxygen uptake, although a measure of aerobic power and a means of quantifying training load, is more a cardiovascular than a metabolic variable. Factors contributing to the improvement of $\dot{V}O_2max$ and the use of $\%\dot{V}O_2max$ reserve as an overload technique are therefore primarily discussed in the section on application of the cardiorespiratory training principles (see Chapter 13).

The Time or Distance Technique

The *time or distance technique* involves performing continuous and/or interval training. As the name implies, continuous training occurs when an individual selects a distance or a time to be active and continues uninterrupted to

TABLE 5.1	Examples of Time-Distance Interval Training for Runners*						
Energy System	Competitive Distance	Best Time	Training Distance	Training Time	Repetitions	Recovery Time	Recovery Type
ATP-PC	100 (m)	0:15	100 (m)	0:18	8	(1:3) 0:54	Rest
LA	1500 (m)	5:16	400 (m)	1:20[†]	5	(1:2) 2:40	Work
O_2	1500 (m)	5:16	1200 (m)	4:24[‡]	3	(1:1/2) 2:12	Rest

*This is not intended to be one workout, although the 100- and 400-m training sets could constitute one workout and the 1200-m repeats another. Each would then total approximately 2 mi of intervals.

[†]Based on 1–4 seconds faster than average 400 m during the 1500–1600-m race. (1500 m ÷ 100 m = 15; 5:16 = 316 seconds ÷ 15 = 0:21·100 m^{-1} × 4 = 1:24·400 m^{-1}; 1:24−0:04 = 1:20.)

[‡]Based on 1–4 seconds slower than average 400 m during 1500-m–1600-m race. (0:21·100 m^{-1} × 12 = 252 s·1200 m^{-1} = 4:12 + 0:12 = 4:24.)

the end, typically at a steady pace. For example, a runner who completes an 8-mi training run at a 7:30-min·mi^{-1} pace has done a continuous workout. If such a continuous steady-state aerobic training session is maintained for an extended period of time or distance, it is sometimes called a **long slow distance (LSD) workout**. If several periods of increased speed are randomly interspersed in a continuous aerobic workout, the term *fartlek* is used. Thus, a **fartlek workout**, named from the Swedish word meaning "speed play," combines the aerobic demands of a continuous run with the anaerobic demands of sporadic speed intervals. The distance, pace, and frequency of the speed intervals can vary depending on what the individual wishes to accomplish that day.

Interval training is an aerobic and/or anaerobic workout that consists of three elements: a selected work interval (usually a distance), a target time for that distance, and a predetermined recovery or relief period before the next work interval. The target time for any given distance should be based on the time trials or past performance of the individual at that distance. The time period of the work interval determines the energy system that is stressed. A work time of less than 30 seconds stresses the ATP-PC system; one between 30 seconds and 2 minutes stresses the LA system. Anything over 2–5 minutes primarily stresses the O_2 system. The choice of length

Long Slow Distance (LSD) Workout A continuous aerobic training session performed at a steady-state pace for an extended time or distance.

Fartlek Workout A type of training session, named from the Swedish word meaning "speed play," that combines the aerobic demands of a continuous run with the anaerobic demands of sporadic speed intervals.

Interval Training An aerobic and/or anaerobic workout that consists of three elements: a selected work interval (usually a distance), a target time for that distance, and a predetermined recovery period before the next repetition of the work interval.

and type of recovery period also depends on the energy system to be stressed. Its length is typically between 30 seconds and 6 minutes, and the type may be rest-relief (which can include light aerobic activity and flexibility exercises) or work-relief (moderate aerobic activity). Examples of ATP-PC, LA, and O_2 interval sets are presented in **Table 5.1** (Fox and Mathews, 1974). Note that the three sets are not intended to be combined. In addition, other techniques for determining interval times can, of course, result in different target and recovery times for the same distance and ability level.

ATP-PC SYSTEM In this example of the ATP-PC set, the runner is doing 100-m sprints. Each repetition is to be run at 3 seconds slower (0:18) than her best time (0:15). A total of eight repetitions are to be completed with 0:54 of rest recovery (which may involve no or mild activity) between repetitions.

The amount of time required to restore half of the ATP-PC used—that is, the half-life restoration period for ATP-PC—is approximately 20–30 seconds, with full restoration taking at least 2 minutes to possibly 8 minutes (Fox and Mathews, 1974; Harris et al., 1976; Hultman et al., 1967). Thus, this individual should restore over half her ATP-PC while she rests.

During the same recovery time, myoglobin O_2 replenishment is also taking place. The amounts replenished and restored are influenced by the individual's activity during the recovery phase, with the greatest restoration occurring with rest during recovery (Dupont et al., 2004).

Because the ATP-PC stores recover so quickly, they can be called upon repeatedly to provide energy. Repeatedly stimulating the ATP-PC system should bring about an increase in its capacity. Any major involvement of the LA system is avoided by keeping the work intervals short so that little lactate accumulation occurs.

LA SYSTEM Stressing the LA system requires work durations of 30 seconds to 2 minutes. In this example, the runner is asked to perform five repetitions of 400 m in 1:20, with a work-relief recovery (which should include mild to moderate exercise) of 2:40 between repetitions.

Lactic acid/lactate is produced in excess of clearance amounts during heavy work of this duration, resulting in an accumulation of lactate in the blood. Because lactate has a half-life clearance time of 15–25 minutes, with full clearance taking almost an hour, it is neither practical nor beneficial to allow for clearance of even half the accumulated lactate between repetitions.

Tolerance to lactate is increased by incomplete recovery periods of 1 minute 30 seconds to 3 minutes. This amount of rest allows the replenishment of myoglobin O_2 as well as most of the ATP-PC, thus allowing the high-intensity work in the next work interval to be partially supplied by the ATP-PC energy system before stressing the LA system again (Fox et al., 1969). Of the three overload factors of frequency, intensity, and duration, intensity is most important for improving the capacity of the LA system. Work-relief recovery is typically used at these work times, since active recovery does speed up lactate clearance.

O_2 **SYSTEM** Long work bouts that are a portion of the competitive event (e.g., 0.5–1-mi [800–1600 m] repeats for a 10-km runner) can be performed to stress the O_2 system. The pace is typically close to average pace during competition and may exceed it. The smaller the proportion of the competitive distance that is performed with each repetition, the faster the pace and the more repetitions performed. The intent is for the intervals to be done aerobically, however. The example in **Table 5.1** is for 1200 m. Note that the time is longer than simply triple the 400-m time (4:12 versus 4:24) and that the recovery time is proportionally very short. The 2:12 recovery allows for a large portion of ATP-PC restoration before the start of the next repetition. Because this pace is already relatively low-intensity work, a rest or walking recovery is best.

The distance for an interval workout (excluding warm-up and cooldown) should rarely exceed 2–5 mi (3.2–8 km) with a frequency of 1–3 d·wk^{-1} (Costill, 1986; Rennie, 2007). High-intensity interval training taxes the muscles and joints, and one must be careful to avoid injury or overtraining. (Chapter 22 lists the signs and symptoms

of overtraining.) Continuous work at lower intensities allows for greater frequency and longer durations, both of which lead to a greater volume of training. A higher training volume is particularly important to endurance athletes.

The Lactate Monitoring Technique

Assessing blood lactate concentration ([La$^-$]) is the second common technique for monitoring overload. Ideally, this technique involves the direct measurement of blood lactate levels from a given workout. Currently, there is no general agreement about how best to use blood lactate values to design and monitor training programs. Nomenclature also varies greatly. Generally, however, six categories of workouts or training zones are useful (**Table 5.2**). These training zones are based on the lactate thresholds (LT1 and LT2) obtained during incremental exercise to maximum. The zones overlap considerably. The three lower zones (recovery, extensive aerobic, and intensive aerobic) involve predominantly low- to moderate-intensity aerobic activity, whereas the three higher zones (threshold, $\dot{V}O_2$max, and anaerobic) represent the transition from aerobic to anaerobic energy supply at progressively higher intensities until both aerobic and anaerobic energy productions are maximized (Anderson, 1998; Bourdon, 2000).

Although it is done for elite athletes, direct measurement of [La$^-$] during training for others is not very practical because of the special equipment needed and the cost of taking multiple blood samples. Some studies (Stoudemire et al., 1996; Weltman, 1995) have demonstrated a reasonably stable relationship between blood lactate values and Borg's rating of perceived exertion (RPE) 6–20 scale. Borg's RPE scale is described fully in Chapter 13. The range of RPE values corresponding approximately to lactate values for each training zone is presented in **Table 5.2**.

A better method to individualize the use of RPE is to test the individual in a laboratory and record both RPE and lactate values at each progressive work rate.

TABLE 5.2	Training Zones Based on Lactate Thresholds and Values					
	Recovery	**Extensive Aerobic**	**Intensive Aerobic**	**Threshold**	**$\dot{V}O_2$max**	**Anaerobic**
Relation to LT1 and LT2	<LT1	LT1 to halfway to LT2	>LT1 but <LT2	LT2	>LT2	Maximal
Lactate values mmol·L^{-1}	<2.0	1.0–3.0	1.5–4.0	2.5–5.5	>5.0	>7.0
RPE	<11–12	11–15	12–15	14–17	17–20	17–20
Workout example	Low-intensity aerobic; e.g., 20–30 min continuous	LSD; e.g., 30 min to 2 hr continuous	Tempo runs; e.g., 10–12 sec slower than 10-km race pace	Fartlek; e.g., 1-min bursts	High-intensity intervals; e.g., 6–8 reps 0:30–3:00	Interval repetitions at maximum; e.g., 2–4 reps 0:45–1:30

Sources: Based on information from Anderson (1998), Bourdon (2000).

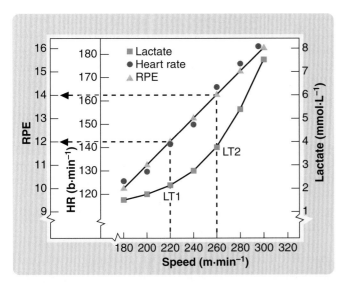

FIGURE 5.1 Heart Rate, Lactate, and Perceived Exertion Responses to Incremental Exercise as a Basis for Exercise Prescription.
LT1 occurred at 220 m·min⁻¹ and LT2 at 260 m·min⁻¹ for the individual whose data are plotted. See text for the explanation of how these points are used to prepare an exercise prescription.

Figure 5.1 presents an example of such results. This individual reached his LT1 at 220 m·min⁻¹. At that speed, he reported an RPE of 12. He reached LT2 at a speed of 260 m·min⁻¹ with an RPE of 14. Combining these results with the guidelines from **Table 5.2** means that his recovery workouts should be performed at an RPE of 9–12, extensive aerobic workouts at 12 or 13, intensive aerobic at 13–14, threshold workouts at 14, and $\dot{V}O_2$max at an RPE of at least 15. The test results presented in **Figure 5.1** do not represent a maximal test for this individual. Maximal workouts should elicit at least an RPE of 17 for everyone. Thus, an individual can be given a workout and an RPE value and adjust his or her intensity accordingly. An alternative method, when a laboratory testing facility is available, is to determine the relationship between [La⁻] and HR values. Then, HR can be used to estimate the [La⁻] level during training sessions, and the intensity modified accordingly (Dwyer and Bybee, 1983; Gilman and Wells, 1993).

In our example, now reading the rectilinear plot as heart rate, the individual would perform recovery activity between approximately 110 and 140 b·min⁻¹; extensive aerobic exercise bouts between 110 and 155 b·min⁻¹; intensive aerobic exercise between 120 and 165 b·min⁻¹; threshold workouts between 157 and 173 b·min⁻¹; $\dot{V}O_2$max workouts close to 170 b·min⁻¹; and maximal activity at least at 185 b·min⁻¹.

Heart rate reflects primarily the functioning of the cardiovascular system, but lactate levels reflect the metabolic energy system. Fox et al. (1988) estimate that if the HR-[La⁻] relationship is not individually determined

to ensure that all individuals are working at or above their "anaerobic threshold," heart rate would have to be greater than 90% of the maximal heart rate or equal to or greater than 85% of the heart rate reserve in order to use it for anaerobic exercise prescription. Experimental data reported by Weltman (1995) confirm that techniques for exercise prescription involving percentages of heart rate maximum or heart rate reserve do not reflect specific blood lactate concentrations. Thus, unless individually correlated with lactate values, heart rate cannot be used for anaerobic exercise prescriptions.

Regardless of the system used to prescribe an individual's training session, a mixture of workout types should be used to maximize the possibility for improvement and prevent boredom.

Rest/Recovery/Adaptation

Adaptation is evident when a given distance or workload can be covered in a faster time with an equal or lower perception of fatigue or exertion and/or in the same time span with less physiological disruption (lower [La⁻] values) and faster recovery. The key to adaptation for energy production in muscles appears to be allowing for sufficient recovery time between hard-intensity workouts. Periodized training programs that alternately stress the desired specific energy system on a hard day and allow it to recover on an easy day lead to optimal adaptation (Bompa, 1999; McCafferty and Horvath, 1977; Weltman et al., 1978). Too many successive hard days working the same muscles and same energy system can lead to a lack of adaptation because of overtraining, and too many successive easy days can lead to a lack of adaptation because of undertraining.

Recently, there has been much interest in the use of modalities to enhance recovery between training sessions or within tournament structures requiring multiple competitions. Overall, the few studies conducted so far have not found massage, hyperbaric oxygen therapy (exposure to whole-body pressure >1 atmosphere while breathing 100% oxygen), stretching, or electromyostimulation (the transmission of electrical impulses through surface electrodes to stimulate motor neurons and induce muscle contraction) advantageous. There appears to be no harm in using water immersion, and this modality may be of benefit if the temperature of the water is thermoneutral to cold. Studies have not supported the use of contrast (alteration of hot and cold) water immersion. Nonsteroidal anti-inflammatory drugs have potential negative health outcomes (cardiovascular, gastrointestinal, and renal) and may negatively affect muscle repair and adaptation to training. Insufficient data are available to evaluate compression garments (stockings, sleeves, tights, and tops) (Barnett, 2006; King and Duffield, 2009; Montgomery et al., 2008; Wilcock et al., 2006).

Progression

Once adaptation occurs, the workload should be progressed if maximizing improvement is desired (McNicol et al., 2009). Progression can involve increasing the distance, speed, workload, number of repetitions, or sessions; decreasing the length of the relief interval; or changing the frequency of the various types of workouts per week. The key to successful progression is an increase in intensity and total **training volume**. The progression should be gradual. A general rule of thumb is that training volume—the total amount of work done, usually expressed as mileage or load—should not increase more than 10% per week. For example, for an individual currently cycling 60 mi·wk^{-1}, the distance should not be increased by more than 6 mi the following week. Steploading, as described in Chapter 1, should be used.

Often in fitness work the challenge is to prevent an individual from doing too much too soon. For example, a 50-year-old man remembers being a high school star athlete and wants to regain that feeling and physique—now! Fitness leaders must gently help such participants be more realistic and should err, if at all, on the side of caution in exercise prescription and progression.

Metabolic adaptation appears to plateau in approximately 10 days to 3 weeks if training is not progressed (Hickson et al., 1981). The ultimate limit may be set by genetics.

Individualization

The first step in individualizing training is to match the sport, event, fitness, or health goal of the participant with the specific mix of energy system demands. The second step is to evaluate the individual. The third step is to develop a periodization sequence for general preparation, specific preparation, competitive, and transition phases. The fourth step is to develop a format: the number of days per week for each type of training or energy system to be stressed. The fifth step is to determine the training load (distance, workload, repetitions, or the like) based on the individual's evaluation and adjusted according to how he or she responds and adapts to the program. Interpreting and adjusting to an individual's response is the art of being a coach or fitness leader.

Maintenance

Once a specific level of endurance adaptation has been achieved, it can be maintained by the same or a reduced volume of work. How the volume is reduced is critical. When training intensity is maintained, reductions of one third to two thirds in frequency and duration have been shown to maintain aerobic power (V̇O$_2$max), endurance performance (at a given absolute or relative submaximal workload), and lactate accumulation levels at submaximal loads. This maintenance may last for at least several months. One day per week may be sufficient for short periods of time (such as during a 1-wk vacation) if intensity is maintained (Chaloupka and Fox, 1975; Neufer, 1989; Weltman, 1995). Conversely, a reduction in intensity brings about a decrease in training adaptation.

It also seems to be important that the mode of exercise is consistent with or closely simulates an athlete's activity because many training adaptations are specific to the muscles involved. Thus, cross training—the use of different modalities to reduce localized stress but increase the overall training volume—is likely to be more beneficial for the cardiovascular system than the metabolic system.

The level of maintenance training necessary for the anaerobic energy systems to keep operating at maximal levels is unknown. Sprint performances are known to deteriorate less quickly than endurance performances, however, with a decrease in training (Wilmore and Costill, 1988).

Many fitness participants are primarily in a maintenance mode after the initial several months or the first year of participation. The appropriate level for maintenance should be based on the individual's goals. For athletes, maintenance should occur primarily during the competitive training cycle.

A special kind of maintenance called tapering is often used by athletes in individual sports such as swimming, cycling, and running. A **training taper** is a reduction in training load before an important competition that is intended to help the athlete recover from previous hard training, maintain physiological conditioning, and improve performance. Athletes often fear that if they taper more than just a few days, their competitive fitness and performance will suffer. However, studies consistently show that if intensity is maintained while training volume is reduced, physiological adaptations are retained and performance either stays the same or improves after a taper (Bosquet et al., 2007; Costill et al., 1985; Houmard et al., 1990; Johns et al., 1992; Mujika and Padilla, 2003; Shepley et al., 1992; Zehsaz et al., 2011). **Figure 5.2** presents a schematic of the four different possible types of taper. Two of the variations are linear—one a gradual decrease in training load and the other making one large step down in training load and remaining at that level throughout the taper. Two of the variations are exponential, with either a large initial drop (fast decay) or slow initial drop (slow decay). Exponential techniques have been shown to be more effective than linear ones, and fast decay more beneficial than slow decay. Optimal tapering strategies include the following:

1. Using a progressive, fast decay exponential taper
2. Maintaining training intensity
3. Reducing training volume by 41–60%, preferably by a decrease in the duration of each training session

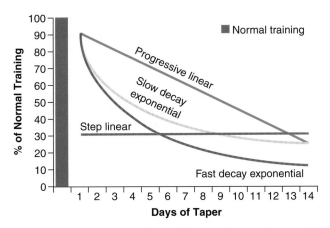

FIGURE 5.2   Representation of Taper Types: Progressive Linear, Step Linear, Slow Decay Exponential, and Fast Decay Exponential.
Source: Modified from Mujika, I. & S. Padilla: Scientific bases for precompetition tapering strategies. *Medicine & Science in Sports & Exercise*. 35(7):1182–1187 (2003), with permission.

4. Maintaining training frequency in highly trained athletes but reducing it 50–70% for moderately trained individuals
5. Continuing the tapering intervention for 2 weeks although effective tapers have varied from 4 days to 28 days
6. Ingesting a high-carbohydrate diet matched to the decrease in energy expenditure to avoid weight gain

The art of tapering involves balancing the goals of minimizing fatigue but not compromising previously acquired adaptations and fitness level. Tapering appears to be beneficial to both males and female athletes. Done properly, tapering strategies can result in an improved performance of approximately 2–3% (range 0.5–6.0%) (Bosquet et al., 2007; Mujika and Padilla, 2003).

Retrogression/Plateau/Reversibility

Coaches and fitness leaders anticipate and react to, rather than apply, the training principles of retrogression, plateau, and reversibility. At one or more times in the process of training, an individual may fail to improve with progression and will either stay at the same level (plateau) or show a performance or physiological decrement (retrogression). When such a pattern of nonimprovement occurs, it is important to check for other signs of overtraining. Changing the training emphasis or

Training Volume The total amount of work done, usually expressed as mileage or load.

Training Taper A reduction in training load before an important competition that is intended to allow the athlete to recover from previous hard training, maintain physiological conditioning, and improve performance.

including more easy days may be warranted. Remember that reducing training load does not necessarily lead to detraining. Of course, not all plateaus can be explained as overtraining; sometimes there is no explanation.

If an individual ceases training completely, for whatever reason, detraining or reversibility of the achieved adaptations will occur.

Warm-up and Cooldown

Information about the effects of warm-up on metabolic function is sparse, but several generalizations can be made. An elevated body temperature—and more specifically an elevated muscle temperature (T_m)—increases the rate of metabolic processes in the cells. This increase occurs largely because enzyme activity is temperature-dependent, exhibiting a steady rise from 0°C to approximately 40°C before plateauing and ultimately declining. At the same time, at elevated temperatures, oxygen is more readily released from the red blood cells and transported into the mitochondria. Therefore, one consequence of an increased T_m is a greater availability of oxygen to the muscles during work. When more oxygen is available sooner, there is less reliance on anaerobic metabolism, and less lactate accumulates at any given heavy workload. At lighter endurance workloads, a greater utilization of fat for energy is possible earlier in the activity. This early use of fat spares carbohydrate and allows a high-intensity effort to be continued longer. Other metabolic benefits of an increased T_m include increased glycogenolysis, glycolysis, and ATP-PC degradation (Bishop, 2003). These beneficial metabolic effects of a warm-up appear to occur in children and adolescents as well as adults (Bar-Or, 1983).

As with the other training principles, to be effective, the warm-up needs to match the intensity and duration of the intended activity. In general, a warm-up should consist of three elements in this order: a period of aerobic exercise, stretching, and a period of activity similar to the event to be performed (Fradkin et al., 2010). In addition, the structure of the warm-up should depend on the participant's fitness level, the environmental conditions, and specific constraints of the situation in which the warm-up will occur. Several guidelines are available for devising a warm-up to achieve these metabolic benefits and possibly improved performance (Bar-Or, 1983; Bishop, 2003; Franks, 1983; Tomaras and MacIntosh, 2011).

1. For a short-term (<10 seconds) high-intensity activity, the goal is to increase T_m but allow time for resynthesis of ATP-PC immediately before the activity. Research suggests a warm-up performed at approximately 40–60% $\dot{V}O_2max$ (~60–70% HRmax) for 5–10 minutes followed by a 5-minute recovery period is optimal.
2. Explosive tasks (such as long or high jumping) at full speed should be used sparingly during warm-up even

FOCUS ON APPLICATION: *Clinically Relevant*

The Effect of Warm-Up on Metabolism

Twelve female ballet dancers (age = 13.7 ± 10 years; HT = 1.61 ± 0.05 m; WT = 45 ± 7 kg; and $\dot{V}O_2$max = 46 ± 2 mL·kg^{-1}·min^{-1}) at the Italian National Academy of Dance were tested to determine the effects of active warm-up on energy cost and energy source. As in classical dance practice, the warm-up consisted of 3 minutes of free jogging (25–35% $\dot{V}O_2$max), 15 minutes of stretching (10–20% $\dot{V}O_2$max), 2 minutes of *pre barre,* and 2:40 of *plié* dance exercises. The ballet dance exercise consisted of a sequence of 25 *tours piques* on full *pointe* performed on diagonal continuously for 30 seconds to music.

The total energy requirement ($\dot{V}O_2$ equivalent) was determined by adding the amount of measured $\dot{V}O_2$ during exercise above resting ($\dot{V}O_2$ aerobic) to the $\dot{V}O_2$ from the fast component of recovery ($\dot{V}O_2$ alactic) and the energy equivalent of peak lactate accumulation ($\dot{V}O_2$ lactic).

The metabolic demand was 1.6 times the dancers' $\dot{V}O_2$max both with and without warm-up, so the energy cost of the activity (graph below, $\dot{V}O_2$ equivalent) did not change. The anaerobic systems were taxed more in both conditions. Relatively (right side of the graph), the anaerobic systems ($\dot{V}O_2$ alactic + $\dot{V}O_2$ lactic) provided 74% of the energy without warm-up and 61% with warm-up. The decreases in anaerobic energy sources (both alactic and lactic, absolute and relative) following warm-up were significant. Conversely, the aerobic component increased significantly.

Source: Guidetti et al. (2007).

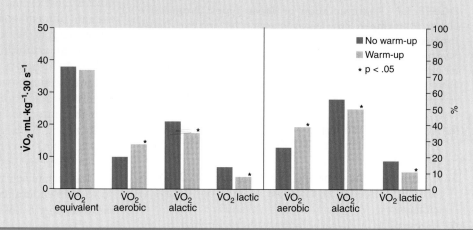

if they are to be performed during exercise or competition. However, a brief, task-specific burst of activity may be beneficial, or the action can be patterned at lower levels.

3. For an intermediate or long-term high-intensity activity, the goal is to elevate baseline oxygen consumption without either causing fatigue or imposing a high thermal load. Research suggests a warm-up performed at approximately 60–70% $\dot{V}O_2$max (~70–80% HRmax) for 5–10 minutes, followed by approximately 5 minutes of recovery for moderately trained individuals.

4. The warm-up for endurance activities generally can occur at a lower intensity (25–30% $\dot{V}O_2$max or <35% HRmax) than for short or intermediate high-intensity activities. The warm-up may be built into an endurance workout if the participant begins at a low intensity and progresses nonstop into higher levels of work.

5. Very fit individuals can use longer, more intense warm-ups than less fit individuals. Higher intensity may be needed by well-conditioned athletes to elevate their core temperature, but fatigue should be avoided. It is probably best to stay below the first lactate threshold and to avoid impacting glycogen stores negatively.

6. An intermittent or interval-type warm-up has been found to be more beneficial for children than a continuous warm-up.

The primary metabolic value of a cooldown lies in the fact that lactate is dissipated faster during an active recovery. As described in Chapter 3, the lactate removal rate is maximized if the cooldown activity is of moderate intensity (a little higher than an individual tends to self-select) and continues for approximately 20 minutes.

In general, all training principles appear to apply to both sexes and, except where noted, to all ages. At the very least, there is insufficient evidence for modifying any of the general concepts based on age or sex, although individual differences should always be kept in mind.

CHECK YOUR COMPREHENSION: CLINICALLY RELEVANT

The metabolic changes described in the Focus on Application: Clinically Relevant box above are considered beneficial. Why?
Check your answer in Appendix C.

Metabolic Adaptations to Exercise Training

When the training principles discussed above are systematically applied and rigorously followed, a number of adaptations occur relative to the production and utilization of energy. The extent to which adaptations occur depends on the individual's initial fitness level and genetic potential. **Figure 5.3** is an expanded version of **Figure 2.4**, showing the metabolic pathways you studied earlier. Numbers have been inserted on the figure to indicate sites where these adaptations occur. The following discussion will follow that numerical sequence. Refer to **Figure 5.3** as you read.

Substrate or Fuel Supply

Regulatory Hormones

Primary among the metabolic adaptations to a training program are changes that occur in the hormones responsible for the regulation of metabolism (see Chapters 2 and 21, **Figure 2.17**, and **Table 2.3**). Although little is known about the impact of training on the hypothalamic-releasing factors and adrenocorticotrophic hormone, a definite pattern occurs with the five hormones directly involved in carbohydrate, fat, and protein substrate regulation. That pattern is one of a blunted response in which the amount of hormone secreted during submaximal aerobic activity is reduced. This pattern occurs whether the load is absolute or relative and in both the fast-responding and slow-responding hormones. Thus, the rise in epinephrine and norepinephrine is less in the trained state. As a result, the rise in glucagon (stimulated by epinephrine) is lower and there is less suppression of insulin (caused by norepinephrine). Similarly, the rise in growth hormone and cortisol is less during submaximal exercise in trained individuals than in untrained individuals (Galbo, 1983; Talanian et al., 2007). Because of these smaller disruptions at submaximal levels, more work can be done before maximum is reached.

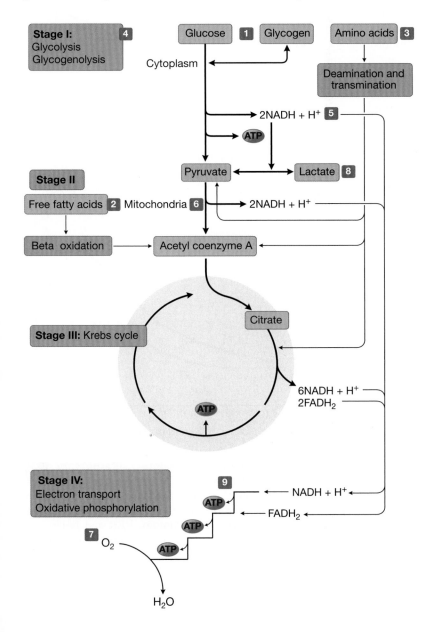

FIGURE 5.3 Metabolic Training Adaptations. The numbers in squares indicate sites where training changes occur. The blue boxes indicate processes. The green boxes indicate important substrates.

Carbohydrate (1)

The rate-limiting step for glucose utilization in muscles is glucose transport, and glucose transport is primarily a function of GLUT-4 transporters. Exercise training increases the GLUT-4 number and concentration in skeletal muscle, especially slow-twitch oxidative fibers (Daugaard et al., 2000; Perry et al., 2008; Sato et al., 1996; Seki et al., 2006). This results in a greater uptake of glucose under the influence of insulin. Thus, at any resting insulin level, the whole-body glucose clearance is enhanced. This occurs in both young and older healthy individuals as well as in individuals with non–insulin-dependent diabetes (Dela, 1996). Despite this increase in the number of GLUT-4 transporters, endurance exercise training reduces glucose utilization during both absolute and relative, moderate-intensity submaximal exercise. This occurs because the translocation of GLUT-4 decreases during exercise. As a result, trained muscles take up and utilize less glucose than untrained muscles during moderate exercise (Mougios, 2006).

Both endurance and sprint training increase muscle and liver glycogen reserves. In addition, at the same absolute submaximal workload (the same rate of oxygen consumption), muscle and liver glycogen depletion occurs at a slower rate in trained individuals than in untrained individuals (Abernethy et al., 1990; Gollnick et al., 1973; Holloszy, 1973; Holloszy and Coyle, 1984; Karlsson et al., 1972). Thus, the trained individual uses less total carbohydrate in his or her fuel mixture. These changes result in lower respiratory exchange ratio (RER) values (**Figure 5.4A**). Because glycogen is the primary source of fuel for high-intensity work, a larger supply of glycogen used less quickly enables an individual to participate in fairly intense activities at submaximal levels longer before fatigue occurs. On the other hand, sprint training can also increase the rate of glycogenolysis at higher levels of work, giving the exerciser a fast supply of energy when needed for short bursts of maximal or supramaximal activity.

Fat (2)

A trained individual can use his or her carbohydrate stores more slowly than an untrained individual because of the changes that occur in fat metabolism. Both trained and untrained individuals have more than adequate stores of fat. However, the rate of free fatty acid oxidation is determined not by the storage amount but by the concentration of free fatty acids in the bloodstream and the capacity of the tissues to oxidize the fat. Training brings about several adaptations in fat metabolism, including the following:

1. Increased mobilization or release of free fatty acids from the adipose tissue
2. Increased level of plasma free fatty acids during submaximal exercise
3. Increase in fat storage adjacent to the mitochondria within the muscles
4. Increased capacity to utilize fat at any given plasma concentration

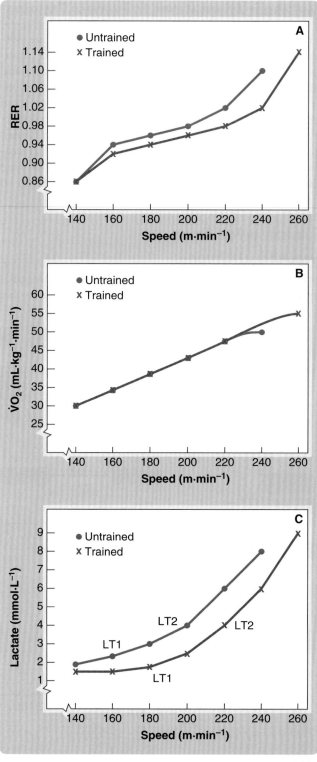

FIGURE 5.4 Metabolic Responses (Respiratory Exchange Rate (RER) in panel A; Oxygen consumption $\dot{V}O_2$ ml·kg^{-1}·min^{-1}, in panel B; lactate accumulation in panel C) of Endurance Trained versus Untrained Individuals to Incremental Exercise to Maximum. RER and lactate are lower in trained individuals; submaximal oxygen consumption is unchanged but maximal is increased in trained individuals. See animation, Oxygen Consumption, at http://thePoint.lww.com/Plowman4e.

The rise in the capacity of the muscle to oxidize lipids is larger than the rise in its capacity to oxidize glycogen. This in conjunction with the lower plasma glucose uptake because of the decreased translocation of the GLUT-4 receptors, leads to the larger contribution of fat to energy production. The increased reliance on fat as a fuel is said to have a *glycogen-sparing effect* and is responsible for lowered RER values (**Figure 5.4A**) at the same absolute and same relative ($\%\dot{V}O_2$max) work intensities. Because glycogen supplies last longer, fatigue is delayed allowing greater endurance at submaximal work levels. Both endurance and sprint training have glycogen-sparing effects (Abernethy et al., 1990; Gollnick et al., 1973; Holloszy, 1973; Holloszy and Coyle, 1984; Mougios, 2006; Perry et al., 2008; Scharhag-Rosenberger et al., 2010; Stisen et al., 2006; Talanian et al., 2007).

Protein (3)

Although proteins are the least important energy substrate, changes do occur as a result of endurance training that enhance their role in metabolism. Adaptations in protein metabolism include an increased ability to utilize the branched chain amino acid leucine and an increased capacity to form alanine and release it from muscle cells. This increased production of alanine is accompanied by decreased levels in the plasma, probably indicating an accelerated removal for gluconeogenesis. In ultraendurance events, this increased gluconeogenesis effect is beneficial for maintaining blood glucose levels (Abernethy et al., 1990; Holloszy and Coyle, 1984; Hood and Terjung, 1990).

Enzyme Activity

The key to increasing the production of ATP is enzyme activity. Since every step in each metabolic pathway is catalyzed by a separate enzyme, the potential for this training adaptation to influence energy production is great. However, it appears that not all enzymes respond to the same training stimulus nor change to the same extent.

Glycolytic Enzymes (4)

The results of studies on the activity of the glycolytic enzymes have historically been contradictory, but a pattern is emerging. Glycolysis is involved in both the aerobic and anaerobic production of energy, and it may be that high-intensity training is required for some glycolytic enzymes to adapt while others respond better to endurance training. Strength and sprint training appear to increase glycolytic enzyme activity (Mougios, 2006). These changes are generally less than the activity increases seen in aerobic enzymes, and the functional significance in terms of actual performance remains questionable (Ross and Leveritt, 2001). Three key enzymes have shown significant training changes: glycogen phosphorylase, phosphofructokinase (PFK), and lactate dehydrogenase (LDH).

GLYCOGEN PHOSPHORYLASE Glycogen phosphorylase catalyzes the breakdown of glycogen stored in the muscle cells for use as fuel in glycolysis. An increase in this enzyme's activity has been found with high-intensity sprint training consisting of either short- (<10 seconds) or long- (>10 seconds) sprint intervals (Mougios, 2006; Ross and Leveritt, 2001). The ability to break down glycogen quickly is important in near-maximal, maximal, and supramaximal exercises.

PHOSPHOFRUCTOKINASE PFK is the rate-limiting enzyme of glycolysis. Results of endurance and sprint training studies are inconsistent but tend to suggest an increase in this enzyme activity with adequate levels of training especially consisting of long-duration sprint repetitions or a combination of long- and short-sprint efforts (Ross and Leveritt, 2001). Increased PFK activity leads to a faster and greater quantity of ATP being produced glycolytically.

LACTATE DEHYDROGENASE LDH catalyzes the conversion of pyruvate into lactate. It exists in several discrete forms, including a cardiac muscle form (LDH 1) that has a low affinity for pyruvate (thus making the formation of lactate less likely) and a skeletal muscle form (LDH 5) that has a high affinity for pyruvate (thus making the formation of lactate more likely). Endurance training tends to have two effects on LDH. It lowers the overall activity of LDH, and it causes a shift from the skeletal muscle to the cardiac muscle form. Thus, lactate is less likely to be produced in the skeletal muscle, and pyruvate is more likely to enter the mitochondria for use as an aerobic fuel. Both of these changes are beneficial to endurance performance (Abernethy et al., 1990; Gollnick and Hermansen, 1973; Holloszy and Coyle, 1984; Sjödin et al., 1982). Strength and sprint training (consisting of both short- and long-sprint intervals) show opposite effects from endurance training, increasing the overall amount of LDH and favoring the LDH skeletal muscle form because of the changes in fast-twitch muscle hypertrophy (Mougios, 2006; Ross and Leveritt, 2001).

Shuttles (5)

The hydrogen ions removed in glycolysis must be transported across the mitochondrial membrane by a shuttle because that membrane is impermeable to $NADH + H^+$. No training changes have been found in the glycerol-phosphate shuttle enzymes that predominate in the skeletal muscle. Conversely, training leads to large increases in the enzymes of the cardiac muscle's malate-aspartate shuttle in both the cytoplasm and the mitochondria, thus increasing shuttle activity. This increase enhances aerobic metabolism in the heart (Holloszy and Coyle, 1984).

Mitochondrial Enzymes (6)

Changes in the mitochondrial enzymes of beta-oxidation, the Krebs cycle, electron transport, and oxidative phosphorylation are coupled with changes in the mitochondria themselves. Both the size and the number of the mitochondria increase with training. In adults these mitochondrial adaptations of increased density and oxidative enzyme activity, known as *mitochondrial biogenesis*, can be on the magnitude of 30–40%. Thus, mitochondria occupy a proportionally larger share of the muscle fiber space. The sarcolemmal mitochondria are affected more than the interfibrillar mitochondria. The stimulus for these increases appears to be a contractile activity itself, rather than any external stimulus such as hormonal changes, since only those muscles directly involved in the exercise training show these changes. For example, runners have an increase in mitochondrial size and number only in the legs, whereas cross-country skiers have mitochondrial increases in both arms and legs.

Within limits, the extent of the augmentation in the mitochondria seems to be a function of the total amount of contractile activity. That is, the more contractions, the greater the change in the mitochondria. It does not seem to matter whether the increase in contractile activity is achieved by completing more contractions per unit of time (speed work) or by keeping the rate of contractions steady but increasing the duration (endurance training). In general, as noted above, the physiological consequence of mitochondrial adaptations in trained distance runners favors a greater reliance on lipid, rather than carbohydrate metabolism. However, when individuals regularly train at high exercise intensity mitochondrial adaptations seem to favor the CHO pathway over the fatty acid lipid pathway for the highest energy production through improvement in Complex I (see **Figure 2.10**) rather than Complexes II and IV (Daussin et al., 2008). Resistance training does not appear to enhance mitochondria.

With larger mitochondria, more transport sites are available for the movement of pyruvate into the mitochondria. The enzymatic activity per unit of mitochondria appears to be the same in trained and untrained individuals; however, the greater mitochondrial protein content means an overall greater enzyme activity to utilize the pyruvate that has been transported there. Interestingly, although most mitochondrial enzymes increase in activity, not all do; nor is the rate of change the same for all. The overall effect of the increased enzyme activity and the increased availability of pyruvate is an enhanced capacity to generate ATP by oxidative phosphorylation. This augmented capacity is more important for supplying energy for submaximal exercise than for maximal exercise (Abernethy et al., 1990; Gollnick et al., 1986; Hawley and Spargo, 2007; Holloszy, 1973; Holloszy and Coyle, 1984; Mougois, 2006; Wibom et al., 1992).

Oxygen Utilization (7)

Maximal Oxygen Uptake

Maximal oxygen uptake ($\dot{V}O_2$max) increases with training (**Figure 5.4B**). Even though this is a measure of the amount of oxygen utilized at the muscle level, $\dot{V}O_2$max is determined more by the cardiovascular system's ability to deliver oxygen than by the muscle's ability to use it. Evidence for

the subsidiary role of muscle in determining $\dot{V}O_2$max includes the fact that individuals can have essentially the same mitochondrial content but very different $\dot{V}O_2$max values. Conversely, individuals with equivalent $\dot{V}O_2$max values can have quite different mitochondrial enzyme levels. Additionally, small training changes can occur in one factor (mitochondrial activity or $\dot{V}O_2$max) without concomitant changes in the other—although, typically, both will increase. These differences probably explain why some runners are more economical (use less oxygen at a given pace than others do) and others possess a greater aerobic power (have a higher $\dot{V}O_2$max) (Holloszy and Coyle, 1984).

Submaximal Oxygen Cost

The oxygen cost ($\dot{V}O_2$ in mL·min^{-1} or mL·kg^{-1}·min^{-1}) of any given absolute submaximal workload is the same before and after the training, assuming that no skill is involved where efficiency would change (Gollnick et al., 1986; Holloszy and Coyle, 1984) (**Figure 5.4B**). For example, if an individual has a smooth, coordinated front crawl stroke but has not participated in lap swimming, the oxygen cost of covering any given distance at a set pace will remain the same as this person trains. However, in an individual who is just learning the front crawl stroke, the oxygen cost could actually go down. It decreases not because of a change in the oxygen requirements but because extraneous inefficient movements that add to the oxygen cost are eliminated as skill is improved (Daniels et al., 1978; Ekblom et al., 1968; Gardner et al., 1989).

Running economy depends both on the energy needed to move at a particular speed (external energy) and on the energy used to produce that energy (internal energy). Specifically, internal energy is associated with oxygen delivery (ventilation and heart rate in particular), thermoregulation, and substrate metabolism (remember that it takes more oxygen to utilize fat as a fuel than to burn carbohydrate). Theoretically, internal energy demand can be lowered by decreasing the ventilation and the heart rate costs and by increasing the percentage of carbohydrate utilized. The first two changes do occur typically with training, but the last one does not. Indeed, the trained individual utilizes a higher percentage of fat at any given submaximal load than does an untrained individual. The primary possibility for improving external energy demand is stride length. However, studies have shown that experienced runners freely select the optimal stride length, so additional improvements in training status do little to change the stride length. The influence of training on running economy is controversial. Cross-sectional studies generally have reported no economy advantage in trained runners over untrained individuals. Longitudinal studies using a running training modality have shown mixed results (Beneke and Hütler, 2005). If anything, improvements in running economy are more likely to occur in less trained than highly trained runners.

High-intensity interval training or continuous running above 4 mmol·L^{-1} has produced improvements in running economy, but the evidence is not strong (Bailey and Pate, 1991; Conley et al., 1981; McCann and Higginson, 2008; Sjödin et al., 1982). Recent evidence suggests that running economy may be improved by the addition of resistance training to the normal aerobic endurance regime of runners. Both traditional weight training and plyometric training have been shown to be effective. Conversely, stretching does not appear to alter running economy. It has been speculated that a combination of improved running mechanics and neuromuscular function results in a decreased oxygen consumption, but many questions remain unanswered (Bonacci et al., 2009; Jung, 2003; Millet et al., 2002; Saunders et al., 2006; Spurrs et al., 2003; Turner et al., 2003). Decreased efficiency or economy can also occur. If so, it should be interpreted as a symptom of overtraining (Fry et al., 1991).

If an individual increases his or her $\dot{V}O_2max$ and yet the oxygen cost of any given (absolute) workload remains the same, then the % $\dot{V}O_2max$ at which that individual is doing the given workload will go down. The task will be relatively easier for the individual, and endurance performance will be greatly enhanced. This improvement results from the biochemical adaptations in the muscle rather than changes in oxygen delivery.

The myoglobin concentration in the muscles increases with endurance training in the muscles directly involved in the activity. As a consequence, the rate of oxygen diffusion through the cytoplasm into the mitochondria increases, making more oxygen available quickly.

Oxygen Deficit and Drift

The oxygen deficit at the onset of activity is smaller, but is not eliminated, in trained individuals. The primary reason for this reduction is that oxidative phosphorylation is activated sooner because of the greater number of mitochondria that are sensitive to low levels of ADP and P_i. This result is advantageous to the exerciser because less lactic acid/lactate is produced and less creatine phosphate depleted (Holloszy, 1973; Holloszy and Coyle, 1984; Krustrup et al., 2004).

The magnitude of oxygen drift is also less after training. This change may be caused by concomitant reductions in epinephrine, norepinephrine, lactate, and body temperature rise during any given submaximal workload (Casaburi et al., 1987; Hagberg et al., 1978).

Excess Postexercise Oxygen Consumption

Excess postexercise oxygen consumption (EPOC) is a function of the intensity and duration of the previous exercise bout. Aerobic endurance training has been shown (Sedlock et al., 2010) to significantly decrease the magnitude of EPOC after exercise at the same absolute submaximal intensity but to result in no change after exercise of the same relative submaximal intensity. This is because the same (pretraining) absolute intensity is a lower relative intensity after training. The mechanisms appear to be the same as for the changes in oxygen drift. These factors include training-induced decreases in blood lactate concentration, body temperature, epinephrine-mediated glucose production, and insulin-mediated glucose uptake. The training-induced shift toward greater fat utilization during exercise continues into the postexercise period.

Lactate Accumulation (8)

Lactic acid/lactate is produced when the hydrogen atoms carried on NADH + H$^+$ are transferred to pyruvic acid in a reaction catalyzed by lactic dehydrogenase. Lactate accumulates when the rate of production exceeds the rate of clearance. Although it is known that a trained individual accumulates less lactate at the same absolute workload than an untrained individual, whether the rate of lactate production decreases or the rate of clearance increases more with training is under debate.

Factors that lead to a decrease in lactic acid/lactate production following training include:

1. Fuel shifts
2. Enzyme activity changes
3. Blunted neurohormonal responses

Pyruvate is the end product of carbohydrate metabolism (glycolysis). Less carbohydrate is utilized at an absolute submaximal workload after training; therefore, less pyruvate is available for conversion into lactate. At the same time, pyruvate dehydrogenase activity increases following training, causing more pyruvate to be converted to acetyl CoA. LDH enzyme shifts from the skeletal muscle form, which favors lactate production, to the cardiac muscle form, which has a lower affinity for pyruvate. In addition, following training, glycolysis is inhibited by several factors, two of which relate to the increased utilization of fat during submaximal exercise. The first is a high concentration of free fatty acid in the cytoplasm; the second is a high level of citrate (the first product in the Krebs cycle). Both factors cause the rate-limiting enzyme PFK to slow down glycolysis and thus decrease the possible production of lactate. Finally, a smaller increase in the concentration of epinephrine and norepinephrine has been found at the same absolute and relative workloads in trained individuals. This decreased sympathetic stimulation may also decrease the activation of glycogenolysis and the potential production of lactate (Gollnick et al., 1986; Holloszy and Coyle, 1984; Messonnier et al., 2006).

Several other changes lead to higher rates of clearance in trained individuals. These can be classified into two main factors:

1. Enhanced lactate transport
2. Enhanced lactate oxidation

Oxygen–Free Radicals, Exercise, Exercise Training Adaptations, and Antioxidant Supplements

Cancer, atherosclerosis, cataracts, Alzheimer's disease, diabetes, loss of memory, Parkinson's disease, and aging may all, in part, be caused by free radical damage (Keith, 1999). What are free radicals? How can they cause so many different problems? What is the link between oxygen-free radicals, exercise, and exercise training adaptations? Should antioxidant supplements be taken by individuals involved in exercise training?

Under normal conditions, electrons orbiting in the shells of a molecule are in pairs. If a single electron is added or removed, instability occurs. The resulting structure is called a *free radical*. Free radicals have a drive to return to a balanced stable state and attempt to do so by taking an electron from, giving an electron to, or sharing an electron with another atom. *Reactive oxygen species (ROS)* contain free radicals and reactive forms of oxygen.

ROS can be produced from sources originating outside the body, such as x-rays, UV rays in sunlight, air pollutants (ozone and nitric oxide in car exhaust), cigarette smoke, toxic chemicals (some pesticides), and physical injury (from contact sports or concussions). They may also result from sources within the body, specifically as part of normal immune function or as a normal by-product of the production of energy (Finaud et al., 2006; Keith, 1999).

Acute exercise produces free radicals. During the aerobic production of ATP, single electrons leak from electron transport in stage IV in the mitochondria. The principal locations of this continuous electron leak are complexes I and III and involve coenzyme Q. The higher the rate of metabolism (as in moving from rest to submaximal to maximal exercise), the more free radicals are produced. Possibly as much as 4–5% of the oxygen consumed is converted to free radicals. Anaerobic energy production provides an abundance of hydrogen ions that can react with an oxygen-free radical to form a ROS, such as hydrogen peroxide, H_2O_2. Hypoxia leads to freeing of metals (Fe, Cu, and Mg) that are needed to catalyze free radical production. Exercise-induced hyperthermia may trigger free radical proliferation. Any damage to muscle fibers leads to increased immune response and free radical production (Finaud et al., 2006). Exercises that result in alterations of blood flow and oxygen supply such as weight lifting trigger free radical production.

ROS have numerous negative effects. If the production of free radicals exceeds that of components called *antioxidants* that suppress them and their harmful effects, *oxidative stress* occurs. Often, a chain reaction occurs that results in damage to lipids (especially the lipid bilayer of cell membranes), proteins (in enzymes, immune cells, joints, and muscles), DNA (breaking strands or shifting bases, thus influencing the genetic code), and, in excess, decreases muscular contractile force. These changes ultimately can lead minimally to muscular fatigue or more seriously to the diseases listed earlier (Alessio and Blasi, 1997; Finaud et al., 2006; Gross et al., 2011; Jenkins, 1993; Keith, 1999).

Conversely, ROS have several positive roles in the body including involvement in the immune system, cellular signaling, enzyme activation, facilitation of glycogen replenishment, and muscle fiber contractile force. Among the cellular signaling done by ROS after aerobic endurance training are the pathways that enhance mitochondrial biogenesis, capillarization, muscle and heart hypertrophy, and glucose transport ability. They can act as a vasodilator and optimize both blood flow and the velocity of blood flow (Gross et al., 2011).

Despite the increased production of free radicals resulting from exercise, it is unlikely that exercise results in substantial damages to a normal healthy individual. The body has a number of natural (endogenous) defenses, and antioxidants ingested in food provide additional (exogenous) defenses. Each cell contains a variety of antioxidant scavenger enzymes, predominantly superoxide dismutase, catalase, and glutathione peroxidase. Antioxidant vitamins, minerals, and phytochemicals include vitamin E, vitamin C, beta carotene (precursor of vitamin A), selenium, coenzyme Q (ubiquinone) and flavonoids.

Acute exercise has been shown to selectively enhance the antioxidant enzymes. In addition, most exercise training studies have shown increased antioxidant levels following both aerobic endurance exercise and dynamic resistance exercise. Part of the training adaptation may be due to increases in the cytochromes in electron transport, which reduces electron leakage (Alessio and Blasi, 1997; American College of Sports Medicine, American Dietetic Association, Dietitians of Canada, 2009).

Recent consensus reports (American College of Sports Medicine et al., 2009; Kreider et al., 2004; Pendergast et al., 2011) do not support the idea that ingested supplementation of Vitamins A, C, or E improve performance, delay fatigue, or protect against muscle damage in adequately nourished individuals. Indeed, several recent exercise studies have provided evidence that high supplementation of antioxidants may actually be counterproductive both acutely and in terms of blunted training adaptations (Peternelj and Coombes, 2011). Acute exercise responses to antioxidant supplementation indicate that the elevated oxidative defenses via the normal upregulation of the antioxidant enzymes may be suppressed. For example, Knez et al. (2007) reported significantly greater oxidative damage in half and full ironman triathletes who took antioxidant supplements than in those who did not. Chronic training adaptations with antioxidant supplementation include evidence of suppressed capillarization and mitochondrial biogenesis (Gross et al., 2011).

However, this is not to say that all antioxidant supplementation should be avoided. Individual athletes and circumstances must be taken into account. Athletes at greatest risk for poor antioxidant intakes include those doing high-intensity training, following a low-fat diet, restricting energy intake, or limiting dietary intakes of fruits, vegetables, and whole grains. In addition, athletes training at high altitude (where free radical

Oxygen-Free Radicals, Exercise, Exercise Training Adaptations, and Antioxidant Supplements (*Continued*)

production is intensified and internal defenses are weakened by hypoxia) could benefit from supplementation. All individuals should make sure that their diets contain large amounts of antioxidant-rich foods, primarily fruits and vegetables. Prunes, raisins, blueberries, strawberries, oranges, spinach, broccoli, beets, onions, corn, eggplant, nuts, and whole grains are particularly beneficial. If vitamin supplements are ingested they should not exceed recommended upper limits such as 1000 mg of vitamin C daily or 400 IU per day for vitamin E. More is not better and in excessive amounts antioxidants can actually act as pro-oxidants with potential negative effects. Supplementation with coenzyme Q is not recommended at all. The search for the optimal balance between the beneficial and harmful effects of ROS

and antioxidant supplementation continues (American College of Sports Medicine et al., 2009; Finaud, 2006; Gross et al., 2011; Jenkins, 1993; Keith, 1999; McGinley et al., 2009; Stear et al., 2010).

Sources: American College of Sports Medicine et al. (2009), Alessio and Blasi (1997), Finaud et al. (2006), Jenkins (1993), Keith (1999), Knez et al. (2007), Kreider et al. (2004), McGinley et al. (2009), Pendergast et al. (2011), Peternelj and Coombes (2011), Stear et al. (2010).

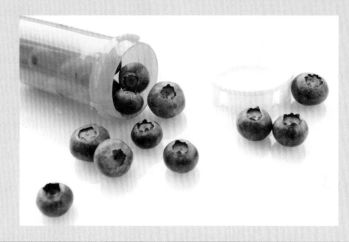

Lactate transport is enhanced by a combination of increased substrate affinity (the ability of the lactate to bind to the transporter), increased intrinsic activity of the enzymes involved, and increased density of the mitochondrial membrane and cell membrane MCT1 lactate transporters (Juel et al., 2004; Thomas et al., 2005). At the same time, mitochondrial size, number, and enzyme concentrations are increased. Taken together, these changes enable muscle cells to increase both the extracellular and intracellular lactate shuttle mechanisms. There is an overall uptake of lactate by muscles, and as a result, more lactate can be oxidized more rapidly during exercise. Concomitantly, blood flow to the liver is enhanced, which aids in overall lactate removal (Bonen, 2000; Brooks, 2000; Brooks et al., 2000; Gladden, 2000; Pilegaard et al., 1994). Training at the velocity of maximal lactate steady-state (MLSSv) has been shown to increase both time to exhaustion at MLSSv and $\dot{V}O_2$max without modifying either [La⁻] or reliance on carbohydrate fuel indicating an increased lactate clearance (Billat et al., 2004). These adaptations in the rate of lactate clearance are probably greater than the changes in the rate of lactate production although both contribute to the reduction in lactate accumulation (Brooks, 1991; Donovan and Brooks, 1983; Mazzeo et al., 1986). The result is a decreased concentration of lactate in the muscles and blood at the same relative workload ($\dot{V}O_2$max) after training.

As a consequence of the change in the ratio of lactate clearance to production after training, a higher workload (both in absolute and relative terms) is required to reach lactate levels in the 2- to 4-mmol·L⁻¹ range (**Figure 5.4C**). This means that an individual can exercise at a higher relative intensity for a given period of time and yet delay the onset of fatigue because the lactate thresholds (LT1 and LT2) have been raised (Allen et al., 1985; Henritze et al., 1985; Holloszy and Coyle, 1984; Londeree, 1997; Skinner and Morgan, 1985; Williams et al., 1967; Yoshida et al., 1982).

At maximal aerobic/anaerobic endurance exercise, the level of lactate accumulation is higher as a result of training. The higher level probably results from the greater glycogen stores and increased activity of some of the glycolytic enzymes other than LDH (Abernethy et al., 1990; Gollnick et al., 1986). It may also be more a psychological than a physiological adaptation, in that the trained individual is more motivated and can better tolerate the pain caused by lactic acid (Galbo, 1983) when working at a higher absolute load.

Resistance training has been shown to affect lactate response to both weight-lifting exercise and dynamic aerobic exercise. For example, after 10 weeks of strength training (3 sets of 7 exercises at 8–12 repetitions with 60–90 seconds of rest between sets, 3 d·wk⁻¹), college females significantly improved their squat 1-RM. When blood lactate values were compared before and after training at the same absolute load (70% and 50% of pretraining 1-RM), there was a significant reduction in blood lactate from 8 to 6 mmol·L^{-1}. When the same relative load was compared (70% and 50% of pretraining 1-RM versus 70% and 50% of posttraining 1-RM), there was no significant difference in blood lactate levels (8 mmol·L^{-1} versus 7.5 mmol·L^{-1}). These results indicate that after training more work could be done before the same accumulation of lactate occurred than before training. Interestingly, the heart rate responses did not vary among the three testing conditions (before, after absolute loads, and after relative loads), but RPE responses paralleled the changes in blood lactate (Reynolds et al., 1997).

In a 12-week study, young adult males trained using a circuit of three sets of 10 exercises, doing 8–10 repetitions with 30 seconds of rest between exercises, 3 d·wk^{-1}. As anticipated, the experimental group significantly improved in both 1-RM upper and lower body strength and leg peak torque, while the controls did not. Neither group changed their treadmill $\dot{V}O_2$max or the cycle ergometer $\dot{V}O_2$peak. However, the experimental subjects cycled 33% longer at 75% $\dot{V}O_2$peak after training, and blood lactate concentrations were significantly reduced at all submaximal intensities tested. Lactate threshold (defined as an absolute value of 3.3 mmol·L^{-1}) increased by 12% following resistance training. These results support the generalization that a higher intensity of endurance exercise can be accomplished before reaching the same level of blood lactate concentration, whether the training modality is dynamic aerobic endurance or dynamic resistance activity (Marcinik et al., 1991). There appears to be a dose-response relationship between the frequency of interval training and the magnitude of lactate threshold improvement (expressed as %$\dot{V}O_2$max) (Dalleck et al., 2010).

ATP Production, Storage, and Turnover

ATP-PC (9)

Although exercise training increases the potential for the production of larger quantities of ATP by oxidative phosphorylation, it does not change the efficiency of converting fuel to ATP or ATP to work. Thirty-two actual ATP molecules are still produced from glucose in skeletal muscle, and the potential energy per mole of ATP is still between 7 and 12 kcal (Abernethy et al., 1990; Gollnick and Hermansen, 1973; Gollnick et al., 1986; Holloszy, 1973; Karlsson et al., 1972; Skinner and Morgan, 1985).

However, the amount of ATP and PC stored in the resting muscle is higher in trained than in untrained individuals, especially if muscle mass increases. Whether this amount is large enough to markedly increase anaerobic capacity is questionable. The resting PC/ATP ratio does not differ among sprint-trained runners, endurance-trained runners, and untrained individuals (Johansen and Quistorff, 2003). At the same absolute workload, there is less depletion of the PC and degradation of ATP levels after training. At the same relative workload, PC depletion and ATP degradation do not change with training. However, the activity of the enzymes responsible for the breakdown of ATP to ADP and the regeneration of ADP and ATP increase. Therefore, the rate of turnover of ATP and PC increases and may be as much as double that of untrained individuals in both sprint- and endurance-trained runners (Johansen and Quistorff, 2003). Taken together, the ATP-PC-LA changes indicate an increased anaerobic power and capacity with sprint type training (Medbø and Burgers, 1990). Values for the ATP-PC, LA, and O$_2$ systems are presented in **Table 5.3**. The values for the untrained were previously presented in **Table 3.1** but are now contrasted with trained males. The LA system changes much more with training than the ATP-PC system, but the greatest change is in the O$_2$ system (Bouchard et al., 1982, 1991).

Work (power) Output

Work (power) output—measured as watts or kilocalories per kilogram of body weight on a bicycle test such as the 10- or 30-second Wingate Anaerobic Test and/or a 90-second test—improves with training. This is evidenced by higher scores of athletes than nonathletes and by higher posttraining than pretraining scores in all populations. Furthermore, sprint- or power-type athletes typically have higher anaerobic values and greater adaptations than endurance athletes. Elite sprinters and power

TABLE 5.3	Estimated Maximal Power and Capacity for Untrained (UT) and Trained (TR) Males							
	Power				**Capacity**			
	kcal·min^{-1}		kJ·min^{-1}		kcal·min^{-1}		kJ·min^{-1}	
System	UT	TR	UT	TR	UT	TR	UT	TR
Phosphagens (ATP-PC)	72	96	300	400	11	13	45	55
Anaerobic glycolysis (LA)	36	60	150	250	48	72	200	300
Aerobic glycolysis plus Krebs cycle plus ETS/OP (O$_2$)	7–19	32–37	30–80	135–155	360–1270	10,770–19,140	1500–5300	45,000–80,000
Source: Modified from Bouchard et al. (1982, 1991).								

athletes score higher than less successful competitors (Bar-Or, 1987; Beld et al., 1989; Horswill et al., 1989; Patton and Duggan, 1987).

Aerobically, a trained individual can continue any given submaximal workload longer than an untrained individual. The trained individual can also accomplish more total work and a higher absolute maximum than an untrained individual. Overall, the trained individual has a metabolic system capable of supporting enhanced performance, both at submaximal and at maximal levels. These changes, summarized in **Table 5.4**, depend on the type of training used.

TABLE 5.4 Metabolic Training Adaptations
1. Fuel Supply
a. Carbohydrate
(1) ↑ GLUT-4 transporter number and concentration; ↓ exercise induced translocation
(2) ↓ Glucose utilization
(3) ↑ Muscle and liver glycogen reserves
(4) ↓ Rate of muscle and liver glycogen depletion at absolute submaximal loads, that is, glycogen sparing
(5) ↑ Velocity of glycogenolysis at maximal work
b. Fat
(1) ↑ Mobilization, transportation, and beta-oxidation of free fatty acids
(2) ↑ Fat storage adjacent to mitochondria
(3) ↑ Utilization of fat as fuel at the same absolute and the same relative workloads
c. Protein
(1) ↑ Ability to utilize the BCAA leucine as fuel
(2) ↑ Gluconeogenesis from alanine
2. Enzyme Activity
a. ↑ Selected glycolytic enzyme activity: glycogen phosphorylase and probably phosphofructokinase
b. ↓ LDH activity with some conversion from the skeletal muscle to cardiac muscle form with endurance training but ↑ with strength/sprint training
c. ↑ Activity of the malate-aspartate shuttle enzymes but not the glycerol-phosphate shuttle enzymes
d. ↑ Number and size of mitochondria
e. ↑ Activity of most, but not all, of the enzymes of beta-oxidation, the Krebs cycle, electron transport, and oxidative phosphorylation due to greater mitochondrial protein amount
3. O_2 Utilization
a. ↑ $\dot{V}O_2$max with aerobic endurance training but not with dynamic resistance training
b. = $\dot{V}O_2$ cost at absolute submaximal workload unless neuromuscular skill aspects improve
c. ↑ Myoglobin concentration
d. ↓ Oxygen deficit
e. ↓ Oxygen drift
f. ↓ EPOC at same absolute submaximal workload
4. LA Accumulation
a. ↑ MCT1 lactate transporters
b. ↑ Intracellular and extracellular lactate shuttle activity
c. ↓ La⁻ accumulation at the same absolute workload and % $\dot{V}O_2$max relative intensity for endurance activity
d. ↓ La⁻ accumulation at the same absolute workload but = La⁻ accumulation at the same relative intensity for resistance exercise
e. ↑ Workload to achieve lactate thresholds
f. ↑ Velocity at maximal lactate steady state (MLSSv) and time to exhaustion at MLSSv
g. ↑ [La⁻] at maximum
5. ATP Productions, Storage, and Turnover
a. = ATP from gram of precursor fuel substrate
b. ↑ ATP-PC storage
c. ↓ Depletion of PC and degradation of ATP at the same absolute workload
d. = Depletion of PC and degradation of ATP at the same relative workload
e. ↑ ATP-PC turnover
↑, increase; ↓, decrease; =, no change.

Substrate Training Adaptations in Children

As has been described, it is clear that in adults the primary substrate utilized to fuel exercise depends on the modality, intensity, and duration of the activity as well as the individual's training status. The "crossover" concept states that at some point, as the intensity increases during incremental exercise, the predominant fuel source shifts from fat to carbohydrate. The crossover point is the power output at which this occurs.

This study by Duncan and Howley shows that the same processes occur in children. Twenty-three volunteer boys and girls (ages 7–12 years) were divided into a training group (N = 10) and a control group (N = 13). All were tested for $\dot{V}O_2$peak on a cycle ergometer and then at five power outputs designed to elicit approximately 35%, 45%, 55%, 65%, and 75% of $\dot{V}O_2$peak. RER values were determined by open-circuit spirometry for the five-stage submaximal test before and after 4 weeks of training. Training consisted of three 10-minute work bouts separated by 1–2 minutes of rest at roughly 50% $\dot{V}O_2$peak, three times per week.

The results, presented in the graph below, clearly show that as the intensity of the submaximal exercise increased, so did the percentage of carbohydrate utilized as fuel, both before and after the training. Furthermore, the crossover point was delayed or shifted to the right in the training group (data for the control group are not shown). This means that

the trained children could work harder while using fat as the predominant fuel. Training apparently has the same carbohydrate-sparing benefit for children as for adults.

Source: Duncan, G. E. & E. I. Howley: Metabolic and perceptual responses to short-term cycle training in children. *Pediatric Exercise Science*. 10:110–122 (1998).

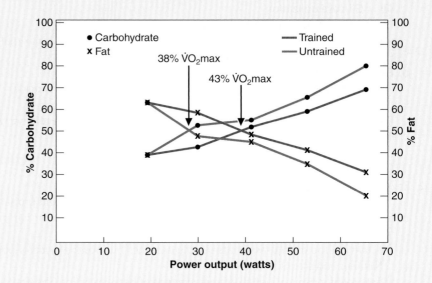

The Influence of Age and Sex on Metabolic Training Adaptations

With the exception of $\dot{V}O_2$max there is little research data on most of the metabolic variables across the age spectrum. The scattered evidence that is available indicates that training and detraining changes in children, adolescents, and older adults are similar in direction and magnitude to changes in adults in the 20- to 50-year range. This is especially true when changes are considered relative to baseline values (i.e., as a percentage of change) rather than as absolutes (Adeniran and Toriola, 1988; Bar-Or, 1983; Clarke, 1977; Eriksson, 1972; Gaisl and Wiesspeiner, 1986; Massicotte and MacNab, 1974; Rotstein et al., 1986; Rowland, 1990).

The one remarkable exception to the above generalization is the uncoupling of endurance performance changes and maximal oxygen uptake changes in youth (**Figure 4.14**) such that children exhibit a limited capacity to improve $\dot{V}O_2$max; despite being able to improve endurance exercise performance. That is, the same exercise training program that would generate a 15–20%

improvement in adults in $\dot{V}O_2$max typically results in only a 5% increase in prepubertal children of both sexes. The question, of course, is why. Rowland (2009) has put forth the *crowded cell hypothesis*. In the skeletal muscle cell there is only so much space and that space is shared by the contractile apparatus, the sarcoplasmic reticulum that regulates each contraction-relaxation cycle, and the mitochondria that provides the energy. Adaptations of cellular elements to training are limited by cell space. The space allocated to the contractile apparatus and sarcoplasmic reticulum cannot be compromised. Children have less space for expansion than adults because before training their muscle fibers have a higher mitochondrial density (~+30–50%) and oxidative enzyme activity than adults. The limited change in mitochondria results in $\dot{V}O_2$max increases with endurance training that are typically a lower percentage in children than adults. Further research is needed to confirm or modify this hypothesis.

There is also minimal data on metabolic adaptations in females of all ages, again with the exception of $\dot{V}O_2$max (Shepard, 1978; Tlusty, 1969; Wells, 1991). Studies have shown the following adaptations in females as a result of appropriate specific training:

1. Fuel utilization shifts in favor of fat both in younger and older women (Johnson et al., 2010).
2. Lactate levels decrease during submaximal work and increase at maximal effort.
3. Some glycolytic enzyme and most oxidative enzymes increase in activity.
4. Submaximal $\dot{V}O_2$max consumption remains stable or decreases slightly.
5. Anaerobic power and capacity increase (Slade et al., 2002; Wells, 1991; Weltman et al., 1978).

In short, both males and females respond to the same training with the same adaptations. Sex differences in the metabolic variables are not obliterated in equally trained males and females, but both sexes are trainable and probably to the same extent.

Detraining in the Metabolic System

Detraining is the partial or complete loss of training-induced anatomical, physiological, and performance adaptations in response to an insufficient training stimulus (Mujika and Padilla, 2000a). If an individual ceases training or reduces training beyond that of a planned taper, detraining or reversibility will occur. This reversibility of training adaptations in metabolic potential occurs within days to weeks after training ceases. A reduction in both maximal and submaximal performance ultimately follows. Those metabolic factors that improve the most with training, that is, those involved with aerobic energy production, also show the greatest reversal. Within 3 to 6 weeks after the cessation of training, the individual typically returns to pretraining levels, especially if the training program was of short duration. Individuals with a long and established training history, however, tend to have an initial rapid decline in some aerobic variables but then level off at higher-than-pretraining levels. Anaerobic metabolic variables have less incremental increase with training and less loss with detraining. This fact may explain why sprint performance is more resistant to inactivity than endurance performance. Complete bed rest or immobilization accelerates detraining (Coyle et al., 1984; Neufer, 1989; Ready and Quinney, 1982; Wilmore and Costill, 1988).

The following specific detraining effects have been documented in detraining studies (Mujika and Padilla, 2000a,b, 2001):

1. Fuel supply:
   a. Both short-term (<4 weeks) and long-term (>4 weeks) detraining are characterized by an increased RER during exercise, indicating a shift toward an increased reliance on carbohydrates as an energy substrate and a decreased reliance on lipid metabolism.
   b. A reduced (17–33% in 6–10 days) muscle GLUT-4 transporter content occurs with detraining. Possibly as a result, insulin-mediated glucose update also decreases rapidly with detraining. Accompanying this is an increase in epinephrine and norepinephrine during submaximal exercise.
   c. Decreases in intracellular glycogen storage have also been reported with as little as 1 week of detraining. Reductions of approximately 20% have been reported in 4 weeks in highly trained athletes, and the level may completely revert to the pretraining level shortly after that.
2. Enzyme activity:
   a. Oxidative enzyme activity decreases between 25% and 45% with both short-term and long-term detraining in highly conditioned individuals and after short-term training programs.
   b. Small, nonsystematic changes in glycolytic enzymes may occur.
3. O_2 utilization:
   a. $\dot{V}O_2$max has been reported to decline 4–14% with short-term (<4 weeks) detraining and 6–20% with long-term detraining (>4 weeks). The decline in trained individuals tends to be progressive and directly proportional to the $\dot{V}O_2$max during the first 8 weeks and then to stabilize at levels higher or equal to that of sedentary individuals. Recently trained individuals may decline a lesser amount in the initial weeks, but with long-term detraining, they tend to revert to pretraining levels.
4. Lactate accumulation:
   a. Increased blood lactate levels during submaximal exercise occur in both the short and the long term with detraining.
   b. Detraining leads to a decrease in maximal lactate values.
   c. LT1 and LT2 occur at a lower percentage of $\dot{V}O_2$max with detraining.
5. ATP production, storage, and transport:
   a. Mitochondrial ATP production rate decreases 12–28% during 3 weeks of detraining after 6 weeks of training in previously sedentary individuals but still remains above pretraining levels.

Retraining does not occur as rapidly as detraining and is not easier or more rapid than the initial training (Wilmore and Costill, 1988). Although direct experimental evidence is scanty, the consequences of detraining and retraining appear to be similar for adults, children, and adolescents of both sexes (Bar-Or, 1983).

FOCUS ON RESEARCH

Detraining and Retraining

This case study of detraining and retraining was conducted on a 49.5-year-old female elite competitive cyclist. Two days after undergoing testing for a research project, the cyclist sustained a right clavicular fracture during a criterion race. She continued a modified training regime until 22 days after the injury, when she developed loss of motion in the shoulder and pain and numbness in the hand. Surgery was performed 26 days after the injury for brachial plexus impingement. Thus, the detraining period began approximately 4 weeks after the injury. Retraining began the 32nd day after surgery (0 on the *X*-axis). Results for her metabolic variables are presented in the accompanying graphs. The baseline represents the values obtained 2 days before the injury. Retesting was done approximately every 2 weeks (0, 14, 28, 42, 56, and 70 days) for 6 weeks and then again at week 11 of retraining (77 days).

$\dot{V}O_2$max decreased approximately 25% during detraining, but by week 11, it was within 2 mL·kg·min^{-1} of preinjury values. The improvement was steady over the first 6 weeks of retraining.

Power output decreased 18.2% at peak, 16.7% at LT1, and 18.9% at 4 mM lactate. Peak lactate decreased by a comparable 19.1%. Although peak power output increased during the first 2 weeks, power output at LT1 and 4 mM lactate did not. This probably occurred because high-intensity work was not included in the initial retraining weeks as is appropriate given the progression principle. By week 11, peak power output and power output at LT1 had returned to baseline values. However, at that point neither peak power output at 4 mM nor peak lactate had regained preinjury levels.

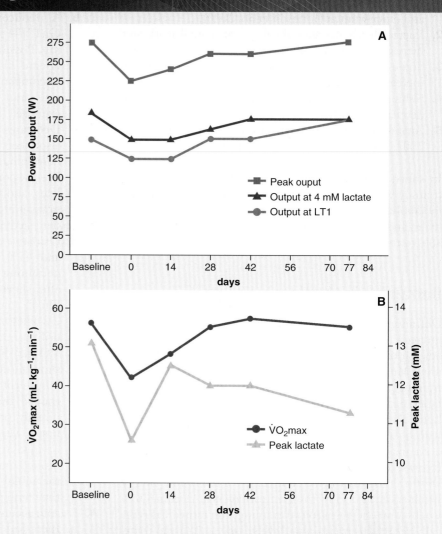

Source: Nichols, J. F., D. Robinson, D. Douglass, & J. Anthony: Retraining of a competitive master athlete following traumatic injury. A case study. *Medicine & Science in Sports & Exercise.* 32(6):1037–1042 (2000).

Summary

1. The most important considerations for applying each training principle to achieve metabolic adaptations are as follows:
   a. For specificity, match the energy system of the activity.
   b. For overload, manipulate time and distance or lactate level.
   c. For rest/recovery/adaptation, alternate hard and easy days.
   d. For progression, re-overload if additional improvement is desired.
   e. For individualization, evaluate the individual according to the demands of the activity and develop a periodization training sequence, system, and load on the basis of this evaluation.
   f. For maintenance, emphasize intensity.
   g. For retrogression, plateau, and reversibility, evaluate the training adaptations and modify as indicated.
   h. For warm-up and cooldown, include activities that will actually elevate and reduce body temperature, respectively.

2. Properly prescribed training programs bring about positive adaptations in fuel supply, enzyme activity, oxygen utilization, lactate accumulation, and ATP production, storage, and turnover.

REVIEW QUESTIONS

1. Name and briefly describe the eight training principles. Select a sport or fitness activity and show how each of the training principles can be specifically applied to that activity.

2. Describe and explain the metabolic adaptations to exercise training for each of the following factors:
   a. Substrate or fuel supply
   b. Enzyme activity
   c. Oxygen utilization
   d. Lactate accumulation
   e. ATP production, storage, and turnover

3. Describe and explain the effect of detraining on each of the following factors:
   a. Substrate or fuel supply
   b. Enzyme activity
   c. Oxygen utilization
   d. Lactate accumulation
   e. ATP production, storage, and turnover

For further review and additional study tools, visit the website at http://thePoint.lww.com/Plowman4e ✳ 🔘

REFERENCES

Abernethy, P. J., R. Thayer, & A. W. Taylor: Acute and chronic responses of skeletal muscle to endurance and sprint exercise: A review. *Sports Medicine.* 10(6):365–389 (1990).

Adeniran, S. A. & A. L. Toriola: Effects of continuous and interval running programmes on aerobic and anaerobic capacities in schoolgirls aged 13 to 17 years. *Journal of Sports Medicine and Physical Fitness.* 28:260–266 (1988).

Alessio, H. & E. R. Blasi: Physical activity as a natural antioxidant booster and its effect on a healthy life span. *Research Quarterly for Exercise and Sport.* 68(4):292–302 (1997).

Allen, W. K., D. R. Seals, B. F. Hurley, A. A. Ehsani, & J. M. Hagberg: Lactate threshold and distance-running performance in young and older endurance athletes. *Journal of Applied Physiology.* 58(4):1281–1284 (1985).

American College of Sports Medicine, American Dietetic Association, Dietitians of Canada: Nutrition and Athletic Performance. *Medicine & Science in Sports & Exercise.* 41(3):709–731 (2009).

Anderson, O.: The rise and fall of tempo training. *Running Research.* 14(8):1, 4–5 (1998).

Bailey, S. P. & R. R. Pate: Feasibility of improving running economy. *Sports Medicine.* 12(4):228–246 (1991).

Barnett, A.: Using recovery modalities between training sessions in elite athletes: Does it help? *Sports Medicine.* 36(9):781–796 (2006).

Bar-Or, O.: *Pediatric Sports Medicine for the Practitioner: From Physiological Principles to Clinical Applications.* New York, NY: Springer-Verlag, 1–65 (1983).

Bar-Or, O.: The Wingate Anaerobic Test: An update on the methodology, reliability and validity. *Sports Medicine.* 4:381–394 (1987).

Beld, K., J. Skinner, & Z. Tran: Load optimization for peak and mean power output on the Wingate Anaerobic Test. *Medicine and Science in Sports and Exercise (Suppl. 164).* 21(2):S28 (1989).

Beneke, R. & M. Hütler: The effect of training on running economy and performance in recreational athletes. *Medicine & Science in Sports & Exercise.* 37(10):1794–1799 (2005).

Billat, V., P. Sirvent, P-M. Lepretre, & J. P. Koralsztein: Training effect of performance, substrate balance and blood lactate concentration at maximal lactate steady state in master endurance-runners. *Pflugers Archives-European Journal of Physiology.* 447:875–883 (2004).

Bishop, D.: Warm up II: Performance changes following active warm up and how to structure the warm up. *Sports Medicine.* 33(7):483–498 (2003).

Bompa, T. O.: *Periodization: Theory and Methodology of Training.* Champaign, IL: Human Kinetics (1999).

Bonacci, J., A. Chapman, P. Blanch, & B. Vicenzino: Neuromuscular adaptations to training, injury and passive interventions: Implications for running economy. *Sports Medicine.* 39(11): 903–921 (2009).

Bonen, A.: Lactate transporters (MCT proteins) in heart and skeletal muscles. *Medicine & Science in Sports & Exercise.* 32(4):778–789 (2000).

Bosquet, L., J. Montpetit, D. Arvisais, & I. Mujika: Effects of tapering on performance: A meta-analysis. *Medicine & Science in Sports & Exercise.* 39(8): 1358–1365 (2007).

Bouchard, C., A. W. Taylor, & S. Dulac: Testing maximal anaerobic power and capacity. In MacDougall, J. D., H. W. Wenger, & H. J. Green (eds.): *Physiological Testing of the High-Performance Athlete* (2nd edition). Champaign, IL: Human Kinetics, 175–221 (1991).

Bouchard, C., A. W. Taylor, J. A. Simoneau, & S. Dulac: Testing anaerobic power and capacity. In MacDougall, J. D., H. A. Wenger, & H. J. Green (eds.): *Physiological Testing of the Elite Athlete* (1st edition). Hamilton, ON: Canadian Association of Sport Sciences Mutual Press Limited, 61–73 (1982).

Bourdon, P.: Blood lactate transition thresholds: Concepts and controversies. In Gore, C. J. (ed.): *Physiological Tests for Elite Athletes.* Champaign, IL: Human Kinetics, 50–65 (2000).

Brooks, G. A.: Current concepts in lactate exchange. *Medicine Science and in Sports and Exercise.* 23(8):895–906 (1991).

Brooks, G. A.: Intra- and extra-cellular lactate shuttles. *Medicine & Science in Sports & Exercise.* 32(4):790–799 (2000).

Brooks, G. A., T. D. Fahey, T. P. White, & K. M. Baldwin: *Exercise Physiology: Human Bioenergetics and Its Applications* (3rd edition). Mountain View, CA: Mayfield (2000).

Casaburi, R., T. W. Storer, I. Ben-Dov, & K. Wasserman: Effect of endurance training on possible determinants of VO_2 during heavy exercise. *Journal of Applied Physiology.* 62(1):199–207 (1987).

Chaloupka, E. C. & E. L. Fox: Physiological effects of two maintenance programs following eight weeks of interval training. *Federation Proceedings (abstract).* 34(3):443 (1975).

Clarke, H. H. (ed.): *Exercise and Aging. Physical Fitness Research Digest*. Washington, DC: President's Council on Physical Fitness and Sports, 7(2):1–27 (1977).

Conley, D., G. Krahenbuhl, & L. Burkett: Training for aerobic capacity and running economy. *Physician and Sportsmedicine*. 9(4):107–115 (1981).

Costill, D. L.: *Inside Running: Basics of Sport Physiology*. Indianapolis, IN: Benchmark Press (1986).

Costill, D. L., D. S. King, R. Thomas, & M. Hargreaves: Effects of reduced training on muscular power in swimmers. *Physician and Sportsmedicine*. 13:94–101 (1985).

Coyle, E. F., W. H. Martin, D. R. Sinacore, M. J. Joyner, J. M. Hagberg, & J. O. Holloszy: Time course of loss of adaptations after stopping prolonged intense endurance training. *Journal of Applied Physiology: Respiratory, Environmental and Exercise Physiology*. 57(6):1857–1864 (1984).

Dalleck, L., T. T. Bushman, R. D. Crain, M. M. Gajda, E. M. Koger, & L. A. Derksen: Dose-response relationship between interval training frequency and magnitude of improvement in lactate threshold. *International Journal of Sports Medicine*. 31(8):567–571 (2010).

Daniels, J., N. Oldridge, F. Nagle, & B. White: Differences and changes in VO_2 among young runners 10 to 18 years of age. *Medicine and Science in Sports and Exercise*. 10(3):200–203 (1978).

Daugaard, J. R., J. N. Nielsen, S. Kristiansen, J. L. Andersen, M. Hargreaves, & E. A. Richter: Fiber type-specific expression of GLUT4 in human skeletal muscle: influence of exercise training. *Diabetes*. 49(7):1092–1095 (2000).

Daussin, F. N., J. Zoll, E. Ponsot, S. P. Dufour, S. Doutreleau, E. Lonsdorfer, et al.: Training at high intensity promotes qualitative adaptations of mitochondrial function in human skeletal muscle. *Journal of Applied Physiology*. 104: 1436–1441 (2008).

Dela, F.: Carbohydrate metabolism in human muscle studied with the glycemic clamp technique: The influence of physical training. In R. J. Maughan, & Shirreffs, S. M. (eds.): *Biochemistry of Exercise IX*. Champaign, IL: Human Kinetics, 13–26 (1996).

Donovan, C. M. & G. A. Brooks: Endurance training affects lactate clearance, not lactate production. *American Journal of Physiology*. 244:E83–E92 (1983).

Duncan, G. E. & E. I. Howley: Metabolic and perceptual responses to short-term cycle training in children. *Pediatric ExerciseS Science*. 10:110–122 (1998).

Dupont, G., W. Moalla, C. Guinhouya, S. Ahmaidi, & S. Berthoin: Passive versus active recovery during high-intensity intermittent exercises. *Medicine & Science in Sports & Exercise*. 36(2):302–308 (2004).

Dwyer, J. & R. Bybee: Heart rate indices of the anaerobic threshold. *Medicine and Science in Sports and Exercise*. 15(1):72–76 (1983).

Ekblom, B., P.-O. Åstrand, B. Saltin, J. Stenberg, & B. Wallström: Effect of training on circulatory response to exercise. *Journal of Applied Physiology*. 24(4):518–528 (1968).

Eriksson, B. O.: Physical training, oxygen supply and muscle metabolism in 11–13 year old boys. *Acta Physiologica Scandinavica*. 384(Suppl.):1–48 (1972).

Finaud, J., G. Lac, & E. Filaire: Oxidative stress: Relationship with exercise and training. *Sports Medicine*. 36(4):327–358 (2006).

Fox, E. L., R. W. Bowers, & M. L. Foss: *The Physiological Basis of Physical Education and Athletics* (4th edition). Philadelphia, PA: Saunders College (1988).

Fox, E. L. & D. K. Mathews: *Interval Training: Conditioning for Sports and General Fitness*. Philadelphia, PA: W. B. Saunders (1974).

Fox, E. L., S. Robinson, & D. L. Wiegman: Metabolic energy sources during continuous and interval running. *Journal of Applied Physiology*. 27(2):174–178 (1969).

Fradkin, A. J., T. R. Zazryn, & J. M. Smoliga: Effects of warming-up on physical performance: A systematic review with meta-analysis. *Journal of Strength Conditioning Research*. 24(1): 140–148 (2010).

Franks, B. D.: Physical warm-up. In M. H. Williams (ed.): *Ergogenic Aids in Sport*. Champaign, IL: Human Kinetics, 340–375 (1983).

Fry, R. W., A. R. Morton, & D. Keast: Overtraining in athletics: An update. *Sports Medicine*. 12(1):32–65 (1991).

Gaisl, G. & G. Wiesspeiner: Training prescriptions for 9- to 17-year-old figure skaters based on lactate assessment in the laboratory and on the ice. In Rutenfranz, J., R. Mocellin, & F. Klimt (eds.): *Children and Exercise XII*. Champaign, IL: Human Kinetics, 17:59–65 (1986).

Galbo, H.: *Hormonal and Metabolic Adaptation to Exercise*. New York, NY: Thieme-Stratton, Inc. (1983).

Gardner, A. W., E. T. Poehlman, & D. L. Corrigan: Effect of endurance training on gross energy expenditure during exercise. *Human Biology*. 61(4):559–569 (1989).

Gilman, M. B. & C. L. Wells: The use of heart rates to monitor exercise intensity in relation to metabolic variables. *International Journal of Sports Medicine*. 14(6):3334–3339 (1993).

Gladden, L. B.: Muscle as a consumer of lactate. *Medicine & Science in Sports & Exercise*. 32(4):764–771 (2000).

Gollnick, P. D., W. M. Bayly, & D. R. Hodgson: Exercise intensity, training, diet, and lactate concentration in muscle and blood. *Medicine and Science in Sports and Exercise*. 18(3): 334–340 (1986).

Gollnick, P. D. & L. Hermansen: Biochemical adaptations in exercise: Anaerobic metabolism. In J. H. Wilmore (ed.): *Exercise and Sport Sciences Reviews*. New York, NY: Academic Press (1973).

Gross, M., O. Baum, & H. Hoppeler: Antioxidant supplementation and endurance training: Win or loss? *European Journal of Sport Science*. 11(1):27–32 (2011).

Guidetti, L., G. P. Emerenziani, M. C. Gallotta, & C. Baldari: Effect of warm-up on energy cost and energy sources of a ballet dance exercise. *European Journal of Applied Physiology*. 99:275–281 (2007).

Hagberg, J. M., J. P. Mullin, & F. J. Nagle: Oxygen consumption during constant-load exercise. *Journal of Applied Physiology: Respiratory, Environmental and Exercise Physiology*. 45(3): 381–384 (1978).

Harris, R. C., R. H. T. Edwards, E. Hultman, L.-O. Nordesjo, B. Nylind, & K. Sahlin: The time course of phosphorylcreatine resynthesis during recovery of the quadriceps muscle in man. *Pflugers Achives*. 36:137–142 (1976).

Hawley, J. A. & F. J. Spargo: Metabolic adaptations to marathon training and racing. *SportsMedicine*. 37(4–5):328–331 (2007).

Henritze, J., A. Weltman, R. L. Schurrer, & K. Barlow: Effects of training at and above the lactate threshold on the lactate threshold and maximal oxygen uptake. *European Journal of Applied Physiology*. 54:84–88 (1985).

Hickson, R. C., J. M. Hagberg, A. A. Ehsani, & J. O. Holloszy: Time course of the adaptive response of aerobic power and heart rate to training. *Medicine and Science in Sports and Exercise*. 13(1):17–20 (1981).

Holloszy, J. O.: Biochemical adaptations to exercise: Aerobic metabolism. In Wilmore, J. H. (ed.): *Exercise and Sport Sciences Reviews*. New York, NY: Academic Press, 1:45–71 (1973).

Holloszy, J. O. & E. F. Coyle: Adaptations of skeletal muscle to endurance exercise and their metabolic consequences. *Journal of Applied Physiology: Respiratory, Environmental and Exercise Physiology*. 56:831–838 (1984).

Hood, D. A. & R. L. Terjung: Amino acid metabolism during exercise and following endurance training. *Sports Medicine*. 9(1):23–35 (1990).

Horswill, C. A., J. R. Scott, & P. Galea: Comparison of maximum aerobic power, maximum anaerobic power, and skinfold thickness of elite and nonelite junior wrestlers. *International Journal of Sports Medicine*. 10:165–168 (1989).

Houmard, J. A., D. L. Costill, J. B. Mitchell, S. H. Park, R. C. Hickner, & J. M. Roemmich: Reduced training maintains performance in distance runners. *International Journal of Sports Medicine*. 11:46–52 (1990).

Hultman, E., J. Bergstrom, & N. McLennan-Anderson: Breakdown and resynthesis of phosphorylcreatine and adenosine triphospate in connection with muscular work in man. *Scandinavian Journal of Clinical Investigation*. 19:56–66 (1967).

Jenkins, R. R.: Exercise, oxidative stress, and antioxidants: A review. *International Journal of Sport Nutrition*. 3:356–375 (1993).

Johansen, L. & B. Quistorff: 31P-MRS characterization of sprint and endurance trained athletes. *International Journal of Sports Medicine*. 24(3):183–189 (2003).

Johns, R. A., J. A. Houmard, R. W. Kobe, T. Hortobagyi, N. J. Bruno, J. M. Wells, & M. H. Shinebarger: Effects of taper on swim power, stroke distance, and performance. *Medicine and Science in Sports and Exercise*. 24(10):1141–1146 (1992).

Johnson, M. L., Z. Zarins, J. A. Fattor, M. A. Horning, L. Messonnier, S. L. Lehman, & G. A. Brooks: Twelve weeks of endurance training increases FFA mobilization and reesterification in postmenopausal women. *Journal of Applied Physiology*. 109: 1573–1581 (2010).

Juel, C., M. K. Holten, & F. Dela: Effects of strength training on muscle lactate release and MCT1 and MCT4 content in healthy and type 2 diabetic humans. *Journal of Physiology*. 556 (Pt 1):297–304 (2004).

Jung, A. P.: The impact of resistance training on distance running performance. *Sports Medicine*. 33(7):539–552 (2003).

Karlsson, J., L.-O. Nordesjö, L. Jorfeldt, & B. Saltin: Muscle lactate, ATP, and CP levels during exercise after physical training in man. *Journal of Applied Physiology*. 33(2):199–203 (1972).

Keith, R. E.: Antioxidants and Health. Alabama Cooperative Extension System. HE-778 (1999).

King, M. & R. Duffield: The effects of recovery interventions on consecutive days of intermittent sprint exercise. *Journal of Strength and Conditioning Research*. 23(6):1795–1802 (2009).

Knez, W. L., D. G. Jenkins, & J. S. Coombes: Oxidative stress in half and full ironman triathletes. *Medicine & Science in Sports & Exercise*. 39(2):283–288 (2007).

Kraemer, W. J. & A. L. Gómez: Establishing a solid fitness base. In: Foran, B. (ed.): *High-Performance Sports Conditioning: Modern Training for Ultimate Athletic Development*. Champaign, IL: Human Kinetics, 3–17 (2001).

Kreider, R. B., A. L. Almada, J. Antonio, C. Broeder, C. Earnest, M. Greenwood, et al.: ISSN exercise and sport nutrition review: Research and recommendations. *Sports Nutrition Review Journal*. 1:1–44 (2004).

Krustrup, P., Y. Hellsten, & J. Bangsbo: Intense interval training enhances human skeletal muscle oxygen uptake in the initial phase of dynamic exercise at high but not low intensities. *Journal of Physiology*. 559(1):335–345 (2004).

Londeree, B. R.: Effect of training on lactate/ventilatory thresholds: A meta-analysis. *Medicine & Science in Sports & Exercise*. 29(6):837–843 (1997).

Marcinik, E. J., J. Potts, G. Schlabach, S. Will, P. Dawson, & B. F. Hurley: Effects of strength training on lactate threshold and endurance performance. *Medicine and Science in Sports and Exercise*. 23(6):739–743 (1991).

Massicotte, D. R. & R. B. J. MacNab: Cardiorespiratory adaptations to training at specified intensities in children. *Medicine and Science in Sports*. 6(4):242–246 (1974).

Mazzeo, R. S., G. A. Brooks, D. A. Schoeller, & T. F. Budinger: Disposal of blood [$1^{2}13$C] lactate in humans during rest and exercise. *Journal of Applied Physiology*. 60(1):232–241 (1986).

McCafferty, W. B. & S. M. Horvath: Specificity of exercise and specificity of training: A subcellular review. *Research Quarterly*. 48(2):358–371 (1977).

McCann, D. J. & B. K. Higginson: Training to maximize economy of motion in running gait. *Current Sports Medicine Reports*. 7(3):158–162 (2008).

McGinley, C., A. Shafat, & A. E. Donnelly: Does antioxidant vitamin supplementation protect against muscle damage? *Sports Medicine*. 29(12):1011–1032 (2009).

McNicol, A. J., B. J. O'Brien, C. D. Paton, & W. L. Knez: The effects of increased absolute training intensity on adaptations to endurance exercise training. *Journal of Science and Medicine in Sport*. 12(4):485–489 (2009).

Medbø, J. I. & S. Burgers: Effect of training on the anaerobic capacity. *Medicine and Science in Sports and Exercise*. 22(4): 501–507 (1990).

Messonnier, L., H. Freund, C. Denis, L. Féasson, & J. R. Lacour: Effects of training on lactate kinetics parameters and their influence on short high-intensity exercise performance. *International Journal of Sports Medicine*. 27(1):60–66 (2006).

Millet, G. P., B. Jaouen, F. Barrani, & R. Candau: Effects of concurrent endurance and strength training on running economy and $\dot{V}O_2$ kinetics. *Medicine & Science in Sports & Exercise*. 34(8):1351–1359 (2002).

Montgomery, P. G., D. B. Pyne, A. J. Cox, W. G. Hopkins, C. L. Minahan, & P. H. Hunt: Muscle damage, inflammation, and recovery interventions during a 3-day basketball tournament. *European Journal of Sport Science*. 8(5):241–250 (2008).

Mougios, V.: *Exercise Biochemistry*. Champaign, IL: Human Kinetics (2006).

Mujika, I. & S. Padilla: Detraining: Loss of training-induced physiological and performance adaptations. Part I. *Sports Medicine*. 30(2):79–87 (2000a).

Mujika, I. & S. Padilla: Detraining: Loss of training-induced physiological and performance adaptations. Part II. *Sports Medicine*. 30(3):145–154 (2000b).

Mujika, I. & S. Padilla: Cardiorespiratory and metabolic characteristics of detraining in humans. *Medicine & Science in Sports & Exercise*. 33(3):413–421 (2001).

Mujika, I. & S. Padilla: Scientific bases for precompetition tapering strategies. *Medicine & Science in Sports & Exercise*. 35(7): 1182–1187 (2003).

Neufer, P. D.: The effect of detraining and reduced training on the physiological adaptations to aerobic exercise training. *Sports Medicine*. 8(5):302–321 (1989).

Nichols, J. F., D. Robinson, D. Douglass, & J. Anthony: Retraining of a competitive master athlete following traumatic injury: A case study. *Medicine & Science in Sports & Exercise*. 32(6):1037–1042 (2000).

Pendergast, D. R., K. Meksawan, A. Limprasertkul, & N. M. Fisher: Influence of exercise on nutritional requirements. *European Journal of Applied Physiology*. 111(3):379–390 (2011).

Perry, C. G. R., G. J. F. Heigenhauser, A. Bonen, & L. L. Spriet: High-intensity aerobic interval training increases fat and carbohydrate metabolic capacities in human skeletal muscle. *Applied Physiology Nutrition and Metabolism*. 33(6):1112–1123 (2008).

Peternelj, T.-T. & J. S. Coombes: Antioxidant supplementation during exercise testing. *Sports Medicine*. 41(12):1043–1069 (2011).

Pilegaard, H., J. Bango, E. A. Richter, & C. Juel: Lactate transport studied in sarcolemmal giant vesicles from human muscle biopsies: Relation to training status. *Journal of Applied Physiology*. 77(4):1858–1862 (1994).

Patton, J. F. & A. Duggan: An evaluation of tests of anaerobic power. *Aviation and Space Environmental Medicine*. 58: 237–242 (1987).

Ready, A. E. & H. A. Quinney: Alternations in anaerobic threshold as the result of endurance training and detraining. *Medicine in Sports and Exercise*. 14(4):292–296 (1982).

Rennie, D.: Your ultimate 10-K plan. Runner's World online: www.runnersworld.com.article. Accessed October 10, 2007.

Reynolds, T. H., P. A. Frye, & G. A. Sforzo: Resistance training and the blood lactate response to resistance exercise in women. *Journal of Strength and Conditioning Research*. 11(2):77–81 (1997).

Ross, A. & M. Leveritt: Long-term metabolic and skeletal muscle adaptations to short-sprint training: Implications for sprint training and tapering. *Sports Medicine*. 31(15):1063–1082 (2001).

Rotstein, A., R. Dotan, O. Bar-Or, & G. Tenenbaum: Effect of training on anaerobic threshold, maximal aerobic power and anaerobic performance of preadolescent boys. *International Journal of Sports Medicine*. 7(5):281–286 (1986).

Rowland, T. W.: *Exercise and Children's Health*. Champaign, IL: Human Kinetics (1990).

Rowland, T. W.: Aerobic (un)trainability of children: Mitochondrial biogenesis and the "crowded cell" hypothesis. *Pediatric Exercise Science*. 21:1–9 (2009).

Sato, Y., Y. Oshida, I. Ohsawa, et al.: The role of glucose transport in the regulation of glucose utilization by muscle. In Maughan, R. J. & S. M. Shirreffs (eds.): *Biochemistry of Exercise IX*. Champaign, IL: Human Kinetics (1996).

Saunders, P. U., R. D. Telford, D. B. Pyne, E. M. Peltola, R. B. Cunningham, C. J. Gore, & J. A. Hawley: Short-term plyometric training improves running economy in highly trained middle and long distance runners. *Journal of Strength and Conditioning Research*. 20(4):947–954 (2006).

Scharhag-Rosenberger, F., T. Meyer, S. Walitzek, & W. Kindermann: Effects of one year aerobic endurance training on resting metabolic rate and exercise fat oxidation in previously untrained men and women: Metabolic endurance training adaptations. *International Journal of Sports Medicine*. 31(7): 498–504 (2010).

Sedlock, D. A., M.-G. Lee, M. G. Flynn, K.-S. Park, & G. H. Kamimori: Excess postexercise oxygen consumption after aerobic exercise training. *International Journal of Sport Nutrition and Exercise Metabolism*. 20:336–349 (2010).

Seki, Y., J. R. Berggren, J. A. Houmard, & M. J. Charron: Glucose transporter expression in skeletal muscle of endurance-trained individuals. *Medicine & Science in Sport & Exercise*. 38(6):1088–1092 (2006).

Shepard, R. J.: *Physical Activity and Aging*. Chicago, IL: Year Book Medical Publishers (1978).

Shepley, B., J. D. MacDougall, N. Cipriano, J. R. Sutton, G. Coates, & M. Tarnopolsky: Physiological effects of tapering in highly trained athletes. *Journal of Applied Physiology*. 72:706–711 (1992).

Sjödin, B., I. Jacobs, & J. Svedenhag: Changes in onset of blood lactate accumulation (OBLA) and muscle enzymes after training at OBLA. *European Journal of Applied Physiology*. 49:45–57 (1982).

Skinner, J. S. & D. W. Morgan: Aspects of anaerobic performance. In Clarke, D. H., & H. M. Eckert (eds.): *Limits of Human Performance*. Champaign, IL: Human Kinetics, 131–144 (1985).

Slade, J. M., T. A. Miszko, J. H. Laity, S. K. Agrawal, & M. E. Cress: Anaerobic power and physical function in strength-trained and non-strength trained older adults. *Journals of Gerontology Series A: Biological Sciences and Medical Sciences*. 57(3):M168–M172 (2002).

Spurrs, R. W., A. J. Murphy, & M. L. Watsford: The effect of plyometric training on distance running performance. *European Journal of Applied Physiology*. 89(1):1–7 (2003).

Stear, S. J., L. M. Castell, L. M. Burke, N. Jeacocke, B. Ekblom, C. Shing, et al.: A-Z of nutritional supplements: Dietary supplements, sports nutrition foods and ergogenic aids for health and performance—part 10. *British Journal of Sports Medicine*. 44:688–690 (2010).

Stisen, A. B., O. Stougaard, J. Langfort, J. W. Helge, K. Sahlin, & K. Madsen: Maximal fat oxidation rates in endurance trained and untrained women. *European Journal of Applied Physiology*. 98(5):497–506 (2006).

Stoudemire, N. M., L. Wideman, K. A. Pass, C. L. McGinnes, G. A. Gaesser, & A. Weltman: The validity of regulating blood lactate concentration during running by ratings of perceived exertion. *Medicine and Science in Sports and Exercise*. 28(4):49–495 (1996).

Talanian, J. L., S. D. Galloway, G. J. Heigenhauser, A. Bonen, & L. L. Spriet: Two weeks of high-intensity aerobic interval training increases the capacity for fat oxidation during exercise in women. *Journal of Applied Physiology*. 102(4):1439–1447 (2007).

Thomas, C., S. Perrey, K. Lambert, G. Hugon, D. Mornet, & J. Mercier: Monocarboxylate transporters, blood lactate removal after supramaximal exercise, and fatigue indexes in humans. *Journal of Applied Physiology*. 98(3):803–809 (2005).

Tlusty, L.: Physical fitness in old age. II. Anaerobic capacity, anaerobic work in graded exercise, recovery after maximum work performance in elderly individuals. *Respiration*. 26: 287–299 (1969).

Tomaras, E. K. & B. R. MacIntosh: Less is more: Standard warm-up causes fatigue and less warm-up permits greater cycling power. *Journal of Applied Physiology*. 111(1):228–235 (2011).

Turner, A. M., M. Owings, & J. A. Schwane: Improvement in running economy after 6 weeks of plyometric training. *Journal of Strength and Conditioning Research*. 17(1):60–67 (2003).

Wells, C. L.: *Women, Sport and Performance: A Physiological Perspective* (2nd edition). Champaign, IL: Human Kinetics (1991).

Weltman, A.: *The Blood Lactate Response to Exercise*. Champaign, IL: Human Kinetics (1995).

Weltman, A., R. J. Moffatt, & B. A. Stamford: Supramaximal training in females: Effects on anaerobic power output, anaerobic capacity, and aerobic power. *Journal of Sports Medicine and Physical Fitness*. 18(3):237–244 (1978).

Wibom, R., E. Hultman, M. Johansson, K. Matherei, D. Constantin-Teodosiu, & P. G. Schantz: Adaptation of mitochondrial ATP production in human skeletal muscle to endurance training and detraining. *Journal of Applied Physiology*. 73:2004–2010 (1992).

Wilcock, I. M., J. B. Cronin, & W. A. Hing: Physiological response to water immersion: A method for sport recovery? *Sports Medicine*. 36(9):747–765 (2006).

Williams, C. G., C. H. Wyndham, R. Kok, & M. J. E. von Rahden: Effect of training on maximal oxygen intake and on anaerobic metabolism in man. *Internationale Zeitschrift fuer Angewandte Physiologie Einschliesslich Arbeitsphysiologie*. 24:18–23 (1967).

Wilmore, J. H. & D. L. Costill: *Training for Sport and Activity: The Physiological Basis of the Conditioning Process* (3rd edition). Dubuque, IA: Brown (1988).

Yoshida, T., S. Yoshihiro, & N. Takeuchi: Endurance training regimen based upon arterial blood lactate: Effects on anaerobic threshold. *European Journal of Applied Physiology*. 49:223–230 (1982).

Zehsaz, F., M. A. Azarbaijani, N. Farhangimaleki, & P. Tiidus: Effect of tapering period on plasma hormone concentration, mood state, and performance in elite male cyclists. *European Journal of Sport Science*. 11(3):183–190 (2011).

6

Nutrition for Fitness and Athletics

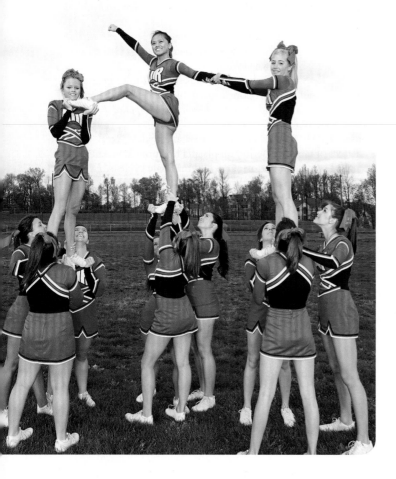

OBJECTIVES

After studying the chapter, you should be able to:

› List the goals for nutrition during training and for nutrition during competition, and explain why they are different.

› Compare a balanced diet for sedentary individuals with a balanced diet for active individuals in terms of caloric intake; carbohydrate, fat, and protein intake; and vitamin, mineral, and fluid requirements.

› Discuss the positive and negative aspects of a high-carbohydrate diet.

› Explain the glycemic index; identify common high-, moderate-, and low-glycemic foods; and explain the best use of each classification. Describe a training situation when fat intake can be too low.

› Compare the theory of carbohydrate loading for endurance athletes to its use for body builders.

› Compare the classic, modified, and short techniques of carbohydrate loading in terms of diet and exercise for endurance event competitors.

› Develop a pre-event meal plan for athletic competition.

› Develop a plan for feeding and drinking during an endurance event, and defend it.

› Judge the value of commercially available sports drinks.

› Differentiate among the eating disorders anorexia nervosa, bulimia nervosa, and anorexia athletica in terms of definitions and characteristics.

› Identify the risk factors for developing an eating disorder.

› Construct guidelines to help prevent or manage eating disorders in exercise settings.

Introduction

Proper nutrition and exercise are natural partners for health, fitness, and athletic performance. Consequently, many fitness enthusiasts pursue healthy diets, and athletes try to optimize their performance by implementing appropriate diets. Although these are very positive trends, they also have the potential to be taken to an extreme, which may simply involve spending money needlessly on "nutritional supplements" or may actually be harmful, as with eating disorders. It is the responsibility of all physical educators, athletic personnel, rehabilitation clinicians, and fitness professionals to understand what constitutes optimal nutrition for fitness and athletics.

Nutrition education should be a part of physical fitness classes, community adult fitness and rehabilitation programs, and athletic training. Most individuals who train regularly want to eat right, but they may confuse advertisements and media hype with factual information.

Optimal nutrition for fitness and athletics must be considered for two different situations. The first is training, and the second competition, whether on the "fun run" fitness or elite competitive level. With the exception of some youth sports, individuals typically spend more total time training than competing, making daily nutritional practices critical. No amount of dietary manipulation the day of or the day before a competition can make up for otherwise poor nutritional habits (Burke and Read, 1989).

Nutrition for Training

Individuals in exercise training need to match their training regimen with an appropriate diet. This often involves consultation with a fitness professional, a complete diet analysis by a nutritionist, and, many times, a trial-and-error approach to find what works best for a given individual.

The goals of an optimal training diet are to:

1. Provide caloric and nutrient requirements
2. Incorporate nutritional practices that promote good health
3. Achieve and maintain optimal body composition and competition weight
4. Promote recovery from training sessions and physiological adaptations
5. Try variations of precompetition and competition fuel and fluid intake to determine the body's responses (Burke and Read, 1989)

There is almost universal agreement that poor nutritional status impairs work performance. There is also considerable, although not universal, agreement that good general nutrition (the balanced diet recommended for just about everyone, as shown in **Table 6.1**) is adequate and probably even optimal for most active individuals as well as sedentary individuals.

TABLE 6.1 Balanced Diets	
For Sedentary Individuals	**For Active Individuals**
Calories Calorie balance of intake and expenditure to maintain acceptable body composition and weight	Adequate caloric intake to balance caloric expenditure of training and competition in excess of normal living while maintaining optimal body composition and playing weight
Protein 5–20% protein (0.95 g·kg^{-1}·d^{-1}), 1–3 yr; 10–30%,(0.85 g·kg^{-1}·d^{-1}), 4–18 yr; 10–35% (0.8 g·kg^{-1}·d^{-1}), adults 19+ yr	10–35% protein (1.2–2 g·kg^{-1}·d^{-1}) adults 19+ yr
Fat 30–40% fat, 1–3 yr; 25–35% 4–18 yr; 20–35%, adults 19+ yr. (<10% saturated; <300 mg cholesterol; trans fats as low as possible) 65 g·2000 kcal^{-1}; 80 g·2500 kcal^{-1} or 0.5–1.5 g·kg^{-1}·d^{-1}	20–35% fat (0.8–1.0 g·kg^{-1})
Carbohydrate 45–65% carbohydrate all ages (130*–300 g·d^{-1}) (4.5 g·kg^{-1}·d^{-1})	58–68% carbohydrate (8–10 g·kg^{-1}·d^{-1})
Vitamins and Minerals DRI/RDA for vitamins and minerals	DRI/RDA for vitamins and minerals
Fluids Total water† 2700–3700 mL·d^{-1}(80–110 fluid oz·d^{-1}) or 2200–3000 mL·d^{-1} (74–100 fluid oz·d^{-1}) drinking water + beverages	Fluids adequate to prevent dehydration: baseline values plus (if needed) 5–7 mL·kg^{-1} (0.2–0.25 fluid oz·kg^{-1}) 4 hr and 3–5 mL·kg^{-1} (0.1–0.2 fluid oz·kg^{-1}) 2 hr prior to exercise; as during exercise, 1.5 L (50 fluid oz) postexercise for each kg of body weight lost

*The RDA value of 130 g·d^{-1} is based on the amount of carbohydrate needed for brain function; the % is based on the role of carbohydrate as an energy source to maintain body weight.

†Total water includes drinking water, water in beverages, and water that is part of food.

Sources: Based on information from American College of Sports Medicine (2007), American College of Sports Medicine et al. (2009), Brotherhood (1984), Dietary Guidelines for Americans (2010), Haymes (1983), Kreider et al. (2010), and Venkatrauman and Pendergast (2002).

Unfortunately, a typical American does not eat the recommended healthy balanced diet. Many people still consume too much fat (37–42% of the daily caloric intake) and too little carbohydrate (43–48%). If the recommended percentages (20–35% fat and 45–65% carbohydrate) from a healthy variety of foods are consumed, the vast majority of youth sport, middle and secondary school, and college athletes, as well as fitness participants of all ages, will not need any modification in their diet. For those athletes or fitness participants training very long, hard, and often competing at an elite level, a few modifications may be beneficial (Allen et al., 1979; American College of Sports Medicine et al., 2009; American Dietetic Association, 1987; Belko, 1987; Brotherhood, 1984; Burke and Read, 1989; Lemon and Nagle, 1981; Nieman, 1990). **Table 6.1** summarizes these recommendations, which are discussed in the following sections.

The United States Department of Agriculture's (USDA) food icon, called MyPlate (**Figure 6.1**), symbolizes healthy nutrition. There are four primary messages to the ChooseMyPlate campaign (ChooseMyPlate.gov):

1. Build a healthy plate that is filled one half with fruits and vegetables and the other half with whole grains and lean protein; add a side of low-fat dairy.

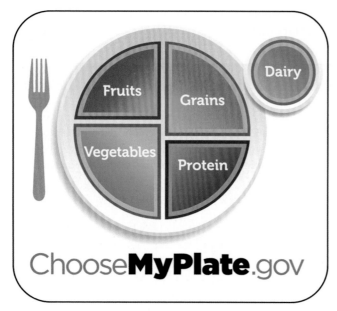

FIGURE 6.1 Food Guide for Sedentary and Active Individuals. This new 2011 plate icon from the U.S. Department of Agriculture emphasizes that one half of your plate should be filled with fruits and vegetables, with whole grains and lean protein on the other half. Low-fat dairy on the side is also suggested. The website MyPlate.gov offers resources for both individuals and professionals teaching others about the concepts based on the *2010 Dietary Guidelines for Americans* to help meet nutrient and caloric needs and make positive eating choices. *Source*: From the U.S. Department of Agriculture website: www.choosemyplate.gov.

2. Cut back on foods high in solid fats, added sugars, and salt (SoFAS).
3. Eat the right amount of calories for you.
4. Be physically active your way.

Individuals are encouraged to go to www.choosemyplate. gov, create a profile, and obtain a daily physical activity target and nutrition plan based on age, sex, height, current weight, and current physical activity. For example, for a 21-year-old female who is 5'8" tall and weighs 145 lb, the food recommendations would be 8 oz of grains, 3 cups of vegetables, 2 cups of fruit, 3 cups of dairy, 6.5 oz. of protein, and 7 tsp of oil. This would leave approximately 330 kcal of empty calories that could be ingested from the limit list of solid fats and added sugars. If this individual were male, the only changes are that he is allotted 9 oz of grains, 3.5 cups of vegetables, 8 tsp of oil, and approximately 362 empty calories. Fruit, dairy, and protein amounts remain the same. Each plan gives examples of what foods count as that category and tips to help make healthy choices. If you have not yet visited this website, it might be an interesting exercise to do. Information for professionals is also included on the website.

Figure 6.2 shows the usual intake in a typical American diet as a percent of goal or limit recommendations and how far typical Americans are from eating the recommended healthy balanced diet. Even more disconcerting are the top five sources of calories among Americans. These are, for 2–18 year olds, grain-based deserts, pizza, soda/energy/sports drinks, yeast breads, and chicken and chicken mixed dishes. For individuals 19+, they are grain-based deserts, yeast breads, chicken and chicken mixed dishes, soda/energy/sports drinks, and alcoholic beverages. Pizza is number six (Dietary Guidelines for Americans, 2010). How does your diet compare? The Focus on Application box provides information on nutrition label information that can be useful in developing a balanced diet.

Kilocalories

The most obvious dietary distinction between active and inactive individuals is the number of calories required per day. Everyone needs sufficient calories to support their daily needs, and children need adequate calories for growth. In addition, an active individual can expend several hundred to several thousand kilocalories more per day than a sedentary individual. The actual amount depends on the individual's size and the intensity, duration, and frequency of the workouts. Large football players doing two-a-day workouts and smaller endurance athletes expend large amounts of energy, but golfers or softball and baseball players of any size expend much smaller amounts (American College of Sports Medicine et al., 2009; American Dietetic Association, 1987; Brotherhood,

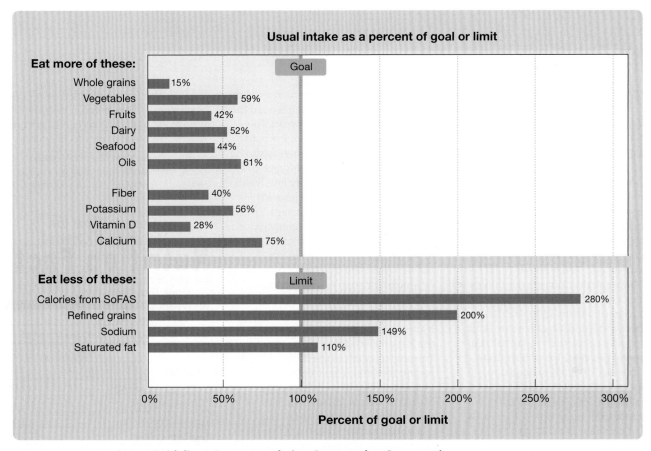

FIGURE 6.2 2010 Dietary Guidelines: Recommendation Compared to Consumption.
The bars show the percentage of key dietary categories in the typical American diet compared with the recommended goal or limit. These vary from a low of 15% for whole grains to a high of 280% from Solid Fat and Added Sugar (SoFAS).
Source: From the U.S. Department of Agriculture website: www.choosemyplate.gov.

1984; Burke and Read, 1989; Kreider et al., 2010; Leaf and Frisa, 1989). Costill (1988) cites figures of 900–2400 kcal·d⁻¹ expended in activity for elite distance runners, 6000 kcal·d⁻¹ for cyclists, and 1250–3750 kcal·d⁻¹ for swimmers during training. These calories must be replaced.

Published reports indicate that male basketball and football players may consume as many as 9000–11,000 kcal·d⁻¹, triathletes 3500–6400 kcal·d⁻¹ (female and male), cross-country skiers 4000–5500 kcal·d⁻¹ (female and male), and track and field athletes (male) 3500–4700 kcal·d⁻¹, depending on the event. It is highly likely that these athletes are adequately resupplying their energy needs (Burke and Read, 1989).

However, competitors in other sports (long-distance running, gymnastics, wrestling, and dance) often attempt to maintain extremely low and, in some cases, "unnatural" body fat and body weight. Intake values as low as 600 kcal·d⁻¹ for male gymnasts and 900 kcal·d⁻¹ for female ballet dancers have been reported. It is likely that these athletes are not adequately resupplying their energy needs (Burke and Read, 1989).

Table 6.2 presents caloric levels based on estimated energy requirements (EER) and activity levels

for males and females from 2 to 76+ years. The EER is the average dietary energy intake that is predicted to maintain energy balance consistent with good health, that is, with a BMI of 18.5–25 kg·m⁻² and a reduced risk of cardiovascular disease. Note that there are separate columns for sedentary, moderately active, and active individuals. Moderate physical activity in this table is defined as activity equivalent to walking 30 minutes or 1.5–3 mi·d⁻¹ at 3–4 mi·hr⁻¹ in addition to daily activities. Active is defined as the equivalent of walking 60 minutes or more than 3 mi·d⁻¹ at 3–4 mi·hr⁻¹ in addition to the light physical activity associated with typical daily life. These caloric values should be sufficient for most individuals engaging in physical activity for health and fitness.

If the relative proportion of nutrients obtained from a healthy diet remained the same as the calories are increased to support training, the active individual would have an acceptable diet. However, some subtle shifting of percentages and/or amounts can be of benefit in certain situations. Chief among them is an increased percentage of carbohydrate ingestion for endurance athletes.

FOCUS ON APPLICATION

Food Label Interpretation

The dietary recommendations presented in **Table 6.1** are expressed as percentages and $g \cdot kg^{-1} \cdot d^{-1}$. Information about both of these measures can be obtained from reading the "Nutrition Facts" label found on most foods. Content of these labels is regulated by the U.S. Food and Drug Administration (FDA).

Serving size is expressed in familiar units such as cups, containers, or pieces and grams. For the accompanying macaroni and cheese label, the serving size is one cup, which equals 228 g and 250 (kilo) calories. Individual nutrients are also given in grams. One cup of macaroni and cheese contains 12 g of fat, 31 g of carbohydrate, and 5 g of protein. Fat is not usually calculated in $g \cdot kg^{-1} \cdot d^{-1}$, but to obtain this value for carbohydrate and protein, all that is needed is to divide by body weight in kilograms. For example, for a 154 lb (70 kg) individual, this represents $0.44 \ g \cdot kg^{-1} \cdot d^{-1}$ of carbohydrate and $0.07 \ g \cdot kg^{-1} \cdot d^{-1}$ of protein. Obviously, this does not satisfy the daily recommendations, but it does illustrate how these values can be obtained. All that is needed would be to total the carbohydrate and protein intake for all the food ingested during the day and divide it by body weight. Thus, if this individual ate 310 g of carbohydrate during the day, it would result in $4.43 \ g \cdot kg^{-1} \cdot d^{-1}$, very close to the recommended $4.5 \ g \cdot kg^{-1} \cdot d^{-1}$.

The % daily value (%DV) column is based on a 2000-kcal diet and shows what percentage of the daily recommendation is achieved by eating one cup of macaroni and cheese. The fat content represents 18% DV and carbohydrate 10% DV. A %DV for protein is not required by the FDA unless a claim is made such as "high in protein" or the product is intended for children under the age of 4 years. This is because protein intake is not a public health concern. Note that there is also no %DV for *trans* fat because this type of fat should be kept as low as possible. Foods that are "low" in a nutrient generally contain ≤ 5% DV; foods that are a "good" source of a nutrient generally contain 10–19%DV; foods that are a "high/rich/excellent" source of a nutrient generally contain ≥20%DV.

The information in a food label is based in large part on the Dietary Reference Intakes (DRIs) established by the Food and Nutrition Board of the National Academy of Sciences. The primary goals of the basic recommendations are to prevent nutrient deficiencies and to reduce the risk of chronic diseases such as cardiovascular disease, cancer, and osteoporosis. The two DRI reference values used in this text are:

1. **Recommended Daily Allowance (RDA)**—the average daily intake level that is sufficient to meet the nutrient requirement of 97–98% of healthy individuals by age and sex

2. **Adequate Intake (AI)**—used when an RDA cannot be determined. The AI is based on observation or is experimentally determined and is an estimate of intake by healthy individuals.

Most vitamin and mineral percentages presented in food labels are based on DRI/RDA values. In the label presented, one serving of macaroni and cheese supplies 4% of the RDA of vitamin A, 2% of vitamin C, 20% of calcium, and 4% of iron. Obviously, if one were to eat both servings in this container, all of the nutrient values would double.

Sources: Dietary Guidelines for Americans (2010), International Food Information Council (2002), U.S. Food and Drug Administration (2004).

Sample label for Macaroni & Cheese

Nutrition Facts

Serving Size 1 cup (228g)
Servings Per Container 2

Amount Per Serving

Calories 250   Calories from Fat 110

	% Daily Value*
Total Fat 12g	**18%**
Saturated Fat 3g	**15%**
Trans Fat 3g	
Cholesterol 30mg	**10%**
Sodium 470mg	**20%**
Total Carbohydrate 31g	**10%**
Dietary Fiber 0g	**0%**
Sugars 5g	
Protein 5g	

Vitamin A	**4%**
Vitamin C	**2%**
Calcium	**20%**
Iron	**4%**

* Percent Daily Values are based on a 2,000 calorie diet. Your Daily Values may be higher or lower depending on your calorie needs.

		Calories:	2,000	2,500
Total Fat	Less than		65g	80g
Sat Fat	Less than		20g	25g
Cholesterol	Less than		300mg	300mg
Sodium	Less than		2,400mg	2,400mg
Total Carbohydrate			300g	375g
Dietary Fiber			25g	30g

Carbohydrates

The discussion of carbohydrate metabolism in Chapter 2 pointed out several important facts about carbohydrates as a fuel for exercise (American College of Sports Medicine et al., 2009; American Dietetic Association, 1987; Burke and Read, 1989; Costill, 1988; Nieman, 1990):

1. The higher the intensity of exercise (whether continuous or intermittent; aerobic, anaerobic, or aerobic-anaerobic), the more important glycogen is as a fuel.

2. The body can only store limited amounts of carbohydrates. Training increases the ability to store carbohydrate and to spare carbohydrate. However, 60–90 minutes of heavy endurance work seriously depletes glycogen stores, and depletion can be

TABLE 6.2   Estimated Calorie Needs per Day by Age, Sex, and Physical Activity Level

Males	Activity level			Females	Activity level		
Age	Sedentary*	Mod. Active*	Active*	Age	Sedentary*	Mod. Active*	Active*
2	1000	1000	1000	2	1000	1000	1000
3	1200	1400	1400	3	1000	1200	1400
4	1200	1400	1600	4	1200	1400	1400
5	1200	1400	1600	5	1200	1400	1600
6	1400	1600	1800	6	1200	1400	1600
7	1400	1600	1800	7	1200	1600	1800
8	1400	1600	2000	8	1400	1600	1800
9	1600	1800	2000	9	1400	1600	1800
10	1600	1800	2200	10	1400	1800	2000
11	1800	2000	2200	11	1600	1800	2000
12	1800	2200	2400	12	1600	2000	2200
13	2000	2200	2600	13	1600	2000	2200
14	2000	2400	2800	14	1800	2000	2400
15	2200	2600	3000	15	1800	2000	2400
16	2400	2800	3200	16	1800	2000	2400
17	2400	2800	3200	17	1800	2000	2400
18	2400	2800	3200	18	1800	2000	2400
19–20	2600	2800	3000	19–20	2000	2200	2400
21–25	2400	2800	3000	21–25	2000	2200	2400
26–30	2400	2600	3000	26–30	1800	2000	2400
31–35	2400	2600	3000	31–35	1800	2000	2200
36–40	2400	2600	2800	36–40	1800	2000	2200
41–45	2200	2600	2800	41–45	1800	2000	2200
46–50	2200	2400	2800	46–50	1800	2000	2200
51–55	2200	2400	2800	51–55	1600	1800	2200
56–60	2200	2400	2600	56–60	1600	1800	2200
61–65	2000	2400	2600	61–65	1600	1800	2000
66–70	2000	2200	2600	66–70	1600	1800	2000
71–75	2000	2200	2600	71–75	1600	1800	2000
76 and up	2000	2200	2400	76 and up	1600	1800	2000

*Calorie levels are based on the Estimated Energy Requirements using reference weights for age and sex and activity levels from the Institute of Medicine Dietary Reference Intakes Macronutrients Report, 2002.

Sedentary = only the light physical activity associated with typical day-to-day life.

Moderately Active = equivalent to walking 1.5–3 mi·d^{-1} at 3–4 mi·hr^{-1} in addition to daily activities.

Active = equivalent to walking more than 3 mi·d^{-1} at 3–4 mi·hr^{-1} in addition to daily activities.

Source: U.S. Department of Agriculture Dietary Guidelines for Americans (2010).

complete in 120 minutes. Muscle glycogen can also be depleted by 15–30 minutes of near-maximal– or supramaximal-intensity interval work.

Recommended Daily Allowance (RDA) The average daily intake level that is sufficient to meet the nutrient requirement of 97–98% of healthy individuals by age and sex.

Adequate Intake (AI) Used when an RDA cannot be determined. The AI is an estimate of intake by healthy individuals.

3. Fat metabolism is linked to carbohydrate metabolism. Fatigue, "hitting the wall," and exhaustion are related to glycogen depletion during high-intensity, long-duration activity. Thus, having an adequate supply of muscle glycogen is necessary to avoid fatigue. Whatever glycogen is utilized, in training or competition, must be replenished before more heavy work can be done.

How much carbohydrate should be included in the diet to accomplish these goals? The RDA of carbohydrate (**Table 6.1**) for the average sedentary individual is

4.5 g·kg^{-1}·d^{-1}. For an individual utilizing high amounts of carbohydrate in training, 8–10 g·kg^{-1}·d^{-1} is recommended. In some cases, this may increase the percentage of carbohydrate to 58–68% of the dietary intake.

Which carbohydrates should be eaten? All carbohydrates are not the same, and the traditional classification of CHO into "simple" or "complex" carbohydrates according to chemical structure is not useful in terms of

TABLE 6.3   Glycemic Index of Selected Foods

High-Glycemic Food (HGI) (85 or Greater)	Moderate-Glycemic Food (MGI) (60–85)	Low-Glycemic Food (LGI) (Under 60)
Sugars, Syrups, and Jellies		
White table sugar		Fructose
Maple syrup		M&M peanuts
Honey		Nutella
Sports drinks (6–20% CHO concentration)		
Cereal Products		
Bagel	Rice	Barley
Bread (white and wheat)	Pasta (spaghetti and macaroni)	All-Bran cereal
Cornflakes/Cheerios	Bread (whole grain and rye)	Wheat tortilla
Shredded wheat	Corn tortilla	9 grain bread
Crackers	Oatmeal (cooked)	Brown rice
Puffed wheat and rice	Pita bread	
Fruits		
Raisins	Grapes	Apples/apple juice
Watermelons	Orange juice	Cherries
Cranberry juice	Bananas	Dried apricots
	Kiwi	Peaches
	Mangos	Pears
		Plums/prunes
		Grapefruits
		Strawberries
Vegetables		
Potatoes (baked, microwaved, mashed, and French fried)	Yams/sweet potatoes	Tomato soup/juice
Carrots	Sweet corn (frozen)	
Parsnips	Potato chips	
Sweet corn (fresh)	Peas	
	Popcorn	
Legumes		
	Baked beans	Beans (butter, green), chickpeas kidney, navy, and pinto (dried)
	Beans (kidney and pinto, canned)	Lentils (green and red, dried)
	Peas (chick and green, canned or frozen)	Peanuts/cashews
	Lentils (red and green, canned)	Hummus
Dairy Products		
Ice cream	Ice cream (low fat)	Milk (skim, whole) and Yogurt Custard
Convenience Foods		
Kraft macaroni and cheese	Snickers bar	Fish fingers
Angel food cake	Chicken nuggets	Pizza Hut Supreme
	Peanut butter sandwich	Ironman bar (chocolate)
	Ensure	
	Instant noodles	
	Power Bar (chocolate)	

Sources: Compiled from Coyle and Coyle (1993), Foster-Powell et al. (2002), Jenkins et al. (1981), Singh et al. (1994), Wolever (1990), and Walton and Rhodes (1997).

the "healthfulness" and impact on glucose and insulin levels. To solve this dilemma, the concept of the glycemic index is used.

Glycemic Index

The **glycemic index (GI)** categorizes foods based on the glucose response they produce, using a numerical value for comparing foods. The GI compares the elevation in blood glucose caused by the ingestion of 50 g of any carbohydrate food with the elevation caused by 50 g of white bread or glucose (dextrose) (Foster-Powell et al., 2002; Wolever, 1990; Wong and Chung, 2003). Thus, the GI value of any given food depends on the speed at which it is digested and absorbed compared with a reference food. When white bread is used as the reference carbohydrate, it has a GI of 100. High-glycemic foods have a rating of 85 or greater, moderate-glycemic foods rate from 60 to 85, and low-glycemic foods have a rating less than 60. Values above 100 are possible; for example, glucose has a value of 143 compared to white bread. When glucose is used as the reference food, the values of all other foods are lower than when white bread is the reference. When referring to tables of GI, it is important to note whether white bread or glucose is the reference value. All the values in **Table 6.3** use white bread as the reference food.

Foods with a high GI (HGI) cause a fast elevation in glucose and subsequently in insulin; foods with lower indices cause a slower rise in both glucose and insulin. **Table 6.3** gives examples of high-, moderate-, and low-glycemic foods. In general, sugars and sports drinks, syrups and jellies, and grain, pasta, and cereal products have high or moderate glycemic indices (MGI). Most fruits, legumes, and dairy products have low glycemic indices (LGI). Meat, poultry, fish, avocados, salad vegetables, cheese, and eggs do not have GI values because these foods contain little or no carbohydrate and when eaten alone do not usually cause a meaningful increase in blood glucose. A food's GI value also depends on where it is grown, its variety (with foods such as rice), and how it is processed (Foster-Powell et al., 2002).

In addition to the GI of specific foods, how an individual's body responds to CHO ingestion depends also, in part, on the person's fitness level (Manore, 2002). **Figure 6.3** shows the typical response pattern of a sedentary individual, a moderately active individual, and a trained endurance runner. In general, trained individuals have a lower glycemic (and hence lower insulin) response to food than untrained individuals.

The GI compares food containing the same amount of CHO. It does not take into account the serving size. To do

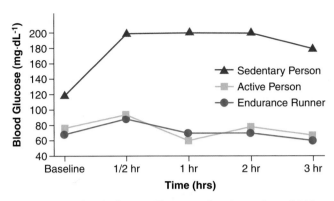

FIGURE 6.3 Blood Glucose Changes after Ingestion of 100 g of Glucose in Sedentary, Active, and Endurance-Trained Individuals.
Source: Manore, M. M.: Carbohydrate: Friend or Foe? Part II: Dietary carbohydrate and changes in blood glucose. *ACSM's Health and Fitness Journal.* 6(3):26–29 (2002). Reprinted with permission.

this, the glycemic load (GL) must be calculated. The GL is the product of the amount of available carbohydrate (g) and the GI divided by 100 (Manore et al., 2004; Wong and Chung, 2003). Thus, eating a large portion of any food produces a higher GL than a small portion. The higher the GL is, the greater the elevation in blood glucose and insulin. The premise of GL is that the effect, if any, on exercise performance is determined by the overall glycemic effect of a diet and not by the amount of CHO alone (O'Reilly et al., 2010). The following section will concentrate on glycogen replenishment, called resynthesis, because of the importance of adequate glycogen levels to training.

CHECK YOUR COMPREHENSION

Rank these CHO foods (normal serving of each) from low to high on the basis of Glycemic Load (GL)

Food	Glycemic Index (GI)	CHO (g)
Bagel	103	35
Snickers Bar	59	35
Banana	79	32
Gatorade	111	15
Pizza (supreme)	52	72
Power Bar (chocolate)	83	47

How does the calculation of the GL affect the impact of the GI of foods? Support your answer.
Check your answer in Appendix C.

Glycemic Index (GI) A measure that compares the elevation in blood glucose caused by the ingestion of 50 g of any carbohydrate food with the elevation caused by the ingestion of 50 g of white bread or glucose.

Glycogen Resynthesis

The storage of carbohydrate in liver and muscles depends primarily on the severity of glycogen depletion resulting from activity, the extent of muscle trauma, and the amount of dietary carbohydrate. Muscle glycogen resynthesis is fastest when the muscle has been depleted, but not necessarily exhausted, and the diet is high in carbohydrate. Muscle fiber damage associated with exhaustive eccentric exercise (in which a contracting muscle is forcibly lengthened), such as running marathon distances especially if downhill running is involved, may delay resynthesis for as long as 7–10 days despite elevated dietary carbohydrate (Burke and Read, 1989; Costill, 1988).

Given optimal amounts of dietary carbohydrate, muscle glycogen resynthesis is faster (per muscle mass per hour) after short-term, high-intensity exercise than after long-term, submaximal endurance exercise. Rates of muscle glycogen resynthesis following dynamic resistance exercise are slower than after short-term, high-intensity exercise but may be less than, equal to, or slightly faster than resynthesis following prolonged endurance exercise. The rate at which glycogen resynthesis occurs largely depends on the blood lactate concentration (higher levels result in faster rates of synthesis) and eccentric loading (higher levels result in slower rates of resynthesis) (Pascoe and Gladden, 1996).

Glycogen resynthesis occurs at about 5–6% per hour under optimal dietary conditions, thus requiring approximately 17–20 hours for complete recovery (Coyle, 1991; Coyle and Coyle, 1993). Optimal conditions involve both the timing and the type of CHO ingestion. Glycogen resynthesis postexercise occurs in two physiological phases: early (<4 hours), which appears to be noninsulin dependent, and late (>4 hours), which shows a period of enhanced insulin sensitivity. Consuming CHO immediately after exercise results in higher glycogen levels 4 hours after exercise than if CHO ingestion is delayed 2 hours. Thus, when the interval between exercise sessions is short (<8 hours), carbohydrate ingestion (50–100 g at the rate of 1.2 $g \cdot kg \cdot BW^{-1} \cdot hr^{-1}$) should begin as soon after the workout or competition as is practical (15–30 minutes), continue at that rate every 15–60 minutes until a larger meal of solid food (150–250 g of carbohydrate) is desired and possible, and be maintained for at least 4–6 hours (Betts and Williams, 2010; Coyle and Coyle, 1993; Jentjens and Jeukendrup, 2003). However, when a longer recovery time is available, the consumption of CHO immediately is not as important. As long as 7–10 $g \cdot kg \cdot BW^{-1}$ of CHO is consumed over 24 hours at a rate of at least 50 $g \cdot hr^{-1}$ muscle and liver glycogen will be replaced over this time (Donaldson et al., 2010). There may be a ceiling effect of 500–600 g of CHO consumed in a day, above which no further resynthesis occurs (Millard-Stafford et al., 2008).

Selection of the type of postexercise CHO should be based on the time available for replenishment and GI of the food (Coyle, 1991; Coyle and Coyle, 1993; Donaldson et al., 2010; Manore et al., 2004; Singh et al., 1994; Wong and Chung, 2003). In general, this means high-glycemic foods should be ingested immediately after exercise, high-glycemic CHO and a mixed balanced meal when solid food is ingested, and high-glycemic foods during recovery (Manore et al., 2004) when time is relatively short. Moderate-glycemic foods may also be useful, however, because they appear to promote glycogen resynthesis just about as effectively (Coyle and Coyle, 1993). The CHO consumed during the immediate postexercise period might not be as important as simply ingesting a sufficient amount of CHO when a full 24 hours of recovery is possible. Ingestion of glucose and sucrose results in a faster replenishment than ingestion of fructose, primarily because glucose and sucrose promote muscle glycogen resynthesis, whereas fructose promotes liver glycogen resynthesis. A combination of glucose and fructose can be an effective combination for the resynthesis of both muscle and liver glycogen. The optimal combination for liver glycogen resynthesis, however, may be maltodextrin drinks with added fructose or galactose. These have been shown to be twice as effective as maltodextrin plus glucose drinks in restoring liver glycogen during short-term postexercise recovery (DéCombaz et al., 2011). Fructose alone is not recommended because it must first be converted to glucose in the liver before muscles can store it as glycogen (Betts and Williams, 2010; Blom et al., 1987; Costill, 1988; Coyle, 1991; Poole et al., 2010). This conversion delays the process of replenishing muscle glycogen stores.

The addition of amino acids and/or protein to a carbohydrate supplement can potentially increase muscle glycogen synthesis because of an enhanced insulin response. Insulin stimulates both glucose uptake and activation of glycogen synthase—the rate-limiting enzyme for glycogen synthesis. When carbohydrate is ingested at the rate of ≥1.2 $g \cdot kg^{-1} \cdot hr^{-1}$ at regular intervals, however, higher insulin concentrations do not further increase the rate of muscle glycogen resynthesis. Conversely, when carbohydrate intake is insufficient (<1.2 $g \cdot kg^{-1} \cdot hr^{-1}$), the addition of amino acids and/or protein can be beneficial. It may not always be possible for an athlete to consume this much CHO, or the athlete may simply prefer a moderate CHO intake (0.8 $g \cdot kg^{-1} \cdot hr^{-1}$) in combination with amino acids or protein at the rate of ≥0.3 $g \cdot kg^{-1} \cdot hr^{-1}$. This should result in the same amount of glycogen resynthesis as the high CHO alone. The combination may have an additional advantage of stimulating postexercise protein anabolism, thus stimulating tissue growth and repair. Thus, the combination of CHO and protein may be particularly beneficial after heavy resistance training (Betts and Williams, 2010; Donaldson, et al., 2010; Jentjens and Jeukendrup, 2003; Manninen, 2006; O'Reilly et al., 2010; Poole et al., 2010).

Interestingly, chocolate milk has been shown to be beneficial as a recovery beverage. Cow's milk provides all the essential amino acids and the CHO content of fat-free chocolate milk exceeds that of white milk. One study compared endurance capacity after a glycogen depletion trial and a 4-hour recovery period during which the participants ingested either chocolate milk (CM), a fluid replacement drink (Gatorade), or a CHO replacement drink (Endurox R4). All three beverages had similar amounts of CHO. The CM and CHO replacement drink had similar amounts of PRO and total kcal. Participants cycled 51% longer after ingesting CM than the CHO replacement alone and 43% longer after ingesting CM than fluid replacement alone (Thomas et al., 2009). Another study compared the effects of fat-free chocolate milk with an equal caloric CHO drink. The milk contained 16 g of protein and the CHO drink had none. The milk was as effective as the CHO drink at maintaining muscle glycogen during recovery and for performance in a subsequent exercise bout. In addition, milk ingested during recovery significantly increased skeletal muscle protein synthesis, decreased whole-body protein breakdown, and suppressed or maintained molecular activity of protein breakdown during the recovery period. These results suggest that chocolate milk supports both skeletal muscle and whole-body protein recovery as well as glycogen resynthesis (Lunn et al., 2012).

Fox et al. (2004) studied the impact of fat calories added to meals after exercise on glycogen resynthesis and glucose tolerance. Seven males performed two trials of cycling for 90 minutes at 66% VO_2peak followed by five high-intensity intervals. Three postexercise meals consisted of either low-fat (5% energy from fat) or high-fat (45% energy from fat) foods with equal protein and carbohydrate. The day after the exercise, intramuscular triglyceride concentration was approximately 20% more during the high-fat trial. However, glucose tolerance and muscle glycogen concentration were identical in both trials. It therefore appears that as long as the meals ingested in the hours after exercise contain the same amount of carbohydrate, the addition of fat does not hinder muscle glycogen resynthesis.

If carbohydrates are not replenished between training bouts, local muscle fatigue will occur, and work output during succeeding training sessions will decline (Costill, 1988; Coyle, 1991). Severe depletion followed by a nonoptimal diet will require more than 1 day of rest, which is one reason to alternate body parts and hard-easy exercise days.

Although most individuals would benefit from increasing their percentage of carbohydrate ingested, levels as high as 58–68% are recommended only for athletes or fitness participants who are actually using high amounts of carbohydrate in their training regimens. Such individuals include long-distance runners, swimmers, cyclists, and soccer, hockey, or lacrosse players (Costill, 1988; Coyle, 1991).

Ingesting 70% carbohydrates has little advantage and possibly some risk, for nonendurance athletes such as golfers, softball or baseball players, fitness walkers, or sedentary individuals, especially if much of this food has a high glycemic index and the diet has a high glycemic load (high GL). As mentioned earlier, a high GL can result in temporary hyperglycemia and an increased insulin response.

Because glycogen storage is limited in sedentary and non–endurance-trained individuals, the glycolytic pathway is overloaded. The result is a greater-than-normal reliance on a side pathway that converts the glucose to free fatty acids (and then triglycerides) and cholesterol (Costill, 1988; Newsholme and Leech, 1983). Absorption of the same amount of low-glycemic carbohydrates results in a smaller blood glucose and insulin rise and thus less lipid formation. High blood levels of triglycerides and more specifically cholesterol are frequently associated with an increased risk of cardiovascular disease. The long-term consumption of a diet with a relatively high GL (adjusted for total energy) is associated with increased risk of type 2 diabetes, cardiovascular disease, breast and colon cancer, and obesity (Foster-Powell et al., 2002).

Endurance-trained individuals demonstrate less hyperglycemia and a lower insulin response to a given glucose load than untrained individuals. Endurance-trained individuals thus appear to convert high dietary levels of carbohydrate, especially high-glycemic foods, into glycogen storage without an elevation of blood lipids. Carbohydrate should be the highest percentage energy substrate for everyone, but an additional 10–20% above the normal 55–58% is not recommended for sedentary individuals or low-intensity nonendurance athletes (Costill, 1988).

Three categories of carbohydrate sources have been developed that are specifically marketed for active individuals and athletes: sports drinks, sports bars, and sports gels.

Sports Drinks

Liquid carbohydrate sources are as effective as solid carbohydrate sources. In fact, liquids may be even more useful, because many individuals are not hungry after an intense bout of exercise but are willing to drink liquid, and fluid replacement is also important (Betts and Williams, 2010; Costill, 1988; Coyle, 1991; Jentjens and Jeukendrup, 2003). **Table 6.4** compares several currently available commercial sports drinks containing carbohydrates. Several drinks also include protein. Note that the drinks have been categorized as fluid/electrolyte replacement drinks, fluid/fuel replacement drinks, and recovery/replenishment drinks. Water is included for comparison. Many more with different formula are available. Note also that sports drinks are not the same as "energy drinks," which are marketed for their mental stimulatory effects and sudden "bursts" of energy. Energy drinks typically contain caffeine and herbal ingredients and may or may not be safe or useful for active individuals (Duchan et al., 2010). Although some sports drinks contain low amounts of the stimulant caffeine, they are designed to maximize fluid absorption and support performance or recovery by delivering water, electrolytes, carbohydrate, and in some cases protein. Sports drinks with appropriate amounts of carbohydrate and electrolytes (especially sodium

TABLE 6.4 Composition of Selected Sports Drinks (per 8 oz or 240 mL)

Name	Type of CHO*	Energy (kcal)	CHO (g)	CHO† Concentration (%)	Na (mg)	K (mg)	Other
Fluid/Electrolyte Replacement Drinks							
Water		0	0	0	Low	Low	Depends on source
Gatorade G Series Fit O$_2$	S	10	2	1	110	30	
Propel Zero		0	0	0	77	0	Vitamin C and E; niacin; B$_6$; pantothenic acid
Fluid/Fuel Drinks							
Accelerade	S, F, GP	80	14	6	125	45	Ca, vitamin E and C; protein; and fat
All Sport	F	60	16	7	55	60	Vitamin C
Clif Shot Electrolyte	Brown rice syrup and cane juice	80	19	8	200	50	Ca, Mg, vitamins A and C
Gatorade Performance	S, G	50	14	6	110	30	Cl
GU Electrolyte Brew	GP, F	50	13	5	125	20	Citric acid
Hydra Fuel	GP, G, F	66	17	7	25	50	Vitamin C, Mg, Cr
Powerade	F, GP	50	14	6	100	25	Vitamin B$_3$, B$_6$, and B$_{12}$ and Mg
Recovery/Replenishment Drinks							
Boost Original	G, F	240	41	17	150	580	Fat, protein, 25 vitamins and minerals
Gatorade Recover 03	S, G	60	7	3	120	45	Protein (8 g; 3%), Ca
GU Recovery Brew	GP, F	125	26	11	80	70	Protein (4 g; 2%), vitamins A, C, and E; Ca; and Mg
Power Bar Ironman Restore	GP, F, G	90	20	8	250	10	Protein (3 g; 1%), Ca, Fe

*F, fructose; G, glucose; GP, glucose polymer; S, sucrose.

†% concentration = [CHO (g)] ÷ [volume (mL)] × 100, rounded to nearest whole percentage.

Note: Some values may vary slightly based on flavors.

Source: Manufacturer's websites and product labels.

and potassium) aid in the maintenance of homeostasis, prevent injuries, delay fatigue, and optimize performance (Coombes and Hamiton, 2000; von Duvillard et al., 2008). Those manufactured by reputable companies have generally been tested and found to be both safe and effective (Seebohar, 2007). Carbohydrate may be in the form of glucose or glucose polymer (maltodextrin), fructose, or sucrose (glucose + fructose), either alone or in combination. The concentration (%) of carbohydrate in these selected sports drinks varies from less than 1 to 17% in the different categories of drink. In general, a CHO concentration of less than 4% is the most useful for workouts lasting less than an hour and in situations where hydration, not substrate availability, is the primary concern. Carbohydrate concentrations of 6–8% are optimum for use during workouts longer than 60 minutes when both fluid and fuel need to be supplied. CHO con-

centrations greater than 8% are best for recovery situations when glycogen replenishment is the primary goal. The key to selecting a sports drink is to find one that tastes good to the individual and is well tolerated.

Sports Bars

Table 6.5 provides the macronutrient breakdown for selected sports bars and a Snickers candy bar for comparison purposes. Sports bars (**Figure 6.4**) provide readily available carbohydrate and fall into two generic categories: high carbohydrate (>60% of total calories) with minimal fat and protein and minimal to moderate carbohydrate (20–55% of total calories) with balanced fat and protein (~22–40% of each) (Applegate, 1998; Manore, 2000). High-carbohydrate bars are suitable for ingestion before, during, and after exercise. CHO in

decreased hemoglobin and red blood cell concentrations. Research supports that blood volume changes do occur. However, the two phenomena, increased dilution and protein degradation, are not mutually exclusive. Furthermore, research evidence suggests that experienced and not just novice endurance athletes may also suffer sports anemia (American Dietetic Association, 1987; Haymes, 1983; Lemon, 1989b; Tarnopolsky et al., 1988).

In addition, high-intensity, long-duration training and competition result in increased amino acid oxidation as fuel, ranging from 5 to 15% of the total calories used, especially if the individual is depleted of carbohydrates (Brotherhood, 1984; Gleeson, 2005). Cool-temperature training (5–20°C or 40–68°F) also utilizes more protein than warm-weather (30°C, or 86°F) training. Females utilize more protein during exercise in the midluteal phase of the menstrual cycle (~ days 14–21) than during the follicular phase (~ days 1–7) (Phillips, 1999).

Finally, skeletal muscle protein turnover increases at rest in healthy adults undergoing an aerobic exercise training program. In contrast to resistance training, a more negative net muscle protein balance (synthesis breakdown) has been shown with endurance training. In addition, plasma amino acid concentration decreases suggesting that 0.85 g·kg^{-1}·d^{-1} is insufficient to optimize muscle protein despite adequate caloric energy intake (Pikosky et al., 2006). Protein availability is critical for maximizing muscle adaptations in response to aerobic endurance training, including increasing synthesis in relation to breakdown, so that the net muscle protein balance is positive, favoring synthesis (Hawley et al., 2006).

For these reasons, a small increase in the intake of dietary protein to 1.2–1.4 g·kg^{-1}·d^{-1} is recommended for high-intensity, long-duration aerobic endurance training (American College of Sports Medicine, 2009). Individuals training at less than 50% $\dot{V}O_2$ max for 20–60 min·d^{-1} do not need to increase their protein intake above the RDA. This increased amount of protein per kilogram of body weight, for high-intensity, long-duration aerobic endurance training, can be achieved without increasing the percentage above the recommended 10–35% of the total calories ingested (Lemon, 1989a; Paul, 1989). Consider, for example, a 56-kg (123-lb) female triathlete. If her caloric intake goes from 1500 kcal·d^{-1} (12% protein) when sedentary to 2250 kcal·d^{-1} during heavy training and if she maintains 12% protein ingestion, her increased caloric consumption now provides her with 1.2 g·kg^{-1} instead of 0.8 g·kg^{-1} of protein. At 15% of her increased calories, 1.5 g·kg^{-1} of protein would be provided daily. The key point is that the total caloric intake must be increased. If the total energy intake is insufficient, then the percentage allotted to protein may be inadequate. For example, if the athlete increased her caloric intake to only 1875 kcal·d^{-1} at 12% protein intake, this increase would amount to only 1 g·kg^{-1}·d^{-1}. Also, if the athlete increased her carbohydrate intake to 70%, she would need to carefully select the remaining 30% of her foodstuffs to get an adequate protein intake.

The problem of ingesting too few calories and thus inadequate protein is especially evident when athletes are concerned with percentage of body fat or making weight in a sport with weight categories. The problem is compounded in children and adolescents. As previously mentioned, individuals at this age need more protein than adults. Inadequate protein intake at this age might adversely affect not only exercise performance but also growth (Lemon, 1991; Steen, 1994). Of course, if the extra protein ingested is also excess calories, body weight and fat will increase, and that also is not usually desirable. For older adults, inadequate nutrition and inadequate protein intake can also be a problem. In addition, the current RDA of 0.8 g·kg^{-1}·d^{-1} seems insufficient to meet the protein needs of most elderly. Endurance training increases the requirement for dietary protein in older adults, but dynamic resistance training has been shown to lower the dietary protein need. However, research has also shown that increasing dietary protein intake up to double the RDA can enhance the hypertrophic response and strength gains of resistance training in older adults (Evans, 2004).

Before the dietary protein is increased, the individual should undergo a complete dietary nutritional analysis under the guidance of a trained nutritionist. It should not be assumed that because an individual is a strength or endurance athlete, he or she needs additional dietary protein or a protein supplement (American College of Sports Medicine, 2009; Lemon, 1991). Ideally the additional protein would be obtained from whole foods. When this is not possible and supplements are ingested, it is recommended that the protein contain both whey and casein components due to their high digestibility, amino acid content, and ability to increase muscle protein. Whey protein elicits a sharp, rapid increase of plasma amino acids following ingestion. Casein protein elicits a moderate, prolonged increase in plasma amino acids that is sustained for hours (Campbell et al., 2007).

Can too much protein in the diet be harmful to a fitness participant or competitive athlete? Although concern has been expressed that excessive protein intake (>3 g·kg^{-1}·d^{-1}) may have negative effects including increased blood lipid levels, kidney damage, and dehydration (Gleeson, 2005), there is no substantive evidence that protein intakes in the suggested ranges for active individuals will have adverse effects in healthy, exercising individuals (Campbell et al., 2007). In individuals with preexisting liver or kidney abnormalities, a high-protein diet can lead to further deterioration of the function (American Dietetic Association, 1987; Campbell et al., 2007; Lemon, 1989b).

Sports Anemia A transient decrease in red blood cells and hemoglobin level (grams per deciliter of blood).

The metabolism of protein requires more water than the metabolism of carbohydrate or fat. Increased excretion of nitrogen in urine increases urinary volume and the risk for dehydration. Therefore, water intake should be increased to avoid dehydration if protein intake is increased.

There is also some concern regarding the impact of high-protein intake on calcium loss. Early studies reported evidence in sedentary individuals that increasing the dietary protein leads to increased calcium excretion, suggesting a loss in bone calcium (Allen et al., 1979; Campbell et al., 2011; Eisenstein et al., 2002; Lemon and Nagle, 1981). It is now known that the phosphate content of protein food and supplements fortified with calcium and phosphorous negates this effect. Data from isotope studies suggest that the main source of the increase in urinary calcium from a high-protein diet is intestinal (dietary) and not from bone resorption. So, as with the concern for kidney function, there appear to be no adverse outcomes to increased protein intake within the recommended levels (up to 2 $g \cdot kg^{-1} \cdot d^{-1}$) in healthy, exercising individuals (Campbell et al., 2007). Similarly, intakes of BCAA supplements of about 10–30 $g \cdot d^{-1}$ seem to be harmless (Gleeson, 2005).

Fat

As discussed in Chapters 2 and 4, fat is a major fuel for exercise of low or moderate intensity, and in most individuals, it is readily available in more-than-adequate stored amounts. In addition, studies have documented (Chapter 5) that with endurance training more fat can be utilized as a fuel, thereby sparing carbohydrate stores, and can be used at higher absolute levels of work intensity.

This increased ability to utilize fat and spare carbohydrate helps postpone fatigue in endurance and ultraendurance events. There has been a great deal of interest in whether a diet high in fat could enhance the glycogen sparing that occurs with training.

To be useful during training, a high-fat diet (defined as 60–70% FAT) must allow continuation of the intended training levels and progression in training adaptation through periodic tests or time trials. There is evidence that a relatively high training intensity has been maintained on a high-fat diet for at least 7 weeks in previously untrained and moderately trained individuals and for at least a short time in elite athletes. However, at all levels of training, higher ratings of perceived exertion (RPE) were reported at constant exercise loads (Fleming et al., 2003; Helge, 2000, 2002). **Figure 6.6** provides an example. At the start of the study (A), both groups had parallel, similar RPE responses to a submaximal (71% $\dot{V}O_2$ max) exercise to exhaustion. After training (B), under different dietary conditions, those on the high-fat diet had a significantly higher RPE at 40 and 60 minutes of the same exercise (Helge, 2000). Heart rate values have also been

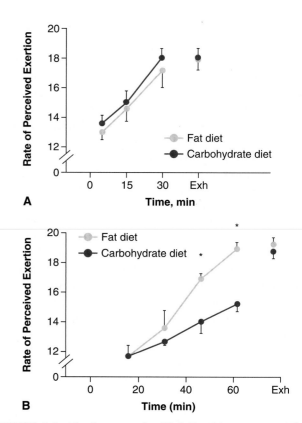

FIGURE 6.6   The Impact of a High-Fat Diet versus a High-Carbohydrate Diet on the RPE before and after 7 Weeks of Training and Dietary Manipulation.
A. Before training and dietary manipulation, there was no significant difference in the RPE between the two groups. **B.** After 7 weeks, the RPE was higher in the high-fat diet group than the high-carbohydrate group prior to exhaustion (*P < 0.05, significant difference).
Source: Helge, J. W.: Long-term fat diet adaptation effects on performance, training capacity, and fat utilization. *Medicine & Science in Sports & Exercise*. 34(9):1499–1504 (2002). Reprinted with permission.

reported to be higher at a given external submaximal workload. In this case, if training is adjusted according to the monitored heart rate, the power output or pace will be lower and the intended training stimulus not achieved (Havemann et al., 2006).

Adaptation to a fat-rich diet does lead to an increased ability to store, mobilize, transport, and utilize fat. There is also evidence that the storage of muscle glycogen and liver glycogen is lower with high-fat diets. As a result, more fat is oxidized during submaximal exercise, presumably sparing carbohydrate compared with an equal-calorie high-carbohydrate diet, even if carbohydrate is ingested immediately before or during the exercise (Burke and Hawley, 2002; Helge, 2000, 2002). However, there generally appears to be no particular performance advantage to these metabolic shifts. The exercise performance of those consuming a high-fat diet is at best equal to, or in some cases lower than, that of those consuming a more

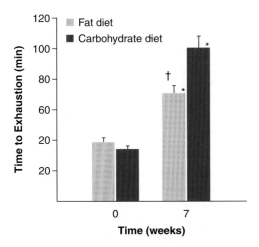

FIGURE 6.7   The Impact of a High-Fat Diet versus a High-Carbohydrate Diet on Submaximal Exercise Performance.
Before training and dietary manipulation, there was no significant difference in the time to exhaustion between the two groups. After 7 weeks, the high-carbohydrate group exercised for significantly longer than did the high-fat group (*P < 0.05, significant difference).
Source: Helge, J. W.: Long-term fat diet adaptation effects on performance, training capacity, and fat utilization. *Medicine & Science in Sports & Exercise*. 34(9):1499–1504 (2002). Reprinted with permission.

traditional high-CHO training diet (American College of Sports Medicine, 2009; Burke and Hawley, 2002; Fleming et al., 2003; Helge, 2000, 2002; Jacobs et al., 2004; Vogt et al., 2003). **Figure 6.7** shows the results of 7 weeks of training on either a high-fat or a high-CHO diet on a time-to-exhaustion test. Performance improved significantly in both groups. However, the high-CHO diet group improved significantly more than the high-fat diet group (Helge, 2002). Within these studies, despite no mean improvements, a few individuals improved performance on the high-fat diet. There may be "responders" and "nonresponders" (Burke and Kiens, 2006).

Obviously, these high-fat diets are far above the recommended daily intake for health. The primary concern is that high-fat diets lead to unhealthy lipid profiles. Surprisingly, based on the few available studies, well-trained individuals who maintain that training seem to have no adverse effects in their lipid/lipoprotein profiles when consuming a high-fat diet over periods of up to 3 months. However, when training is not maintained or when a high-fat diet is consumed for longer, there probably are detrimental effects in general health (Helge, 2000). Thus, given the lack of any beneficial training

> **Vitamins** Organic substances of plant or animal origin that are essential for normal growth, development, metabolic processes, and energy transformations.

effects and the real possibility of eventual negative health effects, a high-fat diet is not recommended for fitness or athletic training.

On the other hand, no attempt should be made to totally remove fat from the diet (American College of Sports Medicine, 2009; Kreider et al., 2010; Sherman and Leenders, 1995). Diets in which less than 20% of the energy is provided from fat increase the risk of inadequate intakes of vitamin E, α-linolenic acid, and linoleic acid and for adverse changes in HDL cholesterol and triglycerides (Dietary Guidelines for Americans, 2005). The recommendation of 20–35% dietary fat for sedentary and moderately active individuals remains the best advice, but it may be that well-trained athletes doing endurance training should not drop below 30% fat in their diet. Most fats should come from polyunsaturated and monounsaturated fatty acid sources such as fish, nuts, and vegetable oils. Adults should consume 5–10% of calories as *n*-6 polyunsaturated fatty acids (linoleic acid) and 0.6–1.2% as *n*-3 polyunsaturated fatty acids (α-linolenic acid) (Dietary Guidelines for Americans, 2005). Two servings of fish per week are recommended—with the caution that women of childbearing age, pregnant women, nursing mothers, and young children should avoid fish and shellfish that are likely to contain high levels of mercury. No more than 10% of dietary fat should be saturated, regardless of the activity level (Burke and Read, 1989; Leaf and Frisa, 1989). In addition, given that *trans fatty acid* and cholesterol intakes are directly and progressively related to LDL cholesterol levels, increasing the risk of coronary heart disease, both of these types of fats should be minimized while consuming a nutritionally adequate diet. For adults with an LDL cholesterol less than 130 mg·dL^{-1}, less than 300 mg of dietary cholesterol per day is recommended. Trans fatty acid consumption should be as low as possible, about ≤1% energy intake (Dietary Guidelines for Americans, 2005). There is no established RDA in g·kg^{-1}·d^{-1} for fat but 0.5–1.5 g·kg^{-1}·d^{-1} has been recommended (Kreider et al., 2010). In addition, as indicated on **Table 6.1**, 65–80 g·d^{-1} is a reasonable level for a total caloric input of 2000–2500 kcal·d^{-1} or proportionally more (~3 g·100 kcal^{-1}) for higher caloric intakes in athletes.

Vitamins

Thirteen compounds are now considered to be vitamins. **Vitamins** are organic substances of plant or animal origin that are essential for normal growth, development, metabolic processes, and energy transformations. The B complex vitamins have two major roles directly related to exercise: (1) involvement in energy production (see Chapter 2 Focus on Application: Metabolic pathways: The vitamin connection) and (2) tissue synthesis and repair. For example, vitamin B$_6$ is important in amino acid metabolism and the breakdown of glycogen to glucose.

Thiamin (B_1) is important in carbohydrate metabolism. Riboflavin (B_2) and niacin are important as the hydrogen carriers FAD and NAD, respectively. B_{12} is needed for the production of red blood cells and protein synthesis. Ascorbic acid (vitamin C) is necessary for the formation of connective tissues and the catecholamines (important in the stress response) and for the maintenance and function of blood vessels. Vitamin E influences the flow of electrons within the mitochondrial respiratory chain. Both C and E are important in protecting cell membranes from oxidative damage (see Chapter 5 Focus on Application: Oxygen-free radicals, Exercise, and Exercise Training Adaptations) (American College of Sports Medicine, 2009; Belko, 1987; vander Beek, 1985, 1991). See animation, Biological Function of Vitamins, at http://thePoint.lww.com/Plowman4e

Some evidence suggests that exercise training may increase the need for vitamin C (especially in hot climates), B complex vitamins (particularly B_6 and B_2, also especially in hot climates), and vitamin E at high altitudes and as antioxidant defense against free radicals (Belko, 1987; Blom et al., 1987; Kreider et al., 2010; vander Beek, 1985, 1991). These increased needs, as with other nutrients, should be adequately covered if the exerciser increases his or her total caloric intake with a balanced diet. The increased needs also mean that athletes who are concerned with restricting body weight or body fat or making weight (gymnasts, dancers, figure skaters, divers, wrestlers, boxers, and jockeys) and who restrict caloric intake could be at risk for an inadequate intake of vitamins. For these individuals, a generic, one-a-day vitamin and mineral tablet might be appropriate to ensure adequate intake (American College of Sports Medicine, 2009; Belko, 1987; Kreider et al., 2010). Athletes who participate in prolonged, strenuous exercise training should consume 100–1000 mg of vitamin C daily (American College of Sports Medicine, 2009).

After decades of research, there is no evidence that vitamin supplementation improves an adequately nourished, healthy individual's exercise or athletic performance, speeds up recovery, or decreases injuries (American College of Sports Medicine, 2009; Belko, 1987; Haymes, 1983; Kreider et al., 2010; Lukaski, 2004). If a deficiency is present, supplementation to the normal physiological level can improve performance. This is another reason for a complete nutritional analysis for anyone training or competing. However, megadoses of vitamins are neither substitutes for vigorous training nor necessary for training adaptations (vander Beek, 1985, 1991). Furthermore, extremely large doses of either water- or fat-soluble vitamins can be toxic, can impair performance, and, more importantly, can cause health problems. Once again, if some is good, more is not necessarily better. For example, very high doses of vitamin C have been linked with the formation of kidney stones and the breakdown of red blood cells, which causes loss of hemoglobin. Megadoses of niacin inhibit fatty acid mobilization and utilization during exercise, thereby increasing the rate of glycogen use (Nieman, 1990). Doses of antioxidants such as vitamin E that are too high could be pro-oxidative instead of antioxidative (American College of Sports Medicine, 2009).

Minerals

Minerals are elements, not of animal or plant origin, that are essential constituents of all cells and for many body functions. Minerals are classified as microminerals (trace elements) or macrominerals based on the amount in the body. Minerals are important for bone density, energy metabolism, enzyme function, muscle contraction, oxygen transport, insulin regulation, and ATP composition, to name just a few functions.

Microminerals

Of the 15 microminerals with DRI/RDAs (Dietary Guidelines for Americans, 2005), only 5 (zinc, chromium, copper, selenium, and iron) have been shown to be affected by or potentially beneficial for exercise training or performance.

Zinc plays a role in repair of muscle tissue and energy production among other things. Low dietary zinc has been shown to impair metabolic responses during exercise (Lukaski, 2005). Because exercise can cause a sizable loss of zinc in sweat and urine, training may lead to a zinc deficiency. However, excess zinc intake above the RDA (11 $mg \cdot d^{-1}$ for adult males and 8 $mg \cdot d^{-1}$ for adult females) can result in an impaired immune response and decreased iron and copper absorption. Two studies with wrestlers have shown that zinc supplementation (3 $mg \cdot kg^{-1} \cdot d^{-1}$) had a positive effect on hematological variables and moderated the inhibition of thyroid hormones and testosterone after exhaustive exercise (Kilic et al., 2004, 2006). Studies also indicate that zinc supplementation during training minimizes exercise-induced changes in immune function (Kreider et al., 2010). Evidence is insufficient, however, to conclude that zinc status or zinc supplementation affects exercise performance (American College of Sports Medicine, 2009; Campbell and Anderson, 1987; Clarkson, 1991b; Lemon, 1989b, 1991; McDonald and Keen, 1988).

Chromium has a role in maintaining proper carbohydrate and lipid metabolism. There is speculation but little evidence that exercise and training may increase the requirements for chromium in part because exercise increases urinary chromium loss. Chromium has no RDA because data are insufficient for establishing these. Instead, daily AI values are 35 $\mu g \cdot d^{-1}$ for adult males and 25 $\mu g \cdot d^{-1}$ for adult females. Speculation that chromium can increase muscle mass and decrease the percentage of body fat in conjunction with resistance training remains just that—speculation (Lefavi et al., 1992). Chromium supplementation (as chromium picolinate) has not been shown to have any positive effect on body composition in healthy individuals when taken alone or used in conjunction with an exercise program (Kreider et al., 2010; Volpe, 2008). Conversely, recent studies suggest potentially deleterious effects (Lukaski et al., 2007; Vincent, 2003).

There is no evidence that either selenium or copper has an impact on acute or chronic exercise responses, although copper may be lost in sweat. The RDA for copper is 890 $\mu g \cdot d^{-1}$ for adolescents and 900 $\mu g \cdot d^{-1}$ for adults. Selenium functions as an antioxidant, so the need for selenium is increased during exercise training without being linearly related to energy expenditure (Margaritis et al., 2005). Suboptimal selenium status has been implicated in a worsening of muscle function following eccentric muscle contractions (Milias et al., 2006), but it does not appear that selenium supplementation would be beneficial for exercise performance (Kreider et al., 2010; Volpe, 2008). The RDA for selenium is 55 $\mu g \cdot d^{-1}$ for male and female adolescents and adults. Intakes of selenium above 1000 $\mu g \cdot d^{-1}$ can be toxic (Campbell and Anderson, 1987; Clarkson, 1991b).

Iron is required for the formation of hemoglobin and myoglobin as well as enzymes involved in energy production. Iron deficiency can be a problem for exercising or training individuals, especially for menstruating females. Iron deficiency occurs in three stages: (1) iron depletion or low-storage levels of iron; (2) iron deficiency erythropoiesis, which is an impairment of the ability to produce red blood cells; and (3) iron deficiency anemia or low hemoglobin levels (<12 $g \cdot dL^{-1}$ for females and <13 $g \cdot dL^{-1}$ for males). Iron deficiency anemia is also characterized by small, pale red blood cells; decreased iron levels in the blood; decreased iron stores; and increased total iron binding capacity as the body attempts to mobilize as much iron as possible. Iron depletion is not associated with reduced performance, and iron deficiency erythropoiesis has marginal impact. However, iron deficiency anemia definitely impairs performance. Lower hemoglobin levels mean lower oxygen transport. Moderate levels of exercise do not appear to affect iron status.

Iron supplementation given to individuals with iron deficiency anemia consistently improves iron status and exercise performance (Kreider et al., 2010). Iron supplementation given to individuals with iron depletion or iron deficiency erythropoiesis shows variable but primarily nonsignificant changes in performance. Iron requirements for endurance athletes are increased by approximately 70% (American College of Sports Medicine, 2009);

Minerals Elements, not of animal or plant origin, that are essential constituents of all cells and of many functions in the body.

however, excessive iron intake can inhibit zinc and copper absorption. The iron status of an individual should be ascertained before supplementation is given that exceeds the RDA (11 $mg \cdot d^{-1}$ for adolescent males; 8 $mg \cdot d^{-1}$ for adult males; 15 $mg \cdot d^{-1}$ for adolescent females; and 18 $mg \cdot d^{-1}$ for adult females) (American College of Sports Medicine, 2009; American Dietetic Association, 1987; Clarkson, 1990; Haymes, 1983; McDonald and Keen, 1988; Zoller and Vogel, 2004).

Macrominerals

Macrominerals include calcium, chlorine, magnesium, phosphorus, potassium, sodium, and sulfur. As macromineral electrolytes, chlorine, potassium, and sodium are discussed in the section "Fluid Ingestion During and After Exercise" in Chapter 14. Sulfur has no direct importance for exercise.

The function of calcium in bone health is directly related to exercise training and is fully described in Chapter 16. Beyond its role in bone health, the relationship between exercise, training, and calcium level and supplementation is largely unknown (Clarkson, 1991a).

Magnesium is involved in oxygen uptake and energy production. Because magnesium is lost in sweat and urine, strenuous exercise may increase the need for magnesium by 10–20%. Some evidence suggests that a marginal magnesium deficit impairs exercise performance and increases oxidative stress (American College of Sports Medicine, 2009). Increased magnesium intake has beneficial effects on exercise performance in magnesium-deficient individuals. However, supplemental magnesium has not been shown to increase performance in active individuals with adequate magnesium status (Kreider, et al., 2010; Nielsen and Lukaski, 2006; Volpe, 2008). Levels above the RDA (400–420 $mg \cdot d^{-1}$ for adolescent and adult males and 360–310 $mg \cdot d^{-1}$ for adolescent and adult females) do not appear to be harmful (McDonald and Keen, 1988).

Several studies have shown that phosphate loading (in the form of sodium phosphate)—increasing phosphate ingestion for several days before an event—may improve performance by delaying the onset of anaerobic metabolism; other studies using a variety of phosphate formula have shown no beneficial effects (Kreider et al., 2010). Because phosphorus supplementation over an extended period of time can result in lowered blood calcium levels, it is not recommended. The RDA for phosphorus is 1200 $mg \cdot d^{-1}$ for adolescents and 700 $mg \cdot d^{-1}$ for adult males and females (Clarkson, 1991a).

In summary, the pattern here is the same for minerals as the one for vitamins. Exercisers should ingest the RDA/AI amounts and, unless diagnosed with a deficiency, only those amounts. For those who are strictly limiting their caloric intake, a generic vitamin-and-mineral, one-a-day pill can be recommended.

Nutrition for Competition

The five goals for an optimal competitive diet are to:

1. Ensure adequate fuel supplies in the pre-event time span
2. Ensure adequate fuel supplies during the event, regardless of its duration
3. Facilitate temperature regulation by preventing dehydration
4. Achieve the desired weight classification while maintaining fuel and water supplies
5. Avoid gastrointestinal discomfort during competition

Depending on the event, an athlete's diet may need to be adjusted during a period of hours or days before competition. Most manipulation focuses on carbohydrate consumption (Burke and Read, 1989).

Carbohydrate Loading (Glycogen Supercompensation)

Individuals competing in continuous endurance events lasting at least 90 minutes at 65–85% $\dot{V}O_2$max may use carbohydrate loading, sometimes called glycogen supercompensation (American Dietetic Association, 1987; Brotherhood, 1984; Hawley et al., 1997). **Carbohydrate loading** is a nutritional modification that results in an additional storage of glycogen in muscle fibers that can be approximately two to three times the normal level. As mentioned previously, the time to exhaustion in long-duration, relatively high-intensity activities is related to initial levels of muscle glycogen. **Table 6.7** details three effective carbohydrate-loading techniques.

Classic Carbohydrate-Loading Technique

The classic carbohydrate-loading technique is based on studies by Swedish investigators in the 1960s (Bergstrom et al., 1967). This technique involves hard exercise to deplete muscle glycogen stores 1 week before the competitive event, followed by 3 days of hard training and 3 days of rest. During the first 3 days after the depletion exercise, the individual eats almost no carbohydrates and then for the next 3 days, eats almost exclusively carbohydrates.

This technique is effective but is not without its problems. The high-fat, high-protein diet after the exercise

> **Carbohydrate Loading (Glycogen Supercompensation)** A process of nutritional modification that results in an additional storage of glycogen in muscle fiber up to two to three times the normal levels.

depletion phase, with less than 5% carbohydrate, means that the individual is ingesting high levels of fat, which is not healthy. This can cause high blood lipid levels. In addition, the ingested fat is incompletely metabolized, and high levels of ketones appear in the blood (ketosis) (Costill, 1988; Newsholme and Leech, 1983). Hypoglycemia (abnormally low blood glucose levels) can also occur, leading to fatigue, restlessness, mental disturbances, irritability, and weakness. At the very least, it is difficult if not impossible to maintain the hard training recommended during this phase. At the same time, the 80–90% carbohydrate diet for the 3 days before the competition can leave the athlete feeling stiff and heavy because of water retention. Since approximately 2.7 g of water are stored with each gram of glycogen, water retention can add approximately 1–2 kg to body weight. Although this water theoretically could help delay or prevent dehydration, it has not been shown to have a beneficial effect on body temperature regulation or dehydration. Overall, an athlete who had trained for months for an event such as a marathon could find himself/herself down both mentally and physiologically in the week before the competition (Sedlock, 2008).

Modified Carbohydrate-Loading Technique

Subsequent research on the classic carbohydrate-loading technique has shown that neither the exhaustive glycogen depletion nor the 3 days of high-protein, high-fat diet is necessary to maximize muscle glycogen storage (Sherman, 1983, 1989). Instead, the modified carbohydrate-loading technique presented in **Table 6.7** emphasizes a slow downward taper in duration and/or intensity of the training regimen. This taper is accompanied by a diet that includes not less than 50% carbohydrate and increases to approximately 70%. An athlete already modifying his or her training diet to include high levels of carbohydrate will have very few changes to make.

Short Carbohydrate-Loading Technique

Both of the carbohydrate-loading techniques described so far require a week to accomplish and a disruption of normal training for an athlete who might not want such a strong taper or rest component. More recently a short technique has been tested. In this version, the athlete either completed a normal training session the day before carbohydrate loading (Bussau et al., 2002) or a supramaximal short depletion routine on the day of carbohydrate loading (Fairchild et al., 2002). The depletion exercise (after a 5 minutes warm-up) consisted of 150 seconds of cycling at 130% $\dot{V}O_2$peak followed by a 30 second all-out sprint. The athletes then ingested either a 10 g·kg·BW^{-1} (Bussau et al., 2002) or 12 g·kg LBM^{-1} of high glycemic index carbohydrates over the next 24 hours. In both studies, the preloaded glycogen level was well within normal concentrations of 80–120 mmol·kg^{-1} wet

TABLE 6.7 Carbohydrate Loading

	Days Prior to Competition							Day of Competition
	-7	-6	-5	-4	-3	-2	-1	
Classic Technique								
Diet	Mixed diet 50% CHO	<5% CHO or <2 g CHO·kg⁻¹·d⁻¹	Continue from previous day	Continue from previous day	80–90% CHO >10–12 g CHO·kg⁻¹·d⁻¹	Continue from previous day	Continue from previous day	High-CHO pre-event meal. Possible during-event CHO feeding
Exercise	Exercise to exhaustion	90–120 min 65–85% V̇O₂max	Continue from previous day	Continue from previous day or exercise to exhaustion	Rest	Rest	Rest	Continuous endurance event lasting 60–90 min, 65–85% V̇O₂max
Modified Technique								
Diet	50% CHO or 4.5 g CHO·kg⁻¹·d⁻¹	Continue from previous day	Continue from previous day	Continue from previous day	70% CHO or 8–10 g CHO·kg⁻¹·d⁻¹	Continue from previous day	Continue from previous day	High-CHO pre-event meal Possible during-event CHO feeding
Exercise	90 min 75% V̇O₂max	Continue from previous day	40 min 75% V̇O₂max	Continue from previous day	20 min 75% V̇O₂max or 30–60 min 50–70% V̇O₂max	Continue from previous day	Rest	Continuous endurance event lasting 60–90 min, 65–85% V̇O₂max
Short Technique								
Diet	Normal training diet →————————————→						10–12 g·kg BW⁻¹ or g·kg LBM⁻¹	High-CHO pre-event meal. Possible during-event CHO feeding
Exercise	Normal training →————————————→						~3 min supramaximal	Continuous endurance event lasting 60–90 min, 60–85% V̇O₂max

weight (95 and 109 mmol·kg⁻¹ wet weight, respectively). Glycogen supercompensation levels are typically close to 200 mmol·kg⁻¹ wet weight. After 24 hours of loading and inactivity, glycogen levels were 180 and 198 mmol·kg⁻¹ wet weight, respectively. Additionally, glycogen supercompensation took place in both fast- and slow-twitch muscle fiber types. **Figure 6.8** shows a scan

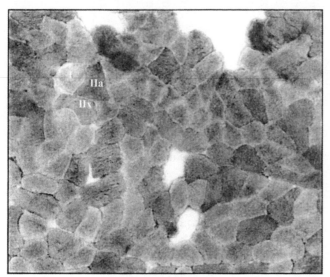

Pre-Loading

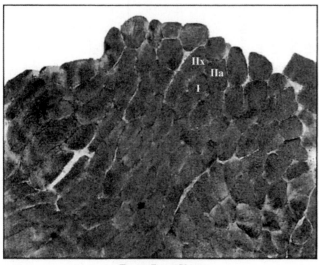

Post-Loading

FIGURE 6.8 Glycogen Supercompensation.
Muscle fiber scan before and after carbohydrate loading. The darker stain in the after scan indicates the increased glycogen storage. Note that glycogen supercompensation occurred in SO (Type 1), FOG (Type 11a), and FG (Type 11x) fibers.
Source: Fairchild, T. J., S. Fletcher, P. Steele, C. Goodman, B. Dawson, & P. A. Fournier: Rapid carbohydrate loading after a short bout of near maximal-intensity exercise. *Medicine & Science in Sports & Exercise*. 34(6):980–986 (2002). Reprinted with permission.

of muscle fibers packed with glycogen following a short CHO loading protocol study (Fairchild et al., 2002). This short technique was effective in achieving glycogen supercompensation. It should be easy for athletes to use and therefore encourages compliance. The Focus on Research: Clinically Relevant box describes the impact of increased glycogen storage on exercise performance. Obviously, each athlete needs to individually determine which technique works best for him/her by trying these techniques during training time trials or in less important competitions.

Fat Plus Carbohydrate-Loading Technique

One technique that does not seem to work is combining 1 day of carbohydrate loading with fat loading. In a simple fat-loading technique, individuals simply ingest a high-fat diet from 1 to 6 days before an endurance event. There is clear evidence (Burke and Hawley, 2002; Helge, 2000) that 1–3 days of fat loading by itself is detrimental to endurance performance. It is too short a time to increase the capacity for fat utilization, and the resting levels of muscle glycogen at the start of an event are lowered. To counteract these shortcomings, a strategy has emerged, which involves 5–6 days of fat loading (60–70% fat in the diet) followed by 1 day of carbohydrate loading (~90% CHO in the diet). This strategy has been shown to increase fat utilization at rest and during exercise, to increase muscle glycogen stores, and to reduce muscle glycogen utilization during exercise. However, as with the studies using high-fat diets in training, there has been no clear evidence of performance improvement.

A study by Havemann et al. (2006) tested the impact of 6 days of a high-fat diet (68% fat) followed by 1 day of high CHO (8–10 g·kg⁻¹) on a 100 km (61 mi) cycling time trial compared with a high-CHO diet (68% CHO + 1 day of 8–10 g·kg⁻¹). The 100-km time trial included five 1-km sprints and four 4-km sprints at 8–19-km intervals. This was an attempt to simulate actual race conditions better than a steady-pace ride would. Overall, in the 100-km time trial, performance was not statistically different between the two dietary manipulations. However, those on the high-fat diet rode 3:44 slower than those on the high-CHO diet. In a competition, almost 4 minutes is a meaningful difference. No significant differences were seen in the 4-km sprints; however, 1-km sprint power output was significantly lower in the fat-loading group. Thus, in those "real world moves" of breakaways, surges, and a sprint to the finish, fat plus carbohydrate loading is a disadvantage. Glycogen sparing after adaptation to fat loading may in fact be glycogen impairment or a downregulation of carbohydrate metabolism at high-intensity exercise (Burke and Kiens, 2006). Current evidence continues to support carbohydrate loading but not fat loading for optimizing performance.

The practice of carbohydrate loading does not appear in any way to adversely affect normal healthy individuals

FOCUS ON RESEARCH: *Clinically Relevant*

The Impact of Increased Glycogen Storage on Exercise Performance

In this study, well-trained male endurance cyclists completed two exercise trials separated by at least 4 days. Each trial consisted first of 2 hours of cycling at approximately 73% $\dot{V}O_2$max. Every 20 minutes, an all-out 60-second sprint followed by 1 minute of unloaded cycling was interspersed. Immediately after the 2-hour ergometer ride, the athlete transferred to his own bike and completed a 1-hour time trial, blind to all data except elapsed time.

Dietary manipulation consisted of either 3 days of each athlete's normal diet or 3 days of a high-carbohydrate diet. A standardized breakfast similar to what they would have eaten before a competition was ingested 3 hours before testing. During the 2-hour ride, each athlete drank 600 mL of a 10% glucose polymer solution and then only water during the time trial.

The results are shown in the accompanying graphs. Although the mean muscle glycogen level after the high-carbohydrate diet was not as high as seen in many studies (151 mmol·kg^{-1} wet weight versus ~200 mmol·kg^{-1} wet weight), it was significantly higher

than after the normal diet. This enabled the cyclists to maintain a significantly higher power output and a faster overall pace during the time trial. Interestingly, muscle glycogen levels after the time trial were similar between groups despite different starting values and different performances. This indicates that the additional stored glycogen was indeed utilized during the time

trial. Furthermore, although the term glycogen depletion is often used, glycogen concentrations do not actually reach zero at exhaustion.

Source: Rauch, H. G. L., A. St. Clair Gibson, E. V. Lambert, & T. D. Noakes: A signaling role for muscle glycogen in the regulation of pace during prolonged exercise. *British Journal of Sports Medicine.* 39:34–38 (2005).

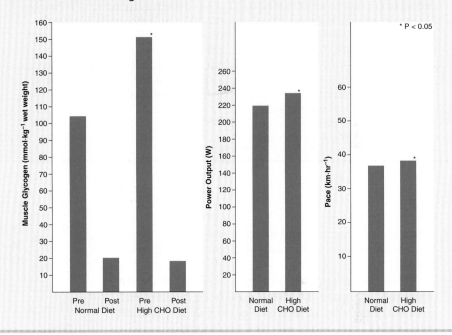

(American Dietetic Association, 1987; Goss and Karam, 1987; Sherman, 1983, 1989). Obviously, individuals with diabetes should consult with a physician before attempting carbohydrate loading. No evidence supports the suggestion that carbohydrate loading is effective only if not done more than once or twice a year. Supercompensation may actually be occurring daily in an athlete undergoing strenuous training who eats 70% carbohydrate. When trained males and females ingest equal amounts of carbohydrate relative to LBM, glycogen supercompensation is equal (James et al., 2001). This means ingesting 10 g·kg LBM^{-1}·d^{-1} (to equal 8 g·kg^{-1}·d^{-1}). Thus, a female must pay close attention to both total energy intake and relative carbohydrate intake when carbohydrate loading to get sufficient other nutrients. Menstrual cycle may influence the effectiveness of carbohydrate loading. Females have a greater capacity for storing glycogen during the luteal phase (days 14–28) than the follicular phase (days 1–14) probably due to the

fluctuations in hormonal levels (Sedlock, 2008). Overall, in the studies cited in this section, there were "responders" (who improved) and "nonresponders" (who did not improve) to both fat loading and carbohydrate loading. Therefore, it must be reemphasized that each athlete should determine what benefits himself or herself most. There is currently not enough evidence to support carbohydrate loading in either children or older adults (Nemet and Eliakim, 2009; Tarnopolsky, 2008).

While carbohydrate loading is intended for endurance athletes, body builders often follow a version of the modified carbohydrate-loading technique (Kroculick, 1988). The primary difference is a restriction of water and sodium intake by body builders during the high-carbohydrate ingestion phase. This water restriction has nothing to do with energy requirements during competition; it is based on the belief that water will be sucked from beneath the skin for storage with glycogen and lead to increased

FOCUS ON APPLICATION: *Clinically Relevant*

The Glycemic Index (GI) of Pre-Event Meals

The GI of food ingested 30–60 minutes before exercise may impact the ensuing performance. A group of cyclists consumed (in random order) either a HGI meal (corn flakes, low-fat milk, and banana), a LGI meal (All-Bran, low-fat yogurt, and apple), or water 30 minutes before cycling 2 hours at 70% $\dot{V}O_2$max followed by cycling to exhaustion at 100% $\dot{V}O_2$max. Compared with the HGI meal, the LGI meal resulted in significantly lower plasma insulin levels during the first 20 minutes of exercise, a significantly lower respiratory exchange ratio (RER) and rating of perceived exertion (RPE) during the 2 hours of cycling, and significantly higher plasma glucose levels at the end of the 2-hour cycling.

Time to exhaustion was 59% longer in the LGI trial than the HGI one and 72% longer than the control ride (DeMarco et al., 1999). Thus, it seems prudent to recommend LGI pre-event meals, especially for an endurance event that does not include CHO ingestion during the race and that might require near maximal performance toward the end (such as sprinting or finishing uphill during a mountain bike race). As always, individuals might respond differently to any given meal, so an athlete should experiment with any food combination before ingesting it before competition.

Source: DeMarco et al. (1999).

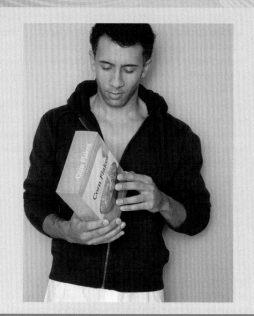

muscle size and definition for competition. In addition, stored glycogen is said to result in a harder muscle. Evidence in support of this consequence is primarily anecdotal.

Results from the only available scientific study are presented in **Figure 6.9**. Nine male body builders had girth measurements taken after a normal dietary routine (55% CHO, 15% PRO, and 30% fat) and after a traditional carbohydrate-loading regimen (3 days of 10% CHO, 33% PRO, and 57% fat, followed by 3 days of 80% CHO, 15% PRO, and 5% fat). Identical weight-lifting workouts were followed during both dietary manipulations and before girth measurement. The trials were randomized. No measurement of muscle definition was made, but as the figure shows, the diet before testing had no effect on muscle girth measurements (Balon et al., 1992). Alarmingly, a case has been reported in which a young body builder in the course of this dietary manipulation developed low blood concentrations of potassium and phosphate, weakness in all four extremities, and rhabdomyolysis (destruction of muscle tissue) (Britschgi and Zünd, 1991).

Pre-Event Meal

Considerations for the pre-event meal involve the meal's timing and nutrient content. Most road races and other endurance events, unless scheduled for the convenience of a television broadcast such as during the Olympics, take place in the morning. Competing after an overnight

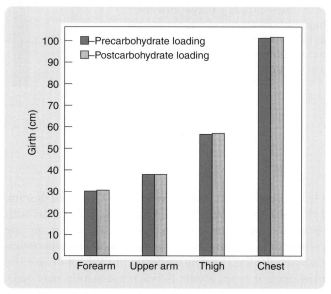

FIGURE 6.9   Girth Measurements in Body Builders with and without Carbohydrate Loading.
Source: Based on data from Balon, T. W., J. F. Horowitz, & K. M. Fitzsimmons: Effects of carbohydrate loading and weight-lifting on muscle girth. *International Journal of Sports Nutrition.* 2(4):328–334 (1992).

fast is probably not effective for an athlete in any sport, but it is most detrimental for endurance athletes. Liver glycogen is the primary endogenous source of blood glucose, and an overnight fast reduces the liver's supply of glycogen. Although it has been demonstrated that fat oxidation can be maximized when an individual exercises in a fasted state, a high-carbohydrate pre-event meal is generally accepted to benefit performance more than fasting (O'Reilly et al., 2010). This is despite the fact that getting up early and eating can be inconvenient. Athletes who compete in the afternoon or evening can more easily time their meals.

It takes about 4 hours for CHO to be digested and begin to be stored as glycogen. Consequently, most evidence supports eating the pre-event meal 4–6 hours before competition (Burke and Read, 1989; Costill, 1988; Coyle, 1991; Kreider et al., 2010; Williams and Serratosa, 2006). For example, when Neufer et al. (1987) fed participants 45 g of either liquid carbohydrate, a candy bar, or flavored water containing no carbohydrate 5 minutes before exercise, total work performed on a cycle ergometer was significantly improved after both the liquid carbohydrate and candy bar compared with the flavored water. When a meal of 200 g of carbohydrate (cereal, bread, and fruit) was eaten 4 hours before exercise in addition to a candy bar 5 minutes before the exercise, total work performed on the cycle ergometer was significantly greater compared with all other trials.

Theoretically, ingestion of carbohydrate from 1 hour to 5 minutes before exercise could be detrimental to performance for the following reasons. The ingestion of carbohydrate causes an increase in blood glucose. The increase of blood glucose causes a concomitant increase in insulin. Insulin favors the removal of blood glucose from the bloodstream, inhibits the release of glucose from the liver, and inhibits the mobilization of free fatty acids, which are used, along with carbohydrate, as fuel for exercise. These actions can cause hypoglycemia and may cause a greater dependency on muscle glycogen stores, depleting them at a faster rate. Despite the popular acceptance of this reasoning, the research literature has not supported the detrimental effects of meals within 1 hour of competition (Burke and Read, 1989; Coyle, 1991; Hawley and Burke, 1997; Williams and Serratosa, 2006). Indeed, ingesting a light snack (50 g CHO + 10 g PRO) 30–60 minutes before exercising is now recommended as a way to increase CHO availability toward the end of an intense exercise bout (Kreider et al., 2010). The physiological changes described above may be nullified by the increased availability of carbohydrate. The individual's glucose or glycogen status before the feeding may also affect whether or not the response is beneficial (Clarkson, 1991b). Fasted individuals may be more sensitive to glucose ingestion within this time span than those who have recently eaten and who had followed a carbohydrate-loading regimen.

What type of carbohydrate should be ingested in the pre-event meal has been extensively investigated. For example, researchers (Stevenson et al., 2006; Wu et al.,

2003) conducted two separate experiments following the same basic protocol to determine the effects of consuming mixed high-carbohydrate meals with different glycemic indices 3 hours before a 60-minute treadmill run at 65% VO_2max on substrate utilization during the run. The HGI meals had a GI of approximately 78, and the LGI meals averaged a GI of approximately 40 in the two studies. As expected, the 2-hour postprandial response showed a higher elevation in glucose and insulin concentration after the HGI meal than the LGI meal. During the exercise, the total fat oxidation was greater in the LGI trial than in the HGI trial in both males and females. Although no performance variable was measured in these two studies, the Focus on Application box on the GI of pre-event meals provides evidence that a LGI but not a high- or a moderate-GI carbohydrate meal improves endurance performance. Note that in the studies comparing HGI to LGI preexercise meals, the meals are often consumed from 30 to 120 minutes before the exercise, not before the recommended 4–6 hours. It is therefore likely that at least some of the food was still being digested during exercise and glucose was released into the circulation throughout the exercise. The common denominator in those studies showing a performance improvement after eating a LGI preexercise meal is a combination of a greater rate of fat oxidation and more stable plasma glucose concentrations during exercise than after a HGI preexercise meal (O'Reilly et al., 2010; Williams and Serratosa, 2006; Wu and Williams, 2006). Additionally, a LGI pre-event meal produces a longer-lasting feeling of satiety than a HGI meal. The GI of a pre-event meal has no effect on hydration during exercise.

Based on the available research, a light meal of 200–500 kcal, including 50–100 g of predominantly LGI carbohydrate and plenty of fluid, is recommended for the pre-event meal. Ideally, this would be ingested 3–6 hours before an endurance event (with the option of a last-minute snack), but it may be eaten as close as 30 minutes to the event if necessary. Athletes should experiment with this timing and content during training. This meal should consist of foods that the individual likes and tolerates well. The absence or presence of gastrointestinal distress can make the difference between a PR (personal record) or a DNF (did not finish). In order to optimize the benefits of a LGI meal, the exercise that follows should occur at an intensity that is conducive to fat oxidation (50–64% VO_2max). Furthermore, if the event is long enough to require the ingestion of large amounts of carbohydrate-electrolyte drinks, the typical LGI preexercise ingestion responses during exercise are overridden to the extent that performance and substrate utilization are similar no matter what CHO type was ingested pre-event (Donaldson et al., 2010; O'Reilly et al., 2010). **Table 6.8** summarizes this information.

TABLE 6.8   Recommended Eating on Game Day

Sport	−3 to −6 hr	−2 hr	−5 to 0 min	Event Begins	+15 to +30 min Repeated for Duration of Event	Recovery (+15 to +30 min post)
Nonendurance	Light balanced meal of high %CHO Fluid ingestion ~5–7 mL·kg^{-1}*	Fluid ingestion ~3–5 mL·kg^{-1}	—	—	Water as desired	Water and normal food some Na$^+$
Endurance	200–500-kcal meal with 50–100 g CHO Fluid ingestion ~5–7 mL·kg^{-1}	-30–60 min 50 g CHO + 10 g PRO Fluid ingestion ~3–5 mL·kg^{-1}	CHO ~50 g (optional)	—	Fluid ingestion CHO [5–10% (6–8% optimal)]† combined types ~20–30 mEq·L^{-1} Na$^+$ ~2–5 mEq·L^{-1} K$^+$	Fluid ingestion ~1.5 L·kg·BW loss + electrolytes CHO + PRO liquid/solid

*If not already adequately hydrated.

†Individually determined during training; marathoners: small or slow ~400 mL·hr^{-1}; big or fast ~800 mL·hr^{-1}.

Feeding during Exercise

When exercise begins, insulin release is suppressed, and catecholamine secretion increases. Thus, the potentially detrimental changes associated with carbohydrate ingestion within 1-hour to 5-minute time span before exercise are no longer a concern. Indeed, both theoretically and experimentally, there is support for the ingestion of carbohydrates once the activity begins, provided the activity is prolonged (>90 minute) and at moderate to high intensities (50–80% VO$_2$max). Even small amounts of carbohydrates (about 25 g·hr^{-1}) taken at 15–30 minute intervals have been found to prevent a decline in blood glucose and to delay fatigue during the latter portion of an endurance event longer than 1 hour. Note that fatigue can be caused by many factors, and carbohydrate feeding merely delays but does not prevent fatigue.

Carbohydrate feedings during intermittent exercise such as soccer or basketball have also been shown to be beneficial (Burke and Read, 1989; Costill, 1988; Coyle, 1991; Phillips et al., 2011; Williams and Serratos, 2006). Eating an orange at half time may thus be more than just a tradition, although modern-day carbohydrate beverages are probably more convenient. In addition, carbohydrates move through the stomach rapidly and are less likely than other nutrients to cause gastrointestinal and abdominal disturbances (Burke and Read, 1989; Coyle, 1991). Approximately 30–90 g of carbohydrates are recommended per hour, with longer, more intense events requiring the higher amounts of carbohydrate, beginning early in the exercise. As previously noted, this can be accomplished at the same time as fluid replenishment.

No differences have been found among glucose, fructose, sucrose, and glucose polymer solutions (maltodextrins) in the rate of gastric emptying or impact on performance. Glucose, sucrose, and glucose polymers stimulate fluid absorption in the stomach, but fructose does not (Coleman, 1988). Fructose ingestion (as the only carbohydrate source) during exercise has been associated with gastrointestinal distress not with improved performance, and the rate of CHO oxidation is unlikely to meet the ideal of 1 g·min^{-1}. The maximal rate at which a single ingested carbohydrate source can be oxidized is about 60–70 g·hr^{-1} because of a limitation in the rate of intestinal absorption. Once transporters become saturated, ingesting more of the same carbohydrate will not be beneficial. However, combinations of carbohydrates, such as glucose plus fructose, maltodextrins plus fructose, or glucose plus sucrose plus fructose, have been shown experimentally to increase oxidation rates. Glucose (HGI CHO) consumed alone or in combination with sucrose does meet the standard of 1 g·min^{-1} and glucose plus fructose exceeds that by 25% or 1.26 g·min^{-1} (Donaldson et al., 2010). Additionally, fluid delivery is greater with a combination of fructose and glucose than with glucose alone (Jeukendrup, 2007). A recent meta-analysis found that a good supplementation regimen is to ingest CHO before and during exercise in many doses with the first dose up to 4 hours before the start of the event. A CHO ingestion regime providing approximately 0.7 g·kg^{-1}·hr^{-1} of glucose polymers, approximately 0.2 g·kg^{-1}·hr^{-1} fructose, and approximately 0.2 g·kg^{-1}·hr^{-1} protein seems to provide the greatest beneficial ergogenic effect (Vandenbogaerde & Hopkins, 2011).

Research shows that beverages containing 2.5–10% carbohydrate are absorbed by the body as rapidly as water. A concentration of 6–8% is thought to be optimal (American College of Sports Medicine, 2009; Kreider et al., 2010). Drinks containing less than 5% carbohydrate do not provide enough energy to enhance performance, and drinks exceeding 10% carbohydrate (such as most soft drinks/soda pop) are often detrimental since they tend to cause abdominal cramps, nausea, and diarrhea (Coleman, 1988). One high-carbohydrate energy bar, 24 oz of sports drink, and two packets of gel are equivalent. Depending on its composition, any of these can provide at least 30–60 g of carbohydrate per hour during endurance exercise.

In general, HGI foods are probably best for ingestion during exercise. They are rapidly digested and absorbed and are thus likely to maintain blood glucose levels. LGI carbohydrates are digested more slowly and thus may cause gastric distress and fail to maintain blood glucose levels (Walton and Rhodes, 1997). The type of GI consumed during exercise has no bearing on performance outcome, per se. The GL may be a better predictor of glycemic responses than GI alone. Some research suggests that it is the amount of CHO rather than the GI type that is the most crucial factor influencing subsequent endurance performance (Donaldson et al., 2010; O'Reilly et al., 2010).

Fluid Ingestion during and after Exercise

The background and guidelines for fluid ingestion during and after exercise are discussed in Chapter 14. Suffice it to say here that fluid intake is important for preserving thermoregulation and avoiding both dehydration and dilutional hyponatremia (loss of sodium). Individuals should develop a customized fluid replacement program during training to prevent dehydration. The goal is a body weight loss of less than 2% during activity. **Table 6.8** summarizes general recommendations as a starting point for an individualized hydration program (American College of Sports Medicine, 2007).

Eating Disorders

Definitions and Diagnostic Criteria

Most individuals participating in fitness programs or athletics view nutrition as a partner with exercise to help them achieve their goals of health or successful competition. Unfortunately, this is not always the case. There appear to be circumstances under which exercise and sport participation constitute a risk factor for disordered eating. Disordered eating exists on a continuum from abnormal eating behaviors to clinically diagnosed eating disorders.

> **Eating Disorders (ED)** Disturbances of eating habits or weight-control behavior that can result in significant impairment of physical health or psychosocial functioning.

Clinically diagnosed **eating disorders** are disturbances of eating habits or weight-control behavior that can result in significant impairment of physical health or psychosocial functioning (Smolak et al., 2000; Sudi et al., 2004).

Of course, eating disorders do not occur only in physically active individuals, nor do all or most physically active individuals have eating disorders. However, symptoms of eating disorders are more prevalent among adult elite athletes than nonathletes. In addition, a higher prevalence of eating disorders has been found among athletes competing in sports where leanness is advantageous compared with both athletes competing in sports where leanness is not particularly relevant and controls (Torstveit et al., 2008). Female athletes struggle more with eating disordered behaviors than male athletes, but this may simply be because eating disorders are an under-recognized problem in male athletes. Male athletes are particularly vulnerable in the same categories of sports as females: sports that emphasize aesthetics (gymnastics, dance, figure skating, diving, and body building), sports where low body fat is advantageous (climbing, long-distance running, road cycling, and ski jumping), and sports in which there is a need to make weight (wrestling, some martial arts, rowing, and horseracing). The culture of the latter sports, in particular, encourages bingeing and purging (Baum, 2006). In the past, males were more likely to actually have been overweight or obese before their eating disorders, whereas females more often simply perceived themselves as such (Sundgot-Borgen, 1993b, 1994a; Thompson and Sherman, 1993). More recently, there has been a rise in the number of young males who are preoccupied with their body image. This preoccupation has been labeled "*muscle dysmorphia*" or "the Adonis complex" (Beals, 2003) and is characterized by a preoccupation with being lean and muscular to the point where it interferes with normal food intake, normal life activities, and reasonable exercise levels. Muscle dysmorphia is not listed by the American Psychiatric Association (1994) and has no formal diagnostic criteria. That does not make it any less of a concern, however. Muscle dysmorphia in males often involves both disordered eating and anabolic steroid abuse (Baum, 2006; Goldfield et al., 2006). Not all males with eating disorders exhibit muscle dysmorphia. Pathological weight control and eating disorders are also evident in fitness instructors, including personal trainers (Höglund and Normén, 2002; Thompson and Sherman, 1993). This not only puts these individuals at personal risk but also jeopardizes the healthy attitudes and sound body ideals they should be communicating to their clients.

The American Psychiatric Association (1994) recognizes three major categories of clinically diagnosed eating disorders:

1. Anorexia nervosa (AN)
2. Bulimia nervosa (BN)
3. Eating disorders not otherwise specified (EDNOS)

TABLE 6.9   Diagnostic Criteria and/or Characteristics for Selected Eating Disorders

Anorexia Nervosa	Bulimia Nervosa	Anorexia Athletica
Refusal to maintain body weight above that considered normal for height and age (>15% below), marked self-induced weight loss	Recurrent episodes of binge eating (rapid consumption of large quantities of calorie-dense food, often secretly), feeling of lack of control while bingeing	Fear of weight gain although lean Weight is ≥5% below specified. Muscular development maintains weight above AN threshold. Distorted body image
Intense fear of weight gain or becoming fat despite being underweight	Purging or compensating for bingeing by self-induced vomiting, use of diuretics or laxatives, vigorous exercise, and strict food restriction or fasting	Restricted calorie intake Often broken by planned binges Excessive or compulsive exercise above normal training needs
Severe body dissatisfaction and body image distortion, denial of seriousness of current low body weight	Exhibiting bingeing or inappropriate compensatory behavior at least twice a week for 3 mo	Menstrual dysfunction Delayed puberty Secondary amenorrhea or oligomenorrhea
Endocrine changes manifested by amenorrhea (for at least three consecutive cycles) in females and loss of sexual interest and potency in males	Severe body dissatisfaction, self-evaluation unduly influenced by body shape and weight	Gastrointestinal complaints

‡Absolute criteria have not been agreed upon.

Sources: Based on *American Psychiatric Association (1994) and †Currie and Morse (2005) and Sundgot-Borgen (1994a,b).

The diagnostic criteria for AN and BN are listed in **Table 6.9**. **Anorexia nervosa**, often referred to as the self-starvation syndrome, is characterized by marked self-induced weight loss accompanied by reproductive hormonal changes and an intense fear of fatness. **Bulimia nervosa** is marked by an unrealistic appraisal of body weight and/or shape and is manifested by alternating bingeing and purging behavior. **Eating disorders not otherwise specified** include conditions of disordered eating when the complete criteria for anorexia nervosa or bulimia nervosa are not met. For example, an eating disorder not otherwise specified is diagnosed if all criteria for BN are met except that binges occur less frequently than 2·week⁻¹ or have occurred for less than 3 months. Note that these definitions are from a psychiatric association, not from a nutritional or exercise professional association. Clinical eating disorders are psychiatric conditions that go beyond body weight/shape dissatisfaction and involve more than abnormal weight-control behaviors (Beals and Meyer, 2007). Specifically perfectionism, obsessiveness, harm avoidance, and low self-esteem have been found to accompany AN (Bachner-Melman et al., 2006). Such individuals have trouble identifying and expressing their emotions and have difficulty forming close interpersonal relationships (Beals and Meyer, 2007).

Other eating problems are considered subclinical: They are a problem but do not meet formal diagnostic criteria for an eating disorder or show significant psychopathology. Athletes with eating disorders have been clinically observed to display less psychopathology than nonathletes with eating disorders. For this reason, eating disorders in athletes may differ from eating disorders in nonathletes. The term **anorexia athletica (AA)** has been proposed to describe a subtype of anorexia, a form of EDNOS, or subclinical disorder that affects athletes or other active individuals (Bachner-Melman et al., 2006; Sudi et al., 2004; Sundgot-Borgen, 1994a, b). Anorexia athletica is characterized by a food intake less than that required to support the training regimen and a body weight at least 5% below normal. Additional characteristics of AA are included in **Table 6.9**. Despite close to 25 years of research in this area, no definite criteria have been established for AA.

Individuals suffering from AA may exhibit a variety of symptoms, some of which are common to AN or BN (Bachner-Melman et al., 2006; Sudi et al., 2004; Sundgot-Borgen, 1994a, b). Typically, the initial reduction in body mass/fat by dieting and/or excessive exercising in AA is based on the performance goals, not body appearance or shape issues. Appearance concerns, however, can develop, especially if the athlete is not as successful in an aesthetic sport as anticipated or desired. The drive to lose weight can become a goal in itself, regardless of the negative impact on athletic performance. Weight cycling (repeated weight loss and regain) may occur, based on different seasonal degrees of training or the necessity to make weight weekly for competition. Finally, the abnormal eating behavior generally disappears when the athlete ends participation (Sudi et al., 2004).

The possible lack of a consistent underlying psychopathology and the possibility of reversal on cessation of competition do not mean that AA is not a serious problem or that it can just be ignored. Nor does it mean that an athlete cannot have AN or BN or underlying psychological issues where exercise dependence becomes an addiction, and obsessive-compulsive traits, body dysmorphic disorder, and substance dependence become apparent (Currie and Morse, 2005). Any and all of these conditions may overlap and coexist. AA is serious and it needs to be dealt with.

Risk Factors

The specific causes of eating disorders are unknown (Sundgot-Borgen, 1994a, b). Psychological, genetic, biological, and sociocultural factors have been implicated but not proven. Individuals who are conscientious and achievement-oriented, who seek perfection, but who, at the same time, have a low self-esteem and a high need for approval seem psychologically predisposed for eating disorders. Eating disorders appear to run in families and are more strongly associated in identical than fraternal twins. By the same token, a cultural obsession with thinness may create a social predisposition, although it is not known why some young girls succumb to the pressure while most do not (Leon, 1991; Sundgot-Borgen, 1994a). Sports and exercise for fitness are not to blame for eating disorders (Currie and Morse, 2005). However, the sport/fitness environment emphasizes performance and often demands, in fact or perception, an ideal body size, shape, weight, or composition both as a means to achieving high performance and, in aesthetic sports, as a major part of the performance itself (Thompson and Sherman, 1993). Once a predisposed individual begins a very restrictive diet, a cycling, self-perpetuating, self-reinforcing process begins, and the individual is at great risk for developing an eating disorder.

Sundgot-Borgen (1994b) identified a series of risk factors or trigger conditions for eating disorders. Their study evaluated 522 elite female Norwegian athletes (out of a possible 603 in the entire country). Ninety-two athletes (17%) were found to have AN (N = 7), BN (N = 43), or AA (N = 42). The six risk factors identified included:

1. *Dieting at an early age.* Dieting is a risk factor, especially if recommended by a coach who indicates that losing weight or fat would enable the athlete to improve performance. Thus, the fact that athletes in weight-dependent sports (judo and karate) and esthetic sports (gymnastics, diving, figure skating, and dancing) have the highest incidence of eating disorders is not unexpected (Sundgot-Borgen, 1993a).
2. *Unsupervised dieting.* Athletes rarely receive guidance from someone trained in nutrition and knowledgeable about their sports' requirements. Those who are given such assistance often do not follow the advice.
3. *Lack of acceptance of pubertal changes.* Young female athletes are often distressed at the bodily changes that occur as they mature—particularly menarche and the increasing levels of body fat. Many young athletes are also aware that a delayed menarche is often associated with athletic success (see Chapter 16).
4. *Early sport-specific training.* Children often specialize in a specific sport at an early age. Being a generalist as a child athlete allows more options later—although realistically, that is harder to do if one wishes to compete on an elite national or international level. An individual's somatotype (body type) greatly influences which sports she can successfully compete in. If this influence is disregarded, a young child may select a sport she enjoys (such as gymnastics) only to find that her body outgrows it.
5. *A large increase in training volume accompanied by a significant weight loss.* Athletes do not always spontaneously increase their energy intake when energy expenditure increases. The athlete sees weight loss as good and has no incentive to eat more. Thus, a pattern of eating less and less to lose more and more weight is initiated.
6. *Traumatic events.* Any traumatic event may be a risk factor, but typically, it is associated with an illness or injury that prevents training (and increases the fear of gaining weight) and/or the loss of a coach who the athlete sees as being vital to her career.

The Consequences of Eating Disorders

The consequences of an eating disorder can be dire. At the very least, the individual's nutritional status is compromised. **Figure 6.10** shows a representative sample of nutrient intake in the Norwegian study of elite female athletes described above (Sundgot-Borgen, 1993a). The control group (C) consisted of 30 athletes not classified

Anorexia Nervosa (AN) An eating disorder characterized by marked self-induced weight loss accompanied by reproductive hormonal changes and an intense fear of fatness.

Bulimia Nervosa (BN) An eating disorder marked by an unrealistic appraisal of body weight and/or shape that is manifested by alternating bingeing and purging behavior.

Eating Disorders Not Otherwise Specified (EDNOS) Conditions of disordered eating that do not meet the complete criteria for AN or BN.

Anorexia Athletica (AA) An eating disorder that is characterized by a food intake less than that required to support the training regimen and by a body weight less than 95% of normal.

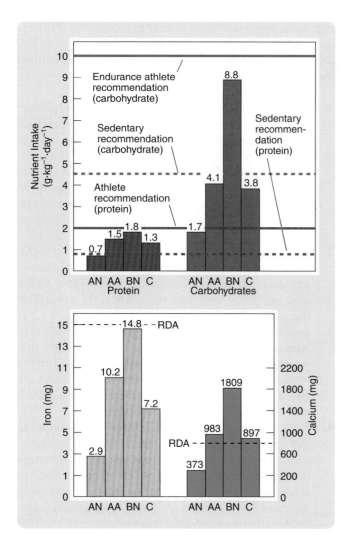

FIGURE 6.10 **Nutrient Intake in Elite Norwegian Female Athletes.**
AN, anorexia nervosa (N = 7); AA, anorexia athletica (N = 43); BN, bulimia nervosa (N = 92), and C = control (N = 30).
Source: Based on data from Sundgot-Borgen, J.: Nutrient intake of female elite athletes suffering from eating disorders. *International Journal of Sport Nutrition.* 3(4):431–442 (1993a).

as at risk for developing an eating disorder. However, 27% of those athletes were on a diet. Except for the bulimic group, all other groups had a lower total energy intake than recommended. The bulimic group's diet also differed in composition from that of the other groups. They ate more fat (30% versus 20%) and less protein (10% versus 20%) than the other groups but an equal amount of carbohydrates. Despite the same percentage of carbohydrates, only the bulimic group took in sufficient amounts of carbohydrates in grams per kilogram per day. Those with AN had the greatest nutritional disturbance. They were simply not ingesting enough of anything.

Although the bulimic group appears to be getting sufficient nutrients in terms of carbohydrates, protein, calcium, and iron, note that these values are prepurging intakes. Most of the BN group and one third of the AA group regularly vomited within 15 minutes of eating. Thus, the nutrients were ingested but they were not absorbed. Individuals who purge by using diuretics or laxatives, in contrast, have minimal caloric loss but lose electrolytes and can become dehydrated.

The loss of electrolytes, especially potassium, can have serious cardiac implications, and dehydration impacts blood pressure levels. Extensive hormonal changes, gastrointestinal complications, skin and hair problems, anemia, disordered thermoregulation, and dental abnormalities are just a few of the other medical problems associated with eating disorders. The impact of disordered eating on menstrual function and bone health is detailed in "The Female Athlete Triad" section in Chapter 16. At times, the medical complications can become severe enough to cause death (Brownell et al., 1992). At the very least, athletes with eating disorders tend to have shorter careers characterized by inconsistent performances and recurrent injuries (Currie and Morse, 2005).

Prevention and Treatment

As a coach, physical educator, athletic trainer, or exercise leader, your role is to be part of the solution, not part of the problem. To this end, it is important to adhere to the following:

1. Encourage youngsters to try a variety of sports. As much as possible, try to guide them into more than one sport experience where they can potentially be successful.

2. Identify realistic, healthy weight goals appropriate for each youngster's stage of maturation. If weight goals are called for at all, provide target weight ranges that allow for growth and development. Allow for individual differences. Male coaches, in particular, must accept that females naturally have a higher percentage of body fat than males, even when both sexes train equally (Thompson and Sherman, 1993).

3. Monitor weight and body composition privately to prevent embarrassment and competitive weight loss. Do not post weights. Avoid all derogatory or teasing remarks about body size, shape, or weight. Coaches should not be directly involved in any decision regarding weight or in actually weighing athletes (International Olympic Committee, 2006; Thompson and Sherman, 1993).

4. Monitor weight and body composition to detect any continued, unwarranted weight loss, weight and fat

fluctuation, or dehydration without always equating weight loss as a positive outcome.

5. Provide proper nutritional guidance—if need be, in conjunction with a nutritionist—and emphasize nutrition for performance, not for weight and fat control.

6. Provide a realistic, progressive training program to which students, athletes, or fitness participants can gradually adjust in terms of energy input and energy output.

7. Provide a realistic, progressive training program to avoid overtraining, illnesses, and injuries.

8. Monitor the relationship between any weight loss and performance. In the early stages of an eating disorder, performance may improve, which in turn may spur the individual on to greater weight loss. However, performance will eventually decline because of malnutrition, depletion of glycogen stores, associated health problems, and the loss of fluid and muscle mass along with decreases in muscular endurance, strength, speed, and coordination.

9. Provide an atmosphere that accepts and supports pubertal changes so that young participants will see them in a positive light.

10. Provide an atmosphere that values the individual and his or her health and well-being above athletic performance or appearance.

11. Be aware of the signs and symptoms of eating disorders. Do not assume that merely educating individuals about eating disorders will be enough to prevent or cure them. Precisely the opposite can occur (Thompson and Sherman, 1993).

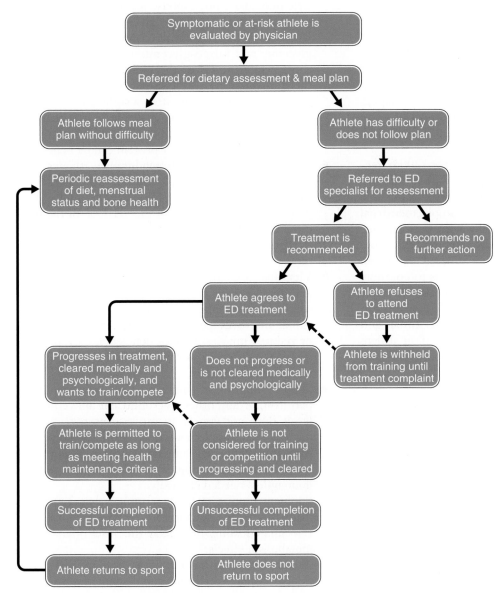

FIGURE 6.11 Decision Tree for Dealing with Athletes Who Exhibit Signs of an Eating Disorder (ED).
Source: International Olympic Committee Medical Commission: Position stand on the female athlete triad (2006). http://multimedia.olympic.org/pdf/en_report_917.pdf. Accessed 8/05/2007.)

12. Seek professional help when dealing with any individual you suspect of having an eating disorder. The first response to being questioned is often denial, and this is best handled by a professional trained in this area. Do not delay. The sooner the treatment is started, the better the chances are for a full recovery (Steen, 1994).

13. Never permit treatment to become secondary to an individual's participation in sports or fitness activities.

Several proactive programs aimed at preventing disordered eating have been studied and shown encouraging results. One such program for fourth to sixth graders, called "Healthy Body Image: Teaching Kids to Eat and Love Their Bodies Too!" consists of 11 lessons. Compared to peers who did not take this class, participants had improved body image, self-image, lifestyle behaviors, awareness of the thinness culture message in the media, understanding of the biology of size and dieting, and awareness of body size prejudices (Kater et al., 2002). Two student-led curricula (Athletes Training and Learning to Avoid Steroids and Athletes Targeting Healthy Exercise and Nutrition Alternatives) for high school males and females, respectively, have shown improved behaviors and intentions related to eating patterns and body-shaping drug use (Elliot et al., 2006; Gabel, 2006). All of these were short-term programs, and follow-up was needed, but they did show promise.

The International Olympic Committee (2006) recommends the decision tree presented in **Figure 6.11** for dealing with athletes with signs or symptoms of a possible eating disorder. Signs may include, for example, menstrual dysfunction, weight loss, suboptimal weight, performance decrement, excessive exercise, stress fractures, etc. Note that this decision tree considers disordered eating an "injury" requiring treatment if the athlete is to continue training and competing. The athlete's health is more important than the athlete's performance. Treatment can be difficult to accept for the athlete whose initial, and often repeated, response is anger. However, if an athlete is diagnosed with disordered eating, treatment is essential (Sherman and Thompson, 2006).

SUMMARY

1. The five goals in an optimal training diet are to:
   a. provide caloric and nutrient requirements
   b. incorporate nutritional practices that promote good health
   c. achieve and maintain optimal body composition and playing weight
   d. promote recovery from training sessions and for physiological adaptations
   e. try variations of precompetition and competition fuel and fluid intake to determine bodily responses

2. A balanced nutritional diet for an adult is composed of sufficient calories to maintain acceptable body weight and composition, with 10–35% protein, 20–35% fat, and 45–65% carbohydrate; the Dietary Reference Intake/Recommended Daily Allowance for vitamins and minerals; and sufficient fluid for hydration. This is also adequate and probably optimal for all but hard-training elite, competitive athletes.

3. Active individuals who are satisfied with their body weight and composition must ingest sufficient calories to balance those expended. This diet should proportionally increase the nutrient intake.

4. For an individual utilizing high levels of carbohydrates in training, $8–10$ $g \cdot kg^{-1} \cdot d^{-1}$ is recommended. This value may increase the intake to 58–68% of carbohydrate.

5. Selection of the type of postexercise CHO should be based on the time available for replenishment and GI. The immediate postexercise feedings should consist of HGI foods to facilitate glycogen replenishment, with the following meals containing both high-glycemic and mixed-glycemic menus when time is short, while the GI of the CHO consumed during the immediate postexercise period might not be as important as simply ingesting a sufficient amount of CHO if a full 24 hours are available. When carbohydrate intake is insufficient (<1.2 $g \cdot kg^{-1} \cdot hr^{-1}$), the addition of amino acids and/or protein can be beneficial.

6. Strength, speed, and ultraendurance athletes may need to consume $1.2–2$ $g \cdot kg^{-1} \cdot d^{-1}$ of protein, up from the RDA of 0.8 $g \cdot kg^{-1} \cdot d^{-1}$ for sedentary adults. This increased intake should not exceed 15% of the total caloric intake.

7. A high-fat diet has no performance advantage for most individuals.

8. Vitamins are important for the production of energy. However, there is no evidence that vitamin supplementation in an adequately nourished individual improves performance, speeds up recovery, or reduces injuries. Where deficiencies are present, supplementation to normal physiological levels can improve performance.

9. Supplementation of zinc, chromium, selenium, copper, iron, or any other micronutrient above normal levels does not appear to increase exercise performance. Iron supplementation given to individuals with iron deficiency anemia consistently improves performance, but supplementation should not be done unless needed clinically.

10. Supplementation of the macrominerals calcium and magnesium does not increase exercise performance. Phosphate loading may delay the onset of anaerobic metabolism effects.

11. A complete nutritional analysis by a trained nutritionist should precede any supplementation to determine need and safety.

12. The five goals of an optimal competitive diet are to:
    a. ensure adequate fuel supplies in the pre-event time span
    b. ensure adequate fuel supplies during the event, regardless of its duration
    c. facilitate temperature regulation by prevention of dehydration
    d. achieve desired weight classifications while maintaining fuel and water supplies
    e. avoid gastrointestinal discomfort during competition

13. Carbohydrate loading is beneficial for individuals competing in endurance events of at least 60–90 minutes at 65–85% VO_2max.

14. The modified carbohydrate-loading technique in which an individual increases the percentage of carbohydrate ingested from 50 to 70% while gradually tapering training the week before competition is safe and effective.

15. The simplified carbohydrate-loading technique requires only a short supramaximal exercise bout followed by approximately 90% carbohydrate ingestion for 24 hours to achieve glycogen supercompensation.

16. A 200–500-kcal light meal composed primarily of low-glycemic index carbohydrate and accompanied by fluids is recommended 4–6 hours before competition; 50 g CHO + 10 g PRO may be ingested closer to the event. During prolonged exercise, either moderate or HGI foods are suggested. Ingestion of CHO during endurance events negates the effect of the consumption of preexercise LGI meals.

17. Carbohydrate beverages ingested in small amounts (200–400 mL) at 15–30-minute intervals during endurance activity can prevent a decline in glucose and delay fatigue. Beverages containing 6–8% of mixed carbohydrate type are recommended for optimal benefit. All carbohydrates ingested during an event should have a high glycemic index.

18. Three types of eating disorders are of great concern for personnel working with active individuals: anorexia nervosa, bulimia nervosa, and anorexia athletica. Although there are technical differences among the three disorders, all involve a restriction of food intake or a purging of food ingested in a binge, a desire for more and more weight loss, and a denial of having a problem.

19. The exact cause of eating disorders is unknown. More athletes than nonathletes suffer from eating disorders, and most cases occur in sports where low weight gives a competitive advantage, in aesthetic sports, or in sports requiring weight classifications. Far more females than males have eating disorders, but prevalence is increasing in males.

20. Personnel working with active individuals between the ages of 10 and 25 should be aware of situations that might trigger an eating disorder, avoid practices that increase the risk, identify problems at an early state, and facilitate appropriate therapy.

REVIEW QUESTIONS

1. List the goals for nutrition during training and the goals for nutrition during competition. Explain why they are different.

2. Make a table comparing a balanced diet for a sedentary individual and one for an active individual. Include caloric intake, percentages, and grams per kilogram per day recommendations for the major nutrients, as well as similarities or differences in vitamin, mineral, and fluid ingestion.

3. Define the GI, and describe how foods are divided into high, moderate, and low categories. Using the GI, design an ideal snack to be eaten approximately 30 minutes after a century bike ride (100 mi), and design an ideal snack to be eaten during a day of hiking on the Appalachian Trail. Explain your choices.

4. Discuss the positive and negative aspects of a high-carbohydrate diet.

5. Discuss the situations in which an increase in protein above the RDA is advisable and situations in which such an increase is not advisable.

6. Describe a training situation and the theory behind when fat intake can be too low in that situation.

7. Compare the theory behind the use of carbohydrate loading for endurance athletes with the theory behind the use of carbohydrate loading for body builders.

8. Compare the classic, modified, and simplified techniques of carbohydrate loading in terms of diet and exercise for endurance athletes. Explain the reasons for the modifications.

9. Make a table of a comprehensive fluid and nutrient intake for pre-event, during the event, and postevent diets for a football player and a triathlete.

10. Define and list the criteria/characteristics of anorexia nervosa, bulimia nervosa, and anorexia athletica.

11. Identify the risk factors for developing an eating disorder. Prepare a set of guidelines that could be used to counteract these risk factors or deal with the disorder early in its progression.

12. Discuss possible consequences of eating disorders.

For further review and additional study tools, visit the website at http://thePoint.lww.com/Plowman4e ✳ ▶

REFERENCES

Allen, L. H., E. A. Oddoye, & S. Margen: Protein-induced hypercalciuria: A longer term study. *The American Journal of Clinical Nutrition.* 32:741–749 (1979).

American College of Sports Medicine: Position stand: Exercise and fluid replacement. *Medicine & Science in Sports & Exercise.* 39(2):377–390 (2007).

American College of Sports Medicine, American Dietetic Association, & Dietitians of Canada: Nutrition and athletic performance. *Medicine & Science in Sports & Exercise*. 41:3: 709–731 (2009).

American Dietetic Association: Nutrition for physical fitness and athletic performance for adults: Technical support paper. *Journal of the American Dietetic Association*. 87(7):934–939 (1987).

American Psychiatric Association: *Diagnostic and Statistical Manual of Mental Disorders* (4th edition). Washington, DC: American Psychiatric Association (1994).

Applegate, L.: Taking the bar. *Runner's World*. 33(10):24–28 (1998).

Bachner-Melman, R., A. H. Zohar, R. P. Ebstein, Y. Elizur, & N. Constantini: How anorexic-like are the symptom and personality profiles of esthetic athletes? *Medicine & Science in Sports & Exercise*. 38:628–636 (2006).

Balon, T. W., J. F. Horowitz, & K. M. Fitzsimmons: Effects of carbohydrate loading and weight-lifting on muscle girth. *International Journal of Sports Nutrition*. 2(4):328–334 (1992).

Baum, A.: Eating disorders in the male athlete. *Sports Medicine*. 36(1):1–6 (2006).

Beals, K. A.: Mirror, mirror on the wall, who is the most muscular one of all? Disordered eating and body image disturbances in male athletes. *ACSM'S Health and Fitness Journal*. 7(2):6–11 (2003).

Beals, K. A., & N. L. Meyer: Female athlete triad update. *Clinics in Sports Medicine*. 26:69–89 (2007).

Belko, A. Z.: Vitamins and exercise—an update. *Medicine and Science in Sports and Exercise*. 19(5 Suppl.):S191–S196 (1987).

Bergstrom, J., L. Hermansen, E. Hultman, & B. Saltin: Diet, muscle glycogen and physical performance. *Acta Physiologica Scandinavica*. 7:140–150 (1967).

Betts, J. A., & C. Williams: Short-term recovery from prolonged exercise: Exploring the potential for protein ingestion to accentuate the benefits of carbohydrate supplements. *Sports Medicine*. 40(1):941–969 (2010).

Bird, S. P., K. M. Tarpenning, & F. E. Marino: Independent and combined effects of liquid carbohydrate/essential amino acid ingestion on hormonal and muscular adaptations following resistance training in untrained men. *European Journal of Applied Physiology*. 97:225–238 (2006).

Blom, P. C. S., A. T. Hostmark, O. Vaage, K. R. Kardel, & S. Maehlum: Effects of different post-exercise sugar diets on the rate of muscle glycogen synthesis. *Medicine and Science in Sports and Exercise*. 19(5):491–496 (1987).

Britschgi, F., & G. Zünd: Body building: Hypokalemia and hypophosphatemia. *Schweizerische Medizinische Wochenschrift*. 121(33):1163–1165 (1991).

Brotherhood, J. R.: Nutrition and sports performance. *Sports Medicine*. 1:350–389 (1984).

Brownell, K. D., J. Rodin, & J. H. Wilmore: *Eating, Body Weight and Performance in Athletics: Disorders of Modern Society*. Philadelphia, PA: Lea & Febiger (1992).

Burke, L. M., & J. A. Hawley: Effects of short-term fat adaptation on metabolism and performance of prolonged exercise. *Medicine & Science in Sports & Exercise*. 34(9):1492–1498 (2002).

Burke, L. M., & B. Kiens: "Fat adaptation" for athletic performance: The nail in the coffin? *Journal of Applied Physiology*. 100:7–8 (2006).

Burke, L. M., & R. S. D. Read: Sport nutrition: Approaching the nineties. *Sports Medicine*. 8(2):80–100 (1989).

Burke, L. M., G. R. Collier, & M. Hargreaves: Muscle glycogen storage after prolonged exercise: Effect of the glycemic index of carbohydrate feedings. *Journal of Applied Physiology*. 75(2):1019–1023 (1993).

Bussau, V. A., T. J. Fairchild, A. Rao, P. Steele, & P. A. Fournier: Carbohydrate loading in human muscle: An improved 1 day protocol. *European Journal of Applied Physiology*. 87(3):290–295 (2002).

Campbell, B., R. B. Kreider, T. Ziegenfuss, P. LaBounty, M. Robers, D. Burke, J. Landis, H. Lopez, & J. Antonio: International Society of Sports Nutrition position stand: Protein and exercise. *Journal of the International Society of Sports Nutrition*. 4(1):8–14 (2007).

Campbell, W. W., & R. A. Anderson: Effects of aerobic exercise and training on the trace minerals chromium, zinc and copper. *Sports Medicine*. 4:9–18 (1987).

Cheuvront, S. N.: The Zone diet and athletic performance. *Sports Medicine*. 27(4):213–228 (1999).

Cheuvront, S. N.: The Zone Diet phenomenon: A closer look at the science behind the claims. *Journal of the American College of Nutrition*. 22(1):9–17 (2003).

Clarkson, P. M.: Minerals: Exercise performance and supplementation in athletes. *Journal of Sports Sciences*. 9:91–116 (1991a).

Clarkson, P. M.: *Tired Blood: Iron Deficiency in Athletes and Effects of Iron Supplementation. Sports Science Exchange*, vol. 3, no. 28. Chicago, IL: Gatorade Sports Science Institute (1990).

Clarkson, P. M.: *Trace Mineral Requirements for Athletes: To Supplement or Not to Supplement. Sports Science Exchange*, vol. 4, no. 33. Chicago, IL: Gatorade Sports Science Institute (1991b).

Coleman, E.: *Sports Drink Update. Sports Science Exchange*, vol. 1, no. 5. Chicago, IL: Gatorade Sports Science Institute (1988).

Coombes, J. S., & K. L. Hamilton: The effectiveness of commercially available sports drinks. *Sports Medicine*. 29(3):181–209 (2000).

Costill, D. L.: Carbohydrates for exercise: Dietary demands for optimal performance. *International Journal of Sports Medicine*. 9(1):1–18 (1988).

Coyle, E. F.: Timing and method of increased carbohydrate intake to cope with heavy training, competition and recovery. *Journal of Sport Sciences*. (9):29–52 (1991).

Coyle, E. F., & E. Coyle: Carbohydrates that speed recovery from training. *The Physician and Sports Medicine*. 21(2): 111–123 (1993).

Cribb, P. J., & A. Hayes: Effects of supplement timing and resistance exercise on skeletal muscle hypertrophy. *Medicine & Science in Sports & Exercise*. 38(11):1918–1925 (2006).

Currie, A. & E. D. Morse: Eating disorders in athletes: Managing the risks. *Clinics in Sports Medicine*. 24:871–883 (2005).

Décombaz, J., R. Jentjens, R. M. Ith, E. Scheurer, T. Buehler, A. Jeukendrup, & C. Boesch: Fructose and galactose enhance postexercise human liver glycogen synthesis. *Medicine & Science in Sports & Exercise*. 43(10):1964–1971 (2011).

DeMarco, H. D., K. P. Sucher, C. J. Cisar, & G. E. Butterfield: Pre-exercise carbohydrate meals: Application of the glycemic index. *Medicine & Science in Exercise & Sports*. 31(1): 164–170 (1999).

Dietary Guidelines for Americans 2010. http://www.dietary-guidelines.gov. Accessed 2/28/2012.

Donaldson, C. M., T. L. Perry, & M. C. Rose: Glycemic index and endurance performance. *International Journal of Sport Nutrition and Exercise Metabolism.* 20:154–165 (2010).

Duchan, E., N. D. Patel, & C. Feucht: Energy drinks: A review of use and safety for athletes. *The Physician and Sportsmedicine.* 38(2):171–179 (2010).

Eisenstein, J., S. B. Roberts, G. Dallal, & E. Saltzman: High-protein weight-loss diets: Are they safe and do they work? A review of the experimental and epidemiologic data. *Nutrition Reviews.* 60(7 Pt 1):189–200 (2002).

Elliot, D. L., E. L. Moe, L. Goldberg, C. A. DeFrancesco, M. B. Durham, & H. Hix-Small: Definition and outcome of a curriculum to prevent disordered eating and body-shaping drug use. *The Journal of School Health.* 76(2):67–73 (2006).

Evans, W. J.: Protein nutrition, exercise and aging. *Journal of the American College of Nutrition.* 23(6):601S–609S (2004).

Fairchild, T. J., S. Fletcher, P. Steele, C. Goodman, B. Dawson, & P. A. Fournier: Rapid carbohydrate loading after a short bout of near maximal-intensity exercise. *Medicine & Science in Sports & Exercise.* 34(6):980–986 (2002).

Fielding, R. A., & J. Parkington: What are the dietary protein requirements of physically active individuals? New evidence on the effects of exercise on protein utilization during post-exercise recovery. *Nutrition in Clinical Care.* 5(4):191–196 (2002).

Fleming, J., M. J. Sharman, N. G. Avery, et al.: Endurance capacity and high-intensity exercise performance responses to a high fat diet. *International Journal of Sport Nutrition and Exercise Metabolism.* 13(4):466–478 (2003).

Foster-Powell, K., S. H. A. Holt, & J. C. Brand-Miller: International table of glycemic index and glycemic load values: 2002. *The American Journal of Clinical Nutrition.* 76:5–56 (2002).

Fox, A. K., A. E. Kaufman, & J. F. Horowitz: Adding fat calories to meals after exercise does not alter glucose tolerance. *Journal of Applied Physiology.* 97(1):11–16 (2004).

Gabel, K. A.: Special nutritional concerns for the female athlete. *Current Sports Medicine Reports.* 5:187–191 (2006).

Gleeson, M.: Interrelationship between physical activity and branched-chain amino acids. *The Journal of Nutrition.* 135:1591S–1595S (2005).

Goldfield, G. S., A. G. Blouin, & D. B. Woodside: Body image, binge eating, and bulimia nervosa in male bodybuilders. *Canadian Journal of Psychiatry.* 51(3):160–168 (2006).

Goss, F. L., & C. Karam: The effects of glycogen supercompensation on the electrocardiographic response during exercise. *Research Quarterly for Exercise and Sport.* 58(1):68–71 (1987).

Havemann, L., S. J. West, J. H. Goedecke, I. A. Macdonald, A. St. Clair Gibson, T. D. Noakes, & E. V. Lambert: Fat adaptation followed by carbohydrate loading compromises high-intensity sprint performance. *Journal of Applied Physiology.* 100:194–202 (2006).

Hawley, J. A., & J. M. Burke: Effect of meal frequency and timing on physical performance. *British Journal of Nutrition.* 77(Suppl. 1):S91–S103 (1997).

Hawley, J. A., E. J. Schabort, T. D. Noakes, & S. C. Dennis: Carbohydrate-loading and exercise performance. *Sports Medicine.* 24(2):73–81 (1997).

Hawley, J. A., K. D. Tipton, M. L. Millard-Stafford: Promoting training adaptations through nutritional interventions. *Journal of Sport Sciences.* 24(7):709–721 (2006).

Haymes, E. M.: Protein, vitamins, and iron. In Williams M. H. (ed.): *Ergogenic Aids in Sports.* Champaign, IL: Human Kinetics, 27–55 (1983).

Helge, J. W.: Adaptation to a fat-rich diet: Effects on endurance performance in humans. *Sports Medicine.* 30(5):347–357 (2000).

Helge, J. W.: Long-term fat diet adaptation effects on performance, training capacity, and fat utilization. *Medicine & Science in Sports & Exercise.* 34(9):1499–1504 (2002).

Höglund, K., & L. Normén: A high exercise load is linked to pathological weight control behavior and eating disorders in female fitness instructors. *Scandinavian Journal of Medicine and Science in Sports.* 12:261–275 (2002).

International Food Information Council: Dietary Reference Intakes: An update. http://ific.org/publications/other/driupdateom.cfm?renderfor print=1. Accessed 8/06/08.

International Olympic Committee Medical Commission: Position stand on the female athlete triad. http://multimedia.olympic.org/pdf/en_report_917.pdf. Accessed 8/05/2007.

Jacobs, K. A., D. R. Paul, R. J. Geor, K. W. Hinchcliff, & W. M. Sherman.: Dietary composition influences short-term endurance training-induced adaptations of substrate partitioning during exercise. *International Journal of Sport Nutrition and Exercise Metabolism.* 14(1):38–61 (2004).

James, A. P., M. Lorraine, D. Cullen, C. Goodman, B. Dawson, T. N. Palmer, & P. A. Fournier: Muscle glycogen supercompensation: Absence of a gender-related difference. *European Journal of Applied Physiology.* 85(6):533–538 (2001).

Jentjens, R., & A. E. Jeukendrup: Determinants of Post-exercise glycogen synthesis during short term recovery. *Sports Medicine.* 33(2):117–144 (2003).

Jeukendrup, A.: Carbohydrate supplementation during exercise: Does it help? How much is too much? *Gatorade Sports Science Institute Sports Science Exchange.* 106:1–5 (2007).

Jenkins, D. J. A., D. M. Thomas, M. S. Wolever, et al.: Glycemic index of foods: A physiological basis for carbohydrate exchange. *American Journal of Clinical Nutrition.* 34:362–366 (1981).

Kater, K., J. Rohwer, & K. Londre: Evaluation of an upper elementary school program to prevent body image, eating and weight concerns. *Journal of School Health.* 72:199–205 (2002).

Kilic, M., A. K. Baltaci, & M. Gunay: Effect of zinc supplementation on hematological parameters in athletes. *Biological Trace Element Research.* 100(1):31–38 (2004).

Kilic, M., A. K. Baltaci, M. Gunay, H. Gökbel, N. Okudan, & I. Cicioglu: The effect of exhaustion exercise on thyroid hormones and testosterone levels of elite athletes receiving oral zinc. *Neuro Endocrinology Letters.* 27(1–2):247–252 (2006).

Kreider, R. B., V. Miriel, & E. Bertun: Amino acid supplementation and exercise performance: An analysis of the proposed ergogenic value. *Sports Medicine.* 16(3):190–209 (1993).

Kreider, R. B., C. D. Wilborn, L. Taylor, B. Campbell, A. L. lmada, R. Collins, et al.: ISSN exercise & sport nutrition review: Research & recommendations. *Journal of the International Society of Sports Nutrition.* 7:7–50 (2010).

Kroculick, S. T.: Carb loading: How to look full and ripped on contest day. *Ironman.* December:152–153 (1988).

Lambert, C. P., L. L. Frank, & W. J. Evans: Macronutrient considerations for the sport of bodybuilding. *Sports Medicine.* 34 (5):317–327 (2004).

Leaf, A., & K. B. Frisa: Eating for health or for athletic performance? *The American Journal of Clinical Nutrition.* 49: 1066–1069 (1989).

Lefavi, R. G., R. A. Anderson, R. E. Keith, G. D. Wilson, J. L. McMillan, & M. H. Stone: Efficacy of chromium supplementation in athletes: Emphasis on anabolism. *International Journal of Sports Nutrition.* 2(2):111–122 (1992).

Lemon, P. W. R.: Beyond the Zone: Protein needs of active individuals. *Journal of the American College of Nutrition.* 19(5):513S–521S (2000).

Lemon, P. W. R.: Effects of exercise on protein requirements. *Journal of Sports Sciences.* 9:53–70 (1991).

Lemon, P. W. R.: Influence of Dietary Protein and Total Energy Intake on Strength Improvement. Sports Science Exchange, 2(14). Chicago: Gatorade Sports Science Institute (1989a).

Lemon, P. W. R.: Nutrition for muscular development of young athletes. In Gisolfi, C. V, & D. R. Lamb (eds.): *Perspectives in Exercise Science and Sports Medicine.* Indianapolis, IN: Benchmark Press, 369–400 (1989b).

Lemon, P. W. R., & F. J. Nagle: Effects of exercise on protein and amino acid metabolism. *Medicine and Science in Sports and Exercise.* 13(3):141–149 (1981).

Leon, G. R.: Eating disorders in female athletes. *Sports Medicine.* 12(4):219–227 (1991).

Lukaski, H. C., W. A. Siders, & J. G. Penland: Chromium picolinate supplementation in women: Effects on body weight, composition, and iron status. *Nutrition.* 23(3):187–195 (2007).

Lukaski, H. C.: Low dietary zinc decreases erythrocyte carbonic anhydrase activities and impairs cardiorespiratory function in men during exercise. *The American Journal of Clinical Nutrition.* 81(5):1045–1051 (2005).

Lukaski, H. C.: Vitamin and mineral status: Effects on physical performance. *Nutrition.* 20(7–8):632–644 (2004).

Lunn, W. R., S. M. Pasiakos, M. R. Colletto, K. E. Karfonta, J. W. Carbone, J. M. Anderson, & N. R. Rodriguez: Chocolate milk and endurance exercise recovery: Protein balance, glycogen, and performance. *Medicine & Science in Sports & Exercise.* 44(4):682–691 (2012).

Manninen, A. H.: Hyperinsulinaemia, hyperaminoacemaemia and post-exercise muscle anabolism: The search for the optimal recovery drink. *British Journal of Sports Medicine.* 40(11):900–905 (2006).

Manore, M. M.: Carbohydrate: Friend or Foe? Part II: Dietary carbohydrate and changes in blood glucose. *ACSM's Health and Fitness Journal.* 6(3):26–29 (2002).

Manore, M. M.: Energy bars: Picking the right one for you. *ACSM's Health and Fitness Journal.* 4 (5):33–35 (2000).

Manore, M. M., M. Mason, & I. Skoog: Applying the concepts of glycemic index and glycemic load to active individuals. *ACSM's Health and Fitness Journal.* 8(5):21–23 (2004).

Margaritis, I., A. S. Rousseau, I. Hininger, S. Palazzetti, J. Arnaud, & A. M. Roussel: Increase in selenium requirements with physical activity loads in well-trained athletes is not linear. *Biofactors.* 23(1):45–55 (2005).

McDonald, R., & C. L. Keen: Iron, zinc and magnesium nutrition and athletic performance. *Sports Medicine.* 5:171–184 (1988).

Milias, G. A., T. Nomikos, E. Fragopoulou, S. Athanasopoulos, & S. Antonopoulou: Effects of baseline serum levels of Se on markers of eccentric exercise-induced muscle injury. *Biofactors.* 26(3):161–170 (2006).

Millard-Stafford, M., W. L. Childers, S. A. Conger, A. J. Kampfer, & S. A. Rahnert: Recovery nutrition: Timing and composition after endurance exercise. *Current Sports Medicine Reports.* 7(4):193–201 (2008).

Nemet, D., & A. Eliakim: Pediatric sports nutrition: an update. *Current Opinion in Clinical Nutrition and Metabolic Care.* 12(3):304–309 (2009).

Neufer, P. D., D. L. Costill, M. G. Flynn, J. P. Kirwan, J. B. Mitchell, & J. Houmard: Improvements in exercise performance: Effects of carbohydrate feedings and diet. *Journal of Applied Physiology.* 62(3):983–988 (1987).

Newsholme, E. A., & A. R. Leech: *Biochemistry for the Medical Sciences.* New York, NY: John Wiley & Sons (1983).

Nielsen, F. H., & H. C. Lukaski.: Update on the relationship between magnesium and exercise. *Magnesium Research.* 19(3):180–190 (2006).

Nieman, D. C.: *Fitness and Sports Medicine: An Introduction.* Palo Alto, CA: Bull Publishing (1990).

O'Reilly, J., S. H. S. Wong, & Y. Chen: Glycaemic index, glycaemic load and exercise performance. *Sports Medicine.* 40(1):27–39 (2010).

Pascoe, D. D., & L. B. Gladden: Muscle glycogen resynthesis after short-term, high intensity exercise and resistance exercise. *Sports Medicine.* 21(2):98–118 (1996).

Paul, G. L.: Dietary protein requirements of physically active individuals. *Sports Medicine.* 8(3):154–176 (1989).

Pfeiffer, B., T. Stellingwerff, E. Zaltas, & A. E. Jeukendrup: CHO oxidation from a CHO gel compared with a drink during exercise. *Medicine & Science in Sports & Exercise.* 42(11):2038–2045 (2010a).

Pfeiffer, B., T. Stellingwerff, E. Zaltas, & A. E. Jeukendrup: Oxidation of solid versus liquid CHO sources during exercise. *Medicine & Science in Sports & Exercise.* 42(11): 2030–2037 (2010b).

Phillips, S. M.: Protein metabolism and exercise: Potential sex-based differences. In Tarnopolsky, M. (ed.): *Gender Differences in Metabolism: Practical and Nutritional Implications.* Boca Raton, FL: CRC Press, 155–178 (1999).

Phillips, S. M., J. Sproule, & A. P. Turner: Carbohydrate ingestion during team games exercise: Current knowledge and areas for future research. *Sports Medicine.* 41(7):559–585 (2011).

Phillips, S. M., & L. J. C. Van Loon: Dietary protein for athletes: From requirements to optimum adaptation. *Journal of Sports Sciences.* 29(S1):S29–S38 (2011).

Pikosky, M. A., P. C. Gaine, W. F. Martin, K. C. Grabarz, A. A. Ferrando, R. R. Wolfe, & N. R. Rodriguez: Aerobic exercise training increases skeletal muscle protein turnover in healthy adults at rest. *Journal of Nutrition.* 136:379–383 (2006).

Poole, C., C. Wilborn, L. Taylor, % C. Kerksick: The role of post-exercise nutrient administration on muscle protein synthesis and glycogen synthesis. *Journal of Sports Science and Medicine.* 9:354–363 (2010).

Price, T. B., S. Krishnan-Sarin, & D. L. Rothman: Smoking impairs muscle recovery from exercise. *American Journal of Physiology Endocrinology and Metabolism.* 285:E116–E122 (2003).

Rauch, H. G. L., A. St. Clair Gibson, E. V. Lambert, & T. D. Noakes: A signaling role for muscle glycogen in the regulation of pace during prolonged exercise. *British Journal of Sports Medicine.* 39:34–38 (2005).

Robinson, Y., E. Cristancho, & D. Boning: Intravascular hemolysis and mean red blood cell age in athletes. *Medicine & Science in Sports & Exercise.* 38(3):480–483 (2006).

Schumacher, Y. O., A. Schmidt, D. Grathwoho, D. Bültermann, & A. Berg: Hematological indices and iron status in athletes of various sports and performances. *Medicine & Science in Sports & Exercise.* 34(5):869–875 (2002).

Sears, B.: *Enter the Zone: A Dietary Road Map to Lose Weight Permanently, Reset Your Genetic Code, Prevent Disease, Achieve Maximal Physical Performance, Enhance Mental Productivity.* New York, NY: Harper Collins (1995).

Sedlock, D. A.: The latest on carbohydrate loading: A practical approach. *Current Sports Medicine Reports.* 7(4):209–213 (2008).

Seebohar, B.: Sports drinks for athletes. http://coaching. usolympicteam.com/coaching/kpub.nsf/v/31nov07. Accessed 11/07/07.

Sherman, R. T., & R. A. Thompson: Practical use of the International Olympic Committee medical commission position stand on the female athlete triad: A case example. *International Journal of Eating Disorders.* 39(3):193–201 (2006).

Sherman, W. M.: Carbohydrates, muscle glycogen, and muscle glycogen supercompensation. In Williams, M. H. (ed.): *Ergogenic Aids in Sport.* Champaign, IL: Human Kinetics, 3–26 (1983).

Sherman, W. M.: *Muscle Glycogen Supercompensation During the Week Before Athletic Competition. Sports Science Exchange,* 2(16). Chicago, IL: Gatorade Sports Science Institute (1989).

Sherman, W. M., & N. Leenders: Fat loading: The next magic bullet? *International Journal of Sport Nutrition.* 5:S1–S12 (1995).

Singh, A., P. A. Pelletier, & P. A. Deuster: Dietary requirements for ultraendurance exercise. *Sports Medicine.* 18(5):301–308 (1994).

Smolak, L., S. K. Murnen, & A. E. Ruble: Female athletes and eating problems: A meta-analysis. *The International Journal of Eating Disorders.* 27:371–380 (2000).

Steen, S. N.: Nutrition for young athelets: special considerations. *Sports Medicine.* 17(7):152–162 (1994).

Stevenson, E. J., C. Williams, L. E. Mash, B. Phillips, & M. L. Nute: Influence of high-carbohydrate mixed meals with different glycemic indexes on substrate utilization during subsequent exercise in women. *The American Journal of Clinical Nutrition.* 84:354–360 (2006).

Sudi, K., K. Öttl, D. Payeri, P. Baumgartl, K. Tauschmann, & W. Müller: Anorexia Athletica. *Nutrition.* 20:657–661 (2004).

Sundgot-Borgen, J.: Eating disorders in female athletes. *Sports Medicine.* 17(3):176–188 (1994a).

Sundgot-Borgen, J.: Nutrient intake of female elite athletes suffering from eating disorders. *International Journal of Sport Nutrition.* 3(4):431–442 (1993a).

Sundgot-Borgen, J.: Prevalence of eating disorders in elite female athletes. *International Journal of Sport Nutrition.* 3(1):29–40 (1993b).

Sundgot-Borgen, J.: Risk and trigger factors for the development of eating disorders in female elite athletes. *Medicine and Science in Sports and Exercise.* 26(4):414–419 (1994b).

Tarnopolsky, M. A.: Nutritional consideration in the aging athlete. *Clinical Journal of Sport Medicine.* 18(6):531–538 (2008).

Tarnopolsky, M. A., J. D. MacDougall, & S. A. Atkinson: Influence of protein intake and training status on nitrogen balance and lean body mass. *Journal of Applied Physiology.* 64(1):187–193 (1988).

Thomas, K., P. Morris, & E. Stevenson: Improved endurance capacity following chocolate milk consumption compare with 2 commercially available sports drinks. *Applied Physiology of Nutrition and Metabolism.* 34:78–82 (2009).

Thompson, R. A., & R. T. Sherman: *Helping Athletes with Eating Disorders.* Champaign, IL: Human Kinetics (1993).

Torstveit, M. K., J. H. Rosenvinge, & J. Sundgot-Borgen: Prevalence of eating disorders and the predictive power of risk models in female elite athletes: A controlled study. *Scandinavian Journal of Medicine and Science in Sports.* 18:108–118 (2008).

U.S. Department of Agriculture, Agriculture Research Service, Dietary Guidelines Advisory Committee: Report of the Dietary Guidelines Advisory Committee on the Dietary Guidelines for Americans, 1995, to the Secretary of Health and Human Services and the Secretary of Agriculture, 58 pp. (1995).

U.S. Food and Drug Administration: How to understand and use the nutrition facts label. http://www.cfsan.fda.gov/~dms/foodlab.html. Accessed 8/06/08.

Vandenbogaerde, T. J., & W. G. Hopkins: Effect of acute carbohydrate supplementation on endurance performance: A meta-analysis. *Sports Medicine* 41:773–792 (2011).

vander Beek, E. J.: Vitamins and endurance training: Food for running or faddish claims? *Sports Medicine* 2:175–197 (1985).

vander Beek, E. J.: Vitamin supplementation and physical exercise performance. *Journal of Sports Sciences.* 9:77–89 (1991).

Vincent, J. B.: The potential value and toxicity of chromium picolinate as a nutritional supplement, weight loss agent and muscle development agent. *Sports Medicine.* 33(3):213–230 (2003).

Vogt, M., A. Puntschart, H. Howald, et al.: Effects of dietary fat on muscle substrates, metabolism, and performance in athletes. *Medicine & Science in Sports & Exercise.* 35(6):952–960 (2003).

Volek, J. S.: Influence of nutrition on responses to resistance training. *Medicine & Science in Sports & Exercise.* 36(4):689–696 (2004).

Volpe, S. L.: Minerals as ergogenic aids. *Current Sports Medicine Reports.* 7(4):224–229 (2008).

von Duvillard, S. P., P. J. Arciero, T. Tietjen-Smith, & K. Alford: Sports drinks, exercise training, and competition. *Current Sports Medicine Reports.* 7(4):202–208 (2008).

Walton, P., & E. C. Rhodes: Glycaemic index and optimal performance. *Sports Medicine.* 23(3):164–172 (1997).

Williams, C., & L. Serratosa: Nutrition on match day. *Journal of Sports Sciences.* 24(7):687–697 (2006).

Wolever, T. M. S.: The glycemic index. In G. H. Bourne (ed.): Aspects of some vitamins, minerals and enzymes in health and disease. *World Review of Nutrition and Dietetics.* 62:120–185 (1990).

Wolfe, R. R.: Skeletal muscle protein metabolism and resistance exercise. *The Journal of Nutrition.* 136:525S–528S (2006).

Wong, H. S., & S. Chung: Glycemic Index: An educational tool for health and fitness professionals? *ACSM's Health and Fitness Journal.* 7(6):13–19 (2003).

Wu, C. L., & C. Williams: A low glycemic index meal before exercise improves endurance running capacity in men. *International Journal of Sport Nutrition and Exercise Metabolism.* 16(5):510–527 (2006).

Wu, C. L., C. Nicholas, C. Williams, A. Took, & L. Hardy: The influence of high-carbohydrate meals with different glycaemic indices on substrate utilization during subsequent exercise. *British Journal of Nutrition.* 90:1049–1056 (2003).

Zoller, H., & W. Vogel: Iron supplementation in athletes—first do no harm. *Nutrition.* 20(7–8):615–619 (2004).

7

Body Composition: Determination and Importance

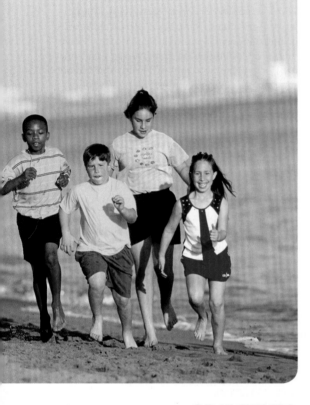

OBJECTIVES

After studying the chapter, you should be able to:

> Detail the extent of the "obesity epidemic."

> Describe the technique of hydrostatic weighing (densitometry) and explain its theoretical basis.

> Calculate body density and percent body fat.

> Discuss variations in the basic assumptions of densitometry related to children, adolescents, and older adults, and describe the practical meaning of these variations.

> List and identify the strengths and weaknesses of the field estimates of body composition.

> Compare the percent body fat estimated by skinfold and bioelectrical impedance measurements with the percent body fat determined by hydrostatic weighing.

> Contrast the percent body fat and the patterns of fat distribution in an average adult male and female.

> Differentiate between overweight and obesity.

> Describe what happens to adipose cells in obesity and the major fat distribution patterns.

> List and discuss the health risks of being overweight or obese and the impact of physical fitness on these risks.

Introduction

Answer the following questions to yourself. Is your body weight just right, a little high, very high, a little low, or very low? Is your percent body fat (%BF) just right, a little high, very high, a little low, or very low? Do you like how you look in a bathing suit? What mental images did you have as you answered these questions?

If you are a female, chances are that regardless of the reality of your body weight, composition, and shape, you feel that your values are too high and you are dissatisfied with how you look. You are probably incorrect in your assessment, but you are certainly not alone. For example, in one study (Lutter, 1994), active women were shown images of five individuals who were 20% underweight, 10% underweight, average weight and size, 10% overweight, and 20% overweight. The subjects were asked to select which image they would like to look like. Only 14% wanted the average shape, 44% wanted to be 10% underweight, and 38% wanted to be 20% underweight!

These feelings are, of course, largely a result of cultural expectations. There have been times in Western civilization (e.g., in the 17th century) when plumpness was the norm for feminine attractiveness. In more modern times, great changes have occurred in the cultural ideal of the female body. An analysis of *Playboy* centerfolds and Miss America Pageant contestants from 1960 to 1980 showed that the percentage of average weight (average weight being based on mean population values at the time) for these individuals declined steadily from approximately 90% to almost 80%. At the same time, average hip and bust sizes for these icons of beauty declined, while waist and height values increased. Thus, the ideal shape changed from the hourglass curve to a more tubular profile (Garner et al., 1980). The concern for the shrinking size of models' figures is so great that at least one country (Italy) has banned from its fashion shows any model with a body mass index (BMI) less than 18.5 kg·m^{-2} (a standard for underweight).

In another study, young and middle-aged males and females were asked to choose, from a range of different body silhouettes, three selections: one that reflected their current shape, the ideal one they would like to look like, and the one considered the most attractive to the opposite sex. A majority of both the young (59%) and the middle-aged (65%) females rated their current figures as being significantly larger than the ideal or attractive shape. However, neither the young nor the middle-aged males reported any significant differences between current, ideal, and most attractive silhouettes. Only 25% of the young and 29% of the middle-aged males expressed a desire to be smaller (Tiggemann, 1992). Thus, if you are a male, chances are that regardless of your real body weight, composition, and shape, you are not concerned with your body weight per se. However, you might like larger muscles and greater muscle definition, which would imply a lower percent body fat and a more triangular shape. Data on Mr. America or Mr. Universe contestants are not available to substantiate this impression, but just look at the muscle magazines at any newsstand. What body shape did you compare yourself with mentally as you considered the opening questions above? Hopefully, you visualized standards that are consistent with good health, but many males as well as females compare themselves to images present in the media that do not represent healthy weights.

Two studies of adolescents suggest that the perception of being overweight leads to unhealthy weight control behaviors. The first study (Talamayan et al., 2006) examined data from the 2003 Youth Risk Behavior study of a total of 9714 normal weight U.S. high school students. A significant portion (25.3% of females and 6.7% of males) misperceived themselves as overweight and engaged (16.8% of all females and 6.8% of all males) in unhealthy weight control behaviors (use of diet pills, laxatives, and fasting) in the 30 days before the study. The second study (Neumark-Sztainer et al., 2006), a 5-year longitudinal study, showed that lower satisfaction with body weight does not serve as a motivator for engaging in healthy weight management behaviors. Rather, it predicts the use of behaviors (unhealthy dieting, binge eating, smoking, lower levels of physical activity, and less fruit and vegetable intake) that place the adolescents at risk for further weight gain and poorer overall health.

An interesting twist regarding body image has recently emerged. In a study of 310 college students, Neighbors and Sobal (2007) confirmed that women are still more dissatisfied with their bodies than men even though in this sample the prevalence of overweight was higher in males (44%) than in females (11%). Most (87%) of the "normal" weight females wanted to weigh less, whereas considerably fewer (24%) of the "not overweight" males wanted to weigh less. Females classified as underweight expressed almost no body weight or shape dissatisfaction. The surprising result was that although both the overweight males and females wanted to lose weight, they did not select an ideal body weight that would move them into a more healthy BMI category. The authors concluded that these results may suggest a shift in body size ideals to more acceptance by many individuals of larger body sizes in an era of prevalent obesity, despite the linkage of obesity and health problems.

Regardless of all of these somewhat conflicting and varied perceptions, the fact is that the prevalence of overweight and obesity is a major worldwide problem. Sixty-five percent of the world's population lives in a country where overweight and obesity kills more people than underweight (World Health Organization, 2011).

In the United States in the early 1970s the prevalence of obesity was 5% for children 2–5 years; 4% for children 6–11 years; and 6% for adolescents 12–19 years. In the late 1970s, 15% of adults were obese. In the early 1990s, zero states had an adult obesity rate of more than 25% (Dietary Guidelines for Americans, 2010).

In 2009–2010, 35.7% of U.S. adults were obese as were 16.9% of U.S. children and adolescents. The rates for boys were 14.4% at 2–5 years, 20.1% at 6–11 years, and 19.6% at 12–19 years. The comparable values for girls were 9.6% (2–5 years), 15.7% (6–11) years, and 17.1% (12–19 years). For adult males the values were 33.2% at 20–39 years, 37.2% at 40–59, and 36.6% over 60 years. The comparable values for adult females were 31.9% (20–39 years), 36% (40–59 years), and 42.3% (≥ 60 years). In 2010, 36 states had an adult obesity rate of more than 25%, with 12 having a prevalence rate of ≥30%. No states had an obesity prevalence less than 20% (Centers for Disease control and Prevention, 2012b; Ogden et al., 2012).

Figure 7.1 shows the latest available (2007–2008) data for both overweight and obesity prevalence based on body mass index from the U.S. National Health and Nutrition Examination Survey (NHANES) study broken down by age, race/ethnicity, and sex (Flegel et al., 2010; Ogden et al., 2010). These data indicate that there is a racial/ethnicity disparity at all ages. The good news is that the prevalence of high BMI in childhood/adolescence has remained relatively steady for 10 years and that for adults the increase in BMI does not appear to be continuing at the same rate as over the past 10 years. The bad news is that the prevalence of high overweight and obesity values has not declined. There is an insidious problem with overweight and an *obesity epidemic*.

As a physical educator/exercise specialist/rehabilitation therapist, you will be dealing with a public that has more questions and concerns about body composition and weight control than just about anything else we deal with. This and the next chapter are designed to present you with an understanding of these crucial areas.

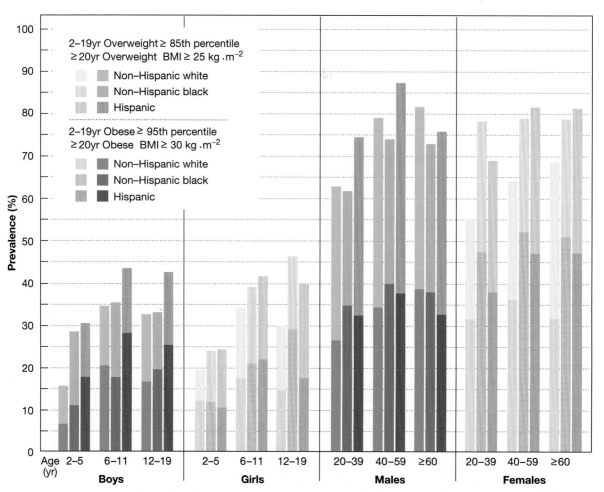

FIGURE 7.1   Prevalence of Overweight and Obesity in the United States by Age, Sex, and Race/Ethnicity.
Source: Based on data from Flegal et al.: Prevalence and trends in obesity among US adults, 1999–2008. *The Journal of the American Medical Association*. 303(3):235–241 (2010) and Ogden et al.: Prevalence of high body mass index in US children and adolescents, 2007–2008. *The Journal of the American Medical Association*. 303(3):242–249 (2010).

Body Composition Assessment

Laboratory Techniques

Although it is unpleasant to think about, the only way to directly assess body composition is by dissection of human cadavers. Few bodies are available for such studies, however, and the technique is difficult and problematic. From 1945 to 1984 (from the earliest to the latest reported studies), body composition has been analyzed in only 40 cadavers. While these studies provided much information, particularly regarding the densities of body tissues, they were not used to determine the accuracy (validity) of the commonly used laboratory techniques for body composition assessment. Theoretically, direct cadaver analysis should be the most accurate technique, but newer cadaver studies were often inconsistent with the results from the earlier studies. Thus, when dealing with body composition analysis, keep in mind that some techniques are better than others, and none is likely to be 100% accurate (Behnke and Wilmore, 1974; Brodie, 1988a).

Many methods are currently available for the laboratory assessment of body composition. Several could possibly serve as criterion measures. Techniques such as densitometry (hydrostatic weight and air displacement plethysmography [Bod Pod]), hydrometry, or dilution to determine total body water (TBW), nuclear techniques such as whole-body counting of potassium 40 or neutron activation, dual-energy X-ray absorptiometry (DXA), computed tomography (CT), magnetic resonance imaging (MRI), ultrasound, and total body electrical conductivity are all accurate enough to be used (Brodie, 1988a,b; Heymsfield et al., 2005). Unfortunately, at this time, these techniques are also often expensive, cumbersome, and/or time-consuming, requiring sensitive instrumentation operated by highly trained technicians. The DXA technique is pictured and described in Chapter 16 because it is considered the "gold standard," or criterion measure, for the assessment of bone mineral density. However, DXA also allows the simultaneous measurement of fat and lean soft tissue for the determination of body composition. In the near future, DXA may become the criterion standard for body composition assessment as well. The Bod Pod also is frequently used. For now, however, pending more research, the criterion measurement for body composition is still hydrostatic, or underwater, weighing (Behnke and Wilmore, 1974; Going, 2005; Goldman and Buskirk, 1961; Lohman and Chen, 2005; Ratamess, 2010).

Hydrostatic Weighing Criterion measure for determining body composition through the calculation of body density.

Archimedes Principle The principle that a partially or fully submerged object will experience an upward bouyant force equal to the weight on the volume of fluid displaced by the object.

Hydrostatic (Underwater) Weighing: Densitometry

Hydrostatic, or underwater, **weighing** determines body composition through the calculation of body density (Behnke and Wilmore, 1974; Going, 2005; Goldman and Buskirk, 1961; Ratamess, 2010). We have Archimedes, a Greek mathematician who lived in the second century BC, to thank for this technique. When King Hieron of Syracuse commissioned a new crown, he suspected that the jeweler substituted silver for pure gold inside the crown. The king asked Archimedes to determine the composition of the crown without harming it in any way. Legend has it that as Archimedes was pondering this question at the public baths, he solved the problem and went running through the streets naked, shouting, "Eureka!" ("I have found it!").

What Archimedes observed was that an amount of water was displaced from the bath equal to the volume of the body entering the bath. Archimedes reasoned that the volume was proportional to the mass of the object and that the object's loss of weight in water equaled the weight of the volume of water displaced. We now define the mass of an object divided by its loss of weight in water as the *specific gravity* of that object. Archimedes also reasoned that the body (or any other object floating or submerged) is buoyed up by a counterforce equal to the weight of the water displaced. Thus, **Archimedes' principle** states that a partially or fully submerged object experiences an upward buoyant force equal to the weight or the volume of fluid displaced by the object. Based on this principle, the volume of any object, including the human body, can be measured by determining the weight lost by complete submersion underwater. In the case of the human body, dividing the mass of the body by its volume defines *body density*. When Archimedes compared the amount of water displaced by a mass of pure gold and a mass of pure silver equal to the mass of the king's crown, he found that the crown displaced more water than the gold, but less than the silver. He confirmed this result by weighing in air and underwater, masses of gold and silver equal to the weight of the crown in air, and found the crown to have an intermediate specific gravity value. Thus, the crown was not pure gold (only about 75%), and we can only speculate as to the fate of the jeweler (Behnke and Wilmore, 1974).

Even if you have never been weighed underwater, you probably have a basic understanding of the principle just described. Think back to a swimming class. Could you float easily, or were you a sinker who could walk on the bottom of the pool? How would you describe floaters and sinkers in terms of being lean or fat? Whether one floats or sinks depends on one's body density, and body density (mass per unit volume) is largely determined by the amount of body fat present. The density of bone and muscle tissue is greater than the density of fat tissue. Thus, the leaner, more muscular individual weighs more underwater and tends to sink, whereas an individual with a large amount of fat weighs less and tends to float.

FIGURE 7.2 Models of Body Composition.

A represents total body weight, *B* is the two-compartment model, *C* lists the tissue components of FFW and of total fat, and *D* indicates the chemical components of FFW and represents a four-component model.

Source: Lohman, T. G.: Applicability of body composition techniques and constants for children and youth. In Pandolf, K. B. (ed.): *Exercise and Sport Sciences Reviews*. New York, NY: Macmillan, 14:325–357 (1986).

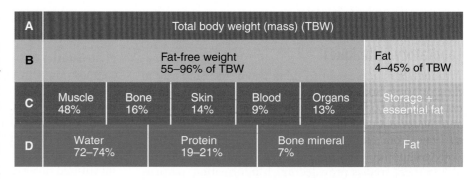

Whole-body **densitometry**, which is the measurement of mass per unit volume, is the foundation of hydrostatic weighing. It is based on dividing the total body weight (**Figure 7.2**, row A) into two compartments: fat and fat-free weight (FFW) (row B). Row C lists the component parts of the **fat-free weight** (all of the tissues of the body minus the extractable fat) as muscle, bone, skin, blood, and organs; this represents a second model. The fat compartment includes both storage and essential fats. *Storage fat* is the fat in the subcutaneous adipose tissues and the fat surrounding the various internal organs (visceral fat). *Essential fat* includes the fat in the bone marrow, central nervous system, cell membranes, heart, lungs, liver, spleen, kidneys, intestines, and muscles.

Note that although the terms *lean body mass* (LBM) and FFW (sometimes called the fat-free body, FFB, or fat-free mass, FFM) are used interchangeably, they are slightly different. Technically, LBM includes the essential fat, but FFW does not. Chemically, FFW is composed of water, proteins, and bone mineral (**Figure 7.2**, row D); this is a third model of compartmentalization or composition (Lohman, 1986). Although each of these models (B, C, and D) describes the composition of the body, when the term body composition is used in exercise physiology, it generally refers to model B. That is, **body composition** is defined as the partitioning of body mass into FFM (weight or percentage) and fat mass (weight or percentage).

Compartmentalizing the body into only fat and FFW (not water, mineral, protein, and fat) and using this two-compartment model to determine percent body fat depends on the following assumptions:

1. The densities of the fat and the FFW are known and additive.
2. The densities of water, bone mineral, and protein that make up the FFW are known and are relatively constant from individual to individual.
3. The percentage of each fat-free component is relatively stable from individual to individual.
4. The individual being evaluated differs from the assumptions of the equation being used only in the amount of storage fat.

Hydrostatic weighing determines body density (D_B), defined as mass (M) or weight (WT) divided by volume (V), according to the following formula where the numerator represents mass and the denominator represents volume (Behnke and Wilmore, 1974):

7.1

body density $(g \cdot cc^{-1})$ = mass in air (g) ÷ {{[mass in air (g) − mass in water (g)] ÷ [density of water $(g \cdot cc^{-1})$]} − [residual volume (L) + volume of gastrointestinal air (0.1 L)]}

or

$$D_B = \frac{M_A}{\dfrac{(M_A - M_W)}{D_W} - (RV + V_G)}$$

The mass of an individual in air (M_A) can be measured either by weighing that individual nude on a sensitive, calibrated scale or by weighing the subject in a bathing suit and then subtracting the weight of the suit. The volume of the human body is obtained by applying Archimedes' principle. In practice, the individual being weighed is submerged in water, attached in some way to a scale or strain gauge instrumentation (**Figure 7.3**). The subject then exhales as much air as possible and sits quietly for 3–7 seconds while the weight is recorded. Multiple trials are usually necessary. The highest consistent weight is selected from the trials, and the weight of the apparatus, called the tare weight, is then subtracted from the scale weight. The resultant weight is the underwater weight (M_W). Body weight may be measured in lb or kg, but calculations are typically done in metric units, so conversion may be necessary. Not all air can be expelled from the body, and air makes the body more buoyant (lighter in weight). Therefore, the underwater weight must be corrected for residual volume (the volume of air remaining in the lungs following maximal expiration) and for gastrointestinal gases, the assumed constant equal to 100 mL or 0.1 L in Equation 7.1. The underwater weight must also be corrected for the density of the water, D_W, which in turn is temperature-dependent.

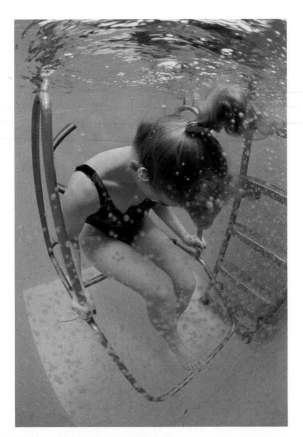

FIGURE 7.3 Hydrostatic Weighing.
The technique for determining body density by hydrostatic (underwater) weighing is based on Archimedes' principle.

EXAMPLE

For example, the following measurements were obtained from a football player:

M_A = 225 lb (102.3 kg) Water Temperature = 34°C
M_W = 6.07 kg Water Density at 34°C = 0.9944
RV = 1.583 L

Substituting into Equation 7.1 we get

$$D_B = \frac{102.3 \text{ kg}}{\left(\dfrac{102.3 \text{ kg} - 6.07 \text{ kg}}{0.9944}\right) - (1.583 \text{ L} + 0.1 \text{ L})}$$

Densitometry The measurement of mass per unit volume.

Fat-free Weight The weight of body tissue excluding extractable fat.

Body Composition The partitioning of body mass into FFM (weight or percentage) and fat mass (weight or percentage).

EXAMPLE (Continued)

Remember that the numerator in this equation represents mass and the denominator represents volume. In the metric system 1 L of water (a volume measure) weighs 1 kg (a mass measure), so conversely 1 kg of water mass occupies 1 L of volume (Appendix A). Therefore, the equation can be solved as written.

$$D_B = \frac{102.3 \text{ kg}}{96.77 - 1.683 \text{ L}}$$
$$= \frac{102.3 \text{ kg}}{95.089 \text{ L}} = 1.0758 \text{ kg} \cdot \text{L}^{-1}$$

Although $\text{kg} \cdot \text{L}^{-1}$ is an accurate unit, the D_B is usually reported in $\text{g} \cdot \text{cc}^{-1}$ units. Dividing the $\text{kg} \cdot \text{L}^{-1}$ unit by 1000 yields $\text{g} \cdot \text{mL}^{-1}$. Then, because 1 mL equals 1 cc (cubic centimeter), the cc designation can easily be substituted for the mL, and typically is. Thus, 1.0758 $\text{kg} \cdot \text{L}^{-1}$ = 1.0758 $\text{g} \cdot \text{cc}^{-1}$

Once body density has been measured, %BF can be calculated. The two most widely used formulas for converting body density to %BF were developed by Siri and Brozek. They have been derived differently but, within the density units of 1.09 and 1.03 $\text{g} \cdot \text{cc}^{-1}$, agree within 1% on the %BF values calculated. At lower densities, the Siri formula gives increasingly higher %BF values than the Brozek formula (Lohman, 1981).

7.2 Brozek: $\%BF = \left[\left(\dfrac{4.570}{D_B}\right) - 4.142\right] \times 100$

7.3 Siri: $\%BF = \left[\left(\dfrac{4.950}{D_B}\right) - 4.5\right] \times 100$

Brozek's formula assumes that the individual has neither lost nor gained substantial amounts of body weight recently.

EXAMPLE

Using the body density results from the football player in the preceding example in Equations 7.2 and 7.3:

Brozek: $\%BF = \left[\left(\dfrac{4.570}{1.0758}\right) - 4.142\right] \times 100 = 10.6\%$

Siri: $\%BF = \left[\left(\dfrac{4.950}{1.0758}\right) - 4.50\right] \times 100 = 10.1\%$

As expected, the %BF values are within 1% of each other with an actual difference of only 0.5% (10.6% − 10.1% = 0.5%).

Once %BF has been determined, body weight at any selected fat percentage can be calculated using the following sequence of formulas. The first formula simply determines the amount of fat-free weight an individual currently has (WT$_1$).

7.4

fat-free weight = current body weight (lb or kg)
$$\times\left(\frac{100\% - \text{percent body fat}}{100}\right)$$

or

$$FFW = WT_1 \times \left(\frac{100\% - BF\%}{100}\right)$$

The second formula calculates the desired weight (WT$_2$).

7.5

body weight at the selected percent of body fat (lb or kg) = [100 × FFW (lb or kg)] ÷ (100% − selected %BF)

or

$$WT_2 = \frac{100 \times FFW}{100\% - \%BF}$$

The third formula calculates the amount of weight to be gained or lost.

7.6

weight to gain or lose (lb or kg) = body weight at selected %BF − current body weight

or

$$\Delta WT = WT_2 - WT_1$$

EXAMPLE

For example, an individual who currently weighs 150 lb at a body fat of 25% wishes to reduce her body fat to 17%. Equation 7.4 is used to calculate her current fat-free weight.

$$FFW = 150\text{ lb} \times \left(\frac{100\% - 25\%}{100}\right) = 112.50\text{ lb}$$

Her current fat-free weight and selected %BF are then substituted into Equation 7.5 to obtain her weight goal.

$$WT_2 = \frac{100 \times 112.50\text{ lb}}{100\% - 17\%} = 135.54\text{ lb}$$

Comparing her current weight to her goal weight in Equation 7.6 we get

$$\Delta WT = 135.5\text{ lb} - 150\text{ lb} = -14.5\text{ lb}$$

This means that to be 17% BF, this individual must reduce her current weight by 14.5 lb. Of course, these calculations assume that in the process of losing weight, muscle mass is maintained. This assumption is not always true.

Now read the Check Your Comprehension box and answer the problems given. The data are presented as they would be recorded during an actual experiment. You will need to do some conversions and analysis to select the correct M$_A$ and M$_W$. As you do each calculation, mentally review the reasons for each step to ensure that you understand the underlying principles.

When the measuring technique is properly conducted, the error of %BF determined by densitometry is approximately ±2.7% for adults. This error range is primarily due to variations in the composition of the FFM (Lohman, 1981). The error is always lowest when the individual being tested closely matches the sample on which the equation was developed (Heyward and Stolarczyk, 1996).

CHECK YOUR COMPREHENSION

1. From the following information, calculate M$_A$.
   Subject name: Phyllis Elizabeth Major
   Sex: F   Age: 18
   Weight with bathing suit: 112.5 lb _____ kg
   Weight of bathing suit: 0.5 lb _____ kg
   Nude weight (M$_A$):   112.0 lb _____ kg (M$_A$)
   Residual volume = 1.2774 L

2. Underwater weighing trials in kg
   Select the representative weight
   a. Highest obtained weight if obtained more than twice.
   b. Second-highest obtained weight if observed more than once.
   c. Third-highest obtained weight.
   Trial   1. 7.8   2. 8.25   3. 8.3   4. 8.35
           5. 8.275   6. 8.325   7. 8.3   8. 8.325
           9. 8.3   10. 8.275
   Tare weight* = 7.06 kg
   Water temperature = 35°C
   Water density (D$_W$) = 0.9941
   Underwater weight (M$_W$)
   = selected weight − tare weight
   M$_W$ = _____ − _____ = _____ kg
   *Tare weight equals the weight of the apparatus without the subject in it.

3. From the information presented and calculated in 1 and 2, use Equation 7.1 to calculate D$_B$ and Equation 7.2 to calculate %BF.

4. Phyllis would like to be 19% BF. Use Equations 7.4, 7.5, and 7.6 to determine whether she needs to gain or lose weight to achieve this goal, and if so, how much.

Answers are presented in Appendix C.

Densitometry: Children and Adolescents and the Older Adult

The previous section outlined the basic assumptions underlying hydrostatic weighing (densitometry). Research has challenged these assumptions with regard to children and adolescents (Lohman et al., 1984).

The values for the FFW or the FFB components for adults (males and females) are assumed to be approximately 73% for water and 7% for mineral content, with an overall density of FFW of 1.100 g·cc⁻¹ (**Figure 7.4**, dashed lines) (Boileau et al., 1984; Lohman, 1986). Protein, not shown on the graph, makes up about 20% of the FFW of adults.

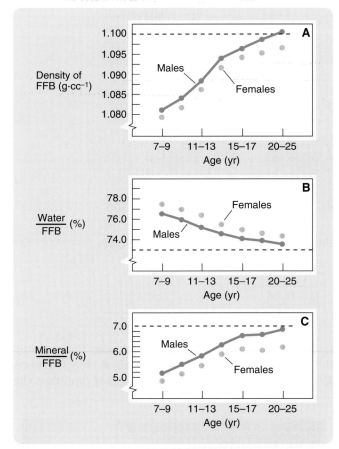

FIGURE 7.4 Estimated Changes in Fat-Free Body (FFB) Composition as a Function of Age.
A. The density of the fat-free body, also known as the FFW, is much lower in both male and female children than in adults. FFB density increases as the child matures, but the female density is lower at each age than the male density and never reaches the assumed adult values of 1.1.
B. The percentage of FFB that is composed of water is higher in both male and female children than in adults. As the child matures, the percentage of water in the FFB declines, but the female percentage is always higher than the male even after adulthood is reached.
C. The percentage of FFB that is composed of minerals is lower in both male and female children than in adults. As the child matures, the percentage of minerals in the FFB increases, but the female percentage is always lower than the male percentage even after adulthood is reached.
Source: Lohman, T. G.: Applicability of body composition techniques and constants for children and youth. In Pandolf, K. B. (ed.): *Exercise and Sport Science Reviews*. New York, NY: Macmillan, 14:325–327 (1986). Reprinted by permission of Williams & Wilkins.

Boileau et al. (1984) have shown that the percentage of water in FFW decreases (**Figure 7.4B**) from 77–78% at ages 7–9 years to 73% at approximately age 20 in a steady but slightly curvilinear fashion. Across the age span, females have a slightly higher percentage of water in FFW than males. Conversely, the percentage of mineral content in FFW (**Figure 7.4C**) increases from approximately 5% at ages 7–9 to 7% at age 20. This change is also slightly curvilinear, and the female values are consistently lower than the male values. The protein change is minimal (and therefore not presented in **Figure 7.4**), varying only about 1% (from 19 to 20%) over the age span. The result of these changes is that body density also increases in a curvilinear fashion from approximately 1.08 to 1.10 g·cc⁻¹ for adult males and from 1.08 to 1.095 g·cc⁻¹ for adult females. This means adult females never meet the 1.10-g·cc⁻¹ assumed value (**Figure 7.4A**) (Lohman, 1986).

Because the components are constantly changing as children mature, no single formula can be used for children of different ages. Nor can one formula be used for boys and for girls. **Table 7.1** shows the array of age and sex formulas needed.

Using the equations developed with assumptions about the composition of adult components will overestimate the %BF of the child or the adolescent. This can be illustrated as follows. If the D_B of a 9-year-old girl is determined to be 1.065 g·cc⁻¹ by hydrostatic weighing, the %BF calculated by the Brozek formula (Equation 7.2) is

$$\left(\frac{4.570}{1.065}\right) - 4.142 \times 100 = 14.9\%$$

The Lohman (1986) age- and sex-specific formula yields

$$\left(\frac{5.350}{1.065}\right) - 4.95 \times 100 = 7.3\% \quad \text{(see Table 7.1)}$$

Most research published to date for children and adolescents has been on normally active nonathletes. Further work is in progress to determine the effects of physical activity and/or athletic participation on bone mineral, hydration, and body density values throughout the growth years. %BF values of young athletes, even if the appropriate age and sex formulas are used, must be interpreted cautiously. Although the pediatric formulas are better than adult formulas, even the pediatric formulas may need to be revised for young athletes. In addition, research in the area of body composition, on both sedentary and active youths, should directly measure water (W) and bone mineral content (M) of the FFW as well as body density to more accurately account for all body compartments. These variables should be used in a more complex formula such as

$$\%BF = \left(\frac{2.747}{D_B}\right) - 0.714(W) + 1.146(M) - 2.0503$$

TABLE 7.1	Formulas for Converting Body Density to Percent Body Fat in Children and Adolescents, by Sex	
Age (Yr)	Male	Female
7–9	$\left(\dfrac{5.38}{D_B} - 4.97\right) \times 100$	$\left(\dfrac{5.43}{D_B} - 5.03\right) \times 100$
9–11	$\left(\dfrac{5.30}{D_B} - 4.89\right) \times 100$	$\left(\dfrac{5.35}{D_B} - 4.95\right) \times 100$
11–13	$\left(\dfrac{5.23}{D_B} - 4.81\right) \times 100$	$\left(\dfrac{5.25}{D_B} - 4.84\right) \times 100$
13–15	$\left(\dfrac{5.07}{D_B} - 4.64\right) \times 100$	$\left(\dfrac{5.12}{D_B} - 4.69\right) \times 100$
15–17	$\left(\dfrac{5.03}{D_B} - 4.59\right) \times 100$	$\left(\dfrac{5.07}{D_B} - 4.64\right) \times 100$
17–20	$\left(\dfrac{4.98}{D_B} - 4.53\right) \times 100$	$\left(\dfrac{5.05}{D_B} - 4.62\right) \times 100$

Note: Calculated from the density FFW constant (D_1) reported by Lohman (1986), and a density of fat constant (D_2) of 0.9 g·cc⁻¹ according to the formula

$$\%BF = \frac{1}{D_B}\left[\left(\frac{D_1 D_2}{D_1 - D_2}\right) - \left(\frac{D_2}{D_1 - D_2}\right)\right] \times 100$$

At the other end of the age continuum, the older adult, the effect of bone mineral density loss (termed osteopenia) should be considered in the determination of %BF. Theoretically, a loss of bone mineral density would cause a decrease in body density and, thus, an overestimation of %BF if not accounted for (Ballor et al., 1988; Brodie, 1988a; Lohman, 1986).

Field Tests of Body Composition

Field methods to determine body composition can be classified as anthropometry (measurement of the human body) or bioelectrical impedance analysis (BIA). Anthropometric techniques include skinfolds, height and weight, BMI, diameters, and circumferences. These techniques are generally practical, require a minimum of equipment, and (if properly applied) can provide useful, reasonably accurate information. They vary in the degree of skill needed by the tester.

Skinfolds

A widely used anthropometric estimation of body size or composition involves the measurement of skinfolds at selected sites. **Skinfolds** (sometimes called fatfolds) are the double thickness of the skin plus the adipose tissue between the parallel layers of the skin (**Figure 7.5**). Because skin thickness varies only slightly among

individuals, skinfold measures generally indicate the thickness of the subcutaneous fat (Behnke and Wilmore, 1974). Technically, however, adipose tissue (and thus the

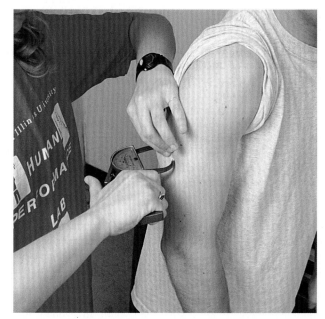

FIGURE 7.5 Measurement of Triceps Skinfold Using a Calibrated Skinfold Caliper.

TABLE 7.2 Percentage of Fat Distribution in a Reference Male and a Reference Female

Distribution Site	70-kg Male Fat (kg)	%	56.8-kg Female Fat (kg)	%
Total body	10.3–10.5	15	13.4–17.2	24–30
Essential	2.1–3.5	3–5	4.5–6.8	8–12
Storage	8.2–8.4	12	8.5–10.4	15–18
Subcutaneous	3.1	4	5.1	9
Intermuscular	3.3	5	3.5	6
Intramuscular	0.8	1	0.6	1
Abdominothoracic cavity	1.0	1	1.2	2

Sources: Modified from Behnke and Wilmore (1974), Going and Davis (2001), and Lohman (1981).

subcutaneous fatfold) has both a fat component and a fat-free component. The fat-free component is composed of water, blood vessels, and nerves. As the fat content of the adipose tissue increases (as in obesity), the water content decreases (Roche, 1987).

The use of skinfold thickness to estimate body composition is based on two assumptions. The first is that selected skinfold sites are representative of the total subcutaneous adipose tissue mass. In general, evidence supports this assumption (Lohman, 1981; Roche, 1987). The second assumption is that the subcutaneous tissue mass has a known relationship with total body fat. **Table 7.2** shows the distribution of total body fat and the relative percentages of each storage site for a reference male and a reference female 20–24 years old.

Most of the values in **Table 7.2** are estimates. They indicate that approximately one-third of the total fat for both males (3.1 kg subcutaneous fat/10.3–10.5 kg total fat) and females (5.1 kg subcutaneous fat/13.4–17.2 kg total fat) is estimated to be subcutaneous. Other estimates put this value as high as 70% and as low as 20%. With advancing age, a proportionally smaller amount of fat is stored subcutaneously. Thus, any given skinfold would then represent a smaller percentage of total body fat. It may also be that lean individuals and fat individuals store their fat in proportionally different ways. Additionally, females may store more or less fat subcutaneously than males (Lohman, 1981). There is little disagreement regarding the differences between essential fat amounts for males and females. The higher essential fat values in females are generally explained as additional storage needed to meet the energy requirements of pregnancy and lactation.

These variations in the estimation of subcutaneous fat percentage mean that the second assumption about the use of skinfolds to estimate body composition is not as firmly

based as the first (Brodie, 1988a). One way of dealing with this problem is to use equations that are age-adjusted or generalized for sedentary individuals and population-specific for various athletic groups (Going, 2006).

When skinfolds are taken by trained professionals and the appropriate equations are used, the variability between appropriate equations and accuracy of skinfold prediction of %BF compared with underwater weighing is approximately ±3–5% (Jackson and Pollock, 1978; Kaminsky and Dwyer, 2006; Lohman, 1992). Improper techniques can result in large prediction errors. The greatest source of error is improper location of the skinfold site. Anyone wishing to use this method to predict %BF should locate the site precisely and practice the technique repeatedly before using it. **Table 7.3** presents equations that can be used to predict %BF from two or three skinfold sites. These equations are specific for sex and age.

Skinfold thickness values may be used in ways other than to predict %BF. First, the millimeter values of several sites (usually 5–7 from anatomically diverse locations) can be added to form a *sum of skinfolds*. Such a sum indicates the relative degree of fatness among individuals. It can also be used to detect changes within a given individual, if measurements are taken repeatedly over time. Second, skinfolds may be used to determine the pattern of distribution of subcutaneous fat. Such a pattern has emerged as an important predictor of the health hazards of obesity (Harrison et al., 1988; Roche, 1987; Van Itallie, 1988). Fat distribution patterns and the associated health problems are discussed later in this chapter.

Height and Weight

In some situations, such as when large numbers of individuals are being evaluated, the only measures of body size that can easily be obtained are height and weight. These values are often used along with height and weight charts that include standards such as acceptable body weight (<10% over the chart weight for a given height), overweight (10–20% over the chart weight), and obese

Skinfolds The double thickness of skin plus the adipose tissue between the parallel layers of skin.

TABLE 7.3   Calculation of %BF from Skinfolds

Group	Equation
Adult males	$\%BF = 0.39287(X_1) - 0.00105(X_1)^2 + 0.15772(X_2) - 5.18845$, where X_1 = sum of abdominal, suprailiac, and triceps skinfolds and X_2 = age
Adult females	$\%BF = 0.41563(X_1) - 0.00112(X_1)^2 + 0.03661(X_2) + 4.03653$, where X_1 = sum of abdominal, suprailiac, and triceps skinfolds and X_2 = age
Male children and adolescents (8–18 yr)	$\%BF = 0.735(X_1) + 1.0$, where X_1 = sum of triceps and calf skinfolds
Female children and adolescents (8–18 yr)	$\%BF = 0.610(X_1) + 5.1$, where X_1 = sum of triceps and calf skinfolds

Note: The last two equations were developed taking into account body density, percentage of water in FFW, and bone mineral content variations by age.

Sources: Based on information in Golding et al. (1989), Jackson and Pollock (1985), and Slaughter et al. (1988).

(>20% over the chart weight) sometimes by frame size. Such use of height and weight charts is minimally acceptable for large group data but is not recommended as a source of what an individual "should" weigh, for the following reasons (Burton et al., 1985; Himes and Frisancho, 1988; Nieman, 1990; Powers and Howley, 1990):

1. The most commonly available height and weight charts from Metropolitan Life Insurance (1959 and 1983) were compiled from the lowest mortality data on individuals who purchased life insurance in non-group situations. The age range was 25–59 years. Some people were included more than once when they purchased more than one policy. Thus, the sample was not randomly drawn, was not statistically valid, and was not truly a representative of the total American population, especially older adults, lower socioeconomic groups, and specific ethnic groups.

2. Individuals with known heart disease, cancer, and/or diabetes were excluded, but smokers were included. Thus, risk factors other than body weight were ignored in determining mortality ratios.

3. Only body weights at the time of purchasing the insurance, not at the time of death, were considered. This omission could greatly affect the categories of acceptable, overweight, and obese weights. In addition, in many cases, height and weight were self-reported and not measured. The accuracy of self-reported data must be questioned.

4. The determination of frame size is not always defined. Even when it is, frame size is very difficult to defend and interpret in relation to body weight.

5. The 1983 Metropolitan Life Insurance height-weight chart shows higher weight values at a given height and frame size than the comparable 1959 chart, reflecting the trend of a national weight gain. The 1959 table values were listed as desirable weights (i.e., weights associated with the lowest mortality), but the 1983 table values were not so listed. If the Metropolitan tables are the only thing available for judging acceptable or unacceptable weights, the 1959 (not the 1983) version should be selected, except for older adults.

Some evidence suggests that desirable weights are slightly higher in older adults. Therefore, the 1983 table values can be used for this population.

6. Weight per se does not provide any information on body composition. What matters is the %BF, not the body weight, because %BF is related to health.

Fortunately, even if height and weight are the only variables known and the use of height and weight charts is not recommended, a reasonable alternative is available: the Body Mass Index.

Body Mass Index

Body Mass Index (BMI) is a ratio of the total body weight to height. Several ratios have been proposed, but the one used most frequently is weight (in kilograms) divided by height (in meters) squared [WT ÷ HT^2 (kg·m^{-2})]. This ratio is also known as the Quetelet index (Brodie, 1988a; Revicki and Israel, 1986; Satwanti et al., 1980). Calculated BMI can then be compared against standard values to determine whether the individual has acceptable body weight, is overweight, or is obese (**Table 7.4**).

EXAMPLE

If a female subject (age = 30 years) weighs 165 lb and is 5 ft 8 in. tall, calculation of her BMI first requires conversion to metric units. Dividing 165 lb by 2.2 kg·lb^{-1} gives a weight of 75 kg. Multiplying 68 in. by 2.54 cm $in.^{-1}$ gives 172.7 cm (1.73 m). Height value squared is 2.98 m^2. Thus, BMI = 75 ÷ 2.98 = 25.2. Check **Table 7.4** to see whether this is an acceptable, overweight, or obesity value for this individual.

The selection of BMI values at the upper limit of acceptable is based on the data relating BMI to morbidity (disease occurrence, particularly cardiovascular disease [CVD]) and mortality (death). For adults there is a J-shaped curvilinear increase in excess mortality (a greater

TABLE 7.4   Commonly Used Body Mass Index (kg·m⁻²) Standards for Acceptable Body Weight, Overweight, and Obesity in Nonathletes

	Acceptable Body Weight		Overweight		Obesity	
Age	Male	Female	Male	Female	Male	Female
<18 yr	5–84th percentile		85–94th percentile		≥95th percentile or BMI ≥30 99th percentile = severe obesity or BMI = 30–32 (10–12 yr) BMI ≥34 (14–16 yr)	
≥18 yr	18.5–24.9 BMI		25.0–29.9 BMI		Class I = 30–34.9 BMI Class II = 35–39.9 BMI Class III = ≤ 40 BMI	

Sources: Based on Barlow and Expert Committee (2007), US Department of Health and Human Services (2000), and World Health Organization (1998).

number of deaths than expected in a given population) with an increasing BMI as initially determined in the now classic study by Bray (1985). He found that BMI values from 15 to 25 kg·m⁻² represented no excess mortality risk. Significant increases in risk were shown to begin at a BMI of 27.3 kg·m⁻² for females and 27.8 kg·m⁻² for males. Therefore, in 1985, the National Institute of Health defined obesity as a BMI of 27.3 kg·m⁻² for females and 27.8 kg·m⁻² for males.

In 1988, the World Health Organization (WHO) adopted BMI standards of less than 18.5 for underweight, 18.5–24.9 for normal weight, 25–29.9 for overweight, and ≥30 for obesity. Obesity was further divided into three classes. Class I obesity is indicated by a BMI of 30–34.9, Class II by a BMI of 35–39.9, and Class III by a BMI ≥40. All values are in kg·m⁻². In 1998, the National Health, Lung, and Blood Institute and the Centers for Disease Control and Prevention (CDC) in the United States concurred with these standards.

Using these WHO cut points, Meyer et al. (2002) also found a J-shaped curvilinear association between BMI and total mortality (**Figure 7.6**) even when stratified based on smoking habits and physical activity, although their data were limited to males. So few deaths occurred in those with a BMI of < 18.5 kg·m⁻² over the length of the study that its influence on the curve has been omitted in **Figure 7.6**.

BMI has been shown to correlate highly with %BF derived from skinfold measures (r = 0.74) and hydrostatic weighing (r = 0.58–0.85). These correlations indicate a moderate relationship, but they also suggest that there is considerable measurement error in using BMI as an estimate of body adiposity (>5%). In situations where the same group of individuals was evaluated, skinfolds generally predicted %BF better than BMI did. Individuals

with a normal BMI can actually have high body fat levels, and individuals with a high BMI (especially those in the 25–27 kg·m⁻² range) may actually have normal, acceptable body fat levels. Individuals who are obviously active and/or muscular should have %BF more directly measured (Gallagher et al., 1996). The Focus on Research box reports a study showing the difficulty with using BMI to classify collegiate athletes and nonathletes as overweight. At any given BMI, females have a higher %BF than males. Older individuals have a higher %BF at any given BMI than younger individuals, and the association with clinical outcomes and mortality is weaker (Gallagher et al., 1996; Sardinha and Teixeira, 2005). The

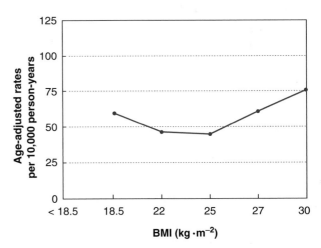

FIGURE 7.6 The Relationship between BMI and Mortality.
Age-adjusted rates of death from all causes based on BMI in 22,304 males without recognized cardiovascular diseases, diabetes mellitus, or cancer at the initial screening followed for an average of 16.3 years. The increasing values for BMI in kg·m⁻² is described as a J-shaped curve.
Source: Meyer, H. E., A. J. Søgaard, A. Tverdal, & R. M. Selmer: Body mass index and mortality: The influence of physical activity and smoking. *Medicine & Science in Sports & Exercise.* 34(7):1065–1070 (2002). Reprinted by permission.

Body Mass Index (BMI) is a ratio of the total body weight to height.

BMI as a Predictor of Percent Fat in College Athletes and Nonathletes

The purposes of this study were to describe the relationship between %BF and BMI in college athletes and nonathletes and to determine the accuracy of the standard of ≥25 kg·m⁻² BMI as defining excessive body fatness in these populations. Data from varsity athletes (149 M and 77 F) and 213 undergraduate students majoring in kinesiology and enrolled in an exercise physiology lab class at a major Midwest university were used in the analyses. The male athletes were involved in basketball, wrestling, ice hockey, and football. The female athletes competed in basketball, crew, and softball.

Overweight was defined as BMI ≥25 kg·m⁻² but <30 kg·m⁻²; obesity was defined as ≥30 kg·m⁻². Overfat was defined as ≥20% BF for males and ≥33% BF for females. No football lineman had a BMI less than 25 kg·m⁻², and only one had a % BF <20%. Therefore, the linemen were separated out from the rest of the male athletes. The results are presented in the figure accompanying: A for males and B for females. FP means false positive—individuals who were classified as

overweight but had normal %BF; FN means false negative—individuals who were classified as normal weight but were overfat; TP means true positive—individuals who were classified as overweight and who were overfat; TN means true negative—individuals who were both normal weight and normal %BF. The concern is for those individuals who are incorrectly classified, that is, the FPs and the FNs.

The scatterplot in Figure A shows that 67% of the male athletes and 25% of the male nonathletes fell within the FP quadrant. The scatterplot in Figure B shows that 31% of the female athletes and 7% of the female nonathletes fell within the FP quadrant. There were no FN in either the male or the female athletes, but 44% of the female athletes and 6% of male nonathletes fell within the FN quadrant. These results indicate that BMI misclassifies normal fat individuals a large percentage of the time. Conversely, a large percentage of overfat female nonathletes were classified as normal weight by BMI.

Statistically determined optimal BMI cut points to minimize the false classifications and maximize the specificity (identification of normal weight individuals as such) and sensitivity (identification of overfat individuals as overweight by BMI) were determined to be 27.9 kg·m⁻² for male athletes, 34.1 kg·m⁻² for football linemen, 26.5 kg·m⁻² for male nonathletes, 27.7 kg·m⁻² for female athletes, and 24.0 kg·m⁻² for female nonathletes. Interestingly, these optimal cut points are consistent with the 1985 NIH recommendations of ≥27.3 kg·m⁻² for females and ≥27.8 kg·m⁻² for males to define overweight (the 85th percentile of BMI distribution in young adults 20–29 years). Optimal cut points for the nonathletes are lower than the athletes at least in part because of less muscle mass in the nonathletes. These results illustrate the limitations in the BMI classification when using one standard for all adults.

Source: Ode, J. A., J. M. Pivarnik, M. J. Reeves, & J. L. Knous: Body mass index as a predictor of percent fat in college athletes and nonathletes. *Medicine & Science in Sports & Exercise.* 39(3):403–409 (2007).

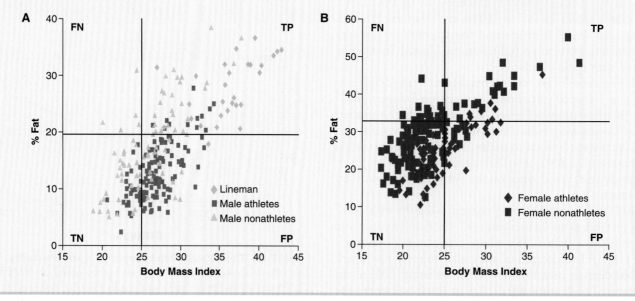

degree of adiposity associated with a given level of BMI varies by racial group/ethnicity as well. At the same BMI black males and females tend to have higher lean body mass and lower fat mass than white males and females. Conversely, Asian populations may have higher body fat

percentages at a given BMI although this is still under debate (Flegal et al., 2010). Finally, BMI gives no indication of fat distribution. The importance of fat distribution is discussed later in this chapter. Nevertheless, BMI is often (and acceptably) used as indication of overweight or obesity and risk stratification in the absence of more specific methods to estimate total body fat, particularly when mass screening is done (Sardinha and Teixeira, 2005).

Table 7.4 presents commonly used BMI standards for acceptable body weight, overweight, and obesity in nonathletic individuals. Note that for adults the values are those presented in the paragraph above. However, for children and adolescents specific values are not given; instead, age- and sex-specific percentiles are used. These require the use of charts such as the CDC BMI Growth charts presented in **Figure 7.7A** (boys) and **B** (girls).

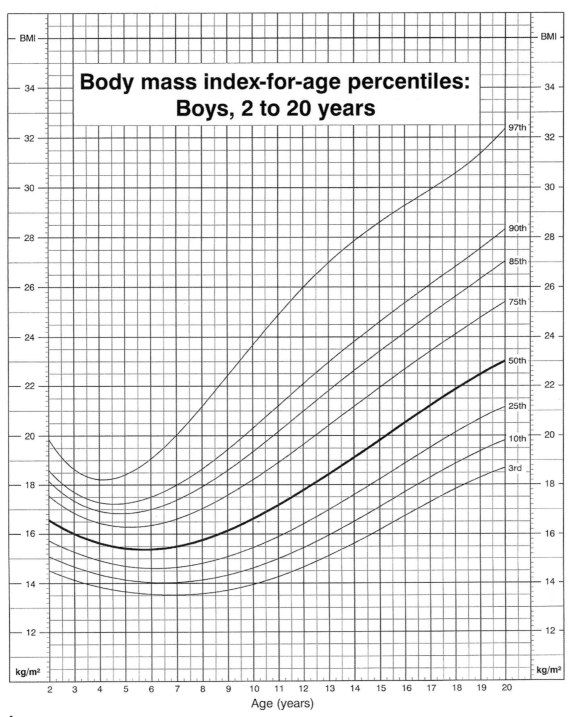

A

FIGURE 7.7 CDC BMI Growth Charts.
A. BMI percentiles by age for boys 2–20 years.

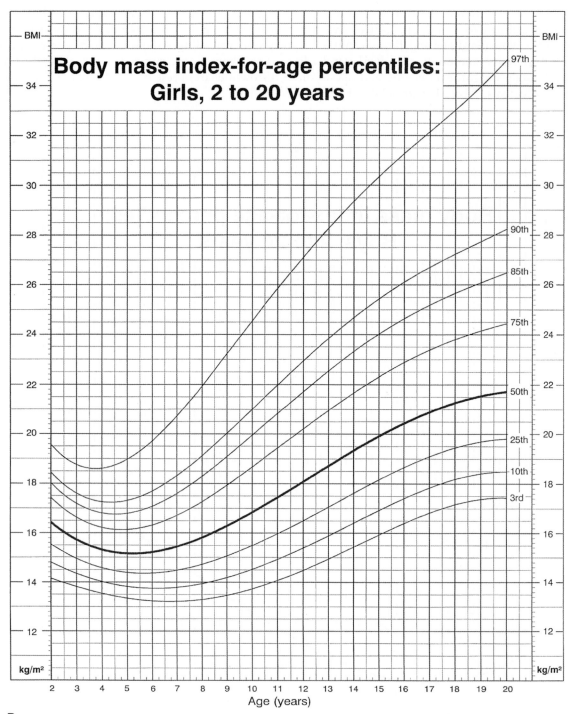

B

FIGURE 7.7 (Continued).
B. BMI percentiles by age for girls 2–20 years.

Recently, FITNESSGRAM® presented new standards for %BF and BMI for children and adolescents (Meredith and Welk, 2010) based on health not population percentiles. Data from over 12,000 white, black, and Mexican American children and adolescents from NHANES surveys were used to assess the relationship between percent body fat and chronic disease risk factors, especially those related to metabolic syndrome. These %BF values also took into account the normal changes in growth and maturation in which boys gain muscle and girls gain fat throughout adolescence (Going et al., 2011). For boys %BF values indicating the threshold of health risk were found to range from 18.9 to 22.3%; for girls the comparable values were 20.9 to 31.4%. These %BF values were then equated to corresponding BMI values (Laurson et al., 2011). The values indicating the threshold of health risk for BMI range from 16.7 to 25.1 kgm·m^{-2} for both boys and girls 5 to 17+ years. Zones are used to indicate "healthy fitness," "leanness," "needs improvement-some risk," and "needs improvement-high risk." The risk refers to developing health problems, especially metabolic syndrome, now and as the individual ages and matures if changes are not made. The "some risk" threshold falls at the CDC 83rd percentile for boys and the 80th for girls. The "high risk" threshold falls at the CDC 92nd and 90th percentiles for boys and girls, respectively. These are not very different from the CDC cut points for overweight and obesity. Further research is needed to determine if the two sets of BMI standards can be used interchangeably as BMI health standards.

Waist-to-Hip Ratio/Waist Circumference

Waist-to-hip (W/H) ratio is another way to estimate health risk based on the individual's pattern of fat distribution. Research has shown that the W/H ratio is a stronger predictor for diabetes, coronary artery disease, and overall death risk than body weight, BMI, or %BF in adults (Brownell et al., 1987; Folsom et al., 1993). In the absence of large total fat stores, the W/H can aid in the identification of certain hormonal and metabolic abnormalities associated with a relative increase in abdominal size but not total fat mass. However, for any given W/H ratio there can be considerable variability in total body fat. Additionally, increases in body fat including intra-abdominal fat may not be detected if a corresponding increase occurs in hip circumference (Sardinha and Teixeira, 2005).

Waist circumference is measured with a tape measure, to the nearest centimeter, at the level of the natural indentation or at the navel if no indentation is apparent. Hip circumference is measured at the largest site. Both measures should be taken while the individual is standing and without clothes. The average value for females aged 17–39 years is 0.80, and this value increases with age to above 0.90. Comparable averages for males range from 0.90 to 0.98. Values ≥ 0.84 for females and 0.99 for males 20–60 years and ≥0.90 and 1.03 for females and males, respectively, 60–69 years indicate a high risk for metabolic disease (Ratamess, 2010; Stamford, 1991).

In 1998, the National Heart, Lung, and Blood Institute's expert panel on obesity concluded that waist circumference (also known as waist girth) alone was more strongly related to visceral abdominal adipose tissue and more predictive of disease risk than the W/H ratio in adults. Similarly, W/H ratio is not a good index of intra-abdominal fat deposition in children and adolescents (Sardinha and Teixeira, 2005; Semiz et al., 2007).

A high waist circumference is associated with an increased risk for Type 2 diabetes, a poor blood lipid profile, high blood pressure, and CVD. It is a stronger predictor of diabetes than is BMI; it can identify those who are at greater cardiometabolic risk better than can BMI; it is consistently related to the risk of developing coronary heart disease; and it is strongly associated with all-cause mortality and selected cause-specific mortality rates (Klein et al., 2007). American College of Sports Medicine (ACSM) now endorses high risk as a waist measure greater than 99 cm (>39 in.) for males and greater than 89 cm (>35 in.) for females (American College of Sports Medicine, 2010) but the traditional values of >102 cm (40 in.) for males and 88 cm (35 in.) for females are still sometimes used as cutoff points (National Heart, Lung, and Blood Institute, 1998; U.S. Department of Health and Human Services, 2000).

Bioelectrical Impedance (Impedance Plethysmography)

Determining body composition by Bioelectrical Impedance (BIA) has gained a great deal of acceptance in fitness facilities primarily because the procedure can easily be done. In many BIA analyzers, four electrodes are attached to a quietly resting supine subject's hands and feet (two per limb either ipsilaterally or contralaterally) (Figure 7.8). Some BIA equipment simply requires the individual to either stand on an electronic digital platform scale with built-in footpad electrodes or to hold the analyzer in both hands. In all types of BIA equipment, a harmless, sensationless, low-amperage (80 mA), radio frequency (50 kHz) electrical current is passed between the electrodes, and the resistance (in ohms) to the current is recorded. Body volume is assumed to be a cylinder of constant cross-sectional area with uniform density distribution. Body

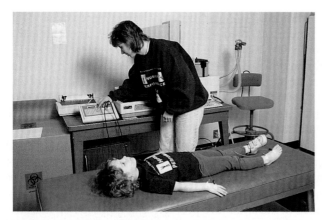

FIGURE 7.8 Determination of Body Composition by Bioelectrical Impedance.

volume is more often defined as height squared divided by resistance (HT² ÷ R) (Baumgartner et al., 1990; Brodie, 1988b; Van Loan, 1990).

The ability to conduct the electrical current is directly related to the amount of water and electrolytes in the various body tissues. Electrical current flows more easily in fat-free tissue (which offers less resistance) than in fat tissue (which acts as an *impedance*) because the fat-free tissue has a higher percentage of water and electrolytes. Therefore, individuals with more fat free weight (FFW) have lower resistance values, and those with more fat weight have higher resistance values.

Because the BIA technique actually measures total body water (TBW), estimates can be made of body density and FFW on the basis of the obtained TBW and the known percentages of water in the body and in the FFW. Another technique is to derive regression equations from height, resistance, and/or other anthropometric variables (such as weight, age, sex, skinfolds, or circumferences) to directly predict FFW or %BF. Hydrostatic weighing is usually used as the criterion measure. As with skinfolds, a number of equations have been generated in this manner.

As you might suspect, the accuracy of BIA measurement depends highly on a normal level of hydration. Either too much fluid (hyperhydration) or too little fluid (hypohydration or dehydration) will affect the readings. The exact effect is controversial. Theoretically, an increase in body water should decrease resistance and %BF. Some experimental evidence supports this theory, but other studies have shown the opposite result. That is, dehydration caused by exercise has decreased resistance, and hyperhydration from ingestion of replacement supplements has increased resistance. This variance may be related to whether the electrolyte content changes proportionally to water and to the shift in water between compartments. What is clear is that individuals should be measured 3–4 hours after the ingestion of a meal or after an exercise session and should not be under the influence of substances, such as caffeine that might act as a diuretic (Baumgartner et al., 1990; Deurenberg et al., 1988; Stump et al., 1988; Van Loan, 1990).

The accuracy of BIA also depends on both ambient and skin temperatures. Resistance is higher in cool temperatures than warm ones. Thus, if an individual is tested repeatedly over a period of 15–20 minutes in an environment where body cooling occurs, the %BF estimate will go up as the skin temperature goes down. Care must therefore be taken that testing is done at a neutral temperature (27–29°C; 80–84°F) when the subject is neither overheated nor chilled (Caton et al., 1988; Stump et al., 1988).

The accuracy of BIA estimates of body composition is also influenced by the equation used. These equations include those for body geometry, cross-sectional area, and current distribution, as well as those used to convert resistance to TBW, body density, and %BF, and are generally closely guarded secrets by the manufacturers. Each of the electrical assumptions is violated by the human body, but the discrepancies are apparently not enough to rule out their use in BIA. However, these violations do limit the accuracy for estimating TBW, FFW, and %BF to individuals not at the extremes of leanness or fatness. Furthermore, if the criterion measure upon which the equation was based did not take into account the age-related differences in TBW, these inaccuracies would be confounded (Baumgartner et al., 1990; Brodie, 1988a; Chumlea and Sun, 2005; Hodgdon and Fitzgerald, 1987).

BIA values under standard conditions will be consistent, but the accuracy is probably no better than that achieved by skinfolds (Baumgartner et al., 1990). The error of the estimate has been reported to range from approximately 3 to 6% BF (Ratamess, 2010).

In summary, %BF and fat-free mass can be estimated adequately for screening and tracking moderate changes in body composition through field measures. On a scale of 1 (excellent) to 5 (unacceptable) based on precision, objectivity, and accuracy, Going and Davis (2001) have ranked the different techniques as follows:

> Skinfolds 2.5 (good to very good)
> Bioelectrical impedance 2.5 (good to very good)
> Circumferences 3.0 (good)
> BMI 4.0 (fair)

Overweight and Obesity

Although being overweight is what bothers most people, it is really the amount and location of fat (%BF, abdominal fat mass) that should be of concern. Excess weight can be caused by high levels of lean muscle mass, but additional muscle mass is beneficial. Except in rare instances, such as providing protection from the cold water for an English Channel swimmer or certain wasting diseases, excess fat is generally not beneficial.

There are no universally agreed upon acceptable %BF standards. The most typically used normal values for young adults (20–29 years) are 12–15% for males and 22–25% for females with an allowance of an additional 2% for each decade of age. Obesity is defined as +5% BF above the normal value (Kaminsky and Dwyer, 2006).

Figure 7.9 shows a wider range of standards based on age, sex, and athletic participation (Lohman et al., 1997). Note that some increase in %BF with age has also been built in for individuals ≥35 years. This was based on studies showing that low or reduced body fat (especially in middle-aged females) is associated with lower bone mineral content. Thus, to maximize the goal of overall health, a balance must be reached between protecting against heart disease (associated with excessive fatness) and osteoporosis and bone fractures (associated with excessive leanness) (Kaminsky and Dwyer, 2006). Note also that there is no category representing overweight in this figure (because this is based on body fat not weight), but there is a break between each recommended range and the start of the corresponding obesity range. Individuals whose %BF falls in this area (as well as the obese range) should reduce %BF.

Figure 7.10 shows average %BF values for males and females across the age spectrum from 12 to 80 years. These data represent averages of non-Hispanic whites, non-Hispanic blacks, and Mexican Americans by sex. The means were computed from BIA data collected during the third National Health and Nutrition Survey (NHANES III) 1988–1994 (Chumlea et al., 2002). Note that even by the generous age-adjusted upper limits for adults presented in **Figure 7.9**, these means are almost borderline obese.

What Happens to Adipose Cells in Obesity? The Cellular Basis of Obesity

Adipose tissue is composed of a matrix of connective tissue in which white adipose cells (adipocytes) appear singularly or in small clusters. A typical cell (**Figure 7.11**) looks something like a signet ring, a metal band with a stone or jewel at the top. The nucleus of the cell appears as the stone or jewel of the ring in the cell membrane, which forms the band of the ring. The triglyceride drop-

Hyperplasia Growth in a tissue or organ through an increase in the number of cells.

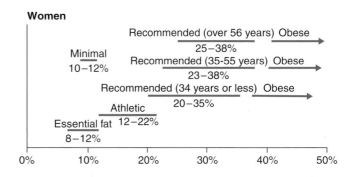

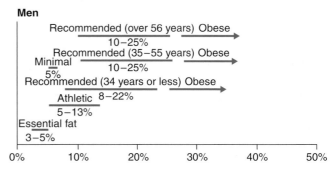

FIGURE 7.9 Percent Body Fat Standards for Adult Males and Females.
Ranges of acceptable %BF and %BF values representing obesity are presented for adult women and men by age and athletic status. Note that the athletic standards begin at the upper limit of essential fat: 5% for men and 12% for women. This coincides with the acceptable minimal value for men. Women have an acceptable minimal range that encompasses part of the essential fat range.
Source: Lohman, T. G., L. B. Houtkooper, & S. B. Going: Body composition assessment: Body fat standards and methods in the field of exercise and sports medicine. *ACSM's Health Fitness Journal.* 1:30–35 (1997). Reproduced with permission.

lets are stored in the space within the confines of the cell (Marieb and Hoehn, 2010). The brown adipose cell in **Figure 7.11** is discussed later.

An adult of acceptable weight has about 30–50 billion fat cells. Females have approximately 50% more fat cells than males. Adipocytes can become up to 10 times larger if needed to store triglycerides. Apparently, this increase in size (hypertrophy) is how increasing levels of fat are first stored. Sometimes when the fat cell size is enlarged, the increased size causes a bulging between the fibrous tissue strands, causing a dimply, waffled appearance. These lumpy areas are often referred to as *cellulite*. Cellulite, however, is simply fat (Björntorp, 1987, 1989).

Once the upper limit of fat storage by hypertrophy is approached (somewhere around 30 kg of fat), fat cell hyperplasia occurs. **Hyperplasia** in general is growth in a tissue or organ through an increase in the number of cells. Fat tissue hyperplasia involves the development of new adipocytes from immature precursor cells. Adipocytes

FIGURE 7.10 Average %BF for Americans Aged 12–80 years.
At all ages, females have a higher %BF than males. The trend is for a steady rise in %BF with age except for males between the ages 12 and 16 years and males and females over the age of 60 years. *Source*: Based on data from Chumlea, W. C., S. S. Guo, R. J. Kuczmarski, et al.: Body composition estimates from NHANES III bioelectrical impedance data. *International Journal of Obesity*. 26(12):1596–1609 (2002).

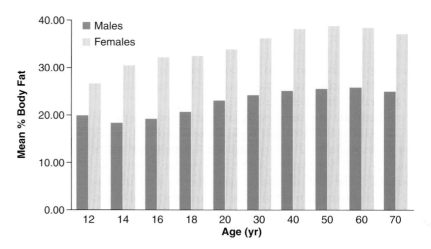

themselves do not divide and multiply, but hypertrophy in adipocytes stimulates cell division and maturation in precursor cells (Malina and Bouchard, 1991). Thus, a newly overweight adult is likely to have the same number of fat cells as when he or she was of normal weight, but

these adipocytes will be larger than before. An obese individual may have enlarged adipocytes, an increased number of adipocytes, or both. Obese individuals may have as many as 75–80 billion fat cells. Once created, fat cell numbers are not naturally reduced, even if body weight and body fat are lost (Sjöström and Björntorp, 1974). Liposuction—the surgical removal of adipose tissue—is the only way to get rid of adipocytes. The maintenance of large numbers of adipocytes may be one reason why it is so difficult for obese individuals to maintain a weight/fat loss once it has been achieved.

These facts emphasize the importance of preventing the maturation of extra fat cells. Overweight or obese infants, children, or adolescents tend to become overweight or obese adults, although adolescent obesity is more predictive of adult obesity than is obesity at birth or in infancy (Charney et al., 1975; Dietz, 1987; Lohman, 1989).

Figure 7.12 indicates the typical pattern of changes in adipose cell size (**Figure 7.12A**) and number (**Figure 7.12B**) that occurs in normal (nonobese) children and adolescents (Malina and Bouchard, 1991). From birth to young adulthood the average adipose cell size doubles or even triples. Most of this increase in size happens during the first year after birth. From 1 year to the onset of puberty there is no significant increase in size and no sex difference. At puberty, adipose cell size increases in females but remains fairly constant in males. Not all adipose cells are of the same size; internal (visceral) fat cells are generally smaller than subcutaneous fat cells. Furthermore, not all subcutaneous cells are equal in size. For example, gluteal adipocytes tend to be larger than abdominal adipocytes, which in turn are larger than subscapular cells.

At birth, the number of adipocytes is approximately 5 billion. For the number to increase to the average adult value of 30 billion, considerable change must occur. However, little increase in number occurs during the first year after birth when the cell size is changing so drastically (**Figure 7.12B**). From 1 year to the onset of puberty, there is a gradual but steady increase in the number of adipocytes, with no difference appearing between the

White Adipose Cell

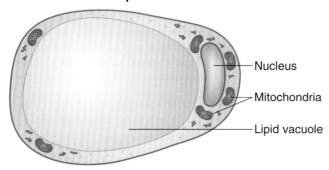

Brown Adipose Cell

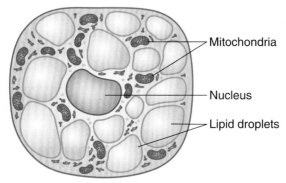

FIGURE 7.11 Adipose Cells.
White and brown adipose cells both store lipid as triglyceride, but do so in slightly different ways. White adipose cells contain one large fat droplet; brown adipose cells contain many small fat droplets. Most of the fat stored in the human body is stored in white adipose cells. *Source:* Malina, R. M., C. Bouchard, & O. Bar-Or: *Growth, Maturation and Physical Activity* (2nd edition). Champaign, IL: Human Kinetics, 163 (2004). Reprinted by permission.

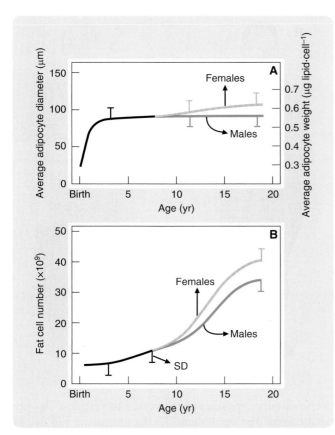

FIGURE 7.12 Adipose Cell Size and Number Changes with Growth.

A. The greatest change in adipose cell size occurs between birth and 1 year. Until approximately age 10, cell size is similar in males and females. After age 10, the difference between males and females gradually widens, and individual variations (indicated by the vertical lines) become more apparent. **B.** The number of adipose cells gradually increases through the childhood years in males and females at a similar rate. At approximately age 10, in both sexes, the rate of increase in fat cell number accelerates, but females far exceed males. Individual differences indicated by vertical bars (labeled SD for standard deviation) increase considerably with age. *Source*: Malina, R. M., C. Bouchard, & O. Bar-Or: Growth, Maturation and Physical Activity (2nd edition). Champaign, IL: Human Kinetics. 166–167 (2004). Data from Bonnet and Rocour-Brumioul (1981), Boulton et al. (1978), Chumlea et al. (1981), Hager (1981), Hager et al. (1977), Knittle et al. (1979), Sjöström (1980), and Soriguer Escofet et al. (1996). Reprinted with permission.

sexes. This gradual increase can double or even triple the number of fat cells. At puberty, the number of adipose cells increases greatly in both males and females, but the female increase far exceeds the male increase. This increase in fat cell number plateaus in late adolescence and early adulthood ideally remains at that level. In reality, however, hyperplasia can and often does occur in adulthood (Malina and Bouchard, 1991). Thus, although there are two critical periods—infancy and adolescence—in the development of adipocytes, this should not be interpreted as meaning that fat cells cannot be added during adulthood.

Some individuals produce more adipocytes than others during growth, and this can amount to billions of cells. During the growth changes, males tend to accumulate more subcutaneous fat on the trunk and females on the extremities.

Fat Distribution Patterns

The location of fat storage varies among individuals. In general, fat is distributed in three basic patterns: android, gynoid, and intermediate patterns (**Figure 7.13**). The *android pattern* (**Figure 7.13A**), also known as the abdominal or apple pattern, is predominately found in males. It is characterized by the storage of fat in the nape of the neck, shoulders, and abdomen (upper part of the body). In this pattern, the largest quantity of fat is stored internally, not subcutaneously, and the trunk area has the greatest amount of subcutaneous fat. The result is the classic potbelly shape. Individuals with potbellies often make the claim they are not fat and occasionally challenge others to hit them in the stomach as hard as possible to prove their superior musculature. In fact, the hardness of the abdominal region is caused by the excess fat in the abdominal cavity pushing against the abdominal muscles and stretching them taut, not by muscle tone or hypertrophy. The amount of intra-abdominal (visceral) fat is twice as high in android obesity as gynoid obesity (Blouin et al., 2008; Campaigne, 1990; Stamford, 1991).

The *gynoid pattern* (**Figure 7.13B**), also called the gluteofemoral or pear pattern, is found predominantly in females. It is characterized by the storage of fat in the lower part of the body, specifically, in the thighs and buttocks, with the largest quantity being stored subcutaneously. No pseudohardness is apparent. These sites tend to be soft and tend to jiggle (Campaigne, 1990; Stamford, 1991).

It is thought that the deposition of fat in the gluteal-femoral region in females is linked to the reproductive function. In particular, gluteal-femoral fat may furnish energy for the development of the fetus, primarily during the latter stages of pregnancy, and for the newborn child during lactation. As would be expected, these fat deposits are controlled by the steroid hormones.

The third type of fat pattern is known simply as the *intermediate pattern* (**Figure 7.13C**). In this pattern, fat is stored in both the upper and the lower parts of the body, giving a somewhat rectangular cubic appearance. Note that all three patterns are found in both males and females, despite the sex-specific predominance associated with android and gynoid shapes (Campaigne, 1990; Stamford, 1991). With menopause, female fat distribution typically changes from a gynoid to an android pattern (Després and Lamarche, 2000; Rosano et al., 2007).

Abdominal fat deposits are easily mobilized; therefore, it is possible to reduce fat accumulation in this area relatively easily (assuming a caloric deficit). Conversely, gluteal-femoral fat deposits are not easily mobilized,

FIGURE 7.13 Patterns of Fat Distribution.
A. Android; **B.** Gynoid; and **C.** Intermediate.

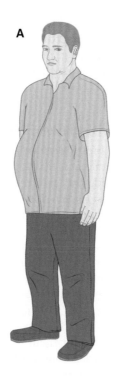 A

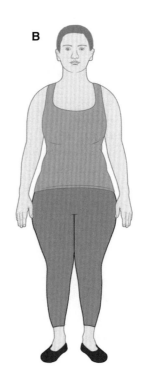 B

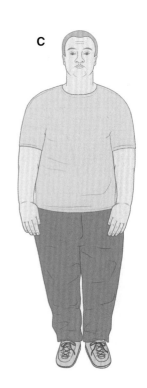 C

and so it is not possible to reduce fat accumulation in these areas easily. The potential for reshaping the gluteofemoral fat pattern is extremely limited (Campaigne, 1990; Stamford, 1991). In one study that measured areas of fat loss from caloric restriction in overweight young females, those with an android distribution of fat lost more weight and showed a greater decrease in waist circumference and a greater intra-abdominal fat loss than those with a gynoid fat distribution (Jones and Edwards, 1999).

The reason behind the variation in the fat deposit mobilization is hormonally based (Wong et al., 2003). Two different receptors, alpha and beta, have been identified in fat cells; they vary in their ability to facilitate or inhibit fat incorporation into the cell or fat mobilization out of the cell. Alpha-receptors inhibit fat transfer to and from the adipocytes, and beta-receptors enhance these transfers. Enzyme activity is concomitantly increased or decreased. Alpha-receptors predominate in the lower body and are thus more abundant in the gynoid pattern. Beta-receptors are concentrated in the upper body and are more abundant in the android pattern. Thus, the adipose cells in the abdominal region are more unstable.

Epinephrine (released from the adrenal medulla) binds to beta-receptors on adipose tissue and causes lipids (fatty acids) to be mobilized from the abdominal cells and released into the circulatory system. If the free fatty acids and glycerol can be used (directly or indirectly) as fuel to support exercise, there is no problem. However, when epinephrine is released in times of emotional stress and there is no need for the excess fuel, the fatty acids and glycerol are then routed to the liver, where they are detrimentally deposited or converted to very low-density lipoproteins and small dense LDLs increasing the risk of coronary heart disease (Després and Lamarche, 2000).

In addition, abdominal fat cells tend to be larger than the fat cells found in other parts of the body. Larger abdominal (android) fat cells are associated with glucose intolerance (the inability to dispose of a glucose load effectively), coupled with insulin resistance, hyperglycemia, and an excess of insulin in the blood (hyperinsulinemia). These conditions are associated with diabetes mellitus (a coronary heart disease [CAD] risk factor) and hypertension (a CAD risk factor). The latter occurs because of the action of insulin in promoting reabsorption of sodium by the kidneys (Brownell et al., 1987; Campaigne, 1990; Stamford, 1991). Conversely, the smaller thigh-hip (gynoid) fat cells are highly insulin sensitive. After a fatty meal when circulating triglycerides are broken down by these cells, the resulting fatty acids tend to be stored immediately. This keeps them out of circulation and avoids the conversion to low-density lipoproteins (LDL) (McCarty, 2003). Finally, visceral adipose tissue releases over 120 hormones and factors called adipokines or adipocytokines. Most of these factors are involved in the pathological development of inflammation, atherosclerosis, hypertension, endothelial dysfunction, and insulin resistance. These are important components in the development of the metabolic syndrome (discussed in Chapter 15) (Hutley and Prins, 2005; Lyon et al., 2003; Wong et al, 2003). Between the two major fat distribution types these factors result in the gynoid pattern being associated with a lower risk and the android pattern with a higher risk of myocardial infarctions, stroke, and metabolic syndrome components (Kang et al., 2011; Toss et al., 2011;

TABLE 7.5 Patterns of Fat Distribution		
Factor	**Android**	**Gynoid**
Sex it predominates in	Males	Females
Regional fat storage	Upper body (neck and abdomen)	Lower body (thighs and buttocks)
Fat storage site	Internal	Subcutaneous
Characteristic of fat deposit	Hard	Soft
Adipose tissue receptors	Beta	Alpha
Mobilizing hormone	Epinephrine	Reproductive, especially prolactin
Adipose cell size	Large	Small
Fat mobilization	Easy	Difficult
Major risk	Coronary artery disease, glucose intolerance, diabetes, and hypertension	Psychological

Wiklund et al., 2010). **Table 7.5** summarizes the differences between android and gynoid fat patterns.

Simply looking in the mirror while naked is probably the best way to determine whether you are android, gynoid, or intermediate in terms of fat distribution, although the calculation of the W/H ratio might also be useful. High ratios reflect a larger waist and thus more upper body fat deposition (android shape) than lower body hip fat deposition.

Health Risks of Overweight and Obesity

Individuals who are overweight from an excess of body fat but who are not obese incur mild to moderate health risks. Individuals who are obese possess an excess of body fat that represents a significant health risk, particularly if that excess fat is visceral. **Figure 7.14** presents an image of visceral abdominal tissue. This particular image was produced by a CT scan. MRI is also frequently used in laboratory studies. These imaging techniques directly

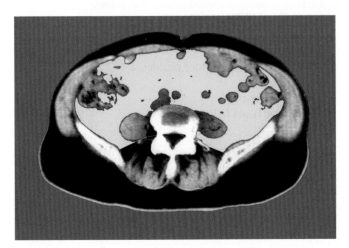

FIGURE 7.14 Visceral Abdominal Tissue.
CT scan at the L4–L5 intravertebral space. The abdominal visceral fat depot is in yellow; the subcutaneous fat depot (both outside the muscle wall and below the skin) is in black.

measure fat tissue. As previously mentioned, measuring waist circumference is the best field technique for estimating abdominal obesity.

Figure 7.15 presents the results of three national surveys conducted on 23,654 adults aged 20–79 years indicating the mean waist circumference and prevalence of age-adjusted abdominal obesity. Abdominal obesity was defined as greater than 102 cm for males and greater than 88 cm for females. Both males and females show a steady increase in the average waist circumference over the approximately 40 years' time span. The male average has remained below the cutoff for abdominal obesity but the female averages for 1988–1994 and 1999–2000 are both above the cutoff. The age-adjusted prevalence has also steadily increased in both males and females, with approximately 40% of males and 60% of females exhibiting abdominal obesity in the 1999–2000 survey (Okosun et al., 2004). The prevalence of abdominal obesity also exceeds that of general obesity in young people (Okosun et al., 2006).

The amount of fat and the distribution of fat are linked to higher risks of major diseases. In 2008, medical costs associated with obesity were estimated at $147 billion total or $1429 higher per person than for nonobese individuals (CDC, 2012a). **Table 7.6** provides a listing of risk factors and diseases divided into those that result from metabolic changes caused by obesity and those that results from the increased mass of fat per se (Bray, 2000). Among equally obese individuals, those with the highest accumulation of visceral adipose tissue (VAT) show the severest deterioration in metabolic variables (Després and Lamarche, 2000). VAT appears to have a stronger relationship with physiological and pathological processes, metabolic syndrome, and cardiometabolic risk factors than total body fat and/or abdominal subcutaneous adipose tissue does (Demerath et al., 2008; Liu et al., 2010; Sardinha and Teixeira, 2005).

Hypertension (High Blood Pressure)

Excess body weight and fat has a strong direct relationship with elevated blood pressure (Bray, 1987; Burton et al.,

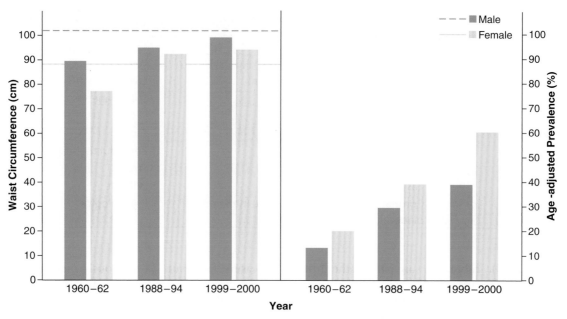

FIGURE 7.15   Abdominal Obesity in U.S. Adult Males and Females, 1960–2000.
The graph on the left presents actual waist circumference measures. Average values for males are below the 102 cm cutoff for abdominal obesity over this time span, but average female values are above the cutoff of 88 cm for abdominal obesity. As shown in the graph on the right, the prevalence (%) of abdominal obesity has climbed steadily in both males and females from 1960 to 2000, with almost 40% of males and 60% of females now considered to exhibit abdominal obesity.

1985; Pi-Sunyer, 1993). A BMI > 23 kg·m⁻² has been shown to be an independent predictor of hypertension in elderly black females (Javed et al., 2011). Hypertension is also a very strong and independent risk factor for coronary heart disease.

Cardiovascular-Respiratory Diseases

A longitudinal study has been investigating the risk factors for heart disease in more than 5000 residents of Framingham, Massachusetts. Data from 26 to 30 years of follow-up have shown that overweight or obesity is

TABLE 7.6 Health Risks Associated with Overweight/Obesity	
From Metabolic Changes	**From Mass of Fat per se**
Diabetes Mellitus type 2; insulin resistance	Osteoarthritis
Gallbladder disease	Sleep apnea
Hypertension	Breathlessness/respiratory problems
Coronary heart disease; stroke	Low back pain
Certain cancers (breast, colon, endometrial, pancreatic prostate, and uterine)	Skin stretch marks
Dyslipidemia/hyperlipidemia (↑LDL, ↑TG, and ↓HDL) LDL, low-density lipoproteins; TG, triglycerides; HDL, high-density lipoproteins	Congestive heart failure
Impaired fertility; other reproductive problems	
Gout	
Digestive diseases	
Impaired kidney function	
Liver malfunction	
Stroke	

FOCUS ON RESEARCH: *Clinically Relevant*
Childhood Obesity and CVD Risk Factors

A total of 1166 White (C) and 1213 African American (AA) girls were tested in the National Heart, Lung, and Blood Institute Growth and Health Study annually between ages 9 or 10 years and 18 years and were contacted for self-reported measures at age 21–23 years. At the time the study began, BMI values above the CDC's age-specific 95th percentile were labeled as overweight. Because these values are now labeled obese, the term obesity will be used here. Young adult obesity was defined as a BMI ≥ 30 kg·m^{-2}.

The rate of obesity increased throughout adolescence from 7% to 10% in the C girls and from 17 to 24% in the AA girls (not shown). Graph A shows the percent of new onset cases (incidence) of obesity by race over the age span. The incidence ranged from 2 to 5% through age 12, after which the annual increase was generally in the 1–2% range. The important part of this information is the fact that it is the so-called "tween" years (ages 9–12 years) when girls are especially at risk of getting fat. Thus, particular attention and intervention should be directed toward this age group to prevent the increase in body weight and fat.

Graph B shows the percentage of selected cardiovascular risk factors in the C and AA groups combined, based on being or not being obese. Girls who were obese were 3–10 times as likely as those who were not obese to be assessed as "at

risk" on four of the six cardiovascular risk factors: unhealthful levels of systolic and diastolic blood pressure (SBP and DBP), high-density lipoproteins (HDL), and triglyceride levels. The increased risk was already evident at age 9 years. Thus, there are meaningful health reasons for not delaying interventions.

Graph C shows the percentage of obese girls in young adulthood who were obese or not at each age in childhood. For example, 71.3% of the obese 9-year-olds were obese at approximately 21 years, but only 10.3% of the nonobese at age 9 were obese at approximately 21 years. Overall, girls who were obese during childhood were 11 to 30 times more likely to be obese in young adulthood. Given that the height and weight values were self-reported by the young adults, and underreporting weight is a known problem, the risk could be even greater. These data clearly show that obesity tracks from childhood to adulthood and needs to be addressed with children.

Source: Thompson, D. R., E. Obarzanek, D. L. Franko, et al.: Childhood overweight and cardiovascular disease risk factors: The National Heart, Lung, and Blood Institute Growth and Health Study. *Journal of Pediatrics.* 150:18–25 (2007).

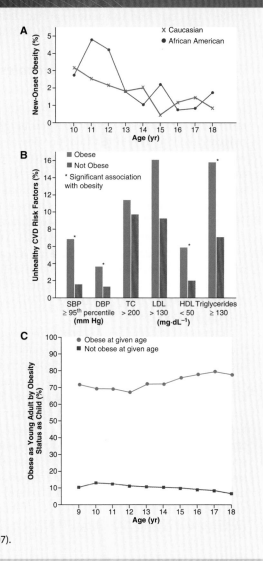

a significant predictor of cardiovascular disease (CVD), independent of age, cholesterol levels, systolic blood pressure, cigarette smoking, and glucose tolerance. Based on this extensive data set, the Framingham investigators have concluded that if everyone were at or within 10% of his or her desirable weight, there would be 25% less coronary heart disease and 35% less congestive heart failure and stroke. The risk is greater for those who become obese early in life, as in childhood, rather than in old age (Bray, 1987; Burton et al., 1985; Pi-Sunyer, 1993; Simopoulos, 1987). A study of 276,835 Dutch children showed that higher BMI vales during childhood (7–13 years of age) were associated with an increased risk of coronary heart disease in adulthood. The associations were stronger in boys than girls and increased as the child became older in both sexes (Baker et al., 2007). Among other things,

the Focus on Research: Clinically Relevant box provides evidence of increased CVD risk factors in female children and adolescents with BMI values greater than the 95th percentile (Thompson et al., 2007).

As mentioned previously, the risk is higher for those who store their fat in the android pattern than in the gynoid pattern. While coronary heart disease is linked to diabetes mellitus, hypertension, and hyperlipidemia (primarily metabolic changes), congestive heart failure is more related to the increase in total fat mass per se. A larger body mass increases circulatory demand, including an elevation in the cardiac output often operating against an elevated systemic vascular resistance induced by hypertension (Arciero and Nindl, 2004).

The increased sizes of the chest and abdomen in obese individuals alter respiratory patterns leading to ventilation-perfusion mismatches and predisposing the individual to hypoxia (too little oxygen) and carbon dioxide retention. Airway obstruction often leads to sleep apnea (absence of spontaneous breathing). If uncontrolled, this can lead to sudden cardiac death from ventricular arrhythmias (Arciero and Nindl, 2004).

Gallbladder Disease and Hypercholesterolemia (High Cholesterol)

In the Framingham study, individuals who were 20% or more above the average weight for their height were about twice as likely to develop gallbladder disease as those who were 10% less than the average weight. In another study, the frequency of gallbladder disease was largely explained by weight, age, and, in females, the number of viable pregnancies (parity). Obese females between ages 20 and 30 years had a 600% greater chance of having gallbladder disease than average-weight females. Within all age groups, the frequency of gallbladder disease increased with body weight. The body weight of males with gallstones has also been shown to be significantly more than the body weight of males without gallstones (Bray, 1987; Pi-Sunyer, 1993).

Increased gallbladder disease in overweight or obese individuals can be at least partly explained by the effect of increased body weight and fat on cholesterol. Fatness has a significant positive relationship with cholesterol level. Cholesterol production is also related to body weight, such that 1 excess kg of body weight increases cholesterol production by 20–22 mg·dL^{-1}. Bile is produced in the liver and stored in the gallbladder and always contains some cholesterol. The bile of obese individuals is more saturated with cholesterol than that of nonobese individuals. This increased presence of cholesterol in bile is the likely cause of the increased risk of gallbladder disease (Arciero and Nindl, 2004; Bray, 1987).

Diabetes Mellitus

Diabetes is a disorder of carbohydrate (glucose) metabolism. Overweight or obesity appears to cause an increase in insulin resistance and deterioration in glucose tolerance (leading to high levels of blood glucose) and to aggravate the appearance of diabetes. The risk for developing diabetes mellitus increases with the degree of obesity and age of the individual. This is also linked to the increased levels of circulating fatty acids that are evident in the obese. Visceral abdominal tissue is more strongly associated with insulin resistance than abdominal subcutaneous fat (Arciero and Nindl, 2004; Bray, 1987; Burton et al., 1985; Pi-Sunyer, 1993; Preis et al., 2010).

Cancer

The American Cancer Society has published data on 750,000 individuals studied between 1959 and 1972. In these studies, as BMI increased, so did the incidence of death from cancer, even independent of cigarette smoking. Overweight males were particularly susceptible to prostate and colorectal cancer; overweight females showed increased rates of breast, cervical, endometrial, uterine, and ovarian cancer. The suspected link, at least for females, is the level of estrogen. Adipose tissue is a site for estrogen formation in all females and the major site in postmenopausal females. Estrogen formation is increased in overweight and obese individuals owing to the increased number of adipose cells (Bray, 1987; Charney et al., 1975; Pi-Sunyer, 1993; Simopoulos, 1987).

Miscellaneous Disorders

In addition to the specific diseases just discussed, overweight or obesity has been linked to kidney and liver dysfunction, joint problems (osteoarthritis) and gout, endocrine disorders including reproductive problems, problematic response to anesthetics for surgery, and an impaired physical work capacity (American College of Sports Medicine, 1983; Pi-Sunyer, 1993). The increased prevalence of these diseases and problems applies to adults, but overweight or obese children also show increased risk factors, though not the actual diseases, compared with normal-weight children (Williams et al., 1992).

The diseases discussed in the preceding sections lead to increased mortality or decreased longevity. In and of itself, visceral fat is an independent predictor of all-cause mortality in males (Kuk et al., 2005). The associations between underweight, overweight, and obesity per se with these diseases and mortality are somewhat more complex. Flegal et al. (2005) estimated the relative risk of mortality (death) associated with different levels of BMI (underweight = BMI < 18.5 kg·m^{-2}; overweight = BMI 25 to <30 kg·m^{-2}; obese = BMI ≥ 30 kg·m^{-2}) using data from NHANES I (1971–1975), II (1976–1980 with follow-up through 1992), and III (1988–1994 with follow-up through 2000). Underweight and obesity were associated with increased mortality relative to normal weight. However, overweight was not associated with excess mortality. The authors speculated that improvements in public health and medical care may have been responsible for this positive outcome for those who are overweight. Two subsequent studies extended the follow-up to 2004 and found similar results. In the first study (Flegal et al., 2007), which used the same databases with a longer follow-up, underweight was linked with increased mortality from noncancer or non-CVD (primarily respiratory-related) but not with cancer or CVD mortality. Obesity was linked with significantly increased mortality from CVD and obesity-related cancers (colon, breast, esophageal, uterine, ovarian, kidney, and pancreatic), but not with other cancers, noncancer, or non-CVD mortality. Overweight and obesity combined were linked with *increased* mortality from diabetes and kidney disease.

Physical Activity/Physical Fitness and the Health Risks of Obesity

Epidemiological evidence indicates that there is a relationship between high physical activity/physical fitness and lower health risks of overweight/obesity. The health risks of overweight and obesity have been detailed in this chapter. It is well established that one way to reduce these health risks is to lose body weight and, more specifically, body fat. However, it is also well established that this is easier said than done, and the same is true for maintaining a weight loss that has been achieved. So, the question becomes whether physical activity or physical fitness can weaken or blunt the increased risk of morbidity or mortality in overweight/obese individuals who remain overweight or obese.

The compiled results of three studies shed some light on this question. These studies were conducted at the Institute for Aerobics Research, Cooper Clinic (Dallas, TX), and are based on approximately 22,000 males aged 20–60 years and 2600 males and females over the age of 60 years. The results presented in the accompanying graph for males aged 20–60 years clearly show that regardless of how body composition is measured (BMI—using 27.8 kg·m^{-2} as the cutoff between normal and obese males %BF, or waist girth), overweight or obese males who are fit have a lower risk of all-cause mortality (early death from all causes) than unfit males (Blair and Brodney, 1999; Welk and Blair, 2000). Indeed, the fit obese males had much less risk of early death than unfit lean males. This can be seen in the figure by comparing the red bars (fit), which have a relative risk (RR) of approximately 1.0, to the blue bars (unfit), where the

RR ranges from 1.62 to 4.88. These higher risk ratios mean that the unfit are 62% to almost 500% more likely to suffer early death than the fit, regardless of body composition. In addition, the risk of all-cause mortality is similar for fit individuals, regardless of their body composition: lean, normal, or obese; that is, the adjusted RR for the fit groups deviated only slightly from 1.0 (0.8 to 1.08, which indicates no excessive risk), regardless of body composition (Blair and Brodney, 1999; Welk and Blair, 2000).

Fitness in these studies was determined by a maximal treadmill test, and only the individuals in the bottom 20% (by age-specific distribution) were classified as unfit. In absolute values, this level of cardiovascular fitness is equivalent to a $\dot{V}O_2$max of 35 mL·kg^{-1}·min^{-1} for 20- to 39-year-old males and 33 mL·kg^{-1}·min^{-1} for 40- to 59-year-old males. These fitness levels can be achieved by as little as 400–1650 kcal of activity per week. This energy expenditure is consistent with 30 minutes of moderate activity on most days of the week.

A 2007 study (Sui et al., 2007) from the same laboratory using the same testing procedures extended these results to individuals more than 60 years of age including approximately 20% females. One change was that individuals were divided into four groups by BMI to match the new standards: 18.5–24.9 kg·m^{-2} (normal), 25.0–29.9 kg·m^{-2} (overweight), 30–34.9 kg·m^{-2} (level I obesity), and greater than 35 kg·m^{-2} (level II and III obesity). The upper limit of %BF was maintained at 25% for males and set at 30% for females. Death rates per 1000 person-years, adjusted for age, sex, and examination year were 32.6, 16.6, 12.8, 12.3, and 8.1

from the lowest to the highest quintiles of fitness. That is, the lowest 20% of this population based on $\dot{V}O_2$max mL·kg·min^{-1} had the highest death rate. Higher fitness was linked to lower risk of death due to all causes. This was true in both normal and overweight BMI groups, for participants with normal waist size, abdominal obesity, normal %BF, and excessive fat. However, fit individuals who were obese (BMI = 30–34.9 kg·m^{-2}, had abdominal obesity, or had excessive %BF) had a lower risk of all-cause mortality than unfit, normal weight, or lean individuals.

The implications for health promotion are clear. There are health risks associated with overweight and obesity, and the advice to lose weight remains sound. Weight loss remains one of the primary reasons individuals join a health club or exercise program. Many overweight/obese individuals, however, become frustrated when the desired weight loss does not happen or does not happen rapidly enough for whatever reason, and they quickly drop out of the exercise regimen. These individuals should be encouraged to remain or become more active in order to reap the physiological benefits of regular activity. The process of being active, rather than the product of changes in body weight or percent fat, should be stressed. Emphasizing the process is more likely to motivate overweight/obese individuals because participation in activity is within each person's control (Welk and Blair, 2000). If the process (regular physical activity) is accomplished, the product (lower health risks) will follow.

Sources: Blair and Brodney (1999), Sui et al. (2007), Welk and Blair (2000).

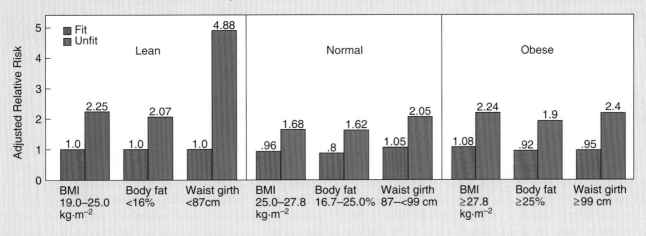

FOCUS ON APPLICATION

The Impact of Fatness on Fitness

While the previous Focus on Application box has shown that cardiovascular fitness positively impacts the health risks of overweight and obesity, the interaction of these two variables can be viewed in another way: how does fatness impact fitness? More specifically, do the increasing overweight/obesity levels of children and adolescents explain the decline in cardiovascular fitness that is now evident? Considerable evidence worldwide supports the contention that aerobic fitness is decreasing and body fatness increasing in children and adolescents. Variability in fatness is known to account for approximately 20% of the variability in running performance, but are the changes in fatness totally responsible for the changes in aerobic fitness?

In this report, Australians aged 10–12 tested in 1985 were matched by age, sex, BMI, and triceps skinfold to children tested in 1997 (N = 279 matched pairs from a total sample of 2748 participants) on the 1.6-km run (also known as the metric mile). Similarly, 12–15-year olds tested in 1995–1996 were matched with adolescents tested in 1999–2000 on the 20-m shuttle run (20 MST) (also known as the PACER) (N = 2834 matched pairs from a total sample of 7938 participants).

The accompanying graph shows the decrement in performance in the total samples for both of the fitness run tests. The values for the 1.6-km run were approximately −7% to −8%, and those for the 20 MST −2% to −3%. The lesser decline for the 20 MST is undoubtedly due to the shorter time between the testing sessions (4 years versus 12 years)

for that test compared with the 1.6-km run. The differences for the matched samples are less than the total samples. In the 1.6-km run, the differences in fitness performance were reduced by 61% and 37% for boys and girls, respectively, by matching for BMI and skinfold thickness. For the 20 MST, the reductions for matching were 46% for boys and 29% for girls. In the matched sample statistical technique, if the declines in running performance seen in the total group had been eliminated in the matched sample, then these fitness declines could have been attributed solely to increases in fatness. However, this clearly did not happen.

These results are of more than just theoretical interest. If the goal is to reverse the decline in fitness (which it certainly should be), it is important to know whether it is due only to increases in fatness, in which case weight reduction strategies alone are called for, or whether other factors are also important. The data indicate that other factors, such as reduced physical activity and a subsequent detraining effect, are likely to have contributed to the decline. This suggests that increasing physical activity levels in conjunction with dietary strategies is needed to improve aerobic fitness.

Source: Olds et al. (2007).

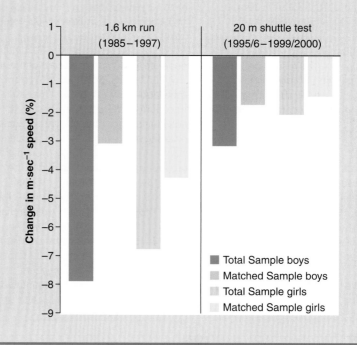

However, overweight and obesity combined were also linked with *decreased* mortality from noncancer or non-CVD causes. Overweight in and of itself was not linked with cancer or CVD mortality and was linked significantly with decreased mortality from noncancer or non-CVD causes. This time the authors speculated that the greater nutritional reserves of being moderately overweight may be associated with improved survival during recovery from situations such as infections or surgeries.

Additionally, some proportion of the individuals classified as overweight based on BMI could actually be in a healthy range for %BF due to a larger amount of LBM. The second study (McAuley et al., 2007) using data from military veterans found that obesity was associated with substantially lower mortality risk in non–heart failure individuals. Higher cardiorespiratory fitness and obesity later in life were suggested as accounting for this "obesity paradox."

SUMMARY

1. In the United States in the early 1970s the prevalence of obesity was 4–6% for children/adolescents and 15% for adults. In 2009–2010, 35.7% of U.S. adults were obese as were 16.9% of U.S. children and adolescents.

2. Hydrostatic, or underwater, weighing is generally considered to be the laboratory criterion measure for the determination of body composition. It is based on densitometry. Recently, air displacement plethysmography (Bod Pod) and dual-energy X-ray absorptiometry (DXA) have emerged as important laboratory techniques.

3. Densitometry usually divides the body into two components, fat and fat-free weight (FFW). FFW is composed of water, protein, and bone mineral. The components are known and are relatively stable in adults but not in children and adolescents. Thus, no single equation, and especially not the adult equations of Brozek or Siri, can be used for children.

4. Important field tests for assessing body composition and/or abdominal obesity include skinfolds (good to very good assessments), bioelectrical impedance (good to very good), height and weight indices (especially body mass index [BMI]) (fair), and waist circumference (good). BMI is associated with, but does not actually measure, %body fat and lean body mass.

5. Waist circumference is strongly related to visceral abdominal obesity, which in turn is predictive of morbidity and mortality.

6. The size and the number of adipocytes increase as a child grows to adulthood. Adult fat gain first involves hypertrophy of the adipocytes and then hyperplasia of precursor cells.

7. Fat is typically distributed in an android (abdominal), gynoid (hips and thighs), or intermediate pattern. The android pattern is more strongly linked with cardiovascular disease (CVD) risk. Visceral adipose tissue appears to have a stronger relationship with physiological and pathological process than total body fat does.

8. The health risks of overweight and obesity include CVD, hypertension, gallbladder disease, hypercholesterolemia, diabetes mellitus, and cancer. Physical fitness can blunt these risks in overweight and obese individuals.

REVIEW QUESTIONS

1. Defend or refute: Obesity has reached epidemic proportions.

2. Define densitometry. Relate densitometry to hydrostatic weighing.

3. Explain the assumptions that must be met in order for hydrostatic weighing to be accurate. What variations in these basic assumptions occur with children, adolescents, and the older adults? State two practical applications of this information.

4. List and identify the strengths and weaknesses of the different field techniques for estimating overweight and obesity. Which technique would you select to use in a field setting? Explain why.

5. Compare the accuracy of %BF determined by skinfolds and bioelectrical impedance with %BF determined by hydrostatic weighing.

6. Compare and contrast the %BF, %BF distribution, and patterns of fat distribution between males and females.

7. Differentiate between overweight and obesity. What are the advantages and disadvantages of determining overweight and obesity by BMI?

8. What happens to adipose cells as an individual becomes overweight and then obese?

9. List and briefly discuss the health risks of being overweight or obese.

10. Describe the interrelationships between cardiovascular fitness and overweight/obesity.

For further review and additional study tools, visit the website at http://thePoint.lww.com/Plowman4e ☀ ◉

REFERENCES

American College of Sports Medicine: Proper and improper weight loss programs. *Medicine and Science in Sports and Exercise.* 15:xi–xiii (1983).

American College of Sports Medicine: *ACSM's Guidelines for Exercise Testing and Prescription* (8th edition). Philadelphia, PA: Lippincott Williams & Wilkins (2010).

Arciero, P. J. & B. C. Nindl: Obesity. In LeMura L. M. & S. P. von Duvillard (eds.): *Clinical Exercise Physiology: Application and Physiological Principles.* Philadelphia, PA: Lippincott Williams & Wilkins. 303–318 (2004).

Baker, J. L., L. W. Olsen, & T. I. Sørensen. Childhood body-mass index and the risk of coronary heart disease in adulthood. *The New England Journal of Medicine.* 357(23): 2329–2337 (2007).

Ballor, D. L., V. L. Katch, M. D. Becque, & C. R. Marks: Resistance weight training during caloric restriction enhances lean body weight maintenance. *American Journal of Clinical Nutrition.* 47:19–25 (1988).

Barlow, S. E. & The Expert Committee: Expert Committee recommendations regarding the prevention, assessment, and treatment of child and adolescent overweight and obesity: Summary report. *Pediatrics.* 120:S164–S192 (2007).

Baumgartner, R. N., W. C. Chumlea, & A. F. Roche: Bioelectrical impedance for body composition. In Pandolf, K. B. (ed.): *Exercise and Sport Sciences Reviews.* Baltimore, MD: Williams & Wilkins, 18:193–224 (1990).

Behnke, A. R. & J. H. Wilmore: *Evaluation and Regulation of Body Build and Composition.* Englewood Cliffs, NJ: Prentice-Hall (1974).

Björntorp, P. A.: Fat cell distribution and metabolism. In Wurtman, R. J. & J. J. Wurtman (eds.): *Annals of the New*

York Academy of Science. New York, NY: New York Academy of Science, 499:66–72 (1987).

Björntorp, P. A.: Sex differences in the regulation of energy balance with exercise. *American Journal of Clinical Nutrition*. 49:958–961 (1989).

Blair, S. N. & S. Brodney: Effects of physical inactivity and obesity on morbidity and mortality: Current evidence and research issues. *Medicine & Science in Sports & Exercise*. 31(Suppl. 11):S646–S662 (1999).

Blouin, K., A. Boivin, & A. Tchernof: Androgens and body fat distribution. *Journal of Steroid Biochemistry and Molecular Biology*. 108(3–5):272–280 (2008).

Boileau, R. A., T. G. Lohman, M. H. Slaughter, T. E. Ball, S. B. Going, & M. K. Hendrix: Hydration of the fat-free body in children during maturation. *Human Biology*. 56(4):651–666 (1984).

Bonnet, F. P., D. Rocour-Brumioul: Normal growth of human adipose tissue. In F. P. Bonnet (ed.): *Adipose Tissue in Childhood*. Boca Raton, FL: CRC Press. 81–107 (1981).

Boulton, T. J. C., M. Dunlop, & J. M. Court: The growth and development of fat cells in infancy. *Pediatric Research*. 12:908–911 (1978).

Bray, G. A.: Complications of obesity. *Annals of Internal Medicine*. 103(6 Pt 2):1052–1062 (1985).

Bray, G. A.: Overweight is risking fate: Definition, classification, prevalence, and risks. *Annals of the New York Academy of Science*. New York, NY: New York Academy of Science, 499:14–28 (1987).

Bray, G. A.: Overweight, mortality and morbidity. In C. Bouchard (ed.): *Physical Activity and Obesity*. Champaign, IL: Human Kinetics, 31–53 (2000).

Brodie, D. A.: Techniques of measurement of body composition: Part I. *Sports Medicine*. 5:11–40 (1988a).

Brodie, D. A.: Techniques of measurement of body composition: Part II. *Sports Medicine*. 5:74–98 (1988b).

Brownell, K. D., S. N. Steen, & J. H. Wilmore: Weight regulation practices in athletes: Analysis of metabolic and health effects. *Medicine and Science in Sports and Exercise*. 19(6):546–556 (1987).

Burton, B. T., W. R. Foster, J. Hirsch, & T. B. van Itallie: Health implications of obesity: An NIH consensus development conference. *International Journal of Obesity*. 9:155–169 (1985).

Campaigne, B. N.: Body fat distribution in females: Metabolic consequences and implications for weight loss. *Medicine and Science in Sports and Exercise*. 22(3):291–297 (1990).

Caton, J. R., P. A. Mole, W. C. Adams, & D. S. Heustis: Body composition analysis by bioelectrical impedance: Effect of skin temperature. *Medicine and Science in Sports and Exercise*. 20(5):489–491 (1988).

Centers for Disease Control and Prevention (a): Adult Obesity. http:www//.cdc.gov/obesity/data/adult.html. Accessed 4/03/2012.

Centers for Disease Control and Prevention (b): U.S. obesity trends. http:www//.cdc.gov/obesity/data/trends.html. Accessed 4/03/2012.

Charney, E., H. C. Goodman, M. McBride, B. Lyon, & R. Pratt: Childhood antecedents of adult obesity. *New England Journal of Medicine*. 295(1):6–9 (1975).

Chumlea, W. C., R. M. Siervogel, A. F. Roche, D. Mukherjee, & P. Webb: Changes in adipocyte cellularity in children 10 to 18 years of age. *International Journal of Obesity*. 6:383–389 (1981).

Chumlea, W. C., S. S. Guo, R. J. Kuczmarski, et al.: Body composition estimates from NHANES III bioelectrical impedance data. *International Journal of Obesity*. 26:1596–1609 (2002).

Chumlea, W. C. & S. S. Sun: Bioelectrical impedance analysis. In Heymsfield, S. B., T. G. Lohman, Z. Wang, & S. B. Going (eds.): *Human Body Composition* (2nd edition). Champaign, IL: Human Kinetics, 79–88 (2005).

Demerath, E. W., D. Reed, N. Rogers, S. S. Sun, M. Lee, A. C. Choh, W. Couch, S. A. Czerwinski, W. C. Chumlea, R. M. Siervogel, & B. Towne: Visceral adiposity and its anatomical distribution as predictors of the metabolic syndrome and cardiometabolic risk factor levels. *American Journal of Clinical Nutrition*. 88(5):1263–1271 (2008).

Després, J.-P. & B. Lamarche: Physical activity and the metabolic complications of obesity. In Bouchard, C. (ed.): *Physical Activity and Obesity*. Champaign, IL: Human Kinetics, 331–354 (2000).

Deurenberg, P. W., I. Paymans, & K. vander Kooy: Factors affecting bioelectrical impedance measurements in humans. *European Journal of Clinical Nutrition*. 42:1017–1022 (1988).

Dietary Guidelines for Americans 2010. http://www.dietary-guidelines.gov. Accessed 2/28/2012.

Dietz, W. H.: Childhood obesity. In Wurtman, R. J. & J. J. Wurtman (eds.): *Annals of the New York Academy of Science*. New York, NY: New York Academy of Science, 499:47–54 (1987).

Flegal, K. M., M. D. Carroll, C. L. Ogden, & L. T. Curtin: Prevalence and trends in obesity among US adults, 1999–2008. *JAMA*. 303(3):235–241 (2010).

Flegal, K. M., B. I. Graubard, D. F. Williamson, & M. H. Gail: Excess deaths associated with underweight, overweight, and obesity. *The Journal of the American Medical Association*. 293(15):1861–1867 (2005).

Flegal, K. M., B. I. Graubard, D. F. Williamson, & M. H. Gail: Cause-specific excess deaths associated with underweight, overweight, and obesity. *The Journal of the American Medical Association*. 298(17):2028–2037 (2007).

Folsom, A. R., S. A. Kaye, T. A. Sellers, C.-P. Hong, J. R. Cerhan, J. D. Potter, & R. J. Prineas: Body fat distribution and 5-year risk of death in older women. *The Journal of the American Medical Association*. 269(4):483–487 (1993).

Gallagher, D., M. Visser, D. Sepulveda, R. N. Pierson, T. Harris, & S. B. Heymsfield: How useful is body mass index for comparison of body fatness across age, sex and ethnic groups? *American Journal of Epidemiology*. 146:228–239 (1996).

Garner, D. M., P. E. Garfinkel, D. Schwartz, & M. Thompson: Cultural expectations of thinness in women. *Psychological Reports*. 47:483–491 (1980).

Going, S. B.: Hydrodensitometry and air displacement plethysmography. In Heymsfield, S. B., T. G. Lohman, Z. Wang, & S. B. Going (eds.): *Human Body Composition* (2nd edition). Champaign, IL: Human Kinetics, 17–33 (2005).

Going, S.: Optimizing techniques for determining body composition. Gatorade Sports Science Institute Sports Science Exchange #101. 19(2):1–5+supplement (choosing the best equation for estimating body composition) (2006).

Going, S. B. & R. Davis: Body composition assessment. In *ACSM's Resource Manual for Guidelines for Exercise Testing and Prescription* (4th edition). Baltimore, MD: Lippincott Williams & Wilkins, 391–400, (2001).

Going, S. B., T. G. Lohman, E. C. Cussler, D. P. Williams, J. A. Morrison, & P. S. Horn: Percent body fat and chronic disease risk factors in U.S. children and youth. *American Journal of Preventive Medicine.* 41(4 Suppl. 2):S77–S86 (2011).

Golding, L. A., C. R. Myers, & W. E. Sinning: *The Y's Way to Physical Fitness* (3rd edition). Champaign, IL: Human Kinetics (1989).

Goldman, R. F. & E. R. Buskirk: Body volume measurement by under water weighing: Description of a method. In J. Brozek & A. Henschel (eds.): *Techniques for Measuring Body Composition.* Washington, DC: National Academy of Sciences—National Research Council, 78–89 (1961).

Hager, A.: Adipose tissue cellularity in childhood in relation to the development of obesity. *British Medical Bulletin.* 37:287–290 (1981).

Hager, A., L. Sjöström, B. Arvidsson, P. Bjorntorp, & U. Smith: Body fat and adipose tissue cellularity in infants: A longitudinal study. *Metabolism.* 26:607–614 (1977).

Harrison, G. G., E. R. Buskirk, J. E. L. Carter, et al.: Skinfold thickness and measurement technique. In T. G. Lohman, A. F. Roche, & R. Martorell (eds.): *Anthropometric Standardization Reference Manual.* Champaign, IL: Human Kinetics, 55–70 (1988).

Heymsfield, S. B., T. G. Lohman, Z. Wang, & S. B. Going: *Human Body Composition* (2nd edition). Champaign, IL: Human Kinetics (2005).

Heyward, V. H. & Stolarczyk, L. M.: *Applied Body Composition Assessment.* Champaign, IL: Human Kinetics (1996).

Himes, J. H. & R. A. Frisancho: Estimating frame size. In Lohman, T. G., A. F. Roche, & R. Martorell (eds.): *Anthropometric Standardization Reference Manual.* Champaign, IL: Human Kinetics, 122–124 (1988).

Hodgdon, J. A. & P. I. Fitzgerald: Validity of impedance predictions at various levels of fatness. *Human Biology.* 59(2):281–298 (1987).

Hutley, L. & J. B. Prins: Fat as an endocrine organ: Relationship to the metabolic syndrome. *American Journal of Medical Science.* 330(6):280–289 (2005).

Jackson, A. S. & M. L. Pollock: Generalized equations for prediction body density of men. *British Journal of Nutrition.* 61:497–504 (1978).

Jackson, A. S. & M. L. Pollock: Practical assessment of body composition. *Physician and Sportsmedicine.* 13:76–90 (1985).

Javed, F., E. F. Aziz, M. S. Sabharwal, G. N. Nadkarni, S. A. Kahn, J. P. Cordova, A. M. Benjo, D. Gallagher, E. Herzog, F. H. Messerli, & F. X. Pi-Sunyer: Association of BMI and cardiovascular risk stratification in the elderly African-American Females. *Obesity* 19(6):1182–1186 (2011).

Jones, P. R. & D. A. Edwards: Areas of fat loss in overweight young females following an 8-week period of energy intake reduction. *Annals of Human Biology.* 26(2):151–162 (1999).

Kaminsky, L. & G. Dwyer: Body Composition. In Kaminsky, L. (ed.): *ACSM's Resource Manual for Guidelines for Exercise Testing and Prescription* (5th edition). Philadelphia, PA: Lippincott Williams and Wilkins, 195–205 (2006).

Kang, S. M., J. W. Yoon, H. Y. Ahn, et al.: Android fat depot is more closely associated with Metabolic Syndrome than adipose visceral fat in elder people. *Plos One.* 6(11):e27694 (2011).

Klein, S., D. B. Allison, S. B. Heymsfield, D. E. Kelley, R. L. Leibel, C. Nonas, & R. Kahn: Waist circumference and cardiometabolic risk: A consensus statement from Shaping America's Health Association for Weight Management and Obesity Prevention; NAASO, The Obesity Society; the American Society for Nutrition; and the American Diabetes Association. *American Journal of Clinical Nutrition.* 85:1197–1202 (2007).

Knittle, J. L., K. Timmers, F. Ginsberg-Fellner, R. E. Brown, & D. P. Katz: The growth of adipose tissue in children and adolescents. *Journal of Clinical Investigation.* 63:239–246 (1979).

Kuk, J. L., P. T. Katzmarzyk, M. Z. Nichaman, T. S. Church, S. N. Blair, & R. Ross: Visceral fat is an independent predictor of all-cause mortality in men. *Obesity.* 14(2):336–341 (2005).

Laurson, K. R., J. C. Eisenmann, & G. J. Welk: Body mass index standards based on agreement with health-related body fat. *American Journal of Preventive Medicine.* 41(4 Suppl. 2):S100–S105 (2011).

Liu, J. K., C. S. Fox, D. A. Hickson, W. D. May, K. G. Hairston, J. J. Carr, & H. A. Taylor: Impact of abdominal visceral and subcutaneous adipose tissue on cardiometabolic risk factors: The Jackson Heart Study. *Journal of Clinical Endocrinology & Metabolism.* 95(12):5419–5426 (2010).

Lohman, T. G.: Skinfolds and body density and their relation to body fatness: A review. *Human Biology.* 53(2):181–225 (1981).

Lohman, T. G.: Applicability of body composition techniques and constants for children and youth. In Pandolf, K. B. (ed.): *Exercise and Sport Sciences Reviews.* New York, NY: Macmillan, 14:325–357 (1986).

Lohman, T. G.: Assessment of body composition in children. *Pediatric Exercise Science.* 1:19–30 (1989).

Lohman, T. G.: *Advances in Body Composition Assessment.* Champaign, IL: Human Kinetics (1992).

Lohman, T. G., R. A. Boileau, & M. H. Slaughter: Body composition in children and youth. In Boileau, R. A. (ed.): *Advances in Pediatric Sport Sciences.* Champaign, IL: Human Kinetics, 29–57 (1984).

Lohman, T. G. & Z. Chen: Dual-energy X-ray absorptiometry. In Heymsfield, S. B., T. G. Lohman, Z. Wang, & S. B. Going (eds.): *Human Body composition* (2nd edition). Champaign, IL: Human Kinetics, 66–77 (2005).

Lohman, T. G., L. B. Houtkooper, & S. B. Going: Body composition assessment: Body fat standards and methods in the field of exercise and sports medicine. *ACSM's Health Fitness Journal.* 1:30–35 (1997).

Lutter, J. M.: Is your attitude weighing you down? *Melpomene Journal.* 13(1):13–16 (1994).

Lyon, C. J., R. E. Law, & W. A. Hsueh: Minireview: Adiposity, inflammation, and atherogenesis. *Endocrinology.* 144(6):2195–2200 (2003).

Malina, R. M., C. Bouchard, O. Bar-Or: *Growth, Maturation and Physical Activity* (2nd edition). Champaign, IL: Human Kinetics (2004).

Marieb, E. N. & K. Hoehn: *Human Anatomy and Physiology* (8th edition). San Francisco, CA: Benjamin Cummings (2010).

McAuley, P., J. Myers, J. Abella, & V. Froelicher: Body mass, fitness and survival in veteran patients: Another obesity paradox. *The American Journal of Medicine.* 120:518–524 (2007).

McCarty, M. F.: A paradox resolves: The postprandial model of insulin resistance explains why gynoid adiposity appears to be protective. *Medical Hypotheses.* 61(2):173–176 (2003).

Meredith, M. D. & G. J. Welk (eds.): *FITNESSGRAM® & ACTIVITYGRAM® Test Administration Manual* (4th edition updated). Champaign, IL: Human Kinetics (2010).

Meyer, H. E., A. J. Søgarrd, A. Tverdal, & R. M. Selmer: Body mass index and mortality: The influence of physical activity and smoking. *Medicine & Science in Sports & Exercise.* 34(7): 1065–1070 (2002).

National Heart, Lung, and Blood Institute: Executive summary of the clinical guidelines on the identification, evaluation, and treatment of overweight and obesity in adults. *Journal of the American Dietetic Association.* 98(10):1178–1191 (1998).

Neighbors, L. A. & J. Sobal: Prevalence and magnitude of body weight and shape dissatisfaction among university students. *Eating Behaviors.* 8(4):429–439 (2007).

Neumark-Sztainer, D., S. J. Paxton, P. J. Hannan, J. Haines, & M. Story: Does body satisfaction matter? Five-year longitudinal associations between body satisfaction and health behaviors in adolescent females and males. *Journal of Adolescent Health.* 39(2):244–251 (2006).

Nieman, D. C.: *Fitness and Sports Medicine: An Introduction.* Palo Alto, CA: Bull Publishing (1990).

Ode, J. J., J. M. Pivarnik, M. J. Reeves, & J. L. Knous: Body mass index as a predictor of percent fat in college athletes and nonathletes. *Medicine & Science in Sports & Exercise.* 39(3):403–409 (2007).

Ogden, C. L., M. D. Carroll, L. R. Curtin, M. M. Lamb, K. M. Flegal: Prevalence of high body mass index in US children and adolescents, 2007–2008. *The Journal of the American Medical Association.* 303(3):242–249 (2010).

Ogden, C. L., M. D. Carroll, B. K. Kit, & K. M. Flegal: Prevalence of Obesity in the United States, 2009–2010. *NCHS Data Brief.* 82:1–7 (2012).

Okosun, I. S., J. M. Boltri, M. P. Eriksen, & V. A. Hepburn: Trends in abdominal obesity in young people: United States 1988–2002. *Ethnicity & Disease.* 16(2):338–344 (2006).

Okosun, I. S., K. M. Chandra, A. Boev, J. M. Boltri, S. T., Choi, D. C. Parish, & G. E. Dever: Abdominal adiposity in U.S. adults: Prevalence and trends, 1960–2000. *Preventive Medicine.* 39(1):197–206 (2004).

Olds, T. S., K. Ridley, & G. R. Tomkinson: Declines in aerobic fitness: Are they only due to increasing fatness? *Medicine and Sport Science.* 50:226–240 (2007).

Pi-Sunyer, F. X.: Medical hazards of obesity. *Annals of Internal Medicine.* 119(7 Pt 2):655–660 (1993).

Powers, S. K. & E. T. Howley: *Exercise Physiology: Theory and Application to Fitness and Performance.* Dubuque, IA: Brown (1990).

Preis, S. R., J. M. Massaro, S. J. Robins, U. Hoffmann, R. S. Vasan, T. Irlbeck, J. B. Meigs, P. Sutherland, R. B. D'Agostino, C. J. O'Donnell, & C. S. Fox: Abdominal subcutaneous and visceral adipose tissue and insulin resistance in the Framingham Heart Study. *Obesity.* 18(11):2191–2198 (2010).

Ratamess, N.: Body composition status and assessment. In Erhman, J. K. (ed.): *ACSM's Resource Manual for Guidelines for Exercise Testing and Prescription* (6th edition). Philadelphia, PA: Lippincott Williams & Wilkins, 264–281 (2010).

Revicki, D. A. & R. G. Israel: Relationship between body mass indices and measures of body adiposity. *American Journal of Public Health.* 76:992–994 (1986).

Roche, A. F.: Some aspects of the criterion methods for the measurement of body composition. *Human Biology.* 59(2):209–220 (1987).

Rosano, G. M., C. Vitale, G. Marazzi, & M. Volterrani: Menopause and cardiovascular disease: The evidence. *Climacteric.* 10(Suppl. 1):19–24 (2007).

Sardinha, L. B. & P. J. Teixeira: Measuring adiposity and fat distribution in relation to health. In Heymsfield, S. B., T. G. Lohman, Z. Wang, & S. B. Going (eds.): *Human Body Composition* (2nd edition). Champaign, IL: Human Kinetics, 177–201 (2005).

Satwanti, B. S., I. P. Singh, & H. Bharadwaj: Body fat from skinfold thicknesses and weight-height indices: A comparison. *Zeitschrift für Morphologie und Anthropologie.* 71(1):93–100 (1980).

Semiz, S., E. Ozgören, & N. Sabir: Comparison of ultrasonographic and anthropometric methods to assess body fat in childhood obesity. *International Journal of Obesity.* 31(1): 53–58 (2007).

Simopoulos, A. P.: Characteristics of obesity: An overview. In Wurtman, R. J. & J. J. Wurtman (eds.): *Annals of the New York Academy of Science.* New York, NY: New York Academy of Science, 499:4–13 (1987).

Sjöström, L: Fat cells and body weight. In Stunkard, A. J. (ed.): *Obesity.* Philadelphia, PA: Saunders, 72–100, (1980).

Sjöström, L. & P. Björntorp: Body composition and adipose tissue cellularity in human obesity. *Acta Medica Scandinavica.* 195:201–211 (1974).

Slaughter, M. H., T. G. Lohman, R. A. Boileau, C. A. Horswill, R. J. Stillman, M. D. Van Loan, & D. A. Bemben: Skinfold equation for estimation of body fatness in children and youth. *Human Biology.* 60(5):709–723 (1988).

Soriguer Escofet, F. J., I. Esteva de Antoni, F. J. Tinahone, & A. Parej: Adipose tissue fatty acids and size and number of fat cells from birth to 9 years of age—a cross-sectional study in 96 boys. *Metabolism.* 45:1395–1401 (1996).

Stamford, B.: Apples and pears: Where you "wear" your fat can affect your health. *The Physician and Sportsmedicine.* 19(1):123–124 (1991).

Stump, C. S., L. B. Houtkooper, M. H. Heweitt, S. B. Going, & T. G. Lohman: Bioelectrical impedance variability with dehydration and exercise. *Medicine and Science in Sports and Exercise.* 20(2):S82 (1988).

Sui, X., M. J. LaMonte, J. N. Laditka, J. W. Hardin, N. Chase, S. P. Hooker, & S. N. Blair: Cardiorespiratory fitness and adiposity as mortality predictors in older adults. *The Journal of the American Medical Association.* 298(21):2507–2516 (2007).

Talamayan, K. S., A. E. Springer, S. H. Keider, E. C. Gorospe, & K. A. Joye: Prevalence of overweight misperception and weight control behaviors among normal weight adolescents in the United States. *Scientific World Journal.* 6:365–373 (2006).

Thompson, D. R., E. Obarzanek, D. L. Franko, B. A. Barton, J. Morrison, F. M. Biro, S. R. Daniels, & R. H. Striegel-Moore: Childhood overweight and cardiovascular disease risk factors: The National Heart, Lung, and Blood Institute Growth and Health Study. *Journal of Pediatrics.* 150:18–25 (2007).

Tiggemann, M.: Body-size dissatisfaction: Individual differences in age and gender, and relationship with self-esteem. *Personality and Individual Differences.* 13(1):39–43 (1992).

Toss, F., P. Wiklund, P. W. Franks, M. Eriksson, Y. Gustafson, G. Hallmans, P. Nordstrom, & A. Nordstrom: Abdominal and gynoid adiposity and the risk of stroke. *International Journal of Obesity.* 35(11):1427–1432 (2011).

United States Department of Health and Human Services: *Practical Guide to the Identification, Evaluation, and Treatment of Overweight and Obesity.* National Institute of Health Publication No. 00–4084. October 2000 available at: www.nhlbi.nih.gov. Accessed 9/28/2012.

Van Itallie, T. B.: Topography of body fat: Relationship to risk of cardiovascular and other diseases. In Lohman, T. G., A. F. Roche, & R. Martorell (eds.): *Anthropometric Standardization Reference Manual*. Champaign, IL: Human Kinetics, 143–149 (1988).

Van Loan, M. D.: Bioelectrical impedance analysis to determine fat-free mass, total body water and body fat. *Sports Medicine*. 10(4):205–217 (1990).

Welk, G. J. & S. N. Blair: Physical activity protects against the health risk of obesity. *President's Council on Physical Fitness and Sports Research Digest*. 3(12):1–8 (2000).

Wiklund, P., F. Toss, J. H. Jansson, M. Eliasson, G. Hallmans, A. Nordstrom, P. W. Franks, & P. Nordstrom: Abdominal and gynoid adipose distribution and incident myocardial infarction in women and men. *International Journal of Obesity*. 34(12):1752–1758 (2010).

Williams, D. P., S. B. Going, T. G. Lohman, D. P. Harsha, S. R. Srinivasau, L. S. Webber, & G. S. Beneuson: Body fatness and risk for elevated blood pressure, total cholesterol, and serum lipoprotein ratios in children and adolescents. *American Journal of Public Health*. 82:358–363 (1992).

Wong, S. L., I. Janssen, & R. Ross: Abdominal adipose tissue distribution and metabolic risk. *Sports Medicine*. 33(10): 709–726 (2003).

World Health Organization: *Obesity and Overweight. Media centre Fact Sheet*. 311 (2011). Available online http://www.who.int/mediacentre/factsheets/fs311/en/ Accessed 4/03/2012.

World Health Organization: *Obesity: Preventing and managing the global epidemic*. Report of a WHO Consultation on Obesity. Geneva: World Health Organization (1998).

8

Body Composition and Weight Control

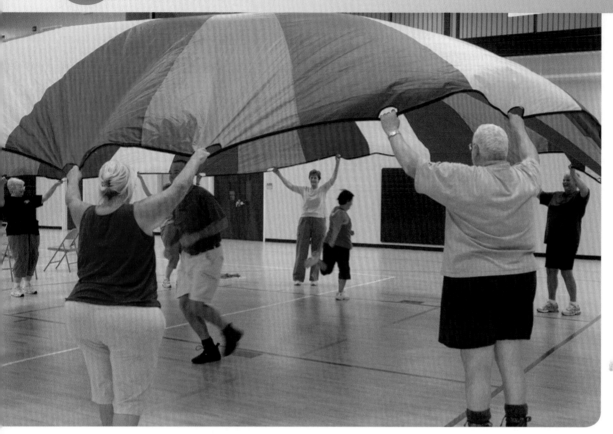

OBJECTIVES

After studying the chapter, you should be able to:

> State the caloric balance equation, and define and explain its components.

> Explain whether more calories are expended at rest or during exercise throughout a normal 24-hour period.

> Discuss the impact of diet, as caloric restriction, on the components of the caloric balance equation.

> Discuss the impact of an exercise session on the components of the caloric balance equation.

> Discuss the impact of exercise training on the components of the caloric balance equation.

> Compare and contrast the effects of diet alone, exercise training alone, and combined diet plus exercise training on body weight and body composition control.

> Apply the training principles to body weight and body composition control.

> Describe possible mechanisms that make maintenance of weight loss difficult.

> Compose guidelines for making weight in a sport.

Introduction

How much an individual weighs and what makes up his or her body mass are the result of the interaction of unmodifiable factors such as age, sex, and heredity and the modifiable factors of energy intake and energy output. Given the concern over the increasing levels of overweight and obesity described in Chapter 7, it is critical to understand these modifiable factors. Literally, hundreds of books and articles are written each year on these topics, often with exaggerated claims and untested suggestions. This chapter provides current scientific knowledge about body composition and weight control.

The Caloric Balance Equation

At its most basic level, weight control follows the first law of thermodynamics. The **First Law of Thermodynamics**, sometimes called the **Law of Conservation of Energy**, states that energy can neither be created nor destroyed, but only changed in form. This law was described fully in Chapter 2.

When the body converts the potential chemical energy of food into other chemical, mechanical, or heat energy, it follows the Law of Conservation of Energy. Theoretically, if the amount of energy taken in equals the amount of energy expended, the body is in balance and the weight (mass) remains stable. If an excess of energy is ingested, that energy is neither destroyed nor lost; rather, weight (mass) is gained. If insufficient energy is ingested in relation to expenditure, the needed energy cannot be created but must be provided from storage sites, and weight (mass) is reduced.

Energy, in the forms involved in the human body, is usually measured in kilocalories (kcal) or kilojoules (kJ). One **kilocalorie** is the amount of heat needed to raise the temperature of 1 kg of water by 1°C at 1 atm. One kilocalorie is equal to 4.186 kJ. A calorie is equal to 0.001 kcal. Calorie with a capital C is equivalent to 1 kcal. To avoid confusion this chapter always uses the unit kilocalorie, not Calorie. The term calorie is often used generically, however, as in the statement "Caloric intake should be equal to caloric output," even though the units would be kilocalories. The caloric equivalent of 1 lb of fat is 3500 kcal.

> **First Law of Thermodynamics or the Law of Conservation of Energy** Energy can neither be created nor destroyed but only changed in form.
>
> **Kilocalorie** The amount of heat needed to raise the temperature of 1 kg of water by 1°C at 1 atmosphere.
>
> **Caloric Balance Equation** The mathematical summation of the caloric intake (+) and energy expenditure (–) from all sources.

The **caloric balance equation**, the mathematical sum of the caloric intake (+) and energy expenditure (–) from all sources, quantifies the law of conservation of energy. It describes the source of potential energy as the food ingested, and the various uses of that energy. As indicated in **Figure 8.1**, input and output can be divided into the following components:

caloric balance = +food ingested (kcal)
- basal or resting metabolic rate (kcal)
- thermogenesis (kcal)
- work or exercise metabolism (kcal)
- energy excreted in waste products (kcal)

Food (and fluid) intake represents the only positive factor in the caloric balance equation. It is the only way that energy can be added to the system (the body). Energy is expended primarily in three ways: the basal or resting metabolic rate, thermogenesis, and work or exercise. These are the primary negative factors in the caloric balance equation. Although also negative, the amount of energy excreted in waste products is insignificant, rarely measured, and need not be considered further here.

Figure 8.2 indicates that the basal or resting metabolic rate accounts for most of the *total energy expenditure* (TEE), varying from approximately 60% to approximately 75% in active and sedentary individuals, respectively. Thermogenesis (the production of heat) accounts for a relatively stable 10% of caloric expenditure in both sedentary and active individuals. The energy expenditure of exercise is obviously higher in active individuals than sedentary ones and depends on the intensity, duration, and frequency of exercise.

If the amount of energy in the food ingested exceeds the energy expended, the body is in a positive balance and body weight will increase. If the amount of energy in the food ingested is less than the energy expended, the body is in a negative balance and body weight will decrease. In the pages that follow, each of the positive (food intake) and negative (basal metabolic rate [BMR], thermogenesis, and physical activity) components of the caloric balance equation will be defined and discussed. (The impact of diet, exercise, and exercise training on each of the components is systematically addressed and summarized in **Table 8.3** at the end of the discussion.)

Food Ingested

Little needs to be said about food intake per se. We all eat, and lists of the potential energy (kilocalorie) content of foods are readily available. Packaged food labels (described in Chapter 7) include kilocalorie values as well as nutrient contents. Getting into the habit of reading food labels is a good idea and should enable you to make wise food choices in terms of both nutritional and energy content.

FIGURE 8.1 Caloric Balance.
Caloric balance is the mathematical sum of the caloric intake (+food and drink) and energy expenditure (-BMR/RMR, -thermogenesis, -exercise/work, -waste products).

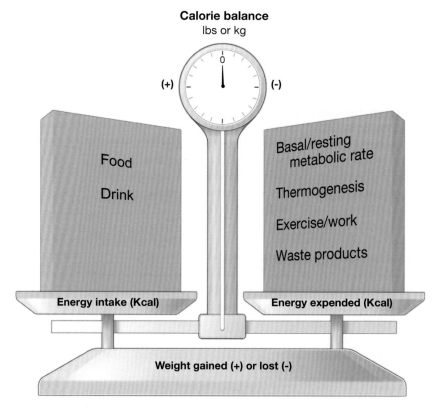

The Impact of Diet on Food Intake

The term **diet** is used in many ways and often refers to the food regularly consumed during the course of normal living. It is also used to mean an intentional restriction of caloric intake. This second meaning is how the term is being used in this chapter. Therefore, "going on a diet," by definition, means reducing food intake.

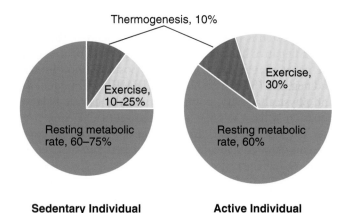

FIGURE 8.2 Energy Expenditure.
Resting metabolic rate accounts for the largest percentage of energy expended in both inactive and active individuals, although the exact percentage varies between the two groups. The percentage of energy expended during exercise is higher in active than inactive individuals. Thermogenesis accounts for about 10% of the energy expended in both active and inactive individuals.

The Impact of Exercise and Exercise Training on Food Intake

The relationships among exercise, exercise training, appetite, and energy intake are complex and often difficult to discern. Appetite and the amount of food ingested are influenced by physiological, nutritional, behavioral, and psychological factors in humans. It is not as simple as a physiological drive to balance energy demand and supply. People eat or do not eat for a variety of reasons. For example, when you are upset, do you cease eating, or do you consume everything in sight?

It is also very difficult to accurately measure food intake. The act of feeding individuals in a controlled setting where food can be measured may cause changes in eating behavior. Asking individuals to write down everything they eat requires faith that they are neither overreporting nor (more likely) underreporting their consumption. For these reasons, conducting studies on the effects of exercise and/or exercise training on appetite in humans is difficult. Despite the difficulties, the following generalizations can be drawn from available studies:

1. There is no effect of exercise on either appetite or energy intake in the short term—depending on the definition of short term. An immediate transient decrease in appetite for 20–30 minutes after aerobic exercise at greater than 60% $\dot{V}O_2$max (but not resistance exercise) has been seen relatively consistently, but not always. This is often termed "exercise-induced

anorexia" (Laan et al., 2010). However, neither a reduction nor an increase in energy intake after the immediate transient decrease for up to 48 hours following a single bout of exercise has been clearly established (Balaguera-Cortes et al., 2011; Blundell and King, 1999; Titchenal, 1988; Wilmore, 1983). In one study, the subjective rating of appetite was lowered in female subjects following 30 minutes of exercise at 50% $\dot{V}O_2$max. Despite this decreased subjective rating, food intake at the postexercise meal and for 2 days after was not affected. Other studies (Maraki et al., 2005; Martins et al., 2007; Moore et al., 2004; Weigle et al., 2005) have shown a decreased appetite during exercise, an increased appetite after exercise, and an increased energy intake at the next meal, but either no change or a decrease in total energy balance for the day. The dietary composition of the meals may impact which of these occurs before the next meal, as can be seen in the Focus on Research box (Luscombe-Marsh et al., 2005). When increased energy intake follows an exercise bout, it typically occurs only with heavy exercise and the compensation is often incomplete. For example, when six young lean (BMI = 21.4 kg·m^{-2}) females exercised moderately (2, 40 minutes cycling sessions that burned 454 kcal), no significant increase occurred in daily energy intake above a no exercise condition. However, when the exercise was heavy (3, 40 minutes cycling sessions that burned 812 kcal), energy intake increased but only compensated for approximately 30% of what had been expended, resulting in a negative energy balance (Stubbs et al., 2002). Another exception to the lack of an effect of exercise on appetite seems to occur in swimming, depending on water temperature. Energy intake has been shown to be as much as 44% higher after exercising in cold water (20°C) than in thermoneutral (33°C) water and 41% higher than under nonexercise conditions (White et al., 2005).

2. An activity-induced negative energy balance can be tolerated without compensation for approximately 1–2 weeks. However, subsequently, food intake spontaneously increases and compensates for approximately 30% of the energy expended in exercise. Thus, this compensation is partial and remarkably similar to that seen after heavy exercise on the same day. Furthermore, individuals tend to either be compensators or noncompensators, for unknown reasons (Blundell et al., 2003). The difference may depend on the fitness and body composition status of the individual. Highly trained athletes and lean individuals usually increase their energy intake in response to increased training loads. Untrained and/or obese individuals often do not initially change energy intake in response to exercise training (Jokisch et al., 2012).

3. The response of appetite to exercise may be sex specific. Evidence is now available that shows that in response to exercise that produces an energy deficit, males show no change in energy-regulating hormones and experience a decreased appetite whereas females show large changes in the energy-regulating hormones but no change in appetite. The primary energy-regulating hormones are *ghrelin*, *leptin*, and *insulin*. Ghrelin is classified as an episodic or short-term energy-regulating hormone that literally operates meal to meal. An increase in ghrelin stimulates an increase in energy intake. Leptin and insulin are classified as tonic or long-term energy-regulating hormones that operate over days or weeks. The reaction of leptin and insulin may be best described as an inverted U response. That is, low and very high levels of these stimulate appetite and food intake whereas moderate levels are suppressive. With a decrease in appetite and no change in energy-regulating hormones, males tend not to change their energy intake, the energy deficit is maintained, and body fat is decreased. Conversely with no decrease in appetite but large changes in the energy-regulating hormones (increased ghrelin and decreased insulin), females tend to increase their energy intake, energy balance is maintained, and no change occurs in body fat. The better matching between energy intake and expenditure in females is thought to be driven by the critical relationship between energy balance and reproductive success that does not operate in males. However, it does mean that regular exercise, with no deliberate dietary changes in females, results in greater body fat loss in males than females (Hagobian and Braun, 2010).

4. Physically active males, females, adults, and children—such as heavy manual laborers and athletes—consume more calories than sedentary individuals. Yet active individuals generally maintain their body weight and composition at or below normal levels.

5. When chronic exercise training ceases, energy intake in humans is spontaneously reduced. Unfortunately, this reduction does not appear to be matched to the reduced energy expenditure. The result is often a positive energy balance, a regain of lost body weight, and a concomitant increase in body fat (Blundell et al., 2003; Stubbs et al., 2004).

Thus, it appears that the physiological factors that modify appetite/food intake in response to hunger or a deficit energy intake are more finely tuned or are more efficient than those factors that respond to satiety or an increase in energy intake. This concept is presented in **Figure 8.3**. It has been speculated that this response to food may have been a survival of the species mechanism in days

Diet (a) The food regularly consumed during the course of normal living; (b) a restriction of caloric intake.

before modern agriculture provided more than enough food for much of the world (Prentice and Jebb, 2004). In other words, humans may have evolved to eat more than needed in times of plenty, in expectation of coming times of less food availability. Thus, it truly may be easier to gain weight than to lose weight.

Resting or Basal Metabolism

Basal energy expenditure, more commonly called **basal metabolic rate (BMR)**, is the level of energy required to sustain the body's vital functions in the waking state. Technically, this definition means that the individual is resting quietly in a supine position, not having eaten for 8–18 hours, is at normal body temperature (37°C) in a neutral ambient temperature (27–29°C; 80–84°F), and is not experiencing any psychological stress. Because of the difficulty of achieving truly basal conditions in laboratory settings, the term **resting metabolic rate (RMR)** is probably a more accurate descriptor. RMR is the energy expended while an individual is resting quietly in a supine position. These two terms are often used interchangeably, since the measured differences are small. That practice will be followed here, with the term RMR used primarily but not exclusively (Bursztein et al., 1989).

Many organs and processes are responsible for energy consumption at rest. The liver is the largest consumer of

energy at rest (29–32%), followed by the brain (19–21%), muscles (18%), heart (10%), lungs (9%), and kidneys (7%). Resting muscle energy is primarily for the maintenance of tonus or tension, necessary even in sleep. On the cellular level, the energy is used to fuel ion pumps (particularly the sodium-potassium pump), synthesize and degrade cellular constituents, conduct electrical impulses, and secrete various substances, including hormones (Bogert et al., 1973; Bursztein et al., 1989).

Basal or resting metabolism is usually determined in relation to body surface area (BSA) and expressed in kcal·m^{-2}. It may also be expressed in kcal·d^{-1} or $\dot{V}O_2$ mL·min^{-1}. The choice of measurement unit depends on how the information will be used. To compare with submaximal or maximal oxygen values, the choice is $\dot{V}O_2$ mL·min^{-1}. To express caloric needs, the kilocalorie unit is used. Tables and graphs are available that allow one to estimate BSA (in square meters) from an individual's height and weight (**Table 8.1**) and standard BMR values per BSA (**Figure 8.4**). From these values, BMR (in kcal·d^{-1}) can be computed.

8.1 basal metabolic rate (kcal·d^{-1}) = standard basal metabolic rate (kcal·m^{-2}·hr^{-1}) × body surface area (m^2) × 24 hr·d^{-1}

or

BMR = standard BMR × BSA × 24

TABLE 8.1	**Surface Area in Square Meters for Different Heights and Weights**																
Height (cm)	**Weight (kg)**																
	25	**30**	**35**	**40**	**45**	**50**	**55**	**60**	**65**	**70**	**75**	**80**	**85**	**90**	**95**	**100**	**105**
200							1.84	1.91	1.97	2.03	2.09	2.15	2.21	2.26	2.31	2.36	2.41
195							1.73	1.80	1.87	1.93	1.99	2.05	2.11	2.17	2.22	2.27	2.32	2.37
190				1.56	1.63	1.70	1.77	1.84	1.90	1.96	2.02	2.08	2.13	2.18	2.23	2.28	2.33
185				1.53	1.60	1.67	1.74	1.80	1.86	1.92	1.98	2.04	2.09	2.14	2.19	2.24	2.29
180				1.49	1.57	1.64	1.71	1.77	1.83	1.89	1.95	2.00	2.05	2.10	2.15	2.20	2.25
175	1.19	1.28	1.36	1.46	1.53	1.60	1.67	1.73	1.79	1.85	1.91	1.96	2.01	2.06	2.11	2.16	2.21
170	1.17	1.26	1.34	1.43	1.50	1.57	1.63	1.69	1.75	1.81	1.86	1.91	1.96	2.01	2.06	2.11	
165	1.14	1.23	1.31	1.40	1.47	1.54	1.60	1.66	1.72	1.78	1.83	1.88	1.93	1.98	2.03	2.07	
160	1.12	1.21	1.29	1.37	1.44	1.50	1.56	1.62	1.68	1.73	1.78	1.83	1.88	1.93	1.98		
155	1.09	1.18	1.26	1.33	1.40	1.46	1.52	1.58	1.64	1.69	1.74	1.79	1.84	1.89			
150	1.06	1.15	1.23	1.30	1.36	1.42	1.48	1.54	1.60	1.65	1.70	1.75	1.80				
145	1.03	1.12	1.20	1.27	1.33	1.39	1.45	1.51	1.56	1.61	1.66	1.71					
140	1.00	1.09	1.17	1.24	1.30	1.36	1.42	1.47	1.52	1.57							
135	0.97	1.06	1.14	1.20	1.26	1.32	1.38	1.43	1.48								
130	0.95	1.04	1.11	1.17	1.23	1.29	1.35	1.40									
125	0.93	1.01	1.08	1.14	1.20	1.26	1.31	1.36									
120	0.91	0.98	1.04	1.10	1.16	1.22	1.27										

Source: Dubois, D. & E. F. DuBois: Clinical calorimetry: A formula to estimate the approximate surface area if height and weight be known. *Archives of Internal Medicine.* 17:863–871 (1916). Reprinted by permission of Archives of Internal Medicine.

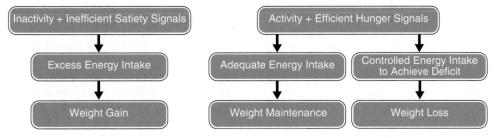

FIGURE 8.3 The Impact of Satiety and Hunger Signals on Body Weight.
If the individual is inactive and satiety signals are inefficient, an excess of energy intake occurs and weight gain follows. If the individual is active and hunger signals are efficient, the individual will maintain weight with adequate energy intake or lose weight with a deficit energy intake.

EXAMPLE

A 22-year-old female is 5 ft 5 in. (165 cm) tall and weighs 143 lb (65 kg). According to **Table 8.1**, her BSA is 1.72 m². The number closest to her age in **Figure 8.3** is 20. For females, the lower line is used to estimate a standard BMR, in her case 35.1 kcal·m⁻²·hr⁻¹. These values are substituted into Equation 8.1:

$$BMR\ kcal \cdot d^{-1} = 35.1\ kcal \cdot m^{-2} \cdot hr^{-1}$$
$$\times 1.72\ m^2 \times 24\ hr \cdot d^{-1}$$
$$BMR = 1448\ kcal \cdot d^{-1}$$

Somewhat less cumbersome is the use of prediction equations such as those presented in **Table 8.2**. For the individual in the previous example, the calculation is RMR = 447.593 + (3.098 × 165) + (9.247 × 65) − (4.330 × 22) = 1464.6 kcal·d⁻¹. Although results from the two techniques do not agree exactly, they are comparable for practical use.

Eighty-five percent of all normal subjects have estimated RMR values within 10% of their measured values. The other 15% of the population have either higher or lower values. The range of variation may exceed 20%. Thus, an individual with an RMR 20% higher than average can ingest more calories without gaining weight, but an individual with a 20% lower RMR must ingest less or gain weight (Bursztein et al., 1989; Guyton and Hall, 2011).

Two criterion measures are available for RMR. The first is open-circuit indirect calorimetry, described in Chapter 4. The second is a blood test for the determination of protein-bound iodine. The iodine comes from thyroxine (T₄), the hormone secreted by the thyroid gland, which has the greatest impact on BMR. This test gives a relative indication of BMR, not a direct kcal·d⁻¹ value (Bogert et al., 1973).

The prediction equations in **Table 8.2** give an indication of the primary nonhormonal factors that influence RMR. What are they? If you said body size, age, and sex, you are absolutely correct. RMR is related strongly to BSA externally and to cell mass internally, so, of course, what that cell mass is composed of (fat or muscle) will have an influence. Obese individuals have a larger surface area and a larger cell mass (both fat and fat-free) than average-weight individuals. Therefore, not surprisingly, the RMR of obese individuals is higher than that of normal-weight individuals (Jequier, 1987).

The influence of age and sex can be seen in **Figure 8.4**. RMR is highest in infants and young children. The decline from age 6 to 18 is approximately 25%, or 2% per year. The decline then slows to about 2–3% per decade after that age. Part of this decline in RMR may be attributed to and be responsible for the increment in %BF that usually occurs as people age.

Figure 8.4 also clearly shows that, at all ages, average-weight females have lower RMR than average-weight males. The difference, which is least in young children, is accentuated at puberty and then tends to remain at

---

Basal Metabolic Rate (BMR) The level of energy required to sustain the body's vital functions in the waking state, when the individual is in a fasted condition, at normal body and room temperature, and without psychological stress.

Resting Metabolic Rate (RMR) The energy expended while an individual is resting quietly in a supine position.

TABLE 8.2	Estimation of Basal (Resting) Metabolic Rate
Males	RMR = 88.362 + (4.799 × HT) + (13.397 × WT) − (5.677 × AGE)
Females	RMR = 447.593 + (3.098 × HT) + (9.247 × WT) − (4.330 × AGE)

HT, height (in centimeters); WT, weight (in kilograms); AGE, age (in years).
Source: Based on Roza, A. M. & H. M. Shizgal: The Harris Benedict equation reevaluated: Resting energy requirements and the body cell mass. *American Journal of Clinical Nutrition.* 40:168–182 (1984).

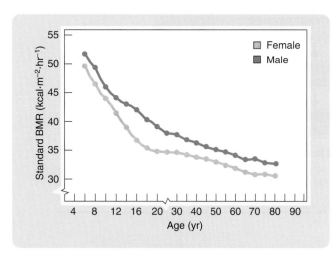

FIGURE 8.4 Standard Basal Metabolic Rate across the Age Span.
Standard basal metabolic rates decline steeply during childhood and adolescence and then more gradually during the adult years. At every age, male values are higher than female values, despite being prorated to body surface area.
Sources: Calculated from Brownell et al. (1987) and Bursztein et al. (1989).

about 5–6% through middle age and old age. In terms of calories, the RMR of adult males averages between 1500 and 1800 kcal·d⁻¹, and the RMR of adult females averages between 1200 and 1450 kcal·d⁻¹. Female values are lower partially because females have smaller internal organs than males and tend to have less total body mass, on average, than males. However, the most obvious explanation is the difference in body cell mass, particularly muscle tissue. Females on average have a higher %BF than do males. At any body weight, for each 1% increase in percent body fat, the RMR decreases 0.6 kcal·hr⁻¹ or 14.4 kcal·d⁻¹. If we assume a 10% difference in %BF between the average male and average female, the result can amount to 144 kcal·d⁻¹. When RMR is expressed relative to fat-free weight (FFW), the sex differences disappear (Bogert et al., 1973; Bursztein et al., 1989).

Another factor that influences RMR is core body temperature. For each degree increase in Celsius or Fahrenheit temperature, metabolic rate increases to 13% or 7.2%, respectively. This holds true even when the core temperature increases due to acute illness (pyrogenesis). Similarly, a decrease in body temperature, at least until the point where shivering is induced, reduces energy expenditure.

The Impact of Diet on Resting Metabolic Rate

Both the amount and the type of food ingested affect RMR. The effect of caloric restriction on RMR is well documented and clear-cut. Severe caloric restriction decreases RMR possibly as much as 10–20% after several weeks (Apfelbaum et al., 1971; Bray, 1969; Brownell et al., 1987; Grande et al., 1958a; Mole et al., 1989; Stiegler

and Cunliffe, 2006). This is shown experimentally in the Focus on Research box where RMR decreased approximately 80 kcal·d⁻¹, regardless of the composition of the diet (Luscombe-Marsh et al., 2005). Because resting metabolism represents the greatest percentage of daily caloric expenditure in sedentary individuals, the discouraging result is a slowing of the weight loss that would be expected from the amount of dietary restriction and negative balance.

EXAMPLE

1 lb (0.45 kg) of body fat contains the energy equivalent of approximately 3500 kcal. For a person to lose 1 lb of weight according to the caloric balance equation, the number of calories expended must exceed the number ingested by 3500 kcal. If an individual expends 2000 kcal·d⁻¹ and ingests 2000 kcal·d⁻¹, weight should be maintained. If that same individual maintains this activity level but reduces his/her caloric intake to just 1000 kcal·d⁻¹, a weight loss of 2 lb·wk⁻¹ would be anticipated (2000 kcal·d⁻¹ – 1000 kcal·d⁻¹ = –1000 kcal·d⁻¹; –1000 kcal·d⁻¹ × 7 d·wk⁻¹ = –7000 kcal; –7000 kcal ÷ 3500 kcal = –2 lb), assuming that approximately 75% of the 2000 kcal·d⁻¹ expenditure or 1500 kcal·d⁻¹ is expended by RMR.

However, within 2–3 weeks of such a restricted diet, the RMR will have been reduced by approximately 15% (the range is typically 10–20%) to 1275 kcal·d⁻¹. The difference is now –1775 kcal·d⁻¹ expended + 1000 kcal·d⁻¹ ingested = –775 kcal·d⁻¹; –775 kcal·d⁻¹ × 7 d·wk⁻¹ = –5425 kcal; –5425 kcal ÷ 3500 kcal·lb⁻¹ = –1.5 lb instead of –2 lb·wk⁻¹. As the drop in RMR continues with severe caloric restriction, the weight loss becomes progressively slower (Mole et al., 1989).

Researchers speculate that this decline in RMR is the body's protective response to energy restriction (Speakman and Selman, 2003). Conversely, a short-term excessive ingestion of food and calories results in an elevation of RMR (Apfelbaum et al., 1971; van Zant, 1992). This elevation has been seen as protection against an increase in the body's "natural" weight (Brownell et al., 1987).

Maintenance of a "natural" weight or body composition is often attributed to an individual's genetically determined set point. According to the *set-point theory*, changes in body mass or fat content are perceived in the periphery and appropriate signals sent to the hypothalamus. The hypothalamus integrates and interprets the incoming feedback and in turn sends out signals that modify food intake or energy expenditure (including but not limited to RMR) to correct any deviations in weight or fat from the set point. The existence of a set point for homeostatic control of human body weight/fat is uncertain and under debate. At the very least, a set point cannot be a fixed permanent value, as it is necessary to allow for such things as growth and development. It may be that the set point actually functions as a "settling point" with new levels set after continuous demands on the outer limits of the acceptable range. These demands may arise from a variety of influences including overfeeding or underfeeding without changes in activity level (Harris, 1990; Macias, 2004).

The Impact of Exercise on Resting Metabolic Rate

The energy cost of exercise (**Figure 8.5**), in oxygen or calorie units, includes a resting component. Metabolic equivalents (METs) (Chapter 4) express the energy cost of activity in multiples of the RMR. Therefore, although metabolism is definitely elevated by exercise, it is not the resting metabolism itself that is elevated. The resting metabolism is assumed to remain constant; the increase in energy consumption is attributed solely to the activity demands and responses.

Immediately after exercise, the metabolic rate remains elevated. This rate is called the excess postexercise oxygen consumption (EPOC) and was discussed in Chapter 3. This recovery oxygen utilization represents additional calories that are expended as a direct result of the response to exercise. These calories are typically not included in the measured caloric cost of the activity. Thus, if an individual expends 250–300 kcal walking or jogging 3 mi, an extra 20–30 kcal may be expended during the hour or two after exercise until complete recovery occurs. Additionally, a slow component that may last up to 48 hours expends even more calories (Speakman and Selman, 2003). These expenditures, however, also do not mean that the RMR itself has been affected.

For it to be concluded that the resting metabolism is changed by exercise, the change would have to be evident 24 or 48 hours after exercise. Research evidence for such a change is mixed and difficult to interpret. The inconsistency of the evidence can partially be attributed to the intensity and duration of the exercise involved. Mild to heavy exercise of moderate duration (35–86% $\dot{V}O_2$max for 20–80 minutes) has generally been shown to cause no long-term metabolic elevation in RMR, whereas longer, moderate exercise (50–70% $\dot{V}O_2$max; 80–180 minutes) has.

There is a problem, however, in interpreting metabolic changes greater than 48 hours after exercise as being caused by the exercise. Studies showing an increase in RMR over the long term, even after heavy exercise, have not controlled for the ingestion of food during the intervening 48 hours. The elevated metabolism observed was probably due, at least in part, to the thermic effect of the meals taken. (The TEM will be fully explained later in this chapter.) Consequently, it is unlikely that exercise causes any permanent change in RMR per se—at least not light or moderate aerobic endurance exercise or dynamic resistance activity (Bingham et al., 1989; Horton, 1985; Melby et al., 1993; Stiegler and Cunliffe, 2006).

The Impact of Exercise Training on Resting Metabolic Rate

The effect of exercise training on RMR is controversial. Results of cross-sectional studies involving RMR and training/fitness status have reported higher, lower, or the same values between trained-untrained and high fit-low fit groups. Similarly, training studies have produced inconsistent results ranging from an increase, to no change, to a decrease. One recent study (Lee et al., 2009) found that after a 12-week treadmill jogging/running program, the RMR of the training group stayed the same, but that of the control group decreased. They concluded that the training program may have prevented a seasonal decline (RMR is highest in winter and lowest in summer) in the training group.

A significant, direct rectilinear relationship has been shown between the level of training or fitness as measured by $\dot{V}O_2$max and RMR (Sullo et al., 2004). Thus, one reason why some studies have not revealed differences between trained and untrained individuals may be that the trained individuals were simply not trained enough. In these studies, neither the trained nor the untrained individuals were restricted calorically. Therefore, what is occurring may be a last-bout effect by those training at high levels (Melby et al., 1993). Or it may be that a high-energy flux (heavy training volume with caloric balance) is the cause. Individuals in a high-energy flux condition have shown higher levels of norepinephrine and RMR than when they were in a state of low-energy flux (sedentary but in caloric balance) (Bullough et al., 1995).

Longitudinal studies investigating the impact of exercise training on RMR often add the exercise component after several weeks of severe caloric restriction in an attempt to reverse the decline in RMR. Others simply

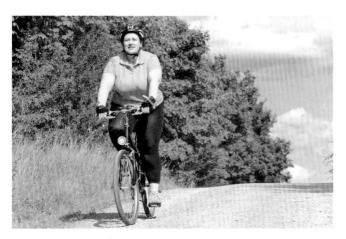

FIGURE 8.5 Exercise Is an Important Component of Body Weight/Body Composition Control.

Macronutrient Impact on Appetite and Thermic Effect of a Meal during Caloric Restriction

Fifty-seven individuals, aged 20–65 years, with BMI values between 27 and 40 kg·m⁻², completed 12 weeks of caloric restriction and 4 weeks of maintenance. The purpose was to determine the effects of two calorically equal diets that differed in protein and fat content on weight loss, appetite regulation, and the thermic effect of test meals. The low-fat, high-protein (LF-HP) diet consisted of 29% fat, 34% protein, and 37% carbohydrate. The high-fat, standard-protein (HF-SP) diet consisted of 45% fat (~29% monounsaturated), 18% protein, and 37% carbohydrate. Caloric intake was set at approximately 1400 kcal·d⁻¹ for both groups during weight loss and at energy balance during maintenance.

Hunger, fullness, satiety, desire to eat, and the amount of food desired were measured before and at 30, 60, 120, and 180 minutes after the test meal. Participants desired less to eat after the LF-HP meal than after the HF-SP meal both before and after the 16 weeks of dieting and maintenance. This indicates a greater satiety with a high protein content despite equal total calories.

Total body weight loss, total fat mass loss, and abdominal fat mass loss are shown in the accompanying graph (A). The males lost more in each category than the females; however, there was no significant difference between the diet groups. This is consistent with the conclusion of most caloric restriction studies. That is, it is the energy intake and not macronutrient composition that primarily determines total weight and fat loss.

The differences in energy expenditure are presented in graphs B and C. The decrease in RMR (B) was not significantly different between diet groups. However,

the decrease in the thermic effect of a meal (TEM) with weight loss (C) was smaller in the LF-HP groups than in the HF-SP group. The authors concluded that although over the short term of the study this difference did not appear to enhance weight loss, it might have some small effect on weight maintenance later.

Thus, a high-protein diet, still within the recommended level of 10–35%, had the advantage over a high

monounsaturated fat diet of blunting both the appetite and the dietary-induced decrease in the TEM.

Source: Luscombe-Marsh, N. D., M. Noakes, G. A. Wittert, J. B. Keogh, P. Foster, and P. M. Clifton: Carbohydrate-restricted diets high in either monounsaturated fat or protein are equally effective at promoting fat loss and improving blood lipids. *American Journal of Clinical Nutrition.* 81:762–772 (2005).

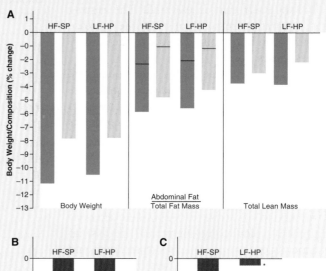

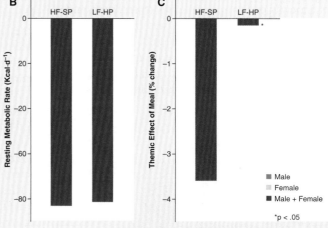

examine the impact of training on RMR during a calorically balanced state. High-intensity programs performed daily have not only brought about a return to baseline in RMR but also, in some instances, caused an elevation of 7–10%. In those studies showing a reversal of the decline in RMR, the change began within just a few days, which is well before any change would be expected in body composition. Thus, the conclusion again is that the effect of

training on RMR is over and above any change in muscle mass. The increases in RMR above pretraining levels in nondieting individuals could also reflect increased norepinephrine levels (Brownell et al., 1987; Mole et al., 1989; Nieman et al., 1988).

In those studies showing an additional decline in RMR when exercise was added to caloric restriction, the decline is often explained as part of the body's protective mechanism. If RMR declines when calories are restricted, burning additional calories in activity simply makes matters worse. Therefore, it is logical that the RMR would decrease even further. It has been suggested that this decline occurs in individuals (such as some athletes) who are attempting to maintain body weights below their natural level (Brownell et al., 1987).

If diet and/or exercise results in a loss of body weight (mass), then a proportional long-term reduction in RMR should be expected. Despite the claims of many overweight individuals to the contrary, overweight or obese people typically have a higher RMR than normal-weight individuals of similar age, sex, and height to begin with. With weight loss, this higher RMR should not be expected to be maintained (Garrow, 1987; Stiegler and Cunliffe, 2006; Wadden et al., 1990).

Because RMR is highly correlated with or related to FFW, but not entirely dependent on it, it might be expected that resistance weight training would bring about an increase in RMR. Again, the data are not definitive. Perhaps the most impressive evidence for this idea comes from a study with males 50–65 years old. After 16 weeks of heavy resistance strength training, these subjects had no change in total body weight but showed a decrease in %BF, an increase in FFW, and an increase in RMR. This increase in RMR remained significant even when expressed per kilogram of FFW. Resting norepinephrine levels also increased. The researchers concluded that the increase in RMR with strength training was only partially due to the increased FFW and may also have been linked to an increase in basal sympathetic nervous system activity (Pratley et al., 1994). This conclusion reinforces the idea that RMR does not totally depend on muscle mass.

A 24-week strength-training study resulted in significant increases in RMR in young and old males, but not in females, perhaps reflecting sex differences in sympathetic nervous activity (Lemmer et al., 2001). Conversely, a 9-week study by Byrne and Wilmore (2001) found that both FFW and RMR (measured 72 hours after the last exercise session) increased in resistance-trained females. A second group who did a combination of aerobic endurance and resistance weight training increased their FFW equally, but their RMR decreased. The control group did not change significantly. When RMR was expressed relative to FFW, there was no significant change in the resistance-trained individuals (indicating that all the increase in RMR could be attributed to changes in FFW for this group), but there was an even greater decrease for the combined training group. The reasons for the decline in RMR are unclear. As noted above, this may simply be a compensatory response to an exercise program that is too intensive.

Thermogenesis The production of heat.

Thermic Effect of a Meal (TEM) The increased heat production as a result of food ingestion.

Thermogenesis

Think about this. The temperature is 38°C (100°F) with a relative humidity of 80%. Your apartment air conditioner is not working. You are hungry but cannot afford to eat out. In your food stock are ground beef, red beans and rice, tuna, and the ingredients for a fruit salad and a tossed salad. Which do you select? In all probability you will pick one or both of the salad options, intuitively choosing a meal you assume will not add to your heat load. Actually, though, following ingestion of any meal, metabolism is elevated.

The production of heat is called **thermogenesis**. The increased heat production as a result of ingesting a meal, such as seen in **Figure 8.6**, is called the **thermic effect of a meal (TEM)** or *dietary-induced thermogenesis (DIT)*. TEM has two components: obligatory and facultative. *Obligatory* thermogenesis is due to the energy-requiring processes of digestion, absorption, assimilation, and synthesis of protein, fat, and carbohydrate. However, more energy is expended than can be accounted for by these processes. The extra energy expenditure is the *facultative* portion of TEM. Facultative thermogenesis usually peaks in 30–90 minutes but, depending on the size and content of the meal, may last as long as 4–6 hours. This energy all appears in the form of heat and has been attributed to sympathetic nervous system activity (Acheson et al., 1984; Blanchard, 1982; Dulloo et al., 2004). Convincing evidence is available for sympathetic activation after carbohydrate-rich meals, but similar evidence is currently lacking after protein and fat ingestion (van Baak, 2008). Cumulatively, the energy expenditure associated with the ingestion of all food during a day is called the *thermic effect of feeding (TEF)*. TEF is what is depicted as thermogenesis in **Figure 8.1** as constituting approximately 10% of daily energy expenditure (Blanchard, 1982; van Baak, 2008).

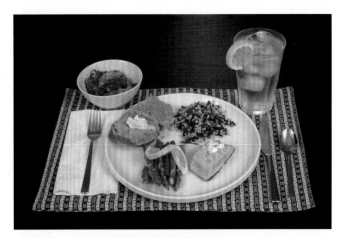

FIGURE 8.6 The Thermic Effect of a Meal.
The thermic effect of a meal is dependent upon the macronutrient content and total kilocalories ingested.

There is some evidence for a link between thermogenesis and the control of body weight (van Zant, 1992). TEF is thought to be a survival technique. When stimulated, TEF allows the individual to adapt to a diet low in nutrients by ingesting more food without gaining weight. When suppressed, TEF allows the body to slow down weight loss during fasting or starvation situations.

Precisely how thermogenesis occurs has not been determined, but probably some mechanism for the uncoupling of oxidative phosphorylation is involved. That is, energy substrates are oxidized but ATP is not produced. Instead, heat is produced. This process may occur at specific steps in the metabolic pathways (known as substrate or futile cycling) or in brown adipose tissue (BAT) (Himms-Hagen, 1984; van Baak, 2008) (see **Figure 7.11**). Brown adipose cells originate from myocytes (muscle cells). They contain a protein called uncoupling protein 1 (UCP1) that appears to be responsible for adaptive thermogenesis. The term **adaptive thermogenesis** is used two ways in the literature, to indicate either an increase or decrease in the efficiency of energy utilization. The first, an *adaptive increase in thermogenesis*, is what is operating here. It indicates a change in the efficiency of energy utilization resulting in increased heat production as the result of some uncoupling of oxidative phosphorylation (Erlanson-Albertsson, 2003; Mozo et al., 2005). In stimulated brown adipocytes, protons move through the alternative UCP1 channel instead of the ATP synthase complex in electron transport, thus producing only heat and not ATP (see **Figure 2.10**). BAT appears to be under adrenergic sympathetic nervous control (specifically norepinephrine) and leptin may play a role. Conditions such as cold exposure or overfeeding increase norepinephrine activity in BAT. Until very recently, it had been thought that only human newborns had any BAT. It has now been demonstrated that substantial amounts of metabolically active BAT are present in healthy adult humans. The main BAT depots are in the neck and shoulder region of the upper torso, along the vertebrae, in the thoracic cavity, and around the renal glands. All individuals do not exhibit defined regions of functionally active BAT. Such tissue is most frequently seen in young, lean females. The search for the precise role of BAT in human energy balance regulation, if any, is actively ongoing (Cypess et al., 2009; Nedergaard and Cannon, 2010; Richard et al., 2010; Virtanen et al, 2009).

Dulloo et al. (2004) have postulated an adipose-specific control of thermogenesis operating as a feedback loop between the white adipose tissue and skeletal muscles. Changes in the sodium-potassium pump activity have also been proposed (Blanchard, 1982).

All or some of these mechanisms may be partly responsible for why some individuals can seemingly eat everything in sight and not gain weight, while others eat much less proportionately and gain weight. Most studies comparing the thermic response of lean and obese individuals to a test meal do indeed show a blunted TEM in the obese (Blanchard, 1982; Jequier, 1987; Newsholme, 1980; Schutz et al., 1984; Schwartz, 1983; Segal et al., 1984, 1985, 1987; Shetty et al., 1981).

The Impact of Diet on the Thermic Effect of a Meal

Both the total caloric content and the percent composition of a meal impact the thermic effect of the meal. The thermic effect of the macronutrients, as a percentage of their energy content, is 2–3% for fat, 6–8% for carbohydrate, and 25–30% for protein (Jequier, 2002). These differences seem to suggest that a high-protein diet would be valuable for individuals wishing to expend extra calories. Indeed, the study (Luscombe-Marsh et al., 2005) presented in the Focus on Research box earlier bears this out partially. Although both the group eating a high monounsaturated fat, standard-protein diet and the group eating a low-fat, high protein diet exhibited a decrease in the thermic response to a standard meal, the decrease with weight loss was smaller in the group on the high-protein diet. However, the total weight loss did not differ between the groups. The authors did suggest that this difference could be beneficial in maintenance, but it was not experimentally tested.

If the percentages of protein, fat, and carbohydrate are kept constant and close to those values recommended for a healthy diet, a direct relationship is found between the caloric content of a meal and TEM; that is, higher caloric meals cause a higher thermic effect. As a result, an individual on a restricted caloric diet will burn fewer calories through dietary-induced thermogenesis than when eating larger meals (Belko et al., 1986; Burstzein et al., 1989).

The Impact of Exercise on the Thermic Effect of a Meal

Both meal ingestion and exercise stimulate the sympathetic nervous system and thermogenesis. Because many people wish to maximize energy expenditure, researchers have tried to determine whether a combination of exercise plus a meal in close temporal proximity would potentiate (or increase) the singular effect of either exercise or food. A number of studies have been completed following two basic sequences. After a period of rest, the subjects eat a meal and then exercise. Or conversely, after a period of rest, the subjects exercise and then eat a meal. In both sequences, some studies have shown that TEM was enhanced due to exercise (Belko et al., 1986; Denzer and Young, 2003; Segal et al., 1984, 1985, 1987; Zahorska-Markiewiez, 1980), while others have shown that TEM was not enhanced due to exercise (Dallasso and James, 1984; Pacy et al., 1985; Welle, 1984; Willms and Plowman, 1991). The studies have been so diverse in terms of subjects, meal composition and energy value, exercise mode, intensity, and duration, however, that it is impossible to determine a pattern for when the effect is additive and when it is not.

The Impact of Exercise Training on the Thermic Effect of a Meal

Both cross-sectional and longitudinal studies investigating the effects of training have shown that aerobic-trained individuals have a larger (Davis et al., 1983; Hill et al., 1984; Lundholm et al., 1986), smaller (LeBlanc et al., 1984a,b; Tremblay et al., 1983, 1985), or similar (Owen et al., 1986; Ratcliff, et al., 2011) TEM response. As in the studies dealing with the acute effects of exercise, these studies involve a wide diversity of subjects (especially in training level), meal composition, and meal energy value. The reasons for these inconsistent findings are presently unknown (Sullo et al., 2004). However, there does appear to be a relationship between $\dot{V}O_2$max and TEF (Davis et al., 1983; Hill et al., 1984; LeBlanc et al., 1984b; Tagliaferro et al., 1986) although whether this is positive or negative may depend on where (high or low) along the continuum of aerobic fitness one falls.

As with aerobic endurance training, study results using resistance-trained individuals are inconsistent. One study compared individuals with similar $\dot{V}O_2$max values within the range of the moderately fit just cited [resistance trained (52 mL·kg⁻¹·min⁻¹) and untrained (51.1 mL·kg⁻¹·min⁻¹)] and found that the untrained subjects had a significantly higher TEM than the resistance trained (Gilbert et al., 1991). A second study compared the response of resistance-trained and sedentary individuals to a high carbohydrate (79%) versus moderate fat (45%), similar protein (18–20%) meal. The resistance-trained individuals had a higher TEM in reaction to the high-CHO meal, but there was no significant difference in response between groups to the moderate-fat meal (Thyfault et al., 2004). Still a third study (Ratcliff et al., 2011) found no difference between the TEM in resistance-trained, endurance-trained, and sedentary individuals although there were difference between groups in response to whether the meal was liquid or solid. Obviously the impact of training on the TEM has yet to be determined.

Exercise/Activity Energy Expenditure

The last element in the caloric balance equation is the amount of energy expended in manual work or exercise (**Figure 8.7**). Restricting calories does not change the energy expended in any activity except as it influences body weight. However, individuals on calorically restrictive diets may have insufficient energy and may not be able to do as much physical work or exercise (Westerterp, 2003).

By definition, exercise increases energy expenditure and the effects of training are cumulative. Unless efficiency and/or body weight changes, the caloric expenditure of any activity does not change with exercise training.

Adaptive Thermogenesis Either an increase or decrease in the efficiency of energy utilization.

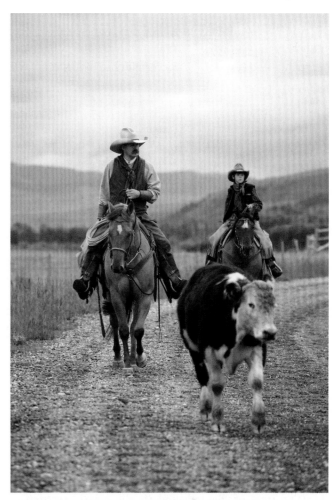

FIGURE 8.7 Energy Expended in Manual Labor Is an Important Component of Total Energy Expenditure.

Table 8.3 summarizes the impact of diet, exercise, and exercise training on all of the elements of the caloric balance equation.

The Effects of Diet, Exercise Training, and Diet Plus Exercise Training on Body Composition and Weight

Many people wish to lose weight strictly for aesthetic reasons (to look better) without caring where this weight comes from. From a physiological standpoint, however, there are four goals for weight loss:

1. To lose body fat with special consideration to visceral abdominal fat
2. To preserve fat free weight (FFW)
3. To maintain or improve health
4. To maintain or improve performance in athletes

TABLE 8.3   Impact of Diet, Exercise, and Exercise Training on the Caloric Balance Equation

Caloric Balance Factor	Diet	Exercise Response	Training Adaptation
Food ingested (+)	By definition, a reduction occurs	No clearly established effect; appetite may transiently decrease immediately, but not over an entire day	Energy intake increases (highly trained and lean individuals) or remains constant (untrained and obese individuals); when training ceases, food intake spontaneously decreases but does not match the decrease in expenditure
BMR and/or RMR (−)	Severe caloric restriction causes a 10–20% decrease; weight cycling does not decrease	Unchanged per se, but metabolic rate postexercise remains elevated	No consistent effect is evident
Thermogenesis (TEM) (−)	Decreases because fewer calories are being ingested; dependent on composition of meals	No consistent additive effect in either a sequence of food-exercise or exercise-food	No consistent effect; may be related to aerobic fitness level
Work or exercise expenditure (−)	If calories are insufficient, may voluntarily do less exercise; but no direct effect on caloric cost	By definition, an increase occurs	A cumulative increase occurs; relatively constant per kg BW

Many factors influence whether these goals can be and are met, including the following:

1. The initial status of the individual (Is he or she a few pounds overweight, or obese?)
2. The type of diet selected (Is the caloric restriction minimal, moderate, severe, or maximal? What percentages of the basic nutrients are included in the diet?)
3. The duration of the weight-reducing program (24–48 hours, 5–20 weeks, or longer)
4. Whether or not exercise training is included as part of the program, and if so, the amount and type of exercise (dynamic aerobic endurance, weight-bearing or non–weight-bearing, or dynamic resistance training)

The American College of Sports Medicine (2001) recommends that adults with a BMI ≥ 25 kg·m⁻² consider reducing their body weight, especially if their waist circumference indicates an excess of visceral abdominal fat. Adults with a BMI of ≥30 kg·m⁻² are encouraged to seek weight loss assistance. The Obesity Evaluation and Treatment Expert Committee (Barlow and Dietz, 2007) recommends that children aged 2–7 years with a BMI in the 85th–94th percentile range according to the CDC growth charts and those greater than the 95th percentile without health complications maintain their weight. Weight loss is recommended for children above the 95th percentile with health complications. Children and adolescents over the age of 7 years with a BMI in the 85th–94th percentile range and no health complications are advised to maintain their weight. Weight loss is recommended for children between the 85th and 94th percentile with health complications and for all individuals with a BMI above the 95th percentile. The following discussion is primarily intended for these individuals for whom weight loss is recommended.

Exact responses to all possible combinations of the above factors (initial status of the individual, type of diet selected, duration of the weight loss program, inclusion or exclusion of exercise, type of exercise program) are not available. But some generalizations can be made. Chief among them is that weight reduction requires that energy expenditure exceed dietary energy intake. Excluding surgical and pharmacological manipulations, this means diet restriction, exercise, or a combination of both. Separately and collectively, diet and exercise affect body composition and body weight.

The Effects of Diet on Body Composition and Weight

The vast majority of individuals wanting to lose weight choose to diet. Caloric restriction may be minimal (a deficit of about 250–500 kcal·d⁻¹), moderate (a total intake of 1200–1500 kcal·d⁻¹), severe (a total intake of 400–800 kcal·d⁻¹), or maximal (fasting, or zero caloric intake). Assuming adherence, all of these will result in a weight loss.

Figure 8.8 shows that with dietary restriction, approximately 28% of the lost total body weight is FFW, and 72% is fat weight. These values, however, are composites primarily from studies with severe caloric restriction. The percentages will vary based on the caloric content of the diet. Thus, body weight loss from total

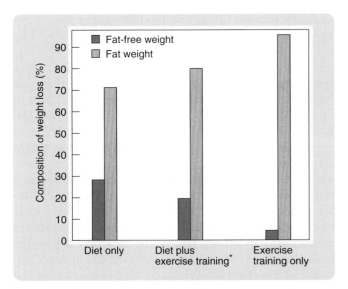

FIGURE 8.8 Effects of Diet, Exercise Training, and Diet plus Exercise on the Composition of Weight Loss.
Almost 30% of the weight lost by dietary restriction is fat free weight (FFW). When exercise is added to dietary caloric restriction, the loss of FFW is reduced. The smallest loss of FFW occurs if the caloric deficit is achieved by exercise alone.
*Diets were generally very low calorie or low calorie (400–1000 kcal·d⁻¹).
Sources: Based on data from Donnelly et al. (1991), Walberg (1989), Hagan (1988), Heymsfield et al. (1989), Zuti and Golding (1976), Hagan et al. (1986), Despres et al. (1985), Bouchard et al. (1990), Ballor et al. (1988).

fasting is split equally between body fat (50%) and FFW (50%); from very low (400–800 kcal·d⁻¹) or low- (800–1200 kcal·d⁻¹) calorie diets, the split is approximately 75% body fat and 25% FFW and from 1200 to 1500 kcal·d⁻¹ diets 90% body fat and only 10% FFW (Nieman, 1990). Fasting, which is obviously incompatible with life over the long haul, is not recommended as a dietary technique. Low-calorie and very low calorie diets (VLCDs) should be undertaken only in extreme situations under the direct supervision of a physician. This technique is typically reserved for extremely obese individuals and is often conducted in a live-in metabolic ward of a hospital. VLCDs result in larger, more rapid reductions in weight, and weight maintenance may be greater with this technique. However, neither the long-term health effects nor the effects of the rate of weight loss on body composition or regional fat loss have been determined (Volek et al., 2005). The 1200–1500 kcal·d⁻¹ regimen is often recommended, but even that does not totally preserve lean body mass (American College of Sports Medicine, 1983). Furthermore, it is better to individualize this approach to a reduction in energy intake of 500–1000 kcal·d⁻¹. With this level of energy deficit, a weight loss of approximately 1–2 lb (0.5–0.9 kg) per week is realistic. A faster rate of weight loss or more initial weight loss has not been shown to improve long-term weight loss compared with this conservative approach (American College of Sports Medicine, 2001).

The importance of the FFW loss may depend on how much excess weight the individual started with. Obese individuals have an excess of both body fat and FFW; their excess body weight is composed of 62–78% fat and 22–38% FFW. The excess FFW is necessary to support and move their larger mass. Therefore, as one loses total body weight, less FFW is needed, and its loss therefore is not unexpected or particularly harmful. The loss of some FFW in such an individual may not be critical, but its preservation would also not be detrimental from a health standpoint. Individuals with less weight to lose need to protect their FFW more (Brown et al., 1983; Donnelly et al., 1991; Jequier, 1987; Pacy et al., 1986).

Recall that FFW is composed of water, protein, and bone mineral (see **Figure 7.2** in Chapter 7). Bone loss often accompanies weight loss brought about by caloric restriction alone (McTigue et al., 2006; Villareal et al., 2006). The key to maintaining bone density may be the intake of adequate or higher calcium (Riedt et al., 2007) or exercise to achieve the negative energy balance (Villareal et al., 2006).

The relative proportions of water and protein loss when dieting vary with the duration of the diet. During the first several days of a diet, most weight loss (55–70%) is water loss. But by the end of the first month, this percentage is considerably reduced (to ~40%), and after 7 to 8 months, it may be as low as 5%. The protein (primarily the component of muscle tissue) loss is a consistent 5% in a nonexercising dieter (Grande et al., 1958a; Heymsfield et al., 1989). What does this say about the proportion of fat loss? Simply that the percentage of fat loss is a mirror image of the percentage of water loss: Little fat is lost at first and then progressively more fat is lost as caloric restriction continues.

Strangely enough, restricting water intake while dieting causes a higher proportion of water to be lost, not less, which could lead to dehydration. More total weight is lost if water is restricted, but not more fat. Water intake should not be restricted when dieting (Grande et al., 1958b; Heymsfield et al., 1989).

The Effects of Exercise Training on Body Composition and Weight

Little evidence suggests that exercise alone produces weight losses as great as what can be achieved with dietary modification alone. Results from short-term studies lasting ≤16 weeks have shown that increased physical activity is positively associated with a reduction in total fat in a dose-response relationship; that is, the more calories expended in exercise, the greater the fat loss. In long-term studies (≥26 weeks), however, no dose-response is seen. On average, the weight loss attained in short-term studies is approximately 85% of that expected (based on caloric expenditure) and is composed almost entirely of fat. Research evidence does not support resistance exercise as effective for weight loss with or without dietary restriction (American College of Sports Medicine, 2009). The failure of exercise to produce weight losses similar to those induced by dietary control may result from individuals compensating for the increased energy expenditure during exercise by decreasing energy expenditure the rest of the day (sometimes called nonexercise activity thermogenesis or NEAT), or from failing to achieve adequate levels of energy expenditure. The study presented in **Figure 8.9** reveals that NEAT changes actually do occur. Thirty-four overweight or obese females (age = 32 years; BMI = 29.3 kg·m^{-2}) exercised for 150 min·wk^{-1} for 8 weeks expending a *net* total of 30.2 ± 12.6 MJ (7724.7 ± 3014.3 kcal) for a predicted fat loss of 0.8 ± 0.2 kg (1.76 ± 0.44 lb). Food intake was not controlled. For the group as a whole, no change in body fat mass occurred. However, there was a large individual variation. The range of fat loss can be seen in **Figure 8.9A**. The 11 individuals who achieved more than the predicted fat loss were classified as "responders," and the 23 individuals who achieved less than the predicted fat loss were classified as "nonresponders." There were no significant differences in the energy intake or macronutrient percentages between responders and nonresponders. Responders increased their daily caloric intake by 0.86 ± 0.75 MJ (206 ± 179.4 kcal) and nonresponders by 1.03 ± 0.53 MJ (246 ± 126.8 kcal) per day. **Figure 8.9B** shows the changes in daily energy expended by responders and nonresponders categorized as total energy expenditure (TEE), activity energy expenditure (AEE, calculated as the energy expenditure of all active activities except the structured exercise sessions), sedentary energy expenditure (SEDEE), and sleeping energy expenditure (SEE). The only significant change was in the AEE with responders showing an increase of 0.79 ± 0.5 MJ (+189 kcal) and the nonresponders a decrease of 0.62 ± 0.39 MJ (–148.3 kcal). Given that both groups expended approximately the same amount of energy during exercise [28.55 MJ ± 2.14 (6830 ± 523 kcal) responders; 30.29 ± 1.76 (7246.3 ± 421 kcal) nonresponders] and increased their energy intake approximately equally, these data indicate that the lower than predicted fat mass loss in the "nonresponders" can be attributed, to some extent, to a compensatory reduction in physical activity outside the supervised exercise sessions.

When the energy deficit is held constant and other factors affecting energy balance are controlled, dynamic aerobic exercise can induce meaningful weight loss. Increases of less than 150 min·wk^{-1} of exercise result in minimal weight loss. Exercise increases between 150 and 225 min·wk^{-1} result in modest weight loss (~2–3 kg/4–7 lb) whereas 225–420 min·wk^{-1} result in 5–7.5 kg (~11–17 lb) weight loss over months to years of activity. Obviously there is a dose-response relationship operating in that higher doses can potentially provide larger losses from initial weight (American College of Sports Medicine, 2009; Hansen et al., 2007; Ross and Janssen, 2001).

Realistically, few people wishing to lose body weight set out to do it entirely by exercising. You may encounter some of these people in health clubs, but they are a minority. On the other hand, there are many individuals who consciously or unconsciously do control their body weight through exercise training. These are, of course, athletes. If we ignore the fact that some athletes also closely watch their caloric intake, indirect evidence of the effect of exercise on body composition can be inferred from the %BF values measured in various groups of athletes. **Figure 8.10** presents a compilation of available data.

Keeping in mind that the %BF for an average young adult male should be 12–15% and that for a young adult female it is 22–25%, several conclusions can be made from this graph. First, even among athletes, the male-female difference in %BF is maintained. Second, male and female athletes in different sports vary considerably in their %BF, from much leaner than average to slightly above average. Third, the %BF values appear to have a direct relationship to the demands of the sport. Athletes in sports where body aesthetics play a part in success (dance, figure skating, body building, gymnastics) tend to have low %BF values. Endurance athletes (cyclists, cross-country skiers, distance runners, and triathletes) also tend to have low %BF values. Athletes in predominantly motor skill sports (baseball, golf, and volleyball) tend to be about average. The only athletes consistently at or above average %BF values are the field event participants.

These data tend to support the value of exercise training in maintaining a low %BF, because athletes in activities known to have high caloric costs and engaged in for long periods of time have the lowest %BF. However, the problem of self-selection is present in studies of this type; that is, we do not know whether individuals who are genetically programmed for leanness and success in these sports naturally gravitate to them, or whether the training demands of the sport determine the body composition of the performer. Both factors are probably operating.

Although the mean values in this graph show a definite pattern, a wide range of variability exists among successful athletes in any given event. For example, successful female distance runners have an average measured %BF value of 16.5%. Included in that group, however, is an athlete who won six consecutive

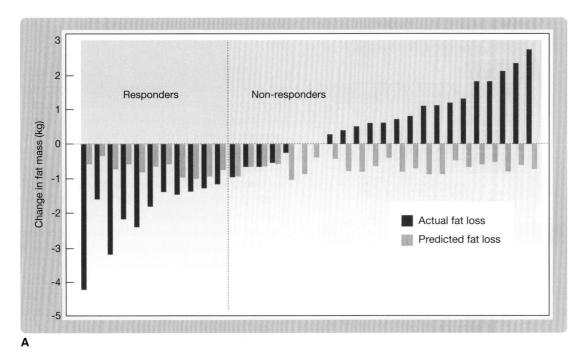

A

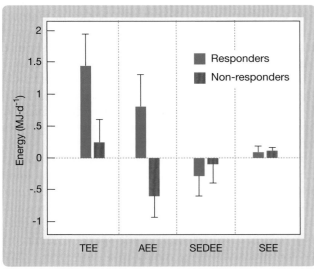

B

FIGURE 8.9 Behavioral Compensation during Exercise Training and Individual Fat Loss.

Graph A compares the predicted and actual changes in body fat mass in individual overweight females who participated in an 8-week exercise training program. Few lost the calculated amount and as a group were divided in "responders" (those that actually lost fat) and "nonresponders" (those who did not lose fat). Graph B shows that the nonresponders compensated for the energy expended during the exercise training by significantly decreasing all other active energy expenditure (AEE) during the day.

TEE = Total Energy Expenditure; AEE = Active Energy Expenditure excluding Exercise Expenditure; SEDEE = Sedentary Energy Expenditure; SEE = Sleeping Energy Expenditure.

Source: Manthou, E., J. M. R. Gill, A. Wright, D. Malkova: Behavioral compensatory adjustments to exercise training in overweight women. *Medicine & Science in Sports & Exercise.* 42(6):1221–1228 (2010).

international cross-country championships and another who held the 1972 world best time for the marathon; both of these runners had only 6% BF. At the other end of the range, the mid-1970s world record holder for the 50-mi run tested at 35.8% BF (Brownell et al., 1987). These extremes point out the importance of not establishing a specific %BF value for all athletes in any sport. The average values should not be interpreted as optimal values for all athletes competing in a particular sport. If %BF values are suggested to athletes, they should be in the form of a range of values. The health and the performance of the athlete need to be monitored within that range, and individual adjustments made based on this monitoring. Eating disorders,

which are sometimes associated with attempts to control body composition for sport, are discussed fully in Chapter 6.

Figure 8.8 includes the results of three studies designed to determine whether weight could be lost but FFW maintained by exercise training without caloric restriction. The column is labeled "exercise training only." In these studies, less than 5% of the weight lost could be attributed to FFW. Indeed, only one study showed any FFW loss. In the other two, FFW was gained.

Wilmore (1983) compiled a list of body weight and body composition changes from 55 training studies whose general purpose was to improve physical fitness.

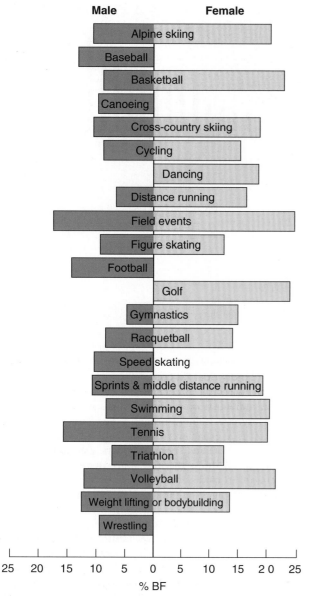

FIGURE 8.10 Average Percent Body Fat of Male and Female Athletes (17–35 years) in Selected Sports.
Source: Wilmore and Costill (1988).

loss; however, there is a volume effect in short-term studies, as more exercise equates to greater caloric expenditure (Hansen et al., 2007).

A 1995 meta-analysis (Garrow and Summerbell, 1995) of 28 studies found that aerobic exercise without dietary restriction led to weight loss but had little effect on FFW (meaning at least that it was maintained). Conversely, resistance exercise had little effect on weight loss but increased FFW by approximately 2–5 lb (1–2 kg). Regression analysis showed that for a weight loss of 10 kg by diet alone, the expected loss of FFW would be approximately 3 kg for males and approximately 2 kg for females. A recent review (Stiegler and Cunliffe, 2006) suggests that exercise training can reduce the loss of FFW during energy restriction.

More importantly, recent evidence has shown that overweight/obese individuals benefit from exercise even if they remain overweight/obese. The Focus on Application box in Chapter 7 discusses some of this evidence from dynamic aerobic exercise. Active overweight/obese persons have better risk profiles for the diseases identified earlier and lower rates of morbidity and mortality than their sedentary counterparts. These health gains are related to the beneficial changes in glucose-insulin responses, lipoprotein values, and cardiovascular function. There is also some evidence that resistance training improves high-density lipoprotein cholesterol (HDL-C), low-density lipoprotein cholesterol (LDL-C), insulin, and blood pressure risk factors. Thus, the value of exercise training for overweight individuals goes far beyond the sometimes minor contribution to weight loss (American College of Sports Medicine, 2009).

Children and adolescents appear similar to adults in relation to the influence of exercise training on body composition. Comparisons of young athletes with their sedentary counterparts typically show that both boy and girl athletes have a lower percent body fat and higher FFW values. The variation among sports is similar to that for adults. Training studies also show that a decrement in percent body fat results from systematically applied exercise programs (Boileau et al., 1985; Epstein and Goldfield, 1999; Plowman, 1989). Two separate systematic reviews (Atlantis et al., 2006; Watts et al., 2005) both concluded that exercise training does not consistently decrease body weight in children and adolescents but that exercise is associated with beneficial changes in fat (decreases) and fat-free mass (increases). The National Heart, Lung, and Blood Institute's Growth and Health Study reported that at ages 18–19 years, BMI was 2.10 kg·m⁻² less for active white girls and 2.98 kg·m⁻² less for active black girls than their sedentary counterparts. Similarly, the sum of skinfolds was 15.04 and 13.54 mm less for the active white and black girls, respectively, than their inactive counterparts. Active girls were doing only the equivalent of 30 minutes of brisk walking 5 d·wk⁻¹. The change in reported energy intake ranged from 17 to 121 kcal·d⁻¹ (Kimm et al., 2005).

The average body fat change was a decrease of only 1.6%, but at the same time a 1% increase occurred in FFW. No information was provided about the caloric balance in these studies. It must be emphasized that the key to weight and fat loss is not exercise per se but the achievement of a caloric deficit through exercise (American College of Sports Medicine, 2009; Donnelly et al., 1991; Walberg, 1989). Diet alone can also achieve a caloric deficit, but when weight is lost through dieting alone, it includes a greater percentage of FFW. Dynamic aerobic endurance activity is most helpful for increasing caloric expenditure; dynamic resistance activity (which is low in caloric cost) acts more directly to increase muscle mass. There seems to be no direct influence of training intensity on fat mass

FOCUS ON RESEARCH: *Clinically Relevant*

The Effect of Increased and Decreased Exercise on Weight Loss and Gain

Even those individuals who routinely use exercise, whether intentionally (many fitness participants) or unintentionally (athletes), to control body weight have variations in their exercise routines. The off-season transition phase, illness/injury, family obligations, work or school demands, aging, weather, travel, holidays, or simply motivational lags often result in temporary or gradual decreases in overall physical activity. Williams investigated the impact of decreases in exercise and contrasted them with changes in body weight and waist circumference with equal amounts of exercise increase.

Data from 4632 males (M) and 1953 females (F) whose running distances increased 2 km·wk⁻¹ (1.25 mi·wk⁻¹) or more and 17,280 M and 5970 F whose running distances decreased by the same amount during 7.7 years of follow-up were analyzed. All data were self-reported and collected nationally at races and through a popular running magazine. Baseline values for BMI (M = 23.9 versus 23.8 kg·m⁻²; F = 21.2 versus 21.3 kg·m⁻²) and waist circumference (M = 84.3 versus 84.4 cm; F = 68.5 versus 68.6 cm) were all in the normal range and similar between those who increased and decreased their running distance, respectively. The groups differed slightly by age (M = 43.6 versus 44.8 years; F = 37.8 versus 38.2 years). Running distances were divided into six intervals (0–8, 8–16, 16–32, 32–48, 48–64, and 64–80 km·wk⁻¹ [~0–5, 5–10, 10–20, 20–30, 30–40, and 40–50 mi·wk⁻¹]).

The accompanying graph presents the results for BMI. Look first at the right axis and the line labeled "weight loss from initiating running."

Read this line from left to right and note that the axis has a loss in BMI (numerically negative changes) above the zero point. At the lowest levels of running (<20 km·wk⁻¹), BMI actually increases. As previously noted, this could be because of increases in FFW, a compensatory decrease in other daily activity, or

a combination of both. It is not until a man runs 25 km·wk⁻¹ (15.5 mi·wk⁻¹) and a woman 48 km·wk⁻¹ (30 mi·wk⁻¹) that a reduction in BMI is expected. For example, a male nonrunner who at follow-up was running 41 km·wk⁻¹ (25.5 mi·wk⁻¹) would have an expected change of −0.23 kg·m⁻² in his BMI.

Now look at the left axis and the line labeled "weight gain from running cessation." Read this line from right to left and note that the axis has a gain in BMI (numerically positive changes) above the zero point. Decreasing running distance causes significant weight gain at all running levels, but the gain becomes progressively greater (the slope of the line steeper) with the fewer kilometers (miles) run. Thus, a man who reduced his running from 16 km·wk⁻¹ to nothing would expect to see a gain in BMI of 0.81 kg·m⁻². If an individual male reduced his running from 32 km·wk⁻¹ to nothing, he would expect to see a gain in BMI of 1.26 kg·m⁻².

However, if this individual male reduced his distance run from 32 to 16 km·wk⁻¹, his increase in BMI would only be 0.45 kg·m⁻² (1.26–0.81 kg·m⁻²).

The most striking aspect of the overall graph interpretation is the asymmetry between the changes in BMI loss with increasing exercise and BMI gain with decreasing exercise. Above 32 km·wk⁻¹ (the equivalent of 30 kcal·kg·wk⁻¹) for men and 16 km·wk⁻¹ (the equivalent of 15 kcal·kg·wk⁻¹) for women, the effects of training and detraining are comparable. The weight gains and losses associated with changes in energy expended in exercise above this threshold are probably reversible. However, at exercise levels below this, an interruption in exercise would be expected to produce a weight gain that is not reversed simply by resuming the prior exercise level. Changes for waist circumference parallel these for BMI.

Food intake data were not available for the study participants, but clearly there was an imbalance between intake and output. Recall that appetite does not automatically adjust in proportion to energy expenditure decrement. Obviously, the duration of detraining was quite long in this study. However, the process of energy imbalance begins immediately. Unfortunately, what happens to many of us is that a temporary decrease in exercise (think of holidays) is accompanied by excess food intake. These results suggest:

1. Weight gains from becoming inactive may not be reversible simply by resuming prior activity levels. This depends on the accustomed level of activity and is most evident in the least active.

2. It is important to minimize exercise variation and/or to match exercise variation with conscious equal adjustment in energy intake for long-term weight control.

Source: Williams, P. T.: Asymmetric weight gain and loss from increasing and decreasing exercise. *Medicine & Science in Sports & Exercise.* 40(2):296–302 (2008).

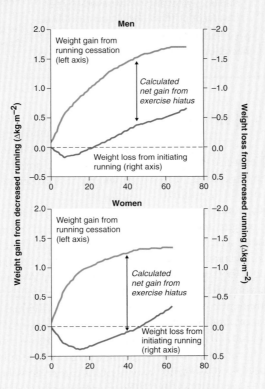

Increase (initiation) or decrease (cessation) in weekly running distance (km)

FOCUS ON APPLICATION

Guidelines for Evaluating a Weight Loss Diet

Throughout this chapter, guidelines are presented for developing and evaluating exercise programs through the use of the training principles. Because the most effective technique for weight loss and control is a combination of diet and exercise, the following guidelines can assist in the development and evaluation of diets intended for weight loss. An acceptable diet should meet the following standards (American College of Sports Medicine, 2000, 2007; Dietary Guidelines for Americans, 2005; van Horn et al., 1998). The diet should:

1. Provide a daily energy intake of approximately 500–1000 kcal below normal prediet intake, but not lower than RMR (approximately 1200 kcal·d^{-1} for females and 1500 kcal·d^{-1} for males), or the total calories halfway between RMR and 30% above RMR

2. Meet the nutritional requirements of 45–65% carbohydrate, 10–35% protein, and 20–35% total fat (<10% saturated, transfats as low as possible, <300 mg cholesterol) and the Dietary Reference Intakes/Recommended Daily Allowance for vitamins and minerals

3. Emphasize a variety of food choices and allow for individual and cultural preferences in terms of acquisition, taste, preparation, and cost

4. Not be based on some "secret" ingredient or "magic" combination of foods, or require the simultaneous ingestion of "fat burning" or other supplements. Taking a daily multivitamin may be acceptable.

5. Be backed by credible scientific or medical organizations (e.g., the American Dietetic Association or the American Heart Association) and/or well-designed research published in peer-reviewed journals that supports both the effectiveness and safety of the diet. Anyone may write a diet book; the publication of diet books is not regulated by any governmental agency or professional society. If someone intends to make money with the diet, "let the buyer beware."

6. Include at least three meals per day (more frequent smaller meals are also acceptable) and 74–100 fluid oz of drinking water and other beverages per day. Alcohol intake should be controlled.

What about the manipulation of macronutrients in diets? Claims that the ingestion of a low-glycemic-index diet (as opposed to a high-glycemic-index diet) will increase the weight loss have generally not been supported. Calorie-restricted diets differing substantially in glycemic load can result in comparable long-term weight loss. If anything, a reduced calorie intake may be harder to sustain on a low-glycemic diet over time (Das et al., 2007). Low-carbohydrate/high-fat diets and high-protein diets can be successful for weight loss but are probably based on water loss, ketosis-induced appetite suppression, and high satiety. Long-term health risks are a concern, and such low-carbohydrate diets are not recommended (Astrup et al., 2004). Similarly, high-carbohydrate diets have been shown to have unfavorable effects on blood lipid levels (Volek et al., 2005). Moderate levels of fat (20% to <30%) as recommended by American College of Sports Medicine (2001) often represent a decrease in fat intake in overweight/obese individuals. However, it is probably not fat restriction per se that results in weight loss but the decrease in total caloric intake (American College of Sports Medicine,

The Effects of Diet Plus Exercise Training on Body Composition and Weight

Studies that have combined diet and exercise seem to suggest that this approach is best for positive, long-term changes. Body weight is not lost faster in combined exercise-plus-diet programs than in diet alone programs because, as has been said several times, weight loss is all about achieving a negative caloric balance and changes in fat mass exceeding changes in FFW (Hansen et al., 2007; Stiegler and Cunliffe, 2006; Wing, 1999). Exercise training, whether alone or in combination with dietary restriction, achieves the desirable maintenance of FFW. **Figure 8.8** shows (from a composite of studies) that when exercise is added to caloric restriction, 20% of the total weight loss is FFW and 80% is fat. This is more FFW loss than when exercise alone is used to achieve the caloric deficit, but less than when diet is used alone. In some cases, muscle mass can actually be gained, despite very similar total weight loss (Zuti and Golding, 1976). Furthermore, the addition of an exercise component to

a weight control program carries several additional benefits. These include improved dietary compliance, the numerous fitness benefits mentioned throughout this chapter, and the possibility of more effective maintenance of weight loss (discussed later in this chapter) (Hansen et al., 2007).

The key to weight loss while maintaining FFW is probably the total caloric deficit, the inclusion of resistance training, and the nutrient content (PRO and CHO) of the calories ingested (American College of Sports Medicine, 2009; Walberg, 1989). One advantage of adding exercise to a weight loss regimen may simply be that it allows an individual to ingest more kilocalories and still be in a negative caloric balance. Eating a moderately restricted diet allows for adequate nutrition and lifestyle changes that can be tolerated for a lifetime; by contrast, a VLCD can seldom be sustained for a prolonged time. Furthermore, physical activity will increase weight loss if dietary restriction is moderate, but not if severe, that is, less than the number of calories equal to RMR (American College of Sports Medicine, 2009).

2001; Volek et al., 2005). Fat restriction avoids the increase in ghrelin caused by dietary energy restriction (Weigle et al., 2003). In addition, a fat intake less than 30% could have beneficial health effects as well that result from the fat restriction per se. Some theoretical and experimental evidence suggests that diets high in protein are beneficial for weight loss and weight maintenance (American College of Sports Medicine, 2001; Layman, 2004; Volek et al., 2005). A high-protein diet can be defined as 18–30% or a ratio of 1 g PRO/1.5 g CHO. A high-protein, moderate-fat, moderate-carbohydrate diet has been shown to be better than a low-protein, moderate-fat, high-carbohydrate diet of equal caloric restriction either alone or when combined with an aerobic plus resistance exercise program for promoting weight loss (Meckling and Sherfey, 2007). Similarly, a high-protein diet has been shown to maintain weight after weight loss with or without controlling for the percentage of carbohydrate in the diet (Weigle et al., 2005; Westerterp-Plantenga et al., 2004). Finally, a high-protein diet was shown to maintain FFW, even when weight was regained (Leidy et al., 2007a;

Westerterp-Plantenga et al., 2004). The benefits of high-protein diets have been attributed in these experimental studies to decreased food efficiency, decreased ghrelin rise, increased leptin sensitivity, increased thermogenic effects of feeding, and increased satiety. A recent study (Dansinger et al., 2005) of four popular diets (Atkins = carbohydrate restriction; Zone = 40–30–30 macronutrient balance; Weight Watchers [caloric restriction]; Ornish = fat restriction]) found that after a year each diet modestly reduced body weight by approximately 2–3 kg (~4–7 lb) and improved several cardiac risk factors. The amount of weight lost was related to adherence to the diet but not to the diet type.

Above all, it must be remembered that the macronutrient content of any diet will affect body weight only when there is a reduction in caloric intake that results in a negative caloric balance. The health costs or benefits of any diet must also be considered. The optimal levels of each macronutrient beyond those established in the current dietary guidelines, if optimal levels actually exist, remain to be determined.

Sources: American College of Sports Medicine (2000, 2001, 2007); Astrup et al. (2004); Dansinger et al. (2005); Das et al. (2007); Dietary Guidelines for Americans (2005); Layman (2004); Leidy et al. (2007a); Meckling and Sherfey (2007); van Horn et al. (1998); Volek et al. (2005); Weigle et al. (2003); Westerterp-Plantenga et al. (2004).

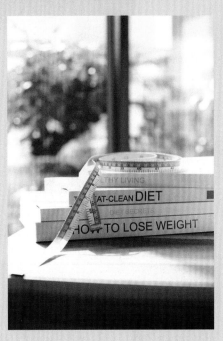

The Effects of Diet, Exercise Training, and Diet Plus Exercise Training on Abdominal Obesity

Of special concern is the impact of diet, exercise training, and diet plus exercise training on abdominal fat, both subcutaneous abdominal adipose tissue (SAAT) and visceral adipose tissue (VAT) as illustrated in **Figure 8.11**. The concern is that abdominal fat is known to be an independent predictor of the metabolic risk factors that are the antecedents for type II (non–insulin-dependent) diabetes and various cardiovascular diseases.

A review of studies investigating the impact of diet alone on VAT found that for every kilogram of weight loss, VAT was reduced 3–4 cm², or approximately 2–3% of the total VAT. Furthermore, there appeared to be a preferential reduction in VAT (which is desirable) over subcutaneous fat loss (Ross, 1997). The degree of caloric restriction (low-calorie or very low calorie diet) does not appear to have any influence on the ratio of the % change in VAT to the % change in total fat. Individuals with the

most VAT lose the greatest amount of VAT (Smith and Zachwieja, 1999).

The impact of exercise training alone on abdominal obesity in adults has been confounded by what measure was used to evaluate it and whether or not a weight loss was achieved. In general, in the absence of weight loss, abdominal fat levels are not reduced if measured by waist-to-hip ratio or waist circumference. Waist circumference is responsive to exercise training, but a change in waist circumference is not always evident when imaging methods show decreased abdominal obesity. Conversely, physical activity with or without weight loss is associated with reductions in visceral and abdominal subcutaneous fat loss when measured by techniques such as MRI or computerized tomography (CT) scan (Ross and Janssen, 1999). The fact that changes in SAAT and VAT can occur without changes in body weight is important because it means that individuals using exercise to lose weight need to be informed of this possibility and appropriate measures taken so that they can see that positive changes

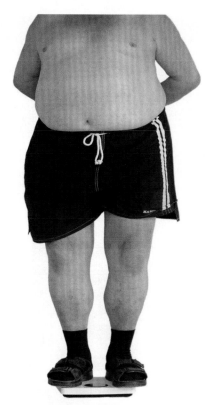

FIGURE 8.11 Abdominal Obesity.
While many individuals are concerned with scale weight, the amount of visceral abdominal fat is more important for health.

are taking place despite what the scale may indicate. On the other hand, both total and abdominal fat are generally much more reduced when weight is lost. Limited evidence from randomized trials shows that reductions occur in abdominal (SAAT and VAT) fat when moderate-to high-intensity exercise interventions of at least 8 weeks duration are undertaken by middle- to older-aged, overweight or obese males and females (Kay and Fiatarone Singh, 2006; Ross and Janssen, 1999).

A systematic review of clinical trials (Ohkawara et al., 2007) reinforced the conclusions that in obese adults with no metabolic disorders there is (a) a significant relationship between aerobic exercise training and visceral fat reduction and (b) that although visceral fat reduction is significantly related to weight reduction during the aerobic exercise training, a significant reduction in visceral fat can occur without significant weight loss. Moreover, there is a dose-response relationship between the amount of aerobic exercise and the amount of visceral fat reduction. At least 10 MET-hr·wk^{-1} of aerobic activity appears to be the threshold to achieve visceral fat reduction. Brisk walking at 3.0 mi·hr^{-1} represents 3.3 METs. Thus, it would take roughly 182 minutes of walking at this pace to achieve the threshold—very comparable to current exercise recommendations (American College of Sports Medicine, 2009).

Although some evidence shows that the average % change in VAT to the % change in fat ratio is higher as a result of exercise training than caloric restriction (CR) alone, it is insufficient to regard exercise training as a more specific therapy for visceral fat loss than dietary restriction (Smith and Zachwieja, 1999). This is shown by a randomized controlled trial conducted on 48 healthy males and females with an initial BMI of 27.3 kg·m^{-2}. Participants were assigned either to a 20% CR diet, an exercise program (EX) designed to produce a similar energy deficit, or healthy lifestyle control group (HL). After 1 year, weight changes corresponding to –10.7%, –8.4%, and –1.7% occurred in the CR, EX, and HL groups, respectively. Whole-body fat mass as well as visceral and SAAT decreased significantly and comparably in the CR and EX group but did not change in the HL group (Racette et al., 2006).

Despite a paucity of research, the interactions between exercise training/physical fitness and abdominal adiposity seem to extend to children and adolescents as well. A cross-sectional study of 9- and 15-year-old students has shown that cardiovascular fitness is inversely associated with abdominal adiposity independently of the time spent at different intensities of physical activity and total physical activity. However, in the low fit group, time spent in vigorous physical activity was related to lower abdominal adiposity. Suggested cutoff values for the inclusion of vigorous physical activity are ≥40 minutes and ≥25 minutes for boys and girls and ≥20 minutes and ≥15 minutes for adolescent males and females (Ortega et al., 2007, 2010). The Focus on Application: Clinically Relevant box shows that exercise training can reduce subcutaneous adipose tissue and retard visceral adipose tissue increase in children (Owens et al., 1999).

The few studies that have investigated the impact of diet plus exercise training on VAT have shown that the relative reduction in VAT is similar to the response induced by diet alone; that is, the addition of exercise training did not provide any preferential benefit for the reduction of VAT (Ross, 1997). This may or may not be true for subcutaneous adipose tissue, as seen by the results from a 20-week intervention study (You et al., 2006). Forty-five obese (BMI = 33 kg·m^{-2}) middle-aged females were assigned to one of three groups, each intended to achieve a 2800-kcal·wk^{-1} deficit: diet only, diet plus low-intensity exercise, and diet plus high-intensity exercise. All three interventions reduced body weight, fat mass, % BF, waist circumference, and hip girth similarly. However, only the diet plus exercise interventions significantly reduced subcutaneous abdominal adipose cell size. Whether this is another case where the use of waist circumference to reflect changes in VAT masked results that imaging might have shown was unknown.

A study by Redman et al. (2007) provides some insight. This study directly compared the effects of equal amounts of exercise increase and caloric reduction on weight loss, total fat mass (measured by dual-energy X-ray absorptiometry) and visceral fat mass (measured by computed tomography). Participants were randomized into a control group ([C] who ingested a healthy weight maintenance diet), a caloric restriction group ([CR] who had a 25% reduction in energy intake), or a caloric restriction plus exercise group ([CR + EX] who had a 12.5% caloric restriction and 12.5% increase in energy expenditure). No significant changes occurred in the control group. The CR group lost 8.3% body weight and the CR + EX group lost 8.1% body weight. These losses were not different between groups. Fat losses are presented in **Figure 8.12**. They represented losses of 27% and 22% for total fat mass, 31% and 24% for VAT mass, and approximately 30% and 25% for subcutaneous abdominal adipose tissue in males and females, respectively. Males showed a significant preferential reduction in VAT. These data suggest that exercise training plays the same role as caloric restriction in terms of changes in total fat mass and abdominal visceral fat mass. However, the addition of exercise did improve the aerobic fitness of the participants more, and this has important additional health implications. The pattern of fat distribution throughout the whole body and within the abdominal compartment was not altered by caloric restriction, reinforcing the idea that individuals are genetically programmed for fat storage in a particular pattern.

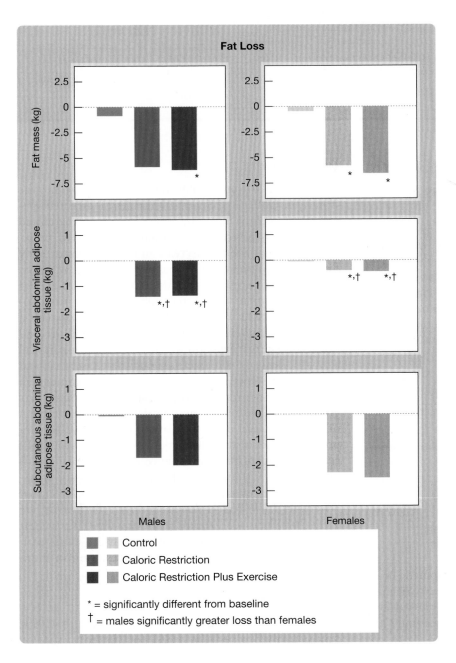

FIGURE 8.12 The Effect of Caloric Restriction with or without Exercise on Fat Loss.

Individuals were randomly assigned to a control group, a 25% caloric restriction group or a 12.5% caloric restriction and 12.5% exercise training group. After 6 months, both groups lost significant and similar amounts of fat mass and visceral abdominal adipose tissue and nonsignificant amounts of subcutaneous abdominal adipose tissue. Males showed a significant preferential lost of VAT compared with females.

Source: Based on data from Redman, L. M., L. K. Heilbronn, C. K. Martin, A. Alfonso, S. R. Smith, & E. Ravussin: Effect of calorie restriction with or without exercise on body composition and fat distribution. *The Journal of Clinical Endocrinology and Metabolism.* 92(3):865–872 (2007).

FOCUS ON APPLICATION

Exercise Training and Visceral Fat in Obese Children

High levels of total body fat mass and visceral adipose tissue (VAT) increase the likelihood that children will develop other coronary artery disease risk factors and non–insulin-dependent diabetes mellitus. Owens et al. (1999) conducted this study to determine if controlled physical training would have a favorable impact on VAT and % body fat in obese children. These authors assigned volunteers to a control group or a physical training group. The physical training group exercised for 40 minutes, at an average heart rate of 157 b·min⁻¹, 5 days a week, for 4 months. The accompanying graph presents the percent change in several variables in the training group and in the control group after 4 months.

These data indicate that obese children:

1. were capable of participating in a high-intensity exercise training program

2. experienced a loss in fat mass, % body fat, and SAAT, whereas the control group experienced a gain in fat mass and SAAT over the same period

3. experienced a smaller increase in VAT than the control group

This study indicates that increasing physical activity of obese children, even without dietary intervention, can improve the aspects of body composition related to cardiovascular risk factors.

Source: Owens et al. (1999).

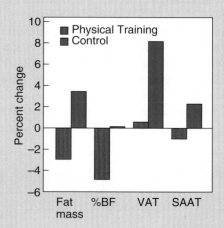

Application of the Training Principles for Weight and Body Composition Loss and/or Control

Based on the previously described impact of diet, exercise training, and diet plus exercise training on body weight and composition, the training principles can be applied to achieve weight and body composition loss, change, and/or control using the following guidelines. These guidelines are intended for the mildly or moderately overweight and overfat individuals whom physical educators and fitness leaders are likely to encounter; they are not meant for more severely obese individuals, who require more drastic reductions and medical supervision.

Specificity

In reality, weight/body composition control are important in three situations:

1. When the goal is to lose weight
2. When the goal is to prevent weight gain, particularly that which tends to occur as individuals age
3. When the goal is to maintain weight loss

Table 8.4 presents physical activity recommendations for weight loss and maintenance from several organizations. The principles for weight loss are discussed first; those for weight maintenance will be discussed under the maintenance training principle.

Weight Loss

Only the 2001 and 2009 recommendations by the American College of Sports Medicine are directed specifically at weight loss. The general goals of weight and body composition control should be (as stated previously) to maximize the decrease in body weight or body fat while minimizing FFW loss and supplying adequate nutrition. To accomplish this, American College of Sports Medicine (2001) recommends a caloric deficit of 500–1000 kcal·d⁻¹ achieved by a combination of decreased energy intake (dietary restriction) and increased energy expenditure (exercise and/or physical activity). Both dynamic aerobic endurance exercise and dynamic resistance training exercise are recommended. The endurance exercise modality selected (walking, jogging, cycling, swimming, aerobic dancing, stair stepping, or stair climbing) does not matter. The aerobic activity produces most of the caloric deficit while the resistance activity helps in the maintenance of fat free weight. A minimum of 150 min·wk⁻¹ of moderate-intensity physical activity is encouraged. Because 1 lb (0.45 kg) of fat equals 3500 kcal, a deficit of 500–1000 kcal·d⁻¹, or 3500–7000 kcal·wk⁻¹, should achieve a 0.5–1 kg weight loss per week. A dose-response relationship exists with more physical activity/caloric deficit resulting in more weight loss.

Spot Reduction

Another way to interpret specificity in relation to weight control might be a desire to reduce body fat from a specific

TABLE 8.4   Physical Activity Recommendations for Weight Loss and Maintenance

Source	Focus	Recommendation
ACSM (2001, 2009)	Weight loss	1. A caloric deficit of 500–1000 kcal·d⁻¹ achieved by a combination of decreased energy intake and increased energy expenditure 2. A minimum of 150 min·wk⁻¹ of moderate-intensity physical activity progressing to 250 min·wk⁻¹ 3. Resistance exercise should supplement aerobic endurance exercise.
ACSM (2009)	Maintenance of normal weight	150–250 min·wk⁻¹ with an energy expenditure of 1200–2000 kcal·wk⁻¹
IOM (2002)	Maintenance of BMI 18.5–25 kg·m⁻²	≥ 60 min·d⁻¹ of moderately intense physical activity for a PAL of 1.6–1.7
IOTF (Erlichman et al., 2002)	Minimize weight gain/ maintain normal weight	60–90 min·d⁻¹ to achieve a PAL ≥ 1.8
IASO (Saris et al., 2003)	Maintenance of normal weight Prevention of weight regain	45–60 min·d⁻¹ or PAL of 1.7 60–90 min·d⁻¹ of moderate-intensity physical activity or fewer of vigorous intensity
ACSM/AHA (Haskell et al., 2007)	Maintenance of normal weight Prevention of weight regain	~60 min·d⁻¹ of moderate to vigorous activity most days of week while not exceeding caloric intake requirements 60–90 min·d⁻¹ of moderate activity while not exceeding caloric intake requirements
ACSM (2009)	Prevention of weight regain	~200–300 min·wk⁻¹; "more is better"

ACSM, American College of Sports Medicine; IOM, Institute of Medicine; IOTF, International Obesity Task Force, 2002; IASO, International Association for Study of Obesity; AHA, American Heart Association; PAL= physical activity level.

body location called spot reduction. The idea behind spot reduction is that fat will be selectively mobilized and thus reduced from the area exercised. For example, as seen in **Figure 8.13**, individuals wishing to reduce his or her abdominal region would concentrate on pelvic tilts, curls, and sit-ups.

Consistent training of specific muscles can increase muscle tone, which may give a slimming appearance (or if hypertrophy occurs, give a more defined appearance). However, no experimental evidence shows that fat (in the form of fatty acids) is mobilized preferentially from adipose cells located near active muscles; that is, spot reducing may be an attractive idea but in reality does not work for either males or females. In one study, 27 women who performed calisthenics for the abdomen, hips, and thighs were compared with 29 women who performed aerobic activities (Noland and Kearney, 1978). Both groups worked out three times per week for 30 minutes for 10 weeks. Although %BF did not decrease significantly in either group, several girth and skinfold measures did decrease in both groups. There was no indication of any preferential site reduction in the specifically selected areas, however. Likewise, when 13 men underwent a 27-day training program during which 5004 sit-ups were performed, no significant changes occurred in %BF, skinfold, or girth measurements either as a result of training or in comparison

with six nonexercising controls. Adipose biopsy measures did show significant decreases in fat cell diameters, but there was no significant difference in these changes between the heavily exercised abdominal site and nonexercised gluteal and subscapular locations (Katch et al., 1984). A newer study involving 24 males and females 18–40 years divided into either a control group or an abdominal exercise group confirmed these results. The exercise group performed seven abdominal exercises, for

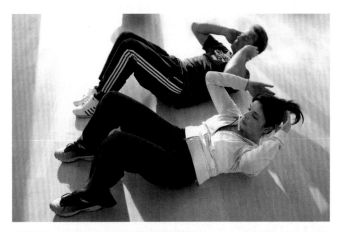

FIGURE 8.13 Anatomically Specific Exercises Do Tone Muscles but Do Not Reduce Fat in That Area.

2 sets of 10 reps, 5 days per week for 6 weeks. There was no significant effect on body weight, %BF, android fat, abdominal circumference, and abdominal or suprailiac skinfold measurements although the exercise group did significantly increase the number of curl-ups performed (Vispute et al., 2011).

Fat is mobilized to be used as a fuel by hormonal action. Hormones circulate to all parts of the body via the bloodstream. The distribution of body fat in the android (abdominal), gynoid (gluteofemoral), or intermediate pattern does not appear to affect the amount of weight lost by caloric deficit, nor is the relative distribution of fat altered by the weight loss. That is, the general shape of the individual is preserved despite a reduction in the total amount of fat and despite any attempt at spot reduction. Because spot reduction does not work, any activity that burns enough calories to cause a negative caloric balance can be used.

Weight Gain Prevention

Five of the other recommendations from national and international organizations (American College of Sports Medicine, 2009; Erlichman et al., 2002; Haskell et al. (ACSM/AHA), 2007; Institute of Medicine, 2002; Saris et al. (IASO), 2003; **Table 8.4**) deal with strategies to prevent weight gain [defined by American College of Sports Medicine (2009) as an increase of >3%] in an individual initially of normal weight. All of these have concluded that a minimum of 45–60 min·d^{-1} or 150 min·wk^{-1} of physical activity are needed for adults, and probably more for children. In 1995, the Centers for Disease Control and Prevention and the American College of Sports Medicine issued a public health recommendation that every US adult should accumulate at least 30 minutes of moderate-intensity physical activity on most, if not all, days of the week. The clear intent was that individuals could reasonably achieve a level of activity that had been shown to be important in limiting health risks for a number of chronic diseases including coronary heart disease and diabetes mellitus. There is now sufficient prospective epidemiological evidence that this guideline (which amounts to approximately 150–200 kcal·d^{-1}) is insufficient for many individuals to prevent weight gain. In these studies, an increase of approximately 350 kcal·d^{-1} (0.25 PAL units) or 50–60 minutes of moderate-intensity activity was needed to prevent weight gain over the years. Therefore, the original recommendation has been amended and clarified (Haskell et al., 2007; Saris et al., 2003).

The reports cited above introduced another way of quantifying physical activity—**physical activity level (PAL)**. The PAL is defined as the ratio of total energy expenditure (TEE) to 24-hour resting or basal/resting energy expenditure (BMR/RMR), that is, TEE/RMR. Four categories of PAL are frequently used: sedentary (1.0–1.39), low active (1.4–1.59), active (1.6–1.89), and very active (1.9–2.5) (Ross and Janssen, 2007). By definition, RMR alone is equal to a PAL of 1.0. The sedentary category includes the energy expenditure required for BMR/RMR, TEF, and maintenance activities of daily independent living (ADL). Because everyone has some values for TEF and ADL, a baseline of approximately 1.4 is typically the starting point for calculating additional needed energy expenditure. Thus, if an individual had an RMR of 1400 kcal·d^{-1}, the difference between PALs of 1.4 and 1.7 is an additional 420 kcal of activity (1.7–1.4 = 0.30; 0.30 × 1400 kcal = 420 kcal) (Saris et al., 2003). This can be achieved by a combination of exercise and other physical activities such as mowing the grass, cleaning house, occupational demands, etc., during the day.

CHECK YOUR COMPREHENSION 2

Danladi is a 48-year-old male professor. He weighs 191 lb and is 6′2″ tall. How many calories does he need to expend in activity to achieve a PAL of 1.6? Use the RMR equation in **Table 8.2** to calculate the baseline PAL of 1.4, ignoring the minor variation from BMR caused by TEM and ADL. He likes to play recreational basketball at noon (6 METs) for 3 days a week and walk with his family (3.3 METs) on Saturdays and Sundays. What is the minimum number of minutes he should do each of these activities on any given day to achieve his goal? How many miles should he walk? Why should most of his additional caloric expenditure come from his planned activity and sport? Check your answer in Appendix C. Then use the MET levels in **Table 4.7** to find the values for your favorite activity, and do the calculation for yourself.

Overload

When weight loss is the goal, overload really means the attainment of a net deficit. However, the general guidelines for the application of the training principles for dynamic aerobic endurance training outlined in Chapters 5 and 13 also apply here. The one exception is a shift in the importance of intensity and duration. The bottom line is that burning large numbers of calories is what is most important.

Previously sedentary, unfit, and overweight or overfat individuals cannot work at high-intensity levels for even short periods of time, and they should not try to. They do not tolerate high-intensity exercise well, risk injury and the inability to then continue exercising, and, at the very least, often dislike the exercise and/or feelings associated with fatigue so much that they will stop. Instead, low-intensity activities continued for a long duration are recommended. The American College of Sports

Medicine (ACSM) recommended duration of exercise for weight loss is presented in **Table 8.4**. Note that this recommendation is for a minimum of 150 min·wk⁻¹ of moderate-intensity exercise progressing to greater than 250 min·wk⁻¹ of endurance and resistance training. This can be broken up into sessions in any number of different ways. The bottom line is that any combination of frequency, duration, and intensity of exercise that burns sufficient calories to obtain a deficit is the goal for weight loss.

This recommendation is contrary to a common misconception that the best way to lose fat is to burn fat doing long-duration, low-intensity exercise. Although it is true that fat is the dominant fuel in long-duration, low-intensity exercise, the important factor in weight loss is to establish a caloric deficit, regardless of the fuel being used. This principle is exemplified in a study by Ballor et al. (1990) of two groups of obese women on equally restricted caloric intakes (1200 kcal·d⁻¹). One group exercised on a cycle ergometer at 51% of their peak $\dot{V}O_2$max for 50 minutes and the other at 85% of their peak $\dot{V}O_2$max for 25 minutes. The low-intensity group expended an average of 283 kcal per session at an RER of 0.80, and the high-intensity group expended an average of 260 kcal per session at an RER of 0.92. The estimated fat utilization was 26% for the high-intensity group and 66.6% for the low-intensity group. Although the high-intensity group did improve their cardiovascular fitness more, both groups lost equal amounts of body weight, fat-free mass, fat mass, and percent body fat and had the same decrease in the sum of five-skinfold thicknesses.

The advantage of the low-intensity exercise was not an increased loss of fat but a better initial tolerance to the exercise sessions. Individuals who are overweight or obese are also frequently out of shape, and low-intensity work at the initiation of an exercise program is more appropriate and less likely to bring about muscle and joint problems than a high-intensity program. On the other hand, more active or higher fit individuals need not be concerned about decreasing exercise intensity in order to reap the weight control benefits of exercise. The intensity and duration can be manipulated to best suit each individual interested in body weight or composition control.

Increasing caloric expenditure per session and increasing the frequency of the exercise both enhance fat and weight loss. An individual combining dynamic aerobic endurance and resistance weight training can alternate days (three each) and still have a rest day, or can combine sessions on each of 3 or 4 days. The caloric cost of dynamic resistance exercise is less than that of dynamic endurance exercise, and this difference needs to be taken into account when designing the exercise program for weight loss or maintenance.

In calculations of the energy cost of an activity session, the *net* value rather than the *gross* value should be used. That is, the calories that would have been burned anyway, had the individual been sedentary, should be subtracted from the cost of the exercise (American College of Sports Medicine, 2000; Pacy et al., 1986). For example, if the energy cost of playing tennis is 7.1 kcal·min⁻¹ but the individual would have expended 1.3 kcal·min⁻¹ at rest, the net cost is 5.8 kcal·min⁻¹. Thus, it would take almost 52 minutes of tennis to burn 300 excess calories, not 42 minutes.

Rest/Recovery/Adaptation

The importance of adaptation in caloric deficit lies in the fact that the composition of the weight loss varies the longer the deficit is maintained. One consistent, moderate-deficit diet is therefore better than a series of short, very calorically restricted diets, especially in light of the concerns about weight cycling described under maintenance. The individual must get past the early water loss stages and into the stage where fat loss is proportionally the greatest. This adaptation will occur in addition to the specific adaptations to the exercise training. There is no rest or recovery specific for weight loss beyond that built into any exercise program.

Progression

The greatest progression is made in the number of calories that can be expended in exercise as the individual adapts to the training. When the calories expended in exercise increase, the amount of food ingested can be kept at the same level, thereby increasing the deficit and/or possibly offsetting any decrease in RMR that may occur. Another possibility is to proportionally increase the amount of food ingested to maintain the same relative deficit. Progression should not be interpreted as an attempt to exercise more and more while eating less and less beyond a reasonable point.

Individualization

To tailor a weight or fat loss program for an individual, several evaluations and calculations are helpful. The first is the direct measurement or estimation of the person's RMR. Formulas such as those presented earlier in the chapter (**Table 8.2**) can be used to estimate RMR fairly easily. Second, the nutrient and caloric intake of the individual should be analyzed. Computer programs are available for this analysis. Third, the number of calories normally expended in daily activity needs to be calculated. Lists of the caloric cost per kilogram of activities, such as that in **Table 4.7** in Chapter 4, can be used for this calculation.

> **Physical Activity Level (PAL)** The ratio of total energy expenditure (TEE) to 24-hour resting or basal/resting energy expenditure (RMR), that is, TEE/RMR.

Once these numbers are known, the relative proportions of the caloric deficit to come from food intake and from energy expenditure can be determined. How much comes from which category should depend on the current caloric intake and fitness level of the individual.

If a sedentary, unfit female ingests 2000 kcal·d⁻¹ and expends 1800 kcal·d⁻¹, 1200 kcal of which is RMR, then an initial 650-kcal decrement makes sense (2000−1800 = 200 kcal to get to a caloric balance, and a 450-kcal deficit for a 1.3-lb weight loss per week). If the individual is really unfit, 100 kcal·d⁻¹ of exercise may be all he or she can do; the other 550 kcal needs to come from decreasing the calories ingested. This diet would still allow for daily caloric ingestion of 1350 kcal. If, however, the individual is relatively fit, more calories can be expended in exercise and either a greater intake of food allowed or a greater deficit achieved.

The caloric ingestion should not fall below the RMR. Although the flat values of 1200 for females and 1500 kcal·d⁻¹ for males are often suggested as a lower limit of caloric intake (American College of Sports Medicine, 1983), a more individualized system is to calculate a value halfway between RMR and 30% above RMR as used in the above example (Schelkun, 1991).

Retrogression/Plateau/Reversibility

Weight loss tends to be uneven, even when caloric intake and output remain the same. Weight loss is fastest in the early stages of caloric deficit and then tends to level off. This pattern occurs, at least in part, because of the early loss of large amounts of glycogen and water. Later, RMR may decrease, and food efficiency and adaptive decreases in exercise energy expenditure may become a factor (Astrup et al., 1999; Bray, 1969; Major et al., 2007). Although few who are attempting to lose weight want to hear about these patterns, they need to be informed so that they are mentally prepared to deal with them. Reverting to old habits of food intake and a sedentary lifestyle (in a sense, detraining) will result in a rapid retrogression or complete reversal, exemplified by regaining lost weight.

Maintenance

As stated previously, many more people manage to lose weight than to maintain that weight loss. The key to the maintenance of a weight or fat loss may be exercise training (American College of Sports Medicine, 2009; Saris et al., 2003; Tate et al., 2007; Wing, 1999). As can be seen in **Table 8.4**, the major public policy organizations in this area universally recommend exercise/physical activity to maintain weight loss. Evidence is compelling that

prevention of weight regain in formerly obese individuals requires at least 60–90 minutes daily of moderate-intensity activity (or lesser amounts of vigorous-intensity activity) or approximately 200–300 min·wk⁻¹ (Saris et al., 2003). This International Association for the Study of Obesity (IASO) recommendation and the remarkably consistent recommendations from the other reports all assume that caloric intake will not exceed that required to maintain weight. More activity does seem to be better than minimal activity (American College of Sports Medicine, 2009). The level of food intake and exercise output at the weight the individual wishes to maintain must be continued for life.

Weight Cycling

Individuals who fail to maintain a weight loss often find themselves weight cycling. **Weight cycling** is repeated bouts of weight loss and regain. Sometimes this cycling is called the "rhythm method of girth control" or the "yo-yo effect."

In addition to nonmaintaining dieters, some athletes (wrestlers, jockeys, ski jumpers, and the like) (**Figure 8.14**) lose and gain weight purposely as they make weight for competition and then make up for missed meals by eating large quantities. Dieters may take months or years to complete each cycle; weight class athletes will do the same thing in 2 or 3 days. Furthermore, dieters may lose and gain 20–100 lb or more in each cycle, but athletes generally lose or gain less than 20 lb.

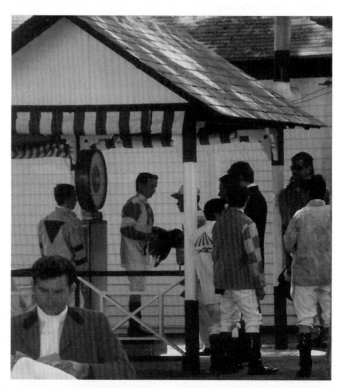

FIGURE 8.14 Some Athletes, Such as Jockeys, Undergo Repeated Bouts of Weight Cycling to Make Weight in Their Sport.

While weight cycling is undoubtedly frustrating to dieters and possibly inconvenient for weight class athletes, there have also been concerns about how it affects the health of the individuals involved. It has been theorized that weight cycling slows down the RMR, increases the difficulty of subsequent weight loss, and enhances abdominal fat (Blackburn et al., 1989; Nash, 1987). Despite the theory, experimental evidence from studies testing the influence of weight cycling on RMR has had inconclusive results. High school wrestlers who weight cycled exhibited a 15% lower RMR than those who did not (Steen et al., 1988). However, college wrestlers who weight cycled had RMRs similar to those of non–weight-cycling wrestlers, and both wrestling groups had higher RMR values than nonwrestling controls (Schmidt et al., 1993). Studies of dieters who were initially obese or overweight are also conflicting, with only one (Strychar et al., 2009) of four studies finding evidence (Beeson et al., 1989; van Dale and Saris, 1989; Wadden et al., 1992) that a history of weight cycling affected RMR.

One study did find that prior weight cycling made subsequent weight loss harder (Blackburn et al., 1989). However, three other studies found no relationship between weight loss in one cycle and the subsequent rate or amount of weight loss in later cycles (Beeson et al., 1989; van Dale and Saris, 1989; Wadden et al., 1992).

Higher android (upper-body) fat deposition, increased adiposity in normal weight, and greater weight gain have been found in several studies of individuals who weight cycled (Anastasiou, et al., 2010; Field et al., 2004; Rodin et al., 1990; Saarni et al., 2006; Strychar et al., 2009; Wallner et al., 2004). Conversely, similar studies have found no difference in fat distribution, waist-to-hip ratio, or increased long-term weight gain as a function of weight-cycling history (Graci et al., 2004; Jeffery et al., 1992; Mason et al., 2010; van Dale and Saris, 1989; van Wye et al., 2007; Wadden et al., 1992). There is no direct magnetic resonance imaging (MRI) evidence that weight cycling leads to increased abdominal visceral fat deposition (Montani et al., 2006). Thus, neither body fat distribution nor body composition in humans is conclusively affected by a history of weight cycling (National Task Force on the Prevention and Treatment of Obesity, 1994).

Another area of controversy involves evidence of increased cardiovascular risk factors, cardiovascular disease mortality, and all-cause mortality associated with weight cycling (Diaz et al., 2005; Montani et al., 2006; Olson et al., 2000; Rzehak et al., 2007). It has yet to be determined if this relationship is directly or indirectly linked to fat accumulation or other factors such as the effects of preexisting disease and smoking. There is no firm evidence that weight loss or weight fluctuation in otherwise healthy individuals is hazardous (Graci et al., 2004; Strychar et al., 2009; Wannamethee et al., 2002). It is, of course, preferable to lose weight into a healthy zone and/or maintain a healthy weight rather than to weight cycle. This is unfortunately easier said than done.

Why is it So Hard to Keep Weight Off Once it has been Lost?

If a change in RMR brought about by weight cycling is not the reason for the difficulty in maintaining a weight/fat loss, what is? There is no definite answer to that question. Interest is currently centered on compliance, lipoprotein lipase, ghrelin and leptin, and adaptive decreases in thermogenesis.

COMPLIANCE The most obvious reason for the difficulty in maintaining weight loss, at least in part, is failure of compliance—the failure to maintain a regular exercise program of sufficient energy expenditure and/or a healthy calorically controlled dietary intake. Sooner or later, many individuals revert back to the same lifestyle that made their weight loss necessary initially. For example, Tate et al. (2007) randomly assigned 202 overweight adults into either 18 months of standard behavioral treatment (SBT) with an exercise goal of 1000 kcal·wk^{-1} or a high physical activity (HPA) group with an exercise goal of 2500 kcal·wk^{-1} in addition to the SBT. The HPA group achieved significantly greater exercise levels and weight loss than the SBT group at 12 and 18 months of follow-up. At 30 months, the average exercise levels were no longer different between the groups, nor did weight loss differ. Participants who reported continuing to engage in high levels of exercise maintained a significantly larger weight loss.

Even those who are extremely conscientious and restrained may suffer lapses. There seems, however, to be more to the problem than a lack of compliance. Will power may be counteracted by powerful internal signals that sense deviations in body weight and trigger compensatory mechanisms such as those discussed below (Dulloo, 2007; Major et al., 2007).

LIPOPROTEIN LIPASE One possible internal signal is lipoprotein lipase. Lipoprotein lipase is the enzyme responsible for fat synthesis and storage in adipose tissue. It has been theorized that lipoprotein lipase notifies the brain when fat cells have shrunk, as they would when the body is losing weight. In response, appetite increases and fat cells refill. In other words, "starving leads to stuffing." The appetite not only increases but also seems selectively predisposed to disproportionately increase the amount of fat ingested. Fat, of course, is calorically dense. Furthermore, after restrictive dieting, the body can more easily convert other excess food nutrients to fatty acids.

Previously or currently obese individuals seem to be more susceptible to the stimulus and response of

Weight Cycling Repeated bouts of weight loss and regain.

lipoprotein lipase. In these individuals, lipoprotein lipase activity may be twice as high as in nondieting individuals. That is the bad news. The good news is that when people who are not obese are put on a mildly or moderately restricted diet, the changes in lipoprotein lipase activity are minimal. It may be that a certain amount of weight (approximately 15% of total body weight) must be lost before lipoprotein lipase activity becomes a counterproductive factor (Gershoff, 1991, 1992; Nash, 1987; Schelkun, 1991).

GHRELIN AND LEPTIN Accumulating evidence suggests that leptin and more especially ghrelin may be involved in regaining weight. Leptin, an appetite-suppressing (anorexigenic) agent primarily secreted by adipose tissue, is part of a negative feedback loop regulating the size of energy stores and energy balance over the long term (2–4 days). The release of leptin signals satiety, decreases food intake, and increases energy expenditure, thereby inducing weight loss. Ghrelin is an appetite-stimulating (orexigenic) agent secreted primarily by endocrine cells in the gastrointestinal tract. Ghrelin is fast acting such that its levels increase before meals and decrease after meals and show additional daily variations (Kalra et al., 2005; Klok et al., 2007; Popovic and Duntas, 2005). Given the respective roles of leptin and ghrelin, it would be expected that in obese individuals leptin levels would be decreased and ghrelin levels increased. Precisely the opposite is true. Obese individuals exhibit high levels of leptin and low levels of ghrelin. Obese individuals seem to be leptin resistant—exhibiting high levels of leptin whose function is blocked. At the same time, obese individuals seem to be overly sensitive to ghrelin, and the decreased levels may represent a physiological adaptation to the positive energy balance of obesity (Huda et al., 2006; Klok et al., 2007).

When an individual loses weight, ghrelin levels increase. Conversely, ghrelin levels decrease when anorexia nervosa patients gain weight. These opposing responses suggest that ghrelin levels change in response to energy intake variations to maintain the current body weight. Increasing ghrelin, therefore, might be a compensation for weight loss, making maintenance of that loss difficult (Hansen et al., 2002; Klok et al., 2007; Leidy et al., 2007b; Romon et al., 2006). The good news is that the rise in ghrelin with weight loss may be transient and may eventually decrease with weight maintenance if that can be achieved. In a randomized clinical trial using diet, exercise, and the weight loss drug orlistat, a group of obese females lost 8.5% of their body weight in 6 months. They had the expected rise in ghrelin. However, when they maintained their weight loss for 6 months, their ghrelin levels returned to baseline (Garcia et al., 2006). Thus, ghrelin may be a counterregulatory mechanism in the short but not long term. In addition, a low-fat diet seems to have an inhibitory effect on ghrelin levels (Klok et al., 2007). Protein consumption results in ghrelin

suppression over a long period of time. Carbohydrate consumption results in an initial suppression of ghrelin more than protein, but then ghrelin rebounds to a higher than baseline level within hours (Foster-Schubert et al., 2008). Exercise training protocols that result in reduced fat mass are generally accompanied by lower leptin concentrations (Bouassida et al., 2010). Weight reduction is also associated with a condition of relative leptin insufficiency, which in turn may increase skeletal muscle work efficiency, thus reducing exercise energy expenditure (Rosenbaum et al., 2005).

ADAPTIVE DECREASES IN THERMOGENESIS An *adaptive decrease in* (or suppression of) *thermogenesis* indicates a change in the efficiency of energy utilization that results in a reduction of energy expenditure in any or all components of TEE including resting, TEF, and exercise expenditure. Experimental evidence is available to support these adaptive reductions (Major et al., 2007).

A residual reduction (adaptive decrease) in RMR is well documented. The impact on RMR is particularly important because it accounts for the highest percentage of daily energy expenditure. When data from 124 formerly obese and 121 control subjects were compared, it was determined that RMR adjusted for fat mass and fat-free mass was 2.9% lower in the formerly obese than the never obese. In addition, a larger percentage (15.3% versus 3.3%) of the formerly obese had a low RMR. When 12 studies were combined in a traditional meta-analysis, relative RMR was 5.1% lower in the formerly obese group than the control group. The authors concluded that the cause of the lower RMR remained unknown; however, the implication was clear. A low RMR is likely to contribute to the formerly obese individual's difficulty in maintaining a weight loss (Astrup et al., 1999; Doucet et al., 2001; Leibel et al., 1995).

As described earlier, the TEF depends on macronutrient and caloric content of the food ingested. When caloric input goes down in dieting, so does the TEF. Further, as was seen in the Focus on Research box, the TEM of a meal decreases with a reduction in body weight. In addition, the adaptive decrease in TEF may be linked to a change in food efficiency. **Food efficiency** is an index of the number of calories an individual needs to ingest to maintain a given weight or percent body fat and probably results from hormonal, neural, and enzyme actions. Food efficiency *increases* when the calories needed to sustain a certain weight (or percent fat) decrease. This response could be protective if food were scarce. Food efficiency *decreases* when the number of calories needed to sustain a certain weight (or percent fat) increases. Being able to eat more to maintain a given weight is what every dieter would like to have happen, but which does not happen (Brodie, 1988).

For example, in one study, a group of obese individuals lost an average of 52 kg (114.4 lb) but remained

60% overweight (39 kg or 85.8 lb, excess) compared with a normal-weight control group. The daily caloric needs (2171 kcal·d⁻¹) of the reduced-weight obese individuals to maintain their weight were found to be 25% lower than the values estimated from their body size and almost 5% lower than the values needed by much lighter normal-weight controls (2280 kcal·d⁻¹) (Leibel and Hirsch, 1984). Their food efficiency had increased.

Finally, an adaptive decrease in exercise energy expenditure has also been documented (Major et al., 2007). Several studies involving dietary and activity analysis indicate that some female distance runners ingest only between 1400 and 1990 kcal·d⁻¹ while training as much as 65 mi·wk⁻¹. These caloric intake values are much lower than those for comparably sized, inactive females of the same age (Brownell et al., 1987). Similar discrepancies have been shown in obese adult males walking on the treadmill (Doucet et al., 2003).

Making Weight for Sport

Although athletes in many sports are concerned with maintaining a low body weight and/or a low percent body fat, only a few sports organize the competition around weight classes. The original intention was to make the competitions as fair as possible by matching individuals of approximately the same size. However, in practice, many participants manipulate their body weight to drop down to a lower-weight class on the assumption that they will then have an advantage over their opponents. One wonders, however, what possible advantage there can be when both competitors are following the same strategy (although each athlete will always think he or she can drop down more than his or her opponent) and, more importantly, the health and performance implications are ignored. Despite these concerns, dropping into a lower-weight class is routinely done, often by individuals in their growth years. Boxers, wrestlers, rowers, and jockeys all engage in making weight, but by far, most research attention involves wrestlers (**Figure 8.15**).

The American College of Sports Medicine (1996) has published several versions of the "Position Stand on Weight Loss in Wrestlers," the latest in 1996. The techniques typically used by wrestlers and the physiological consequences were detailed in the 1976 version, as well as suggestions for "making weight" in a healthier manner. Unfortunately, these early recommendations appear to have had little impact on the patterns of weight loss and regain in wrestlers. In 1997 in one 5-week period, three collegiate wrestlers died from complications caused

> **Food Efficiency** An index of the number of calories an individual needs to ingest to maintain a given weight or percent body fat.

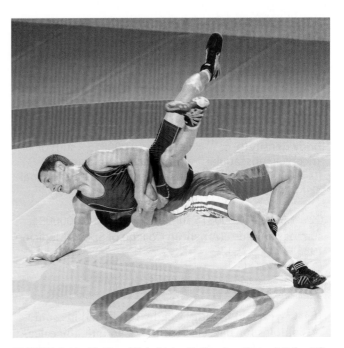

FIGURE 8.15 Making Weight by Following Sound Scientific Guidelines Should Be an Important Goal for Wrestlers at All Levels of Competition.

by rapid weight loss (Centers for Disease Control and Prevention, 1998). These tragedies brought about rule changes from the NCAA (and adopted by many high school associations) that included adding 7 lb to each weight class, moving weigh-ins to 1 hour before the competition; requiring preseason assessment of body composition, hydration, and weight by a member of the school's athletic medical staff; a minimal weight for each wrestler; and regulation of weight loss/gain. The raw data from the preseason assessments are entered into the online National Wrestling Coaches Association Optimal Performance Calculator. An ideal minimal competition weight and a safe weight loss/gain plan are established, and athletes are assigned to daily nutrient goals based on their weight loss/gain plan. This plan mandates that a wrestler may not lose more than 1.5% of body weight per week while descending to the lowest certified weight class. The ACSM guidelines of not less than 7% BF for male competitors younger than 16 years and not less than 5% BF for males 16 years or older are part of this mandated plan. Female wrestlers are required to have a minimum of 12–14% BF. Total body weight loss cannot exceed 7%. The use of laxatives, emetics, excessive fluid and food restriction, self-induced vomiting, hot environments (including practice rooms of >80°F), saunas, steam rooms, diuretics, vapor-impermeable suits, and intravenous rehydration are prohibited (National Collegiate Athletic Association, 2007). Hydrostatic (underwater) weighing, displacement plethysmography (Bod Pod), and skinfolds using the Lohman (1981) equation are approved by the NCAA. Several high school associations allow bioelectrical impedance analysis (BIA) as well, although BIA has been shown to have a high prediction error in wrestlers and research indicates that skinfolds and BIA body composition values cannot be used interchangeably (Clark et al., 2002, 2005).

The Lohman skinfold equation is as follows:

body density $(g \cdot cc^{-1}) = 1.0982 - \{[0.000815 \times$ sum of triceps + subscapular + abdominal skinfolds (mm)] + $[0.0000084 \times$ sum of triceps + subscapular + abdominal skinfolds squared (mm)]$\}$

$D_B = 1.0982 - (0.000815$ sum of skinfolds $+ 0.0000084$ sum of skinfolds^2)(American College of Sports Medicine, 1983)

EXAMPLE

If a 17-year-old wrestler weighs 165 lb and his sum of skinfolds for the selected sites is 46 mm, the calculation would be

$$D_B = 1.0982 - [0.000815 (46) + 0.0000084 (2116)]$$
$$= 1.0429 g \cdot cc^{-1}$$

The D_B value is then substituted into the age-appropriate formula presented in Table 7.1 in Chapter 7 for a male adolescent to determine %BF. For a 17-year-old this is

$$\%BF = \left[\frac{5.03}{D_B} - 4.59\right] \times 100 = 23.31$$

Equations 7.4, 7.5, and 7.6 are then used to determine the wrestler's most appropriate competitive weight. Using Equation 7.4,

$$FFW = 165\,lb \times \left[\frac{100\% - 23.3\%}{100}\right] = 126.6\,lb$$

Using Equation 7.5,

$$WT_2 = \left[\frac{100 \times 126.6}{100\% - 16.3\%}\right] = 151.3\,lb$$

Note: 16% is used here as the desirable %BF, not 5%, which is the lowest recommended %BF for a wrestler of this age. The 16.3% complies with the recommendation that weight loss not exceed 7% of body weight.

To get down to 5% BF, this wrestler would need to lose 18.3% of his body weight, and that is too much. Using Equation 7.6,

$$151.3\,lb - 165\,lb = -13.7\,lb$$

To achieve his recommended body weight, this wrestler needs to lose 13.7 lb.

Complete the problem in the Check Your Comprehension 2 box.

Specific guidelines for making weight have not been established for other sports, but the principles discussed here can and should be applied.

CHECK YOUR COMPREHENSION 2

Calculate the weight at which the following 14-year-old wrestler should compete.

Name: Zachary   Triceps skinfold: 8 mm
Weight: 138 lb   Subscapular skinfold: 9 mm
                  Abdominal skinfold: 12 mm

How much weight does Zachary need to gain or lose to achieve this weight?
Check your answer in Appendix C.

Several studies have investigated compliance with the new regulations. A 1999 survey of 43 collegiate teams (Oppliger et al., 2003) found that the most weight lost during the season was 6.9% of body weight, but average weekly weight loss was 4.3%. Although 40.2% indicated that the then-new NCAA rules deterred extreme weight loss behaviors, approximately 55% fasted, approximately 28% used saunas, and approximately 27% used vapor-barrier suits at least once a month. Overall, however, compared to college wrestlers in the 1980s, weight behavior was less extreme. A follow-up study (Oppliger et al., 2006) of 811 competitors in Division I, II, and III national championship tournaments from 1999 to 2004 showed that weight and %BF decreased from preseason to postseason competition. However, the preseason certified minimum weight remained unchanged (68.0 ± 9.2 kg versus 67.9 ± 9.1 kg), thus showing good agreement between the preseason recommendations and the actual end-of-season weights. Rapid weight loss before weigh-in was found to be statistically significant but small (~1.7% of body weight). The average wrestlers at the tournaments were competing at 9.5% BF, down from the preseason average of 12.3 ± 3.4%, but well above the minimum of 5%. The investigators concluded that the NCAA weight management program appears to be effective in reducing unhealthy weight-cutting behaviors (although the wrestlers were not asked how they achieved weight goals) and promoting competitive equity.

This is an example of very successful cooperation between science and sport for the benefit of the participants, but it needs to be extended to all levels and types of wrestling and modified appropriately for use in all weight-category sports.

SUMMARY

1. Weight gain, loss, and stabilization follow the First Law of Thermodynamics as expressed in the caloric balance equation. The components of this equation are food ingestion (+), resting or basal metabolic rate (−), thermogenesis (−), and exercise (−).

2. Diet, acute exercise, and exercise training can have an impact on the components of the caloric balance equation.

3. The goal of weight or fat control should be to lose body fat (especially visceral abdominal fat), to preserve fat-free weight (FFW), to maintain or improve health, and for athletes to maintain or improve performance.

4. Twenty-eight percent of the total weight lost by diet alone is FFW, and 72% is fat; 20% of the total weight loss by diet plus exercise is FFW, and 80% is fat; only 4.5% of the weight lost by exercise alone is FFW, and 95.5% is fat. Thus, exercise helps to preserve FFW during times of caloric deficit.

5. A combination of diet plus exercise is the preferred technique for body composition and body weight control both to accomplish an initial loss and to maintain a weight loss.

6. The exercise training component of weight and fat control should include both an aerobic endurance portion (to expend 1200–2000 kcal·wk⁻¹) and a resistance weight training portion (to maintain and/or build FFW).

7. Although there is no definite answer as to why the maintenance of weight loss is so difficult, current interest is centered on compliance, lipoprotein lipase, ghrelin and leptin, and adaptive decreases in thermogenesis.

8. Proper weight for all sports should be determined based on %BF and safe weight loss procedures.

REVIEW QUESTIONS

1. State the caloric balance equation, and relate it to the First Law of Thermodynamics. Define and explain the components of the caloric balance equation.

2. Discuss the impact of dietary restriction on the components of the caloric balance equation.

3. Discuss the impact of exercise on the components of the caloric balance equation.

4. Discuss the impact of exercise training on the components of the caloric balance equation.

5. Compare and contrast the effects of diet alone, exercise training alone, and diet and exercise training combined on body weight and composition control.

6. List and explain how each of the training principles should be specifically applied for body weight or body composition control or maintenance.

7. Defend or refute the following statements, using evidence provided in this chapter.
   a. Weight cycling makes subsequent weight loss physiologically more difficult.
   b. The most important reason to add exercise or exercise training to a weight loss or maintenance program is that exercise decreases appetite.
   c. If food is eaten near the time of exercise (either directly before or after), the thermic response is potentiated (made more effective) so that more calories are burned and weight is lost faster.
   d. The maintenance of, increase in, or decrease in resting metabolic rate depends on the maintenance or change in lean body mass.
   e. To lose fat, burn fat by doing long-duration, low-intensity exercise.

8. Describe the possible roles of compliance, lipoprotein lipase, ghrelin and leptin, and adaptive decreases in thermogenesis on the maintenance of weight loss.

9. Prepare a set of weight control guidelines for a jockey.

For further review and additional study tools, visit the website at http://thePoint.lww.com/Plowman4e ✳ ◯

REFERENCES

Acheson, K. J., E. Ravussin, J. Wahren, & E. Jéquier: Thermic effect of glucose in man. Obligatory and facultative thermogenesis. *Journal of Clinical Investigation.* 74:1572–1580 (1984).

American College of Sports Medicine: Proper and improper weight loss programs. *Medicine and Science in Sports and Exercise.* 15:xi–xiii (1983).

American College of Sports Medicine: Position stand on weight loss in wrestlers. *Medicine and Science in Sports.* 28(2):ix–xii (1996).

American College of Sports Medicine: *ACSM's Guidelines for Exercise Testing and Prescription* (6th edition). Philadelphia, PA: Lippincott Williams & Wilkins (2000).

American College of Sports Medicine: Appropriate intervention strategies for weight loss and prevention of weight regain for adults. *Medicine & Science in Sports & Exercise.* 33(12):2145–2156 (2001).

American College of Sports Medicine: Position stand: Exercise and fluid replacement. *Medicine & Science in Exercise & Sports.* 39(2):377–390 (2007).

American College of Sports Medicine: Appropriate physical activity intervention strategies for weight loss and prevention of weight regain for adults. *Medicine & Science in Sports & Exercise.* 41(2):459–471 (2009).

Anastasiou, C. A., M. Yannakoulia, V. Pirogianni, G. Rapti, L. S. Sidossis, & S. A. Kavouras: Fitness and weight cycling in relation to body fat and insulin sensitivity in normal-weight young women. *Journal of the American Dietetic Association.* 110:280–284 (2010).

Apfelbaum, M., J. Bostarron, & D. Lacatis: Effect of caloric restriction and excessive caloric intake on energy expenditure. *American Journal of Clinical Nutrition.* 24:1405–1409 (1971).

Astrup, A., P. C. Gotzsche, K. vandeWerken, C. Ranneries, S. Toubro, A. Raben, & B. Buemann: Meta-analysis of resting metabolic rate in formerly obese subjects. *American Journal of Clinical Nutrition.* 69:1117–1122 (1999).

Astrup, A., T. Meinert-Larsen, A. Harper: Atkins and other low-carbohydrate diets: Hoax or an effective tool for weight loss? *Lancet.* 364:897–899 (2004).

Atlantis, E., E. H. Barnes, & M. A. Singh: Efficacy of exercise for treating overweight in children and adolescents: A systematic review. *International Journal of Obesity.* 30(7):1027–1040 (2006).

Balaguera-Cortes, L., K. E. Wallman, T. J. Fairchild, & K. J. Guelfi: Energy intake and appetite-related hormones following acute aerobic and resistance exercise. *Applied Physiology Nutrition and Metabolism.* 36(6):958–966 (2011).

Ballor, D. L., V. L. Katch, M. D. Becque, & C. R. Marks: Resistance weight training during caloric restriction enhances lean body weight maintenance. *American Journal of Clinical Nutrition.* 47:19–25 (1988).

Ballor, D. L., J. P. McCarthy, & E. J. Wilterdink: Exercise intensity does not affect the composition of diet- and exercise-induced body mass loss. *American Journal of Clinical Nutrition.* 51:142–146 (1990).

Barlow, S. E. & W. H. Dietz: Obesity evaluation and treatment: Expert Committee Recommendations. *Pediatrics.* 120:S164–S192 (2007) http://www.periatrics.org/cgi/content/full/102/3/e29. Accessed 12/12/2007.

Beeson, V., C. Ray, R. A. Coxon, & S. Kreitzman: The myth of the yo-yo: Consistent rate of weight loss with successive dieting by VLCD. *International Journal of Obesity.* 13:135–139 (1989).

Belko, A. Z., T. F. Barbier, & E. C. Wong: Effect of energy and protein intake and exercise intensity on the thermic effect of food. *American Journal of Clinical Nutrition.* 43:863–869 (1986).

Bingham, S. A., G. R. Goldberg, W. A. Coward, A. M. Prentice, & J. H. Cummings: The effect of exercise and improved physical fitness on basal metabolic rate. *British Journal of Nutrition.* 61:155–173 (1989).

Blackburn, G. L., G. T. Wilson, B. S. Kanders, et al.: Weight cycling: The experience of human dieters. *American Journal of Clinical Nutrition.* 49:1105–1109 (1989).

Blanchard, M. S.: Thermogenesis and its relationship to obesity and exercise. *Quest.* 34(2):143–153 (1982).

Blundell, J. E. & N. A. King: Physical activity and regulation of food intake: Current evidence. *Medicine & Science in Sports & Exercise.* 31(Suppl. 11):S573–S583 (1999).

Blundell, J. E., R. J. Stubbs, D. A. Hughes, S. Whybrow, & N. A. King: Cross talk between physical activity and appetite control: Does physical activity stimulate appetite? *Proceedings of the Nutrition Society.* 62(3):651–661 (2003).

Bogert, L. J., G. M. Briggs, & D. H. Calloway: *Nutrition and Physical Fitness* (9th edition). Philadelphia, PA: W. B. Saunders (1973).

Boileau, R. A., T. G. Lohman, & M. H. Slaughter: Exercise and body composition in children and youth. *Scandinavian Journal of Sport Sciences.* 7:17–27 (1985).

Bouassida, A., K. Chamari, M. Zaouali, Y. Feki, A. Zbidi, & Z. Tabka: Review of leptin and adiponectin responses and adaptations to acute and chronic exercise. *British Journal of Sports Medicine.* 44:620–630 (2010).

Bouchard, C. T., et al.: Fournier: Long-term exercise training with constant energy intake. 1. Effect on body composition. *International Journal of Obesity.* 14:57–73 (1990).

Bray, G. A.: Effect of caloric restriction on energy expenditure in obese patients. *Lancet.* 2:397–398 (1969).

Brodie, D. A.: Techniques of measurement of body composition: Part I. *Sports Medicine.* 5:11–40 (1988).

Brown, M. R., W. J. Klish, J. Hollander, M. A. Campbell, & G. B. Forbes: A high protein, low calorie liquid diet in the treatment of very obese adolescents: Long-term effect on lean body mass. *The American Journal of Clinical Nutrition.* 38:20–31 (1983).

Brownell, K. D., S. N. Steen, & J. H. Wilmore: Weight regulation practices in athletes: Analysis of metabolic and health effects. *Medicine and Science in Sports and Exercise.* 19(6):546–556 (1987).

Bullough, R. C., C. A. Gillette, M. A. Harris, & C. L. Melby: Interaction of acute changes in exercise energy expenditure and energy intake on resting metabolic rate. *American Journal of Clinical Nutrition.* 61:473–481 (1995).

Burszstein, S. E., D. H. Elwyn, J. Askanazi, & J. M. Kinney: *Energy Metabolism, Indirect Calorimetry and Nutrition.* Baltimore, MD: Lippincott Williams & Wilkins (1989).

Byrne, H. K. & J. H. Wilmore: The effects of a 20-week exercise training program on resting metabolic rate in previously sedentary, moderately obese women. *International Journal of Sports Nutrition and Exercise Metabolism.* 11:15–31 (2001).

Centers for Disease Control and Prevention: Hyperthermia and dehydration-related deaths associated with intentional rapid weight loss in three collegiate wrestlers-North Carolina, Wisconsin, and Michigan, November-December 1997. *JAMA.* 279:824–825 (1998).

Clark, R. R., C. Bartok, J. C. Sullivan, & D. E. Schoeller: Is leg-to-leg BIA valid for predicting minimum weight in wrestlers. *Medicine & Science in Sports & Exercise.* 37(6):1061–1068 (2005).

Clark, R. R., R. A. Oppliger, & J. C. Sullivan: Cross-validation of the NCAA method to predict body fat for minimum weight in collegiate wrestlers. *Clinical Journal of Sports Medicine.* 12(5):285–290 (2002).

Cypess, A. M., S. Lehman, G. Williams, I. Tal, D. Rodman, A. B. Goldfine, et al.: Identification and importance of brown adipose tissue in adult humans. *New England Journal of Medicine.* 360:1509–1517 (2009).

Dallasso, H. M. & W. P. James: Whole-body calorimetry studies in adult men. 2. The interaction of exercise and over-feeding on the thermic effect of a meal. *British Journal of Nutrition.* 52:65–72 (1984).

Dansinger, M. L., J. A. Gleason, J. L. Griffith, H. P. Selker, & E. J. Schaefer: Comparison of the Atkins, Ornish, Weight Watchers, and Zone diets for weight loss and heart disease risk reduction: A randomized trial. *The Journal of the American Medical Association.* 293(1):43–53 (2005).

Das, S. K., C. H. Gilhooly, J. K. Golden, et al.: Long-term effects of 2 energy-restricted diets differing in glycemic load on dietary adherence, body composition, and metabolism in CALERIE: A 1-y randomized controlled trial. *American Journal of Clinical Nutrition.* 85(4):1023–1030 (2007).

Davis, J. R., A. R. Tagliaferro, R. Kertzner, T. Gerardo, J. Nichols, & J. Wheeler: Variations in dietary-induced thermogenesis and body fatness with aerobic capacity. *European Journal of Applied Physiology.* 50:319–329 (1983).

Denzer, C. M. & J. C. Young: The effect of resistance exercise on the thermic effect of food. *International Journal of Sport Nutrition and Exercise Metabolism.* 13(3):396–402 (2003).

Despres, J. P., C. Bouchard, A. Tremblay, R. Savard, & M. Marcotte: Effects of aerobic training on fat distribution in male subjects. *Medicine and Science in Sports and Exercise.* 17(1):113–118 (1985).

Diaz, V. A., A. G. Mainous, C. J. Everett: The association between weight fluctuation and mortality: Results from a population-based cohort study. *Journal of Community Health.* 30(3):153–165 (2005).

Dietary Guidelines for Americans: http://www.health.gov/dietary guidelines/dga2005. Accessed 9/03/2007 (2005).

Donnelly, J. E., J. Jakicic, & S. Gunderson: Diet and body composition: Effect of very low calorie diets and exercise. *Sports Medicine.* 12(4):237–249 (1991).

Doucet, E., P. Imbeault, S. St. Pierre, et al.: Greater than predicted decrease in energy expenditure during exercise after body weight loss in obese men. *Clinical Science.* 105:89–95 (2003).

Doucet, E., S. St. Pierre, N. Almeras, J. P. Despres, C. Bouchard, & A. Tremblay: Evidence for the existence of adaptive thermogenesis during weight loss. *British Journal of Nutrition.* 85:715–723 (2001).

Dulloo, A. G.: Suppressed thermogenesis as a cause for resistance to slimming and obesity rebound: Adaptation or illusion? *International Journal of Obesity.* 31:201–203 (2007).

Dulloo, A. G., J. Seydoux, & J. Jacquet: Adaptive thermogenesis and uncoupling proteins: A reappraisal of their role in fat metabolism and energy balance. *Physiology and Behavior.* 83:587–602 (2004).

Epstein, L. H. & G. S. Goldfield: Physical activity in the treatment of childhood overweight and obesity: Current evidence and research issues. *Medicine & Science in Sports & Exercise.* 31(Suppl. 11):S553–S559 (1999).

Erlanson-Albertsson, C.: The role of uncoupling proteins in the regulation of metabolism. *Acta Physiologica Scandinavica.* 178(4):405–412 (2003).

Erlichman, J., A. L. Kerbey, & W. P. T. James: Physical activity and its impact on health outcomes. Paper 2: Prevention of unhealthy weight gain and obesity by physical activity: An analysis of the evidence. *Obesity reviews.* 3:273–287 (2002).

Field, A. E., J. E. Manson, C. B. Taylor, W. C. Willett, & G. A. Colditz: Association of weight change, weight control practices, and weight cycling among women in the Nurses' Health Study II. *International Journal of Obesity.* 28:1134–1142 (2004).

Foster-Schubert, K. E., J. Overduin, C. E. Prudom, et al.: Acyl and total ghrelin are suppressed strongly by ingested proteins, weakly by lipids, and biphasically by carbohydrates. *The Journal of Clinical Endocrinology and Metabolism.* 93:1971–1979 (2008); Online rapid release: http://jcem.endojournals.org/cgi/ Accessed 1/31/2008.

Garcia, J. M., D. Iyer, W. S. Poston, M. Marcelli, R. Reeves, J. Foreyt, & A. Balasubramanyam: Rise of plasma ghrelin with weight loss is not sustained during weight maintenance. *Obesity.* 14:1716–1723 (2006).

Garrow, J. S.: Energy balance in man: An overview. *American Journal of Clinical Nutrition.* 45:1114–1119 (1987).

Garrow, J. S. & C. D. Summerbell: Meta-analysis: Effect of exercise, with or without dieting, on the body composition of overweight subjects. *European Journal of Clinical Nutrition.* 49(1):1–10 (1995).

Gershoff, S. N. (ed.): Ask the experts. *Tufts University Diet and Nutrition Letter.* 9(7):8 (1991).

Gershoff, S. N. (ed.): Ask the experts. *Tufts University Diet and Nutrition Letter.* 9(11):7 (1992).

Gilbert, J. A., J. E. Misner, R. A. Boileau, L. Ji, & M. H. Slaughter: Lower thermic effect of a meal post-exercise in aerobically trained and resistance-trained subjects. *Medicine and Science in Sports and Exercise.* 23(7):825–830 (1991).

Graci, S., G. Izzo, S. Savino, et al.: Weight cycling and cardiovascular risk factors in obesity. *International Journal of Obesity.* 28:65–71 (2004).

Grande, F. A., J. T. Anderson, & A. Keys: Changes of basal metabolic rate in man in semistarvation and refeeding. *Journal of Applied Physiology.* 12(2):230–238 (1958a).

Grande, F. T., H. L. Taylor, J. T. Anderson, E. Buskirk, & A. Keys: Water exchange in men on a restricted water intake and a low calorie carbohydrate diet accompanied by physical work. *Journal of Applied Physiology.* 12(2):202–210 (1958b).

Guyton, A. C. & J. E. Hall: *Textbook of Medical Physiology* (12th edition). Philadelphia, PA: W. B. Saunders (2011).

Hagan, R. D.: Benefits of aerobic conditioning and diet for overweight adults. *Sports Medicine.* 5:144–155 (1988).

Hagan, R. D., S. J. Upton, L. Wong, & J. Whittam: The effects of aerobic conditioning and/or calorie restriction in overweight men and women. *Medicine and Science in Sports and Exercise.* 18(1):87–94 (1986).

Hagobian, T. A. & B. Braun: Physical activity and hormonal regulation of appetite: Sex differences and weight control. *Exercise and Sport Sciences Reviews.* 38(1):25–30 (2010).

Hansen, T. K., R. Dall, H. Hosoda, M. Kojima, K. Kangawa, J. S. Christiansen, & J. O. L. Jergensen: Weight loss increases circulating levels of ghrelin in human obesity. *Clinical Endocrinology.* 56:203–206 (2002).

Hansen, D., P. Dendale, J. Berger, L. J. C. van Loon, & R. Meeusen: The effects of exercise training on fat-mass loss in obese patients during energy intake restriction. *Sports Medicine.* 37(1):34–46 (2007).

Harris, R. B. S.: Role of set-point theory in regulation of body weight. *FASEB Journal.* 4:3310–3318 (1990).

Haskell, W. L., I.-M. Lee, R. R. Pate, et al.: Physical activity and public health: Updated recommendation for adults from the American College of Sports Medicine and the American Heart Association. *Medicine & Science in Sports & Exercise.* 39(8):1423–1434 (2007).

Heymsfield, S. B., K. Casper, J. Hearn, & D. Guy: Rate of weight loss during underfeeding: Relation to level of physical activity. *Metabolism.* 38(3):215–233 (1989).

Hill, J. O., S. B. Heymesfield, C. McMannus III, & M. DeGirolamo: Meal size and thermic response to food in male subjects as a function of maximum aerobic capacity. *Metabolism.* 33:743–749 (1984).

Himms-Hagen, J.: Thermogenesis in brown adipose tissue as an energy buffer. *The New England Journal of Medicine.* 311(24):1549–1558 (1984).

Horton, E. S.: Metabolic aspects of exercise and weight reduction. *Medicine and Science in Sports and Exercise.* 18(1):10–18 (1985).

Huda, M. S., J. P. Wilding, & J. H. Pinkney: Gut peptides and the regulation of appetite. *Obesity Reviews.* 7(2):163–182 (2006).

Institute of Medicine: *Dietary Reference Intake for Energy, Carbohydrate, Fiber, Fat, Fatty Acids, Cholesterol, Protein and Amino Acids.* Washington, DC: National Academy Press (2002).

Jeffery, R. W., R. R. Wing, & S. A. French: Weight cycling and cardiovascular risk factors in obese men and women. *American Journal of Clinical Nutrition.* 55:641–644 (1992).

Jequier, E.: Energy, obesity, and body weight standards. *The American Journal of Clinical Nutrition.* 45:1035–1047 (1987).

Jequier, E.: Pathways to obesity. *International Journal of Obesity Related Metabolic Disorders.* 26 (Suppl. 2):S12–17 (2002).

Jokisch, E., A. Coletta, H. A. Raynor: Acute energy compensation and macronutrient intake following exercise in active and inactive males who are normal weight. *Appetite.* 58(2):722–729 (2012).

Kalra, S. P., N. Ueno, & P. S. Kalra: Stimulation of appetite by ghrelin is regulated by leptin restraint: Peripheral and central sites of action. *Journal of Nutrition.* 135(5):1331–1335 (2005).

Katch, F. I., P. M. Clarkson, W. Kroll, T. McBride, & A. Wilcox: Effects of sit-up exercise training on adipose cell size and adiposity. *Research Quarterly for Exercise and Sport.* 55(3):242–247 (1984).

Kay, S. J. & M. A. Fiatarone Singh: The influence of physical activity on abdominal fat: A systematic review of the literature. *Obesity Reviews.* 7:183–200 (2006).

Kimm, S. Y. S., N. W. Glynn, E. Obarzanek, et al.: Relation between the changes in physical activity and body-mass index during adolescence: A multicentre longitudinal study. *Lancet.* 366:301–307 (2005).

Klok, M. D., S. Jakobsdottis, & M. L. Drent: The role of leptin and ghrelin in the regulation of food intake and body weight in humans: A review. *Obesity Reviews.* 8(1):21–34, 2007.

Laan, D. J., H. J. Leidy, E. Lim, & W. W. Campbell: Effects and reproducibility of aerobic and resistance exercise on appetite and energy intake in young, physically active adults. *Applied Physiology, Nutrition, and Metabolism.* 35:842–847 (2010).

Layman, D. K.: Protein quantity and quality at levels above the RDA improves adult weight loss. *Journal of the American College of Nutrition.* 23(6):631S–636S (2004).

LeBlanc, J., P. Diamond, J. Côté, & A. Labrie: Hormonal factors in reduced postprandial heat production of exercise-trained subjects. *Journal of Applied Physiology.* 56:772–776 (1984a).

LeBlanc, J., P. Mercier, & P. Samson: Diet-induced thermogenesis with relation to training state in female subjects. *Canadian Journal of Physiology and Pharmacology.* 62:334–337 (1984b).

Lee, M.-G., D. A. Sedlock, M. G. Flynn, & G. H. Kamimori: Resting metabolic rate after endurance exercise training. *Medicine & Science in Sports & Exercise.* 41(7):1444–1451 (2009).

Leibel, R. L. & J. Hirsch: Diminished energy requirements in reduced-obese patients. *Metabolism.* 33(2):164–170 (1984).

Leibel, R. L., M. Rosenbaum, & J. Hirsch: Changes in energy expenditure resulting from altering body weight. *The New England Journal of Medicine.* 332:621–628 (1995).

Leidy, H. J., N. S. Carnell, R. D. Mattes, W. W. Campbell: Higher protein intake preserves lean mass and satiety with weight loss in pre-obese and obese women. *Obesity.* 15(2):421–429 (2007a).

Leidy, H. J., K. A. Dougherty, B. R. Frye, K. M. Duke, & N. I. Williams: Twenty-four-hour ghrelin is elevated after calorie restriction and exercise training in non-obese women. *Obesity.* 15(2):446–455 (2007b).

Lemmer, J. T., F. M. Ivey, A. S. Ryan, et al.: Effect of strength training on resting metabolic rate and physical activity: Age and gender comparisons. *Medicine & Science in Sports & Exercise.* 33(4):532–541 (2001).

Lohman, T. G.: Skinfolds and body density and their relation to body fatness: A review. *Human Biology.* 53(2):181–225 (1981).

Lundholm, K., G. Holm, L. Lindmark, B. Larsson, L. Sjostrom, & P. Bjorntorp. Thermogenic effect of food in physically well-trained elderly men. *European Journal of Applied Physiology.* 55:486–492 (1986).

Luscombe-Marsh, N. D., M. Noakes, G. A. Wittert, J. B. Keogh, P. Foster, & P. M. Clifton: Carbohydrate-restricted diets high in either monounsaturated fat or protein are equally effective at promoting fat loss and improving blood lipids. *American Journal of Clinical Nutrition.* 81:762–772 (2005).

Macias, A. E.: Experimental demonstration of human weight homeostasis: Implication for understanding obesity. *British Journal of Nutrition.* 91(3):479–484 (2004).

Major, G. C., E. Doucet, P. Trayhurn, A. Astrup, & A. Tremblay: Clinical significance of adaptive thermogenesis. *International Journal of Obesity* 31:204–212 (2007).

Manthou, E., J. M. R. Gill, A. Wright, D. Malkova: Behavioral compensatory adjustments to exercise training in overweight women. *Medicine & Science in Sports & Exercise.* 42(6): 1221–1228 (2010).

Maraki, M., F. Tsofliou, Y. P. Pitsiladis, D. Malkova, N. Mutrie, & S. Higgins: Acute effects of a single exercise class on appetite, energy intake and mod. Is there a time of day effect? *Appetite.* 45(3):272–278 (2005).

Martins, C., L. M. Morgan, S. R. Bloom, & M. D. Robertson: Effects of exercise on gut peptides, energy intake and appetite. *Journal of Endocrinology.* 193(2):251–258 (2007).

Mason, C., L. Xiao, I. Imayama, A. Kong, K. Foster-Schubert, C. R. Duggan, et al.: Influence of past weight cycling on weight loss and physiological changes during a 12-month randomized controlled trial of diet and/or exercise in overweight post-menopausal women. *Obesity.* 18 (Suppl. 2): S228 (2010) (abstract).

McTigue, K. M., R. Hess, & J. Ziouras: Obesity in older adults: A systematic review of the evidence for diagnosis and treatment. *Obesity.* 14(9):1485–1497 (2006).

Meckling, K. A. & R. Sherfey: A randomized trial of a hypocaloric high-protein diet, with and without exercise, on weight loss, fitness, and markers of the Metabolic Syndrome in overweight and obese women. *Applied Physiology of Nutrition and Metabolism.* 32(4):743–752 (2007).

Melby, C., C. Scholl, G. Edwards, & R. Bullough: Effect of acute resistance exercise on postexercise energy expenditure and resting metabolic rate. *Journal of Applied Physiology.* 75(4):1847–1853 (1993).

Mole, P. A., J. S. Stern, C. L. Schultz, E. M. Bernauer, & B. J. Holcomb: Exercise reverses depressed metabolic rate produced by severe caloric restriction. *Medicine and Science in Sports and Exercise.* 21(1):29–33 (1989).

Montani, J-P., A. K. Viecwlli, A. Prévot, & A. G. Dulloo: Weight cycling during growth and beyond as a risk factor for later cardiovascular diseases: The 'repeated overshoot' theory. *International Journal of Obesity.* 30:S58–S66 (2006).

Moore, M. S., C. J. Dodd, J. R. Welsman, & N. Armstrong: Short-term appetite and energy intake following imposed exercise in 9- to 10-year-old girls. *Appetite.* 43(2):127–134 (2004).

Mozo, J., Y. Emre, F. Bouillaud, D. Ricquier, & F. Criscuolo: Thermoregulation: What role for UCPs in mammals and birds? *Bioscience Reports*. 25(3–4): 227–249 (2005).

Nash, J. D.: Eating behavior and body weight: Physiological influences. *American Journal of Health Promotion*. 1(3):5–15 (1987).

National Collegiate Athletic Association: *NCAA Wrestling Rules and Interpretations*. Indianapolis, IN: NCAA, WR-27-WR-35 (2007).

National Task Force on the Prevention and Treatment of Obesity: Weight cycling. *Journal of the American Medical Association*. 272(15):1196–1202 (1994).

Nedergaard, J. & B. Cannon: The changed metabolic world with human brown adipose tissue: therapeutic visions. *Cell Metabolism*. 11:268–272 (2010).

Newsholme, E. A.: A possible metabolic basis for the control of body weight. *New England Journal of Medicine*. 302(7):400–405 (1980).

Nieman, D. C.: *Fitness and Sports Medicine: An Introduction*. Palo Alto, CA: Bull Publishing (1990).

Nieman, D. C., J. L. Haig, E. D. DeGuis, G. P. Dizon, & U. D. Register: Reducing diet and exercise training effects on resting metabolic rates in mildly obese women. *Journal of Sports Medicine and Physical Fitness*. 28(1):79–88 (1988).

Noland, M. & J. T. Kearney: Anthropometric and densitometric responses of women to specific and general exercise. *Research Quarterly*. 49(3):322–328 (1978).

Ohkawara, K., S. Tanaka, M. Miyachi, K. Ishikawa-Takata, & I. Tabata: A dose-response relation between aerobic exercise and visceral fat reduction: Systematic review of clinical trials. *International Journal of Obesity*. 31:1786–1797 (2007).

Olson, M. B., S. F. Kelsey, V. Bittner, S. E. Reis, N. Reichek, E. M. Handberg, et al.: Weight cycling and high-density lipoprotein cholesterol in women: Evidence of an adverse effect: A Report from the NHLBI-sponsored WISE Study. *Journal of the American College of Cardiology*. 36(5):1565–1571 (2000).

Oppliger, R. A., S. A. Steen, & J. R. Scott: Weight loss practices of college wrestlers. *International Journal of Sport Nutrition and Exercise Metabolism*. 13(1):29–46 (2003).

Oppliger, R. A., A. C. Utter, J. R. Scott, R. W. Dick, & D. Klossner: NCAA rule change improves weight loss among national championship wrestlers. *Medicine & Science in Sports & Exercise*. 38(5):963–970 (2006).

Ortega, F. B., J. R. Ruiz, A. Hurtiz-Wennlöf, G. Vincente-Rodríguez, N. S. Rizzo, M. J. Castillo, & M. Sjöström: Cardiovascular fitness modifies the associations between physical activity and abdominal adiposity in children and adolescents: The European Youth Heart Study. *British Journal of Sports Medicine*. 44:256–262 (2010).

Ortega, F. B., J. R. Ruiz, & M. Sjöström: Physical activity, over-weight and central adiposity in Swedish children and adoles-cents: the European Youth Heart Study. *International Journal of Behavioral Nutrition and Physical Activity*. 4:61 (2007).

Owen, O. E., E. Kavle, R. S. Owen, et al.: A reappraisal of caloric requirements in healthy women. *American Journal of Clinical Nutrition*. 44(1):1–19 (1986).

Owens, S., B. Gutin, J. Allison, S. Riggs, M. Ferguson, M. Litaker, & W. Thompson: Effect of physical training on total and visceral fat in obese children. *Medicine & Science in Sport & Exercise*. 31(1):143–148, 1999.

Pacy, P. J., N. Barton, J. D. Webster, & J. Garrow: The energy cost of aerobic exercise in fed and fasted normal subjects. *American Journal of Clinical Nutrition*. 42:764–768 (1985).

Pacy, P. J., J. Webster, & J. S. Garrow: Exercise and obesity. *Sports Medicine*. 3:89–113 (1986).

Plowman, S. A.: Maturation and exercise training in children. *Pediatric Exercise Science*. 1:303–312 (1989).

Popovic, V. & L. H. Duntas: Brain somatic cross-talk: Ghrelin, lep-tin and ultimate challengers of obesity. *Nutrition Neuroscience*. 8(1):1–5 (2005).

Pratley, R., B. Nicklas, M. Robin, et al.: Strength training increases resting metabolic rate and norepinephrine levels in healthy 50- to 65-yr-old men. *Journal of Applied Physiology*. 76(1):133–137 (1994).

Prentice, A. & S. Jebb: Energy intake/physical activity interac-tions in the homeostasis of body weight regulation. *Nutrition Reviews*. 62(7):S98–S104 (2004).

Racette, S. B., E. P. Weiss, D. T. Villareal, et al.: One year of caloric restriction in humans: Feasibility and effects on body composition and abdominal adipose tissue. *Journals of Gerontology Series A: Biological Sciences and Medical Sciences*. 61(9):943–950 (2006).

Ratcliff, L., S. S. Gropper, D. White, D. M. Shannon, K. W. Huggins: The influence of habitual exercise training and meal form on diet-induced thermogenesis in college-age men. *International Journal of Sport Nutrition and Exercise Metabolism*. 21:11–18 (2011).

Redman, L. M., L. K. Heilbronn, C. K. Martin, A. Alfonso, S. R. Smith, & E. Ravussin: Effect of calorie restriction with or without exercise on body composition and fat distribution. *The Journal of Clinical Endocrinology and Metabolism*. 92(3):865–872 (2007).

Richard, D., A. C. Carpenter, G. Doré, V. Ouellet, & F. Picard: Determinants of brown adipocyte development and ther-mogenesis. *International Journal of Obesity*. 34:S59–S66 (2010).

Riedt, C. S., Y. Schlussel, N. von Thun, et al.: Premenopausal overweight women do not lose bone during moderate weight loss with adequate or higher calcium intake. *American Journal of Clinical Nutrition*. 85(4):972–980 (2007).

Rodin, J., N. Radke-Sharpe, M. Rebuffe-Scrive, & M. R. C. Greenwood: Weight cycling and fat distribution. *International Journal of Obesity*. 14:303–310 (1990).

Romon, M., S. Gomila, P. Hincker, B. Soudan, & J. Dallongeville: Influence of weight loss on plasma ghrelin responses to high-fat and high-carbohydrate test meals in obese women. *Journal of Clinical Endocrinology and Metabolism*. 91(3):1034–1041 (2006).

Rosenbaum, M., R. Goldsmith, D. Bloomfield, et al.: Low-dose leptin reverses skeletal muscle, autonomic, and neuroendo-crine adaptations to maintenance of reduced weight. *Journal of Clinical Investigations*. 115(12):3579–3586 (2005).

Ross, R.: Effects of diet- and exercise-induced weight loss on visceral adipose tissue in men and women. *Sports Medicine*. 24(1):55–64 (1997).

Ross, R. & I. Janssen: Is abdominal fat preferentially reduced in response to exercise-induced weight loss? *Medicine & Science in Sports & Exercise*. 31(Suppl. 11):S568–S572 (1999).

Ross, R. & I. Janssen: Physical activity, total and regional obe-sity: Dose-response considerations. *Medicine & Science in Sports & Exercise*. 53(6 Suppl.): S521–S527 (2001).

Ross, R. & I. Janssen: Physical activity, fitness, and obesity. In Bouchard, C., S. N. Blair, W. L. Haskell (eds.): *Physical Activity and Health*. Champaign, IL: Human Kinetics, 173–189 (2007).

Roza, A. M. & H. M. Shizgal: The Harris Benedict equation reevaluated: Resting energy requirements and the body cell mass. *American Journal of Clinical Nutrition*. 40:168–182 (1984).

Rzehak, P., C. Meisinger, G. Woelke, S. Brasche, G. Strube, & J. Heinrich: Weight change, weight cycling and mortality in the ERFORT Male Cohort Study. *European Journal of Epidemiology*. 22:665–673 (2007).

Saarni, S. E., A. Rissanen, S. Sarna, M. Koskenvuo, & J. Kaprio: Weight cycling of athletes and subsequent weight gain in middle age. *International Journal of Obesity*. 30:1639–1644 (2006).

Saris, W. H. M., S. N. Blair, M. A. van Baak, et al.: How much physical activity is enough to prevent unhealthy weight gain? Outcome of the IASO 1st Stock Conference and consensus statement. *Obesity Reviews*. 4:101–114 (2003).

Schelkun, P. H.: The risks of riding the weight-loss roller coaster. *The Physician and Sportsmedicine*. 19(6):149–156 (1991).

Schmidt, W. D., D. Corrigan, & C. L. Melby: Two seasons of weight cycling does not lower resting metabolic rate in college wrestlers. *Medicine and Science in Sports and Exercise*. 25(5):613–619 (1993).

Schutz, Y. B., T. Bessard, & E. Jequier: Diet-induced thermogenesis measured over a whole day in obese and nonobese women. *American Journal of Clinical Nutrition*. 40:542–552 (1984).

Schwartz, R. S., J. B. Halter, & E. L. Bierman: Reduced thermic effect of feeding in obesity: Role of norepinephrine. *Metabolism*. 32:114–117 (1983).

Segal, K. R., B. Gutin, J. Albu, & F. Pi-Sunyer: Thermic effects of food and exercise in lean and obese men of similar lean body mass. *American Journal of Physiology*. 252:E110–E117 (1987).

Segal, K. R., B. Gutin, A. M. Nyman, & F. X. Pi-Sunyer: Thermic effect of food at rest, during exercise, and after exercise in lean and obese men of similar body weight. *Journal of Clinical Investigation*. 76:1107–1112 (1985).

Segal, K. R., E. Presta, & B. Gutin: Thermic effect of food during graded exercise in normal weight and obese men. *American Journal of Clinical Nutrition*. 40:995–1000 (1984).

Shetty, P. S., R. T. Jung, W. P. James, M. A. Barrand, & B. A. Callingham: Postprandial thermogenesis in obesity. *Clinical Science*. 60:519–525 (1981).

Smith, S. R. & J. J. Zachwieja: Visceral adipose tissue: A critical review of intervention strategies. *International Journal of Obesity*. 23:329–335 (1999).

Speakman, J. R. & C. Selman: Physical activity and resting metabolic rate. *Proceedings of the Nutrition Society*. 62:621–634 (2003).

Steen, S. N., R. A. Oppliger, & K. D. Brownell: Metabolic effects of repeated weight loss and regain in adolescent wrestlers. *Journal of the American Medical Association*. 260(1):47–50 (1988).

Stiegler, P. & A. Cunliffe: The role of diet and exercise for the maintenance of fat-free mass and resting metabolic rate during weight loss. *Sports Medicine*. 36(3):239–262 (2006).

Strychar, I., M.-E. Lavoie, L. Messier, A. D. Karelis, E. Doucet, D. Prud'Homme, et al.: Anthropometric, metabolic, psychosocial, and dietary characteristics of overweight/obese postmenopausal women with a history of weight cycling: A MONET (Montreal Ottawa New Emerging Team) Study. *Journal of the American Dietetic Association*. 109:718–724 (2009).

Stubbs, R. J., A. Sepp, D. A. Hughes, A. M. Johnstone, N. King, G. Horgan, & J. E. Blundell: The effect of graded levels of exercise on energy intake and balance in free-living women. *International Journal of Obesity*. 26:866–869 (2002).

Stubbs, R. J., D. A. Hughes, A. M. Johnstone, G. W. Horgan, N. King, & J. E. Blundell: A decrease in physical activity affects appetite, energy, and nutrient balance in lean men feeding ad libitum. *American Journal of Clinical Nutrition*. 79(1):62–69 (2004).

Sullo, A., P. Cardinale, G. Brizzi, B. Fabbri, & N. Maffulli: Resting metabolic rate and post-prandial thermogenesis by level of aerobic power in older adults. *Clinical and Experimental Pharmacology and Physiology*. 31(4):202–206 (2004).

Tagliaferro, A. R., R. Kertzer, J. R. Davis, C. Janson, & S. K. Tse: Effects of exercise-training on the thermic effect of food and body fatness of adult women. *Physiology and Behavior*. 38(5):703–710 (1986).

Tate, D. F., R. W. Jeffery, N. E. Sherwood, & R. R. Wing: Long-term weight losses associated with prescription of higher physical activity goals. Are higher levels of physical activity protective against weight regain? *American Journal of Clinical Nutrition*. 85(4):954–959 (2007).

Thyfault, J. P., S. R. Richmone, M. J. Carper, J. F. Potteiger, & M. W. Hulver: Postprandial metabolism in resistance-trained versus sedentary males. *Medicine & Science in Sports & Exercise*. 36(4):709–716 (2004).

Titchenal, C. A.: Exercise and food intake: What is the relationship? *Sports Medicine*. 6:135–145 (1988).

Tremblay, A., J. Côté, & J. LeBlanc: Diminished dietary thermogenesis in exercise-trained human subjects. *European Journal of Applied Physiology*. 52:1–2 (1983).

Tremblay, A., E. Fontaine, & A. Nadeau: Contribution of postexercise increment in glucose storage to variation in glucose-induced thermogenesis in endurance athletes. *Canadian Journal of Physiology and Pharmacology*. 63:1165–1169 (1985).

Van Baak, M. A.: Meal-induced activation of the sympathetic nervous system and its cardiovascular and thermogenic effects in man. *Physiology and Behavior*. Doi: 10.1016/j.physbeh.2007.12.020 (2008).

van Dale, O. & W. H. M. Saris: Repetitive weight loss and weight regain: Effects on weight reduction, resting metabolic rate, and lipolytic activity before and after exercise and/or diet treatment. *American Journal of Clinical Nutrition*. 49:409–416 (1989).

van Horn, L., K. Donato, S. Kumanyika, M. Winston, T. E. Prewitt, & L. Snetselaar: The dietitian's role in developing and implementing the first federal obesity guidelines. *Journal of the American Dietetic Association*. 98(10):1115–1117 (1998).

van Wye, G., J. A. Dubin, S. N. Blair, & L. DiPietro: Weight cycling and 6-year change in healthy adults: The Aerobics Center Longitudinal Study. *Obesity*. 15(3):731–739 (2007).

Van Zant, R. S.: Influence of diet and exercise on energy expenditure—a review. *International Journal of Sport Nutrition*. 2(1):1–19 (1992).

Villareal, D. T., L. Fontana, E. P. Weiss, et al.: Bone mineral density response to caloric restriction-induced weight loss or exercise-induced weight loss: A randomized controlled trial. *Archives of Internal Medicine*. 166(22):2502–2510 (2006).

Virtanen, K. A., M. E. Lidell, J. Orava, M. Heglind, R. Westergren, T. Niemi, et al.: Functional brown adipose tissue in healthy adults. *New England Journal of Medicine*. 360:1518–1525 (2009).

Vispute, S. S., J. D. Smith, J. D. LeCheminant, & K. S. Hurley: The effect of abdominal exercise on abdominal fat. *Journal of Strength and Conditioning Research*. 25(9):2559–2564 (2011).

Volek, J. S., J. L. van Heest, & C. E. Forsythe: Diet and exercise for weight loss: A review of current issues. *Sports Medicine*. 35(1):1–9 (2005).

Wadden, T. A., S. Bartlett, & K. A. Letizia: Relationship of dieting history to resting metabolic rate, body composition, eating behavior and subsequent weight loss. *American Journal of Clinical Nutrition*. 56:206S–211S (1992).

Wadden, T. A., G. D. Foster, K. A. Letizia, & J. L. Mullen: Long-term effects of dieting on resting metabolic rate in obese outpatients. *Journal of the American Medical Association*. 264(6):707–711 (1990).

Walberg, J. L.: Aerobic exercise and resistance weight-training during weight reduction: Implications for obese persons and athletes. *Sports Medicine*. 47:343–356 (1989).

Wallner, S. J., N. Luschnigg, W. J. Schnedl, et al.: Body fat distribution of overweight females with a history of weight cycling. *International Journal of Obesity*. 28:1143–1148 (2004).

Wannamethee, S. G., A. G. Shaper, & M. Walker: Weight change, weight fluctuation, and mortality. *Archives of Internal Medicine*. 162(22):2575–2580 (2002).

Watts, K., T. W. Jones, E. A. Davis, & D. Green: Exercise training in obese children and adolescents: Current concepts. *Sports Medicine*. 35(5):375–392 (2005).

Weigle, D. S., P. A. Breen, C. C. Mattys, H. S. Callahan, K. E. Meeuws, V. R. Burden, & J. Q. Purnell: A high-protein diet induces sustained reduction in appetite, adlibitum caloric intake, and body weight despite compensatory changes in diurnal plasma leptin and ghrelin concentrations. *American Journal of Clinical Nutrition*. 82(1):41–48 (2005).

Weigle, D. S., D. E. Cummings, P. D. Newby, et al.: Roles of leptin and ghrelin in the loss of body weight caused by a low fat, high carbohydrate diet. *Journal of Clinical Endocrinology and Metabolism*. 88(4):1577–1586 (2003).

Welle, S.: Metabolic response to a meal during rest and low intensity exercise. *American Journal of Clinical Nutrition*. 40:990–994 (1984).

Westerterp, K. R.: Impacts of vigorous and non-vigorous activity on daily energy expenditure. *Proceedings of the Nutritional Society*. 62:645–650 (2003).

Westerterp-Plantenga, M. S., M. P. Lejeune, I. Nijs, M. van Ooijen, & E. M. Kovacs: High protein intake sustains weight maintenance after body weight loss in humans. *International Journal of Obesity*. 28(1):57–64 (2004).

White, L. J., R. H. Dressendorfer, E. Holland, S. C. McCoy, & M. A. Ferguson: Increased caloric intake soon after exercise in cold water. *International Journal of Sport Nutrition and Exercise Metabolism*. 15(1):38–47 (2005).

Willms, W. L. & S. A. Plowman: The separate and sequential effects of exercise and meal ingestion on energy expenditure. *Annals of Nutrition and Metabolism*. 35(6):347–356 (1991).

Wilmore, J. H.: Appetite and body composition consequent to physical activity. *Research Quarterly for Exercise and Sport*. 54(4):415–425 (1983).

Wilmore, J. H. & D. L. Costill: *Training for Sport and Activity: The Physiological Basis of the Conditioning Process* (3rd edition). Dubuque, IA: Brown (1988).

Wing, R. R.: Physical activity in the treatment of the adulthood overweight and obesity: Current evidence and research issues. *Medicine & Science in Sports & Exercise*. 31(Suppl. 11): S547–S552 (1999).

You, T., K. M. Murphy, M. F. Lyles, J. L. Demons, L. Lenchik, & B. J. Nicklas: Addition of aerobic exercise to dietary weight loss preferentially reduces abdominal adipocyte size. *International Journal of Obesity*. 30(8):1211–1216 (2006).

Zahorska-Markiewicz, B.: Thermic effect of food and exercise in obesity. *European Journal of Applied Physiology*. 44:231–235 (1980).

Zuti, W. B. & L. A. Golding: Comparing diet and exercise as weight reducing tools. *The Physician and Sports medicine*. 4:49–53 (1976).

Cardiovascular-Respiratory System Unit

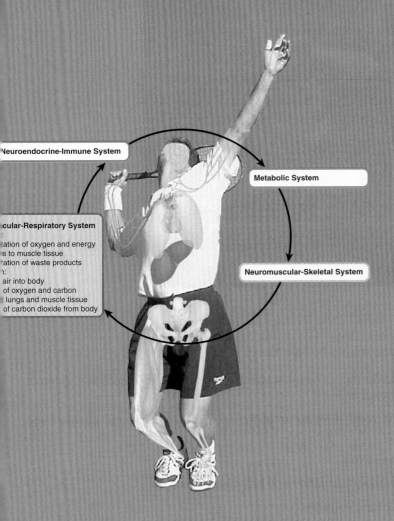

Neuroendocrine-Immune System

Metabolic System

cular-Respiratory System

tation of oxygen and energy
s to muscle tissue
ation of waste products
:
air into body
of oxygen and carbon
lungs and muscle tissue
of carbon dioxide from body

Neuromuscular-Skeletal System

The cardiorespiratory system brings oxygen into the body (respiratory system) and transports it to the cells (cardiovascular system), which use the oxygen in the production of energy through the process of cellular respiration. Thus, the respiratory and cardiovascular systems are functionally linked and often referred to collectively as the cardiovascular-respiratory, or cardiorespiratory, system. The cardiorespiratory system directly supports metabolism by delivering oxygen and nutrients to the cells of the body. The metabolic production of ATP from oxygen and foodstuffs then directly supports the neuromuscular system by providing the energy for muscle contraction. The neuroendocrine-immune system plays an important role in regulating both the respiratory and the cardiovascular systems.

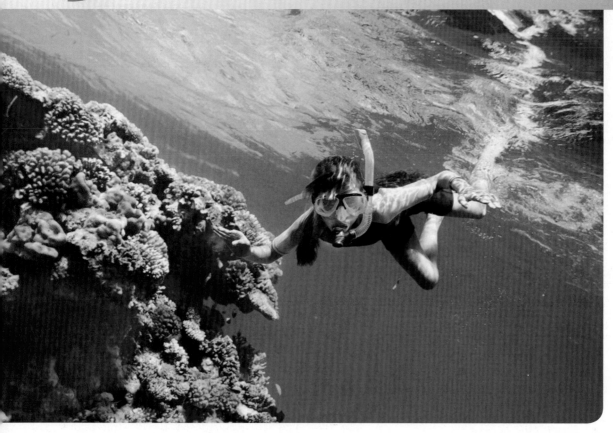

9 Respiration

OBJECTIVES

After studying the chapter, you should be able to:

❯ Distinguish among and explain the component variables of pulmonary ventilation, external respiration, and internal respiration.

❯ Identify the conductive and respiratory zones of the respiratory system and compare the functions of the two zones.

❯ Explain the mechanics of breathing.

❯ Differentiate between pulmonary circulation and bronchial circulation.

❯ Describe static and dynamic lung volumes.

❯ Distinguish between the conditions under which respiratory measures are collected and reported.

❯ Calculate minute and alveolar ventilation, the partial pressure of a gas in a mixture, the amount of oxygen carried per deciliter of blood, and the arteriovenous oxygen difference.

❯ Explain how respiration is regulated at rest and during exercise.

❯ Explain how oxygen and carbon dioxide are transported in the circulatory system and how oxygen is released to the tissues.

❯ Explain the role of respiration in acid-base balance.

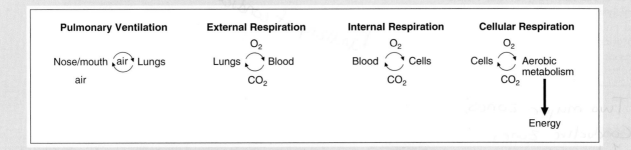

FIGURE 9.1 Overview of Respiration.
Respiration consists of four separate processes. The first is pulmonary ventilation, in which air is moved into and out of the body. The second, external respiration, involves the exchange of oxygen and carbon dioxide between the lungs and the blood. The third is internal respiration, which involves the exchange of oxygen and carbon dioxide at the cellular or tissue level. Finally, cellular respiration is the utilization of oxygen to produce energy, which also produces carbon dioxide as a by-product.

Introduction

The common denominator for all sports, exercise, and physical activity is muscle action. For muscles to be able to act, energy must be provided. The first link in the chain supplying a large portion of this energy is respiration, which provides oxygen to and removes carbon dioxide from the body. In reality most of us take respiration for granted (we don't have to think to do it), and we are unaware of it until something like hard exercise increases the sensation. Thus, it comes as quite a surprise to many exercise physiology students that respiration is relatively complex physiologically. In addition, there are a great many abbreviations used for the multitude of respiratory terms. The reader is referred to the two pages entitled "Commonly used symbols and abbreviations" directly inside the front of the textbook as a quick reference to help keep these terms straight. In addition, summaries of the variables important for the major divisions of respiration (pulmonary ventilation, external respiration, and internal respiration) are provided at the end of the appropriate sections of text.

Although it is typical to think of respiration as being the same as breathing and/or ventilation, technically, it is not. **Figure 9.1** presents an overview of respiration. The volume of air flowing into the lungs from the external environment through either the nose or the mouth is called **pulmonary ventilation**. Ventilation is accomplished by breathing, the alternation of inspiration and expiration that causes the air to move. The actual exchange of the gases oxygen (O_2) and carbon dioxide (CO_2) between the lungs and the blood is known as **external respiration**. At the cellular level, oxygen and carbon dioxide gases are again exchanged; this exchange is called **internal respiration**. **Cellular respiration** is the utilization of oxygen by the cells to produce energy with carbon dioxide as a by-product. Cellular respiration includes both aerobic (with O_2) and anaerobic (without O_2) energy production and is discussed in Chapter 2. This chapter concentrates on pulmonary ventilation, external respiration, and internal respiration.

Structure of the Pulmonary System

The respiratory system consists of two major portions: (1) the conductive zone, which transports the air to the lungs, and (2) the respiratory zone, where gas exchange takes place.

The Conductive Zone

The basic structure of the conductive zone is shown in **Figure 9.2**. The structures from the nose or mouth to the terminal bronchioles comprise the *conductive zone*. The primary role of the conductive zone is to transport air. Because no exchange of gases takes place here, this zone is also called *anatomical dead space*. As a general guideline, the amount of anatomical dead space can be estimated as 1 mL for each 1 lb of "ideal" body weight (Slonim and Hamilton, 1976). Hence, a 130-lb female who is at her ideal weight has an estimated 130 mL of anatomical dead space. However, if this individual were to gain 20 lb, she would still have

Pulmonary Ventilation The process by which air is moved into and out of the lungs.

External Respiration The exchange of gases between the lungs and the blood.

Internal Respiration The exchange of gases between the blood and the tissues at the cellular level.

Cellular Respiration The utilization of oxygen by the cells to produce energy.

FIGURE 9.2 Anatomy of the Pulmonary System.

The pulmonary system is divided into two zones: the conductive zone transports air to the lungs and the respiratory zone where gas exchange takes place.

[Handwritten notes:]

Two major zones:
- Conductive Zones
  1. transport air
  2. Humidify air
  3. Filter air
- Respiratory Zones

Physiological dead space = ana. + ave.
alveolar deadspace = no capillaries
anatomical dead space =
    1 mL per 1 lb of bodyweight

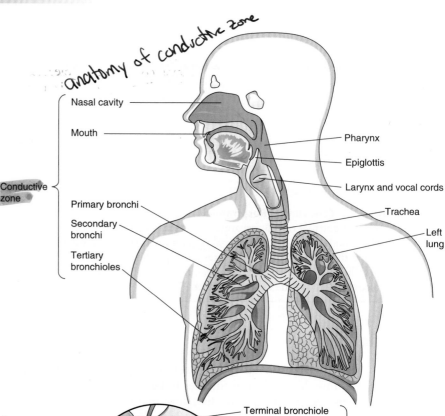

[Handwritten labels on figure:] anatomy of conductive zone; anatomy of Resp. Zone

Nasal cavity
Mouth
Pharynx
Epiglottis
Larynx and vocal cords
Conductive zone
Primary bronchi
Secondary bronchi
Tertiary bronchioles
Trachea
Left lung
Terminal bronchiole
Pulmonary arteriole
Pulmonary venule
Respiratory bronchiole
Alveolar sacs
Respiratory zone

the same anatomical dead space and that estimate would remain at 130 mL. Anatomical dead space is important in determining the alveolar ventilation, as discussed later.

The second important role of the conductive zone is to warm and humidify the air. By the time the air reaches the lungs, it will be warmed to body temperature (normally ~37°C) and will be 99.5% saturated with water vapor. This protective mechanism helps maintain core body temperature and protects the lungs from injury (Slonim and Hamilton, 1976). The warming and humidifying of air is easily accomplished over a wide range of environmental temperatures under resting conditions, when the volume of air transported is small and the air is inhaled through the nose. During heavy exercise, however, large volumes of air are inhaled primarily through the mouth, thus bypassing the warming and moisturizing sites of the nose and nasal cavity. As a result, the mouth and the throat may feel dry. If heavy exercise takes place in cold weather (especially at subzero temperatures), dryness increases and throat pain may be felt. These uncomfortable feelings are not a symptom of freezing of the

lungs; rather, they are the result of the drying and cooling of the upper airway. The lower portions of the conductive zone still moisturize and warm the air sufficiently before it reaches the lungs. A scarf worn across the mouth will trap moisture and heat from the exhaled air and thereby decrease or eliminate the uncomfortable sensations.

The third role of the conductive zone is to filter the incoming air. The nasal cavity, pharynx, larynx, trachea, and bronchial system are all lined with ciliated mucous membranes (**Figure 9.2**). These membranes with their hair-like projections trap impurities and foreign particles (particulates) that are inhaled. Both smoke and environmental air pollutants diminish ciliary activity and can ultimately destroy the cilia.

The Respiratory Zone

The *respiratory zone* consists of the respiratory bronchioles, the alveolar ducts, alveolar sacs (grape-like clusters), and the alveoli (**Figure 9.2**). The alveoli are the actual site of gas exchange between the pulmonary system and the cardiovascular system. At birth, humans have about 24 million alveoli. This number increases to about 300 million by 8 years of age and remains constant until age 30, when it begins a gradual decline. Although each individual alveolus is small, only about 0.2 mm in diameter, collectively the alveoli in a young adult have a total surface area of 50–100 m² (West, 2005). This area would cover a badminton court or even a tennis court if flattened out. Despite this large surface area, the lungs weigh only about 2.2 lb (1 kg). The volume of the respiratory zone is about 2.5–3.0 L·min⁻¹ (West, 2005). The membrane between the alveoli and the capillaries is actually composed of five very thin layers, two of which are the endothelial cells of the alveoli and the capillaries. The endothelium of the alveoli produces a substance called surfactant that reduces surface tension and helps prevent alveoli from collapsing (Seifter et al., 2005). Despite the number of layers, the thickness is less than the paper this book is printed on, and gas exchange takes place easily (West, 2005).

In addition to the anatomical dead space where no exchange takes place, some alveoli have no capillary blood supply or the capillaries are pathologically blocked and therefore cannot participate in gas exchange; these alveoli make up an *alveolar dead space*. The anatomical plus the alveolar dead space combined make up the *physiological dead space*. Because alveolar dead space is minimal in healthy individuals, the physiological dead space is only slightly larger than the anatomical dead space (West, 2005).

Mechanics of Breathing

The movement of air into the lungs from the atmosphere depends on two factors: pressure gradient (ΔP) and resistance (R). The relationship between these factors is expressed by the equation for *airflow* (V̇):

9.1

$$\text{airflow (L·min}^{-1}) = \frac{\text{pressure gradient (mmHg)}}{\text{resistance (R unit)}}$$

or

$$\dot{V} = \frac{\Delta P}{R}$$

A *pressure gradient* is simply the difference between two pressures. Difference is represented by the Greek capital letter delta: Δ. The larger the differences in pressure, the larger the pressure gradient is. Gases—in this case, air which is a mixture of gases—move from areas of high pressure to areas of low pressure.

Resistance is the sum of the forces opposing the flow of the gases. About 20% of resistance to airflow is caused by tissue friction as the lungs move during inspiration and expiration. The remaining 80% is due to the friction between the gas molecules and the walls of the airway (airway resistance) and the internal friction between the gas molecules themselves (viscosity). Airway resistance is determined by the size of the airway and the smoothness or turbulence of the airflow.

As Equation 9.1 shows, in order for air to flow, the pressure gradient must be greater than the resistance to the flow. Thus, for inspiration to take place, pressure must be higher in the atmosphere than in the lungs; for expiration, pressure in the alveoli of the lungs must be higher than in the atmosphere. **Figure 9.3** shows how the inspiratory pressure gradient is created.

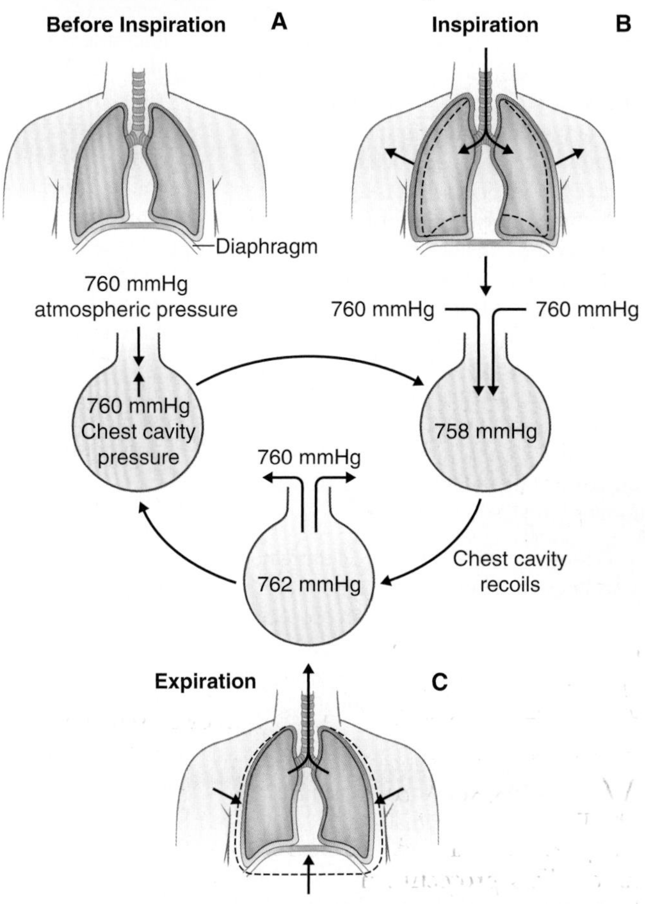

FIGURE 9.3 Inspiratory and Expiratory Pressure Gradients. Inspiration and expiration are accomplished through pressure gradients. **A.** The respiratory musculature is relaxed, and the atmospheric pressure equals the chest cavity pressure, so no air movement occurs. **B.** The external intercostals and diaphragm contract, moving the ribs up and out and the diaphragm down, respectively. This muscle action enlarges the chest cavity laterally, anteroposteriorly, and downward, increasing the volume. Chest cavity pressure is therefore lower than atmospheric pressure, and air flows in. **C.** The inspiratory muscles relax, and the chest cavity recoils, creating a pressure higher than atmospheric pressure. Air flows out. The respiratory cycle then begins again.

FOCUS ON APPLICATION

External Nasal Dilators   *myth debunked*

Originally intended as a sleep aid, the Breathe Right strip external nasal dilator (END) has been embraced by a broad range of exercisers, including professional athletes from football players to marathoners. This device is a flexible "spring-like" band worn externally over the bridge of the nose as in the accompanying photo. It has been shown to increase nasal valve area and to decrease air resistance in the nasal cavity (Gehring, 2000; Portugal et al., 1997). The question is whether this larger area and decreased resistance result in a higher tidal volume (V_T), lower frequency of breathing (f), or changes in minute ventilation—the amount of air exhaled each minute ($\dot{V}_E$). Such changes, in turn, could result in a reduction in the respiratory muscle work (less oxygen consumption, $\dot{V}O_2$) and ultimately a better athletic performance or faster recovery from exercise.

Experimental studies provide at least a partial answer. In each of the first four experiments, participants underwent three trials: control (C), normal breathing; placebo (P), wearing an inoperable END; and experimental (E), wearing an active functioning END.

1. O'Kroy et al. (2001) tested 14 untrained college students during randomly assigned C, P, and E trials. An esophageal balloon measured the inspiratory elastic work, the inspiratory resistive work, and the expiratory resistive work. $\dot{V}O_2$, $\dot{V}_E$, V_T, and f of breathing were also monitored. No significant differences were found in any variable either at submaximal (70% $\dot{V}O_2$max) or at maximal work.

2. In another study (O'Kroy, 2000), 15 participants performed three incremental exercise tests to volitional fatigue on a cycle ergometer. Maximal power output (a performance variable) was not significantly different among the

three trials (C = 256 ± 73W, P = 255 ± 70W, and E = 257 ± 74W). Neither the total body perception of effort nor the perceived effort of breathing differed among these trials.

3. In a series of field tests of maximal performance, Macfarlane and Fong (2004) studied 30 male adolescents in a short-term anaerobic power test (40-m sprint), a long-term anaerobic power test (shuttle sprint), and an incremental aerobic test (20-m shuttle/PACER) under C, P, and E conditions. The rate of perceived breathing effort was significantly reduced in the long anaerobic tests and aerobic tests in the E trial over the C trial but not the P trial. No significant differences were seen in the actual performances of either anaerobic test. In the 20-m shuttle aerobic test, performance was improved in the E condition 3.2% over the C trial and 2.9% over the P trial, but no change occurred in the perception of breathing effort.

4. Thomas et al. (2001) examined the effect of END on recovery from an anaerobic treadmill test under C, P, and E conditions. No differences were found for recovery in heart rate, $\dot{V}O_2$, or $\dot{V}_E$.

In a fifth study, three separate groups of females participated: a sedentary group, preseason college athletes, and in-season college rowers. Each individual performed two incremental exercise tests, one with and one without an END. No significant differences were found in blood lactate concentration at the lactate threshold in any group. Thus, there was no improvement

in either the exercise intensity at the lactate threshold or lower blood lactate levels during moderate- to high-intensity exercise (Boggs et al., 2008).

These combined experimental results indicate that the work of breathing, anaerobic performance, and recovery from anaerobic performance are not changed by wearing an END. In the one study showing an improvement in incremental aerobic and a decrease in perception of breathing effort, the changes were minimal. Based on these studies, the use of nasal dilators during exercise does not appear to be warranted.

Sources: Boggs et al. (2008), Gehring et al. (2000), O'Kroy (2000, 2001), Macfarlane and Fong (2004), Portugal et al. (1997), Thomas et al. (2001).

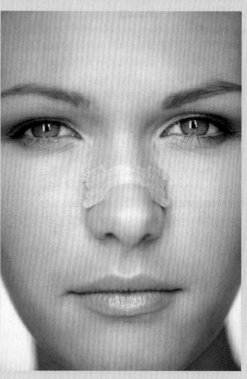

A key to understanding **Figure 9.3** is Boyle's law. *Boyle's law* states that the pressure of a gas is inversely related to its volume (or vice versa) under conditions of constant temperature: Low pressure is associated with large volume, and high pressure is associated with small volume.

For pulmonary ventilation, an increase in chest cavity volume is accomplished by muscle contraction for inspiration. This increase in volume leads to an internal lung pressure decrease according to Boyle's law. As a result, a negative pressure exists in the chest cavity relative to the atmosphere outside the body. Thus, a pressure gradient has

[Handwritten annotations at top:
Boyle's Law =
Low pressure / High volume
High pressure / Low volume
Volume change per unit of pressure = compliance]

been created. Air flows into the chest cavity in an attempt to equalize this pressure difference. The volume change per unit of pressure is called *compliance* (West, 2005).

The main inspiratory muscle is the dome-shaped diaphragm. With neural stimulation, the diaphragm contracts and moves downward, elongating the chest cavity (**Figure 9.3B**). In normal resting breathing, the diaphragm moves about 1 cm; in heavy or forced breathing, it may move as much as 10 cm (West, 2005). During exercise, the chest cavity is further enlarged by the action of the external intercostal muscles and others, known collectively as the accessory muscles, which elevate the rib cage and cause expansion both laterally (side to side) and anteroposteriorly (front to back). The extent of accessory muscle activity and the resultant drop in pressure depend on the depth of the inspiration.

These changes in the chest cavity volume transfer themselves to the lungs through the pleura. Pleurae are thin, double-layered membranes that line both the chest cavity (the inner surfaces of the thorax, sternum, ribs, vertebrae, and diaphragm) and the external lung surfaces. The portion covering the chest cavity is called the parietal pleura; the portion covering the external lung surfaces is called the visceral or pulmonary pleura. A fluid secreted by the pleura fills the space between the pleurae (the intrapleural space), allowing the lungs to glide smoothly over the chest cavity walls. It also causes the parietal and the pulmonary pleurae to adhere to each other in the same way that two pieces of glasses are held together by a thin film of water. Because of this adhesion, the lungs themselves move when muscle actions move the chest cavity (Guyton and Hall, 2011; Martin et al., 1979).

During normal resting conditions, expiration occurs simply because the diaphragm and other inspiratory muscles relax. When these muscles relax, both the lungs and the muscles, which are highly elastic, recoil to their original positions. This elastic recoil decreases lung volume and thus creates a pressure inside the chest cavity that is higher than the atmospheric pressure. As the chest cavity volume decreases, the intrathoracic pressure increases slightly above that of the atmosphere. The result is that the air moves out of the lungs into the atmosphere. The pressures equalize again, and the cycle repeats with the next inspiration. A complete respiratory cycle includes both inspiration and expiration.

During heavy breathing, as in exercise, expiration is an active process. The primary expiratory muscles are the abdominals and the internal intercostals. The abdominals (rectus abdominus, the obliques, and the transverse abdominus) push the abdominal organs—and hence the diaphragm—upward; the internal intercostals pull the ribs inward and down. This decrease in chest volume increases

intrathoracic pressure more quickly than passive elastic recoil alone, and the air is forced out of the lungs faster.

The pleurae also serve a purpose during expiration. Pressure in the intrapleural space fluctuates with breathing in a way that parallels pressure within the lungs. However, the intrapleural pressure is always negative (24–28 mmHg) relative to the intrapulmonary (lung) pressure. This negative pressure protects the lungs from collapsing. If the intrapleural pressure were equal to the atmospheric pressure, the lungs would collapse at the end of expiration because of the elastic recoil.

Because muscle activity is involved during the respiratory cycle of inhalation and exhalation, energy is consumed. During rest, however, this energy consumption (restricted to inspiratory muscles) amounts to only 1–2% of the total body energy expenditure in nonsmokers (Pardy et al., 1984).

[Handwritten annotations:
Pleurae = thin double layered
Parietal pleura = covers chest
Visceral / pulmonary = covers externally]

Respiratory Circulation

The lung has two different circulatory systems. Pulmonary circulation serves the external respiratory function, and bronchial circulation supplies the internal respiratory needs of the lung tissue (**Figure 9.4**). *[Handwritten: Two circulatory systems]*

The structure of the pulmonary circulation parallels the divisions of the structures in the conductive zone, branching in a tree-like manner called *arborization* (**Figure 9.5**). Arborization ends in a dense alveolar capillary network, blanketing most but not all alveoli. The capillary blood flow through this network is called perfusion of the lung (Guyton and Hall, 2011; West, 2005).

The pulmonary artery exits the right ventricle of the heart and gives rise to the capillary network in the lungs (**Figure 9.4A**). The pulmonary vein originates from this capillary network and enters the heart at the left atrium. As with pulmonary airflow and the rest of the circulatory system, blood flows through this circuit due to differences in pressure that produce a pressure gradient large enough to overcome resistance to the flow. Normal pulmonary artery blood pressure is low, only 25/10 mmHg, but venous pulmonary blood pressure is even lower, only 7 mmHg. Although this pressure gradient between the pulmonary artery and vein is not large, it is enough to bring about the blood flow. Because of the low gradient, however, gravity affects the pulmonary circulation more than the systemic or total body circulation. The lowest portion of the lungs, therefore, is perfused best. The portion of the lungs that is best perfused with blood is also ventilated best (Guyton and Hall, 2011; Leff and Schumacker, 1993; Martin et al., 1979). Which portion it is varies with the body posture. *[Handwritten: Normal 25/10, Venous 7 mmHg]*

The bronchial circulation (**Figure 9.4B**) consists of relatively small systemic arteries that originate from the descending portion of the aorta, called the thoracic artery, travel through the lungs, and return as veins that empty

Perfusion of the Lung Pulmonary circulation, especially capillary blood flow.

FIGURE 9.4 Lung Circulatory Systems.
Pulmonary circulation **(A)** serves the process of external respiration, picking up oxygen for and unloading carbon dioxide from the body as a whole at the alveoli. Bronchial circulation **(B)** serves the process of internal respiration, unloading oxygen to and picking up carbon dioxide from the lung tissue. *Source*: Modified from Germann, W. J. & C. L. Stanfield: *Principles of Human Physiology*. San Francisco, CA: Benjamin Cummings (2002).

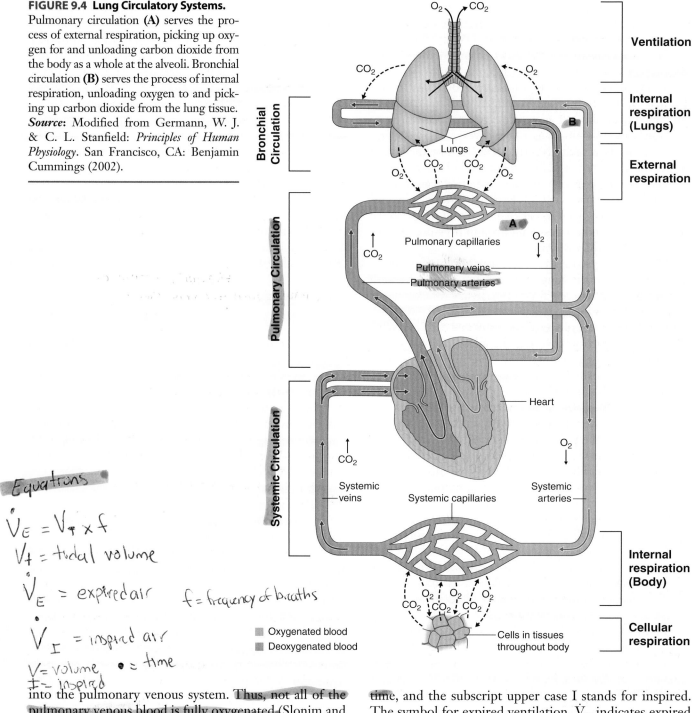

Equations

$$\dot{V}_E = V_t \times f$$
V_t = tidal volume
$\dot{V}_E$ = expired air
f = frequency of breaths
$\dot{V}_I$ = inspired air
V = volume, $\bullet$ = time
f = inspired

into the pulmonary venous system. Thus, not all of the pulmonary venous blood is fully oxygenated (Slonim and Hamilton, 1976).

Minute Ventilation/Alveolar Ventilation

The amount of air inspired or the amount of air expired in 1 minute is known as **minute ventilation or minute volume.** The most common units of measurement are liters per minute ($L \cdot min^{-1}$) and milliliters per minute ($mL \cdot min^{-1}$). Inspired minute ventilation is symbolized as $\dot{V}_I$, where V is volume, the "dot" indicates per unit of

time, and the subscript upper case I stands for inspired. The symbol for expired ventilation, $\dot{V}_E$, indicates expired rather than inspired air.

Minute ventilation depends on **tidal volume (V_T)**, the amount of air inhaled or exhaled per breath, and the frequency (f) of breaths per minute ($b \cdot min^{-1}$). The equation is

9.2 minute ventilation ($mL \cdot min^{-1}$)
= tidal volume ($mL \cdot br^{-1}$) × frequency ($br \cdot min^{-1}$)

or

$$\dot{V}_E = V_T \times f$$

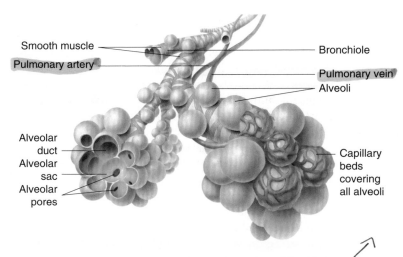

Smooth muscle

Pulmonary artery

Bronchiole

Pulmonary vein

Alveoli

Alveolar duct

Alveolar sac

Alveolar pores

Capillary beds covering all alveoli

FIGURE 9.5 Pulmonary Circulation Showing Arborization around the Alveoli.
Source: Asset provided by Anatomical Chart Co.

amount   example

$$\dot{V}_E = V_T \cdot \times f$$
$$= 400 mL \times 15\ br \cdot min$$
$$= \frac{6000\ mL \cdot min}{1000} \quad \text{convert to Liters}$$
$$= 6.0\ L \cdot min^{1}$$

Milliliters per minute are then commonly converted to liters per minute by dividing by 1000.

At rest, a normal young adult breathes at a frequency of 12–15 times per minute and has a tidal volume of 400–600 mL. Children ventilate at a much faster rate but with a smaller tidal volume.

EXAMPLE

Compute $\dot{V}_E$ when f = 15 br·min⁻¹ and V_T = 400 mL. You should set up and solve the equation as follows:

$$\dot{V}_E = (400\ mL \cdot br^{-1}) \times (15\ br \cdot min^{-1})$$
$$= 6000\ mL \cdot min^{-1}$$

$$\frac{6000\ mL \cdot min^{-1}}{1000\ mL \cdot L^{-1}} = 6.0\ L \cdot min^{-1}$$

Because minute ventilation represents the total amount of air moved into or out of the lungs per minute, it includes the portion of air that fills the conduction zone. Thus, minute ventilation does not represent the amount of air that is available for gas exchange. The amount of air that is available for gas exchange is termed **alveolar ventilation** (or *anatomical effective ventilation*). Alveolar ventilation ($\dot{V}_A$) takes into account tidal volume (V_T), dead space (V_D), and the frequency (f) of breathing. The equation for calculating $\dot{V}_A$ is

---

Minute Ventilation or Minute Volume ($\dot{V}_I$ or $\dot{V}_E$)
The amount of air inspired or expired each minute, or the pulmonary ventilation rate per minute; calculated as tidal volume times frequency of breathing.

Tidal Volume (V_T) The amount of air that is inspired or expired in one breath.

Alveolar Ventilation ($\dot{V}_A$) The volume of air available for gas exchange; calculated as tidal volume minus dead space volume times frequency.

9.3 alveolar ventilation (mL · min⁻¹)
= [tidal volume (mL · br⁻¹) − dead space (mL · br⁻¹)] × frequency (br · min⁻¹)

or

$$\dot{V}_A = (V_T - V_D) \times f$$

alveolar vent = (Tidal volume − dead space) × frequency of breath

Typically, approximately 70% of $\dot{V}_I$ reaches the alveoli for gas exchange. The ratio of anatomical dead space (V_D) to tidal volume (V_T) is abbreviated as V_D/V_T. This is not a mathematical constant because both factors can change. The dead space actually increases from some stretching of the respiratory passages as breathing becomes deeper and the deeper breathing increases the inspired volume of air. The increase in dead space is only a very small portion of the increase in the volume of air inspired.

$$V_A = (400 mL - 130 mL) \times 15$$
$$= 4050 \div 1000\ mL = 4.05L$$

EXAMPLE

Calculate alveolar ventilation using the values of f and V_T given in the previous example, for a female who is at her ideal weight of 130 lb. Also calculate the percent of $\dot{V}_I$ that is available for gas exchange. This problem becomes

$$\dot{V}_A = [(400\ mL \cdot br^{-1}) - (130\ mL \cdot br^{-1})]$$
$$\times (15\ br \cdot min^{-1})$$
$$= 4050\ mL \cdot min^{-1} \div 1000\ mL \cdot L^{-1}$$
$$= 4.05\ L \cdot min^{-1}$$

The percentage is 67.5% [(4050 mL·min⁻¹)/(6000 mL·min⁻¹)].

As with minute ventilation, alveolar ventilation can be calculated from either $\dot{V}_E$ or $\dot{V}_I$. The alveolar dead space is so negligible in normal healthy individuals that it does not need to be considered in these calculations. To be sure you understand the implications of this concept, complete the problems in the Check Your Comprehension 1 box.

CHECK YOUR COMPREHENSION 1

1. Given two breathing patterns, A and B, in the accompanying table, calculate the alveolar ventilation.

	Breathing Pattern	
	A	**B**
$\dot{V}_E$ (L·min^{-1})	6	6
V_T (mL·br^{-1})	600	200
f (br·min^{-1})	10	30
V_D (mL·br^{-1})	150	150
$\dot{V}_A$ (mL·min^{-1})	?	?

On the basis of your calculations, is it better to breathe fast and shallowly or slowly and deeply?

2. Individuals learning the front crawl swimming stroke are often reluctant to exhale air while their faces are in the water. They then try to inhale more air when their faces are turned to the side or to both exhale and inhale in the short time available during the head turn. Why is this not an effective breathing technique?

3. What is the effect of using a snorkel on the dead space? What implication does this effect have for breathing through a snorkel?

Check your answers in Appendix C.

In summary, the major variable for pulmonary ventilation are minute ventilation ($\dot{V}_E$ or $\dot{V}_I$), dead space (V_D), tidal volume (V_T), frequency of breathing (f), and the ratio of dead space to tidal volume (V_D/V_T). Alveolar ventilation ($\dot{V}_A$) is considered part of external respiration.

Measurement of Lung Volumes

Lung volumes can be measured either statically or dynamically. Static lung volumes are anatomical measures, are independent of time, and thus do not measure flow. Dynamic lung volumes depend on time and measure both airflow and air volume.

Static Lung Volumes

Take as deep a breath as you can. At this point, your lungs contain the maximum amount of air they can hold. This amount of air is called total lung capacity (TLC). TLC can be divided into four volumes and three other capacities, as depicted in **Figure 9.6**. Note that the four capacities are combinations of two or more volumes. All of these volumes and capacities have clinical significance, but only those important in the study of exercise physiology are discussed briefly here.

As mentioned previously, tidal volume (V_T) is the amount of air either inhaled or exhaled in a single breath. A normal V_T inflates the lungs to about half of the TLC

when sitting erect or standing and only about a third when lying supine (Slonim and Hamilton, 1976). When the demand for energy increases during exercise, V_T increases by expanding into both the inspiratory reserve volume (IRV) and expiratory reserve volume (ERV). Thus, the limits of vital capacity (VC = IRV + V_T + ERV) represent the absolute limit of the tidal volume increase during exercise.

Residual volume (RV) is the amount of air left in the lungs following a maximal exhalation. This leftover air is important because it allows for a continuous gas exchange between the alveoli and the capillaries between breaths. If all air were forced out of the lungs, no gas would be available for exchange. During exercise, when V_T expands, the functional residual capacity (FRC) helps maintain a smooth exchange, in the following way. The V_T can and does expand into both the IRV and the ERV, but it expands more into the IRV than the ERV, leaving a relatively large FRC intact. This large FRC dilutes the gas changes (the decrease in oxygen and increase in carbon dioxide) caused by the increased energy production and expenditure of exercise. By reducing fluctuation, the FRC stabilizes and smoothes the gas exchange.

Despite its beneficial physiological aspects, RV presents a measurement difficulty. When body composition is determined by hydrostatic (underwater) weighing (see Chapter 7), RV must be measured or estimated. Residual air makes the body more buoyant; if not accounted for, it would reduce the underwater weight. The less an individual weighs underwater, the higher the measured percentage of body fat. Thus, if RV were not accounted for, it would erroneously increase the measurement of fat. This is the most common reason for determining RV in exercise physiology. Sometimes RV is estimated from VC; however, it is more accurate if measured directly either outside or inside the tank (Wilmore, 1969). RV is estimated as 24% of VC for males and 28% of VC for females.

Vital capacity (VC) is simply the largest amount of air that can be exhaled following a maximal inhalation. The common way of testing VC is to ask the individual to inhale maximally and then forcefully exhale all of the air as quickly as possible. Because the exhalation is forced, the designation forced vital capacity, FVC, is used.

Dynamic Lung Volumes

When volumes are measured at specified time intervals (usually 1 and 3 seconds) during a forced VC test, the name is changed to *forced expiratory volume*, specifically, FEV_1 and FEV_3. This provides information not only about the total volume of air moved but also the rate of flow. Normal healthy individuals should be able to exhale at least 80% of their FVC in 1 second; this measurement is labeled FEV_1. FEV_1 values below 65–70% indicate moderate to severe restriction to airflow (Adams, 1994).

The second commonly measured dynamic lung volume is a test of ventilatory capacity called *maximal voluntary*

must know for the test

VC = max in, max out
RV = max out
TLC = max in

Inspiratory reserve volume IRV: *normal* *spiro*
The greatest amount of air that can be inspired at the end of a normal inspiration

Tidal volume V_T: *spiro*
The amount of air that is inspired or expired in a normal breath

Expiratory reserve volume ERV: *spiro*
The greatest amount of air that can be expired at the end of a normal expiration

Residual volume RV:
The amount of air that is left in the lungs following a maximal exhalation

IRV   IC

VT

ERV

FRC

RV   RV

VC

TLC

Inspiratory capacity IC: *spirometer*
The greatest amount of air that can be inspired from a resting expiratory level
$IC = IRV + V_T$

Vital capacity VC: *spirometer*
The greatest amount of air that can be exhaled following a maximal inhalation
$VC = IRV + V_T + ERV$

Functional residual capacity FRC:
The amount of air left in the lungs at the end of a normal expiration
$FRC = ERV + RV$

Total lung capacity TLC:
The greatest amount of air that can be contained in the lungs
$TLC = VC + RV$
$= IC + FRC$
$= IRV + V_T + ERV + RV$

FIGURE 9.6 Static Lung Volume Spirogram.
TLC can be subdivided into four volumes (IRV, V_T, ERV, and RV) and into three other capacities (IC, FRC, and VC). From the normal resting depth of inspiration and expiration (indicated by the wavy line moving up and down, respectively, in the box labeled V_T), both inspiration and expiration can be expanded into the IRV and ERV until all possible air is inhaled and exhaled (VC). The RV remains in the lungs at all times.

ventilation (MVV). In this test, a timed maximal ventilation of either 12 or 15 seconds is recorded and then multiplied by 5 (if 12 seconds) or 4 (if 15 seconds) to extrapolate to the volume that could be ventilated in 1 minute. This value is usually higher than what can actually be achieved during exercise in untrained individuals, but it gives a rough estimate of exercise ventilation potential. Low values may reflect airway resistance and poorly conditioned or poorly functioning ventilatory muscles.

Both FEV and MVV tests are often used as screening tests before maximal exercise tests of oxygen consumption.

Spirometry

All of the lung volumes and capacities described previously—except for TLC, FRC, and RV—can be measured using a spirometer. Historically, most spirometers had an inverted container, called a bell, that fit inside another container usually filled with water. When air is exhaled into the tube, the bell is pushed up; inhalation moves the bell down. In this way, the volumes of air inspired and expired can be measured, and the various volumes, capacities, and flow rates can be calculated. A spirometer that

measures air volumes over water is called a wet spirometer. Newer dry spirometers are often digital and do not use water (**Figure 9.7**).

Gas Dilution

TLC, FRC, and RV cannot be measured by simple spirometry because these involve air that cannot be exhaled voluntarily from the lungs. Thus, it is necessary to determine the volume of air that remains in the lungs. The most common technique for this measurement is gas dilution. One technique involves the dilution of an inert, insoluble, foreign gas such as helium (He). A second technique involves the dilution of medical grade oxygen and the measurement of nitrogen (N_2) and is called the nitrogen

Total Lung Capacity (TLC) The greatest amount of air that the lungs can contain.

Residual Volume (RV) The amount of air left in the lungs following a maximal exhalation.

Vital Capacity (VC) The greatest amount of air that can be exhaled following a maximal inhalation.

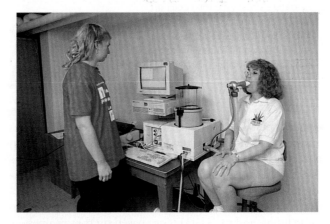

FIGURE 9.7 A Spirometer.

The Relationship between Forced Expiratory Volume and Health

Evidence is mounting that forced expiratory volume in one second (FEV_1) is related to health.

An epidemiological study by Schunemann et al. (2000) explored the link between low values of FEV_1 (expressed as a *percentage of predicted FEV₁* [FEV_1%pred]) and mortality (death from all causes).

A randomly selected sample of 554 adult men and 641 adult women were part of a 29-year follow-up. During that time, 302 (54.5%) of the men and 278 (43.4%) of the women died. Only 39 of these deaths (29 males and 10 females) were directly attributed to respiratory disease. Nevertheless, pulmonary function was a significant predictor of all-cause mortality: Each 1% increase in FEV_1%pred (pred = predicted) was associated with a 1–1.5% decrease in all-cause mortality. The risk of an early death for individuals scoring in the lowest quintile (≤ 80.2 FEV_1%pred for males and ≤ 80.5 FEV_1%pred for females) was approximately twice as great (2.24 for males and 1.81 for females) as the risk in the highest quintile (≥ 108.8 FEV_1%pred for males and ≥ 113.6 FEV_1%pred for females).

The reasons for these results are unknown. It was initially thought that FEV_1%pred was simply a proxy for smoking status, but other research has shown that this association is independent of smoking status. Possible explanations for the association include the following:

1. Impaired pulmonary function could lead to a decreased tolerance against environmental toxins.

2. Oxidative stress (see the Focus on Application box in Chapter 5 for a discussion of oxidative stress), which is negatively related to FEV_1%pred, could adversely affect the overall health status. Conversely, reduced pulmonary function could be an underlying factor responsible for increased oxidative stress.

3. Low FEV_1 values may simply adversely affect physical activity patterns, such that inactivity is the true causal factor.

Exploring the idea of environmental toxins, a study by Aronson et al. (2006) investigated whether a decline in lung function (defined as FEV_1) in apparently healthy individuals was associated with systemic inflammation as measured by C-reactive protein (CRP). The immune system and inflammation are detailed in Chapter 22, but briefly, the lungs are a major location for immune cell function. During breathing and gas exchange, the lungs must protect themselves against a variety of infectious agents, noxious gases, and various particulates (Look ahead to Figure 9.13 and note the macrophage immune cell). Thus, the investigators speculated that lung function could indicate an immune response occurring, along with resultant low-grade inflammation, before any overt disease appeared. Participants were 1131 individuals without known pulmonary disease. Median values for CRP by FEV_1%pred are presented in the graph for smokers and nonsmokers. The lowest quartile (<93% FEV_1pred) contained 96 individuals with below normal (defined as < 80% FEV_1pred) values. The association between CRP and FEV_1 was highly significant and remained so even after adjustment for age, sex, body mass index, metabolic abnormalities, and cardiorespiratory fitness level. These results indicate that systemic inflammation may be linked to early declines in pulmonary function.

These combined results may mean that FEV_1 can be used as a convenient health assessment tool.

Sources: Aronson, D., I. Roterman, M. Yigia, et al.: Inverse association between pulmonary function and C-reactive protein in apparently healthy subjects. *American Journal of Respiratory and Critical Care Medicine.* 174(6):626–632 (2006); Schunemann, H. J., J. Dorn, B. J. B. Grant, W. Winkelstein, & M. Trevisan: Pulmonary function is a long-term predictor of mortality in the general population: 29-year follow-up of the Buffalo Health Study. *Chest.* 118(3):656–664 (2000).

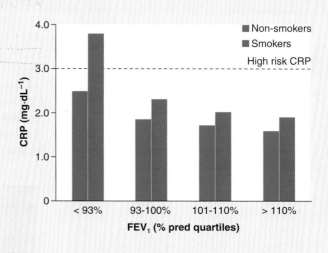

washout technique. In each case, the participant inhales a known volume of either helium or oxygen and then rebreathes the gas mixture. Helium ultimately equilibrates with the gases in the lungs and spirometer, and calculations are based on the dilution of the original helium mixture. Oxygen dilutes the original nitrogen concentration in the lungs, and calculations are based on these values.

Standardization

The respiratory measurements detailed above are performed under ambient or atmospheric conditions. This means that the temperature measured is the temperature in the room or in the spirometer just before testing, and the pressure is the barometric pressure of the room. Because the air is exhaled from inside the human body, which is a wet environment, the air is saturated with water vapor. These measurements are therefore designated as *ATPS*: ambient (A) temperature (T) and pressure (P) saturated (S). Because ATPS volumes vary by environmental conditions, they must be converted to standardized conditions for purposes of comparison and assessment. Standardization is based on the known effects of pressure, temperature, and water vapor on gas volumes. **Figure 9.8** illustrates these three effects, which are as follows:

1. The volume of a given quantity of gas is inversely related to the pressure exerted on it when the temperature remains constant. This effect is described by Boyle's law and was discussed previously in the section on the mechanics of breathing. As shown in **Figure 9.8A**, when pressure is reduced from 760 to 600 mmHg, 5 L of air expands to 6.3 L. The reverse is also true. If the pressure increases from 600 to 760 mmHg, the volume is reduced from 6.3 to 5.0 L (Slonim and Hamilton, 1976; West, 2005).

2. The volume of a given quantity of gas is directly related to the temperature of the gas when the pressure remains constant. This relationship is described by *Charles's law*. As shown in **Figure 9.8B**, if the temperature is reduced from 37°C to 0°C, the volume of the gas is reduced from 5 to 4.4 L. The reverse is also true. If the temperature rises from 0°C to 37°C, the volume also rises from 4.4 to 5.0 L.

3. Water molecules evaporate into a gas, such as air, and are responsible for part of the pressure of that gas. The amount of pressure accounted for by the water vapor is related exponentially to temperature. As shown in **Figure 9.8C**, when a volume of air is converted from saturated to dry air at a constant temperature, the volume is reduced from 5.0 to 4.7 L. Once again, the reverse is also true. If a gas volume goes from dry to wet at a given temperature, the volume increases (Slonim and Hamilton, 1976; West, 2005).

The numbers for temperature and pressure in **Figure 9.8** were not chosen arbitrarily. They are involved in the two standardized conditions to which ATPS lung volumes are converted: BTPS and STPD. The abbreviation *BTPS* means body (B) temperature (T) (37°C), ambient pressure (P), and fully saturated (S) with water vapor. Remember that in its passage through the conduction zone, the air is both warmed and humidified to achieve these values. When converting from ATPS to BTPS, the temperature increases and the pressure, adjusted for the effects of temperature on water vapor pressure, decreases. Because of Charles's law (an increase in temperature causes an increase in volume) and Boyle's law (a decrease in pressure causes an increase in volume), the volume expressed as BTPS has to be larger than the volume originally measured as ATPS.

BTPS is typically used when the anatomical space from which the volume of gas originated is of primary importance. Thus, most lung volumes and capacities are conventionally expressed as BTPS.

STPD means standard (S) temperature (T) (0°) and pressure (P) (760 mmHg), dry (D). The STPD volume is smaller than the originally measured ATPS volume because under typical testing conditions, temperature decreases from ATPS (~20°C) to STPD (0°C) and, by Charles's law, so does volume. Unless the testing is done at sea level, pressure increases from ATPS (variable, but around 735–745 mmHg before considering the influence of water vapor) to STPD (760 mmHg), and according to Boyle's law, volume decreases. Going from wet to dry conditions also decreases the volume.

STPD volumes are used when it is necessary to know the amount of gas molecules present. Inspired or expired minute ventilation is typically converted and reported in STPD conditions, although sometimes it may be expressed as BTPS.

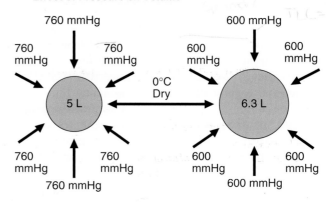

A Effect of Pressure on Volume

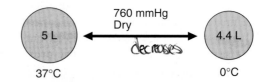

B Effect of Temperature on Volume

C Effect of Water Vapor on Volume

FIGURE 9.8 Effects of Pressure, Temperature, and Water Vapor on Air Volume.
A. The volume of a given quantity of a gas is inversely related to the pressure exerted on it, if the temperature remains constant (Boyle's law). **B.** The volume of a given quantity of gas is directly related to the temperature of the gas if the pressure remains constant (Charles's law). **C.** The volume of a gas increases as the content of water vapor increases.

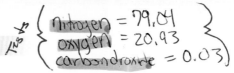

(handwritten note at top right)

Test
{ nitrogen = 79.04
oxygen = 20.93
carbondioxide = 0.03 }

Partial Pressure of a Gas: Dalton's Law

Dry, unpolluted atmospheric air is a mixture of gases including oxygen, carbon dioxide, nitrogen, argon, and krypton. Because the last three are considered inert in humans, they are generally grouped together and labeled simply as nitrogen (the largest component). Thus, air is said to be composed of 79.04% nitrogen, 20.93% oxygen, and 0.03% carbon dioxide. These percentages are also referred to as fractions of each gas and are given in decimal form: 0.7904 nitrogen, 0.2093 oxygen, and 0.0003 carbon dioxide. Another way to describe the composition of a gas mixture such as air is by the partial pressures exerted by each gas (Leff and Schumacker, 1993).

All gases exert pressure. In a mixture of gases, the total pressure is the sum of the pressure of individual gases making up the mixture. Total pressure is standardized to the sea-level barometric pressure of 760 mmHg, but at altitudes above sea level, the actual barometric pressure, P_B, must be used. The **partial pressure of a gas (P_G)** is that portion of the total pressure exerted by any single gas in the mixture. The partial pressure of any gas is proportional to its percentage in the total gas mixture. These relationships are described by *Dalton's law of partial pressures*.

The partial pressure of any gas is the product of the total pressure and the fraction of the gas (expressed as a decimal).

9.4   partial pressure of a gas (mmHg) = total pressure (mmHg) × fraction of the gas

or

$$P_G = P_B \times F_G$$

(handwritten) Partial pressure of gas = barometric pressure × fraction of gas (F_G) (P_B) (P_G)

For example, the standardized partial pressure of nitrogen, PN_2, is 760 × 0.7904 mmHg = 600.7 mmHg.

Substituting the appropriate fractions, calculate the PO_2 and PCO_2 of dry atmospheric air. **Table 9.1**, column (a), shows the answers. For extra practice, also calculate the partial pressure of dry atmospheric air at altitude and of alveolar air. Look first at **Table 9.1**, columns (a) and

(b). Notice that the gas percentages are the same at sea level and at altitude, in this case 4268 m (14,000 ft). These percentages remain the same at any altitude. Conversely, the barometric pressure (P_B) is lower at both the selected altitude and any other altitude in comparison with sea level. Exactly how much lower than sea level the P_B is depends on how high the altitude is. At 4268 m (14,000 ft), P_B is 440 mmHg. As the altitude increases, the barometric pressure decreases. Now, compare **Table 9.1**, columns (a) and (c). Notice that now the barometric pressure values are the same; that is, they are both standardized to 760 mmHg. However, the fractions of the gases are different. This difference between alveolar air and atmospheric air occurs because the percentage of oxygen in the alveoli is decreased by diffusion of oxygen into the capillary blood. Similarly, the percentage of carbon dioxide is increased by the diffusion of carbon dioxide out of the capillary blood. In addition, water vapor now occupies a percentage of the total air mixture. At normal body temperature (37°C), water vapor exerts a pressure of 47 mmHg. This value must be subtracted from 760 mmHg prior to multiplying by the fraction of each gas to determine the partial pressure of each gas.

Knowledge of the partial pressure of gases is important for at least two reasons. The first is that the partial pressures of oxygen (PO_2) in the blood and more specifically the partial pressure of carbon dioxide (PCO_2) help to regulate pulmonary ventilation to bring air into the lungs. The PO_2 and PCO_2 are sensed by various chemoreceptors and influence respiratory centers in the brain (see full discussion later in this chapter). The second reason is that both external and internal respiration depend on pressure gradients.

Regulation of Pulmonary Ventilation

Breathing, or pulmonary ventilation, results from inspiratory and expiratory muscle contraction and relaxation. The muscle action—and therefore the rate, depth, and

(handwritten note at bottom left) ⚹ Know for the test

TABLE 9.1	Approximate Gas Partial Pressures in Ambient Air and Selected Ventilatory and Respiratory Sites								
	(a) Dry Atmospheric Air, Sea Level			**(b) Dry Atmospheric Air, Altitude = (4268 m) 14,000 ft (Pike's Peak)**			**(c) Alveolar Air, Sea Level**		
Gases	%	P_B (mmHg)	P (mmHg)	%	P_B (mmHg)	P (mmHg)	%	P_B (mmHg)	P (mmHg)
O_2	20.93	760	159	20.93	440	92.0	13.7–14.6	760 − 47 =713	104–98*
CO_2	0.03	760	0.3	0.03	440	0.1	5.3	760 − 47= 713	40
N_2	79.04	760	600.7	79.04	440	348.0	78.7–79.8	760 − 47 = 713	561–569
H_2O	0.00	760	0.0	0.00	440	0.0			47†
						440			760

*Owing to minor variations in percentage, the PO_2 in alveolar air is often rounded to 100 mmHg.

†Assumes a body temperature of 37°C and PH_2O of 47 mmHg, which must be subtracted from 760 mmHg before determining PO_2, PCO_2, PN_2.

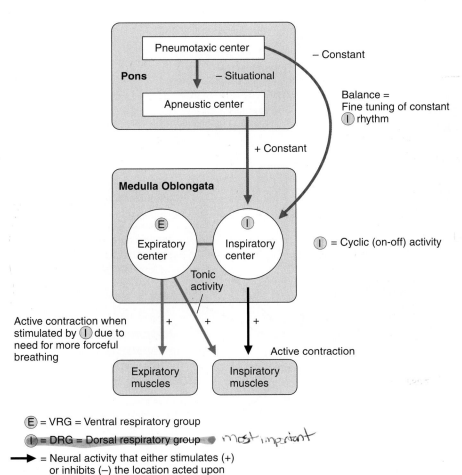

FIGURE 9.9 Brain Stem Control of Pulmonary Ventilation.
Schematic representation of the respiratory centers that control ventilation.

at rest = 12–15 br·min

E = VRG = Ventral respiratory group

I = DRG = Dorsal respiratory group ● *most important*

→ = Neural activity that either stimulates (+) or inhibits (−) the location acted upon

rhythm of breathing—is controlled by the brain and nervous system and is tightly coupled to the body's overall need for oxygen and the subsequent production of energy and carbon dioxide. The coordinated control of respiratory muscles, especially during exercise, is a very complex process that is not yet fully understood.

The Respiratory Centers

There are four respiratory centers in the brain that function together to control breathing; two are located in the medulla oblongata and two are located in the pons. These four centers are schematically diagramed in **Figure 9.9**.

The two respiratory centers located within the medulla oblongata of the brain stem are composed of anatomically distinct neural networks. The inspiratory center (I), also called the dorsal respiratory group, is the most important. The other center is the expiratory center (E), sometimes

Partial Pressure of a Gas (P_G) The pressure exerted by an individual gas in a mixture; determined by multiplying the fraction of the gas by the total barometric pressure.
Respiratory Cycle One inspiration and expiration.
Eupnea Normal respiration rate and rhythm.

called the ventral respiratory group. The nerves of the inspiratory center depolarize spontaneously in a cyclic, rhythmical on-off pattern. During the "on" portion of the cycle, nerve impulses traveling via motor neurons in the phrenic nerve stimulate the diaphragm and the external intercostal inspiratory muscles to contract. Inhalation occurs when the thoracic cavity is enlarged and intrathoracic pressure decreases. During the "off" portion of the cycle, the nerve impulses are interrupted, the inspiratory muscles relax, and exhalation occurs. Without outside influence and at rest, the inspiratory center causes a respiratory cycle of approximately 2 seconds for inspiration and 3 seconds for exhalation (for a rate of 12–15 br·min⁻¹). This normal respiratory rate and oscillating rhythm is known as eupnea (Leff and Schumacker, 1993).

The expiratory center is quiet during normal resting breathing. However, it causes active contraction of the expiratory muscles (internal intercostals and abdominals) when forceful breathing is required, such as during moderate to heavy exercise (Leff and Schumacker, 1993; West, 2005).

Two neural centers in the pons area of the brain stem (pneumotaxic and apneustic centers) also act as respiratory centers. They seem to be important for ensuring that the transitions between inhalation and exhalation are smooth. The pneumotaxic center constantly transmits

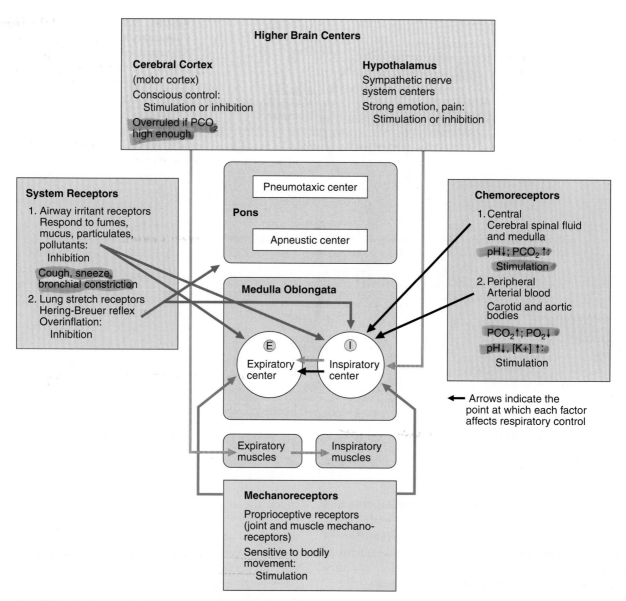

FIGURE 9.10 Anatomical Sensors and Factors That Influence the Control of Pulmonary Ventilation.
Schematic representation of the pathways of action of factors influencing the brain stem control of ventilation.

inhibitory (indicated on the diagram by a minus sign, –) neural impulses directly to the inspiratory center and situationally to the apneustic center. This limits or in some cases shortens inspiration and promotes expiration—thus, fine tuning the breathing pattern and preventing lung overinflation. The apneustic center continually stimulates (indicated on the diagram by a plus sign, +) the inspiratory center unless inhibited situationally by the pneumotaxic center (Leff and Schumacker, 1993; West, 2005).

Anatomical Sensors and Factors Affecting Control of Pulmonary Ventilation

The inspiratory, expiratory, pneumotaxic, and apneustic centers are influenced by a number of factors through a variety of anatomical sensors that are important during exercise (Dempsey et al., 1985).

Figure 9.10 schematically presents the major factors and where each factor operates. Without outside influences, the rate (frequency) of breathing and the depth (tidal volume) of breathing exhibit the greatest changes. A disruption in rhythm rarely occurs except under voluntary control (Guyton and Hall, 2011; Leff and Schumacker, 1993; Whipp et al., 1982).

Higher Brain Centers

Both the hypothalamus and the cerebral cortex can influence breathing. The first operates involuntarily and the second voluntarily.

HYPOTHALAMUS The sympathetic nervous system centers in the hypothalamus are activated by pain or strong emotions. In turn, they send neural messages to the respiratory centers. The reaction can either stimulate or inhibit breathing. Hyperventilation by an individual who is emotionally upset is an example of hypothalamic stimulation. Feeling your breath taken away when you jump into very cold water exemplifies hypothalamic inhibition. This hypothalamic control mechanism may be very important for increasing respiration on initiation of movement and sustaining the increase throughout the duration of an activity (Eldridge, 1994).

CEREBRAL CORTEX Cerebral control of breathing originates in the motor cortex. Such voluntary control is important to musicians, singers, and athletes such as swimmers, weight lifters, archers, and shooters, to name just a few. The motor cortex may also operate such that the conscious anticipation of exercise unconsciously increases ventilation. Neural impulses from the motor cortex pass directly to the respiratory muscles, bypassing the control centers in the medulla. Voluntary control is limited, however (Leff and Schumacker, 1993; West, 2005). If you doubt this, take a reading break at the end of this paragraph and jog in place at a fast pace for 3 minutes. Then sit down immediately and try holding your breath for 1 minute. If you can do that, great; but even if you can, you will probably feel a desire to breathe. More than likely, the automatic drive to breathe will overrule your conscious signal not to, and at some point before the end of the minute, you will gasp for air.

Systemic Receptors

The lungs themselves contain several types of receptors that provide sensory information to the respiratory control centers and result in reflex action. Chief among them are irritant receptors and stretch receptors (Leff and Schumacker, 1993; Martin et al., 1979; West, 2005). Both of these receptors are more important for protection than for regulating normal resting or exercise ventilation.

IRRITANT RECEPTORS Irritant receptors within the conduction zone respond to foreign substances such as chemicals, noxious gases, cold air, mucus, dust, and other pollutant particulates. They cause a reflex response. Depending on the irritating substance and the anatomical location, the response may be a cough, a sneeze, or a bronchial constriction, all of which disrupt the normal breathing pattern (Leff and Schumacker, 1993; West, 2005).

STRETCH RECEPTORS Stretch receptors in the airway smooth muscle respond to deep, fast inflation. Increases in the lung volume stimulate the stretch receptors, which send inhibitory impulses to both the apneustic center and the inspiratory center. As a result, respiratory frequency is slowed because of the increased expiratory time (inflation reflex). An opposing deflation reflex tends to increase inspiratory activity. These reflexes are called the *Hering-Breuer reflexes*. The threshold for these is quite high. They do not appear to function in adults at rest and play a minor role in exercise only if tidal volume exceeds 1 L (Leff and Schumacher, 1993; West, 2005).

Mechanoreceptors

Specific mechanoreceptors called proprioceptors exist in skeletal muscles (including respiratory muscles) and joint capsules. These receptors provide information to a variety of sites in the brain about movement and body position in space. Input from these receptors probably plays some minor role in the stimulation of respiration during exercise, but they are not involved in respiration during rest (Leff and Schumacker, 1993).

Chemoreceptors

Chemoreceptor sensors that respond to fluctuations in chemical substances important to respiration are found in two major anatomical locations. Central chemoreceptors are located in the medulla oblongata (but not in the respiratory control centers); these are sensitive to an increased partial pressure of carbon dioxide ($\uparrow PCO_2$) and increased acidity ($\downarrow pH$). Peripheral chemoreceptors are located in large arteries, specifically, at the aortic body and the carotid body. In addition to being sensitive to $\uparrow PCO_2$ and $\downarrow pH$, these receptors are also sensitive to a decrease in the partial pressure of oxygen ($\downarrow PO_2$) and an increase in the concentration of potassium ions ($\uparrow[K^+]$). Each of these factors is explained in the following subsections.

INFLUENCE OF PO₂ The peripheral carotid body chemoreceptors are the main oxygen sensors. Under normal circumstances, a decline in PO_2 has very little impact on minute ventilation other than enhancing sensitivity to PCO_2 (Leff and Schumacker, 1993).

Figure 9.11 shows that from the normal arterial PO_2 (PaO_2) of 95 mmHg (**Table 9.1**) to a value of about 60 mmHg, minute ventilation does not change if the arterial PCO_2 ($PaCO_2$) remains normal (~36–42 mmHg). However, if the PaO_2 decreases below 50 mmHg, minute ventilation is stimulated to rise exponentially. Such a large decrease is not a normal physiological event at sea level, even at very heavy levels of exercise, because the PaO_2 mmHg is maintained within narrow limits. However, PaO_2 may fall below 50 mmHg at altitudes at or above 4268 m (14,000 ft), triggering the graphically depicted increase in minute ventilation (Leff and Schumacker, 1993; West, 2005).

INFLUENCE OF PCO₂ Both the central and the peripheral chemoreceptors are sensitive to an increase in the $PaCO_2$. However, the peripheral chemoreceptors respond more directly to PCO_2 than the central chemoreceptors do. The central chemoreceptors respond initially to rising PCO_2 levels but thereafter primarily to the effect these rising PCO_2 levels have on pH. The ventilatory response

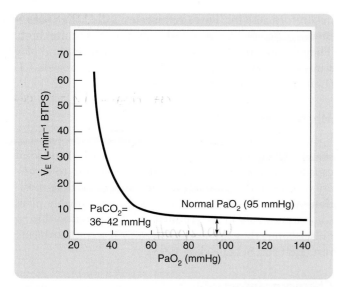

FIGURE 9.11 The Effect of Arterial PO₂ (PaO₂) on Minute Ventilation.
At a normal $PaCO_2$ of 36–42 mmHg, reduced PaO_2 does not stimulate ventilation until the value of PaO_2 is less than 60 mmHg. *Source*: Leff, A. R. & P. T. Schumacker: *Respiratory Physiology: Basics and Applications*. Philadelphia, PA: W. B. Saunders (1993). Reprinted by permission.

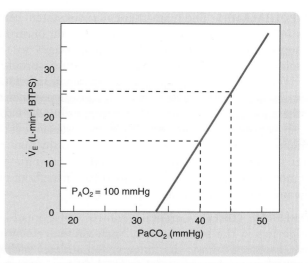

FIGURE 9.12 The Ventilatory Response to Carbon Dioxide.
At a normal P_AO_2 of approximately 100 mmHg, a rise in $PaCO_2$ from the normal value of 40 mmHg to just 45 mmHg almost doubles pulmonary ventilation (from ~15 to 26 L·min⁻¹, as indicated by the dashed lines intersecting the y-axis), showing how sensitive ventilation is to $PaCO_2$.
Source: Modified from Nielsen, M. & H. Smith: Studies on the regulation of respiration in acute hypoxia. *Acta Physiologica Scandinavica*. 4:293–313 (1951). Reprinted by permission.

to PCO_2 is split 40–60% between peripheral and central chemoreceptors, respectively. At rest, the regulation of pH in the cerebrospinal fluid (CSF) is the primary control mechanism (by the central receptors) of ventilation.

Figure 9.12 shows the influence of increasing arterial PCO_2 values on minute ventilation. Even a small deviation from the normal value of $PaCO_2$ of approximately 40 mmHg (**Table 9.1**) causes a large rectilinear increase in minute ventilation when arterial PO_2 is maintained at approximately normal levels (~95 mmHg). The steepness and the immediacy of this rectilinear increase indicate that ventilation is much more sensitive to an increase in PCO_2 than to a decrease in PO_2. Hence, $PaCO_2$ is the strongest regulating factor. An increase as small as 5 mmHg in $PaCO_2$ increases ventilation by approximately 67%. The ventilatory response to CO_2 is reduced in sleep, with increasing age, in trained athletes, and in underwater divers (West, 2005).

Holding your breath will cause an increase in the arterial PCO_2, called *hypercapnia*. Sometimes an excess of CO_2 in the blood can lead to labored or difficult ventilation, which is termed **dyspnea**. Excess CO_2 is not the only possible cause of dyspnea, and this is not a normal exercise response. A buildup of CO_2 is the reason your conscious control of respiration was overruled if you tried not to breathe after the 3-minute jog in place earlier. Conversely, **hyperventilation**—defined as increased pulmonary ventilation, especially ventilation that exceeds metabolic requirements—decreases PCO_2 (called *hypocapnia*) and the drive to breathe. Hyperventilation may be caused by

an altitude response to a decreased PO_2, an involuntary response during an anxiety attack, or a conscious attempt to extend breath-holding time.

INFLUENCE OF pH As with an increase in arterial PCO_2, both the peripheral and the central chemoreceptors are sensitive to the decreases in pH. The pH level is partially related to the CO_2 level. When CO_2 is hydrated, it forms carbonic acid (H_2CO_3), which degrades readily into hydrogen ions (H^+) and bicarbonate (HCO_3^-) according to the following reactions:

$$CO_2 + H_2O \leftrightarrow H_2CO_3 \leftrightarrow H^+ + HCO_3^-$$

Carbon dioxide + water $\leftrightarrow$ carbonic acid $\leftrightarrow$ hydrogen ions + bicarbonate

In blood, the H^+ can be buffered, but if that capacity is exceeded, any change in arterial pH is detected by the aortic and carotid bodies. The brain and the spinal cord are bathed by a protein-free solution known as the cerebrospinal fluid (CSF). CO_2 easily diffuses across the blood-brain barrier and into the CSF. Because brain cells also produce CO_2 and because CSF has no protein buffers, the pH of the CSF is slightly more acidic than that of blood. An excess of H^+ in the CSF acts directly on the central chemoreceptors to increase respiration; a decrease in H^+ suppresses respiration.

All changes in pH, of course, are not caused by CO_2. For example, during high-intensity exercise, large quantities of lactate accumulate. If the blood's ability to buffer the resultant H^+ is exceeded, pH decreases and respiration increases.

FOCUS ON APPLICATION: *Clinically Relevant*
Decreased PCO$_2$ and Drowning

The decrement in PCO$_2$ with hyperventilation can have serious consequences. Many people know that hyperventilating can extend breath-holding time but erroneously believe it does so because more oxygen is taken in. They are unaware that it is CO$_2$ levels that are changing (being blown off), not O$_2$, and that respiration is more sensitive to PCO$_2$ changes than to PO$_2$ changes. Craig (1976) summarized 58 cases of loss of consciousness during underwater swimming and diving following hyperventilation. Of these 58 cases, 23 (40%) ended as fatalities, with most occurring in guarded pools. Because an individual continues patterned motor activity (swimming) for a short time after loss of consciousness caused by a lack of oxygen to the brain, these life-threatening

cases are difficult for a lifeguard to detect quickly. Beginning swimmers frustrated by trying to coordinate their arms, legs, and breathing who simply put their head in the water and try to go as far as possible without breathing are also vulnerable. As a

result of these findings, it is recommended that underwater swimming be limited to one length of a standard 25-yd or 25-m pool.

Source: Craig (1976).

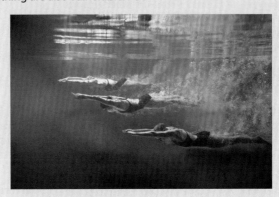

INFLUENCE OF [K⁺] Of the chemical factors mentioned so far (↓PO$_2$, ↑PCO$_2$, and ↓pH), only ↓pH changes enough during exercise to cause the needed increase in ventilation known as hyperpnea. **Hyperpnea is increased pulmonary** ventilation that matches an increased metabolic demand. An increase in the concentration of potassium [K⁺] may be another factor that changes sufficiently in exercise to increase ventilation. Potassium moves from the working muscles to blood during exercise of any intensity. This increased [K⁺], called *hyperkalemia*, directly stimulates the carotid bodies. At rest, [K⁺] is not a factor (Eldridge, 1994; Forster and Pau, 1994; Nye, 1994).

Figure 9.10 earlier schematically depicted factors that control the rate and depth of ventilation. It would be logical to assume that changes in the arterial PO$_2$ and PCO$_2$ occur during exercise and have the primary role in

control. However, this is not what happens. Neither PO$_2$ nor PCO$_2$ change enough, especially early in exercise or at low to moderate to heavy intensities in untrained individuals, to play a major role in ventilatory control during exercise. Exactly which factor is most important is not known precisely. Changes may take place in the sensitivity of the medullary respiratory control centers themselves during exercise. Neural messages from the motor cortex, muscle proprioceptors, and hypothalamic sympathetic nervous system activity, as well as increases in the hydrogen ion and potassium ion concentrations, all appear to have a role during exercise (Eldridge, 1994; West, 2005).

Gas Exchange and Transport

Gas Exchange: Henry's Law

As mentioned previously, knowledge of the partial pressure of gases is important for two reasons. First, the partial pressures of gases play a role in the control of pulmonary ventilation, as discussed above. Second, the movement of O$_2$ and CO$_2$ between the alveoli and the capillaries (external respiration) and between the capillaries and the tissues (internal respiration) occurs by the process of diffusion. **Diffusion is the tendency of gaseous, liquid, or solid molecules to move from an area of higher concentration to an area of lower concentration by constant random action.** Diffusion can occur only if there is a pressure gradient (a difference in the partial pressures of

---

Dyspnea Labored or difficult breathing.

Hyperventilation Increased pulmonary ventilation, especially ventilation that exceeds metabolic requirements; carbon dioxide is blown off, leading to a decrease in its partial pressure in arterial blood.

Hyperpnea Increased pulmonary ventilation that matches an increased metabolic demand, such as during exercise.

Diffusion The tendency of gaseous, liquid, or solid molecules to move from an area of higher concentration to an area of lower concentration by constant random action.

the gas) between the capillary and the tissue. Gases diffuse down the pressure gradient from a higher pressure area to a lower pressure area. The rate of diffusion depends on the magnitude of the pressure gradient (millimeters of mercury at the high end minus millimeters of mercury at the low end), the surface area available for diffusion, the thickness of the barrier between the two locations, and the solubility (ability to be dissolved) of the gas in the barrier liquid. *Henry's law* states that when a mixture of gases is in contact with a liquid, each gas dissolves in the liquid in proportion to its partial pressure and solubility until equilibrium is achieved and the gas partial pressures are equal in both locations (Leff and Schumacker, 1993; Martin et al., 1979).   Henry's law

External Respiration

External respiration is the movement of gases at the alveolar-pulmonary capillary level (**Figure 9.13**). Specifically, oxygen diffuses from the alveoli into the pulmonary capillaries, and carbon dioxide diffuses from the pulmonary capillary into the alveoli. This exchange is diagramed in **Figure 9.14A** and **D**.

Remember that pulmonary circulation originates from the right ventricle of the heart. By definition, an artery is a vessel carrying blood away from the heart. Unlike systemic

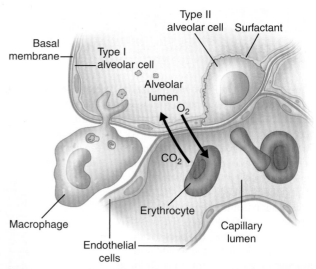

FIGURE 9.13 Anatomical Diagram of External Respiration.
Source: Seifter J., A. Ratner, & D. Sloane: *Concepts in Medical Physiology*. Philadelphia, PA: Lippincott Williams & Wilkins (2005).

arteries, the pulmonary artery carries partially deoxygenated blood. The pulmonary arteries quickly branch into capillaries that parallel the alveoli. While they are small, the capillaries do have a definable length.

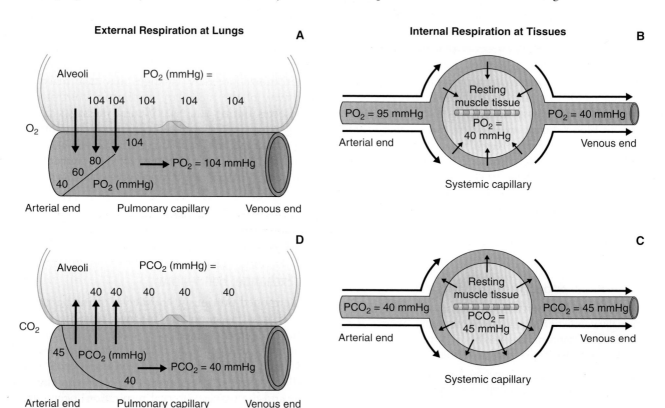

FIGURE 9.14 Oxygen and Carbon Dioxide Exchange.
Gas exchange takes place at two anatomical locations: the alveoli-pulmonary capillary interface (external respiration) and the systemic capillary-tissue interface (internal respiration). **A.** External respiration for oxygen. **B.** Internal respiration for oxygen. **C.** Internal respiration for carbon dioxide. **D.** External respiration for carbon dioxide.

At the arterial end of the capillary, PO_2 in the alveoli (P_AO_2) is high (98–104 mmHg) (**Table 9.1**), and PO_2 in the pulmonary capillary is low (40 mmHg). Oxygen diffuses down the pressure gradient until equilibrium is reached at approximately 104 mmHg. Note in **Figure 9.14A** that this equalization of pressure occurs within the first third of the capillary length.

Refer again to **Table 9.1** and **Figure 9.14A** and **B**. In **Figure 9.14B**, notice that PaO_2 (systemic arterial blood) is listed as 95 mmHg, not as 98–104 mmHg as given in **Table 9.1** and **Figure 9.14A**. The lower value in the systemic arterial blood (95 mmHg) versus the venous pulmonary blood (104 mmHg) results because the fully oxygenated blood in the pulmonary vein is diluted with partially oxygenated venous blood (PvO_2 = 40 mmHg) from the bronchial vein as blood from both the veins flows into the left atrium. Remember that the bronchial artery, the capillaries, and the vein provide blood to and return it from the lungs as part of the systemic circulation and so have the normal systemic gas contents and pressures (**Figure 9.4**). Although blood from the bronchial vein amounts to only about 2% of the total blood returning to the left atrium, it is sufficient to bring the PaO_2 of systemic arterial blood down to approximately 95 mmHg (Guyton and Hall, 2011).

At the same time that oxygen is diffusing from the alveoli to the pulmonary capillaries, carbon dioxide diffuses from the pulmonary capillaries to the alveoli. At the arterial end of the capillary, PCO_2 in the capillary is high (about 45 mmHg) and PCO_2 in the alveoli is low (40 mmHg) (**Table 9.1**). Carbon dioxide also diffuses from high to low pressure down the gradient until equilibrium is reached. Note in **Figure 9.14D** that this equalization of pressure occurs within the first third of the capillary length. Note also that the pressure gradient for CO_2 is not nearly as steep (5 mmHg) as it is for O_2 (64 mmHg). Carbon dioxide diffuses with a lesser pressure gradient because it is more soluble.

Remember that each gas moves down its own concentration gradient, regardless of the concentration of any other gas present.

The major variables that are important in external respiration are alveolar ventilation ($\dot{V}_A$), the partial pressure of oxygen at the alveoli (P_AO_2), partial pressure of oxygen in the arterial blood (PaO_2), oxygen or partial pressure of oxygen gradient between the alveoli and the arteries (A-a) PO_2, the percent saturation of arterial blood with oxygen ($SaO_2\%$), and the partial pressure of carbon dioxide at the alveoli (P_ACO_2).

Internal Respiration

Internal respiration is the movement of gases at the capillary-tissue level. Although the tissue can be any tissue, it is particularly relevant for exercise physiology students to think of the tissue as skeletal muscle tissue. Internal respiration is diagrammed in **Figure 9.14B** and **C**. Skeletal muscle fibers are well supplied with capillaries. When blood enters the arterial end of any systemic capillary, PaO_2 is high (95 mmHg). Within the tissue, PO_2 at rest is low (40 mmHg). Oxygen diffuses from high to low pressure until equilibrium is reached. Blood exiting into the systemic venous system thus has a PvO_2 of 40 mmHg, which is maintained until oxygenation occurs again at the alveoli.

Carbon dioxide is produced at the tissue level as a direct result of cellular respiration. Thus, PCO_2 levels are higher (about 45 mmHg) in the tissues than elsewhere in the system. Diffusion occurs as always from the area of high pressure (45 mmHg in the tissue) to the area of low pressure (40 mmHg in the systemic capillary), once again achieving equilibrium. The venous level of PCO_2 is also maintained until it reaches the alveoli, where the carbon dioxide diffuses out of the bloodstream and is exhaled. To make sure that you understand the movement of respiratory gases during rest, complete the task in the Check Your Comprehension 2 box below.

CHECK YOUR COMPREHENSION 2

Trace the movement of oxygen through the body from the alveoli to the pulmonary capillaries, through the left side of the heart, the systemic arteries, the tissue, the systemic capillaries, the systemic veins, the right side of the heart, and back to the alveoli. Give the PO_2 at each site and any diffusion of oxygen. Do the same thing for carbon dioxide, giving PCO_2, but start at the tissue level where carbon dioxide is produced and follow it through the systemic capillaries and veins, the right side of the heart, the pulmonary capillaries and the alveoli, the pulmonary vein, the left side of the heart, the systemic arterial system, and back to the systemic capillaries at the tissue level.

Check your answer in Appendix C.

The respiratory variables that are important for internal respiration are the partial pressure of oxygen in arterial blood (PaO_2), the partial pressure of oxygen in the venous blood (PvO_2), the amount of oxygen carried in the arteries minus the amount carried in the veins (a-vO_2diff), the partial pressure of carbon dioxide in arterial blood ($PaCO_2$), the partial pressure of carbon dioxide in venous blood ($PvCO_2$), and the percent saturation of venous blood with oxygen ($SvO_2\%$).

Oxygen Transport

Oxygen is carried in two ways in the blood. First, oxygen is transported in a dissolved form in the liquid portion of the blood. The amount of oxygen transported this way is only about 1.5–3% of the total oxygen transported. However, it is this dissolved component that is responsible for the partial pressure of oxygen in the blood (**Figure 9.14**). The dissolved oxygen content is determined by the PO_2 and the solubility of oxygen, which is a constant of 0.00304 mL·dL^{-1}·mmHg at 37°C. The formula is as follows (Guyton and Hall, 2011; Leff and Schumacker, 1993):

9.5   dissolved O_2 content $(mL \cdot dL^{-1}) = PO_2 (mmHg) \times$ solubility $(mL \cdot dL^{-1} \cdot mmHg^{-1})$

EXAMPLE

In normal systemic arterial blood with a PaO_2 of 95 mmHg, the calculation becomes

dissolved O_2 content $= (95\,mmHg)$
$\times (0.00304\,mL \cdot dL^{-1} \cdot mmHg^{-1})$
$= 0.29\,mL \cdot dL^{-1}$

Thus, only 0.29 mL of oxygen is dissolved in a deciliter of arterial blood. You may also see this result expressed in units of milliliters per 100 milliliters (mL·100 mL^{-1}) of blood or as milliliters percent (mL %). All are comparable.

The second way oxygen is transported in the blood is bound to hemoglobin. The vast majority, 97–98.5%, of the oxygen in the bloodstream is transported this way.

Red Blood Cells and Hemoglobin

Red blood cells (RBCs), or erythrocytes, are small, flexible cells shaped like biconcave disks, or miniature doughnuts, with an area where the hole would be just squished in (**Figure 9.15**). Females typically have a RBC count of 4.3–5.2 million per cubic milliliter of blood; the male count is generally 5.1–5.8 million per cubic milliliter of blood. The average person has about 35 trillion RBCs, which have a total surface area of about 2000 times the body's total surface area. Hemoglobin, which is the protein portion of the RBC that binds with oxygen, constitutes about one third of a RBC by weight if water is included or 97% if water is excluded. Normal values for hemoglobin for adult females are 12–16 g·100 mL^{-1} blood (g·dL^{-1}), with a mean of 14 g·100 mL^{-1} blood. For adult males, the values are 14–18 g·100 mL^{-1} blood, with a mean of 16 g·100 mL^{-1} blood. Children have slightly lower values (Guyton and Hall, 2011).

Hemoglobin consists of four iron-containing pigments called *hemes* (**Figure 9.16**) and a protein called *globin*. Each of the four iron atoms in a hemoglobin molecule can combine reversibly with one molecule of oxygen. Therefore, each hemoglobin molecule can transport four molecules of oxygen. The chemical symbol for hemoglobin not bound to oxygen, sometimes called *deoxyhemoglobin* or reduced hemoglobin, is Hb. Hemoglobin bound to oxygen, symbolized HbO$_2$, is called *oxyhemoglobin*. None of the oxygen bound to hemoglobin is used by the RBC.

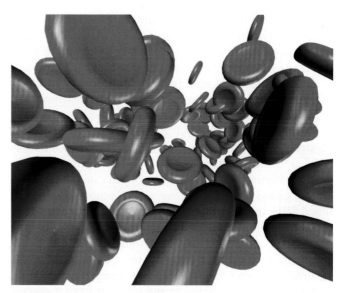

FIGURE 9.15 Red Blood Cells.
An electron micrograph of erythrocytes, or RBCs, showing the biconcave disk shape. See animation, Oxygen Transport, at http://thePoint.lww.com/Plowman4e.

The Binding of Oxygen with Hb: The Oxygen Dissociation Curve

All four oxygen molecules do not bind with the four heme atoms at the same time (**Figure 9.17**). **Figure 9.17A** shows deoxyhemoglobin (Hb). Binding of one oxygen molecule onto a fully deoxygenated hemoglobin

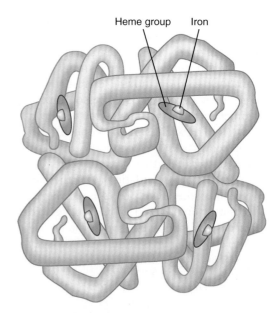

FIGURE 9.16 Hemoglobin.
Hemoglobin consists of four iron-containing heme units and the protein globin (the chains surrounding the heme units).
***Source*:** Seifter, J., A. Ratner, & D. Sloane: *Concepts in Medical Physiology*. Philadelphia, PA: Lippincott Williams & Wilkins (2005).

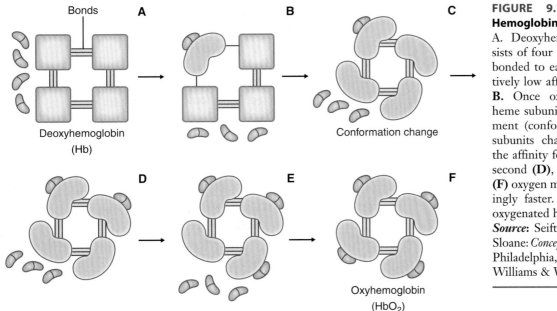

Bonds

A

B

C

Deoxyhemoglobin
(Hb)

Conformation change

D

E

F

Oxyhemoglobin
(HbO₂)

FIGURE 9.17 Oxygenation of Hemoglobin.
A. Deoxyhemoglobin (Hb) consists of four heme subunits tightly bonded to each other with a relatively low affinity for oxygen (O_2). **B.** Once oxygen binds to one heme subunit, the spatial arrangement (conformation) of all other subunits changes **(C)**, increasing the affinity for oxygen. As a result, second **(D)**, third **(E)**, and fourth **(F)** oxygen molecules bind increasingly faster. This results in fully oxygenated hemoglobin (HbO_2). *Source*: Seifter J., A. Ratner, & D. Sloane: *Concepts in Medical Physiology.* Philadelphia, PA: Lippincott Williams & Wilkins (2005).

molecule (**Figure 9.17B**) changes the spatial arrangement (conformation) of all of the other subunits (**Figure 9.17C**). This change increases the binding affinity for oxygen. Thus, each succeeding oxygen molecule binds more easily and quickly than the preceding one (**Figure 9.17D–F**) (Seifter et al., 2005). The result is a fully oxygenated hemoglobin molecule (HbO_2). When graphed, this process of successive molecules of oxygen binding to hemoglobin produces the characteristic sigmoid-shaped curve of oxyhemoglobin shown in **Figure 9.18**. This curve is called the *oxygen dissociation curve*, for reasons that will become clear later.

When all four of its heme groups are bound to oxygen, the hemoglobin molecule is said to be fully saturated. All hemoglobin molecules may not be fully saturated, though. The amount of the oxygen-carrying capacity being used at a given time is referred to as **percent saturation of hemoglobin**, designated as $SbO_2\%$. Percent saturation is calculated as

9.6
$$SbO_2\% = \frac{Hb \text{ combined with } O_2}{Hb \text{ capacity for combining with } O_2} \times 100$$

> **Hemoglobin (Hb)** The protein portion of the red blood cell that binds with oxygen, consisting of four iron-containing pigments called hemes and a protein called globin.
>
> **Percent Saturation of Hemoglobin ($SbO_2\%$)** The ratio of the amount of hemoglobin combined with oxygen to the total hemoglobin capacity for combining with oxygen, expressed as a percentage; indicated generally as $SbO_2\%$ or specifically as $SaO_2\%$ for arterial blood or as $SvO_2\%$ for venous blood.

The symbols $SaO_2\%$ and $SvO_2\%$ may be used to distinguish percent saturation of blood in the arteries and the veins, respectively, whereas Sb refers nonspecifically to blood.

Percent saturation depends primarily on the partial pressure of oxygen. In the arterial blood at a PO_2 of 95 mmHg, the percent saturation is 97%. Find this value on **Figure 9.18**, where PO_2 is on the x-axis and $SbO_2\%$ is on the left y-axis. On the same figure, determine the $SbO_2\%$ in normal venous blood. Since the PO_2 in normal venous blood is 40 mmHg, you should have determined that the $SbO_2\%$ was 75%. This value is also shown in **Figure 9.18**.

In addition to knowing the % saturation of blood with oxygen, it is also useful to know how much oxygen is carried in the blood. The *oxygen content* is the amount of oxygen (in mL) carried in 100 mL (or 1 dL) of blood. The oxygen content of hemoglobin depends upon the hemoglobin level and the physiological oxygen-binding capacity, according to the following formula:

9.7
oxygen content of hemoglobin ($mL \cdot dL^{-1}$) = hemoglobin level ($gm \cdot dL^{-1}$) × oxygen-binding capacity ($mL\ O_2 \cdot gm\ Hb^{-1}$) × percent saturation (expressed as a decimal fraction)

or

$$HbO_2 = Hb \times 1.34 \times SbO_2\%$$

In this equation, the hemoglobin level will, of course, vary from individual to individual. The physiological oxygen-binding capacity is a constant 1.34 mL $O_2 \cdot gm\ Hb^{-1}$, and the percent saturation of hemoglobin will vary between arterial and venous blood and resting and exercise conditions.

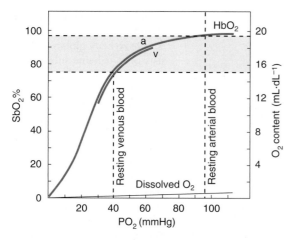

Assumes Hb = 15g·dL⁻¹ blood; Body temperature = 37°C
a = arterial blood; PaCO₂ = 40 mmHg; pH = 7.4
v = venous blood; PvCO₂ = 45 mmHg; pH = 7.38

FIGURE 9.18 Oxygen Dissociation Curve.
Under normal resting conditions, approximately 25% of the oxygen being transported in arterial blood is dissociated (released or exchanged by internal respiration) for use by body tissues. The shaded area at the top of the diagram represents this in percentage on the left y-axis and as an absolute amount on the right y-axis. See text for full explanation and calculations.

Using an average hemoglobin level of 15 gm·dL⁻¹, calculate the oxygen content for arterial blood where the percent saturation is 97%.

$$HbO_2 \, mL \cdot dL^{-1} = 15 \, gm \cdot dL^{-1}$$
$$\times 1.34 \, m \, LO_2 \cdot gm \, Hb^{-1} \times 0.97$$
$$= 19.5 \, mL \cdot dL^{-1}$$

In **Figure 9.18**, look at the right side y-axis. This axis is of O_2 content in mL·dL⁻¹ rounded to the nearest whole number. The value for normal arterial blood at 97% saturation is the value just calculated.

Arteriovenous Oxygen Difference

The amount of oxygen released (dissociated) from the blood during one circuit through the systemic system is called the **arteriovenous oxygen difference (a-vO₂diff)**. That is, the a-vO₂diff is the difference between the amount of oxygen originally carried in the arterial blood and that returned in the venous blood. Before subtracting to obtain the a-vO₂diff, we must calculate the total oxygen in both the arteries and the veins. The amount normally carried in the arterial blood has already been determined. It is

$$
\begin{array}{ll}
\text{dissolved } O_2 = & 0.29 \, mL \cdot dL^{-1} \\
+ HbO_2 = & \dfrac{19.50 \, mL \cdot dL^{-1}}{19.79 \, mL \cdot dL^{-1}} = \text{total } O_2 \text{ content} \\
& \text{in arterial blood} \, (aO_2)
\end{array}
$$

Calculate the dissolved O_2 and HbO_2 in venous blood.

The calculations are as follows:

$$
\begin{aligned}
\text{dissolved } O_2 \, (\text{venous}) &= 40 \, mmHg \\
&\times 0.00304 \, mL \, O_2 \cdot dL^{-1} \cdot mmHg \\
&= 0.12 \, mL \cdot dL^{-1} \\
HbO_2 \, (\text{venous}) &= 15 \, g \cdot dL^{-1} \times 1.34 \, mL \cdot g^{-1} \\
&\times 0.75 = 15.08 \, mL \cdot dL^{-1}
\end{aligned}
$$

Now, add these values:

$$
\begin{array}{ll}
\text{dissolved } O_2 = & 0.12 \, mL \cdot dL^{-1} \\
HbO_2 = & \dfrac{15.08 \, mL \cdot dL^{-1}}{15.20 \, mL \cdot dL^{-1}} = \text{total } O_2 \text{ content in} \\
& \text{venous blood} \, (vO_2)
\end{array}
$$

The a-vO₂diff is calculated by the formula

9.8   a-vO₂diff = O_2 in arterial blood (mL · dL⁻¹) – O_2 in venous blood (mL · dL⁻¹)
or
a-vO₂diff = $aO_2 - vO_2$

Therefore, the difference, using the values already calculated, is

$$
\begin{aligned}
\text{a-vO}_2\text{diff} &= 19.79 \, mL \cdot dL^{-1} - 15.20 \, mL \cdot dL^{-1} \\
&= 4.59 \, mL \cdot dL^{-1}
\end{aligned}
$$

Approximately 5 mL O_2·dL⁻¹ is used by the tissue to support cellular metabolism under normal resting conditions. This means that approximately 25% (4.59 ÷ 19.79 = 0.23 × 100 = 23%) of the oxygen is actually released from the hemoglobin to the tissues and used during rest. And, thus, approximately 75% of the oxygen is held in reserve for use when needed such as during physical exercise. The actual amount of oxygen used, measured as the a-vO₂diff, is called the *coefficient of oxygen utilization*. The normal resting coefficient of oxygen utilization is 4.59 mL·dL⁻¹.

Note that the 75% is also the SbO₂% value for venous blood. Refer to **Figure 9.18** again. The shaded area at the top—between the SbO₂% values of 97% and 75% on the left axis and between the values 19.79 and 15.20 mL·dL⁻¹ on the right axis—represents these relative and absolute amounts of O_2 that have been released or dissociated primarily from the RBCs. The separation or release of oxygen from the RBCs to the tissues is called **oxygen dissociation**, and the curve is called the oxygen dissociation curve. Check your comprehension of oxygen transport in the box.

Carbon Dioxide Transport

Carbon dioxide is carried in three ways in the blood from muscles or other tissues where it is produced to the lungs, where it is eliminated from the body. As with O_2, the first way it is transported is by dissolving in blood plasma. The amount of CO_2 transported in this fashion is only about 5–10% of the total. However, as with dissolved O_2, it is this dissolved CO_2 component that determines the partial pressure of CO_2 in the blood. Because the exchange of CO_2 in internal and external respiration depends largely upon the PCO_2, this is a critical role for dissolved CO_2. The remaining 90–95% of the CO_2 diffuses into the RBCs.

As CO_2 enters the RBC, about 20% combines chemically with the globin portion of the Hb molecule to produce *carbamino hemoglobin* (*HbCO₂*). This is the second form of CO_2 transport. Some small quantity may combine with proteins in the plasma as well. Note that when CO_2 combines with Hb, the CO_2 is not competing with oxygen for space on the heme units, because it combines with the globin portion. However, more CO_2 can combine with Hb if it is deoxygenated. That is, the lower the PO_2 and SbO_2%, the greater is the amount of CO_2 that can be carried in the blood. This reaction is known as the *Haldane effect* (Leff and Schumacker, 1993).

At the lungs, the situation is reversed: As O_2 saturates the Hb, less CO_2 can be bound, so the release of CO_2 is stimulated. Thus, Hb is really a transport vehicle carrying O_2 from the alveoli to the cells and CO_2 from the cells to the alveoli. This task is made easier by the fact that the dissociation (dropping off) of one molecule facilitates the binding (picking up) of the other at both sites.

The third way that CO_2 is transported is as bicarbonate ions. Approximately 70–75% of the CO_2 is transported in

Oxygen Dissociation The separation or release of oxygen from the RBCs to the tissues.

Arteriovenous Oxygen Difference (a-vO₂diff) The difference between the amount of oxygen originally carried in arterial blood and the amount returned in venous blood.

this way. When CO_2 diffuses into the RBCs, it combines with water under the influence of the enzyme carbonic anhydrase and forms carbonic acid (H_2CO_3). Carbonic acid is weak and unstable and quickly dissociates into hydrogen ions (H^+) and bicarbonate ions (HCO_3^-). The chemical reaction is depicted as

$$CO_2 + H_2O \xleftarrow{\text{carbonic anhydrase}} H_2CO_3 \leftrightarrow H^+ + HCO_3^-$$

The H^+ binds to Hb ($H^+ + Hb \rightarrow HHb$), thus preventing much change in pH, and the HCO_3^- diffuses into plasma. To counteract this loss of negative charges, chloride ions (Cl^-) move from plasma to the RBC. This ion exchange is called the *chloride shift*. At the lungs, where PCO_2 is relatively low, the reactions are all reversed. The chemical reactions are

$$O_2 + HHb \rightarrow HbO_2 + H^+$$
$$H^+ + HCO_3^- \rightarrow H_2CO_3 \rightarrow CO_2 + H_2O$$

Once back in the form of CO_2, the CO_2 diffuses along its partial pressure gradient from the blood to the alveoli and is exhaled (Guyton and Hall, 2011; Leff and Schumacker, 1993). See animation, Transport of Carbon Dioxide, at http://thePoint.lww.com/Plowman4e.

Figure 9.19 summarizes the transport of both oxygen and carbon dioxide in arterial and venous blood. Take time to study this in terms of the processes that have been described above.

The Respiratory System and Acid-Base Balance

The ability of hemoglobin to bind the hydrogen ions (H^+) produced during the transport of carbon dioxide and the ability of pulmonary ventilation both to respond to (**Figures 9.9 and 9.11**) and eliminate carbon dioxide are very important for maintaining acid-base balance. These reactions exemplify two of the three lines of defense for regulating acid-base balance: the chemical buffer system and the respiratory system. Furthermore, the partial pressure of carbon dioxide is also directly involved in the third line of defense, renal regulation by the kidneys.

Acid-base balance involves a series of mechanisms that attempt to regulate the concentration of hydrogen ions in body fluids. This balance is vitally important, because virtually all biochemical reactions in the human body require the pH to be maintained within very narrow limits for proper functioning (Guyton and Hall, 2011). Hydrogen ions come from several sources in the human body, but most result from the production of energy when oxygen is used and carbon dioxide is generated or when lactic acid accumulates in energy production without the use of oxygen.

Chemical buffers are either weak acids or weak bases that release or bind hydrogen ions, respectively. They respond instantaneously. Hemoglobin is not the only chemical buffer, but in terms of capacity, it is the most important buffer in the blood. Bicarbonate (HCO_3^-) is another important base.

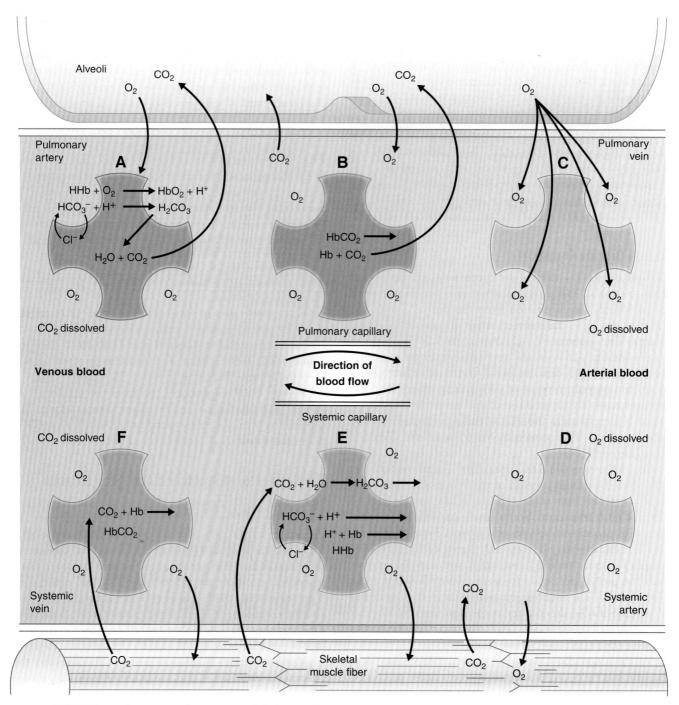

FIGURE 9.19 Summary of Oxygen and Carbon Dioxide Transport.
Oxygen is transported in two ways in the circulatory system—dissolved and bound to the heme units of hemoglobin (RBC). Carbon dioxide is transported in three ways in the circulatory system—dissolved, bound to the globin portion of hemoglobin, and as bicarbonate. **A.** The oxygenation of hemoglobin and diffusion of carbon dioxide from bicarbonate. **B.** The diffusion of carbon dioxide from the globin portion of hemoglobin. **C.** The transport of oxygen on heme portions of hemoglobin. **D.** The diffusion of oxygen from the heme portion of hemoglobin. **E.** The transport of carbon dioxide as bicarbonate. **F.** The transport of carbon dioxide on the globin portion of hemoglobin.

The carbonic acid-bicarbonate system (H_2CO_3/HCO_3^-) provides temporary buffering of hydrogen ions as they travel through the circulatory system. It also provides for the removal from the body of the carbon dioxide formed in the buffering process. The sensitivity of pulmonary ventilation to PCO_2 and pH enables varying amounts of acid production to be dealt with, because increased levels of carbon dioxide can be exhaled as needed. This respiratory compensation reacts within a matter of 1–3 minutes (Slonim and Hamilton, 1976).

The kidney's role in acid-base balance is twofold: (1) to conserve or eliminate bicarbonate ions, thereby stabilizing the amount in the body, and (2) to excrete hydrogen ions. Renal bicarbonate retention or excretion depends on the PCO_2 in arterial blood. The kidneys are the most potent of the acid-base mechanisms. However, they require hours or even days to effectively change pH (Guyton and Hall, 2011).

In the normal resting condition, venous pH is slightly lower than arterial pH (venous = 7.35, arterial = 7.4), but this difference has very little effect on most physiological functions. The key is maintaining arterial pH levels. Overall, then, not only does the respiratory system deliver oxygen for the production of energy and remove carbon dioxide, but it also contributes to the effective functioning of all biochemical reactions in the body through its role in maintaining acid-base balance.

SUMMARY

1. Respiration consists of pulmonary ventilation, and oxygen and carbon dioxide gases exchange at the alveolar (external) and tissue (internal) levels.

2. Structurally, the pulmonary system can be divided into the conductive and respiratory zones. The conductive zone serves to transport air, warm and humidify air, and filter the air. Gas exchange takes place in the respiratory zone.

3. At rest, inspiration is an active process brought about by a pressure gradient that exceeds resistance to the flow of air. Resting expiration is a passive process accomplished primarily by elastic recoil.

4. The conductive zone makes up the anatomical dead space. An alveolar dead space occurs when functional alveoli are not supplied with capillaries or capillaries are pathologically blocked. Together anatomical and alveolar dead spaces are called the physiological dead space.

5. Minute ventilation ($\dot{V}_E$ or $\dot{V}_I$) is the respiratory variable most commonly measured in exercise situations. Alveolar ventilation is the best measure of air available for gas exchange.

6. Residual volume, the amount of air remaining in the lungs after a maximal expiration, must be accounted for when one determines body composition by underwater weighing.

7. Respiratory measures are collected under ambient conditions (ATPS). Most lung volumes and capacities are then converted to body temperature values (BTPS). Minute ventilation may also be converted to standard temperature and pressure, dry (STPD) conditions.

8. Primary control of respiration resides in the medulla oblongata (inspiratory and expiratory centers), with fine tuning provided by the pneumotaxic and apneustic centers in the pons. Factors affecting these centers include:
   a. Conscious thought through the cerebral cortex
   b. Sympathetic nerve reactions through the hypothalamus
   c. Irritants or lung inflammation through systemic receptors in the airways and lungs
   d. PO_2, PCO_2, pH, and K^+ through central and peripheral chemoreceptors
   e. Movement via proprioceptive stimulation from mechanoreceptors and muscles and joints

9. Gases always flow down a pressure gradient. Each gas moves independently. Oxygen moves from the alveoli into arterial blood and red blood cells (RBCs) and then from the RBCs and capillary blood into the muscle tissues. Carbon dioxide moves from the muscle tissues into capillary blood and RBCs and then from the venous blood and RBCs into the alveoli.

10. Hemoglobin is composed of four iron heme units and one globin (a protein). When fully saturated, each hemoglobin molecule will have oxygen bound to each of its four heme structures. Normal arterial saturation (SaO_2%) is 97%; normal resting venous saturation (SvO_2%) is 75%.

11. Oxygen released from the RBCs at the tissue level is said to have been dissociated. At rest, the primary drive for this dissociation is the pressure gradient for oxygen.

12. At rest, only about 25% of circulated oxygen is used; 75% remains saturated in venous blood. These percentages translate into an arteriovenous oxygen difference of approximately 4.6 mL·dL^{-1}.

13. Carbon dioxide is transported from the tissue to the lungs in three ways: dissolved, as carbamino hemoglobin, and as bicarbonate ions. The chemical buffering and removal of carbon dioxide from the body are important for maintaining acid-base balance.

REVIEW QUESTIONS

1. Define pulmonary ventilation, external respiration, and internal respiration. Define the following variables and classify each as involved in pulmonary

ventilation, external respiration, or internal respiration. Some may be classified in more than one way.

(A-a) PO_2 diff	V_T	$PvCO_2$	V_D/V_T
a-vO_2diff	$\dot{V}_A$	PvO_2	
V_D	PaO_2	$SaO_2\%$	
f	P_AO_2	$SbO_2\%$	
$\dot{V}_E$ and $\dot{V}_I$	$PaCO_2$	$SvO_2\%$	

2. Diagram the conductive and respiratory zones of the respiratory system. Compare the function of the two zones.

3. Why does air flow into and out of the lungs?

4. What is the functional difference between pulmonary circulation and bronchial circulation? How does bronchial circulation affect the PaO_2?

5. Identify the three capacities and four volumes into which TLC can be divided. Which is most responsive during exercise? Which must be accounted for when one determines body composition by hydrostatic (underwater) weighing?

6. Explain the conditions represented by the volume designations ATPS, BTPS, and STPD. Where is each condition most appropriately used? Which volume is typically the largest? Which is the smallest? Name and explain the gas laws that cause these differences.

7. Discuss the primary control of respiration and the factors that affect such control.

8. Describe how oxygen and carbon dioxide are transported in the circulatory system. Explain the importance of each transport form and any interaction between the movements of the individual gases.

9. Explain how the transport and removal of carbon dioxide relate to acid-base balance. Why is it important to maintain acid-base balance?

10. Graph a normal resting oxygen dissociation curve. What percentage of the available oxygen is normally dissociated at rest?

For further review and additional study tools, visit the website at http://thePoint.lww.com/Plowman4e ✳ ◉

REFERENCES

Adams, G. M.: *Exercise Physiology Laboratory Manual* (2nd edition). Dubuque, IA: Brown (1994).

Aronson, D., I. Roterman, M. Yigia, et al.: Inverse association between pulmonary function and C-reactive protein in apparently healthy subjects. *American Journal of Respiratory and Critical Care Medicine*. 174(6):626–632 (2006).

Boggs, G. W., J. R. Ward, & S. Stavrianeas: The external nasal dilator: Style over function? *Journal of Strength and Conditioning Research*. 22(1):269–275 (2008).

Craig, A. B.: Summary of 58 cases of loss of consciousness during underwater swimming and diving. *Medicine and Science in Sports*. 8(3):171–175 (1976).

Dempsey, J. A., E. H. Vidruk, & G. S. Mitchell: Pulmonary control systems in exercise: Update. *Federation Proceedings*. 44:2260–2270 (1985).

Eldridge, F. L.: Central integration of mechanisms in exercise hyperpnea. *Medicine and Science in Sports and Exercise*. 26(3):319–327 (1994).

Forster, H. V. & L. G. Pau: The role of the carotid chemoreceptors in the control of breathing during exercise. *Medicine and Science in Sports and Exercise*. 26(3):328–336 (1994).

Gehring, J. M., S. R. Garlick, J. R. Wheatley, & T. C. Amis: Nasal resistance and flow resistive work of nasal breathing during exercise: Effects of a nasal dilator strip. *Journal of Applied Physiology*. 89(3):1114–1122 (2000).

Guyton, A. C. & J. E. Hall: *Textbook of Medical Physiology* (12th edition). Philadelphia, PA: W. B. Saunders (2011).

Leff, A. R. & P. T. Schumacker: *Respiratory Physiology: Basics and Applications*. Philadelphia, PA: W. B. Saunders (1993).

Macfarlane, D. J. & S. K. Fong: Effects of an external nasal dilator on athletic performance of male adolescents. *Canadian Journal of Applied Physiology*. 29(5):579–589 (2004).

Martin, B. J., K. E. Sparks, C. W. Zwillich, & J. V. Weil: Low exercise ventilation in endurance athletes. *Medicine and Science in Sports*. 11(2):181–185 (1979).

Nye, P. C. G.: Identification of peripheral chemoreceptor stimuli. *Medicine and Science in Sports and Exercise*. 26(3):311–318 (1994).

O'Kroy, J. A.: Oxygen uptake and ventilatory effects of an external nasal dilator during ergometry. *Medicine & Science in Sports & Exercise*. 32(8):1491–1495 (2000).

O'Kroy, J. A., J. T. James, J. M. Miller, D. Torok, & K. Campbell. Effects of an external nasal dilator on the work of breathing during exercise. *Medicine & Science in Sports & Exercise*. 33(3):454–458 (2001).

Pardy, R. L., S. N. A. Hussain, & P. T. Macklein: The ventilatory pump in exercise. *Clinics in Chest Medicine*. 5(1):35–49 (1984).

Portugal, L. G., R. H. Mehta, B. E. Smith, J. B. Savnani, & M. J. Matava: Objective assessment of the breathe-right device during exercise in adult males. *American Journal of Rhinology*. 11(5):393–397 (1997).

Schunemann, H. J., J. Dorn, B. J. B. Grant, W. Winkelstein, & M. Trevisan: Pulmonary function is a long-term predictor of mortality in the general population: 29-year follow-up of the Buffalo Health Study. *Chest*. 118(3):656–664 (2000).

Seifter, J., A. Ratner, & D. Sloane: *Concepts in Medical Physiology*. Philadelphia, PA: Lippincott Williams & Wilkins (2005).

Slonim, N. B. & L. H. Hamilton: *Respiratory Physiology* (3rd edition). St. Louis, MO: Mosby (1976).

Thomas, D. Q., B. M. Larson, M. R. Rahija, & S. T. McCaw: Nasal strips do not affect cardiorespiratory measures during recovery from anaerobic exercise. *Journal of Strength and Conditioning Research*. 15(3):341–343 (2001).

West, J. B.: *Respiratory Physiology: The Essentials* (7th edition). Philadelphia, PA: Lippincott Williams & Wilkins (2005).

Whipp, B. J., S. A. Ward, N. Lamarra, J. A. Davis, & K. Wasserman: Parameters of ventilatory and gas exchange dynamics during exercise. *Journal of Applied Physiology: Respiratory, Environmental and Exercise Physiology*. 52(6):1506–1513 (1982).

Wilmore, J. H.: The use of actual, predicted, and constant residual volumes in the assessment of body composition by underwater weighing. *Medicine and Science in Sports*. 1:87–90 (1969).

Respiratory Exercise Response, Training Adaptations, and Special Considerations

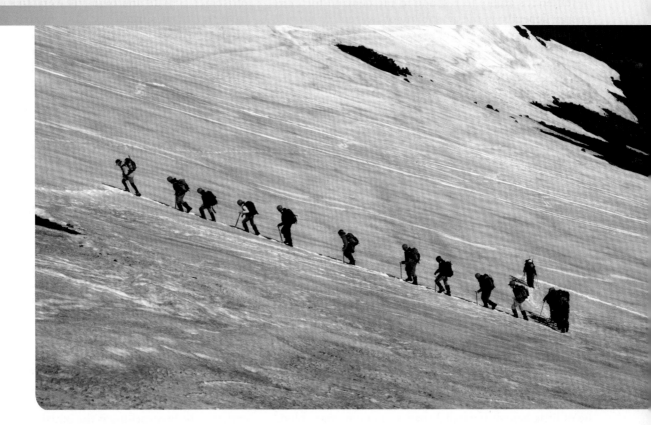

OBJECTIVES

After studying the chapter, you should be able to:

❯ Graph and explain the pattern of response for the major respiratory variables during short-term, light to moderate submaximal aerobic exercise.

❯ Graph and explain the pattern of response for the major respiratory variables during long-term, moderate to heavy submaximal aerobic exercise.

❯ Graph and explain the pattern of response for the major respiratory variables during incremental aerobic exercise to maximum.

❯ Graph and explain the pattern of response for the major respiratory variables during static exercise.

❯ Compare and contrast the pulmonary ventilation, external respiration, and internal respiration responses to short-term, light to moderate submaximal aerobic exercise; long-term, moderate to heavy submaximal aerobic exercise; incremental aerobic exercise to maximum; and static exercise.

❯ Explain why respiration may be a limitation to performance in elite athletes.

❯ Differentiate between respiratory muscle training and adaptations and whole body respiratory training and adaptations.

❯ Identify variations in resting volumes, exercise responses, and exercise training adaptations between males and females and among young adults, children and adolescents, and older adults.

❯ Determine the value of altitude training and training in polluted conditions.

Introduction

During exercise, the demand for energy increases. The demand varies, of course, with the type, intensity, and duration of the exercise. In most exercise situations, much of the body's ability to respond to the demand for more energy depends on the availability of oxygen. To provide the needed oxygen for aerobic energy production, the respiratory system—including pulmonary ventilation, external respiration, and internal respiration—must respond. Pulmonary ventilation increases to enhance alveolar ventilation, external respiration adjusts to maintain the relationship between ventilation and perfusion in most cases, and internal respiration responds with an increased extraction of oxygen by the muscles. These changes in respiration not only provide adequate oxygenation for the muscles but also play a major role in maintaining acid-base balance, which is, in turn, closely related to carbon dioxide levels.

In general, all levels of respiratory activity are precisely matched to the rate of work being done. Furthermore, because of this precise control and the large reserve built into the system, respiration in normal, healthy, sedentary, or moderately fit individuals is generally not a limiting factor in activity. This is true despite the perception of feeling out of breath during exercise. Only occasionally do the capacities of the cardiovascular and metabolic systems exceed that of the respiratory system such that respiration can be considered a limitation to maximal work and, paradoxically, that is generally in elite highly trained athletes.

Of course, changes in pulmonary ventilation would be of little benefit if parallel changes in pulmonary blood volume and flow and total body systemic circulation did not also occur. These accompanying cardiovascular responses will be detailed in the following chapters in the cardiovascular unit.

This chapter concentrates on pulmonary ventilation, external respiration, and internal respiration responses to aerobic activity, including short- and long-term, constant-load submaximal activity and incremental exercise to maximum. The most prominent changes in the respiratory system occur within these classifications of activity. Static exercise responses will also be briefly discussed. However, respiratory responses to dynamic resistance activity and high-intensity anaerobic exercise have not been specifically documented and therefore cannot be discussed here. When reading this discussion and studying the accompanying graphs, you may wish to refer to the glossary of respiratory symbols in **Table 10.1**. Note that several variables are involved in more than one process.

Response of the Respiratory System to Exercise

Short-Term, Light to Moderate Submaximal Aerobic Exercise

The responses to short-term (5–10 minutes), light to moderate submaximal (30–69% of maximal work capacity) aerobic exercise are shown in **Figure 10.1, 10.2** and **10.5**. These responses are discussed in detail in the following subsections.

Pulmonary Ventilation

The most obvious response to an increased metabolic demand, such as exercise, is the increase in pulmonary minute ventilation ($\dot{V}_E$ L·min^{-1}), called hyperpnea. What is perhaps a little surprising is the initial immediate reaction. In **Figure 10.1A**, note that between the onset of exercise at 0 and 2 minutes into the exercise, a triphasic response in $\dot{V}_E$ occurs. Within the first respiratory cycle at the onset of exercise, there is an initial abrupt increase in $\dot{V}_E$, termed phase 1. This increase is maintained for approximately 10–20 seconds. Phase 2 is a slower exponential rise from the initial elevation to a steady-state leveling off. At the

TABLE 10.1 Respiratory Symbols		
Pulmonary Ventilation	**External Respiration**	**Internal Respiration**
$\dot{V}_E$ = minute ventilation	$\dot{V}_A$ = alveolar ventilation	a-vO_2diff = amount of oxygen carried in the arteries minus the amount carried in the veins
V_D = dead space	P_AO_2 = partial pressure of oxygen at the alveoli	PaO_2 = partial pressure of oxygen in the arterial blood
V_T = tidal volume	PaO_2 = partial pressure of oxygen in the arterial blood	$PaCO_2$ = partial pressure of carbon dioxide in the arterial blood
f = frequency	(A-a)PO_2diff = oxygen or PO_2 pressure gradient between the alveoli and the arteries	$PvCO_2$ = partial pressure of carbon dioxide in venous blood
V_D/V_T = ratio of dead space to tidal volume	SaO_2% = percent saturation of arterial blood with oxygen	SvO_2% = percent saturation of venous blood with oxygen
	P_ACO_2 = partial pressure of carbon dioxide at the alveoli	PvO_2 = partial pressure of oxygen in venous blood

low to moderate workload depicted here, this exponential rise is generally completed in 2–3 minutes. At this point, phase 3, a new steady state, is achieved. The actual level of this achieved exercise steady state depends on a number of factors, including the workload, the fitness status of the individual, and the environmental conditions. In the time span depicted in this graph, the steady-state level is maintained. The three-phase response at the onset of activity is typically not seen when $\dot{V}_E$ is reported or graphed minute by minute, rather than second by second or even breath by breath, but it does occur (Bell, 2006; Pardy et al., 1984; Whipp, 1977; Whipp and Ward, 1980; Whipp et al., 1982).

The initial rise in ventilation occurs primarily because of an increase in tidal volume (Leff and Schumacker, 1993). Theoretically, tidal volume ranges from the resting level to the limits of vital capacity (VC). In reality, rarely is more than 50–65% of VC reached before a plateau occurs. Furthermore, although tidal volume encroaches into both the inspiratory reserve volume (IRV) and the expiratory reserve volume (ERV), it encroaches much more into IRV than ERV (Koyal et al., 1976; Pearce and Milhorn, 1977; Turner et al., 1968; Younes and Kivinen, 1984).

At light to moderate workloads, the contribution of increased breathing frequency to minute ventilation is minimal and gradual. Both tidal volume and frequency level off at a steady state that satisfies the oxygen requirements of the short submaximal activity (**Figure 10.1B** and **C**).

Airway resistance decreases because of bronchodilation as soon as exercise begins. Likewise, the ratio of dead space (V_D) to tidal volume (V_T) decreases, and in this case, the largest changes are evident at the lowest work rate (Wasserman et al., 1967; Whipp and Ward, 1980). This result is shown in **Figure 10.1B**. The depth of the drop in V_D/V_T is moderate at low to moderate exercise intensities. The V_D itself changes minimally with bronchodilation, but with the proportionally larger increase in V_T, the ratio declines (Grimby, 1969). This result is important because alveolar ventilation ($\dot{V}_A$) thus increases from about 70% of the total pulmonary ventilation at rest to a higher percentage during exercise. Since $\dot{V}_A$ is the critical ventilation, this reduction in the V_D/V_T ratio means that the appropriate level of $\dot{V}_A$ can be achieved with a smaller rise in $\dot{V}_E$ than would be needed if the ratio did not change (Wasserman and Whipp, 1975).

External Respiration

The $\dot{V}_A$ response to low to moderate exercise is depicted in **Figure 10.2A**. This curve parallels the change in $\dot{V}_E$, except that the initial adjustments seen in $\dot{V}_E$ are not depicted for $\dot{V}_A$. The rise in $\dot{V}_A$ is sufficient to maintain PO_2 at the alveolar level (P_AO_2) during short-term submaximal exercise (**Figure 10.2B**). Maintenance of P_AO_2 is important because it represents the driving force for oxygen transfer across the alveolar-capillary interface (Powers et al., 1993; Wasserman, 1978).

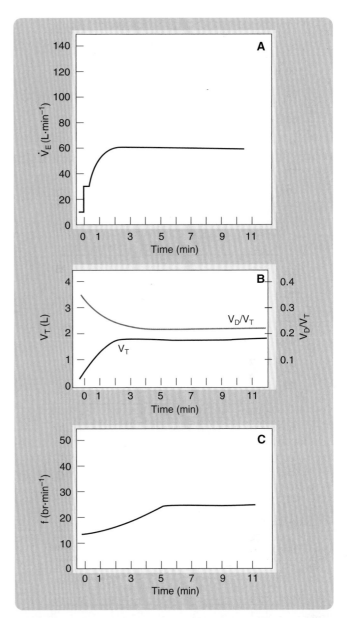

FIGURE 10.1 Responses of Pulmonary Ventilation Variables to Short-Term, Light to Moderate Submaximal Aerobic Exercise. A. Minute ventilation. **B.** Tidal volume (V_T) and ratio of dead space to tidal volume (V_D/V_T). **C.** Frequency.

As explained in Chapter 9, under resting conditions, there is an inequity in PO_2 between the alveoli (P_AO_2) and systemic arterial blood (PaO_2) owing to the dilution of the systemic arterial blood with the bronchial venous blood. During short-term, low-intensity submaximal exercise, PaO_2 is maintained. The alveolar to arterial oxygen partial pressure difference, depicted as (A-a)PO_2diff in **Figure 10.2C**, either does not change or decreases slightly (Jones, 1975; Leff and Schumacker, 1993; Wasserman and Whipp, 1975). At moderate workloads, a slight increase may occur. The (A-a)PO_2diff reflects the efficiency and/or adequacy of oxygen transfer in the

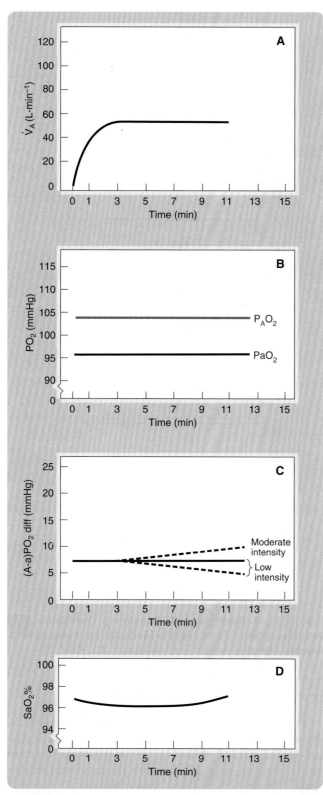

FIGURE 10.2 Responses of External Respiration Variables to Short-Term, Light to Moderate Submaximal Aerobic Exercise. A. Alveolar ventilation. **B.** Partial pressure of oxygen at the alveoli (A) and in arterial blood (a). **C.** Partial pressure of oxygen gradient between the alveoli and the arteries. **D.** Percent saturation of arterial blood with oxygen.

lungs during exercise. At the steady-state submaximal levels described here, there is no noticeable change in this efficiency.

Gas exchange and blood perfusion in the lungs during low to moderate exercise are sufficient to maintain the saturation of red blood cells with oxygen ($SaO_2\%$) within a narrow range approximating resting levels (**Figure 10.2D**) (Gurtner et al., 1975).

Internal Respiration

Recall that internal respiration involves the dissociation of oxygen from the red blood cells so that it may diffuse down the pressure gradient into the muscles and other tissues.

Refer to **Figure 10.3** and refamiliarize yourself with the resting relationships for oxygen dissociation described in Chapter 9 and labeled in this figure. The perpendicular line on the x-axis at 95 mmHg represents the PaO_2 for resting arterial blood. It intersects with the middle curve and indicates a percent saturation of hemoglobin ($SbO_2\%$) of approximately 97% (seen on the left y-axis). The perpendicular line on the x-axis at 40 mmHg represents the PvO_2 for resting venous blood. This line also intersects with the middle curve and indicates a SbO_2 of 75%; that is, at rest, 75% of the oxygen remains associated with the red blood cells in venous blood. Thus, much more oxygen could be extracted at the tissue capillary level and normally is during exercise.

Four factors are involved in increased oxygen extraction during exercise:

1. Increased PO_2 gradient
2. Increased PCO_2
3. Decreased pH
4. Increased temperature

Each of these factors is depicted in the oxygen dissociation curve in **Figure 10.3**. How each factor operates is described below.

INCREASED PO_2 GRADIENT Under resting conditions, sufficient oxygen remains in the muscle tissue to maintain a PO_2 of 40 mmHg. When exercise increases the demand for energy, the oxygen already present in the muscle tissue is used immediately. Since the oxygen is used, the muscle tissue partial pressure is reduced correspondingly. The PO_2 of arterial blood remains unchanged. Therefore, the pressure gradient can widen from 55 mmHg (95 mmHg at the arterial end of the capillary minus 40 mmHg in the muscle tissue) up to possibly 65 mmHg (95 mmHg at the arterial end of the capillary minus 30 mmHg in the muscle tissue) during light submaximal exercise.

Equilibrium is reached between the muscle tissue and the blood by the venous end of the capillary, so the returning venous blood also has the lower PO_2. Refer to **Figure 10.3** and find the line labeled submaximal for venous blood during exercise above the x-axis value of

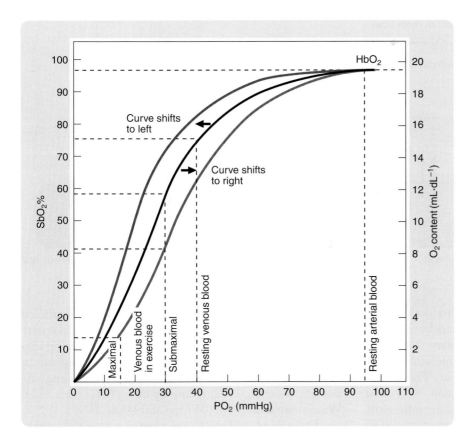

FIGURE 10.3 Oxygen Dissociation during Exercise.

The center curve represents normal resting values: $PaCO_2$ = 40 mmHg, pH = 7.4, body temperature = 37°C. During all intensities and types of exercise, the $PaCO_2$ increases, pH decreases (becomes more acidic), and body temperature increases. Each of these conditions causes the curve to shift to the right, with the result that more oxygen is dissociated from red blood cells to be used by the muscles. Consequently, the higher the intensity of exercise, the lower both the oxygen content of the venous blood and the SbO_2% in venous blood.

30 mmHg. Assume for the moment that this is the only change that occurs (a false assumption, as will be seen later, but which does no harm here). In the figure, you can see the effect this increased pressure gradient has on the dissociation of oxygen. By following this submaximal exercise line to where it intersects the solid line middle curve and then to the left y-axis, you can see that the corresponding SbO_2% (actually SvO_2% now) is approximately 59%, not 75%. Instead of 23% of the oxygen being dissociated as it was at rest (97% SaO_2% – 75% SvO_2% = 22%; 22% ÷ 97% = 23%), now 38% (97% SaO_2% – 59 SvO_2% = 38%; 37% ÷ 97% = 39%) has been released from the red blood cells just because of the change in the pressure gradient. Thus, an additional 16% of the available oxygen (39% – 23% = 16%) has been dissociated and is used for energy production. Because all submaximal exercise does not require the same amount of oxygen, these numbers simply illustrate the effect of a widening pressure gradient.

INCREASED PCO₂ When oxygen is used to provide energy, carbon dioxide is produced as a by-product. Increasing levels of carbon dioxide mean that PCO_2 increases. An increase in PCO_2 shifts the oxygen dissociation curve to the right. This shift occurs in a minimal way even at rest, as seen in the venous curve in **Figure 9.18**. However, during exercise, the shift is further to the right. Exactly how far the curve shifts depends on the intensity of the exercise and how much carbon dioxide is produced. The shift in the curve to the right means that at any given

PO_2, more dissociation occurs, as shown in **Figure 10.3**. Follow the line for venous blood during exercise from the value of 30 mmHg on the PO_2 x-axis until it intersects the right-hand curve. A horizontal line from this intersection to the left y-axis yields a saturation value of about 41%. Thus, more oxygen is dissociated than would have been if the pressure gradient had been operating alone. **Figure 10.4** emphasizes that the actual shift occurs during the red blood cell transit through the capillary before reaching the venous blood vessel.

DECREASED pH OR INCREASED HYDROGEN ION CONCENTRATION Hydrogen ions (H⁺) come from two primary sources during exercise. First, carbon dioxide combines with water to form carbonic acid. The carbonic acid then breaks down into hydrogen ions and bicarbonate. Second, lactic acid breaks down into lactate and hydrogen ions. The presence of increased levels of hydrogen ions lowers the pH to a more acidic level. This more acidic pH shifts the oxygen dissociation curve to the right in the same way that an increased PCO_2 does and with the same results: a greater dissociation of oxygen from red blood cells. How far to the right the curve shifts depends on the amount of hydrogen ions released. As with carbon dioxide, this effect is taking place during the red blood cell's transit through the muscle capillaries (**Figure 10.4**). The interactive effect of carbon dioxide and pH on the affinity of hemoglobin for oxygen is known as the *Bohr effect* (Guyton and Hall, 2011; Kenney, 1982).

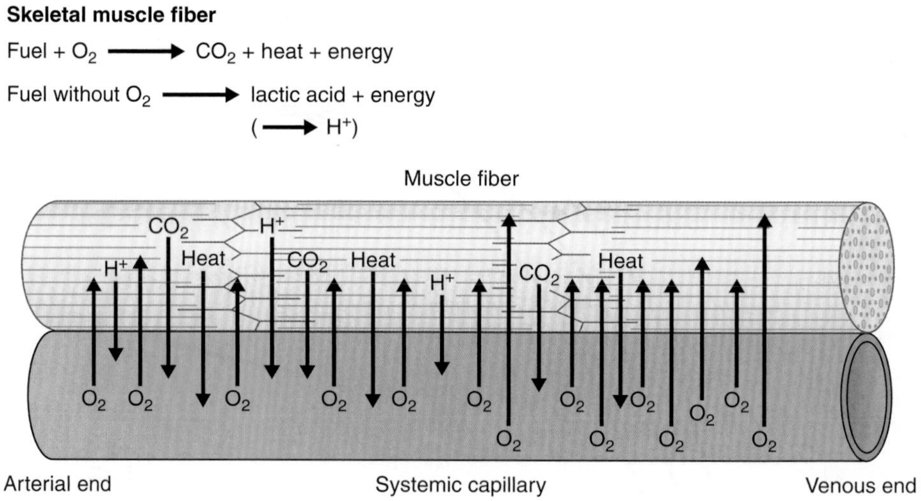

FIGURE 10.4 Factors Influencing Oxygen Dissociation during Exercise. The by-products of the production of energy—namely, carbon dioxide, heat, and hydrogen ions (H^+)—in skeletal muscle fibers stimulate the dissociation of oxygen from red blood cells as they traverse systemic capillaries.

Skeletal muscle fiber

Fuel + O_2 $\longrightarrow$ CO_2 + heat + energy

Fuel without O_2 $\longrightarrow$ lactic acid + energy

($\longrightarrow$ H^+)

Muscle fiber

Arterial end   Systemic capillary   Venous end

INCREASED TEMPERATURE Another by-product of muscle energy production is heat. Heat is transferred from the muscle tissue (high heat) to the capillary (low heat) (**Figure 10.4**). The resultant rise in temperature shifts the oxygen dissociation curve to the right. The action is precisely the same as that of the increased PCO_2 and decreased pH, and so it is again depicted by the same shift in **Figure 10.3**. Thus, the elevation in the use of oxygen to produce energy during exercise and the by-products of that energy production operate together to make the reserves of oxygen available: the first (increased oxygen consumption) by widening the pressure gradient, and the other three (increased PCO_2, decreased pH, and increased body temperature) by shifting the oxygen dissociation curve to the right.

The exercise responses for the variables from the oxygen dissociation curve are depicted in **Figure 10.5**. The best overall indicator of internal respiration is the arteriovenous oxygen difference (a-vO_2diff) (Gurtner et al., 1975). Because PaO_2 (**Figure 10.5A**) and SaO_2% (**Figure 10.2D**) do not change with short-term, low-intensity exercise, the actual amount of oxygen being carried in the arteries (in milliliters per deciliter) also does not change (Wasserman et al., 1967). However, because energy production uses more oxygen even at these low intensities, the venous oxygen value, PvO_2 (**Figure 10.5C**), and SvO_2% (**Figure 10.5F**) decrease. With an equal arterial oxygen and lower venous oxygen content, the a-vO_2diff (**Figure 10.5E**) increases. Because this is a steady-state submaximal situation, the a-vO_2diff will level off when sufficient oxygen is being extracted to supply the needs of the cell (Davies et al., 1972; Dempsey et al., 1977; Kao, 1974).

Because energy production also produces carbon dioxide, it would be anticipated that the $PvCO_2$ would increase. As shown in **Figure 10.5D**, this increase does occur, but it is not particularly large at these low to moderate workloads. The extra carbon dioxide is exhaled easily from the lungs, and the hyperpnea of exercise may even blow off a little extra carbon dioxide, resulting in a slight decrement in $PaCO_2$ (**Figure 10.5B**). Regulation of ventilation maintains $PaCO_2$ very close to resting values (Davies et al., 1972; Dempsey et al., 1977; Kao, 1974; Wasserman et al., 1967; Whipp and Ward, 1980).

These combined responses are well within the reserve capacity of the respiratory system for normal, healthy individuals.

Long-Term, Moderate to Heavy Submaximal Aerobic Exercise

If submaximal aerobic exercise is increased in duration and maintained at high-moderate to heavy intensity (60–75% of maximal working capacity), respiratory responses vary primarily in magnitude compared with the changes just discussed for short-term, light to moderate submaximal exercise. In addition, several of the variables have a drifting pattern.

Pulmonary Ventilation

Figure 10.6A shows that $\dot{V}_E$ increases to a higher level than during light to moderate submaximal exercise before plateauing at a steady state. Achievement of the steady state may take somewhat longer than at lower work intensities and often is not held throughout the duration of the exercise. Note that after about 30 minutes, a gradual rise in $\dot{V}_E$ occurs, despite an unchanging workload, an effect called *ventilatory drift* (Dempsey et al., 1977; Hanson et al., 1982; Wasserman, 1978). The precise reason for this drift is unknown (Sawka et al., 1980), although a rising body temperature is most often speculated as the primary reason. This drift is both inefficient and advantageous. It is inefficient because the extra air breathed is in excess of the workload demand. It is advantageous for gas exchange because alveolar ventilation parallels the drift, and acid-base balance is maintained (Dempsey et al., 1977; Hanson et al., 1982).

As for lower-intensity submaximal exercise, the initial change in $\dot{V}_E$ is due primarily to an increase in V_T (**Figure 10.6B**). However, in the later stages of heavy submaximal work, tidal volume may decrease slightly.

The drift in $\dot{V}_E$ comes about primarily as a result of increased breathing frequency (**Figure 10.6C**). The V_D/V_T ratio (**Figure 10.6B**) still decreases primarily at the onset of activity, but it does so to a greater extent with a heavier workload than at lighter loads. After about an hour of heavy submaximal work, the V_D/V_T ratio may increase very slightly.

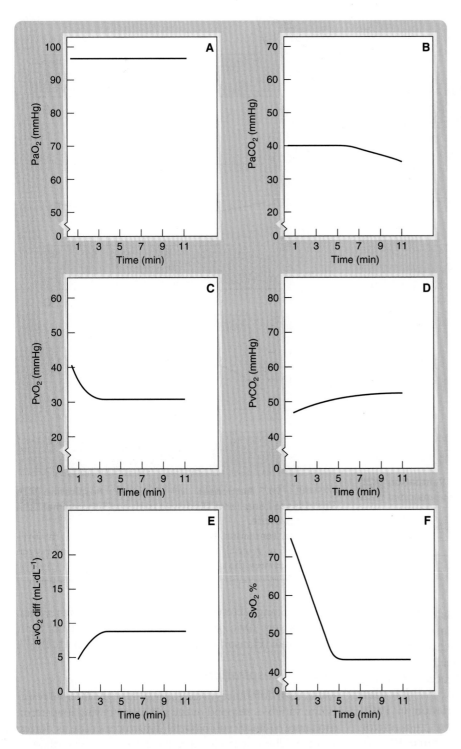

FIGURE 10.5 Responses of Internal Respiration Variables to Short-Term, Light to Moderate Submaximal Aerobic Exercise.
A. Partial pressure of oxygen in arterial blood. **B.** Partial pressure of carbon dioxide in arterial blood. **C.** Partial pressure of oxygen in venous blood. **D.** Partial pressure of carbon dioxide in venous blood. **E.** Arterial-venous oxygen difference. **F.** Percent saturation of venous blood with oxygen.

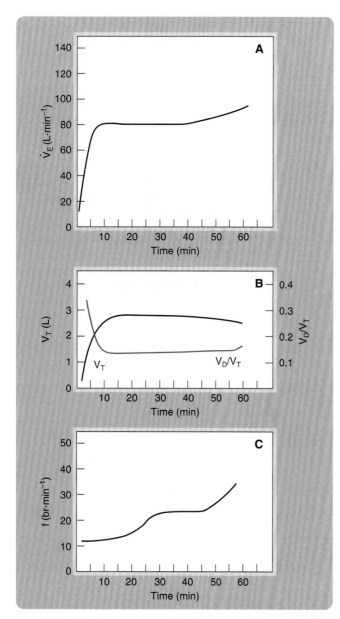

FIGURE 10.6 Responses of Pulmonary Ventilation Variables to Long-Term, Moderate to Heavy Submaximal Aerobic Exercise.
A. Minute ventilation. **B.** Tidal volume (V_T) and ratio of dead space to tidal volume (V_D/V_T). **C.** Frequency.

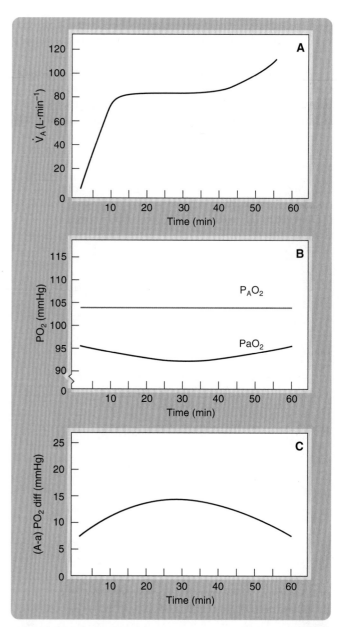

FIGURE 10.7 Responses of External Respiration Variables to Long-Term, Moderate to Heavy Submaximal Aerobic Exercise.
A. Alveolar ventilation. **B.** Partial pressure of oxygen at the alveoli (A) and in arterial blood (a). **C.** Partial pressure of oxygen gradient between the alveoli and the arteries.

External Respiration

As stated earlier, the drift in $\dot{V}_E$ is paralleled by a similar drift in $\dot{V}_A$ (**Figure 10.7A**). P_AO_2 remains constant (**Figure 10.7B**), as it did with lower-intensity submaximal work. However, PaO_2 decreases gradually but slightly until about the time when ventilatory drift occurs, forming a shallow U-shaped curve (Dempsey et al., 1977). It then returns toward baseline values. This variation in PaO_2 while P_AO_2 remains unchanged is reflected in a mirror image relationship in the (A-a)PO_2diff (**Figure 10.7C**), depicted as a truncated, inverted U-shaped curve. The initial increase in the (A-a)PO_2diff indicates inefficiency

in gas exchange. However, the small loss of efficiency seen here has very little practical meaning and does not limit the exercise (Hanson et al., 1982; Wasserman et al., 1967).

Internal Respiration

Other than differences in magnitude, all of the internal respiration variables respond in the same way during long-term, moderate to heavy submaximal dynamic exercise as during shorter, lighter dynamic exercise, as previously described.

Despite the higher workload and the shallow U-shaped response, PaO_2 is relatively constant (**Figure 10.8A**).

Because of the heavier workload, more oxygen is dissociated and used, and the PvO_2 (**Figure 10.8C**) and SvO_2% (**Figure 10.8F**) decrease to lower levels than in shorter, lighter workloads. The result is a widening of the a-vO_2diff (**Figure 10.8E**). The factors responsible for the dissociation of oxygen are the same as those for lower-intensity exercise. $PaCO_2$ (**Figure 10.8B**) decreases slightly due to the increased volume of air being exhaled. $PvCO_2$ (**Figure 10.8D**) increases because the greater use of oxygen to produce energy also results in more carbon dioxide being carried in the venous system to the lungs to be exhaled.

Incremental Aerobic Exercise to Maximum

Incremental aerobic exercise to maximum consists of a series of progressively increasing work intensities, which stop when the individual cannot do any more work. The

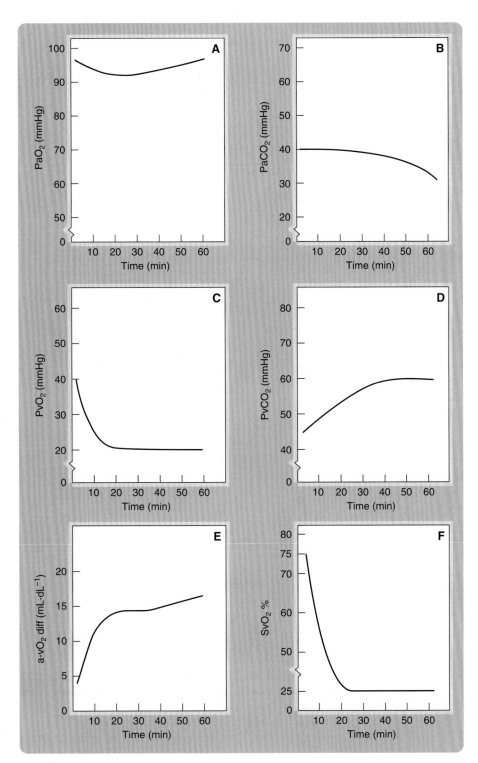

FIGURE 10.8 Responses of Internal Respiration Variables to Long-Term, Moderate to Heavy Submaximal Aerobic Exercise.
A. Partial pressure of oxygen in arterial blood. **B.** Partial pressure of carbon dioxide in arterial blood. **C.** Partial pressure of oxygen in venous blood. **D.** Partial pressure of carbon dioxide in venous blood. **E.** Arterial-venous oxygen difference. **F.** Percent saturation of venous blood with oxygen.

length of each work intensity, often called a stage, generally varies from 1 to 3 minutes to allow for the achievement of a steady state at that level, at least until the higher workloads, when a steady state cannot be either attained or maintained.

Pulmonary Ventilation

It might be anticipated, because $\dot{V}_E$ rises and levels off at submaximal workloads, that this rise would be proportional, direct, and rectilinear throughout the entire range from rest to maximal exercise. However, as shown in **Figure 10.9A**, the response is not a smooth rise. At light to moderate and even heavy intensities, up to approximately 50–75% of maximum workload, $\dot{V}_E$ does increase in a rectilinear fashion. At this point, a break in the linearity occurs, and a second, steeper linear rise ensues. This proportional rise continues until approximately 85–95% of maximum workload, when a second break in linearity occurs. The slope of the third linear rise to maximum that follows is even steeper (Koyal et al., 1976; Powers and Beadle, 1985; Wasserman, 1978). These points where the rectilinear rise in minute ventilation breaks from linearity during incremental exercise to maximum are called **ventilatory thresholds**. The first breakpoint is called the first ventilatory threshold (VT1), and the second breakpoint is called the second ventilatory threshold (VT2).

Precisely what causes these breakpoints is unknown. One theory has linked ventilatory breakpoints with an excess of carbon dioxide resulting from the buffering of lactic acid; this theory calls the breakpoints anaerobic thresholds. Although carbon dioxide is a known respiratory stimulator, this theory is probably not accurate (for reasons that are fully discussed in the unit on metabolism). Therefore, the term "ventilatory threshold" is preferable. Other possible mechanisms—including catecholamine or potassium stimulation of the carotid bodies; limitations in changes in V_T, frequency, and V_D/V_T to maintain $\dot{V}_A$; increasing body temperatures; and feedback from the skeletal muscle proprioceptors—have been suggested as causes of the VTs, but their role remains unproven. A combination of factors likely is responsible (Loat and Rhodes, 1993; Skinner and McLellan, 1980; Walsh and Banister, 1988).

Knowledge of the VTs, regardless of why they occur, has some practical benefit. The workloads at which the VTs occur are related to endurance exercise training and performance. VT1 is thought to indicate the upper boundary of moderate exercise and VT2 to separate heavy but sustainable exercise intensity from very heavy nonsustainable intensity. This means that VT1 and VT2 can be used for exercise prescription. That is, training at work rates between VT1 and VT2 would stimulate aerobic metabolism but allow for activity of long duration (Neder and Stein, 2006). It also means that the VTs can be useful for predicting performance (Amann et al., 2006). The higher the workload where the breaks occur, the greater the intensity of activity that can be sustained (Loat and Rhodes, 1993; Walsh and Banister, 1988).

Once again, the changes in minute ventilation ($\dot{V}_E$) during low to moderate workloads are achieved primarily by an increase in V_T (**Figure 10.9B**). At very heavy workloads, however, the depth of breathing may actually decrease, forming a truncated, inverted U-pattern (Dempsey, 1986; Younes and Kivinen, 1984). When V_T reaches its highest point, any further increase in ventilation can occur only as the result of an increased breathing frequency (Wasserman, 1978). The rise in breathing frequency is exponential at the higher work levels (**Figure 10.9C**). As with submaximal workloads,

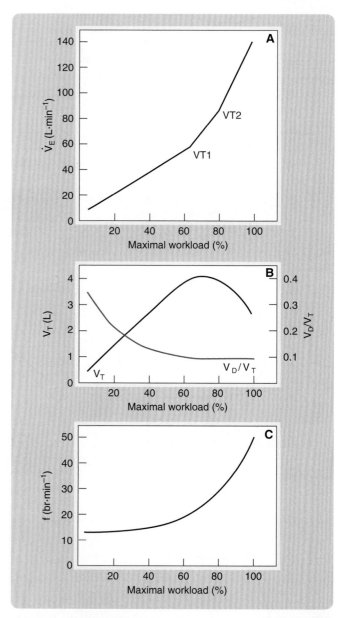

FIGURE 10.9 Responses of Pulmonary Ventilation Variables to Incremental Aerobic Exercise to Maximum. **A.** Minute ventilation. **B.** Tidal volume (V_T) and ratio of dead space to tidal volume (V_D/V_T). **C.** Frequency.

the V_D/V_T ratio decreases the most in the initial light to moderate stages of the incremental work (Grimby, 1969). The maximal reduction is reached at about 60% of maximal work, and this value is maintained to maximum. Since the V_D/V_T ratio is reduced to 0.1 (or 10% of V_T), 90% of V_T is available for exchange at the alveoli ($\dot{V}_A$), providing a more efficient ventilation (Grimby, 1969; Jones, 1975; Wasserman and Whipp, 1975; Wasserman et al., 1967).

External Respiration

Changes in $\dot{V}_A$ parallel the changes in $\dot{V}_E$, including the slope of the rectilinear rises and the two breakpoints (**Figure 10.10A**). The breakpoints in $\dot{V}_A$, however, occur before the breakpoints in $\dot{V}_E$—that is, at slightly lower percentages of maximal work (Jones, 1975; Wasserman, 1978).

The rise in $\dot{V}_A$ is sufficient to maintain P_AO_2 and subsequently PaO_2 through the light to moderate submaximal exercise stages (**Figure 10.10B**). As the workload becomes higher, P_AO_2 rises exponentially to maximum. This rise provides the driving force to reach an equilibrium of alveolar gas with mixed venous blood and, in so doing, maintains PaO_2 and SaO_2% (solid lines) within narrow limits in normal or moderately fit individuals (**Figure 10.10D**) (Dempsey, 1986; Grimby, 1969; Segal, 1992; Wasserman and Whipp, 1975; Wasserman et al., 1967). The (A-a)PO₂diff follows the pattern of the exponential rise in P_AO_2 (**Figure 10.10C**). The increase of the (A-a)PO₂diff to approximately 30 mmHg shown in **Figure 10.10C** is considered a small increase (Amann, 2012; Jones, 1975).

EXERCISE-INDUCED ARTERIAL HYPOXEMIA Refer again to **Figure 10.10B** and **D**. Note the dotted lines, which show steep decreases in PaO₂ and SaO₂%. A decrease of at least 10 mmHg PaO₂ or 4% SaO₂% (if persistent) is called **exercise-induced arterial hypoxemia (EIAH)**. This is a condition in which the amount of oxygen carried in arterial blood is decreased. As shown on the graph in **Figures 10.10B** and **10.11A**, the decline in PaO₂ with EIAH can be considerable, ranging from 18 to 38 mmHg below resting values (96 – 18 = 78 mmHg; 96 – 38 = 58 mmHg). At the same time, the SaO₂% (**Figure 10.10D**) is reduced. Mild EIAH is indicated by a SaO₂% of 93–95%, moderate as 88–93%, and severe as less than 88% (Amann, 2012; Richards et al., 2004).

Surprisingly, 40–50% of highly trained, healthy, elite male cyclists and runners with $\dot{V}O_2$max in excess of 4.5 L·min⁻¹ or 55 mL·kg⁻¹·min⁻¹ exhibit this response at work rates from 60% to 90% of maximum. Although most of

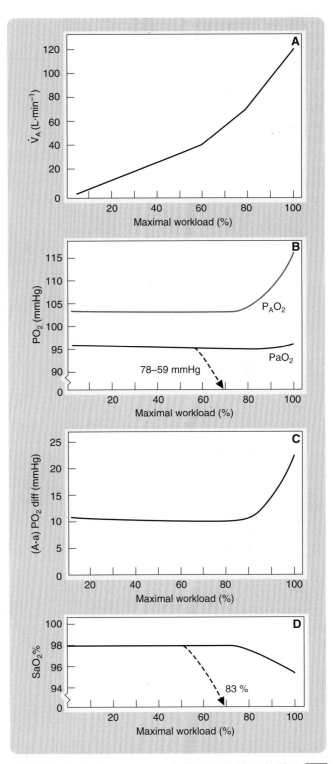

FIGURE 10.10 Responses of External Respiration Variables to Incremental Aerobic Exercise to Maximum. **A.** Alveolar ventilation. **B.** Partial pressure of oxygen at the alveoli (A) and in arterial blood (a). **C.** Partial pressure of oxygen gradient between the alveoli and the arteries. **D.** Percent saturation of arterial blood with oxygen.

Ventilatory Thresholds Points where the rectilinear rise in minute ventilation breaks from linearity during an incremental exercise to maximum.

Exercise-Induced Arterial Hypoxemia (EIAH) A condition in which the amount of oxygen carried in arterial blood is severely reduced by ≥4% consistently.

FIGURE 10.11 Responses of Internal Respiration Variables to Incremental Aerobic Exercise to Maximum.
A. Partial pressure of oxygen in arterial blood. **B.** Partial pressure of carbon dioxide in arterial blood. **C.** Partial pressure of oxygen in venous blood. **D.** Partial pressure of carbon dioxide in venous blood. **E.** Arterial-venous oxygen difference. **F.** Percent saturation of venous blood with oxygen.

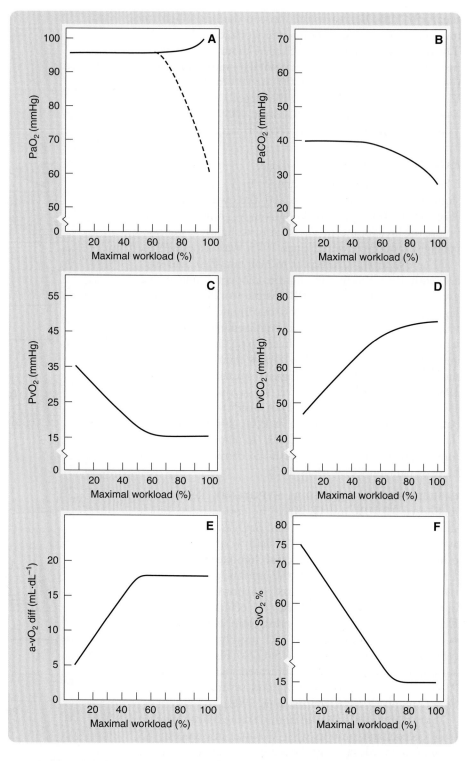

the original data were collected from these elite adult male athletes, there is now evidence of EIAH in females as well as younger and older adult athletes of both sexes (Prefaut et al., 2000). Recently, EIAH has also been reported in untrained, low-fit females (Richards et al., 2004) and nonelite sportsmen and sportswomen following high-intensity interval training (Mucci et al, 2004).

During EIAH, the individual's ability to process oxygen and therefore to perform high-intensity activity is lower than it would be without EIAH, although both may be higher than in untrained or moderately trained individuals. It has been estimated that $\dot{V}O_2$max is reduced by approximately 1.5–2% for each 1% reduction in SaO_2% (Dempsey and Wagner, 1999). One study tested participants with and without EIAH who had similar $\dot{V}O_2$max and power outputs (Legrand et al., 2005). The EIAH athletes, however, had higher muscle deoxygenation. That is, their working muscles had adapted and were able to compensate, at least to some extent, for the reduced oxygen delivery by extracting more oxygen from what was available. Thus, external respiration may be a limitation for exercise in some individuals with full or partial compensation from internal respiration. Athletes who exhibit EIAH at sea level suffer more severe gas exchange impairments during short-term exposure to higher altitudes than athletes who do not exhibit EIAH at sea level (Amann, 2012; Powers et al., 1993).

What causes EIAH? There are apparently two types of EIAH. The first occurs with a fast desaturation ($\downarrow SaO_2\%$) at relatively moderate submaximal workloads. The second occurs with a slow desaturation at high-intensity maximal exercise (Richards et al., 2004).

Evidence suggests that a relative hypoventilation induced by endurance training may be involved if the EIAH occurs at moderate submaximal exercise intensities (Aguilaniu et al., 2002; Prefaut et al., 2000). Although it has been suggested as a possible mechanism, inspiratory muscle fatigue does not appear to be a causal factor in fast desaturation EIAH. Diminished chemical responsiveness (review **Figure 9.10**) has also been speculated as another possible mechanism, but this has not been demonstrated consistently experimentally (Richards et al., 2004).

If the EIAH occurs only at higher intensities, both theoretical and experimental evidence suggest an inequality between respiratory ventilation and circulatory perfusion as the primary cause (Hopkins, 2006). This limits external respiration diffusion. The failure to achieve complete diffusion equilibrium may also be related to a mild, transient extravascular water accumulation and edema, which lengthens the diffusion distance from the alveolar membrane to the red blood cells (Hodges et al., 2006; Powers et al., 1993; Prefaut et al., 2000; Segal, 1992). Alternatively, this could be related to the faster transit time of red blood cells through the capillary bed of athletes with a highly developed cardiovascular system. In normal sedentary or moderately trained individuals, pulmonary capillary blood volume increases with exercise. This increases the surface area for diffusion and slows down the red blood cell transit time sufficiently to allow complete diffusion and equilibration of the gases. In highly trained athletes, pulmonary capillary blood volume reaches its maximum at relatively low workloads (Segal, 1992). When these elite athletes continue to increase their workloads and total body blood flow, pulmonary capillary volume cannot expand further. Instead, blood flow velocity increases, decreasing red blood cell transit time. As a result, the red blood cell transit time in elite endurance athletes is estimated to be considerably less than that required for gas equilibration (Wagner, 1991). This creates an imbalance between respiratory ventilation and circulatory perfusion and results in incomplete diffusion equilibrium. Why EIAH occurs in some individuals and not others has not been determined. Preventive techniques are unknown.

With EIAH, the $(A-a)PO_2$diff curve increases even more than shown in **Figure 10.10C**, and the $SaO_2\%$ curve declines as shown in **Figure 10.10D**. The excessively widened $(A-a)PO_2$diff is the most consistent contributor to EIAH and is also a definite indication of lack of efficiency in respiration (Rowell et al., 1964; Shapiro et al., 1964).

In addition to EIAH there are two other respiratory limitations to exercise. These are most evident in sustained high-intensity endurance exercise performance (>85% $\dot{V}O_2$max). They are respiratory muscle fatigue and positive expiratory intrathoracic pressures that limit cardiac output. High-intensity endurance exercise requires large increases in both inspiratory and expiratory muscle work, often leading to respiratory muscle fatigue. Metabolites accumulate in the respiratory muscles and activate afferent neurons that transport signals to the brain, which in turn increases sympathetic vasoconstrictor activity in the vasculature of the exercising limbs. This vasoconstriction leads to peripheral muscle fatigue, increased perception of effort, and a decrease in exercise performance. Any limitation in cardiac output contributes to a decrease in blood flow to the exercising limbs and brings about the same results. During sustained exercise >85% $\dot{V}O_2$max in a highly trained endurance athlete the respiratory muscles require up to 15–16% $\dot{V}O_2$max and cardiac output versus ≤10% in the untrained individual (Amann, 2012; Dempsey et al., 2008).

Internal Respiration

The dissociation or release of oxygen reaches its limit during incremental exercise to maximum. At low and moderate workloads, more and more oxygen is released according to the sigmoid-shaped curve in **Figure 10.3**. The factors that stimulate the dissociation of oxygen during incremental exercise to maximum are the same as previously described, but they typically are greater in magnitude, that is, the pressure gradient is wider, PCO_2 is higher, pH is lower, and temperature is higher as the exercise load increases (Wagner, 1991). A muscle PO_2 of 3–15 mmHg is considered reasonable for maximal or very heavy dynamic exercise, indicating that almost all of the oxygen can be extracted from the blood perfusing the working muscles. A muscle PO_2 of 15 mmHg has a corresponding pressure gradient of close to 80 mmHg (95 mmHg at the arterial end of the capillary minus 15 mmHg in the muscle tissue). Some oxygen is returned in venous blood. The result is a venous saturation ($SvO_2\%$) of oxygen of approximately 15–35% (**Figure 10.11F**), which exerts a partial pressure of 15–25 mmHg (**Figure 10.11C**) (Richardson et al., 1995a,b; Wagner, 2006).

As more oxygen is used to produce more energy, more carbon dioxide is produced. This metabolic carbon dioxide—as well as nonmetabolic carbon dioxide produced in the effort to buffer the lactic acid that accumulates at the higher workloads—results in the slightly curvilinear rise in $PvCO_2$ shown in **Figure 10.11D**.

	Short-Term, Light to Moderate Submaximal Aerobic Exercise	Long-Term, Moderate to Heavy Submaximal Aerobic Exercise[†]	Incremental Aerobic Exercise to Maximum	Static Exercise
TABLE 10.2 Respiratory Responses to Exercise*				
Pulmonary Ventilation				
$\dot{V}_E$	Increase rapidly; plateaus	Increases rapidly; plateaus; positive drift	Shows initial rectilinear rise; has two breakpoints	Minor gradual increase; rebound rise in recovery
V_D	Decreases	Decreases	Decreases	All responses the same as for short-term, light to moderate submaximal exercise
V_T	Increases rapidly; plateaus	Increases rapidly; plateaus	Has truncated, inverted U-shaped curve; increases greatly; has incomplete reversal	
f	Slowly increases; plateaus	Increases slowly; plateaus; positive drift	Positive curvilinear rise	
V_D/V_T	Decreases initially; plateaus	Decreases rapidly initially; plateaus	Decreases rapidly initially; levels off at 60% of maximum and is maintained	
External Respiration				
$\dot{V}_A$	Increases rapidly; plateaus	Increases rapidly; plateaus; positive drift	Shows initial rectilinear rise; has two breakpoints	
P_AO_2	Shows no change	Shows no change	Shows no change until approximately 75% of maximum; then positive exponential rise	
P_aO_2	Shows no change	Has small U-shaped curve	Shows no change until approximately 75% of maximum; then increases slightly	
(A-a) PO_2diff	Decreases slightly or shows no change (light); increases slightly (moderate)	Has truncated, inverted U-shaped curve; increases rapidly initially; has incomplete reversal	Shows no change until approximately 75% of maximum; then positive exponential rise[‡]	
SaO_2%	Decreases less than 1%; has U-shaped curve	—	—	
Internal Respiration				
$PaCO_2$	Is level; then decreases slightly	Is level; then decreases slightly	Is level; then decreases	
$PvCO_2$	Shows slight linear rise	Shows a gradual linear rise; plateaus	Has sharp rise; levels slightly	
PvO_2	Decreases rapidly; plateaus	Decreases rapidly; plateaus	Decreases sharply; levels off	
SvO_2%	Decreases initially; plateaus	Decreases initially; plateaus	Decreases sharply; never reaches 0	Shows no change or decreases slightly
a-vO_2diff	Increases rapidly; plateaus	Increases rapidly; plateaus; positive drift	Shows rectilinear rise to 40–60% $\dot{V}O_2$max; plateaus	No change during; rebound rise in recovery

*Resting values are taken as baseline.

[†]The difference between leveling during the short-term, light to moderate and long-term, moderate to heavy submaximal exercise responses is one of magnitude; that is, leveling occurs at a higher value with higher intensities.

[‡]Hypoxemia may occur in higher altitudes.

FOCUS ON APPLICATION: *Clinically Relevant*
Breathing Patterns during Exercise

Beginning exercisers often ask how and when they should breathe. The best advice for most land exercise appears to be to breathe in whatever pattern comes naturally, whether spontaneously or in an entrainment pattern. The primary exception is weight training. The static component of weight training can cause the **Valsalva maneuver**, a breath-holding action that involves closing of the glottis (which keeps air in the lungs) and contraction of the diaphragm and

abdominal musculature. The result is an increase in intra-abdominal pressure and a large increase in blood pressure. Individuals may become lightheaded or faint. Blood pressure remains much lower when breathing during the contraction. For this reason, it is generally recommended to inhale during the lowering phase of a resistance exercise and to exhale during the lifting phase of each repetition (Fleck and Kraemer, 2004; Narloch and Brandstater, 1995).

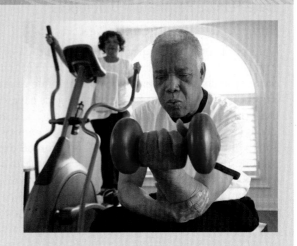

Conversely, PaCO$_2$ (**Figure 10.11B**) is maintained at first and then decreases. This fall in arterial carbon dioxide partial pressure reflects the excess removal of carbon dioxide brought about by alveolar hyperventilation (Dempsey et al., 1977; Grimby, 1969; Jones, 1975). The a-vO$_2$diff (**Figure 10.11E**) parallels the changes in oxygen dissociation, gradually increasing with the incremental workloads until it can increase no more. It plateaus at approximately 50–60% of the maximal workload (Rowell, 1969; Saltin, 1969). Thus, even maximal exercise is well within the respiratory reserves for most individuals.

Static Exercise

Static exercise involves the production of force or tension with no mechanical work being done. Therefore, gradations of static exercise are usually expressed relative to the individual's ability to produce force in a given muscle group (called the maximal voluntary contraction, or MVC) held for a specified period of time. For example, an individual might perform a 30% MVC for 5 minutes.

Figure 4.5 presents respiratory and metabolic responses to heavy static exercise. Note that, despite this being "heavy" static activity, the rise in $\dot{V}O_2$ representing energy cost is minimal. As always, pulmonary ventilation ($\dot{V}_E$) increases to provide the needed additional oxygen. At the onset of static exercise, however, the initial (0–2 minutes) three-phase response in $\dot{V}_E$ that occurs in aerobic exercise is

> **Entrainment** The synchronization of limb movement and breathing frequency that accompanies rhythmical exercise.
>
> **Valsalva Maneuver** Breath holding that involves closing of the glottis and contraction of the diaphragm and abdominal musculature.

absent. The a-vO$_2$diff either remains the same or decreases slightly during static exercise. This is undoubtedly related to the occlusion of blood flow in statically contracting muscles. For both $\dot{V}_E$ and a-vO$_2$diff, a rebound rise occurs in recovery. In all other aspects, the respiratory responses are similar in static exercise and in low-intensity, aerobic exercise. Static exercise does not push the reserve capacity of the respiratory system (Asmussen, 1981).

Table 10.2 summarizes the respiratory responses to exercise discussed in preceding sections.

Entrainment of Respiration during Exercise

In some but not all individuals, the performance of rhythmical exercise (such as walking, running, cycling, and rowing) is accompanied by a synchronization of limb movement and breathing frequency called **entrainment** (Bechbache and Duffin, 1977; Caretti et al., 1992; Clark et al., 1983; Hill et al., 1988; Jasinskas et al., 1980; Kay et al., 1975; Mahler et al., 1991; Sporer et al., 2007). For example, an individual may always inhale during the recovery phase of rowing and always exhale during the drive portion of the stroke. Or a walker, runner, or cyclist may always exhale during the push-off phase of one leg or the other. Unlike swimming, in which breathing coordination is a function of head placement during the stroke as a learned response, entrainment occurs without conscious thought.

Individuals who entrain naturally have a slightly improved ventilatory efficiency (Bonsignore et al., 1998) and a lower energy cost during exercise when they entrain but not when they breathe randomly. However, subjects forced to breathe in specific entrainment patterns rather than being allowed to breathe spontaneously do not exhibit any reduction in energy cost or perceive any less breathing effort with entrained breathing (Maclennan et al., 1994).

The Influence of Sex and Age on Respiration at Rest and during Exercise

Male-Female Respiratory Differences

Lung Volumes and Capacities

Values for total lung capacity (TLC) and each of its subdivisions are, on the average, lower for females than males across the entire age span, with the possible exception of around 12–13 years of age, when most girls have had their pubertal growth spurt but boys have not. These differences carry over into the dynamic measurements of maximal voluntary ventilation (MVV) and forced expiratory volume in one second (FEV_1). Part of these differences can be attributed to the smaller size of females. Males, for example, have larger-diameter airways, more alveoli, and larger diffusion surfaces than females. However, even when values are expressed relative to height, weight, or surface area, some differences in lung capacities remain (Åstrand, 1952; Comroe, 1965; Ferris et al., 1965; Harms, 2006).

Pulmonary Ventilation

At rest, there is no consistent difference in breathing frequency between males and females (Malina et al., 2004). However, at the same submaximal ventilation, females typically display a higher frequency and a lower V_T than males. This pattern is maintained at maximal exercise (Saris et al., 1985) (**Figure 10.12B**). Ventilatory responsiveness during exercise may be influenced in females by levels of circulating estrogen and progesterone (Harms, 2006). Males also exhibit higher $\dot{V}_E$ at most ages than females at maximal exercise, although these differences are narrowed considerably when expressed relative to body weight (**Figure 10.12A**) (Åstrand, 1952, 1960). Surprisingly, experiments have shown that the inspiratory muscles including the diaphragm of females may fatigue at a slower rate than those of males (Gonzales and Scheuermann, 2006; Guenette et al., 2010).

External and Internal Respiration

Data to compare males and females are unavailable for most external and internal respiratory measures (Harms, 2006). The a-vO_2diff has been measured at rest and during submaximal and maximal exercise, but the results show little consistency (Åstrand et al., 1964; Becklake et al., 1965; Zwiren et al., 1983). The (A-a)PO_2diff is higher and the PaO_2 is lower in females compared to males at any given level of oxygen utilization. An excessive widening of the (A-a)PO_2diff occurs in EIAH, and females exhibit this condition at least as often as males (Harms, 2006). $\dot{V}_A$ is equal in males and females. The $PaCO_2$ is slightly lower in females than males at any given $\dot{V}O_2$ (Hopkins and Harms, 2004).

Children and Adolescents

Lung Volumes and Capacities

In general, the TLC and each of its subdivisions increase in a mostly rectilinear pattern for both boys and girls as they progress from about 6 years of age into the late teens or early twenties. The FEV_1 and MVV follow essentially the same incremental pattern in children (Åstrand, 1952; Åstrand et al., 1963; Bjure, 1963; Koyal et al., 1976; Malina et al., 2004). From birth to approximately age 10, these changes depend largely on the growth and development of the respiratory system. After that, cell proliferation ceases and hypertrophy of existing structures occurs until maturity. Thus, these changes result primarily but not exclusively from structural enlargement and are strongly related to body height (Bjure, 1963; Johnson and Dempsey, 1991). When the subdivisions of TLC are expressed as a percentage of the V_T, the proportions remain the same from about age 8 to age 20. The anatomical dead space increases in proportion to maturity (Ashley et al., 1975; Robinson, 1938) and, as in adults, is approximately 1 $mL \cdot lb^{-1}$ of body weight (Rowland, 2005).

Pulmonary Ventilation

The control of ventilation is similar in children and adults, except that there is a lower set point of PCO_2 in children than adults (Rowland, 2005). However, there are some minor differences in $\dot{V}_E$ and its components across the age span (Zauner et al., 1989).

REST The $\dot{V}_E$ at rest is surprisingly consistent regardless of age (Robinson, 1938). **Figure 10.13** shows that $\dot{V}_E$ in males varies less than 2 $L \cdot min^{-1}$ from ages 6 to 76. Comparable data are not available for females. When $\dot{V}_E$ is expressed relative to body weight, younger boys have a higher $\dot{V}_E$ than older adolescents or adults, but from adolescence to old age, there is little change in $\dot{V}_E$.

The remarkably consistent $\dot{V}_E$ is achieved differently by children, however, than by older adolescents and adults. **Figure 10.14A** shows that breathing frequency is higher and V_T lower in youngsters than in older adolescents and adults. From approximately the midteen years until old age, frequency stabilizes at 10 $br \cdot min^{-1}$, and V_T stabilizes at about 500 mL in males (Malina et al., 2004; Robinson, 1938). Younger children use a higher portion of their VC as V_T than older adolescents and young adults (**Figure 10.14B**).

SUBMAXIMAL EXERCISE Children's and adolescents' respiratory responses to exercise are similar to those of adults. $\dot{V}_E$ rises in response to greater oxygen needs at all ages, but it does so faster at the onset of exercise in younger individuals than adults (Rowland, 2005). The higher $\dot{V}_E$ in relation to body weight at rest is maintained, as is the variation in how $\dot{V}_E$ is obtained. That is, children exhibit a higher frequency and lower V_T at any given submaximal

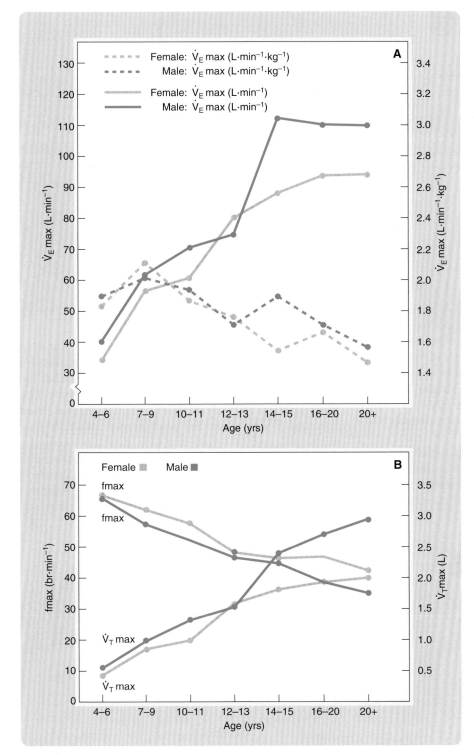

FIGURE 10.12 Pulmonary Ventilation Responses to Maximal Treadmill Exercise as Children Age to Adulthood for Males and Females. *Source:* Based on data from Åstrand (1952).

load than adults. They also respond with a higher $\dot{V}_E$ in relation to body weight at an equal work rate. The ratio of liters of air processed per one liter of oxygen used ($\dot{V}_E/\dot{V}O_2$) is called the **ventilatory equivalent.** Children and adolescents have a higher ventilatory equivalent at all exercise intensities than adults, indicating that they are hyperventilating. Girls hyperventilate more than boys (Rowland, 2005). These differences are considered negative, indicating a wasteful ventilation, and gradually disappear by late adolescence (Bar-Or, 1983; Do Prado et al., 2010; Robinson, 1938; Rowland, 2005; Rowland and Green, 1988; Rowland et al., 1987). **Figure 10.15A**

Ventilatory Equivalent The ratio of liters of air processed per liter of oxygen used ($\dot{V}_E/\dot{V}O_2$).

FIGURE 10.13 Minute Ventilation at Rest and during Maximal Exercise for Males Aged 6–76.
Source: Based on data from Robinson (1938).

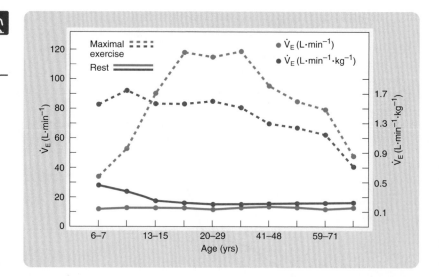

and **B** show differences in frequency (f), V_T, and $\dot{V}_E$ for 11-year-old girls and boys in comparison to 29-year-old adults (Rowland and Green, 1988; Rowland et al., 1987). The speeds are different for males and females, so direct comparison between the sexes cannot be made, but within the sexes, the age differences are similar. In addition to the differences shown in **Figure 10.15**, younger children use a marginally lower proportion of their VC during submaximal exercise than adults.

During prolonged submaximal exercise, children and adolescents have the same ventilatory drift as adults, probably in response to a rising core temperature. Nothing in the respiratory response to prolonged exercise would indicate that children are not suited for such activity (Malina et al., 2004; Rowland, 2005).

MAXIMAL EXERCISE In general, children's responses to maximal exercise parallel the differences seen at rest and during submaximal work rates. The older the child, the higher the $\dot{V}_E$ that can be achieved in absolute terms. The $\dot{V}_E$ in relation to body weight gradually declines from about age 7 until adulthood is achieved at about 20 years of age, although in 4- to 6-year-olds, this value is comparable to that of young adults (**Figure 10.12A**) (Åstrand, 1952; Åstrand et al., 1963; Fahey et al., 1979; Krahenbuhl et al., 1985; Robinson, 1938; Rowland, 1990; Rowland and Green, 1988). Breathing frequency decreases

FIGURE 10.14 Frequency of Breathing, Tidal Volume, and the Percentage of Vital Capacity Used as Tidal Volume at Rest and during Maximal Exercise for Males Aged 6–76.
Source: Based on data from Robinson (1938).

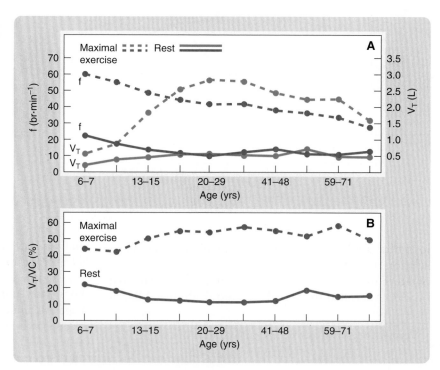

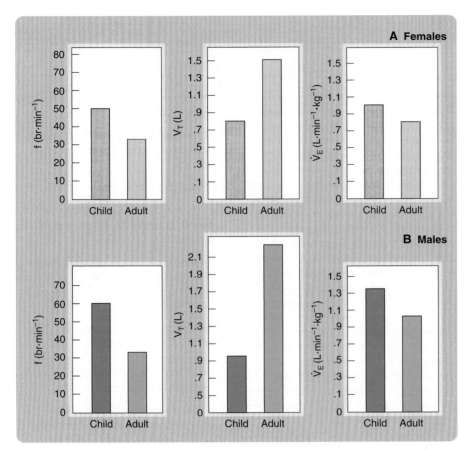

FIGURE 10.15 Pulmonary Ventilation Responses to Submaximal Exercise in Male and Female Children and Adults.
Females: Mean age of child = 11.3 years, adult = 28.7 years; treadmill speed = 7.3 kph (122 m·min⁻¹). Males: Mean age of child = 11.6 years, adult = 29.2 years; treadmill speed = 9.6 kph (160 m·min⁻¹). *Sources*: Based on data from Rowland and Green (1988) and Rowland et al. (1987).

consistently from the youngest children tested to approximately age 20, while V_T shows a steady rise over the same time span (**Figure 10.12B**). The percentage of VC used as V_T rises slightly from childhood to young adulthood. The $\dot{V}_E/\dot{V}O_2$ gradually declines at maximal work in both boys and girls (Rowland, 2005). Children also show ventilatory breakpoints during incremental exercise to maximum. Some inconclusive evidence suggests that VT1 and VT2 (expressed as a percentage of $\dot{V}O_2$max) are higher in younger children than adults and gradually decline as children mature into adults (Do Prado et al., 2010; Mahon and Cheatham, 2002). The physiological mechanisms responsible for the VT1 and VT2 in children are as unclear as they are for adults (Bar-Or, 1983; Rowland and Green, 1988).

External and Internal Respiration

Little is known about the changes in gas exchange and transport that occur during normal growth and maturation. The higher frequency and lower V_T of children in relation to adolescents and adults, at rest and during exercise, seem to be offset by their smaller anatomical dead space. Consequently, $\dot{V}_A$ is more than adequate at all values of $\dot{V}_E$ (Bar-Or, 1983; Malina et al., 2004; Zauner et al., 1989).

Pulmonary diffusion during exercise does not appear to differ by age. Likewise, no meaningful aging trends are apparent for P_AO_2, PaO_2, or $(A-a)PO_2$diff at rest or during exercise. However, PaO_2 decreases slightly and the $(A-a)PO_2$diff increases slightly as children mature to adulthood (Bar-Or, 1983; Eriksson, 1972; Robinson, 1938). As a consequence, SaO_2% is also relatively constant across the age span (Robinson, 1938). EIAH is evident in some trained youth as in some adults, and the causes are also uncertain in this age group (Nourry et al., 2004; Prefaut et al., 2000).

The a-vO_2diff is also very similar at both rest and maximal exercise levels from childhood to maturity. If anything, children may be able to extract about 5% more oxygen during maximal exercise than adults (Eriksson, 1973).

Older Adults

Lung Volumes and Capacities

The effect of aging on TLC is controversial. Inconsistent evidence shows that TLC may decrease or stay the same in individuals over the age of 50 (Berglund et al., 1963; Jain and Gupta, 1974a,b; Johnson and Dempsey, 1991; Kenney, 1982; Stanescu et al., 1974; Storstein and Voll, 1974). However, research has firmly established that VC and inspiratory capacity (IC) decrease with age and that residual volume (RV) and functional residual capacity (FRC) increase, thus changing the percentage of total volume that each occupies (Åstrand, 1952, 1960; Ericsson and Irnell, 1974; Slonim and Hamilton, 1976; Stanescu et al., 1974; Turner et al., 1968). For example, the ratio

FOCUS ON APPLICATION
Side Stitches

The "side stitch," known medically as *exercise-related transient abdominal pain (ETAP)*, is a common, poorly understood, generally self-limiting acute abdominal pain that is difficult to treat (Waterman and Kapur, 2012). Mild ETAP is generally described as cramping, aching, or pulling whereas more severe pain is described as sharp or stabbing. Most stitches occur in the right or left lumbar regions of the abdomen, but occasionally the pain radiates to the shoulder. Although most frequently associated with runners, a high incidence of ETAP has also been reported in other athletes whose sport involves repetitive torso movement and/or jolting such as swimmers and endurance equestrians. Cyclists seem to have a low incidence of ETAP (Morton and Callister, 2000).

Stitches seem to occur more frequently in younger individuals and in individuals with kyphotic or lordotic spinal misalignment (Morton and Callister, 2010). Some studies report more incidences of stitch in females than males, but others do not. ETAP is experienced more commonly when starting a new or increased exercise routine, but training/fitness level is not totally protective (Morton and Callister, 2002; Waterman and Kapur, 2012). The consumption of large amounts of food before or fruit juice that is high in carbohydrate and osmolality both shortly before and during exercise tends to increase the incidence of stitches in individuals susceptible to ETAP (Morton and Callister, 2000; Morton et al., 2004).

Several theories have been postulated to explain the causes of ETAP, but there is no consensus to date (Waterman and Kapur, 2012). Theories include (1) a lack of blood flow to the diaphragm during exercise leading to pain from ischemia; (2) subdiaphragmatic visceral ligament stress; (3) skeletal muscle cramps; and (4) irritation of the parietal peritoneum. Given that the muscles involved in respiration may deprive the rest of the body of blood flow under circumstances of deficit cardiac output and that ETAP is not associated with reduced inspiratory performance it is unlikely that the diaphragm is directly responsible (Morton and Callister, 2000, 2006). Electromyogram (EMG) activity is not elevated during ETAP; therefore it is also highly unlikely that muscle cramps are responsible despite the subjective feeling of cramping (Morton and Callister, 2008). The visceral ligament stress theory is consistent with the influence of increased mass in the gut but does not explain the shoulder-referred pain. The primary function of the parietal peritoneum is to lubricate mobile viscera. Irritation could arise as a result of friction and that in turn could lead to pain. However promising this theory, it has yet to be fully substantiated (Morton and Callister, 2000; Plunkett and Hopkins, 1999; Waterman and Kapur, 2012).

Several practical applications of the collective research have been suggested. To avoid a side stitch, an exerciser can try these recommendations:

1. Do not exercise immediately after eating a big meal or ingesting a large amount of fluid (≥1 L). Wait 2–3 hours.

2. When drinking during exercise, take small amounts (200–400 mL) frequently (at 15- to 30-minutes intervals) rather than a single large drink at a rest stop or aid station.

3. When running downhill, try to keep your breathing regular and your footfalls light.

To deal with a stitch when it occurs:

1. Push in at the location of the pain with your hand, bend forward, and tighten the abdominal muscles.

2. Breathe more deeply to move more air into the lungs at the beginning of each breath, but do not try to force more air out at the end of each breath.

3. Breathe out through pursed lips. This contracts the abdominals. At the same time, if you are an entrainment breather, try to exhale on the opposite foot/side from normal.

4. If you experience side stitches frequently, try wearing a light, wide belt around your waist that can be tightened when necessary.

Sources: Morton and Callister (2000, 2002, 2006, 2008, 2010), Morton et al. (2004), Plunkett and Hopkins (1999), Waterman and Kapur (2012).

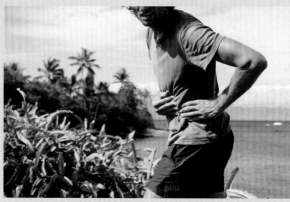

of RV/TLC doubles from about 15 to 30% in the elderly (Comroe, 1965; Johnson and Dempsey, 1991).

FEV_1 and MVV decline steadily after approximately age 35 in both males and females (Ashley et al., 1975; Ericsson and Irnell, 1974; Shepard, 1978; Slonim and Hamilton, 1976; Stanescu et al., 1974). These declines result from a combination of structural and mechanical changes in the respiratory system. These changes include (1) decreased elastic recoil of lung tissue; (2) stiffening of the thoracic cage, which decreases chest mobility and creates a greater reliance on the diaphragm; (3) a decrease in intervertebral spaces, which in turn decreases height and changes the shape of the thoracic cavity; and (4) losses in respiratory muscle force and velocity of contraction. Of all these changes, the loss of elastic recoil appears to be the most important (Johnson and Dempsey, 1991; Turner et al., 1968).

Pulmonary Ventilation

REST Resting $\dot{V}_E$ (**Figure 10.13**) and its components V_T and frequency (**Figure 10.14A**) are remarkably consistent across the entire age span. However, at rest, the percentage of VC used as V_T does show a very slight U-shaped curve (**Figure 10.14B**). Both young children and older adults use slightly more of their VC for V_T at rest than young adults (Robinson, 1938).

SUBMAXIMAL EXERCISE $\dot{V}_E$ rises in older adults in response to increased energy needs. As in young adults, this increase is accomplished mainly by an increase in V_T at lighter work rates and then by an increased frequency, if needed. Like children, older adults seem to have an exaggerated response in $\dot{V}_E$ compared with younger adults. That is, the absolute $\dot{V}_E$ is higher at any given work rate in older than in younger adults. Because the VC decreases with age and V_T remains fairly stable, V_T represents a higher percentage of the older adult's VC (Åstrand, 1952, 1960; Davies, 1972; DeVries and Adams, 1972; Robinson, 1938; Shepard, 1978).

MAXIMAL EXERCISE With aging, both the ability to exercise maximally and the ability to process air decline. The decrement in pulmonary function contributes to the decline in work capacity but probably simply parallels the changes in circulation, metabolism, and muscle function that are occurring.

The highest $\dot{V}_E$ values are typically seen in young adults, and these may decline by almost half by the seventh decade of life (**Figure 10.13**). This decline is evident both in absolute values ($\dot{V}_E$ in liters per minute) and in values adjusted for body weight ($\dot{V}_E$ in liters per kilogram per minute). Most of this decline is brought about by a reduction in V_T, although maximal frequency does decrease slightly.

The percentage of VC used during maximal work is relatively stable with age from young adulthood on. However, the dead space to tidal volume ratio is consistently 15–20% higher in older adults than in younger adults (Robinson, 1938) because dead space increases both at rest and during exercise. The ventilatory breakpoints occur at lower absolute and relative workloads in older adults than in younger adults (Shepard, 1978). Respiratory work and the sensation of dyspnea are increased at maximal work in older adults.

External Respiration

REST The loss of elastic recoil in the lungs not only affects static and dynamic lung volumes but also influences the distribution of air in the lungs. Thus, ventilation may not be preferentially directed to the base of the lung in the upright posture at rest, although most blood flow is still directed there. As a result, there may be an imbalance between alveolar ventilation and pulmonary perfusion (Johnson and Dempsey, 1991).

In addition, structural changes in aging lung tissue decrease the alveolar capillary surface area, which in turn means a decrease in diffusion capacity (Donevan et al., 1959; Johnson and Dempsey, 1991). Furthermore, pulmonary capillary blood volume decreases because of a stiffening of both pulmonary arteries and capillaries. The cumulative effects of these changes are a decrease in PaO_2, but not P_AO_2, and a widening of the $(A-a)PO_2$diff—although these changes are neither inevitable nor large. The saturation of hemoglobin with oxygen in arterial blood declines about 2–3% from age 10 to age 70 (Robinson, 1938; Shepard, 1978).

EXERCISE During exercise, the increased ventilation that is required results in a more homogeneous distribution of ventilation in the lungs. Although the decreases noted at rest in diffusion surface and pulmonary capillary blood volume remain, the matching of ventilation and perfusion improves during exercise as more of the lung is used. The available reserve is sufficient to meet the demands for oxygen transport even to maximal exercise levels.

Nevertheless, $\dot{V}_A$ is a smaller portion of minute ventilation in older adults than in younger adults. This change indicates a slightly decreased efficiency of respiration, but general arterial hypoxemia is prevented, and carbon dioxide elimination is adequate. That is, the PaO_2 and $PaCO_2$ are maintained within narrow limits and are similar to those for younger adults. The $(A-a)PO_2$diff is more variable in older than in younger adults but, on average, is only slightly wider than the usual mean values for younger individuals (Johnson and Dempsey, 1991; Robinson, 1938; Shepard, 1978). Highly fit older adults can, however, exhibit EIAH, as noted previously (Prefaut et al., 2000).

Internal Respiration

At rest and at any given submaximal level of exercise, the a-vO_2diff is greater in older adults than in younger adults. Thus, SvO_2% is lower. Conversely, at maximal exercise, the a-vO_2diff is lower in older individuals than in younger ones. Maximal values average 14–15 mL·dL^{-1} in older adults but average 15–20 mL·dL^{-1} in younger adults. Some of these changes in the a-vO_2diff can be attributed to a shift in the oxygen dissociation curve to the left, which makes the release of oxygen to the tissues more difficult (Kenney, 1982; Shepard, 1978). Refer to **Figure 10.3** to see this effect.

Respiratory Muscle Training Principles and Adaptations

Extensive training principles or guidelines are not included here for the respiratory system because respiratory training for healthy individuals is still rare and requires specialized equipment. Yet the respiratory muscles are muscles and as such are subject to fatigue, especially the diaphragm and as mentioned previously this may cause vasoconstriction in the working musculature. During both short- and long-duration incremental or constant load exercise ≤80% $\dot{V}O_2$max, the diaphragm does not fatigue. However, at more than 80% $\dot{V}O_2$max intensity continued to exhaustion, the diaphragm does fatigue. The consequence of this fatigue is a decrease in exercise tolerance (Sheel, 2002). One study (Enright et al., 2006) documented increased diaphragm thickness with increased performance and power output after high-intensity inspiratory muscle training. There is a growing interest in specific training for the respiratory muscles.

There are three major types of respiratory muscle training (RMT): (1) inspiratory flow resistive loading (IFRL); (2) voluntary isocapnic hyperpnea training (VIHT); and (3) inspiratory pressure-threshold loading (IPTL). Only occasionally has expiratory muscle training been undertaken, most training involves only the inspiratory muscles.

Two techniques for IFRL training are used. The first utilizes equipment that requires the individual to inspire using a variable diameter opening. At any given flow, the smaller the opening, the greater the resistance. The second first tests individuals by having them forcefully exhale to residual volume followed immediately by maximally inhaling against resistance to TLC. An image representing typically 80% of this pressure-time profile effort is presented on the computer screen. The training regime requires the participant to match (or exceed) this onscreen template within a progressively increasing work-rest ratio. For example, the maneuver is initially performed six times with a 60-second recovery. Only 45 seconds of recovery is permitted following the second set of six efforts. This pattern continues for six sets during which recovery is gradually reduced to 5 seconds.

VIHT is performed with a device that uses partial rebreathing and ensures normal CO_2 values. Tidal volume is controlled by feedback and breathing frequency is paced. Training sessions are typically conducted for 30 min·d^{-1}, 3–5 d wk^{-1} at 60–90% of MVV.

IPTL involves inspiration against a resistance at a set percentage of peak inspiratory mouth pressure using a specific muscle trainer. This device requires continuous application of inspiratory pressure during inspiration for the valve to remain open while allowing for unrestricted expiration. Typically 30 inspiratory efforts are performed twice a day.

In general, regardless of the specific type of inspiratory muscle training employed, functional measures of inspiratory muscle strength, endurance, maximal rate of shortening, and power have been increased. The importance of these changes is that they likely prevent or delay exercise-induced diaphragmatic fatigue. Delaying or diminishing respiratory muscle fatigue may attenuate the reflex vasoconstrictor activity in the limbs and help preserve limb blood flow. Whole body training does not provide resistance to inspiratory muscles fatigue. Structurally, significant increases in the proportion of Type I (slow twitch, oxidative) fibers and the size of Type II (fast twitch, oxidative glycolytic) fibers have been observed with RMT. Often, but not always, the perception of dyspnea is decreased. Respiratory values for minute ventilation, alveolar ventilation, breathing frequency, and tidal volume as well as oxygen consumption and lactate concentration are typically lowered and actual performance increased during constant submaximal performances or time trials, whereas no improvement is seen at maximal exercise. The magnitude of performance improvements when compared to control groups ranges from approximately 3 to 36%. The inability of RMT to bring about significant changes in $\dot{V}O_2$max is not really surprising as central circulatory adaptations require sustained and direct cardiovascular stimulation and this does not occur during RMT. In addition, $\dot{V}O_2$max tests only require high respiratory volumes for a brief period at the end of the test. Conversely, endurance time-trial performances require high ventilatory volumes for a long duration placing a greater demand directly on respiratory muscles. These positive changes have been seen in rowers, cyclists, soccer players, swimmers, and runners as well as nonathletes such as the elderly (Edwards and Walker, 2009; Forbes et al., 2011; Griffiths and McConnell, 2007; Inbar et al., 2000; Kilding et al., 2010; Leddy et al., 2007; McConnell and Romer, 2004; Mickleborough et al., 2010; Nicks et al., 2009; Ray et al., 2010; Romer et al., 2002; Verges et al., 2007; Volianitis et al., 2001; Watsford and Murphy, 2008; Williams et al., 2002).

Controlled Frequency Breathing Training

In addition to RMT, swimmers occasionally use a technique called controlled frequency breathing (CFB) as a training technique. As opposed to RMT, which makes the work of breathing harder, CFB restricts the number of breaths from the normal breathing pattern. The original assumption was that if a swimmer inhaled once every third, fifth, or eighth arm stroke, instead of every other arm stroke, then the reduced volume of air taken in would decrease oxygen partial pressure and create hypoxia, a decrease in available oxygen. According to this idea, hypoxia should bring about the same beneficial effects for swimmers as altitude training. Now it is accepted that this does not occur. However, it is theorized that by restricting air exchange at the lungs, oxygen concentrations in pulmonary circulation and at the muscle tissue level allow the swimmer to train at moderate intensity but to mimic the limited oxygen levels characteristic of high-intensity exercise, thus stimulating adaptations to improve oxygen delivery. The long-term benefits of CFB on either sprint or endurance swim performance have yet to be evaluated.

Controlled frequency breathing does reduce $\dot{V}O_2$ somewhat despite compensatory increases in V_T and oxygen extraction. At the same time, CFB as low as every fourth stroke increases the severity of inspiratory muscle fatigue that occurs during high-intensity front crawl swimming. Most importantly, it produces not hypoxia but hypercapnia, an increase in the partial pressure of carbon dioxide. The hypercapnia in turn has been shown to alter the heart rate response to exercise by lowering it. This reduction in exercise HR means that if workouts are monitored by HR intensity, adjustment needs to be made in target values. In addition, hypercapnia often causes headaches that last for 30 minutes or more after the workout ceases. These headaches are painful and may interfere with training. On the positive side, CFB may increase buoyancy and improve body position, enabling the swimmer to concentrate on the biomechanics of the stroke. Despite this, CFB should be used sparingly and be closely monitored (Dicker et al., 1980; Holmer and Gullstrand, 1980; Jakovljevic and McConnell, 2009; Lavoie and Montpetit, 1986; West et al., 2005; Zempel, 1989).

Whole Body Respiratory Training Principles and Adaptations

Other than the specific responses to inspiratory muscle training indicated above, training adaptations that have been documented in the respiratory system occur as a byproduct of whole body training for cardiovascular, neuromuscular, and/or metabolic improvement. Applications of the training principles are presented for these systems in their respective units. The few training adaptations that do occur in the respiratory system are documented in the following section.

Lung Volumes and Capacities

Studies of land training (running, cycling, wrestling, and the like) have found no consistent significant changes in TLC, VC, RV, FRC, or IC in males or females of any age; nor have they found any differences favoring athletes over nonathletes (Bachman and Horvath, 1968; Cordain et al., 1990; Dempsey and Fregosi, 1985; Eriksson, 1972; Kaufmann et al., 1974; Niinimaa and Shepard, 1978; Reuschlein et al., 1968; Saltin et al., 1968). Studies of water-based activities (swimming and scuba diving), however, have shown that swimmers have higher volumes and capacities than both land-based athletes and nonathletes (Cordain et al., 1990; Leith and Bradley, 1976). In addition, swim training studies have demonstrated increases in TLC and VC in both children and young adults. Similar generalizations can be made for the dynamic measures of FEV_1 and MVV

(Andrew et al., 1972; Bachman and Horvath, 1968; Clanton et al., 1987; Vaccaro and Clarke, 1978; Walsh and Banister, 1988).

Precisely why swimmers but not land-based athletes show improvements in static and dynamic lung volumes is not known. However, swimmers doing all strokes except the backstroke breathe against the resistance of water, using a restricted breathing pattern with repeated expansion of the lungs to total lung capacity. Swimming also takes place with the body in a horizontal position, and this posture is optimal for perfusion of the lung and diffusion of respiratory gases (Cordain and Stager, 1988; Mostyn et al., 1963).

Pulmonary Ventilation

Changes in $\dot{V}_E$ are the primary and most consistent adaptations seen in the respiratory system as a result of endurance training. Although $\dot{V}_E$ itself does not change at rest, a shift occurs in its components: V_T increases, and frequency decreases. This shift is maintained during submaximal work but overall V_T is lower during submaximal exercise as a result of the training. At maximal work, $\dot{V}_E$ is higher after training than before, accompanying the ability to do more work. The major component that changes is frequency, but V_T increases as well (Dempsey et al., 1977; Mahler et al., 1991; Rasmussen et al., 1975; Reid and Thomson, 1985; Whipp, 1977; Wilmore et al., 1970). In addition, the capacity for sustaining high levels of voluntary ventilation is improved, reflecting increased strength and endurance of the respiratory muscles (Krahenbuhl et al., 1985; Robinson and Kjeldgaard, 1992).

These adaptations occur within the first 6–10 weeks of a training program (Reid and Thomson, 1985). They result from both land- and water-based activities across the entire age span (Bar-Or, 1983; Fringer and Stull, 1974; Nourry et al., 2004; Pollock et al., 1969; Seals et al., 1984; Zauner and Benson, 1981; Zauner et al., 1989). The ventilatory thresholds shift to a higher workload and oxygen consumption as a result of training both in children and in adults indicating that a greater intensity of exercise can be maintained during endurance exercise performance across this age span (Haffor et al., 1990; Laursen et al., 2005; Loat and Rhodes, 1993; Mahon and Cheatham, 2002; Paterson et al., 1987; Pogliaghi et al., 2006; Poole and Gaesser, 1985).

External and Internal Respiration

In a healthy individual of any age and either sex, gas exchange varies little as a result of training (Reid and Thomson, 1985). Diffusion capacity has been reported to be higher in elite swimmers (Comroe, 1965; Magel and Andersen, 1969; Mostyn et al., 1963; Vaccaro et al., 1977) and runners (Kaufmann et al., 1974), but it does not

Respiratory Training Changes in Older Adults

This study exemplifies several important concepts discussed in this text. Eighteen healthy sedentary males, aged 65–75 years, were divided into three equal groups. One group performed leg training (LT) on a leg ergometer (LE); the second group performed arm training (AT) on an arm ergometer (AE); the third group served as a control (C) and remained sedentary. Pre (before) and post (after) training, all participants performed two incremental exercise tests to maximum: one on the cycle ergometer and one on the arm ergometer. Twelve weeks of training occurred between tests. Training intensity was based on heart rate at the first ventilatory threshold (HR_{VT1}): 7 minutes at 90%; 10 minutes at 100%; 5 minutes at 110%; and 5 minutes at 90% for a total of 30 minutes 3 d·wk^{-1}. This is an example of how VT1 can be used to prescribe exercise. Approximately every 2 weeks, the training load (in watts) was adjusted to maintain the HR_{VT1} percentages.

The results are presented in the accompanying graphs. Panel A presents the results in terms of power output (W). Four conclusions can be drawn:

1. The control group (data not shown) did not change either its maximal power output or the wattage at which the VT1 occurred. Thus, changes in the training groups can be interpreted as being the result of the training.

2. The AT and LT groups significantly improved post training in both modalities of testing and had significantly higher values than the controls. Thus, elderly individuals were trainable.

3. In all three groups, the power outputs were higher at both peak exercise and VT1 for the LE than the AE. This is a good example of large muscle versus small muscle mass differences.

4. The LT group improved more on the LE than the AE; the AT group improved more on the AE than LE. This exemplifies the principle of specificity. Both groups, however, improved in both modalities, indicating a degree of cross-training.

Panels B and C present the results for $\dot{V}_E$ at peak exercise and VT1 during submaximal exercise. Parallel conclusions can be drawn for these variables:

1. Again, the control group (data not presented) did not show any changes.

2. Posttraining increases in both respiratory variables showed significant increases over pretraining values, except for the AT group on $\dot{V}_E$ peak during LE testing. Maximal (or peak) minute ventilation increases are the most consistent pulmonary ventilation adaptation to training. Ventilatory thresholds were also expected to increase and did so consistently.

3. In all three groups, both $\dot{V}_E$ and VT1 were significantly higher for LE than for AE, paralleling the differences in power output.

4. Specificity was again evident for both $\dot{V}_E$ and VT1; the LT group improved more on the LE than the AE, and the AT group improved more on the AE than the LE.

Source: Pogliaghi, S., P. Terziotti, A. Cevese, F. Balestreri, & F. Schena: Adaptations to endurance training in the healthy elderly: Arm cranking versus leg cycling. *European Journal of Applied Physiology.* 97(6):723–731 (2006).

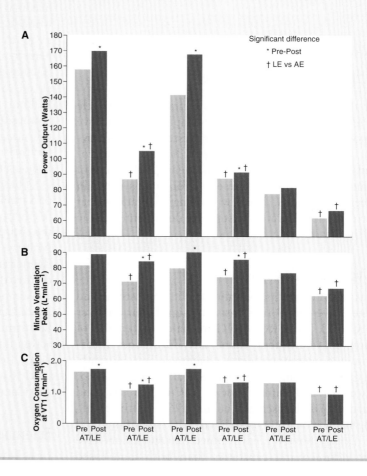

TABLE 10.3 Respiratory Training Adaptations

	Rest	Submaximal Exercise	Maximal Exercise
Lung volumes and capacities	Show no changes from land-based activities; swimming and diving show increases, especially in total lung capacity and vital capacity	—	—
Pulmonary ventilation			
$\dot{V}_E$	Shows no change	Decreases	Increases
V_T	Increases	Increases	Increases
f	Decreases	Decreases	Increases
VT1 and VT2	—	Increase to higher workload/oxygen consumption	—
External respiration			
(A-a)PO$_2$diff	Shows no change	Decreases	Shows no change
Internal respiration			
PvCO$_2$	—	Decreases	—
Oxygen dissociation curve	—	Curve shifts to the right	Curve shifts to the right
a-vO$_2$diff	Shows no change in children; increases in young adults	Shows no change in children; inconsistent changes in adults	Shows no change in children; increases in young adults

consistently increase at either submaximal or maximal work as a result of training (Saltin et al., 1968). Even in studies where diffusing capacity did increase with training, it was most likely due to circulatory changes (an increase in pulmonary capillary volume) rather than any pulmonary membrane change per se. Higher values in diffusion capacity may be an example of genetic selection for specific athletes (Comroe, 1965; Dempsey, 1986; Dempsey et al., 1977; Niinimaa and Shepard, 1978; Reuschlein et al., 1968; Vaccaro and Clarke, 1978; Wagner, 1991).

Arterial values of pH and PCO$_2$ do not change with training, but venous pH levels increase (become less acidic) and PCO$_2$ values decrease (Rasmussen et al., 1975) during the same submaximal exercise. The (A-a)PO$_2$diff decreases at submaximal workloads as a result of training, indicating greater efficiency (Saltin et al., 1968). Training may also cause the oxygen dissociation curve to shift to the right, facilitating the release of oxygen from the blood into the muscle tissue (Rasmussen et al., 1975).

In children, neither the submaximal nor the maximal a-vO$_2$diff adapts as a result of training (Bar-Or, 1983; Eriksson, 1973). In young adults, the a-vO$_2$diff increases at rest (Clausen, 1977; Saltin et al., 1968) and at maximal exercise as a result of training (Blomqvist and Saltin, 1983; Coyle et al., 1984; Saltin et al., 1968). Both increases and decreases in the a-vO$_2$diff have been found during submaximal exercise as a result of endurance training (Clausen, 1977; Ekelund, 1967; Ekelund and Holmgren, 1967; Saltin et al., 1968). Changes in middle-aged and elderly adults are less likely than in younger adults (Green and Crouse, 1993; Saltin, 1969). None of the other partial pressure or saturation variables changes significantly and/or consistently with training.

Table 10.3 summarizes the respiratory training adaptations discussed above.

Why Are There so Few Respiratory Adaptations to Whole Body Exercise Training?

The most commonly accepted answer to the question of why there are so few respiratory adaptations to whole body exercise training is that the pulmonary system is endowed with a tremendous reserve capacity that is more than sufficient to meet the demands of heavy physical exercise. Thus, the various structural and functional components of the respiratory system (lungs and airways) are not stressed to any significant limits during physical training and so do not need to change. At the same time, the cardiovascular and metabolic capacities of muscle are being stressed and do respond by adapting. The adaptations in these systems may ultimately exceed the capability of the respiratory system, as seen with EIAH and diaphragmatic fatigue, and the pulmonary system can become a limiting factor in elite athletes. So, the generalization that the respiratory system is "overbuilt" is accurate but only to a point. There is no need for great changes in the respiratory system in the normal healthy, moderately trained individual (Dempsey, 1986; Dempsey et al., 1977; McKenzie, 2012; Sheel, 2002).

Detraining and the Respiratory System

All available research evidence suggests that any physiological variable that is responsive to exercise training will also respond to detraining. There is no reason to suspect that this is not also true for the respiratory system, although research evidence is sparse for both specific respiratory muscle training and whole body respiratory training adaptations. The most common pattern is a rapid deterioration in maximal $\dot{V}_E$. In addition, detraining is associated with an increase in $\dot{V}_E/\dot{V}O_2$ during standardized submaximal exercise and at maximal exercise. These changes occur rapidly and progress to reductions approximating 10–14% if training is stopped for more than 4 weeks (Mujika and Padilla, 2000a,b).

Special Considerations

Altitude

The effects of altitude were mentioned briefly in Chapter 9. This section details the effects of both acute and chronic exposure to altitude, the exercise response at altitude, and discusses the impact of altitude training on athletic performance. Refer back to **Table 9.1** and Equation 9.4 as background for the following discussion.

The Acute Impact of Altitude

The percentage of oxygen in air remains constant at 20.93% to an altitude of 100,000 m (328,083 ft) (Clausen, 1977). However, the barometric pressure (P_B) decreases exponentially with increasing altitude. Thus, air has a lower density (fewer molecules per volume) at higher altitudes because the gas has expanded. For instance, at Denver (1600 m, or 5280 ft), P_B is 630 mmHg, and at Colorado Springs (2300 m, or 7590 ft), P_B is 586 mmHg (**Figure 10.16**). Therefore, the oxygen partial pressure (PO_2) in atmospheric air is reduced at altitude. At Denver, the PO_2 is 132 mmHg (630 mmHg × 0.2093), and at Colorado Springs, it is 123 mmHg (586 mmHg × 0.2093), compared to 159 mmHg at sea level (760 mmHg × 0.2093). Because the partial pressure of the inspired oxygen decreases with altitude, the P_AO_2 also decreases to 80 and 74 mmHg, respectively, at Denver and Colorado Springs:

$$[(630 \text{ mmHg}) - (47 \text{ mmHg})] \times (0.137 \text{ O}_2) = 80 \text{ mmHg};$$
$$[(586 \text{ mmHg}) - (47 \text{ mmHg})] \times (0.137 \text{ O}_2) = 74 \text{ mmHg}.$$

FIGURE 10.16 The Impact of Altitude on External Respiration.

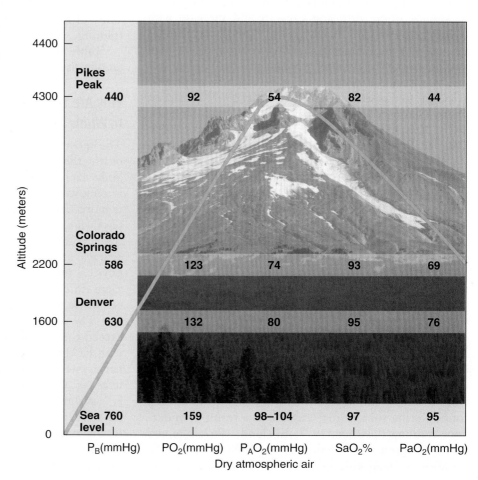

This decrease in P_AO_2 reduces the pressure gradient between the returning venous blood (PvO_2) and the alveoli, resulting in a lower percent saturation ($SaO_2\%$) and arterial partial pressure (PaO_2):

80 mmHg × 0.95 = PaO_2 of 76 mmHg at Denver;
74 mmHg × 0.93 = PaO_2 of 69 mmHg at Colorado Springs

Figure 10.16 summarizes these changes.

Acute Altitude Compensations

The decrease in PaO_2 stimulates an increase in $\dot{V}_E$ via the aortic and carotid body chemoreceptors as compensation to provide more oxygen for alveolar ventilation. The initial increase in $\dot{V}_E$ is hyperventilation (an increase in pulmonary ventilation that exceeds metabolic requirements) and is achieved primarily by an increase in respiratory frequency. Climbers on Mount Everest reportedly averaged 62 br·min^{-1} and a $\dot{V}_E$ of 207 L·min^{-1}, obviously very high values (Armstrong, 2000). Altitude-induced hyperventilation increases the amount of carbon dioxide exhaled. In turn, the increased exhalation of carbon dioxide decreases alveolar and arterial carbon dioxide partial pressure and increases pH. The decrease in $SaO_2\%$ and the other resultant changes at the altitudes of Denver and Colorado Springs are minimal, perhaps 2–5% because of the flatness of the oxygen dissociation curve (**Figure 10.3**) in that range. However, at the top of Pikes Peak (4300 m, or 14,100 ft), $SaO_2\%$ is 82%, and the effect of altitude is very evident (Hannon, 1978; Haymes and Wells, 1986; Ratzin Jackson and Sharkey, 1988). **Table 9.1** and **Figure 10.16** show the external respiration values. The $SaO_2\%$ is approximately 15% less at Pikes Peak than at sea level. **Table 10.4**, first column, summarizes these changes.

Within the red blood cells, a chemical called 2,3-diphosphoglycerate (2,3-DPG) increases at altitude. The effect of increased 2,3-DPG is the same as increased carbon dioxide partial pressure, hydrogen ion concentration, and body temperature on the oxygen dissociation curve (**Figure 10.3**). That is, it shifts the oxygen dissociation curve to the right, offsetting the initial shift to the left (and decreased release of oxygen) that occurs because of the decreased PCO_2 and increased pH brought about by hyperventilation. The result is a diminished ability of O_2 to combine with Hb in the pulmonary circuit. However, at low and moderate altitudes, the increased dissociation at the tissue level is considered more important and beneficial.

Within 2 days of altitude exposure, hemoglobin concentration increases, which in turn increases the amount of oxygen transported per deciliter of blood. Unfortunately, the hemoglobin concentration increases only because total blood volume initially decreases due to mild dehydration. That is, the same number of red blood cells is distributed in a smaller volume of blood, a process called *hemoconcentration*. The blood volume loss reflects a total body water loss through the kidneys and through increased respiratory evaporation because of the compensatory hyperventilation. Such hemoconcentration increases the viscosity of the blood, resulting in greater resistance to blood flow. In an attempt to maintain blood flow, heart rate increases (Haymes and Wells, 1986; Ratzin Jackson and Sharkey, 1988). **Table 10.4**, second column, summarizes these acute responses.

TABLE 10.4 Pulmonary Ventilation and External Respiration Responses to Altitude

Physiological Sequence	Acute Compensation*	Chronic Adaptation*
↑Altitude ↓	↑$\dot{V}_E$ (↑f) → ↑CO_2 blown off ↓	↑$\dot{V}_E$ (↑V_T) (>SL, >Acute) ↓
↓P_B ↓	↓P_ACO_2, $PaCO_2$, pH +	↑P_AO_2 (<SL, >Acute)
↓PO_2 ↓	↑2,3-DPG→O_2 dissociation curve shifts to the right	↑RBC + ↓ →↑ BV† ↓
↓P_AO_2 ↓	↑ [Hb] + ↓BV ↓	↑PaO_2 (~SL, >Acute) +
↓PaO_2 ↓$SaO_2\%$	↑O_2·dL^{-1} blood	↑$SaO_2\%$ (<SL, >Acute)

*At rest and during submaximal aerobic exercise.

†Decrease continues for at least several weeks; by 2 months, blood volume is increasing.

P_B, barometric pressure; PO_2, partial pressure of oxygen; P_AO_2, partial pressure of oxygen at the alveoli; PaO_2, partial pressure of oxygen in arterial blood; $SaO_2\%$, percent saturation of arterial blood with oxygen; $\dot{V}_E$, minute ventilation; f, frequency of breathing; P_ACO_2, partial pressure of carbon dioxide at the alveoli; $PaCO_2$, partial pressure of carbon dioxide in arterial blood; pH, negative logarithm of the hydrogen ion concentration; 2,3-DPG, 2,3-diphosphoglycerate, chemical within red blood cells; [Hb], concentration of hemoglobin; BV, blood volume; O_2, oxygen; V_T, tidal volume; SL, sea level; RBC, red blood cells.

These altitude-induced acute responses are compounded during exercise. The normal exercise increase in diffusion capacity does not exceed that at sea level because PaO_2 is decreased and PvO_2 remains the same. As a result, the normal exercise increase in a-vO$_2$diff is not as great at altitude as it is at sea level.

Cardiovascular changes occur as well. Heart rate and cardiac output increase in an attempt to compensate for the reduced oxygen content of the blood. Stroke volume in only marginally reduced initially but progressively declines for 1–2 weeks before stabilizing (Mazzeo, 2008).

Although the individual probably does not perceive any of the changes described above, except possibly hyperventilation, alterations can also occur in sensory acuity (vision and hearing), motor skills, memory, and mood (increased irritability). Dehydration and weight loss are common, as is sleep disturbance. In addition, some unpleasant sensations including a loss of appetite, dizziness, fatigue, nausea, vomiting, and weakness may mark the onset of altitude sickness (Guyton and Hall, 2011; Haymes and Wells, 1986).

Exercise Responses at Altitude

The acute effects of altitude are experienced most directly in terms of the intensity at which an aerobic endurance activity can be maintained. The higher the altitude and exercise intensity, the greater the impact and the sooner fatigue is felt. Although oxygen diffusion capacity is not a limiting factor, oxygen delivery cannot keep pace with muscle demand. Maximal aerobic power ($\dot{V}O_2$max) declines (Mazzeo, 2008; Wehrlin and Hallén, 2006). Thus any submaximal absolute load represents a higher relative load. The intensity at which any endurance event can be performed is lower, as is the ability to sustain that activity. The blood lactate response for a given power output is greater compared with sea level. These responses are true for all individuals at all ages, although high-altitude mountain climbers are impacted the most simply by virtue of the extreme altitudes at which they perform. Sprints and other muscular strength, muscular endurance, and power events do not appear to be physiologically disadvantaged, and they may even be enhanced because of lower air resistance at higher elevations (Burtscher et al., 2006; Haymes and Wells, 1986; Mazzeo, 2008; Ratzin Jackson and Sharkey, 1988).

Acclimation to Altitude

Acclimation to altitude begins quickly. It involves subtle but important shifts caused by the initial attempts to adjust to the lower oxygen partial pressure. Hemoconcentration continues, but the cause shifts from being a decrease in plasma volume with no change in red blood cell count to an increase in red blood cells under the influence of the hormone erythropoietin (Guyton and Hall, 2011). Blood volume remains depressed for several weeks but then begins to increase (Haymes and Wells, 1986). Likewise, hyperventilation continues, but instead of an increased frequency, an increase in V_T occurs. Increased V_T allows a more effective pulmonary gas exchange. $PaCO_2$ remains depressed, but PaO_2 increases somewhat as acclimation proceeds (Adams et al., 1975; Grover, 1978; Guyton and Hall, 2011; Hannon, 1978; Haymes and Wells, 1986; Ratzin Jackson and Sharkey, 1988). Cardiac output is lower due to the combined reductions in heart rate and stroke volume with acclimation. Muscle blood flow and hence oxygen delivery to the muscles remains unchanged, but to an extent these are compensated for by increased extraction of oxygen [(a-v)O$_2$diff]. $\dot{V}O_2$max remains reduced. In a much debated paradox, after acclimatization, the blood lactate response for the same absolute workload, as well as at maximal exercise, may be reduced from the initial altitude exposure (Mazzeo, 2008). Females seem to acclimatize to altitude more readily than males (Grover, 1978). **Table 10.4**, third column, summarizes the respiratory chronic adaptations.

Training and Competing at Altitude and Sea Level

Athletes who wish to compete at altitude have two choices in attempting to minimize the adverse environmental effects. The first is to arrive at the altitude site 12–18 hours before the activity. Many collegiate and some professional teams do this, even at the moderate altitudes where they compete. Although this strategy does not prevent the effects of altitude, it does minimize the chances that acute altitude sickness will impair performance (Haymes and Wells, 1986; Ratzin Jackson and Sharkey, 1988; Weston et al., 2001).

The second choice is to train at the same altitude as the eventual competition. During training, athletes can acclimate somewhat to the altitude. However, even with extensive acclimation a former sea-level resident will not be as physiologically adapted as the individual who was born and has always lived at altitude.

In 2007, the International Federation of Association Football (Fédération Internationale de Football Association or FIFA) passed a regulation regarding the matches in FIFA competitions at high altitude for both players and officials. The guidelines are as follows:

1. Above 2500 m (~8200 ft), an acclimation period of 3 days is strongly recommended.
2. Above 2750 m (~9000 ft), there is a mandatory acclimation period of 1 week.
3. Above 3000 m (~9800 ft), games are generally not permitted. If a game is permitted, there is a minimum acclimation period of 2 weeks.

Unfortunately, these processes of acclimation do not completely counteract the fundamental hypoxic stress of altitude. Individuals training at altitude cannot train at the same level of intensity for as long as they could at sea level. A reduction of training intensity to 40% of that at sea level may be necessary initially, and intensity can usually be increased only up to 75% of sea-level intensity (Armstrong, 2000). Highly trained athletes (especially those prone to exercise-induced hypoxemia) are likely to benefit the least from altitude training. Untrained or minimally trained individuals, however, may still be doing more training than they did at sea level and reap the benefits of altitude training.

Athletes who train at altitude usually see positive results from that training if the competition is at the same altitude and occurs directly after the training period. The effect of altitude training on later sea-level maximal performance is highly controversial, and shows large individual variations (Mazzeo, 2008).

One group of athletes who must always perform at altitude is mountaineers. They typically follow a pattern of training and acclimation called "work (climb) high, sleep low." Climbers traditionally establish a series of camp sites, each at a higher altitude than the previous one. During the day, they and their porters (**Figure 10.17**). carry supplies up to the higher camp (camp 2) and work at that altitude, and then they descend at night to camp 1 to sleep. This pattern continues for days or weeks, at which time the climbers reestablish themselves between the old high camp (camp 2) and a new higher location (camp 3), progressing then from 3 to 4, 4 to 5) until they are in position for the final ascent of the summit.

The most popular current strategy for nonmountaineer athletes who wish to improve competitive performance at sea level is really a variation of what mountaineers do called "live high, train low" (Brugniaux et al., 2006a,b;

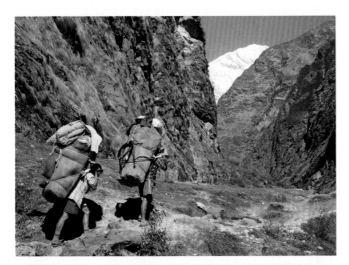

FIGURE 10.17 Mountain Climbers Acclimate to Altitude by Establishing a Series of Camps in Which They Progressively Work High and Sleep Low until Attempting the Summit.

Koistinen et al., 2000; Levine and Stray-Gundersen, 1997; Wehrlin et al., 2006). The goal is to avoid the detrimental effects of altitude (having to train at greatly reduced exercise intensity, with the concomitant detraining effects), while at the same time reaping the benefits of altitude acclimation, which can improve oxygen-carrying capacity and dissociation. The Focus on Research box describes the definitive classic study that evaluated this approach. As is often the case with any training technique, individual reactions to "living high, training low" can vary widely, and some individuals will not respond at all.

Although "living high and training low" might seem to simply require a mountain with a nearby accessible valley, in practice, such geographical features can be difficult to find and access. Another option now being used experimentally is a nitrogen house; an airtight dwelling flushed with air diluted with nitrogen. This reduces the oxygen content from 20.93% to approximately 15% and simulates being at altitude. To train low, athletes simply leave the house (Koistinen et al., 2000). A much less costly option requiring further research is the use of a nitrogen tent. The tent can be set up on any bed or floor and used by an individual when resting and sleeping in his or her own home. Additional simulated situations include the use of hypobaric chambers or hypoxic inhalers.

A recent meta-analysis (Bonetti and Hopkins, 2009) investigated the effects on performance measured at or near sea level and related physiological measures of adaptation to six different variations of altitude training. These were (1) natural live-high, train-high (LHTH); (2) natural live-high, train-low (LHTL); (3) artificial (simulated) LHTL with long (8–18 hours) continuous exposure to "altitude"; (4) artificial LHTL with brief (1.5–5 hours) continuous exposure to "altitude"; (5) brief (<1.5 hours) intermittent periods of artificial hypoxia; and (6) artificial live-low, train-high (LLTH). Subelite athletes were found to achieve substantial enhancement of maximal endurance power output with #2—natural live-high, train-low (4.2%), #5—artificial brief intermittent LHTL (2.6%), and #3—long continuous artificial LHTL (1.4%). Elite athletes benefited only from #2 natural LHTL (4.0%). Thus, LHTL seems best for both nonelite and elite athletes.

For those who choose the "live high, train low" approach, the following guidelines are important (Brugniaux et al., 2006a,b; Rusko et al., 2004):

1. The simulated altitude should be at least between 2100 and 2500 m (~6700–8200 ft) but less than 3000 m (~9800 ft).
2. Hypoxic exposure should be greater than 12 hr·d⁻¹, and preferably 16 hr·d⁻¹.
3. Training should last at least 3 weeks.
4. High-intensity training must be maintained as if altitude were not involved.

FOCUS ON RESEARCH: *Clinically Relevant*

Live High, Train Low

This study was designed to test the hypothesis that acclimation to living at moderate altitude (2500 m, 8260 ft) combined with training at low altitude (1250 m, 4125 ft) (high-low condition) would improve sea-level (5000 m, 3.1 mi) performance in already well-conditioned athletes more than both living and training either at high altitude (2500–2700 m, 8260–8900 ft), called high-high condition, or at sea level, called low-low control condition.

Thirty-nine athletes completed 2 weeks of sea-level familiarization and 4 weeks of sea-level training before being randomized into three groups of 13 athletes (nine males and four females in each group) for 4 weeks of high- or low-altitude or sea-level training and living. Training was periodized and tapered before all tests for all groups. As expected, those training at high altitude did so at a slower speed and at a lower percentage of maximal oxygen uptake than those at sea level. However, the training intensity of the low-altitude training group was reduced by only 6% compared with the sea-level group, whereas that of the high-altitude training group was reduced by 18.5%. Both groups that lived at moderate altitude significantly increased red blood cell mass by 9% and $\dot{V}O_2$max by 5%, while the sea-level group showed neither change. Arterio-venous oxygen difference was significantly higher for both altitude groups at velocities near 5000-m run time trial speeds after altitude training. Velocity at $\dot{V}O_2$max increased only for the high-low group. The only group that significantly improved its 5000-m time was the high-low group, by an average of 13.4 ± 10 seconds. This improvement persisted for at least 3 weeks after the return from altitude, at which point testing stopped.

These results suggest that an improvement in sea-level performance from altitude training is possible if athletes live at moderate altitude but train at lower levels that permit maintaining a high training intensity.

Source: Levine, B. D. & J. Stray-Gundersen: "Living high—training low": Effect of moderate-altitude acclimatization with low-altitude training on performance. *Journal of Applied Physiology*. 83(1):102–112 (1997).

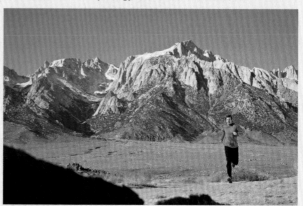

CHECK YOUR COMPREHENSION 1

Rank the following events in order of the impact of altitude (from greatest to least) if the athletic competition were held in Mexico City (~3000 m). Explain your rankings:

(a) Shot put, (b) marathon, (c) 100 m, (d) 10,000 m run, and (e) 400 m hurdles

Check your answer in Appendix C.

Exercise Training and Pollution

Air pollution consists of a mixture of many different chemicals. The major components of automotive pollution include sulfur dioxide (SO_2), nitrogen oxides (NO_x), ozone (O_3), particulates, and carbon monoxide (CO). Cigarette smoke and by-products of the combustion of other fuels also contribute to air pollution.

The impairment of cilia function mentioned in Chapter 9 is not the only respiratory effect of inhaling these pollutants. Sulfur dioxide is absorbed by the moist surfaces of the upper airways and can cause bronchospasm. Sulfur dioxide peaks at midday but is rarely a major problem. Normal values approximate 0.005 ppm and sulfur dioxide does not negatively affect exercise until levels of 0.2 ppm (Marr and Ely, 2010). Nitrogen oxides are absorbed by the mucosal lining of the nose and pharynx and lead to irritation, cough, dyspnea, and diminished resistance to respiratory infection. Levels of NO_x are usually relatively low (~0.001 ppm), but values above 1 ppm would detrimentally affect exercise (Marr and Ely, 2010). Ozone is formed naturally by the action of ultraviolet radiation (UVR) on oxygen as UVR enters the earth's atmosphere and by the action of sunlight UVR on automobile exhaust (Armstrong, 2000). O_3 levels are typically around 0.03 ppm and become a problem for exercise at 0.05 ppm (Marr and Ely, 2010). Ozone causes a decrease in forced vital capacity (FVC) and FEV_1 and an increase in airway resistance. Ozone levels are higher in summer than in winter because of the greater sunlight, and in rural rather than urban areas.

Particulates, also called particulate matter (PM), are solid or liquid materials produced from fuel combustion that remain suspended in air for long periods of time. PM is categorized by size into coarse, fine, and ultrafine. Particulates >10 µm in diameter are not considered harmful to airways since they are generally filtered by the nasal passageways. Coarse particulates are usually between 10 and 2.5 µm in diameter and are labeled as

PM_{10}. Fine particulates are between 0.1 and 2.5 µm in diameter ($PM_{2.5}$) and ultrafine particles are <0.1 µm ($PM_{0.1}$). The smaller the particles the deeper they can penetrate into the lungs. Experiments have shown that the deposit of ultrafine particles is high during mouth breathing in healthy individuals at rest and increases more than 4.5 times as much during moderate exercise (Daigle et al., 2003). As the intensity of exercise increases, the volume, rate, and depth of breathing also increase. An athlete running at 70% $\dot{V}O_2$max for approximately 3 hours during a marathon inhales the same volume of air as a sedentary person would in 2 days! When the ventilatory rate exceeds 30 L·min⁻¹ (which it does easily even in low-intensity submaximal exercise), a combination of nasal and mouth breathing begins. This is important because a portion of the air then bypasses the nasal filtration, warming and humidifying system (Sacha and Quinn, 2011). Additionally, as a result, a greater percentage of inhaled pollutants penetrates more deeply into the respiratory tract than at rest. Particulate pollution is highest in heavy smog, which can also include ozone. Lead is associated with particulates, and a significant relationship has been shown between training duration and blood lead accumulation. The effects of particulates include systemic oxidative stress, airway inflammation, vascular dysfunction, and decreased capacity for oxygen exchange (Carlisle and Sharp, 2001; Rundell, 2012). There is an inverse dose-response relationship between air pollutants and lung function at constant exercise workloads (Marr and Ely, 2010). The prevalence of exercise-induced bronchoconstriction (EIB), asthma, and low resting lung function is high for individuals who train and compete in high PM environments. Indoor winter athletes, especially ice hockey players, figure and speed skaters can be particularly vulnerable. Ice resurfacing by internal combustion fossil fueled machines (gas and/or propane) produces levels of CO, NO_x, and PM 20–30 times greater than outside air. The use of electric-powered ice resurfacers maintains air quality. In addition to these health aspects, inhalation of high levels of PM during exercise has been shown to result in decreased performance in the range of 3–5%. In elite competitions this could be enough to separate the winner and last-place finisher. Even a light 20-minute warm-up or one 6-minute bout of exercise in high-pollution conditions may have a detrimental carry-over effect that could last for 3 days (Haymes and Wells, 1986; McCafferty, 1981; Rundell, 2012).

If the pollutant is CO, it reduces both the ability to carry oxygen and the ability to release oxygen already bound to red blood cells. The affinity of hemoglobin for CO is 210–230 times greater than its affinity for oxygen, and CO binds at the same site where oxygen would. Thus, when carboxyhemoglobin (COHb) is formed, the arterial percent saturation of oxygen decreases. The release of oxygen from hemoglobin is impaired by a shift in the oxygen dissociation curve to the left (see **Figure 10.3**). Myoglobin

(Mb—the oxygen transporting and storage protein of muscles) and its role in assisting oxygen diffusion through the sarcoplasm to the mitochondria are also affected. First, the decreased release of oxygen from the red blood cells reduces the efficiency of Mb for attracting and holding oxygen within the muscle cells. Second, CO binds directly to Mb with approximately the same affinity as to Hb, thereby reducing myoglobin's ability to combine with whatever oxygen is available. The combined result of the effects of elevated CO levels on Hb and Mb is an earlier and possibly greater dependence on anaerobic metabolism.

This is manifested by a lower exercise intensity at which anaerobic metabolism becomes important, a shorter endurance time at submaximal loads, a lower maximal exercise performance, a lower maximal a-vO_2diff, and a lower maximal oxygen consumption ($\dot{V}O_2$max) (McDonough and Moffatt, 1999). As little as a 4% COHb level will have detrimental effects on exercise time and intensity. This level may result if training is done near heavy traffic (**Figure 10.18**). CO inhaled by smoking has additional respiratory impact, including increased pulmonary airway resistance, increased oxygen cost of ventilation, and an increased diffusion distance for oxygen and carbon dioxide across the alveolar walls because of mucosal swelling and bronchial constriction (McDonough and Moffatt, 1999). Individuals smoking 10 or fewer cigarettes per day average approximately 4% COHb, and a two-pack-a-day habit almost doubles this value. A non-smoker riding in a car for 1 hour with a smoker can reach 3% COHb level (Haymes and Wells, 1986). Strenuous exercise near heavy traffic for 30 minutes can increase the level of COHb as much as smoking 10 cigarettes (Carlisle and Sharp, 2001). The half-life of COHb is 3–4 hours, meaning that it takes that long for one half of the CO to become unbound to hemoglobin and be removed.

Athletes are often affected by pollution levels that do not bother spectators. Individuals with cardiovascular and respiratory diseases and children are also particularly

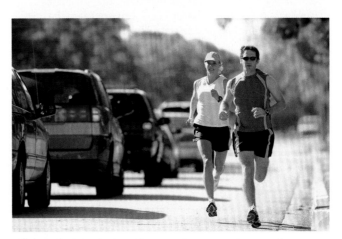

FIGURE 10.18 Training Near Traffic Will Increase COHb Levels.

vulnerable (McCafferty, 1981). The following recommendations are suggested to minimize the impact of pollutants on an exercise training session or competition.

1. Individuals with health problems that make them particularly susceptible to the effects of pollution should not exercise outside during air quality warnings. They should seek sites where the air is filtered.

2. Everyone should avoid prolonged heavy exercise when hazardous air warnings are in effect. Individuals can adapt to breathing pollutants, but in the long term, adaptation is harmful because it suppresses normal defense mechanisms. Therefore, adaptation should not be attempted. Anyone experiencing symptoms such as coughing, wheezing, chest tightness, pain with breathing deeply, or difficulty breathing should reduce their activity level and seek medical attention (Campbell et al., 2005).

3. Atmospheric ozone levels peak at around 1–3 P.M. and are much higher during most of the daylight hours in summer than in winter. CO peaks at approximately 7 A.M. and 8 P.M. and is higher in winter than in summer. Thus, heavy outdoor workouts might be best early in the morning and late evening during the summer and around noontime in the winter (Armstrong, 2000). Runners, cyclists, and in-line skaters should seek locations away from heavy vehicular traffic. Locations upwind with at least 50 ft between motor vehicles and exercisers are best. Avoid trailing close to a pace car or waiting at stoplights behind cars' exhaust pipes.

4. At the very least, smoking should be banned from all indoor training and competition sites. Smoking should be discouraged at all times (McCafferty, 1981).

CHECK YOUR COMPREHENSION 2

Which two of the following conditions/situations that can decrease maximal exercise performance share the same basic physiological causes? Explain your choices.

1. Altitude (>~2500 ft)

2. Breathing polluted air

3. Entrainment

4. Hypoxic swimming (controlled-frequency breathing)

5. EIAH

Check your answer in Appendix C.

SUMMARY

1. During short-term, light to moderate aerobic exercise, minute ventilation, alveolar ventilation, and the arteriovenous oxygen difference (a-vO$_2$diff) increase rapidly and reach a steady state within approximately 2–3 minutes. The partial pressure of oxygen at the alveolar and arterial levels does not change, and, as a result, the alveolar to arterial oxygen pressure gradient and percent saturation of arterial hemoglobin with oxygen are maintained. The ratio of dead space to tidal volume, percent saturation of oxygen in venous blood, and the partial pressure of oxygen in venous blood decrease rapidly and reach a steady state within approximately 2–3 minutes. The partial pressure of carbon dioxide increases in the venous blood as the result of the increased energy production, but the partial pressure of carbon dioxide decreases slightly due to the hyperpnea.

2. During the first 30 minutes of long-term, moderate to heavy aerobic exercise, the only meaningful differences in respiratory responses from short-term, light exercise are in magnitude and a slight drop in the arterial partial pressure of oxygen; this in turn widens the alveolar to arterial oxygen pressure gradient. After approximately 30 minutes, minute ventilation, alveolar ventilation, and the a-vO$_2$diff exhibit an upward drift. This respiratory drift is associated with a rising body temperature.

3. During incremental aerobic exercise to maximum, both minute ventilation and alveolar ventilation exhibit a rectilinear rise interrupted by two breakpoints that change the slope upward. The a-vO$_2$diff rises rectilinearly until approximately 60% of maximal work, where it levels off. The partial pressures of both alveolar and arterial oxygen, and the resultant alveolar to arterial oxygen pressure gradient and percent saturation of arterial blood remain constant until approximately 75% of maximal work. At this point, the first three exhibit a slight exponential rise, and the arterial oxygen saturation percent decreases slightly as a result. Both the percent saturation of oxygen in venous blood and the venous oxygen partial pressure decrease rectilinearly until approximately 60% of maximal work, where they level off. As the oxygen is extracted and used, carbon dioxide is produced so that the partial pressure of carbon dioxide in venous blood rises sharply at first and then more slowly. The arterial partial pressure of carbon dioxide is maintained initially but then declines as additional carbon dioxide is blown off by the increasing hyperpnea.

4. In most healthy sedentary or moderately trained individuals the respiratory system has more than enough reserve for the ventilatory and gas-exchange demands for exercise of any intensity. However, in highly trained endurance athletes participating in sustained high-intensity activity respiration can be a limitation to performance. A primary cause to this exercise-induced arterial hypoxemia is the failure to maintain arterial oxygen saturation. Two additional limitations are respiratory muscle fatigue and positive

expiratory intra-thoracic pressures that limit cardiac output.

5. All of the respiratory responses to static exercise are the same as for short-term, light to moderate submaximal aerobic exercise except that oxygen extraction, as denoted by the a-vO_2diff, either shows no change or decreases slightly and minute ventilation and a-vO_2diff exhibit little, if any, change during exercise, with a rebound rise in recovery.

6. During exercise, oxygen dissociation is increased by a widening of the oxygen pressure gradient, an increase in partial pressure of carbon dioxide, a decrease in pH, and an increase in body temperature. The changes in PCO_2, pH, and body temperature increase oxygen release by causing a shift to the right of the oxygen dissociation curve. At altitude, the tendency for the decrease in PCO_2, caused by the compensatory hyperventilation, to shift the curve to the left and impair oxygen dissociation is counteracted by an increase in 2,3-diphosphoglycerate activity.

7. When exercising, individuals should use either an entrainment or a spontaneous breathing pattern, whichever comes more naturally to them.

8. In general, exercise responses are in the same direction but may vary in magnitude across the age span for both males and females.

9. Many of the differences in respiratory measures when comparing children and adolescents with young adults or males with females are at least partially related to size. Smaller individuals have smaller values.

10. Specific respiratory muscle training results in increases in functional measures of inspiratory muscle strength, endurance, maximal rate of shortening, and power. Structurally, significant increases in the proportion of Type I (slow twitch, oxidative) fibers and the size of Type II (fast twitch, oxidative glycolytic) fibers have been observed. Often, but not always, the perception of dyspnea is decreased. Respiratory values for minute ventilation, alveolar ventilation, breathing frequency, and tidal volume as well as oxygen consumption and lactate concentration are typically lowered and actual performance increased during constant submaximal performances or time trials, whereas no improvement is seen at maximal exercise.

11. Whole body training respiratory adaptations are minimal in land-based athletes or fitness participants. The most consistent change is in minute ventilation, which goes down during submaximal work and increases at maximum. Swimming and diving show increases in most static and dynamic lung volumes and capacities, particularly in total lung capacity and vital capacity.

12. The relative percentages of oxygen, carbon dioxide, and nitrogen remain the same to an altitude of 100,000 m (328,083 ft). However, because barometric pressure goes down exponentially as altitude increases, the partial pressures exerted by oxygen and carbon dioxide also decrease with altitude. The result is a lower percent saturation of oxygen and a decreased ability to maintain high-intensity aerobic exercise.

13. Individuals who must compete at altitude should arrive at the location either 12–18 hours or 3 days to 4 weeks before the event. Acclimation and training at altitude appear to be beneficial for competing at that same altitude. Evidence supports the use of a "live high-train low" regimen for improvement in sea-level performance for endurance athletes. Not everyone will be a responder to altitude training.

14. Exercise in highly polluted air should be avoided. Any adaptation to such conditions is done at the expense of natural defense mechanisms.

REVIEW QUESTIONS

1. List and explain the four factors that increase oxygen dissociation during exercise and how these are related. Describe the additional factor that influences oxygen dissociation at altitude.

2. Compare and contrast the pulmonary ventilation, external respiration, and internal respiration responses to short-term, light to moderate submaximal aerobic exercise; long-term, moderate to heavy submaximal aerobic exercise; incremental aerobic exercise to maximum; and static exercise. Where known, explain the mechanisms for each response.

3. Should fitness participants and athletes be encouraged to practice entrainment rather than spontaneous breathing? Why or why not?

4. Explain EIAH. What other factor may indicate a respiratory limitation to maximal exercise?

5. Compare the procedures and adaptations of specific respiratory muscle training and whole body training for respiratory variables.

6. Defend or refute this statement: "Hypoxic training, whether achieved by training at altitude or by breath holding, is beneficial to an athlete."

7. Explain the impact of environmental pollutants on exercise training.

For further review and additional study tools, visit the website at http://thePoint.lww.com/Plowman4e ✳ ▶

REFERENCES

Adams, W. C., E. M. Bernauer, D. B. Dill, & J. B. Bomar: Effects of equivalent sea-level and altitude training on VO$_2$max and running performance. *Journal of Applied Physiology.* 39(2):262–266 (1975).

Aguilaniu, B., P. Flore, J. Maitre, J. Ochier, J. R. Lacour, & H. Perrault: Early onset of pulmonary gas exchange disturbance during progressive exercise in healthy active men. *Journal of Applied Physiology.* 92(5):1879–1894 (2002).

Amann, M.: Pulmonary system limitations to endurance exercise performance in humans. *Experimental Physiology.* 97(3): 311–318 (2012).

Amann, M., A. W. Subudhi, & C. Foster. Predictive validity of ventilatory and lactate thresholds for cycling time trial performance. *Scandinavian Journal of Medicine & Science in Sports.* 16:27–34 (2006).

Andrew, G. M., M. R. Becklake, J. S. Guleria, & D. V. Bates: Heart and lung functions in swimmers and nonathletes during growth. *Journal of Applied Physiology.* 32(2):245–251 (1972).

Armstrong, L. E.: *Performance in Extreme Environments.* Champaign, IL: Human Kinetics (2000).

Ashley, F., W. B. Kannel, P. D. Sorlie, & R. Masson: Pulmonary function: Relation to aging, cigarette habit and mortality; the Framingham Study. *Annals of Internal Medicine.* 82: 739–745 (1975).

Asmussen, E.: Similarities and dissimilarities between static and dynamic exercise. *Circulation Research.* 48(6 Suppl. I): I-3–I-10 (1981).

Åstrand, I.: Aerobic work capacity in men and women with special reference to age. *Acta Physiologica Scandinavica.* 49(Suppl. 169):1–92 (1960).

Åstrand, P.-O.: *Experimental Studies of Physical Working Capacity in Relation to Sex and Age.* Copenhagen: Munksgaard (1952).

Åstrand, P.-O., T. E. Cuddy, B. Saltin, & J. Stenberg: Cardiac output during submaximal and maximal work. *Journal of Applied Physiology.* 19(2):268–274 (1964).

Åstrand, P.-O., L. Engstrom, B. O. Eriksson, P. Karlberg, I. Nylander, B. Saltin, & C. Thoren: Girl swimmers: With special reference to respiratory and circulatory adaption and gynecological and psychiatric aspects. *Acta Paediatrica.* 147(Suppl.):1–73 (1963).

Bachman, J. C. & S. M. Horvath: Pulmonary function changes which accompany athletic conditioning programs. *Research Quarterly.* 39(2):235–239 (1968).

Bar-Or, O.: *Pediatric Sports Medicine for the Practitioner: From Physiological Principles to Clinical Applications.* New York, NY: Springer-Verlag, 1–65 (1983).

Bechbache, R. R. & J. Duffin: The entrainment of breathing frequency by exercise rhythm. *Journal of Physiology.* 272: 553–561 (1977).

Becklake, M. R., H. Frank, G. R. Dagenais, G. L. Ostiguy, & C. A. Guzman: Influence of age and sex on exercise cardiac output. *Journal of Applied Physiology.* 20(5):938–947 (1965).

Bell, H. J.: Respiratory control at exercise onset: An integrated systems perspective. *Respiratory Physiology and Neurobiology.* 152(1):1–15 (2006).

Berglund, E., G. Birath, J. Bjure, G. Grimby, I. Kjellmer, L. Sandqvist, & B. Söderholin: Spirometric studies in normal subjects. I. Forced expirograms in subjects between 7 and 70 years of age. *Acta Medica Scandinavica.* 173:185–206 (1963).

Bjure, J.: Spirometric studies in normal subjects. IV. Ventilatory capacities in healthy children 7–17 years of age. *Acta Paediatrica.* 52:232–240 (1963).

Blomqvist, C. G. & B. Saltin: Cardiovascular adaptations to physical training. *Annual Review of Physiology.* 45:169–189 (1983).

Bonetti, D. L. & W. G. Hopkins: Sea-level exercise performance following adaptation to hypoxia. *Sports Medicine.* 39(2): 107–127 (2009).

Bonsignore, M. R., G. Morici, P. Abate, S. Romano, & G. Bonsignore: Ventilation and entrainment of breathing during cycling and running in triathletes. *Medicine & Science in Sports & Exercise.* 30(2):239–245 (1998).

Brugniaux, J. V., L. Schmitt, P. Robach, et al.: Living high-training low: Tolerance and acclimatization in elite endurance athletes. *European Journal of Applied Physiology.* 96(1):66–77 (2006a).

Brugniaux, J. V., L. Schmitt, P. Robach, et al.: Eighteen days of "living high, training low" stimulate erythropoiesis and enhance aerobic performance in elite middle-distance runners. *Journal of Applied Physiology.* 100(1):203–211 (2006b).

Burtscher, M., M. Faulhaber, M. Flatz, R. Likar, & W. Nachbauer: Effects of short-term acclimatization to altitude (3200m) on aerobic and anaerobic exercise performance. *International Journal of Sports Medicine.* 27(8):629–635 (2006).

Campbell, M. E., Q. Li, S. E. Gingrich, R. G. Macfarlane, & S. Cheng: Should people be physically active outdoors on smog alert days? *Canadian Journal of Public Health.* 96(1):24–28 (2005).

Caretti, D. M., P. C. Szlyk, & I. V. Sils: Effects of exercise modality on patterns of ventilation and respiratory timing. *Respiration Physiology.* 90:201–211 (1992).

Carlisle, A. J. & N. C. C. Sharp: Exercise and outdoor ambient air pollution. *British Journal of Sports Medicine.* 35(4):214–222 (2001).

Clanton, T. L., G. F. Dixon, J. Drake, & J. E. Gadek: Effects of swim training on lung and inspiratory muscle conditioning. *Journal of Applied Physiology.* 62(1):39–46 (1987).

Clark, J. M., F. C. Hagerman, & R. Gelfand: Breathing patterns during submaximal and maximal exercise in elite oarsmen. *Journal of Applied Physiology.* 55(2):440–446 (1983).

Clausen, J. P.: Effects of physical training on cardiovascular adjustments to exercise in man. *Physiology Reviews.* 57(4): 779–815 (1977).

Comroe, J. H.: *Physiology of Respiration: An Introductory Text.* Chicago, IL: Year Book Medical Publishers (1965).

Cordain, L. & J. Stager: Pulmonary structure and function in swimmers. *Sports Medicine.* 6:271–278 (1988).

Cordain, L., A. Tucker, D. Moon, & J. M. Stager: Lung volumes and maximal respiratory pressures in collegiate swimmers and runners. *Research Quarterly for Exercise and Sport.* 61(1):70–74 (1990).

Coyle, E. F., W. H. Martin III, D. R. Sinacore, M. J. Joyner, J. M. Hagberg, & J. O. Holloszy: Time course of loss of adaptations after stopping prolonged intense endurance training. *Journal of Applied Physiology: Respiratory, Environmental and Exercise Physiology.* 57(6):1857–1864 (1984).

Daigle, C. C., D. C. Chalupa, F. R. Gibb, P. E. Morrow, G. Oberdörster, M. J. Utell, & M. W. Frampton: Ultrafine particle deposition in humans during rest and exercise. *Inhalation Toxicology.* 15:539–552 (2003).

Davies, C. T. M.: The oxygen-transporting system in relation to age. *Clinical Science.* 42:1–13 (1972).

Davies, C. T. M., P. E. DiPrampero, & P. Cerretelli: Kinetics of cardiac output and respiratory gas exchange during exercise and recovery. *Journal of Applied Physiology.* 32(5):618–625 (1972).

Dempsey, J. A.: Is the lung built for exercise? *Medicine and Science in Sports and Exercise.* 18(2):143–155 (1986).

Dempsey, J. A., M. Amann, L. M. Romer, & J. D. Miller: Respiratory system determinants of peripheral fatigue and endurance performance. *Medicine & Science in Sports & Exercise*. 40(3):457–461 (2008).

Dempsey, J. A. & R. F. Fregosi: Adaptability of the pulmonary system of changing metabolic requirements. *American Journal of Cardiology*. 55:59D–67D (1985).

Dempsey, J. A., N. Gledhill, W. G. Reddan, H. V. Foster, P. G. Hanson, & A. D. Claremont: Pulmonary adaptation to exercise: Effects of exercise type and duration, chronic hypoxia and physical training. In P. Milvy (ed.): The Marathon: Physiological, Medical, Epidemiological, and Psychological Studies. *Annals of the New York Academy of Sciences*. 301: 243–261 (1977).

Dempsey, J. A. & P. D. Wagner: Exercise-induced arterial hypoxemia. *Journal of Applied physiology*. 87:1997–2006 (1999).

DeVries, H. A. & G. M. Adams: Comparison of exercise responses in old and young men. II. Ventilatory mechanics. *Journal of Gerontology*. 27(3):349–352 (1972).

Dicker, S., G. K. Lofthus, N. W. Thorton, & G. A. Brooks: Respiratory and heart rate responses to tethered controlled frequency breathing swimming. *Medicine and Science in Sports and Exercise*. 12(1):20–23 (1980).

Donevan, R. E., W. H. Palmer, C. J. Varvis, & D. V. Bates: Influence of age on pulmonary diffusing capacity. *Journal of Applied Physiology*. 14(4):483–492 (1959).

Do Prado, D. M., A. M. Braga, M. U. Rondon, L. F. Azevedo, L. D. Matos, C. E. Negrao, & I. C. Trombetta: Cardiorespiratory responses during progressive maximal exercise test in healthy children. *Arquivos Brasileiros de Cardiologia*. 94(4):493–499 (2010).

Edwards, A. M. & R. E. Walker: Inspiratory muscle training and endurance: A central metabolic control perspective. *International Journal of Sports Physiology and Performance*. 4:122–128 (2009).

Ekelund, L. G.: Circulatory and respiratory adaptation during prolonged exercise. *Acta Physiologica Scandinavica*. 70(Suppl. 292):1–38 (1967).

Ekelund, L. G. & A. Holmgren: Central hemodynamics during exercise. *Circulation Research*. 20–21(Suppl. 1):1–33 (1967).

Enright, S. J., Unnithan, V. B., Heward, C., Withnall, L., & D. H. Davies: Effect of high-intensity inspiratory muscle training on lung volumes, diaphragm thickness, and exercise capacity in subjects who are healthy. *Physical Therapy*. 86(3):345–354 (2006).

Eriksson, B. O.: Physical training, oxygen supply and muscle metabolism in 11–13 year old boys. *Acta Physiologica Scandinavica*. 384(Suppl.):1–48 (1972).

Eriksson, B. O.: Effects of physical training on hemodynamic response during submaximal and maximal exercise in 11–13 year old boys. *Acta Physiological Scandinavica*. 87:27–39 (1973).

Ericsson, P. & L. Irnell: Spirometric studies of ventilatory capacity in elderly people. In J. R. Edge, K. K. Pump, J. Arias-Stella, et al. (eds.): *Aging Lung: Normal Function*. New York, NY: MSS Information Corporation, 209–222 (1974).

Fahey, T. D., A. D. Valle-Zuris, G. Oehlsen, M. Trieb, & J. Seymour: Pubertal stage differences in hormonal and hematological responses to maximal exercise in males. *Journal of Applied Physiology: Respiratory, Environmental and Exercise Physiology*. 46(4):823–827 (1979).

Ferris, B. G., D. O. Anderson, & R. Zickmantel: Prediction values for screening tests of pulmonary function. *American Review of Respiratory Diseases*. 91:252–261 (1965).

Fleck, S. J. & W. J. Kraemer: *Designing Resistance Training Programs* (3rd edition). Champaign, IL: Human Kinetics (2004).

Forbes, S., A. Game, D. Syrotuik, R. Jones, & G. J. Bell: The effect of inspiratory and expiratory respiratory muscle training in rowers. *Research in Sports Medicine*. 19(4):217–230 (2011).

Fringer, M. N. & G. A. Stull: Changes in cardiorespiratory parameters during periods of training and detraining in young adult females. *Medicine and Science in Sports*. 6(1):20–25 (1974).

Gonzales, J. U. & B. W. Scheuermann: Gender differences in the fatigability of the inspiratory muscles. *Medicine & Science in Sports & Exercise*. 38(3):472–479 (2006).

Green, J. S. & S. F. Crouse: Endurance training, cardiovascular function and the aged. *Sports Medicine*. 16(5):331–341 (1993).

Griffiths, L. A. & A. K. McConnell: The influence of inspiratory and expiratory muscle training upon rowing performance. *European Journal of Applied Physiology*. 99(5):457–466 (2007).

Grimby, G.: Respiration in exercise. *Medicine and Science in Sports*. 1(1):9–14 (1969).

Grover, R. F.: Adaptation to high altitude. In Folinsbee, L. J., J. A. Wagner, J. F. Borgia, B. L. Drinkwater, J. A. Gliner, & J. F. Bedi (eds.): *Environmental Stress: Individual Human Adaptations*. New York, NY: Academic Press (1978).

Guenette, J. A., L. M. Romer, J. S. Querido, R. Chua, N. D. Eves, J. D. Road, et al.: Sex differences in exercise-induced diaphragmatic fatigue in endurance-trained athletes. *Journal of Applied Physiology*. 109(1):35–46 (2010).

Gurtner, H. P., P. Walser, & B. Fässler: Normal values for pulmonary hemodynamics at rest and during exercise in man. *Progress in Respiration Research*. 9:295–315 (1975).

Guyton, A. C. & J. E. Hall: *Textbook of Medical Physiology* (12th edition). Philadelphia, PA: Saunders (2011).

Haffor, A. A., A. C. Harrison, & P. A. Catledge Kirk: Anaerobic threshold alterations caused by interval training in 11-year-olds. *Journal of Sports Medicine and Physical Fitness*. 30(1): 53–56 (1990).

Hannon, J. P.: Comparative altitude adaptability of young men and women. In Folinsbee, L. J., J. A. Wagner, J. F. Borgia, B. L. Drinkwater, J. A. Gliner, & J. F. Bedi (eds.): *Environmental Stress: Individual Human Adaptations*. New York, NY: Academic Press (1978).

Hanson, P., A. Claremont, J. Dempsey, & W. Reddan: Determinants and consequences of ventilatory responses to competitive endurance running. *Journal of Applied Physiology: Respiratory, Environmental and Exercise Physiology*. 52(3): 615–623 (1982).

Harms, C. A.: Does gender affect pulmonary function and exercise capacity? *Respiratory Physiology & Neurobiology*. 151: 124–131 (2006).

Haymes, E. M. & C. L. Wells: *Environment and Human Performance*. Champaign, IL: Human Kinetics (1986).

Hill, A. R., J. M. Adams, B. E. Parker, & D. F. Rochester: Short-term entrainment of ventilation to the walking cycle in humans. *Journal of Applied Physiology*. 65(2):570–578 (1988).

Hodges, A. N., J. R. Mayo, & D. C. McKenzie. Pulmonary edema following exercise in humans. *Sports Medicine*. 36(6):501–512 (2006).

Holmer, I. & L. Gullstrand: Physiological responses to swimming with a controlled frequency of breathing. *Scandinavian Journal of Sports Science*. 2(1):1–6 (1980).

Hopkins, S. R.: Exercise induced arterial hypoxemia: The role of ventilation-perfusion inequality and pulmonary diffusion limitation. *Advanced Experimental Medical Biology*. 588:17–30 (2006).

Hopkins, S. R. & C. A. Harms: Gender and pulmonary gas exchange during exercise. *Exercise and Sport Sciences Reviews*. 32(2):50–56 (2004).

Inbar, O., P. Weiner, Y. Azgad, A. Rotstein, & Y. Weinstein: Specific inspiratory muscle training in well-trained endurance athletes. *Medicine & Science in Sports & Exercise*. 32(7):1233–1237 (2000).

International Federation of Association Football: Ex-Co upholds altitude decision, welcomes positive steps. Friday March 14, 2008. http://www.fifa.com/about fifa/federations/bodies/media/newsid=713561.html. Accessed 9/14/2008.

Jain, S. K. & C. K. Gupta: Age, height, and body weight as determinants of ventilatory "norms" in healthy men above forty years of age. In Edge, J. R., K. K. Pump, J. Arias-Stella et al. (eds.): *Aging Lung: Normal Function*. New York, NY: MSS Information Corporation, 190–202 (1974a).

Jain, S. K. & C. K. Gupta: Lung function studies in healthy men and women over forty. In Edge, J. R., K. K. Pump, J. Arias-Stella et al. (eds.): *Aging Lung: Normal Function*. New York, NY: MSS Information Corporation, 182–189 (1974b).

Jakovljevic, D. G. & A. K. McConnell: Influence of different breathing frequencies on the severity of inspiratory muscle fatigue induced by high-intensity front crawl swimming. *Journal of Strength and Conditioning Research*. 23(4):1169–1174 (2009).

Jasinskas, C. L., B. A. Wilson, & J. Hoare: Entrainment of breathing rate to movement frequency during work at two intensities. *Respiration Physiology*. 42:199–209 (1980).

Johnson, B. D. & J. A. Dempsey: Demand vs. capacity in the aging pulmonary system. In Holloszy, J. O. (ed.): *Exercise and Sport Sciences Reviews*. 19:171–210 (1991).

Jones, N. L.: Exercise testing in pulmonary evaluation: Rationale, methods and the normal respiratory response to exercise. *New England Journal of Medicine*. 293(11):541–544 (1975).

Kao, F. F.: *An Introduction to Respiratory Physiology*. New York, NY: American Elsevier (1974).

Kaufmann, D. A., E. W. Swenson, J. Fencl, & A. Lucas: Pulmonary function of marathon runners. *Medicine and Science in Sports*. 6(2):114–117 (1974).

Kay, J. D. S., E. Strange Petersen, & H. Vejby-Christensen: Breathing in man during steady-state exercise on the bicycle at two pedalling frequencies, and during treadmill walking. *Journal of Physiology*. 251:645–656 (1975).

Kenney, R. A.: *Physiology of Aging: A Synopsis*. Chicago, IL: Year Book Medical Publishers (1982).

Kilding, A. E., S. Brown, & A. K. McConnell: Inspiratory muscle training improves 100 and 200 m swimming performance. *European Journal of Applied Physiology*. 108(3):505–511 (2010).

Koistinen, P. O., H. Rusko, K. Irjala, et al.: EPO, red cells, and serum transferrin receptor in continuous and intermittent hypoxia. *Medicine & Science in Sports & Exercise*. 32(4):800–804 (2000).

Koyal, S. N., B. J. Whipp, D. Huntsman, G. A. Bray, & K. Wasserman: Ventilatory responses to the metabolic acidosis of treadmill and cycle ergometry. *Journal of Applied Physiology*. 40(6):864–867 (1976).

Krahenbuhl, G. S., J. S. Skinner, & W. M. Kohrt: Developmental aspects of maximal aerobic power in children. In Terjung, R. L. (ed.): *Exercise and Sport Sciences Reviews*. 13:503–538 (1985).

Laursen, P. B., C. M. Shing, J. M. Peake, J. S. Coombes, & D. G. Jenkins: Influence of high-intensity training on adaptations in well-trained cyclists. *Journal of Strength and Conditioning Research*. 19(3):527–533 (2005).

Lavoie, J.-M. & R. R. Montpetit: Applied physiology of swimming. *Sports Medicine*. 3:165–189 (1986).

Leddy, J. J., A. Limprasertkul, S. Patel, F. Modich, C. Buyea, D. R. Prendergast, & C. E. Lundgren: Isocapnic hyperpnea training improves performance in competitive male runners. *European Journal of Applied Physiology*. 99(6):665–676 (2007).

Leff, A. R. & P. T. Schumacker: *Respiratory Physiology: Basics and Applications*. Philadelphia, PA: Saunders (1993).

Legrand, R., S. Ahmaidi, W. Moalla, D. Chocquet, A. Marles, F. Prieur, & P. Mucci: O_2 arterial desaturation in endurance athletes increases muscle deoxygenation. *Medicine & Science in Sports & Exercise*. 37(5):782–788 (2005).

Leith, D. G. & M. Bradley: Ventilatory muscle strength and endurance training. *Journal of Applied Physiology*. 41(4):508–516 (1976).

Levine, B. D. & J. Stray-Gundersen: "Living high—training low": Effect of moderate-altitude acclimatization with low-altitude training on performance. *Journal of Applied Physiology*. 83(1):102–112 (1997).

Loat, C. E. R. & E. C. Rhodes: Relationship between the lactate and ventilatory thresholds during prolonged exercise. *Sports Medicine*. 15(2):104–115 (1993).

Maclennan, S. E., G. A. Silvestri, J. Ward, & D. A. Mahler: Does entrained breathing improve the economy of rowing? *Medicine and Science in Sports and Exercise*. 26(5):610–614 (1994).

Magel, J. R. & K. L. Andersen: Pulmonary diffusing capacity and cardiac output in young trained Norwegian swimmers and untrained subjects. *Medicine and Science in Sports*. 1(3):131–139 (1969).

Mahler, D. A., C. R. Shuhart, E. Brew, & T. A. Stukel: Ventilatory responses and entrainment of breathing during rowing. *Medicine and Science in Sports and Exercise*. 23(2):186–192 (1991).

Mahon, A. D. & C. C. Cheatham: Ventilatory threshold in children: A review. *Pediatric Exercise Science*. 14:16–29 (2002).

Malina, R. M., C. Bouchards', O. Bar-Or: *Growth, Maturation and Physical Activity* (2nd ed). Champaign, IL: Human Kinetics (2004).

Marr, L. C. & M. R. Ely: Effect of air pollution on marathon running performance. *Medicine & Science in Sports & Exercise*. 42(3):585–591 (2010).

Mazzeo, R. S.: Physiological responses to exercise at altitude: An update. *Sports Medicine*. 38(1):1–8 (2008).

McCafferty, W. B.: *Air Pollution and Athletic Performance*. Springfield, IL: Thomas (1981).

McConnell, A. K. & L. M. Romer: Respiratory muscle training in healthy humans: Resolving the controversy. *International Journal of Sports Medicine*. 25:284–293 (2004).

McDonough, P. & R. J. Moffatt: Smoking-induced elevations in blood carboxyhaemoglobin level. *Sports Medicine*. 27(5):275–283 (1999).

McKenzie, D. C.: Respiratory physiology: Adaptations to high-level exercise. *British Journal of Sports Medicine*. 46(6):381–384 (2012).

Mickleborough, T. D., T. Nichols, M. R. Lindley, K. Chatham, & A. A. Ionescu: Inspiratory flow resistive loading improves respiratory muscle function and endurance capacity in endurance runners. *Scandinavian Journal of Medicine & Science in Sports*. 20:458–468 (2010).

Morton, D. P. & R. Callister: Characteristics and etiology of exercise-related transient abdominal pain. *Medicine & Science in Sports & Exercise*. 32(2):432–438 (2000).

Morton, D. P. & R. Callister: Factors influencing exercise-related transient abdominal pain. *Medicine & Science in Sports & Exercise*. 34(5):745–749 (2002).

Morton, D. P. & R. Callister: Spirometry measurements during an episode of exercise-related transient abdominal pain. *International Journal of Sports Physiology and Performance*. 1(4):336–346 (2006).

Morton, D. P. & R. Callister: EMG activity is not elevated during exercise-related transient abdominal pain. *Journal of Science and Medicine in Sport*. 11:569–574 (2008).

Morton, D. P. & R. Callister: Influence of posture and body type on the experience of exercise-related transient abdominal pain. *Journal of Science and Medicine in Sport*. 13(5):485–488 (2010).

Morton, D. P., L. F. Argon-Vargas, & R. Callister: Effect of ingested fluid composition on exercise-related transient abdominal pain. *International Journal of Sport Nutrition and Exercise Metabolism*. 14:197–208 (2004).

Mostyn, E. M., S. Helle, J. B. L. Gee, L. G. Bentiveglio, & D. V. Bates: Pulmonary diffusing capacity of athletes. *Journal of Applied Physiology*. 18(4):687–695 (1963).

Mucci, P., N. Blondel, C. Fabre, C. Nourry, & S. Berthoin: Evidence of exercise-induced O_2 arterial desaturation in non-elite sportsmen and sportswomen following high-intensity interval-training. *International Journal of Sports Medicine*. 25(1):6–13 (2004).

Mujika, I. & S. Padilla: Detraining: Loss of training-induced physiological and performance adaptations. Part I. Short term insufficient training stimulus. *Sports Medicine*. 30(2):79–87 (2000a).

Mujika, I. & S. Padilla: Detraining: Loss of training-induced physiological and performance adaptations. Part II: Long term insufficient training stimulus. *Sports Medicine*. 30(2):145–154 (2000b).

Narloch, J. A. & M. E. Brandstater: Influence of breathing technique on arterial blood pressure during heavy weight lifting. *Archives of Physical and Medical Rehabilitation*. 76(5):457–462 (1995).

Neder, J. A. & Stein, R.: A simplified strategy for the estimation of the exercise ventilatory thresholds. *Medicine & Science in Sports & Exercise*. 38(5):1007–1013 (2006).

Nicks, C. R., D. W. Morgan, D. K. Fuller, & J. L. Caputo: The influence of respiratory muscle training upon intermittent exercise performance. *International Journal of Sports Medicine*. 30(1):16–21 (2009).

Niinimaa, V. & R. J. Shepard: Training and oxygen conductance in the elderly. I. The respiratory system. *Journal of Gerontology*. 33(3):354–361 (1978).

Nourry, C., Fabre, C., Bart, F., Grosbois, J. M. & P. Mucci: Evidence of exercise-induced arterial hypoxemia in prepubescent trained children. *Pediatric Research*. 55(4):674–681 (2004).

Pardy, R. L., S. N. A. Hussain, & P. T. Macklein: The ventilatory pump in exercise. *Clinics in Chest Medicine*. 5(1):35–49 (1984).

Paterson, D. H., T. M. McLellan, R. S. Stella, & D. A. Cunningham: Longitudinal study of ventilation threshold and maximal O_2 uptake in athletic boys. *Journal of Applied Physiology*. 62(5):2051–2057 (1987).

Pearce, D. H. & H. T. Milhorn: Dynamic and steady-state respiratory responses to bicycle exercise. *Journal of Applied Physiology: Respiratory, Environmental and Exercise Physiology*. 42(6):959–967 (1977).

Plunkett, B. T. & W. G. Hopkins: Investigation of the side pain "stitch" induced by running after fluid ingestion. *Medicine & Science in Sports & Exercise*. 31(8):1169–1175 (1999).

Pogliaghi, S., P. Terziotti, A. Cevese, F. Balestreri, & F. Schena: Adaptations to endurance training in the healthy elderly: Arm cranking versus leg cycling. *European Journal of Applied Physiology*. 97(6):723–731 (2006).

Pollock, M. L., T. K. Cureton, & L. Greninger: Effects of frequency of training on working capacity, cardiovascular function, and body composition of adult men. *Medicine and Science in Sports*. 1(2):70–74 (1969).

Poole, D. C. & G. A. Gaesser: Response of ventilatory and lactate thresholds to continuous and interval training. *Journal of Applied Physiology*. 58(4):1115–1121 (1985).

Powers, S. K. & R. E. Beadle: Onset of hyperventilation during incremental exercise: A brief review. *Research Quarterly for Exercise and Sport*. 56(4):352–360 (1985).

Powers, S. K., D. Martin, & S. Dodd: Exercise-induced hypoxemia in elite endurance athletes: Incidence, causes and impact on VO_2max. *Sports Medicine*. 16(1):14–22 (1993).

Prefaut, C., F. Durand, P. Mucci, & C. Caillaud: Exercise-induced arterial hypoxemia in athletes: A review. *Sports Medicine*. 30(1):47–61 (2000).

Rasmussen, B., K. Klausen, J. P. Clausen, & J. Trap-Jensen: Pulmonary ventilation, blood gases, and blood pH after training of the arms or the legs. *Journal of Applied Physiology*. 38(2):250–256 (1975).

Ratzin Jackson, C. G. & B. J. Sharkey: Altitude, training, and human performance. *Sports Medicine*. 6:279–284 (1988).

Ray, A. D., D. R. Prendergast, & C. E. G. Lundgren: Respiratory muscle training reduces the work of breathing at depth. *European Journal of Applied Physiology*. 108(4):811–820 (2010).

Reid, J. G. & J. M. Thomson: *Exercise Prescription for Fitness*. Englewood Cliffs, NJ: Prentice Hall (1985).

Reuschlein, P. S., W. G. Reddan, J. Burpee, J. B. L. Gee, & J. Rankin: Effect of physical training on the pulmonary diffusing capacity during submaximal work. *Journal of Applied Physiology*. 24(2):152–158 (1968).

Richards, J. C., D. C. McKenzie, D. E. Warburton, J. D. Road, & A. W. Sheet: Prevalence of exercise-induced arterial hypoxemia in healthy women. *Medicine & Science in Sports & Exercise*. 36(9):1514–1521 (2004).

Richardson, R. S., D. R. Knight, D. C. Poole, S. S. Kurdak, M. C. Hogan, B. Grassi, & P. D. Wagner: Determinants of maximal exercise V. O_2 during single leg knee extensor exercise in humans. *American Journal of Physiology*. 268(4 Pt 2):H1453–1461 (1995a).

Richardson, R. S., E. A. Noyszewski, K. F. Kendrick, J. S. Leigh, & P. D. Wagner: Myoglobin O_2 desaturation during exercise. Evidence of limited O_2 transport. *Journal of Clinical Investigation*. 96(4):1916–1926 (1995b).

Robinson, S.: Experimental studies of physical fitness in relation to age. *Arbeitsphysiologie*. 10:251–323 (1938).

Robinson, E. P. & J. M. Kjeldgaard: Improvement in ventilatory muscle function with running. *Journal of Applied Physiology: Respiratory, Environmental and Exercise Physiology*. 52(6):1400–1406 (1992).

Romer, L. M., A. K. McConnell, & D. A. Jones: Inspiratory muscle fatigue in trained cyclists: Effects of inspiratory muscle training. *Medicine & Science in Sports & Exercise.* 34(5):785–792 (2002).

Rowell, L. B.: Circulation. *Medicine and Science in Sports.* 1(1):15–22 (1969).

Rowell, L. B., H. L. Taylor, Y. Wang, & W. S. Carlson: Saturation of arterial blood with oxygen during maximal exercise. *Journal of Applied Physiology.* 19(2):284–286 (1964).

Rowland, T. W.: Developmental aspects of physiological function relating to aerobic exercise in children. *Sports Medicine.* 10(4):255–266 (1990).

Rowland, T. W.: *Children's Exercise Physiology* (2nd edition). Champaign, IL: Human Kinetics (2005).

Rowland, T. W., J. A. Auchmachie, T. J. Keenan, & G. M. Green: Physiologic responses to treadmill running in adult and prepubertal males. *International Journal of Sports Medicine.* 8(4):292–297 (1987).

Rowland, T. W. & G. M. Green: Physiological responses to treadmill exercise in females: Adult-child differences. *Medicine and Science in Sports and Exercise.* 20(5):474–478 (1988).

Rundell, K. W.: Effect of air pollution on athlete health and performance. *British Journal of Sports Medicine.* 46:407–412 (2012).

Rusko, H. K., H. O. Tikkanen, & J. E. Peltonen: Altitude and endurance training. *Journal of Sports Sciences.* 22(10):928–944 (2004).

Sacha, J. J. & J. M. Quinn: The environment, the airway, and the athlete. *Annals of Allergy, Asthma, & Immunology.* 106:81–88 (2011).

Saltin, B.: Physiological effects of physical conditioning. *Medicine and Science in Sports.* 1(1):50–56 (1969).

Saltin, B., G. Bloomqvist, J. H. Mitchell, R. L. Johnson, K. Wildenthal, & C. B. Chapman: Response to exercise after bed rest and after training. *Circulation.* 38(5 Suppl. VII):VII-1–VII-78 (1968).

Saris, W. H. M., A. M. Noordeloos, B. E. M. Ringnalda, M. A. Van't Hof, & R. A. Binkhorst: Reference values for aerobic power of healthy 4- to 18-year-old Dutch children: Preliminary results. In Binkhorst, R. A., H. C. G. Kemper, & W. H. M. Saris (eds.): *Children and Exercise XI.* Champaign, IL: Human Kinetics, 15:151–160 (1985).

Sawka, M. N., R. G. Knowlton, & R. M. Glaser: Body temperature, respiration, and acid-base equilibrium during prolonged running. *Medicine and Science in Sports and Exercise.* 12(5):370–374 (1980).

Seals, D. R., B. F. Hurley, J. Schultz, & J. M. Hagberg: Endurance training in older men and women. II. Blood lactate response to submaximal exercise. *Journal of Applied Physiology: Respiratory, Environmental and Exercise Physiology.* 57(4):1030–1033 (1984).

Segal, S. S.: Convection, diffusion, and mitochondrial utilization of oxygen during exercise. In Lamb, D. R. & C. V. Gisolfi (eds.): *Energy Metabolism in Exercise and Sport.* Dubuque, IA: Brown & Benchmark, 269–338 (1992).

Shapiro, W., C. E. Johnston, R. A. Dameron, & J. L. Patterson: Maximum ventilatory performance and its limiting factors. *Journal of Applied Physiology.* 19(2):197–203 (1964).

Sheel, A. W.: Respiratory muscle training in healthy individuals: Physiological rationale and implications for exercise performance. *Sports Medicine.* 32(9):567–581 (2002).

Shepard, R. J.: *Physical Activity and Aging.* Chicago, IL: Year Book Medical Publishers, 40–44; 85–95 (1978).

Skinner, J. S. & T. H. McLellan: The transition from aerobic to anaerobic metabolism. *Research Quarterly for Exercise and Sport.* 51(1):234–298 (1980).

Slonim, N. B. & L. H. Hamilton: *Respiratory Physiology* (3rd edition). St. Louis, MO: Mosby (1976).

Sporer, B. C., Foster, G. E., Sheel, A. W., & D. C. McKenzie: Entrainment of breathing in cyclists and non-cyclists during arm and leg exercise. *Respiratory and Physiological Neurobiology.* 155(1):64–70 (2007).

Stanescu, S., Q. St. Dutu, Z. Jienescu, L. Hartia, N. Nicolescu, & F. Sacerdoteanu: Investigations into changes of pulmonary function in the aged. In Edge, J. R., K. K. Pump, & J. Aris-Stella et al. (eds.): *Aging Lung: Normal Function.* New York, NY: MSS Information Corporation, 171–181 (1974).

Storstein, O. & A. Voll: New prediction formulas for ventilation measurements: A study of normal individuals in the age group 20–59 years. In Edge, J. R., K. K. Pump, & J. Aris-Stella et al. (eds.): *Aging Lung: Normal Function.* New York, NY: MSS Information Corporation, 156–170 (1974).

Turner, J. M., J. Mead, & M. E. Wohl: Elasticity of human lungs in relation to age. *Journal of Applied Physiology.* 25(6):664–671 (1968).

Vaccaro, P. & D. H. Clarke: Cardiorespiratory alterations in 9 to 11 year old children following a season of competitive swimming. *Medicine and Science in Sports.* 10(3):204–207 (1978).

Vaccaro, P., C. W. Zauner, & W. F. Updyke: Resting and exercise respiratory function in well trained child swimmers. *Journal of Sports Medicine and Physical Fitness.* 17:297–306 (1977).

Verges, S., O. Lenherr, A. C. Haner, C. Schulz, & C. M. Spengler: Increased fatigue resistance of respiratory muscles during exercise after respiratory muscle endurance training. *American Journal of Physiology: Regulatory, Integrative and Comparative Physiology.* 292(3):R1246 (2007).

Volianitis, S., A. K. McConnell, Y. Koutedakis, L. McNaughton, K. Backx, & D. A. Jones: Inspiratory muscle training improves rowing performance. *Medicine & Science in Sports & Exercise.* 33(5):803–809 (2001).

Wagner, P. D.: Central and peripheral aspects of oxygen transport and adaptation with exercise. *Sports Medicine.* 11(3):133–142 (1991).

Wagner, P. D.: The oxygen transport system: Integration of functions. In Tipton, C. M. (ed.): *ACSM's Advanced Exercise Physiology.* Philadelphia, PA: Lippincott Williams & Wilkins, 300–313 (2006).

Walsh, M. L. & E. W. Banister: Possible mechanisms of the anaerobic threshold: A review. *Sports Medicine.* 5:269–302 (1988).

Wasserman, K.: Breathing during exercise. *New England Journal of Medicine.* 298(14):780–785 (1978).

Wasserman, K., A. L. VanKessel, & G. G. Burton: Interaction of physiological mechanisms during exercise. *Journal of Applied Physiology.* 22(1):71–85 (1967).

Wasserman, K. & B. J. Whipp: Exercise physiology in health and disease. *American Review of Respiratory Disease.* 112:219–249 (1975).

Waterman, J. J. & R. Kapur: Upper gastrointestinal issue in athletes. *Current Sports Medicine Reports.* 11(2):99–104 (2012).

Watsford, M. & A. Murphy: The effects of respiratory-muscle training on exercise in older women. *Journal of Aging and Physical Activity.* 16(3):245–260 (2008).

Wehrlin, J. P. & J. Hallén: Linear decrease in V̇O₂max and performance with increasing altitude in endurance athletes. *European Journal of Applied Physiology.* 96(4):404–412 (2006).

Wehrlin, J. P., P. Zuest, J. Hallén, & B. Marti: Live high-train low for 24 days increases hemoglobin mass and red cell volume in elite endurance athletes. *Journal of Applied Physiology.* 100(6):1938–1945 (2006).

West, S. A., M. J. Drummond, J. M. VanNess, & M. E. Ciccolella: Blood lactate and metabolic responses to controlled frequency breathing during graded swimming. *Journal of Strength and Conditioning Research.* 19(4):772–776 (2005).

Weston, A. R., G. MacKenzie, A. Tufts, & M. Mars: Optimal time of arrival for performance at moderate altitude (1700 m). *Medicine & Science in Sports & Exercise.* 33(2):298–302 (2001).

Whipp, B. J.: The hyperpnea of dynamic muscular exercise. In Hutton, R. S. (ed.): *Exercise and Sport Science Reviews* (Vol. 5). Santa Barbara, CA: Journal Publishing Affiliates (1977).

Whipp, B. J. & S. A. Ward: Ventilatory control dynamics during muscular exercise in men. *International Journal of Sports Medicine.* 1:146–159 (1980).

Whipp, B. J., S. A. Ward, N. Lamarra, J. A. Davis, & K. Wasserman: Parameters of ventilatory and gas exchange dynamics during exercise. *Journal of Applied Physiology: Respiratory, Environmental and Exercise Physiology.* 52(6): 1506–1513 (1982).

Williams, J. S., J. Wongsathikun, S. M. Boon, & E. O. Acevedo: Inspiratory muscles training fails to improve endurance capacity in athletes. *Medicine & Science in Sports & Exercise.* 34(7):1194–1198 (2002).

Wilmore, J. H., J. Royce, R. N. Girandola, F. I. Katch, & V. L. Katch: Physiological alterations resulting from a 10-week program of jogging. *Medicine and Science in Sports.* 2(1):7–14 (1970).

Younes, M. & G. Kivinen: Respiratory mechanics and breathing pattern during and following maximal exercise. *Journal of Applied Physiology: Respiratory, Environmental and Exercise Physiology.* 57(6):1773–1782 (1984).

Zauner, C. W. & N. Y. Benson: Physiological alterations in young swimmers during three years of intensive training. *Journal of Sports Medicine and Physical Fitness.* 21:179–185 (1981).

Zauner, C. W., M. G. Maksud, & J. Milichna: Physiological considerations in training young athletes. *Sports Medicine.* 8(1):15–31 (1989).

Zempel, C.: Hypoxic isn't: Exploding the myth. *Triathlete.* Nov/Dec 20–21 (1989).

Zwiren, L. D., K. J. Cureton, & P. Hutchinson: Comparison of circulatory responses to submaximal exercise in equally trained men and women. *International Journal of Sports Medicine.* 4:255–259 (1983).

The Cardiovascular System

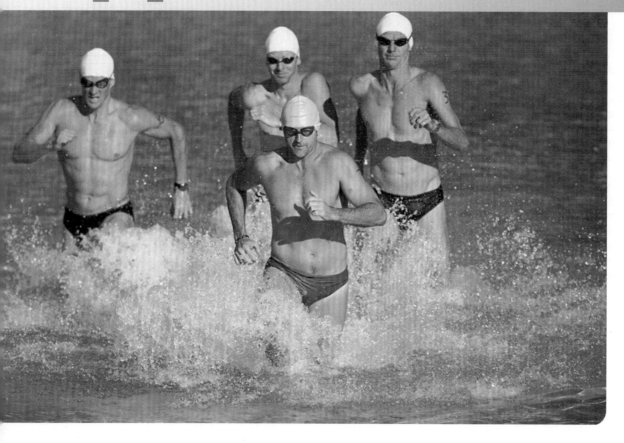

OBJECTIVES

After studying the chapter, you should be able to:

> Explain the functions of the cardiovascular system.

> Identify the various components of the cardiovascular system.

> Distinguish among the vessels that comprise the vascular system, and compare the pressure, velocity, and resistance in each type of vessel.

> Explain how electrical excitation spreads through the conduction system of the heart.

> Explain the relationships among the electrical, pressure, contractile, and volume changes throughout the cardiac cycle.

> Calculate mean arterial pressure, total peripheral resistance, and cardiac output.

> Describe the hormonal mechanisms by which blood volume is maintained.

> Explain how the cardiovascular system is regulated.

> Describe how these variables are measured: maximal oxygen consumption, cardiac output, stroke volume, heart rate, and blood pressure.

Introduction

Chapter 9 described how oxygen is taken into the body for delivery to body cells. The ability to deliver oxygen (and other substances) depends on the proper functioning of the cardiovascular system. In many ways, the cardiovascular system and the respiratory system operate together to accomplish a common mission—to deliver oxygen to working muscles—and they are driven by similar mechanisms. This chapter provides an overview of the cardiovascular system, discusses basic principles of cardiovascular dynamics, and outlines techniques typically used to assess cardiovascular function at rest, during, and following exercise.

Overview of the Cardiovascular System

The *cardiovascular system* includes the heart, blood vessels, and blood. Its primary functions are:

1. To transport oxygen and nutrients to the cells of the body and to transport carbon dioxide and waste products from the cells
2. To regulate body temperature, pH levels, and fluid balance
3. To protect the body from blood loss and infection

The heart is a double pump that provides the force to circulate the blood throughout the vessels of the circulatory system. The blood vessels serve as dynamic conduits for the blood as it travels through the body. The blood transports gases and nutrients within the cardiovascular system.

Figure 11.1 is a schematic overview of the cardiovascular system. *Arteries* carry blood away from the heart, and *veins* return blood to the heart. The *capillary beds* serve as the site of exchange for gases and nutrients between the blood and body tissues. Blood is ejected from the ventricles on both sides of the heart simultaneously. The right ventricle pumps blood through the pulmonary arteries to the lungs, where it is oxygenated and then returned to the left atrium via the pulmonary veins; this is called the *pulmonary circulation*. The left ventricle pumps oxygenated blood through the aorta, which then branches extensively into arteries to carry the blood to body cells through numerous specific circulations. The partially deoxygenated blood returns to the right atrium. Collectively, this route from the left ventricle to the right atrium is known as the *systemic circulation*.

As described in the respiration chapters, *external respiration* is the exchange of gases (O_2, CO_2) between the lungs and blood. *Internal respiration* is the exchange of gases (O_2, CO_2) at the cellular level. The cardiovascular system functions primarily to move the gases (as well as nutrients from the digestive tract to the tissues) between these two exchange sites so that energy can be produced by cellular respiration. *Cellular respiration* is described completely in the Metabolic Unit.

The Heart

The heart is a hollow muscular organ located in the thoracic cavity. It weighs approximately 250–350 g and is 12–14 cm long, about the size of a clenched fist. The heart beats approximately 70 times per minute in a resting adult—or over 100,000 times per day!

Macroanatomy of the Heart

The heart has four chambers and is functionally separated into the right and left heart. The right side pumps blood to the lungs (pulmonary circulation), and the left side pumps blood to the entire body (systemic circulation). Heart muscle is called **myocardium**. The two sides of the heart are separated by the interventricular septum. The upper chambers, called *atria* (*atrium* is the singular), receive the blood into the heart. The lower chambers, called *ventricles*, eject blood from the heart (**Figure 11.2A**). Blood is ejected from the right ventricle to the pulmonary artery and from the left ventricle to the aorta.

One-way valves control blood flow through the heart. The *atrioventricular (AV) valves* separate the atrium and ventricle on each side of the heart. Specifically, the tricuspid valve separates the atrium and ventricle on the right side of the heart, and the bicuspid (or mitral) valve separates the atrium and ventricle on the left side of the heart. The *semilunar valves* control blood flow from the ventricles. Specifically, the aortic semilunar valve allows blood to flow from the left ventricle into the aorta, and the pulmonary semilunar valve allows blood to flow from the right ventricle into the pulmonary artery.

Figure 11.2A shows the chambers and valves of the heart and the flow of blood. **Figure 11.2B** summarizes the blood flow through the heart and body.

See animation, Blood Circulation, at http://thePoint. lww.com/Plowman4e 🐭.

Microanatomy of the Heart

Cardiac muscle cells, called *myocytes,* are the contractile cells that produce the force that ejects blood from the ventricles. Cardiac muscle cells are both similar to and different from skeletal muscle cells. Both are striated in appearance because they contain the contractile proteins actin and myosin. The primary difference between cardiac and skeletal muscle cells is that cardiac muscle cells are highly interconnected; that is, the cell membranes of adjacent cardiac cells are structurally and functionally

Myocardium The heart muscle.

FIGURE 11.1 Schematic Overview of the Cardiovascular System and Interaction with the Respiratory System.

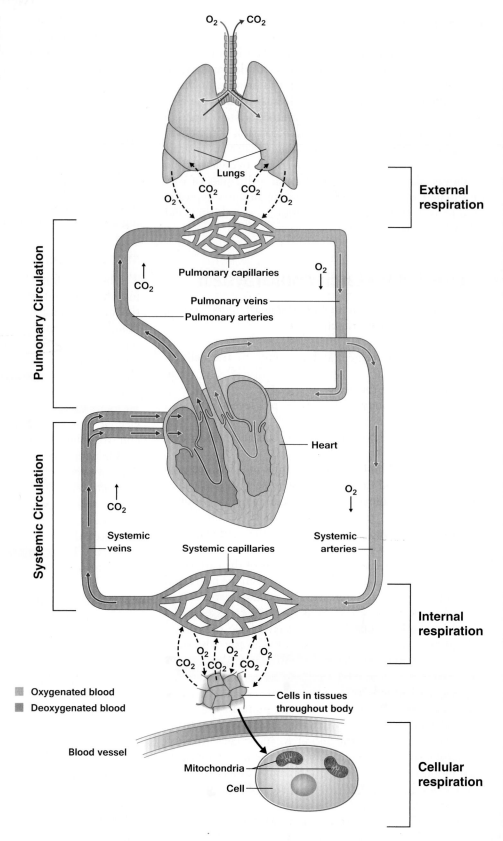

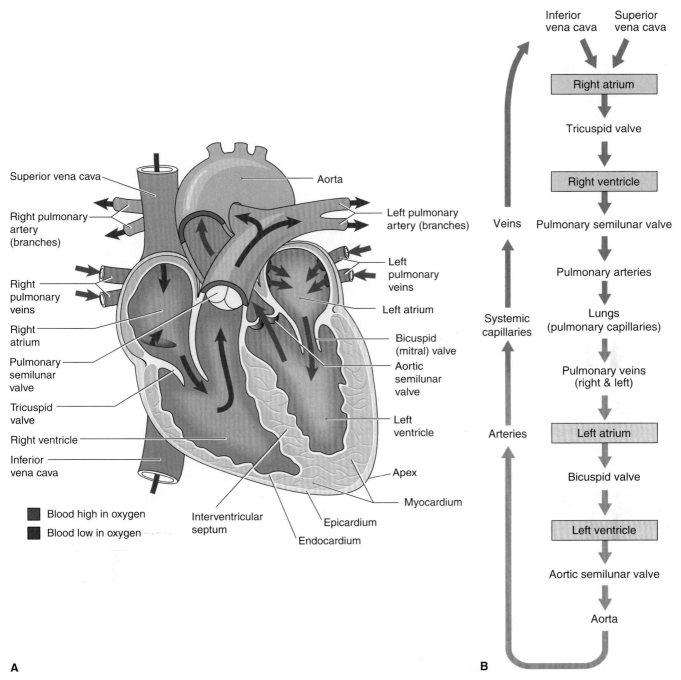

FIGURE 11.2   Blood Flow Through the Heart. A. Schematic of the heart. B. Summary of blood flow through the heart.

linked by **intercalated discs** (**Figure 11.3**). The intercalated discs contain specialized intracellular junctions (gap junctions) that allow the electrical activity in one cell to pass to the next. Thus, the individual cells of the

myocardium function collectively: when one cell is stimulated electrically, the stimulation spreads from cell to cell over the entire area. This electrical coupling allows the myocardium to function as a single coordinated unit, or a functional **syncytium**. Each of the two functional syncytia, the atrial and ventricular, contracts as a unit.

The Heart as Excitable Tissue

Cardiac muscle cells are excitable cells that are polarized (have an electrical charge with the inside being negative relative to the outside of the cell) in the resting state and

Intercalated Discs The junction between adjacent cardiac muscle cells that forms a mechanical and electrical connection between cells.

Syncytium A group of cells of the myocardium that function collectively as a unit during depolarization.

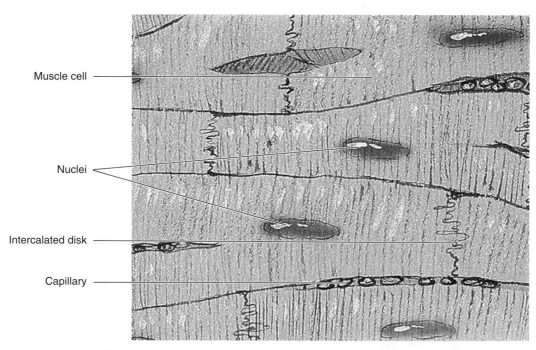

Muscle cell

Nuclei

Intercalated disk

Capillary

FIGURE 11.3 Cardiac Myocyte.

contract when they become depolarized (the charges reverse). Repolarization (the electrical charge returns to resting value) occurs during relaxation of the muscle cells. With each contraction, blood is ejected from the chambers. Individual myocardial cells function together to produce a coordinated contraction of the entire syncytium. Generally, when contraction of the heart is referred to, unless specified otherwise, it means contraction of the ventricles.

In addition to contractile muscle cells, the heart contains specialized conducting cells (**Figure 11.4A**). Although there are far fewer conducting cells than contractile muscle cells, they are essential because they spread the electrical signal quickly throughout the myocardium. The conduction system cells with the fastest spontaneous rate of depolarization are called the *pacemaker* cells. These are located in the *sinoatrial (SA) node* in the right atria. As shown in **Figure 11.4A**, the excitation spreads from the SA node throughout the right atria by internodal tracts and to the left atria by *Bachmann's bundle*. Because the atrial and ventricular syncytia contract separately, excitation in the atria does not lead directly to the contraction of cardiac cells in the ventricles. The electrical signal is spread from the atria to the ventricles via the *atrioventricular (AV) node*. Once the AV node is depolarized, the electrical signal continues down the specialized conduction system consisting of the *bundle of His*, the *left and right bundle branches*, and the *Purkinje fibers*. The electrical excitation then spreads out from the conducting system to excite all of the cardiac muscle cells in the ventricles. Thus, the excitation is spread first by the conduction system and then by cell-to-cell

contact: The excitation must be passed from muscle cell to muscle cell within the ventricles since the conduction system does not reach each individual cell.

As mentioned earlier, the cells of the SA node are considered the pacemaker cells of the heart because they normally have the fastest rate of depolarization. Cells in each area of the conduction system have their own inherent rates of depolarization. For the SA node, the intrinsic rate of depolarization is 60–100 times·min^{-1}. The AV node discharges at an intrinsic rate of 40–60 times·min^{-1}, and the Purkinje fibers at a rate of 15–40 times·min^{-1} (Guyton and Hall, 2011). If the SA node is diseased, the AV node may take over the pacemaking. While it is generally known that endurance training leads to a lower resting heart rate, if the only thing you knew about an individual was that he or she had a resting heart rate of 40 b·min^{-1}, you could not tell whether the person was a highly trained endurance athlete or someone in need of an artificial pacemaker implant because the SA node was not functioning properly.

Electrocardiogram

An **electrocardiogram (ECG)** provides a graphic illustration of the electrical current generated by excitation of the heart muscle. **Figure 11.4B** presents an ECG tracing that is color-coded to match the movement of the electrical current though the conduction system in **Figure 11.4A**. The spread of the electrical signal through the conduction system of the atria is shown in green. The P wave represents atrial depolarization, which causes atrial contraction. Repolarization of the atria, which

QRS depolarization ventricles

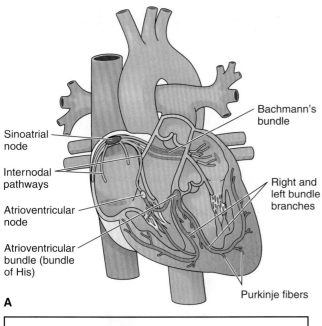

Bachmann's bundle

Sinoatrial node

Internodal pathways

Atrioventricular node

Atrioventricular bundle (bundle of His)

Right and left bundle branches

Purkinje fibers

A

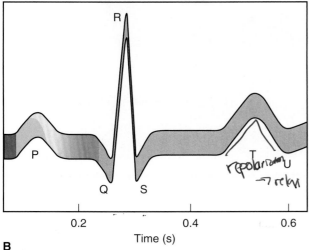

R

P

Q S

T

repolarization U

→ relax

0.2   0.4   0.6

Time (s)

B

FIGURE 11.4 Conduction System of the Heart.
A. Conduction pathway of the heart. **B.** ECG tracing that is color-coded to show movement of the electrical signal through the conduction system and then through the heart.

bundle of His and bundle branches (shown in red) occurs in the middle of the PR interval, followed by excitation of the Purkinje fibers (shown in purple). Note that excitation of the various portions of the conduction system happens very quickly and that activation of the entire conduction system precedes the QRS complex. The QRS complex reflects depolarization of the muscle fibers in the ventricles. It occurs after the electrical signal has traveled through the specialized conduction system in the ventricles and is occurring simultaneously with atrial repolarization. The T wave reflects repolarization of the muscle fibers in the ventricles and is followed by relaxation in preparation to start the cycle all over again. The U wave may or may not be seen in a normal ECG but is often present in the slower cardiac cycle of trained individuals. When present it probably represents the final phase of ventricular repolarization during which the Purkinje system recovers.

Although the SA node can depolarize spontaneously, the firing of the SA node is influenced by neural and hormonal factors. Additionally, heart rate varies with age. **Table 11.1** presents typical resting heart rate (HR) values in healthy individuals of various ages. While the resting heart rate values may not seem impressive when reported on a per minute basis, it is remarkable to consider how many times the heart beats per hour, or per day. Other factors that affect heart rate are discussed later in this chapter.

Cardiac Cycle

To function successfully as a pump, the heart must have alternating times of relaxation and contraction. The relaxation phase, called **diastole**, is the period when the heart fills with blood. The contraction phase, called **systole**, is the period when blood is ejected from the heart. The **cardiac cycle**—one complete sequence of contraction and relaxation of the heart—includes all events associated with the flow of blood through the heart. During the cardiac cycle there are dramatic changes in pressure and blood volume. **Figure 11.5** summarizes the flow of blood in the heart and the position of the heart valves throughout the phases of the cardiac cycle.

The *ventricular-filling period (VFP)* (**Figure 11.5A**) occurs when the ventricles are at rest (ventricular diastole) and the AV valves are open. The ventricles fill as blood is returned to the atria and flows down into the ventricles. Blood flow into the ventricles from the atria is assisted by gravity in an upright person. Atrial contraction also pushes a small volume of additional blood into the ventricles at the end of diastole. Blood volume in the ventricles is greatest at the end of ventricular filling, but pressure remains relatively low because the ventricles are relaxed.

Systole (the contraction phase, shown on the right side of the figure) is divided into two periods, the *isovolumetric contraction period (ICP)* and the *ventricular ejection*

results in a Ta wave, is normally not detectable on a resting ECG, but occurs during the time period concurrent with the QRS complex and may be evident during exercise. The electrical signal reaches the AV node at the end of the P wave (shown in yellow). Excitation of the

Electrocardiogram (ECG) Tracing that provides a graphic illustration of the electrical current generated by excitation of the heart muscle.

Diastole The relaxation phase of the cardiac cycle.

Systole The contraction phase of the cardiac cycle.

Cardiac Cycle One complete sequence of contraction and relaxation of the heart.

FOCUS ON APPLICATION: *Clinically Relevant*
Are All Elevations in Heart Rate Equal?

Heart rate (HR) can be elevated by a variety of factors mediated by the neural and hormonal systems (see Figures 11.16 and 11.17). One of these factors is movement (exercise), but others include emotion and environmental temperatures. Does an individual derive the same benefit from HR elevation caused by emotion or heat as from HR elevation caused by exercise? That is, is it possible to improve one's cardiovascular function while sitting in a sauna or hot tub or when frightened, angry, or anxious?

A regular, sustained elevation in HR is recognized as an important factor for improving cardiovascular fitness (techniques of exercise prescription based on HR are described in Chapter 13). However, the exercise HR responses are primarily an indicator of the training stimulus to the body—the increase in energy expenditure or metabolism (oxygen consumption). Heart rate and oxygen consumption rise in a directly proportional fashion during exercise. When emotion or temperature causes an elevation in HR, however, minimal

changes occur in energy expenditure; hence there is no training stimulus.

The importance of an increase in oxygen consumption has been demonstrated by individuals on medications such as beta blockers, which markedly suppress HR at rest and during exercise, and by those with constant heart-rate pacemakers. Both of these

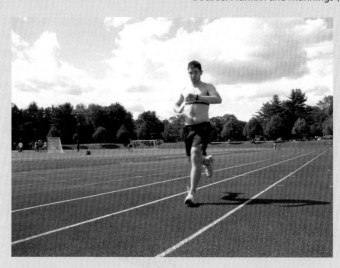

groups routinely show improvements in exercise capacity and fitness as a result of exercise programs, despite the fact that the exercise-induced increase in HR is dampened. Although HR can be elevated by other factors, you do not derive the health-related benefits unless the elevated HR is accompanied by physical activity.

Source: Franklin and Munnings (1998).

---

period (VEP). During the ICP (**Figure 11.5B**) both the AV valves and the semilunar valves are closed. Thus, for this brief time period, blood volume in the ventricles remains constant (isovolumetric) despite the high pressure generated by the contraction of the ventricular myocardium. Once the pressure in the ventricles exceeds the pressure in the aorta, the semilunar valves are forced open and blood is ejected from the ventricles, initiating the VEP. During VEP, ventricular volume decreases as blood exits the ventricles through the open semilunar valves (**Figure 11.5C**).

During the *isovolumetric relaxation period (IRP)* both the AV and the semilunar valves are closed (**Figure 11.5D**). Thus, ventricular volume is again unchanged (isovolumetric), but pressure is low because the ventricles are relaxed.

All these events occur within a single cardiac cycle, which repeats with every beat of the heart. **Figure 11.6** summarizes the cardiac cycle graphically, showing concurrent information about the electrocardiogram; the pressure in the left atrium, the left ventricle, and aorta; the left ventricular volume; the heart phase; the period of the cardiac cycle; and the position of the heart valves.

TABLE 11.1	Typical Resting Cardiovascular Values for Males and Females of Various Ages					
	Age of Males (yr)			**Age of Females (yr)**		
Cardiovascular Value	**10–15**	**20–30**	**50–60**	**10–15**	**20–30**	**50–60**
HR (b·min^{-1})	82	72	80	85	76	82
SV (mL·b^{-1})	50	90	70	40	75	62
Cardiac output (L·min^{-1})	04.0	06.5	05.5	03.4	05.5	05.0
Sources: Åstrand (1952); Fleg et al. (1995); Ogawa et al. (1992); Spina et al. (1992, 1993a,b).						

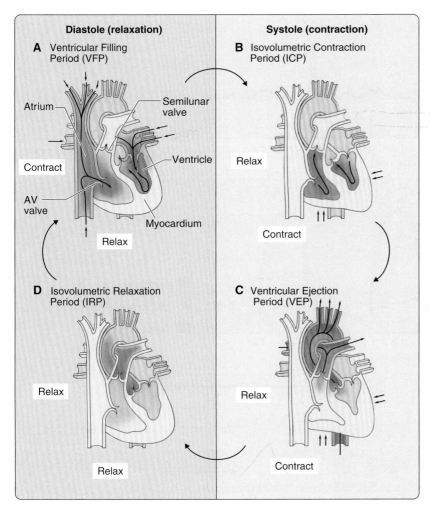

Diastole (relaxation)

A Ventricular Filling
Period (VFP)

Atrium

Semilunar valve

Contract

Ventricle

AV valve

Relax

Myocardium

D Isovolumetric Relaxation
Period (IRP)

Relax

Relax

Systole (contraction)

B Isovolumetric Contraction
Period (ICP)

Relax

Contract

C Ventricular Ejection
Period (VEP)

Relax

Contract

FIGURE 11.5 Periods of the Cardiac Cycle.
A. Ventricular Filling Period (VFP). The ventricles are relaxed. The A-V valves are open and venous blood is filling the ventricles. **B.** Isovolumetric Contraction Period (ICP). The contraction of the myocardium increases intraventricular pressure, but all the valves are closed and blood volume in the ventricles remains constant. **C.** Ventricular Ejection Period (VEP). Increasing ventricular pressure forces the semilunar valves open and blood is ejected from the ventricles. **D.** Isovolumetric Relaxation Period (IRP). The ventricles are relaxed and all the valves are closed, so blood volume in the ventricles remains constant.

As in **Figure 11.5**, diastole is shown in blue and systole is shown in green. The position of the AV and semilunar valves is shown in **Figures 11.5** and **11.6**.

Figure 11.6 begins arbitrarily during the VFP of ventricular diastole (also shown in **Figure 11.5A**). The AV valves are open, allowing blood to flow from the atria into the ventricles; therefore, ventricular volume is increasing. As the atria contract, more blood is forced into the ventricles, causing a small increase in ventricular volume and ventricular pressure.

Following the QRS complex, there is an immediate and dramatic increase in ventricular pressure as the myocardium contracts. Note, however, that the ventricular volume does not immediately change. This is the ICP. Locate Point A on the graph of ventricular pressure in **Figure 11.6**—this is the point where pressure in the ventricle exceeds pressure in the aorta, and the aortic semilunar valve is forced open. Follow the dashed lines downward to the row for the semilunar valves in the chart at the bottom of the figure, and note that these valves are now opened. Also note that this dashed line coincides with the start of a rapid decrease in ventricular volume. Once the valves are open, blood is forced out of the

ventricles; thus, blood volume in the ventricles decreases. This is the VEP.

When pressure in the ventricles falls below pressure in the aorta, the semilunar valves close. Refer to Point B on the pressure curve of **Figure 11.6** and again follow the dashed line downward, noting ventricular volume and valve position. Ventricular pressure is decreasing because the myocardium is relaxed (in diastole). Ventricular volume, however, remains constant, because all the valves are closed and no blood can enter or leave the ventricles. This is known as the IRP.

Following the T wave (ventricular repolarization), the ventricles relax and begin to fill with blood: The AV valves are open, and ventricular volume increases. This is the VFP. This cycle of diastole followed by systole followed by diastole continues with each beat of the heart.

Diastole provides time for the cardiac cells to relax and the ventricles to fill. The length of time spent in diastole thereby directly affects the amount of blood that will be present in the ventricles to be pumped during the subsequent systole. Furthermore, it is during diastole that the myocardium is supplied with blood.

Systole is the contraction period of the heart, first isometrically (ICP) and then dynamically (VEP). The volume

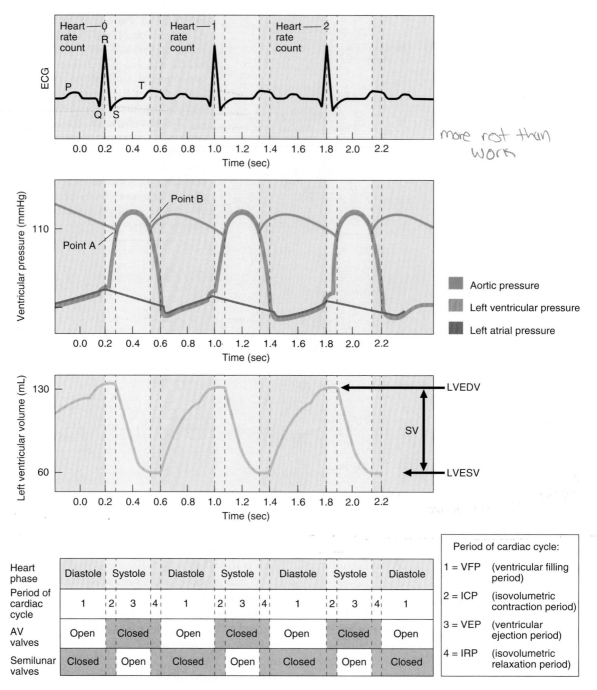

more rest than work

FIGURE 11.6 Graphic Summary of the Cardiac Cycle.
The periods of the cardiac cycle are labeled as 1, VFP; 2, ICP; 3, VEP; and 4, IRP.

of blood ejected from the ventricles directly affects the cardiovascular system's ability to meet the demands of the body. The volume of blood in the ventricles at the end of diastole is termed **end–diastolic volume (EDV)** and is labeled in **Figure 11.6.** Similarly, the volume of blood in the ventricles at the end of systole is termed **end–systolic volume (ESV).** The amount of blood ejected from the ventricles with each beat is called **stroke volume (SV),** which is equal to EDV – ESV. **Figure 11.6** depicts the

volume in the left ventricle (LV), but because both sides of the heart must pump the same amount of blood over any significant period of time, the SV is typically the same for both sides of the heart.

Before going to the next section, study **Figures 11.5** and **11.6.** Be sure you understand what is happening with the ECG, with ventricular, atrial, and aortic pressure, with ventricular volume, and with the heart valves at each period of the cardiac cycle. Now, find your radial pulse and begin

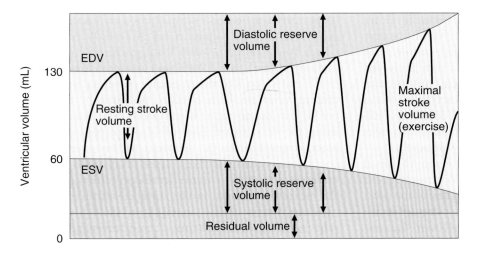

FIGURE 11.7 Subdivisions of Ventricular Volume.
Source: Based on G. A. Brechar & P. M. Galletti. Functional anatomy of cardiac pumping. In Hamilton, W. F. (ed.): *Handbook of Physiology, Section 2: Circulation*. Washington, DC: American Physiological Society (1963).

counting: 0, 1, 2, 3, …. All the events described in this section occur every time you feel a pulse, which occurs once every 0.8 seconds when the heart rate is 75 b·min⁻¹. **Heart rate (HR)** is thus defined as the number of cardiac cycles per minute, expressed as beats per minute (b·min⁻¹).

See animation, Cardiac Cycle, at http://thePoint.lww.com/Plowman4e .

Stroke Volume

As mentioned previously, stroke volume (SV) is the volume of blood ejected from the ventricles with each beat, expressed as milliliters per beat (mL·b⁻¹) or simply in milliliters (mL). The amount of blood ejected from the heart is determined by three primary factors:

1. The volume of blood returned to the heart (preload)
2. The force of myocardial contraction (contractility)
3. The resistance presented to the contracting ventricle (afterload)

The volume of blood returned to the heart is called **preload** and is critical to the stroke volume because the heart cannot eject blood that is not there. Under resting conditions the heart ejects approximately 50–60% of the blood that is returned; this is known as the **ejection fraction (EF)**. Figure 11.7 depicts changes in the volume of blood in the ventricles throughout the cardiac cycle and defines specific volumes associated with the ventricles. In this figure, the EDV is approximately 130 mL of blood, which is typical for an adult male under resting conditions. Following systole the ESV is approximately 60 mL of blood. Stroke volume can then be calculated as

11.1 stroke volume (mL) = end-diastolic volume (mL) − end-systolic volume (mL)

or

$$SV = EDV - ESV$$
$$70\ mL = 130\ mL - 60\ mL$$

(handwritten: Stroke Volume = Endd ventricle minus end systolic)

Thus, 70 mL of blood was ejected from each ventricle during this contraction of the heart.

The ejection fraction (EF) can now be calculated from the information as follows:

11.2 ejection fraction(%) = stroke volume (mL) ÷ end-diastolic volume (mL) × 100

or

$$EF = \frac{SV}{EDV} \times 100$$

(handwritten: $EF\ \frac{SV}{EDV} \times 100$)

EXAMPLE

Calculate the ejection fraction for the previous example.

$$EF = \left[\frac{70\ mL}{130\ mL}\right] \times 100 = 54\%$$

End–Diastolic Volume (EDV) The volume of blood in the ventricle at the end of diastole.

End–Systolic Volume (ESV) The volume of blood in the ventricle at the end of systole.

Stroke Volume (SV) Amount of blood ejected from the ventricles with each beat of the heart.

Heart Rate (HR) The number of cardiac cycles per minute.

Preload Volume of blood returned to the heart.

Ejection Fraction (EF) The percentage of EDV that is ejected from the heart.

Total Heart Volume ≈ 350mL
¼ ≈ 90mL

Note in **Figure 11.7** that the SV can increase by either an increased EDV (which encroaches into diastolic reserve volume) or a decreased ESV (which encroaches into systolic reserve volume) or a combination of the two. However, the entire blood volume cannot be ejected; thus, there is always a residual volume of blood in the heart (Brechar and Galletti, 1963). Because the subdivisions of ventricular volume parallel those of the lungs, it may be helpful to refer back to **Figure 9.6** to fully understand this principle.

Under normal conditions, as the volume of blood returned to the heart (EDV) increases, SV increases. This relationship is known as the Frank-Starling law of the heart (**Figure 11.8**). Increasing EDV, to a point, increases stroke volume because the increased volume of blood in the ventricles provides a preload that stretches the myocardium and enhances the force of contraction by optimizing the overlap of actin and myosin filaments (Levick, 2003).

CHECK YOUR COMPREHENSION 1

Using **Figure 11.8**, answer the following questions under normal conditions and increased sympathetic nervous stimulation:

1. What is the SV associated with an EDV of 150 mL? Of 200 mL? Of 250 mL? Of 300 mL?

2. What is the EF for each SV?

Contractility, the force of contraction of the myocardium, is determined primarily by neural innervation. Sympathetic nervous stimulation causes an increase in the contractility of the myocardium independent of the volume of blood returned to the heart. Circulating catecholamines (hormones) also reinforce the increased contractility caused by sympathetic nerve stimulation. During exercise, the Frank-Starling mechanism (preload) and increased contractility (due to sympathetic nervous stimulation) function together to enhance stroke volume. **Figure 11.8**

(upper curve) shows how sympathetic nervous stimulation can increase stroke volume at any given EDV. Answer the Check Your Comprehension 1 box to ensure your understanding of this figure. Check your answer in Appendix C.

The **afterload**, or the resistance presented to the contracting ventricle, is determined primarily by the blood pressure in the aorta. As blood pressure increases, opposition to the outward flow of blood increases and less blood is ejected from the ventricles for any given force of contraction—that is, stroke volume decreases as afterload increases. The stroke volume decreases in this way because the increased pressure in the aorta causes the semilunar valves to remain closed longer and to close sooner. The valve is thus open for less time, thereby causing a decrease in ejection time and a subsequent decrease in stroke volume. **Table 11.1** presents typical values for stroke volume at rest in healthy individuals of various ages.

Cardiac Output

Cardiac output ($\dot{Q}$) is the amount of blood pumped per unit of time, normally reported in liters per minute. It represents the total blood flow through the entire cardiovascular system and reflects the body's ability to meet changing metabolic needs during rest and exercise. Cardiac output is calculated as

11.3   cardiac output $(mL \cdot min^{-1})$ = stroke volume $(mL \cdot b^{-1}) \times$ heart rate $(b \cdot min^{-1})$

or

$\dot{Q} = SV \times HR$ *Rest cardiac output*

At rest, cardiac output for an adult male is approximately 5 L·min⁻¹. It is interesting to note that resting blood volume, in average-sized adult males, is also approximately 5 L. Thus, at rest, the entire volume of blood is circulated through the body each minute. **Table 11.1** presents typical values for cardiac output at rest in healthy individuals of various ages.

EXAMPLE

Calculate $\dot{Q}$ for an individual with an HR of 64 b·min⁻¹ and an SV of 100 mL of blood.

$\dot{Q} = SV \times HR = (100 \text{ mL} \cdot b^{-1}) \times (64 \text{ b} \cdot min^{-1})$
$= 6400 \text{ mL} \cdot min^{-1}$

Because $\dot{Q}$ is usually reported in liters, this value is divided by 1000 and is reported as 6.4 L·min⁻¹. Note that although SV is usually expressed in milliliters (mL), it is actually measured in milliliters per beat (mL·b⁻¹) since by definition SV must be per beat.

The Check Your Comprehension 2 box asks you to do some calculations to check your understanding of this formula. Check your answers in Appendix C.

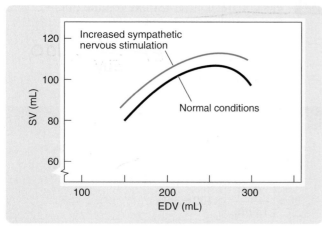

FIGURE 11.8 Frank-Starling Law of the Heart.

CHECK YOUR COMPREHENSION 2

Using your knowledge of the components of cardiac output, perform the necessary calculations to determine the missing values.

	HR (b·min⁻¹)	SV (mL·b⁻¹)	Q̇ (L·min⁻¹)
Mike	80	90	
Keiko	60	120	
Kirk	122	146.5	
Don	72		6.34
Nora		98	5.68

Coronary Circulation

The energy necessary for cardiac function is supplied through aerobic metabolism. Arterial coronary circulation supplies oxygenated blood to the myocardium through two major arteries, the right coronary artery and the left coronary artery (**Figure 11.9**). Both arteries originate at the root of the aorta. The left coronary artery divides into the left circumflex and anterior descending arteries. The right coronary artery divides into the marginal artery and the posterior interventricular artery. The myocardium is supplied with a dense distribution of arterioles and capillaries, approximately 3000–4000 capillaries per square millimeter of cardiac muscle (Rowell, 1986). The venous blood from the coronary circulation is returned to the right atrium via the coronary sinus.

Coronary blood flow is affected greatly by the phase of the cardiac cycle. Because of the high intramyocardial pressure during systole, the coronary arteries are compressed, and blood flow to the myocardium is decreased. Thus, the myocardium receives the largest portion of its blood flow during diastole (Guyton and Hall, 2011). The myocardial blood flow required to provide necessary oxygen at rest is about 250 mL·min⁻¹, which represents approximately 4% of the normal resting cardiac output (Rowell, 1986). The coronary circulation very effectively extracts oxygen as the blood flows through the capillary beds. Under resting conditions, 60–70% of the available oxygen is extracted.

Contractility The force of contraction of the heart.

Afterload Resistance presented to the contracting ventricle.

Cardiac Output (Q̇) The amount of blood pumped per unit of time, in liters per minute.

Myocardial Oxygen Consumption The amount of oxygen used by the heart muscle to produce energy for contraction.

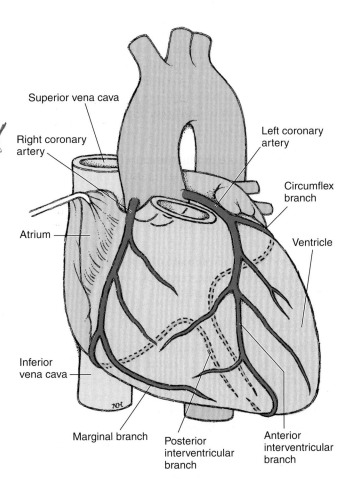

FIGURE 11.9 Coronary Circulation.

Myocardial Oxygen Consumption

myocardial infarction (MI) = heart attack

Because the metabolic demands of the myocardium are increased during exercise, **myocardial oxygen consumption**—the **amount of** oxygen used by the heart muscle to produce energy for contraction—increases during exercise. Myocardial oxygen consumption reflects the work of the heart and is determined by *oxygen extraction (a-vO₂diff)* and *blood flow (Q̇)*. As mentioned previously, oxygen extraction of the coronary circulation is nearly optimal at rest (60–70%) and increases little if at all during exercise. Thus, the increased myocardial oxygen consumption during exercise occurs almost entirely by increased blood flow (Q̇) to the myocardium.

The coronary blood flow must be regulated to meet the demands of the myocardium for oxygen. In addition to a higher heart rate, blood flow is increased by two mechanisms:

1. The greater force of myocardial contraction that results from exercise causes more blood to be forced into the coronary circulation.
2. By-products of cellular work cause vasodilation of the arterioles that supply the myocardium. Thus, as the heart works harder and produces more by-products, the arterioles dilate, which decreases resistance and effectively increases blood flow.

Myocardial oxygen consumption increases as heart rate increases. Because heart rate increases with the intensity of exercise, so also does myocardial oxygen consumption (Kitamura et al., 1972). Myocardial oxygen consumption can be estimated from the <u>rate-pressure product **(RPP)**</u>, which is the product of heart rate (HR) and systolic blood pressure (SBP):

11.4 rate-pressure product (units) = [systolic blood pressure (mmHg) × heart rate (b·min^{-1})] ÷ 100

or

$$RPP = \frac{SBP \times HR}{100}$$

RPP provides a good estimate of myocardial oxygen consumption under a wide range of conditions, including dynamic and static exercise.

The Vascular System

The *vascular system* is composed of vessels that transport the blood throughout the body. Their size and structure vary throughout the vascular tree, with each portion of the vascular system having a specific structure and function related to the overall function of the cardiovascular system. Blood vessels, except for capillaries, have three layers; the adventitia (outer layer), tunica

media (middle layer), and tunica intima (innermost layer) (**Figure 11.10**). The adventitia is composed of connective tissue and attaches the blood vessel to surrounding tissue. The tunica media contains smooth muscle, which is critical for controlling the vessel's diameter, and connective tissue, and gives the vessel elasticity and strength. The intima consists of a single layer of endothelial cells, the **endothelium**, and a thin layer of connective tissue (basal lamina). The endothelium serves as the barrier between blood and underlying tissue and

1. Plays a critical role in the movement of material out of the blood
2. Releases factors that help regulate the contraction of smooth muscle in the tunica media, thus helping to regulate blood flow
3. Helps prevent unnecessary clot formation
4. Interacts with immune cells in the inflammatory process

The vessels of the vascular system, along with various circulations, are illustrated in **Figure 11.11**.

Arteries

The arteries are thick-walled conduits that carry blood from the heart to the body's organs (see **Figure 11.10**). They contain a large amount of elastic tissue that allows

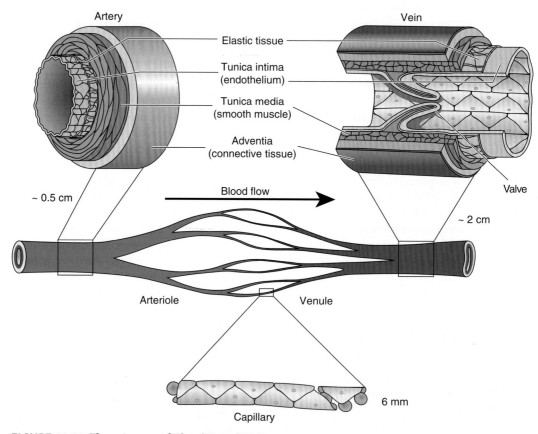

FIGURE 11.10 Three Layers of Blood Vessel Wall.

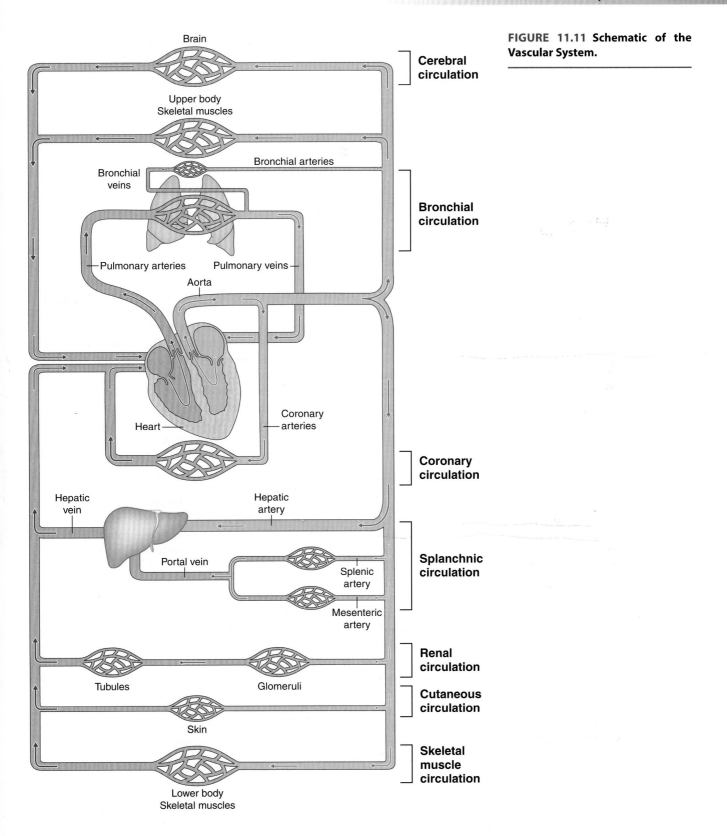

FIGURE 11.11 Schematic of the Vascular System.

Cerebral circulation

Bronchial circulation

Coronary circulation

Splanchnic circulation

Renal circulation

Cutaneous circulation

Skeletal muscle circulation

Brain

Upper body Skeletal muscles

Bronchial arteries

Bronchial veins

Pulmonary arteries   Pulmonary veins

Aorta

Heart

Coronary arteries

Hepatic vein   Hepatic artery

Portal vein   Splenic artery

Mesenteric artery

Tubules   Glomeruli

Skin

Lower body Skeletal muscles

Rate-Pressure Product (RPP) An estimate of the myocardial oxygen consumption, calculated as the product of heart (HR) and systolic blood pressure (SBP).

Endothelium Single layer of epithelial tissue.

them to distend when blood is ejected during systole and to recoil during diastole. Blood flow in the arteries is pulsatile owing to the pumping action of the heart.

As the left ventricle ejects blood into the aorta, the blood stretches the aorta's elastic walls. Blood pressure

$$\boxed{\text{Resting MAP} = (PP / 3) + DBP_2} \quad \boxed{\text{Exercise} \atop \text{MAP} = (PP/2) + DBP_1}$$

TABLE 11.2   Typical Resting Blood Pressure Values for Males and Females of Various Ages

Blood Pressure Value	Age of Males (yr)			Age of Females (yr)		
	10–15	20–30	50–60	10–15	20–30	50–60
Systolic blood pressure SBP (mmHg)	100	120	134	84	120	130
Diastolic blood pressure DBP (mmHg)	60	80	84	40	74	84
Mean arterial pressure MAP (mmHg)	73	93	97	55	88	92

Sources: Fleg et al. (1995); Ogawa et al. (1992); Spina et al. (1993a,b).

$$\underline{PP \text{ (pulse pressure)} = SBP - DBP}$$

(BP) is the force exerted on the wall of the blood vessel by the blood. **Systolic blood pressure (SBP)** is the force exerted on the wall of the blood vessel by blood during systole. During relaxation of the heart (diastole), the arterial walls recoil, maintaining pressure on the blood still in the vessels. As a result, although the blood pressure drops during diastole, there is always some pressure in the arteries. Thus, **diastolic blood pressure (DBP)** is the force exerted on the wall of blood vessels by blood during diastole. **Mean arterial pressure (MAP)** is a weighted average of SBP and DBP, representing the mean driving force of blood throughout the arterial system. Typical resting blood pressure values for males and females at different ages are given in **Table 11.2**.

Arterioles

Arterioles, also called **resistance vessels**, are smaller than arteries and are the major site of resistance in the vascular system. Because of this increased resistance, the pulsatile arterial blood flow becomes continuous before it reaches the capillaries. Arterioles absorb the pulsatile force of blood flow because they contain a large amount of elastic tissue. Imagine bouncing a basketball on a gymnasium floor and on a wrestling mat. The ball rebounds from the gym floor at an angle and height proportional to the force imparted by your muscle action. However, the same force will not produce much (if any) rebound from the wrestling mat. The elastic tissue in the walls of the arteries absorbs the energy from the pulsatile blood flow in a similar way that the mat absorbs energy from the basketball. In an individual with reduced elasticity, or arterial stiffening (sometimes called hardening of the arteries), the arteries, like the gym floor, are not able to distend as readily, resulting in elevated blood pressure.

The smooth muscle surrounding arterioles is able to contract and relax. Contraction of the smooth muscle around an arteriole results in *vasoconstriction*, a decrease in vessel diameter and therefore a decrease in blood flow to a given region. Relaxation of the smooth muscle results in *vasodilation*, an increased vessel diameter and therefore an increase in blood flow to a region. The vasoconstriction and vasodilation of the smooth muscles surrounding the

arterioles is primarily responsible for determining blood flow distribution to various organs.

The degree to which an arteriole vasodilates or vasoconstricts depends on the balance of *extrinsic* (originating outside the part on which it acts) and *intrinsic* (originating within the part on which it acts) mechanisms. Extrinsic mechanisms are geared toward maintaining mean arterial pressure and include nervous stimulation and circulating hormones. Smooth muscle surrounding terminal arteries and arterioles is innervated by sympathetic neurons. Sympathetic stimulation causes most arterioles to vasoconstrict. However, during exercise, when the sympathetic nervous system is clearly activated, arterioles to the working muscles dilate in order to supply the working muscle with increased blood flow. The role of the sympathetic nervous system in accounting for this dilation is controversial. Although sympathetic vasodilatory fibers have been identified in several species, and postulated in humans, there is no direct evidence of vasodilatory sympathetic nerve fibers in humans (Joyner and Dietz, 2003).

Intrinsic (local) mechanisms that control arteriole diameter include myogenic (originating within the muscle) mechanisms, metabolic factors, and shear stress in the blood vessel that causes the release of local vasoactive substances. Myogenic control is accomplished by mechanisms that cause the vessels to dilate in response to decreased stretch (decreased flow) and vasoconstrict in response to increased stretch (increased flow). This reflex action helps to ensure that changes in blood pressure do not lead to dramatic changes in blood flow to a given vascular bed. The metabolic control of vascular diameter plays a critical role in determining the degree of smooth muscle contraction and hence local blood flow. When tissue is metabolically active, such as skeletal muscle during exercise, it produces metabolic by-products that act locally to cause vasodilation, thereby increasing blood flow to the metabolically active area. Thus contracting skeletal muscles act locally (intrinsically) on the smooth muscle surrounding the arterioles to increase blood flow in that region. In the case of exercise, the local vasodilatory effects have a greater effect on vessel diameter in arterioles supplying the skeletal muscle than the sympathetic vasoconstrictor effects, leading to vasodilation in the skeletal muscle. On the other hand, arterioles supplying nonworking muscle and other organs (stomach, kidneys) constrict, resulting in decreased blood flow during exercise due to sympathetic nerve stimulation. The endothelium of the blood vessel also releases vasoactive substances that regulate vascular tone, and hence vessel diameter. For example, an increase in shear stress (caused by blood flow) is associated with the release of nitric oxide (NO) from the endothelium, which causes smooth muscle surrounding the vessel to relax, thus causing vasodilation. Conversely, other substances released from the endothelium, such as endothelin-1, are potent vasoconstrictors.

Capillaries

The *capillaries* perform the ultimate function of the cardiovascular system: transferring gases and nutrients between the blood and tissues. Some exchange of gases occurs in the smallest vessels on both sides of the capillaries (collectively termed the **exchange vessels**) but most of the gas exchange occurs across the capillary wall. The walls of the capillaries are very thin, essentially composed of a single layer of endothelial cells (**Figure 11.10**). Capillaries have a very small diameter, such that red blood cells often must pass through in single file.

Blood flow through capillaries also depends on the other vessels that make up the microcirculation. As shown in **Figure 11.12**, the **microcirculation** includes several vessels: arterioles, venules, arteriovenous anastomoses, metarterioles, and true capillaries. *Anastomoses* are wide, connecting channels that act as shunts between arterioles and venules. These vessels are not common in most tissue but are abundant in the skin and play an important role in thermoregulation (Levick, 2003). When anastomoses are open, large volumes of blood can be directed to blood

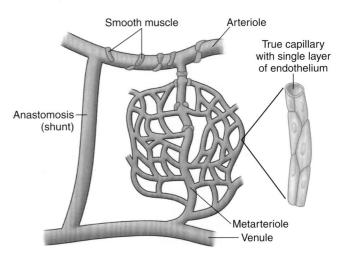

FIGURE 11.12 Anatomy of the Microcirculation.

vessels close to the surface of the skin, facilitating heat dissipation. A *metarteriole* is a short vessel that connects an arteriole with a venule, creating a direct route through the capillary bed. The metarteriole gives rise to the capillaries. *True capillaries* vary in number depending on the capillary bed. Smooth muscles around these vessels that relax or constrict in response to local chemical conditions control blood flow through the capillaries. Thus, a capillary bed can be perfused with blood or be almost entirely bypassed, depending on the needs of the tissue it supplies.

GAS EXCHANGE The exchange of gases and nutrients in the capillaries depends on *diffusion*. For a substance to diffuse from a capillary into a cell, it must cross two membranes: the capillary wall (composed primarily of endothelium) and the cell membrane. Substances pass from the capillary to the interstitial space by the process of diffusion. Movement from the interstitial space into the cell may also occur by diffusion or may require carrier-mediated transport. The movement of gases and nutrients into and out of the capillaries depends on the concentration gradient or pressure gradient of the substance or gas that is diffusing.

As discussed in Chapter 9, oxygen and carbon dioxide diffuse down pressure gradients. Oxygen diffuses down its pressure gradient from systemic capillaries into muscle cells. Therefore, there is less oxygen in the veins draining skeletal muscles than in the arteries supplying them. The difference in the oxygen content of the arteries and veins is termed the *a-vO₂difference*, which reflects the oxygen taken up by the skeletal muscles.

MOVEMENT OF FLUIDS Fluids also pass through the capillary membrane. The movement of fluids is determined by two opposing forces: hydrostatic pressure and osmotic pressure. *Hydrostatic pressure*, created by blood pressure, acts to "push" fluid out of the capillaries. *Osmotic pressure*, caused by the larger concentration of proteins in the capillaries, acts to "pull" water into the

---

Systolic Blood Pressure (SBP) The force exerted on the wall of blood vessels by the blood as a result of contraction of the heart (systole).

Diastolic Blood Pressure (DBP) The force exerted on the wall of blood vessels by blood during relaxation of the heart (diastole).

Mean Arterial Pressure (MAP) The weighted average of SBP and DBP, representing the mean driving force of blood throughout the arterial system.

Resistance Vessels Another name for arterioles because this is the site of greatest resistance to blood flow in the vascular system.

Exchange Vessels Another name for capillaries because this is the site of gas and nutrient exchange between the blood and tissues.

Microcirculation Smallest vessels of the vascular system, including arterioles, venules, arteriovenous anastomoses, metarterioles, and true capillaries.

capillaries. The net result of these opposing forces is the loss of approximately 3 L of fluid a day from the plasma into interstitial spaces (Marieb and Hoehn, 2010). This fluid returns to the blood via the lymphatic system. Any change in hydrostatic pressure or osmotic pressure of the blood will alter the fluid exchange between the blood and the interstitial fluid.

Venules

The venules are small vessels on the venous side of the vascular system. These vessels contain some smooth muscle, which can influence capillary pressure. The venules and capillaries constitute the microcirculation where gas and nutrient exchange occurs. Venules empty into veins.

Veins

Veins, also called **capacitance vessels**, are low-resistance conduits that return blood to the heart (**Figure 11.10**). They contain smooth muscle innervated by the sympathetic nervous system, which can change their diameter. Contraction of smooth muscle around the veins is known as *venoconstriction*; relaxation of the veins is known as *venodilation*. Because veins can expand (distensibility), they can pool large volumes of blood—up to 60% of the total blood volume at rest—and therefore are sometimes referred to as a blood reservoir. The amount of blood in all the veins varies with posture and activity. If blood accumulates in the veins and is not returned to the heart, ventricular end–diastolic volume decreases, and hence stroke volume decreases. Conversely, venoconstriction can significantly increase ventricular end–diastolic volume and thereby lead to an increase in stroke volume, according to the Frank-Starling law of the heart.

The skeletal muscle pump and the respiratory pump help increase venous return by "massaging" blood back toward the heart. The one-way valves in the veins also help regulate venous pressure and are particularly helpful in counteracting the effects of gravity that oppose blood flow back to the heart because they prevent the backward flow of blood. Additionally, the increased sympathetic nervous activity during exercise helps to increase venous return via venoconstriction.

Blood

Blood is the fluid that circulates through the heart and the vasculature to transport nutrients and gases. Blood contains living blood cells suspended in a nonliving fluid matrix called plasma. **Figure 11.13** depicts blood that has been centrifuged to separate the cells and the plasma. Blood cells are classified as erythrocytes (red blood cells, RBC) or leukocytes (white blood cells, WBC). Blood cells account for 38–45% of the total blood volume in adult females and 43–48% of the total blood volume in adult males. The ratio of blood cells to total blood volume is known as **hematocrit** and is usually expressed as a percentage.

As discussed in the respiratory section, the RBCs transport oxygen from the lungs to body cells by binding oxygen to hemoglobin. Leukocytes are less numerous than erythrocytes, accounting for about 1% of total blood volume. Despite their seemingly small number, leukocytes are essential to the body's defense against disease and play a critical role in inflammation.

Plasma accounts for approximately 55% of the volume of blood. It is composed primarily of water, which accounts for approximately 90% of its volume. It also contains over 100 dissolved solutes, including proteins, nutrients, electrolytes, and respiratory gases. The composition of plasma varies greatly, depending on the needs of the body. Plasma also plays an important role in thermoregulation by helping to distribute heat throughout the body.

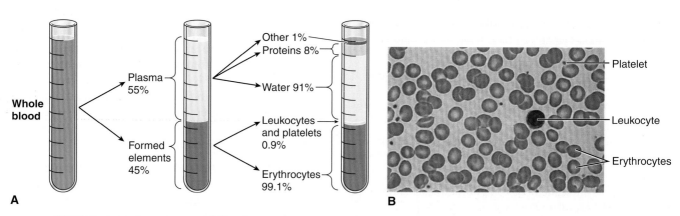

FIGURE 11.13 Components of Blood.
A. Whole blood is composed of formed elements and plasma, which can be separated by "spinning the blood" in a centrifuge. **B.** Formed elements (platelets, leukocytes, and erythrocytes) as seen through a microscope (400×).

Blood Donation and Exercise

When one donates blood, approximately one pint of blood (about 450–500 mL) is typically taken from the body. Because the total blood volume is approximately 5000 mL (5 L), the donation results in roughly a 10% reduction in blood volume, or a greater percentage in small individuals with less blood (typically women). The blood plasma volume is reestablished in approximately 24 hours, and red blood cells are replaced in about 6 weeks. Because of this reduction in plasma volume, it seems prudent for endurance athletes to avoid donating blood during the competitive phases of the training cycle. Strenuous activities should be avoided for 24 hours after giving blood to allow the body to replace the majority of the lost fluids. Plenty of water should be ingested following blood donation.

Training intensity may need to be slightly reduced pending complete RBC replacement for fitness participants or athletes who do donate blood.

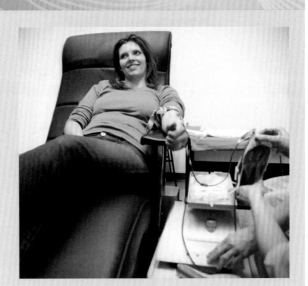

Hormonal Control of Blood Volume

As is discussed in the accompanying Focus on Application: Clinically Relevant Box, blood volume is decreased by blood donation. Decreased blood volume may also result from profuse sweating and/or dehydration. Blood volume varies considerably among individuals and is affected by fitness status. Healthy adult males have an average blood volume of approximately 75 mL of blood per kg of body weight, or a total of approximately 5–6 L of blood. Healthy adult females have approximately 65 mL of blood per kg of body weight, which equals 4–4.5 L of blood for the average-sized woman. Children typically have about 60 mL of blood per kg of body weight, with total volume varying depending on body size.

Blood volume plays an important role in maintaining stroke volume, cardiac output, and blood pressure. Under normal conditions blood volume is maintained within physiological limits by homeostatic mechanisms involving the endocrine system and urinary system. The major hormones involved in maintaining blood volume are antidiuretic hormone (ADH), released from the posterior pituitary gland, and aldosterone, released from the adrenal cortex. **Figure 11.14** outlines the hormonal mechanisms that respond to a reduction in blood volume.

Capacitance Vessels Another name for veins because of their distensibility, which enables them to pool large volumes of blood and become reservoirs for blood.

Hematocrit The ratio of blood cells to total blood volume, expressed as a percentage.

Plasma volume reduction causes a decrease in atrial and arterial pressure. The decrease in pressure is sensed by atrial baroreceptors (*baro* means "pressure") and arterial receptors in the kidneys. Atrial baroreceptor activation leads to the release of ADH from the posterior pituitary gland, which causes the tubules of the kidneys to reabsorb water, thus increasing plasma volume.

A reduction in blood volume is also associated with an increase in plasma osmolarity (solute concentration). For example, with profuse sweating more water than solutes is lost; thus, the osmolarity of the blood increases. An increase in osmolarity of the blood stimulates osmoreceptors in the hypothalamus, which signals the posterior pituitary gland to release ADH. ADH causes the kidneys to retain water, thus leading to an increase in blood volume.

Simultaneously, the receptors in the kidneys respond to decreased arterial pressure by releasing the enzyme renin. Renin is necessary for the conversion of angiotensinogen to angiotensin I, which is then converted to angiotensin II. Angiotensin II signals the adrenal cortex to release aldosterone. Aldosterone causes the kidneys to retain salt and water. Angiotensin II also has a vasoconstrictor effect on arterioles, thus helping to increase blood pressure.

Cardiovascular Dynamics

The different components of the cardiovascular system function together to meet the changing demands of the body. These components are highly integrated and interdependent. Although both the heart and the vasculature

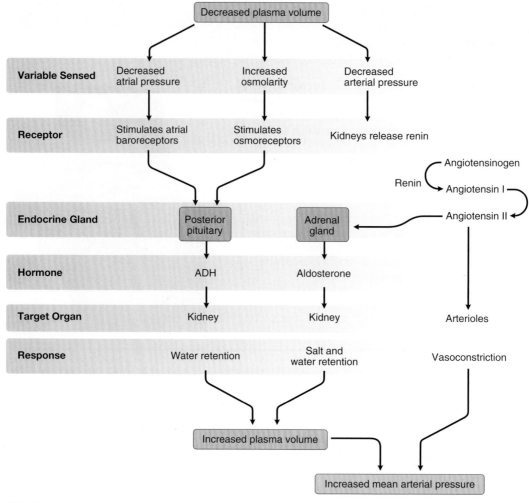

FIGURE 11.14   Hormonal Control of Blood Volume.

respond independently to various conditions, they are interrelated because the response of the heart affects the vessels, and vice versa.

To differentiate the responses of the heart and the vessels, we commonly refer to central and peripheral cardiovascular responses. **Central cardiovascular responses** are those directly related to the heart: heart rate, stroke volume, cardiac output, etc. **Peripheral cardiovascular responses** are those occurring in vessels: vasodilation, vasoconstriction, venous return, etc.

Cardiac Output (Q̇)

As described earlier, cardiac output is the amount of blood ejected from the ventricles each minute. This volume of blood changes constantly to meet the body's metabolic demands. The volume of blood flow can be described using the basic formula presented in Chapter 9 to describe air flow (F = ΔP / R). Applied to the cardiovascular system, this equation is

11.5   cardiac output $(L \cdot min^{-1})$ = mean arterial blood pressure (mmHg) ÷ total peripheral resistance $(mmHg \cdot mL^{-1} \cdot min^{-1})$

or

$$\dot{Q} = \frac{MAP}{TPR}$$

In this formula, cardiac output represents the blood flow for the entire cardiovascular system, mean arterial pressure reflects the pressure gradient driving blood through the vascular system, and total peripheral resistance refers to the factors that oppose blood flow in the entire system. Technically, the equation should use the difference in pressure (ΔP) between mean arterial pressure and the pressure in the right atrium (where blood is flowing to). However, since pressure in the right atrium is so low (<4 mmHg), it is considered negligible and is not usually given in the formula. Thus, mean arterial pressure is used alone in the equation.

Mean Arterial Pressure (MAP)

Mean arterial pressure represents the driving force of blood through the vascular system. Adequate MAP is necessary to ensure adequate perfusion of all the vital organs of the body. On the other hand, excess blood pressure can damage the endothelial lining of the blood vessels. Thus, MAP is a physiological variable that is tightly controlled by homeostatic mechanisms. MAP can be expressed in relation to $\dot{Q}$ and TPR by rearranging the equation above to become

11.6 mean arterial pressure (mmHg) = cardiac output
$(L \cdot min^{-1}) \times$ total peripheral resistance (TPR units)
$MAP = \dot{Q} \times TPR$

Total Peripheral Resistance (TPR)

Total peripheral resistance (TPR), or simply **resistance (R)**, results from factors that oppose blood flow. It is expressed in millimeters of mercury per milliliter per minute ($mmHg \cdot mL^{-1} \cdot min^{-1}$), or more simply as TPR units. Most of the resistance in the vascular tree results from the friction of blood against vessel walls, and it varies depending on the size of the vessel. The three primary factors that affect resistance and their mathematical relationship are described by Poiseuille's law:

11.7
$$resistance = \frac{length \times viscosity}{(radius)^4}$$

Thus, the more viscous the blood is, the greater the resistance to flow. The longer the blood vessel, the greater the friction between the vessel walls and the blood. Under normal conditions, however, a vessel's length and blood viscosity do not change substantially. On the other hand, the vessel's radius can change considerably because of vasodilation or vasoconstriction. Furthermore, because the resistance is inversely related to the fourth power of the radius, a small change in vessel diameter can result in a large change in blood flow. Thus, vessel radius is by far the most important factor determining resistance to blood flow. Recall that vessel diameter is affected by local conditions (local control) and neural innervation (extrinsic control).

Total peripheral resistance (TPR) can be calculated by rearranging the formula $\dot{Q} = MAP \div TPR$ to solve for TPR, provided that the flow rate ($\dot{Q}$) and blood pressure (MAP) are known. The formula for TPR becomes

Central Cardiovascular Responses Responses directly related to the heart.

Peripheral Cardiovascular Responses Responses directly related to the vessels.

Total Peripheral Resistance (TPR) or Resistance (R) The factors that oppose blood flow.

11.8 total peripheral resistance (TPR units) = mean arterial blood pressure (mmHg) ÷ cardiac output
$(L \cdot min^{-1})$

or

$$TPR = \frac{MAP}{\dot{Q}}$$

EXAMPLE

Assume that normal resting blood pressure is 110/80 (MAP = 90 mmHg), normal cardiac output = 5.4 $L \cdot min^{-1}$, and central venous pressure = zero. Calculate TPR for the entire cardiovascular system.

The calculation is

$$TPR = \frac{MAP}{\dot{Q}} = \frac{90 \text{ mmHg}}{5.4 \text{ L} \cdot min^{-1}} = 16.67 \text{ (TPR units)}$$

In Check Your Comprehension 3, calculate the TPR. Check your answer in Appendix C.

CHECK YOUR COMPREHENSION 3

Given the following information, calculate TPR.
SBP = 150 mmHg; DBP = 90 mmHg;
$\dot{Q} = 5.1 \text{ L} \cdot min^{-1}$.

Principles of Blood Flow

Figure 11.15 presents the relationships among the cross-sectional area of the blood vessels, blood pressure, and blood velocity throughout the vascular system. The diameter of the various vessels is shown in **Figure 11.15A**, and the total cross-sectional area of the various vessels is shown in **Figure 11.15B**. Thus, although a single capillary is incredibly small, approximately 6 μm, there are so many capillaries that the total cross-sectional area far exceeds that of the other vessels. **Figure 11.15B** also depicts the velocity of blood in the various vessels—that is, the speed at which blood flows. The velocity of a fluid in a closed system varies inversely with the total cross-sectional area at any given point. Therefore, the velocity of blood flow decreases dramatically in the capillaries. This decreased velocity allows adequate time for the exchange of respiratory gases and nutrients.

Figure 11.15C depicts the blood pressure throughout the vascular system. The driving force for the blood is the contraction of the myocardium. Blood flows because of a pressure gradient. Thus, blood flows through the vascular tree because pressure is highest in the aorta and major arteries and lowest in the great veins and right atrium of the heart. Pressure continues to decrease as the blood travels further from the heart, reaching a low

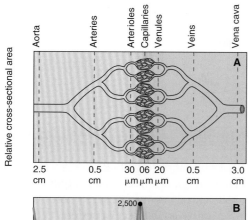

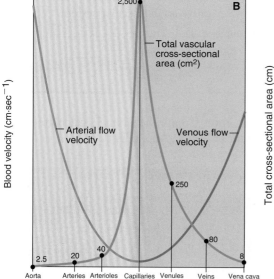

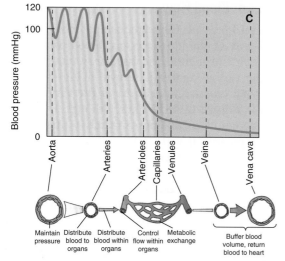

FIGURE 11.15 Relationships among Cross-Sectional Area of Blood Vessels, Blood Pressure, and Resistance.
A. Despite the very small diameter of individual capillaries, relative cross-sectional area (CSA) of the capillaries is much higher than that of other vessels because they are so numerous. **B.** Blood velocity through the vascular system is inversely related to total CSA. **C.** Blood pressure is pulsatile in the aorta and major arteries but becomes continuous as blood travels through the arterioles. Blood pressure in the venous system is very low compared to the arterial system.

of approximately 4 mmHg in the right atrium. In fact, one-way venous valves and muscle and respiratory pump activity are needed to help return blood to the heart.

Regulation of the Cardiovascular System

The cardiovascular system is regulated by interrelated and overlapping mechanisms, including mechanical events, neural control, and neurohormonal control. Mechanical events, such as muscle action, influence venous return and thereby help regulate stroke volume and cardiac output. This regulation is particularly important during exercise. Neural and neurohormonal mechanisms of cardiovascular control are more complex and are discussed in detail in the following sections.

Neural Control

Three cardiovascular centers are located within the medulla oblongata of the brainstem (**Figure 11.16**). These regulatory centers play an important role in controlling the output of the heart and the radius of the blood vessels. The cardioaccelerator and cardioinhibitor centers innervate the heart. As the names imply, the *cardioaccelerator center* sends signals, via sympathetic accelerator nerves, that cause the heart rate to increase and the force of contraction to strengthen. The *cardioinhibitor center*, also called the vagal nucleus, sends signals via the vagus nerve that cause a decreased heart rate and force of contraction. The *vasomotor center* innervates the smooth muscles of the arterioles via sympathetic nerves. Activation of these sympathetic fibers generally causes vasoconstriction (sympathetic fibers to the skin are the only clear exception to this rule in humans).

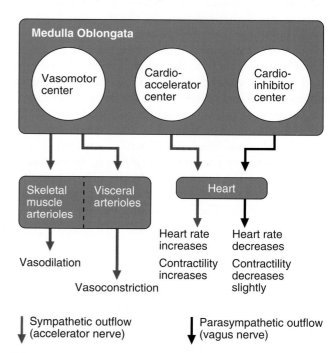

FIGURE 11.16 Neural Control of Cardiovascular Function.

In summary, activation of sympathetic nervous outflow leads to an increased heart rate, increased cardiac contractility, and vasoconstriction in most arterioles. During exercise, there is also vasodilation in the arterioles of skeletal muscle, but the role of the autonomic nervous system in this response is not clear. What is clear is that metabolic (intrinsic) controls lead to a wide spread vasodilation in arterioles supplying skeletal muscle in response to increased metabolic activity during exercise. Activation of the parasympathetic nervous system leads to the opposite responses in each of the above.

See animation, Neural Control of CV System, at http://thePoint.lww.com/Plowman4e.

Anatomical Sensors and Factors Affecting Control of the Cardiovascular System

The cardiovascular centers—and therefore, the sympathetic and parasympathetic outflow from those centers—are influenced by several factors in a variety of circumstances, including exercise. **Figure 11.17** schematically presents the most important factors influencing the cardiovascular centers. These factors are described in detail in the following sections.

Higher Brain Centers

The cardiovascular medullary centers are influenced by several higher brain centers, including the cerebral cortex and the hypothalamus. Emotional influences arising from the cerebral cortex can affect cardiovascular function at rest. Input from the motor cortex, which is relayed

through the hypothalamus, can influence cardiovascular function during exercise, leading to an increase in heart rate and vasodilation in active muscle. The influence of the cortex and hypothalamus on the cardiovascular centers during exercise is often termed "central command," denoting that the signal to alter cardiovascular variables comes from the central nervous system.

Body temperature also affects the cardiovascular centers through the influence of the hypothalamus. An increased body temperature results in an increased heart rate, increased cardiac output, and vasodilation in the arterioles of the active muscles and skin.

Systemic Receptors

Systemic receptors are present in the great veins, the heart, and the arterial system. These receptors provide sensory information to the cardiovascular control centers that leads to reflex action.

BARORECEPTORS Baroreceptors are located in the aorta and carotid bodies. With an increase in mean arterial pressure, these receptors cause a reflex decrease in mean arterial pressure through a decreased heart rate (and thus decreased cardiac output). The decrease in heart rate is mediated through an increased parasympathetic outflow and a simultaneous decrease in sympathetic outflow to the heart. This reflex control of blood pressure is called the *baroreceptor reflex*.

Because this reflex functions to maintain mean arterial blood pressure, you may wonder how someone becomes hypertensive (high blood pressure) or why mean arterial blood pressure goes up during exercise. In someone with hypertension, the action of the baroreceptors is mediated by

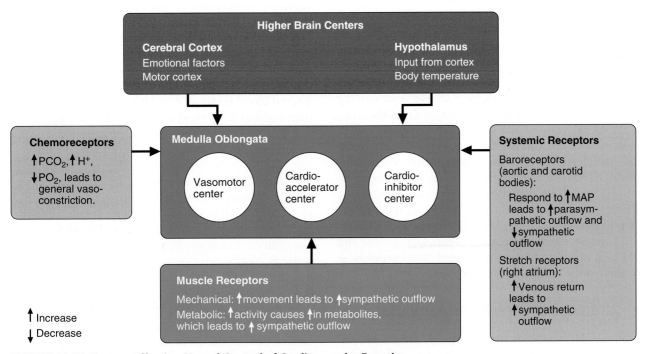

FIGURE 11.17 Factors Affecting Neural Control of Cardiovascular Function.

a set point. If something causes the resting blood pressure to be elevated (and no one knows precisely what causes this elevation), the baroreceptors fire for about 24 hours in an effort to bring down the mean arterial pressure. If this is unsuccessful, the baroreceptors appear to simply reset at a level above the previous value. The baroreceptor reflex is also reset during exercise. The resetting of the barore-flex is in direct proportion to exercise intensity (Raven et al., 2006). The baroreceptor reflex is also very important in achieving recovery to baseline values after exercise.

STRETCH RECEPTORS Stretch receptors, located in the right atrium of the heart, are stimulated by an increase in venous return. The signal is transmitted to the cardiovas-cular centers in the medulla, where they cause an increase in sympathetic outflow and a decrease in parasympathetic outflow. This results in an increased heart rate and force of contraction, increasing cardiac output. This sequence is called the *Bainbridge reflex*.

Chemoreceptors

Chemoreceptors are located in the aortic and carotid arter-ies. They are sensitive to arterial blood PO_2, PCO_2, and H^+. An increase in PCO_2 and H^+ or a decrease in PO_2 causes a reflex vasoconstriction of arterioles.

Muscle Joint Receptors

Muscle receptors include mechanical (*mechanoreceptors*) and metabolic (*metaboreceptors*) receptors located in the joints and muscles. These receptors send impulses to the brain, where the impulses synapse with the cardiovascular cent-ers. When stimulated by muscle contraction, these recep-tors lead to an increased rate and force of heart contraction. Vasoconstriction occurs in inactive skeletal muscles.

Neurohormonal Control

The endocrine system also helps regulate the cardiovas-cular system. Considerable control is exerted by compo-nents of the autonomic nervous system and the hormones of the adrenal medulla. The previous section discussed the influence of the sympathetic nervous system on the heart and the blood vessels. The sympathetic nervous system also innervates the adrenal medulla, causing the adrenal glands to release the hormones epinephrine and norepi-nephrine. These hormones travel in the bloodstream to the heart and the blood vessels. Generally, epinephrine and norepinephrine have the same effect on these target organs as the sympathetic nerve fibers innervating them.

In addition to the adrenal hormones, aldosterone and ADH help maintain blood volume and blood pressure as described in the section on blood volume.

Measurement of Cardiovascular Variables

Cardiovascular variables are routinely measured and monitored in sports, fitness, rehabilitation, and research

settings. The following variables are measured in order to assess fitness, prescribe exercise, and monitor physiologi-cal responses to exercise. Most of these variables can be assessed both at rest and during submaximal or maximal exercise.

Cardiac Output

Recall that cardiac output ($\dot{Q}$) is equal to the product of stroke volume and heart rate (Equation 11.3). However, because stroke volume has historically been very dif-ficult to measure, cardiac output has been calculated from another known relationship described by the **Fick equation:**

11.9 cardiac output $(L \cdot min^{-1})$ = oxygen consumption $(mL \cdot min^{-1})$ ÷ arteriovenous oxygen difference $(mL \cdot L^{-1})$

or

$$\dot{Q} = \frac{\dot{V}O_2}{a\text{-}vO_2\text{diff}}$$

See animation, Fick Principle, at http://thePoint.lww. com/Plowman4e.

The direct determination of cardiac output via the Fick equation requires measurement of both oxygen con-sumption and arteriovenous oxygen difference. Many laboratories can directly measure oxygen consumption (see Chapter 4). The assessment of arteriovenous oxygen difference (a-vO_2diff), however, is more problematic. This invasive test requires a sample of arterial blood from an artery and a sample of mixed venous blood from the vena cava or right atrium. Other invasive tests that are used clinically to measure $\dot{Q}$ include dye-dilution and ther-modilution (Barker et al., 1999; Warburton et al., 1999). Dye-dilution is based on the same principle as the Fick method but instead of measuring O_2 concentrations, the concentration of a dye is measured. A dye is injected into the venous circulation and the concentration of dye in arterial blood is sampled and used to calculate the $\dot{Q}$. The thermodilution method is based on the same principle as dye-dilution except that instead of injecting a dye, this technique uses the injection of a cold fluid on the venous side. Blood in the pulmonary artery is then sampled to determine the extent of cooling. The amount of cooling is inversely proportional to $\dot{Q}$ (Darovic, 1995; Warburton et al., 1999). Although the methods discussed above are considered criterion measures in a clinical setting, they are difficult to obtain in most exercise science research settings. Noninvasive measures of $\dot{Q}$ include variations of acetylene (C_2H_2), nitrous oxide (N_2O), or carbon dioxide (CO_2) gas-rebreathing techniques to estimate $\dot{Q}$. These inert gases rapidly diffuse across the lung blood-gas bar-rier but are limited by capillary perfusion. Thus, the rate of disappearance of the gas is directly proportional to the flow of blood through the pulmonary circulation.

Source: Rowland, T., K. Heffernan, S.Y. Jae, G. Echols, G. Krull, and B. Fernhall: Cardiovascular responses to static exercise in boys: insights from tissue Doppler imaging. *European Journal of Applied Physiology.* 97(5):637–642 (2006).

FOCUS ON RESEARCH
Cardiovascular Responses to Exercise

Researchers interested in quantifying cardiovascular responses to exercise often rely on both easily obtained measurements and measurements requiring sophisticated laboratory equipment. In this study, Doppler echocardiography (an ultrasound system that is typically found only in hospital settings or well-equipped laboratories; see Figure 11.18) was used to investigate the stroke volume response to isometric contraction. Investigators had young boys between the ages of 7 and 12 years perform isometric leg extension exercises at 30% of maximal voluntary contraction (MVC) for 3 minutes. Researchers measured systolic blood pressure (SBP) and diastolic blood pressure (DBP) through standard auscultatory methods (see Figure 11.20) and then calculated mean arterial pressure (MAP). The

results of this study when compared with previous research on young adult males suggest that young boys respond to isometric exercise in much the same way that young adult males do, with an increase in MAP and a small decrease in SV.

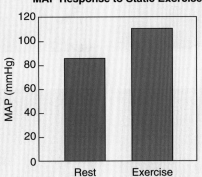
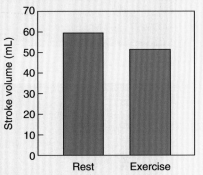

Pulmonary blood flow is equivalent to systemic blood flow ($\dot{Q}$) (Warburton et al., 1999).

Given the difficulties of obtaining a direct measurement of $\dot{Q}$, researchers often take the approach of measuring SV and HR and calculating $\dot{Q}$ ($\dot{Q} = SV \times HR$).

Stroke Volume

Advances in technology have made the assessment of stroke volume (SV) easier, particularly during exercise. Stroke volume can now be measured using **Doppler echocardiography**. This is a technique that calculates stroke volume from noninvasive measurements of aortic cross-sectional area (CSA) and time-velocity integral (TVI) of the blood flow in the ascending aorta (**Figure 11.18**) using this formula:

11.10 stroke volume(mL) = cross-sectional area(cm^2) × time-velocity integrals(cm)

or

SV = CSA × TVI

Note that, for conversion purposes, cm^3 = mL.

Fick Equation An equation used to calculate cardiac output from oxygen consumption ($\dot{V}O_2$) and arteriovenous oxygen difference (a-vO_2diff).

Doppler Echocardiography A technique that calculates stroke volume from measurements of aortic cross-sectional area and time-velocity integrals in the ascending aorta.

Two-dimensional echocardiography is used to measure aortic diameter (**Figure 11.18**). Cross-sectional area is then calculated from a geometric model using the following formula:

11.11 cross-sectional area(cm^2) = diameter(cm^2) × π / 4

or

CSA = d^2 × π / 4

Doppler ultrasound is used to assess blood velocity in the ascending aorta (**Figure 11.18B**). From the Doppler waveforms a time-velocity integral is obtained. Once stroke volume is known, cardiac output can be calculated using the formula $\dot{Q} = SV \times HR$.

EXAMPLE

Using the information provided in **Figure 11.18C** and **D**, calculate SV.

The calculation are:

CSA = 2.57^2 × π / 4 = 5.18 cm^2
SV = (5.18 cm^2) × (25 cm) = 129.5 mL

The Doppler method does not require a steady state and thus is a viable option for assessing stroke volume (and $\dot{Q}$) during maximal exercise. Disadvantages of the Doppler method include the high cost of the equipment and the training required to obtain good time-velocities, especially during heavy exercise (Rowland and Obert, 2002).

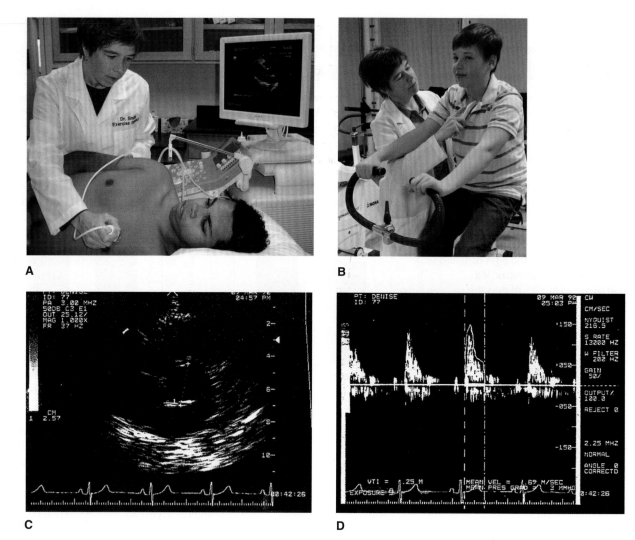

FIGURE 11.18 Doppler Echocardiography.
Ultrasound technician obtains aortic diameter (**A**) and Doppler waveforms from the suprasternal notch (**B**). Printout of aortic diameter (**C**) and Doppler waveforms (**D**).

Heart Rate

In a laboratory, heart rate is often obtained by measuring the R-R interval in an ECG recording (**Figure 11.19**). Although the ECG equipment/computer may be programmed to automatically calculate the HR, it is useful to know how this measure is performed. The first step is to calculate the distance the ECG paper travels in one minute based on the speed of the paper. The distance between cycles is then measured. Because you now know the number of cycles that occurred within the distance measured, you can solve for the b·min⁻¹ by solving for X in the following equation:

11.12   HR (b · min⁻¹) = [number of beats ÷ distance the cycles occupy (mm)] = [X (b · min⁻¹) ÷ distance the paper travels in one minute (mm · min⁻¹)]

EXAMPLE

Using the ECG strip in **Figure 11.19**, calculate the heart rate.

Step 1: Using the paper speed, calculate the distance the paper travels in one minute. Paper speed equals 25 mm·sec⁻¹. Since there are 60 sec·min⁻¹, 25 mm·sec⁻¹ × 60 sec·min⁻¹ = 1500 mm·min⁻¹.

Step 2: Measure the distance between 4 cycles, which in this case is 125 mm.

Step 3: Since 4 cycles (1 box = 5 mm) occurred within the time period required for the ECG paper to travel 125 mm, you calculate how many beats occur in 1 minute by solving for X in the equation:

$$\frac{4}{125} = \frac{X}{1500}$$

125X = 6000, X = 6000/125 = 48 b · min⁻¹

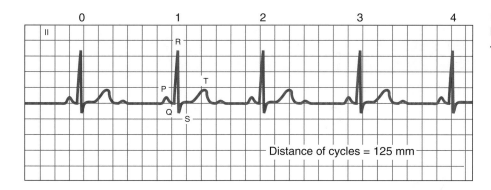

FIGURE 11.19 ECG Used to Calculate Heart Rate.

Heart rate can also be recorded by wireless telemetry. Most often the transmitter is worn around the chest, and the heart rate signal is transmitted to a small receiver that looks very similar to a watch. Many pieces of fitness equipment also have the ability to pick up the HR signal from the transmitter, or to measure heart rate by having the exercisers grasp a sensor built into the exercise equipment.

Heart rate is often measured during exercise to monitor exercise intensity. In some exercise sessions, however, heart rate-measuring devices are not available. Heart rate can then be assessed by counting the pulse—a method called palpation. The pulse can be felt at the carotid or radial artery. This technique requires instruction and practice.

To measure an exercise heart rate, the person usually pauses and finds the pulse as quickly as possible. The pulse count begins with zero and is counted for a set period of time, usually 6, 10, or 15 seconds, using a watch. This pulse count is then multiplied by 10, 6, or 4, respectively, to obtain the per-minute heart rate. A period less than 1 minute is used because the heart rate drops quickly once exercise is paused.

Maximal Oxygen Consumption

Maximal oxygen consumption is the highest amount of oxygen an individual can take in and utilize to produce energy (ATP) aerobically while breathing air during heavy exercise. It is abbreviated as $\dot{V}O_2$max to indicate the maximal volume of oxygen consumed. The respiratory system brings in the oxygen from the environment, the cardiovascular system transports the oxygen, and the cells extract the oxygen and use it in the production of energy (ATP). The assessment of maximal oxygen consumption is therefore a means of quantifying the functional capacity of the entire cardiovascular system. $\dot{V}O_2$max is often considered the single most important variable in describing an individual's fitness level and is routinely used to describe an individual's cardiorespiratory capacity.

The limit of cardiovascular function is reached at the highest attainable oxygen consumption. By rearranging the Fick equation (Equation 11.9), this is expressed:

11.13 $\dot{V}O_2max = (\dot{Q}max) \times (a\text{-}vO_2 diff\ max)$

True for any VO₂ calculation

$VO_2 = HR(SV)(a\text{-}VO_2 \Delta)$

Although $\dot{V}O_2$max can be calculated from the variables in Equation 11.13, it is typically measured in the laboratory using open-circuit indirect spirometry with the equipment often organized into a metabolic cart. The assessment of oxygen consumption is described in detail in Chapter 4. Although oxygen is utilized only in aerobic metabolic production of ATP, the delivery of oxygen is primarily limited by the cardiovascular system. Thus, $\dot{V}O_2$max is considered to be a cardiovascular variable.

Field Tests of Cardiorespiratory Capacity ($\dot{V}O_2$max)

Several field techniques may be used to assess cardiorespiratory endurance and estimate cardiorespiratory capacity ($\dot{V}O_2$max). They include submaximal cycle ergometer tests, step tests, and distance walks or runs. By far the most practical and inexpensive method, especially when large numbers of individuals are tested in a short period of time (such as in a school setting), is the distance run. Walking tests are recommended for testing the elderly or very sedentary adults. Three tests are described here: the 1-mile walk/run, the progressive aerobic cardiovascular endurance run (PACER) (The Cooper Institute, 2010), and the Rockport Fitness Walking Test (RFWT) (Kline et al., 1987).

The mile run test allows the individual to walk if necessary, but the intent is to cover the mile as quickly as possible, and that goal is best accomplished by running the entire distance. Thus, the individual is asked to perform at a high percentage of his or her maximal capacity for the entire test.

The $\dot{V}O_2$max estimate from the mile run is calculated as follows (Cureton et al., 1995):

11.14 $\dot{V}O_2max = 0.21(age \times sex) - 0.84(BMI) -$
$8.41(MT) + 0.34(MT^2) + 108.94$
$SEE = 4.8\ mL \cdot kg^{-1} \cdot min^{-1}$

where age is the age of the individual in years; sex is 0 if female or 1 if male; BMI is the body mass index (weight in kilograms divided by height in meters squared); and MT is the time it takes the individual to run a mile in minutes.

Effect of Firefighting Gear on Maximal Oxygen Consumption

Firefighters perform strenuous physical work in hot and hostile environments. Because of the dangerous environment in which they work, firefighters must wear heavy protective clothing (firefighting gear) and a self-contained breathing apparatus (SCBA). The weight of the gear and SCBA, and restrictions to breathing provided by the SCBA, however, may pose a significant physiological challenge to firefighters who are called upon to work at near-maximal levels.

In this study, researchers asked 12 healthy men familiar with exercise in the firefighting ensemble (mean age = 31.0 years; mean height = 179.8 cm; mean body weight = 83.0 kg) to perform a graded treadmill test to volitional fatigue (a $\dot{V}O_2$max test) under two conditions: once while wearing standard physical training (PT) clothing (shorts and a T-shirt) and once while wearing firefighting gear and SCBA (FFG). The treadmill test required each participant to initially walk at a constant speed (94 m·min⁻¹) while grade increased by 2% every 2 minutes until 10% grade was reached. Subsequently, the grade was increased every 2 minutes until a 20% grade was achieved. After this point, increases in grade (2% increments) and speed (13 m·min⁻¹ increments) were individually selected until volitional fatigue. The table below presents mean values for oxygen consumption and minute ventilation at 6, 12, and 18% grade (the last level that all participants could complete) and maximal values obtained at the end of the test.

Exercise in the firefighting gear led to an earlier onset of fatigue. Hence, the participants exercised longer and achieved a higher $\dot{V}O_2$max in the PT trial (52 mL·kg·min⁻¹) versus the FFG trial (43 mL·kg·min⁻¹). However, at every stage of the graded exercise test (above 4% grade), the oxygen cost of performing the work was greater when wearing the FFG than in the PT trial. Similarly, maximal minute ventilation ($\dot{V}_E$max) was higher in the PT condition (167 versus 143 L·min⁻¹) than in the FFG condition, but submaximal minute ventilation values were higher at each exercise workload when the work was performed in the FFG.

This study documented that there was a substantial (18% reduction) in $\dot{V}O_2$max in the FFG conditions compared to the PT condition. Furthermore, the data suggest that the decrease in maximal minute ventilation was the main reason for the decrease in oxygen consumption. The reason for the decreased minute ventilation at maximal exercise when wearing the SCBA is not clear, but may be related to the increased work of breathing due to expiratory resistance caused by the regulator. Thus, while firefighters require protective equipment to protect them from the environment they face, the protective equipment, especially the SCBA, has a negative effect on maximal oxygen consumption. These data, showing the elevated oxygen cost of doing physical work while wearing heavy protective equipment, highlight the importance of high physical fitness for firefighters.

Source: Dreger, R.W., R. L. Jones and S. R. Petersen. Effects of the self-contained breathing apparatus and fire protection clothing on maximal oxygen uptake. *Ergonomics.* 49(10):911–920 (2006).

		Treadmill Grade		
	6%	**12%**	**18%**	**Maximal Value**
Oxygen consumption (mL·kg·min⁻¹)				
PT	15	28	37	52
FFG	16	32	40	43
Minute ventilation (L·min⁻¹)				
PT	40	60	95	167
FFG	45	80	130	143

Estimate $\dot{V}O_2$max given the following data.

    Age = 15yr; BMI = 24.3

    sex = female; MT = 8.75 minutes

The calculation is

$$\dot{V}O_2max = (0.21)(15 \times 0) - (0.84)(24.3) - (8.41)$$
$$(8.75) + 0.34(8.75^2) + 108.94 = 40.97 \text{ mL} \cdot \text{kg}^{-1} \cdot \text{min}^{-1}$$

Note that the equation includes an indication of the standard error of the estimate (SEE). For $\dot{V}O_2$max, acceptable errors generally range from 3 to 5 mL·kg⁻¹·min⁻¹. The 4.8 mL·kg⁻¹·min⁻¹ for this equation falls within that range. The SEE means that as estimates, not measured values, the calculated results could vary from the measured value by that much. That is, the 40.97 mL·kg⁻¹·min⁻¹ calculated in the example might actually be anywhere from 36.17 to 45.77 mL·kg⁻¹·min⁻¹.

The RFWT also covers a 1-mi distance; however, it is specifically designed for walking, with the fastest sustainable walking speed as the goal. Depending on the age and fitness level of the participant, this speed may or may not represent a high percentage of maximal aerobic capacity (Kline et al., 1987).

Unlike the previous set distance tests, the PACER is a multistage fitness test adapted from the 20-m shuttle run developed in Europe by Léger and his colleagues (1982, 1988). It most closely resembles a graded exercise test that would be performed on a treadmill in a laboratory. It begins with a light workload and progresses, in small increments, until the individual can no longer complete the required number of laps per minute. This test is run between two lines marked 20 m apart on a smooth unobstructed surface. This test does not require a sustained high-intensity effort but a gradual progression from submaximal to maximal effort. Pacing is accomplished by prerecorded music or beeps (The Cooper Institute, 2010)

The equations used to estimate maximal oxygen consumption from the RFWT (Kline et al., 1987; McSwegin et al., 1998) and the PACER test (Leger et al., 1988; Plowman and Liu, 1999) are given in Appendix B. FITNESSGRAM® currently uses a test-equating system to convert the results from the PACER or the 1-mile walk to 1-mile run times and then uses the equation given above to calculate V̇O₂max. This ensures that predicted V̇O₂max and the resultant fitness classification is the same no matter which test a student has taken. Criterion-referenced norms are available for evaluation of the results of all these field tests (The Cooper Institute, 2010).

Blood Pressure

In well-equipped laboratories and hospitals, blood pressure can be measured directly by an intra-arterial transducer. A small transducer is inserted into the artery, and systolic blood pressure and diastolic blood pressure are recorded for every beat of the heart. Although this procedure provides valuable information, it is not

practical for routine use because as an invasive procedure it involves risks.

By far the most common technique for obtaining blood pressure measurements is the auscultation method. The indirect method of auscultation uses a sphygmomanometer and a blood pressure can wrapped around the upper arm (**Figure 11.20A**). For a blood pressure measurement to be accurate and meaningful, the proper cuff size must be used to obtain the measurement. As a general rule, the BP cuff should encircle at least 80% of the arm circumference (American College of Sports Medicine, 2005). The blood pressure cuff is inflated to a pressure greater than systolic pressure (140 mmHg) as shown in **Figure 11.20B**. Note that systolic blood pressure (**Figure 11.20C**) is taken as the First Korotkoff sound (the first loud sound heard through the stethoscope), but that there are two diastolic blood pressures (**Figure 11.20D**). The first diastolic blood pressure (DBP₁) occurs when the sound heard through the stethoscope is muffled (the Fourth Korotkoff sound). The second diastolic blood pressure (DBP₂) occurs when sound disappears through the stethoscope (the Fifth Korotkoff sound). The pressure at the Fifth Korotkoff sound (DBP₂) is considered the best measure of diastolic blood pressure in normal adults at rest. However, DBP₁ is recommended for children, for adults during exercise, and for adults if DBP₂ is lower than 40 mmHg (American

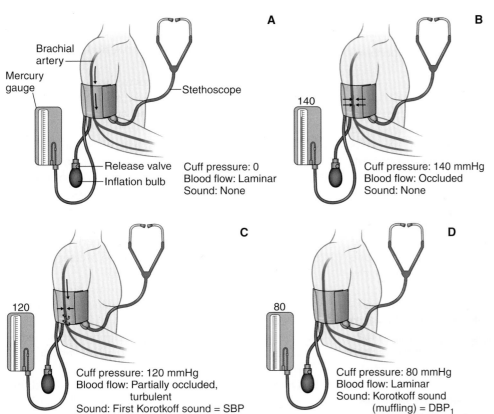

A.

Brachial artery
Mercury gauge
Stethoscope
Release valve
Inflation bulb
Cuff pressure: 0
Blood flow: Laminar
Sound: None

B.

140
Cuff pressure: 140 mmHg
Blood flow: Occluded
Sound: None

FIGURE 11.20 Assessment of Blood Pressure.

A. An appropriate sized blood pressure cuff is placed around the upper arm. **B.** The blood pressure cuff is inflated to approximately 20 mmHg higher than SBP in order to occlude arterial blood flow. **C.** Pressure in the cuff is slowly released until the First Korotkoff sound is heard. **D.** Pressure in the cuff continues to be released until there is a muffling or disappearance of the Korotkoff sounds.

C.

120
Cuff pressure: 120 mmHg
Blood flow: Partially occluded, turbulent
Sound: First Korotkoff sound = SBP

D.

80
Cuff pressure: 80 mmHg
Blood flow: Laminar
Sound: Korotkoff sound
  (muffling) = DBP₁
  Fifth Korotkof sound
  (diappearance) = DBP₂

Society of Hypertension, 1992). This is important for an accurate description of blood pressure and in the calculation of mean arterial pressure (MAP).

In resting and exercise recovery situations, mean arterial pressure is determined by first calculating pulse pressure. Pulse pressure is equal to the difference between SBP and DBP_2 ($PP = SBP-DBP_2$). MAP is then calculated as

11.15a   mean arterial pressure (mmHg) = pulse pressure (mmHg)/3 + diastolic blood pressure$_2$ (mmHg)

or

$$MAP = \frac{PP}{3} + DBP_2$$

MAP is not simply computed as the average of SBP and DBP because diastole lasts longer than systole and is thus weighted more heavily in the computation of MAP.

For adults during exercise or for children at rest, MAP can be computed according to a modified equation that uses DBP_1, (Robinson et al., 1988):

11.15b   mean arterial pressure (mmHg) = pulse pressure (mmHg)/2 + diastolic blood pressure$_1$ (mmHg)

or

$$MAP = \frac{PP}{2} + DBP_1$$

This formula provides a more accurate measurement of MAP during exercise because it gives less weight to DBP. Although both systole and diastole time shorten because of the increased heart rate, diastole shortens proportionally more.

SUMMARY

1. The primary functions of the cardiovascular system are to transport oxygen and nutrients to the cells of the body and transport carbon dioxide and waste products from the cells; to regulate body temperature, pH levels, and fluid balance; and to protect the body from blood loss and infection.

2. The cells of the heart, called cardiac muscle cells or collectively the myocardium, are functionally linked by intercalated discs with gap junctions. When one cell is depolarized, the stimulation spreads over the entire myocardium.

3. The heart has its own conduction system, consisting of the sinoatrial (SA) node, internodal fibers and Bachmann's bundle, the atrioventricular (AV) node, the bundle of His, the left and right bundle branches, and Purkinje fibers, all of which rapidly spread the electrical signal throughout the heart.

4. The cardiac cycle refers to the alternating periods of relaxation and contraction of the heart. The contraction phase is called systole, and the relaxation phase is called diastole. There are known relationships

among the electrical, pressure, volume, and contractile events throughout the cardiac cycle.

5. The volume of blood ejected from the heart with each beat is known as stroke volume. The amount of blood ejected from the heart each minute is called cardiac output. Under resting conditions the heart ejects approximately 60% of the blood that is returned to it; this percentage represents the ejection fraction.

6. The cardiovascular system is primarily controlled by the medulla oblongata (cardioaccelerator, cardioinhibitor, and vasomotor centers). Factors affecting these centers include

   a. Higher brain centers that exert conscious and unconscious control

   b. Baroreceptors that are sensitive to mean arterial pressure

   c. Stretch receptors that sense blood return to the right atrium

   d. Chemoreceptors that sense the PO_2, PCO_2, and H^+

7. Maximal oxygen consumption ($\dot{V}O_2$max) is the highest amount of oxygen that the body can take in, transport, and use. Assessment of $\dot{V}O_2$max allows for quantifying the functional capacity of the entire cardiovascular system.

REVIEW QUESTIONS

1. Describe the primary functions of the cardiovascular system.

2. Diagram the conduction system of the heart, and describe how activation of the SA node leads to contraction of the heart.

3. Describe the electrical events in the heart in relation to pressure in the left ventricle, the volume of blood in the left ventricle, and the position of the heart valves.

4. Describe the major mechanical, electrical, and volume changes that occur throughout the cardiac cycle.

5. Describe how myocardial oxygen consumption changes with exercise. What determines myocardial oxygen consumption and how can it be estimated during exercise?

6. Identify the different vessels of the peripheral circulation, and describe the velocity and pressure in each. What accounts for the differences?

7. Describe the hormonal mechanisms by which the body attempts to compensate for a decrease in plasma volume.

8. Discuss the neurohormonal regulation of the cardiovascular system and the factors that affect such regulation.

9. Describe how cardiac output can be measured and explain why it is not routinely measured in exercise physiology labs or in field settings.

10. Why is maximal oxygen consumption ($\dot{V}O_2$max) considered to be a cardiovascular variable?

11. Explain the steps involved in attaining an accurate measurement of BP.

For further review and additional study tools, visit the website at http://thePoint.lww.com/Plowman4e ✳ ◉

REFERENCES

American College of Sports Medicine.: *ACSM's Health-Related Physical Fitness Assessment Manual*. Philadelphia, PA: Lippincott, Williams & Wilkins (2005).

American Society of Hypertension, Public Policy Position Paper: Recommendations for routine blood pressure measurement by indirect cuff sphygmomanometry. *American Journal of Hypertension*. 5:207–209 (1992).

Åstrand, P.: *Experimental Studies of Physical Working Capacity in Relation to Sex and Age*. Copenhagen, Munksgaurd: University Microfilms International (1952).

Barker, R. C., S. R. Hopkins, N. Kellogg, I. M. Olfert, T. D. Brutsaert, T. P. Gavin, P. L. Entin, A. J. Rice, & P. D. Wagner: Measurement of cardiac output during exercise by open-circuit acetylene uptake. *Journal of Applied Physiology*. 87(4):1506–1512 (1999).

Brechar, G. A. & P. M. Galletti: Functional anatomy of cardiac pumping. In Hamilton, W. F. (ed.): *Handbook of Physiology, Section 2: Circulation*. Washington, DC: American Physiological Society (1963).

Cureton, K. J., M. A. Sloniger, J. P. O'Bannon, D. M. Black, & W. P. McCormack: A generalized equation for prediction of $\dot{V}O_2$ peak from 1-mile run/walk performance. *Medicine and Science in Sports and Exercise*. 27:445–451 (1995).

Darovic, G. O.: *Hemodynamic Monitoring: Invasive and Noninvasive Clinical Application*. Philadelphia, PA: W. B. Saunders Company (1995).

Dempsey, J. A.: Is the lung built for exercise? *Medicine and Science in Sports and Exercise*. 18(2):143–155 (1986).

di Prampero, P. E.: Factors limiting maximal performance in humans. *European Journal of Applied Physiology*. 90:420–429 (2003).

Dreger, R. W., R. L. Jones & S. R. Petersen: Effects of the self-contained breathing apparatus and fire protection clothing on maximal oxygen uptake. *Ergonomics*. 49(10):911–920 (2006).

Fleg, J. L., F. O'Connor, G. Gerstenblith, L. C. Becker, J. Clulow, S. P. Schulman, & E. G. Lakatta: Impact of age on the cardiovascular response to dynamic upright exercise in healthy men and women. *Journal of Applied Physiology*. 78(3):890–900 (1995).

Franklin, B. A., & F. Munnings: A common misunderstanding about heart rate and exercise. *ACSM's Health and Fitness Journal*. 2(1):18–19 (1998).

Guyton, A. C. & J. E. Hall: *Textbook of Medical Physiology* (12th edition). Philadelphia, PA: Saunders (2011).

Joyner, M. J. & N. M. Dietz: Sympathetic vasodilation in human muscle. *Acta physiologica Scandinavica*. 177:329–336 (2003).

Kitamura, K., C. R. Jorgensen, F. L. Gobel, H. L. Taylor, & Y. Wang: Hemodynamics correlates of myocardial oxygen consumption during upright exercise. *Journal of Applied Physiology*. 32:516–522 (1972).

Kline, G. M., J. P. Porcari, R. Huntermeister, P. S. Freedson, A. Ward, R. F. McCarron, J. Ross, & J. M. Rippe: Estimation of VO_2max from a one-mile track walk, gender, age and body weight. *Medicine and Science in Sports and Exercise*. 19:253–259 (1987).

Léger, L. A. & J. Lambert: A maximal multistage 20-m shuttle run test to predict VO2max. *European Journal of Applied Physiology*. 49:1–12 (1982).

Léger, L. A. D. Mercier, C. Gadoury, & J. Lambert: The multistage 20 metre shuttle run test for aerobic fitness. *Journal of Sports Sciences*. 6:93–101 (1988).

Levick, J. R.: *An Introduction to Cardiovascular Physiology* (4th edition). London: Arnold (2003).

Marieb, E. N. & K. Hoehn: *Human Anatomy and Physiology* (8th edition). San Francisco, CA: Benjamin Cummings (2010).

McSwegin, P. J., S. A. Plowman, G. M. Wolff & G. L. Guttenberg: The validity of a one-mile walk test for high school age individuals. Measurement in Physical Education and Exercise Science. 2(1):47–63 (1998).

Ogawa, T., R. J. Spina, W. H. Martin, W. M. Kohrt, K. B. Schechtman, J. O. Holloszy, & A. A. Ehsani: Effects of aging, sex, and physical training on cardiovascular responses to exercise. *Circulation*. 86:494–503 (1992).

Plowman, S. A. & N. Y. S. Liu: Norm-referenced and criterion-referenced validity of the one-mile run and PACER in college age individuals. *Measurement in Physical Education and Exercise Science*. 3:63–84 (1999).

Raven, P. B., P. J. Fadel, & S. Ogoh: Arterial baroflex resetting during exercise: A current perspective. *Experimental Physiology*. 91(1):37–49 (2006).

Robinson, T. E., D. Y. Sue, A. Huszczuk, D. Weiler-Ravell, & J. E. Hansen: Intra-arterial and cuff blood pressure responses during incremental cycle ergometry. *Medicine and Science in Sports and Exercise*. 20(2):142–149 (1988).

Rowell, L. B.: *Human Circulation Regulation During Physical Stress*. New York, NY: Oxford University Press (1986).

Rowland, T., K. Heffernan, S. Y. Jae, G. Echols, G. Krull, & B. Fernhall: Cardiovascular responses to static exercise in boys: insights from tissue Doppler imaging. *European Journal of Applied Physiology*. 97(5):637–642 (2006).

Rowland, T. & P. Obert: Doppler echocardiography for the estimation of cardiac output with exercise. *Sports Medicine*. 32(15):973–986 (2002).

Spina, R. J., T. Ogawa, W. H. Martin III, A. R. Coggan, J. O. Holloszy, & A. A. Ehsani: Exercise training prevents decline in stroke volume during exercise in young healthy subjects. *Journal of Applied Physiology*. 72(6):2458–2462 (1992).

Spina, R. J., T. Ogawa, W. M. Kohrt, W. H. Martin III, J. O. Holloszy, & A. A. Ehsani: Differences in cardiovascular adaptations to endurance exercise training between older men and women. *Journal of Applied Physiology*. 75(2):849–855 (1993a).

Spina, R. J., T. Ogawa, T. R. Miller, W. M. Kohrt, & A. A. Ehsani: Effect of exercise training on left ventricular performance in older women free of cardiopulmonary disease. *American Journal of Cardiology*. 71:99–104 (1993b).

The Cooper Institute. FITNESSGRAM® & ACTIVITYGRAM® Test Administration Manual (4th edition updated). Meredith, M. D. & G. J. Welk (eds.): Champaign, IL: Human Kinetics (2010).

Warburton, D. E. R., M. J. F. Haykowsky, H. A. Quinney, D. P. Humen, & K. K. Teo: Reliability and validity of measures of cardiac output during incremental to maximal aerobic exercise. Part I: Conventional techniques. *Sports Medicine*. 27(1):23–41 (1999).

12 Cardiovascular Responses to Exercise

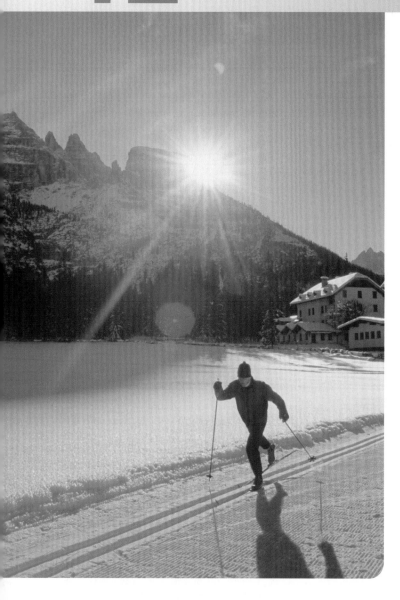

OBJECTIVES

After studying the chapter, you should be able to:

》 Graph and explain the pattern of response for the major cardiovascular variables during short-term, light to moderate submaximal aerobic exercise.

》 Graph and explain the pattern of response for the major cardiovascular variables during long-term, moderate to heavy submaximal aerobic exercise.

》 Graph and explain the pattern of response for the major cardiovascular variables during incremental aerobic exercise to maximum.

》 Explain the importance of measuring maximal oxygen consumption ($\dot{V}O_2max$).

》 Graph and explain the pattern of response for the major cardiovascular variables during dynamic resistance exercise.

》 Graph and explain the pattern of response for the major cardiovascular variables during static exercise.

》 Compare the response of the major cardiovascular variables to short-term, light to moderate submaximal aerobic exercise; long-term, moderate to heavy sub-maximal aerobic exercise; incremental aerobic exercise to maximum; static exercise; and dynamic resistance exercise.

》 Discuss the similarities and differences between the sexes in the cardiovascular responses to the various categories of exercise.

》 Discuss the similarities and differences between children/adolescents and young adults in the cardiovascular responses to the various categories of exercise.

》 Discuss the similarities and differences between young/middle-aged and older adults in the cardiovascular responses to the various categories of exercise.

Introduction

All types of human movement, no matter what the mode, duration, or intensity, require an expenditure of energy above resting values. Much of this energy comes from the use of oxygen. To supply the working muscles with the needed oxygen, the cardiovascular and respiratory systems work together. The responses of the respiratory system during exercise are detailed in Chapter 10. This chapter describes the parallel cardiovascular responses to dynamic aerobic activity, static exercise, and dynamic resistance exercise. Minimal attention is paid here to short-term, high-intensity anaerobic exercise because this type of activity is typically performed to stress the metabolic system and is therefore discussed in detail in the metabolic unit.

Cardiovascular Responses to Aerobic Exercise

Aerobic exercise requires more energy—and therefore more oxygen (remember the term aerobic means "with oxygen")—than either static or dynamic resistance exercise. How much oxygen is needed depends primarily on the intensity of the activity and secondarily on its duration. As in the discussion of respiration, this chapter categorizes exercises as short-term (5–10 minutes), light (30–49% of maximal oxygen consumption, $\dot{V}O_2max$) to moderate (50–74% of $\dot{V}O_2max$) submaximal exercise; long-term (>30 minutes), moderate to heavy (60–85% of $\dot{V}O_2max$) submaximal exercise; or incremental exercise to maximum (increasing from ~30% to 100% $\dot{V}O_2max$).

Short-Term, Light to Moderate Submaximal Aerobic Exercise

Figure 12.1 depicts generalized cardiovascular responses to short-term, light to moderate submaximal aerobic exercise. The actual magnitude of each variable's change depends on the work rate or load, environmental conditions, and the individual's genetic makeup and fitness level. At the onset of light- to moderate-intensity exercise, cardiac output ($\dot{Q}$) initially increases to plateau at a steady state (see **Figure 12.1A**). Cardiac output plateaus within the first 2 minutes of exercise, reflecting

the fact that cardiac output is sufficient to transport the oxygen needed to support the metabolic demands of the activity. Cardiac output increases because of an initial increase in both stroke volume (SV) (**Figure 12.1B**) and heart rate (HR) (**Figure 12.1C**); both level off within 2 minutes.

During exercise of this intensity, the cardiorespiratory system can meet the body's metabolic demands; thus, this type of exercise is often called **steady-state** or steady-rate exercise. During steady-state exercise, energy provided aerobically is balanced with the energy required to perform the exercise. The plateau in cardiovascular variables (in **Figure 12.1**) indicates that a steady state has been achieved.

Stroke volume (SV) increases rapidly at the onset of exercise due to an increase in venous return, which in turn increases the end-diastolic volume (EDV) (preload). The increased preload stretches the myocardium and causes it to contract more forcibly, as described by the Frank-Starling law of the heart (Chapter 11). Contractility of the myocardium is also enhanced by the sympathetic nervous system, which is activated during physical activity. The increase in the EDV and the decrease in the end-systolic volume (ESV) both contribute to the increase in the SV during light to moderate dynamic exercise (Poliner et al., 1980). HR increases immediately at the onset of activity as a result of parasympathetic withdrawal. As exercise continues, further increases in the HR result from the sympathetic nervous system activation (Rowell, 1986).

Systolic blood pressure (SBP) rises in a pattern very similar to that of cardiac output: an initial increase followed by a plateau once steady state is achieved (**Figure 12.1D**). The increase in SBP results from the increased cardiac output. SBP would be even higher if not for the fact that resistance decreases, thereby partially offsetting the increase in cardiac output. When blood pressure (BP) is measured intra-arterially, diastolic blood pressure (DBP) does not change. When it is measured by auscultation, it either does not change or may go down slightly. DBP remains relatively constant because of peripheral vasodilation, which facilitates blood flow to the working muscles. The small rise in SBP and the lack of a significant change in DBP cause the mean arterial pressure (MAP) to rise only slightly, following the pattern of SBP.

Total peripheral resistance (TPR) decreases because of vasodilation in the active muscles (**Figure 12.1E**). This vasodilation results primarily from the influence of local chemical factors (lactate, K^+, and so on), which reflect increased metabolism. The TPR can be calculated using Equation 11.8:

$$TPR = \frac{MAP}{\dot{Q}}$$

Steady-State A condition in which the energy provided during exercise is balanced with the energy required to perform that exercise, and factors responsible for the provision of this energy reach elevated levels of equilibrium.

FIGURE 12.1 Cardiovascular Responses to Short-Term, Light to Moderate Submaximal Aerobic Exercise.
A. Cardiac output ($\dot{Q}$). **B.** Stroke volume (SV). **C.** Heart rate (HR). **D.** Blood pressure (SBP, MAP, and DBP). **E.** Total peripheral resistance (TPR). **F.** Rate-pressure product (RPP).

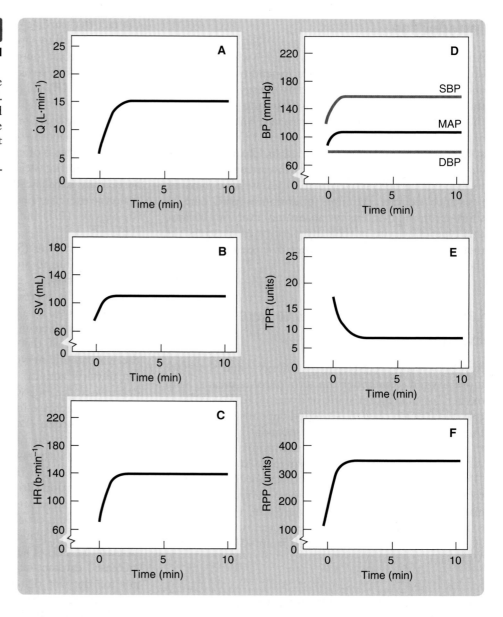

Calculate TPR for an individual doing short-term, light to moderate submaximal aerobic exercise by using the following information from **Figures 12.1A** and **D**:

$$MAP = 110 \text{ mmHg}; \dot{Q} = 15 \text{ L·min}^{-1}$$

The computation is

$$TPR = \frac{110 \text{ mmHg}}{15 \text{ L·min}^{-1}} = 7.33 \text{ (TPR units)}$$

Thus, in this example, TPR is 7.33.

The decrease in TPR has two important implications. First, vasodilation of the vessels supplying the active muscle causes decreased resistance that leads to an increased blood flow, thereby increasing the availability of oxygen and nutrients. Second, the decreased resistance keeps MAP from increasing dramatically. The increase in the MAP is determined by the relative changes in cardiac output and the TPR. Since cardiac output increases more than resistance decreases, the MAP increases slightly during dynamic aerobic exercise.

Myocardial oxygen consumption increases during dynamic aerobic exercise because the heart must do more work to increase cardiac output to supply the working muscles with additional oxygen. The rate-pressure product (RPP) increases due to increases in the HR and the SBP. This increase reflects the greater myocardial oxygen demand of the heart during exercise (**Figure 12.1F**). In the Check Your Comprehension Box 1, calculate cardiovascular variables based on measured values, which are examples of normal responses to several exercise categories. Refer back to these answers as the categories are discussed in this chapter.

CHECK YOUR COMPREHENSION 1

The following measurements were obtained from a 42-year-old man at rest and during several exercise sessions:

Condition	HR (b·min⁻¹)	SBP (mmHg)	DBP (mmHg)	Q̇ (L·min⁻¹)
Rest	80	134	86	6
Short-term, light to moderate submaximal aerobic exercise	130	150	86	10
Long-term, moderate to heavy submaximal aerobic exercise	155	170	88	13
Incremental aerobic exercise to maximum	180	200	88	15
Static exercise	135	210	100	8
Dynamic resistance exercise	126	180	92	10
Calculate MAP, TPR, and RPP for each condition.				

Check your answer in Appendix C.

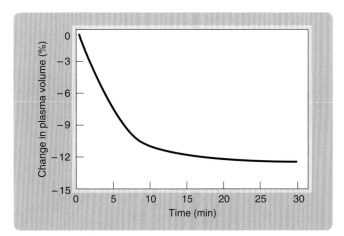

FIGURE 12.2 Percent Reduction of Plasma Volume during 30-minute Moderate Cycle Ergometer Exercise. *Source:* Fortney, S. M., C. B. Wenger, J. R. Bove, & E. R. Nadel: Effect of blood volume on sweating rate and body fluids in exercising humans. *Journal of Applied Physiology.* 51(6):1594–1600 (1981).

Blood volume decreases during submaximal aerobic exercise. **Figure 12.2** shows the reduction of plasma volume during 30 minutes of moderate cycle ergometer exercise (60–70% $\dot{V}O_2$max) in a warm environment (Fortney et al., 1981). The largest decrease occurs during the first 5 minutes of exercise, and then plasma volume stabilizes. This rapid decrease in plasma volume suggests that it is fluid shifts, rather than fluid loss, that account for the initial decrease (Wade and Freund, 1990). The magnitude of the decrease in plasma volume depends on the intensity of exercise, environmental factors, and the individual's hydration status.

Figure 12.3 shows the distribution of cardiac output at rest and during light aerobic exercise. Notice that cardiac output increases from 5.8 to 9.4 L·min⁻¹ in this example (the increase in Q̇ is illustrated by the larger pie chart). The most dramatic change in cardiac output distribution with light exercise is the increased percentage (from 21 to 47%) and the increased blood flow (from 1200 to 4500 mL) to the working muscles to support energy production. Skin blood flow also increases to meet the thermoregulatory demands of exercise. The absolute blood flow to the coronary muscle also increases, although its percentage of cardiac output remains relatively constant. The absolute amount of cerebral blood flow remains constant while the percentage of cardiac output distributed to the brain decreases. Both renal and

splanchnic blood flow are modestly decreased during light exercise. In summary, with aerobic exercise, cardiac output increases and it is redistributed so that tissues that need increased blood flow, such as the muscles and skin, receive it and other tissues receive either equal or less blood flow.

Long-Term, Moderate to Heavy Submaximal Aerobic Exercise

The cardiovascular responses to long-term, moderate to heavy submaximal aerobic exercise (60–85% of $\dot{V}O_2$max) are shown in **Figure 12.4**. Similar to light to moderate workloads, cardiac output increases rapidly during the first minutes of exercise and then plateaus and remains relatively constant throughout the exercise (**Figure 12.4A**). Notice, however, that the absolute cardiac output attained is higher during heavy exercise than during light to moderate exercise. The increase in cardiac output results from increased SV and HR.

SV has an initial increase, plateaus, and then has a negative (downward) drift as exercise duration continues past approximately 30 minutes. SV increases rapidly during the first minutes of exercise and then plateaus after a workload of approximately 40–50% of $\dot{V}O_2$max is achieved (Åstrand et al., 1964) (**Figure 12.4B**). Thus, during work that requires more than 50% of $\dot{V}O_2$max, the SV response does not depend on intensity. SV remains relatively constant during the first 30 minutes of heavy exercise.

As with short-term, light to moderate submaximal aerobic exercise, the increase in SV is believed to result from an increased venous return (leading to the Frank-Starling mechanism) and increased contractility

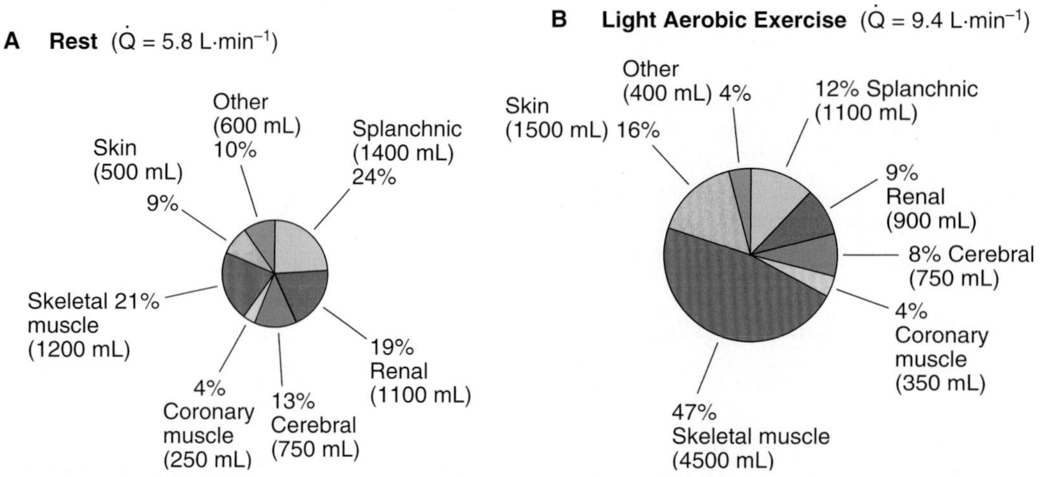

A Rest ($\dot{Q}$ = 5.8 L·min⁻¹)
Other (600 mL) 10%
Splanchnic (1400 mL) 24%
Skin (500 mL) 9%
Skeletal muscle 21% (1200 mL)
19% Renal (1100 mL)
4% Coronary muscle (250 mL)
13% Cerebral (750 mL)
B Light Aerobic Exercise ($\dot{Q}$ = 9.4 L·min⁻¹)
Other (400 mL) 4%
Skin (1500 mL) 16%
12% Splanchnic (1100 mL)
9% Renal (900 mL)
8% Cerebral (750 mL)
4% Coronary muscle (350 mL)
47% Skeletal muscle (4500 mL)

FIGURE 12.3 Distribution of Cardiac Output at Rest and during Light Aerobic Exercise. ***Source*:** Data from Anderson, K. L.: The cardiovascular system in exercise. In Falls, H. B. (ed.): *Exercise Physiology*. New York, NY: Academic Press (1968).

FIGURE 12.4 Cardiovascular Responses to Long-Term, Moderate to Heavy Submaximal Aerobic Exercise. **A.** Cardiac output ($\dot{Q}$). **B.** Stroke volume (SV). **C.** Heart rate (HR). **D.** Blood pressure (SBP, MAP, and DBP). **E.** Total peripheral resistance (TPR). **F.** Rate-pressure product (RPP).

A
$\dot{Q}$ (L·min⁻¹)
Time (min)
B
SV (mL)
Time (min)
C
HR (b·min⁻¹)
Time (min)
D
BP (mmHg)
SBP
MAP
DBP
Time (min)
E
TPR (units)
Time (min)
F
RPP (units)
Time (min)

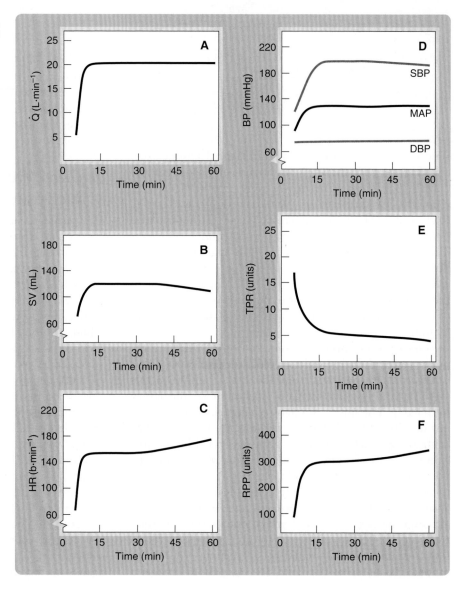

FOCUS ON APPLICATION: *Clinically Relevant*

The Importance of Fluid Ingestion

The magnitude of cardiovascular drift is heavily influenced by fluid ingestion. The accompanying figure presents data from a study in which participants cycled for 2 hours with or without fluid replacement. Values are for minutes 20 through 120; the initial increase in these variables is not shown. When participants consumed enough water to completely replace the water lost through sweat, cardiac output remained nearly constant throughout the first hour of exercise and actually increased during the second hour (panel A). Cardiac output was maintained in the fluid replacement trial because SV did not drift downward (panel B). HR was significantly lower when fluid replacement occurred (panel C). This information is important for coaches and fitness leaders. If your clients exercise for prolonged periods, they must replace the fluids that are lost during exercise, or performance will suffer.

Source: Hamilton et al. (1991).

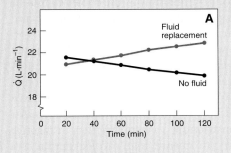
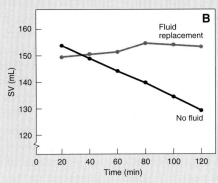
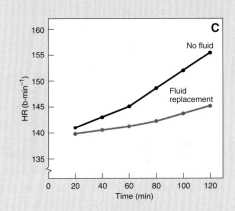

due to sympathetic nerve stimulation. Thus, changes in SV occur because EDV increases and ESV decreases (Poliner et al., 1980). EDV increases primarily because of the increased venous return of blood to the heart by the active muscle pump and increased venoconstriction, which decreases venous pooling. ESV decreases because of augmented contractility of the heart, which effectively ejects more blood.

If the exercise continues beyond approximately 30 minutes, SV gradually drifts downward while remaining above the resting value. This downward shift is most often attributed to thermoregulatory stress, which results in vasodilation, plasma loss, and a redirection of blood to the cutaneous vessels to dissipate heat, effectively reducing venous return and thus SV. This theory suggests that HR increases to compensate for a decrease in SV in order to maintain $\dot{Q}$. An alternate viewpoint suggests that the downward drift in SV is due to an increase in HR (due to augmented sympathetic nerve activity) that leads to a reduced filling time, thus leading to a reduced SV (Rowland, 2005b).

Cardiovascular Drift The changes in observed cardiovascular variables that occur during prolonged, heavy submaximal exercise without a change in workload.

HR initially increases, plateaus at steady state, and then has a positive drift as exercise continues for a prolonged period. HR increases sharply during the first 1–2 minutes of exercise, the magnitude of which depends on the intensity of exercise (**Figure 12.4C**). The increase in HR is brought about by parasympathetic withdrawal and activation of the sympathetic nervous system. After approximately 30 minutes of heavy exercise, HR begins to drift upward. The increase in HR is proportional to the decrease in SV, so cardiac output is maintained during exercise.

These cardiovascular changes, notably in HR and SV, during long-term, moderate to heavy submaximal aerobic exercise without a change in workload are known as **cardiovascular drift**. Cardiovascular drift is probably associated with rising body temperature during prolonged exercise. Exercise and heat stress produce competing regulatory demands, as the skin and the muscles compete for increased blood flow. SV decreases as a result of vasodilation, a progressive increase in the fraction of blood being directed to the skin, and a loss of plasma volume (Rowell, 1974; Sjogaard et al., 1988).

SBP response to long-term, moderate to heavy submaximal aerobic exercise is characterized by an initial increase, a plateau at steady state, and a negative drift. SBP increases rapidly during the first 1–2 minutes of exercise, the magnitude of increase depending on the intensity of the exercise (**Figure 12.4D**). SBP then remains relatively stable or drifts slightly downward as a result of continued vasodilation and a resultant decrease in resistance (Ekelund and Holmgren, 1967). DBP does not change, or changes so little that it has no physiological significance, during prolonged exercise in a thermoneutral environment. But it may decrease slightly in a warm environment because of increased vasodilation resulting from heat production. Because of the increased SBP and the relatively stable DBP, MAP increases modestly during prolonged activity. Again, as in light to moderate exercise, the magnitude of the increase in MAP is mediated by a large decrease in resistance.

TPR decreases rapidly, plateaus, and then has a slight negative drift during long-term heavy exercise (**Figure 12.4E**) because of vasodilation in active muscle and because of vasodilation in cutaneous vessels (Rowell, 1974). Finally, because both HR and SBP increase substantially during heavy work, the rate-pressure product increases markedly with the onset of exercise and then plateaus at steady state (**Figure 12.4F**). An upward drift in rate-pressure product may occur after approximately 30 minutes of exercise because the HR increases more than SBP decreases. The high rate-pressure product reflects the large amount of work the heart must perform to support heavy exercise.

During prolonged exercise, particularly in a warm environment, total body fluid is continually lost due to sweating. This loss typically ranges from 900 to 1300 mL·hr^{-1}, depending on work intensity and environmental conditions (Wade and Freund, 1990). If fluid is not replaced during long-duration exercise, plasma volume will continually be reduced throughout the exercise.

Figure 12.5 shows the distribution of cardiac output at rest and during heavy aerobic exercise. Notice that cardiac output increases from 5.8 L·min^{-1} at rest to 17.5 L·min^{-1} in this example. The most dramatic change here is the increased blood flow to the working muscle, which now receives 71% of cardiac output. Skin blood flow is also increased to meet the thermoregulatory demands. The absolute blood flow to the coronary muscle increases while its percentage of cardiac output remains relatively constant. The absolute cerebral blood flow remains constant, while its percentage of cardiac output decreases. Both renal and splanchnic blood flow are further decreased as exercise intensity increases. Although blood flow to the working muscle increases during aerobic exercise, blood flow to the inactive muscle decreases because of vasoconstriction. Vasoconstriction in inactive muscle is necessary to ensure that cardiac output can supply adequate blood flow to the working muscle. In summary, cardiac output increases and it is redistributed during heavy aerobic exercise so that tissues that need increased blood flow receive it and other tissues receive either equal or less blood flow.

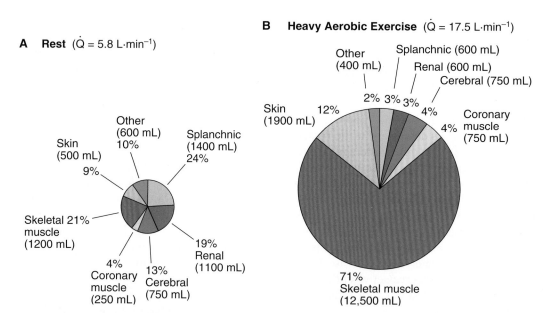

FIGURE 12.5 Distribution of Cardiac Output at Rest and during Heavy Aerobic Exercise.
Source: Data from Anderson, K. L.: The cardiovascular system in exercise. In Falls, H. B. (ed.): *Exercise Physiology*. New York, NY: Academic Press (1968).

Interval Exercise versus Steady-State Exercise

Throughout this book, we examine the exercise response to various categories of exercise, such as the cardiovascular responses in this chapter. Most studies examining cardiovascular responses to exercise have used continuous activity. Yet, many clinical populations (e.g., people undergoing cardiac rehabilitation) and many athletic populations use interval training. Interval workouts generally use repetitions from several seconds to several minutes in length and intensities from light to very hard.

Foster et al. set out to determine the cardiovascular responses to continuous exercise compared to those of very short-term, high-intensity interval exercise when the total power output remained constant. A group of adults (mean age = 52.9 years) participated in two separate 15-minute cycling trials—one involving steady-state exercise, the other using interval exercise. Participants cycled at 170 W for the full 15 minutes in one trial and alternated 1-minute "hard" (220 W) and "easy" (120 W) periods in the second trial, resulting in an equal power output (170 W) for both trials. Cardiovascular measurements were obtained before exercise (0 minute) and after minutes 4, 7, 12, and 15 and are presented in the accompaning graphs.

The results showed no significant difference in any of the variables between the steady-state exercise and the interval exercise. The authors concluded that heart function during interval exercise is remarkably similar to continuous steady-state exercise at the same average power output, when moderate duration and evenly timed hard and easy periods are used. These results are good news for individuals with low levels of fitness who may not be able to perform 15 minutes of continuous activity when starting an exercise program. Even if such individuals are unable to perform the high-intensity interval exercise used in this experiment, fitness professionals can assure them that alternating periods of "hard" and "easy" work results in cardiovascular responses similar to those resulting from sustained exercise of the same average power output.

Source: Foster, C., K. Meyer, N. Georgakopoulos, et al.: Left ventricular function during interval and steady state exercise. *Medicine & Science in Sports & Exercise.* 31(8):1157–1162 (1999).

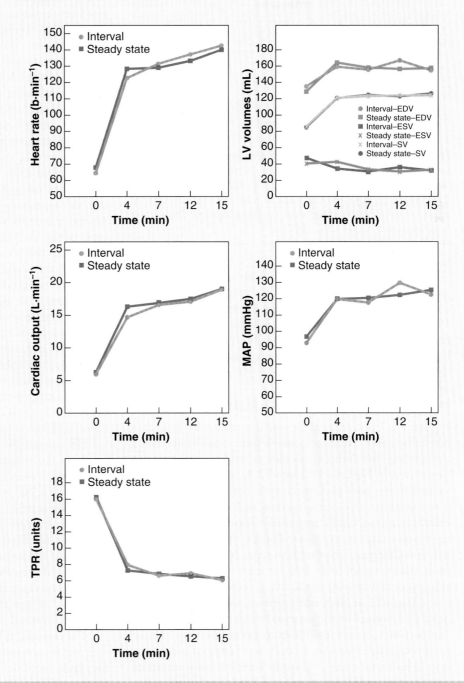

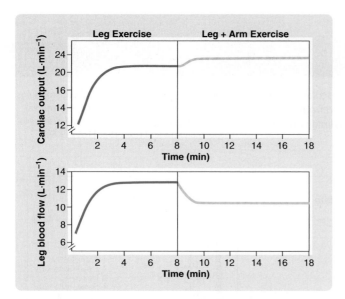

FIGURE 12.6 Effect of Combined Arm and Leg Exercise on Leg Blood Flow.
Source: Based on Secher, N. H., J. P. Clausen, K. Klausen. I. Noer, & J. Trap-Jensen: Central and regional circulatory effects of adding arm exercise to leg exercise. *Acta Physiologica Scandinavica*. 100:288–297 (1977).

Figure 12.6 presents data from a study in which participants exercised on a cycle ergometer for 8 minutes, then added an arm-cranking exercise (Secher et al., 1977). The combination of leg and arm cycling increased cardiac output modestly but actually caused a decrease in leg blood flow because a portion of cardiac output now had to be distributed to the working muscles in the arm.

Incremental Aerobic Exercise to Maximum

Figure 12.7 presents cardiovascular responses to incremental aerobic exercise to maximum. Note that unlike the graphs for light to moderate and heavy exercise (presented in **Figures 12.1** and **12.4**), the cardiovascular variables are now presented with percentage of maximum work on the x-axis. Incremental exercise to maximum (or a max test) consists of a series of work stages, each becoming progressively harder, that continue until volitional fatigue. The duration of each work stage (level of intensity) varies from 1 to 3 minutes to allow a steady state to occur, at least at the lower workloads. Max tests are performed in laboratory settings to quantify physiological responses to the maximal work that an individual can perform. Incremental tests to maximum may or may not include the direct measurement of oxygen consumption. The techniques used in the direct measurement of oxygen consumption are presented in Chapter 4.

During an incremental test, cardiac output has a rectilinear increase and plateaus at maximal exercise (**Figure 12.7A**). The initial increase in cardiac output reflects an increase in the SV and the HR; however, at workloads greater than 40–50% $\dot{V}O_2$max, the

continued increase in cardiac output in untrained individuals is achieved almost completely by an increase in the HR. As shown in **Figure 12.7B**, in untrained individuals, the SV increases rectilinearly initially and then plateaus at approximately 40–50% of $\dot{V}O_2$max (Åstrand et al., 1964; Higginbotham et al., 1986). The exact SV response to incremental exercise continues to be debated (González-Alonso, 2008; Rowland, 2005a,b; Warburton and Gledhill, 2008). As indicated above, it has traditionally been believed that the SV plateaus at approximately 50% of $\dot{V}O_2$max in untrained individuals. However, there appears to be considerable interindividual variability in this response, and many laboratories have reported an increase in the SV at maximal exercise in most endurance athletes and some untrained individuals (Ferguson et al., 2001; Gledhill et al., 1994; Warburton et al., 1999). In contrast, other researchers have documented a decrease in the SV at the maximal exercise (Mortensen et al., 2005; Stringer et al., 1997), and some researchers contend that after an initial increase (due to the skeletal muscle pump returning the pooled venous blood to the heart), the SV remains essentially unchanged during the incremental maximal exercise (Rowland, 2005b). Much of the controversy is undoubtedly associated with difficulties in measuring the SV during maximal exercise (see Chapter 11), with the use of different exercise protocols, and with individual variability.

Figure 12.8 indicates the changes in the EDV and the ESV that account for changes in the SV during progressively increasing exercise (Poliner et al., 1980). The EDV increases largely because of the return of blood to the heart by the active muscle pump and the increased sympathetic outflow to the veins causing venoconstriction and augmenting venous return. ESV decreases because of augmented contractility of the heart, which ejects more blood and leaves less in the ventricle.

HR increases in a rectilinear fashion throughout much of the submaximal (~120–170 b·min⁻¹) portion of incremental exercise and plateaus at maximal exercise (**Figure 12.7C**) (Astrand and Rhyming, 1954; Hale, 2008). Myocardial cells can contract at over 300 b·min⁻¹ but rarely exceed 210 b·min⁻¹ because a faster HR would not allow for adequate ventricular filling. Thus, SV and ultimately cardiac output would decrease. Consider the simple analogy of a bucket brigade. Up to a point it is useful to increase the speed of passing buckets under the water source, but the maximum rate is limited because of the time required for the buckets to be filled with water.

The arterial BP responses to incremental dynamic exercise to maximum are shown in **Figure 12.7D**. SBP increases rectilinearly and plateaus at maximal exercise, often reaching values in excess of 200 mmHg in very fit individuals. This increase is caused by the increased cardiac output, which outweighs the simultaneous decrease in resistance. SBP and HR are routinely monitored during exercise tests to ensure the safety of the participant. If either of these variables fails to rise with an increasing

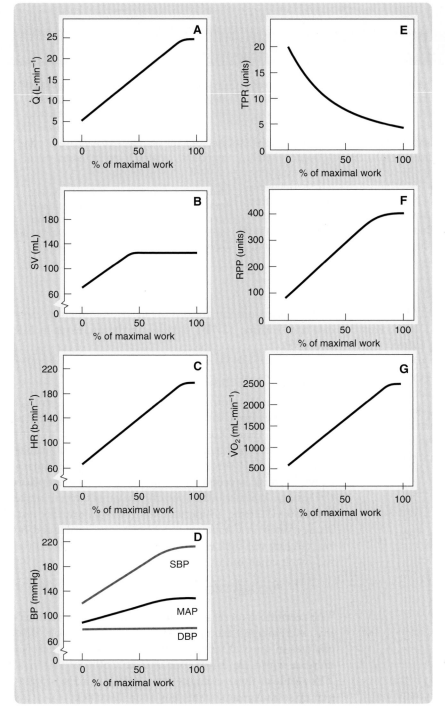

FIGURE 12.7 Cardiovascular Response to Incremental Aerobic Exercise to Maximum.
A. Cardiac output ($\dot{Q}$). **B.** Stroke volume (SV). **C.** Heart rate (HR). **D.** Blood pressure (SBP, MAP, and DBP). **E.** Total peripheral resistance (TPR). **F.** Rate-pressure product (RPP). **G.** Oxygen consumption ($\dot{V}O_2$).

workload, cardiovascular insufficiency and an inability to adequately perfuse tissue may result, and the exercise test should be stopped. A drop in SBP of 10 mmHg or more that occurs despite an increase in workload indicates that the exercise test or session should be discontinued. Similarly a rise in SBP above 250 mmHg or in DBP above 115 mmHg indicates that the exercise test or session should be discontinued.

DBP typically remains relatively constant or changes so little it has no physiological significance, although it may decrease at high levels of exercise. Diastolic pressure remains relatively constant because vasodilation in the vasculature of the active muscle is balanced by vasoconstriction in other vascular beds. Diastolic pressure is most likely to decrease when exercise is performed in a hot environment because skin vessels are more dilated and there is decreased resistance to blood flow. A rise in DBP above 115 mmHg is an indicator that the exercise test or session should be discontinued.

Individuals with an exaggerated BP response to exercise are at greater risk for hypertension, stroke, and cardiovascular disease mortality than those with a normal

FOCUS ON RESEARCH

Exaggerated Blood Pressure Responses and Carotid Atherosclerosis

It has been known for some time that an exaggerated blood pressure response to exercise, in otherwise apparently healthy individuals, is predictive of future hypertension, stroke, and cardiovascular disease mortality. In this study, researchers investigated the hypothesis that an exaggerated SBP response to incremental aerobic exercise to maximum was associated with carotid atherosclerosis (deposition of fatty plaque in the carotid artery) in middle-aged (~48 years) men.

The researchers used data from over 9000 apparently healthy men who had undergone an exercise stress test and a series of cardiovascular tests. No participants had a history of hypertension or cardiovascular disease. Approximately 4% or 375 participants had an exaggerated SBP response to exercise (defined as SBP > 210 mmHg). When the researchers compared the group that had an exaggerated SBP response to exercise to those who had a normal response, they found

that individuals with an exaggerated SBP response to exercise had a 2.02 times increased risk for carotid atherosclerosis.

These results suggest that an exaggerated SBP response to exercise is independently related to an increased risk of carotid atherosclerosis.

Source: Jae, S. Y., B. Fernhall, K. S. Heffernan, et al.: Exaggerated blood pressure response to exercise is associated with carotid atherosclerosis in apparently healthy men. *Journal of Hypertension*. 24:881–887 (2006).

exercise BP response (see Focus On Research) (American College of Sports Medicine, 1993; Jae et al., 2006; Kurl et al., 2001; Miyai et al., 2002; Mundal et al., 1994).

TPR decreases in a negative curvilinear pattern and reaches its lowest level at maximal exercise (**Figure 12.7E**). Decreased resistance reflects maximal vasodilation in the active tissue in response to the need for increased blood flow during maximal exercise. The large drop in resistance is also important for keeping MAP from becoming too high. The rate-pressure product increases in a rectilinear

fashion plateauing at maximum in an incremental exercise test (**Figure 12.7F**), paralleling the increases in HR and SBP.

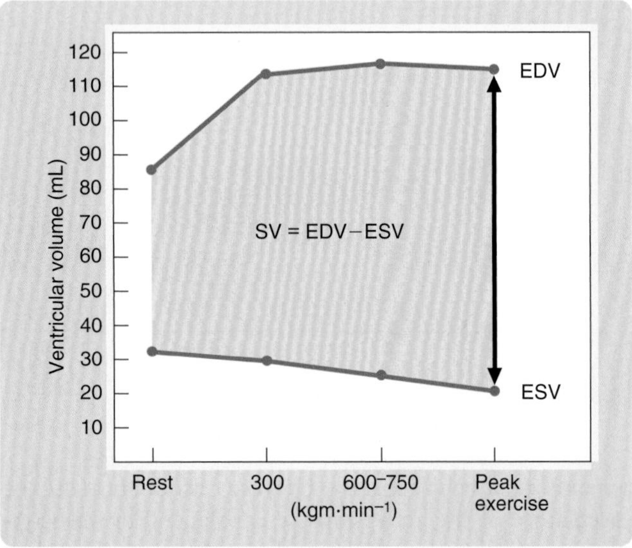

Maximal Oxygen Consumption

Oxygen consumption rises rectilinearly in direct proportion to the exercise intensity during an incremental exercise to maximum (**Figure 12.7G**). The highest amount of oxygen an individual can take in, transport, and utilize to produce ATP aerobically while breathing air during heavy exercise is called **maximal oxygen consumption** ($\dot{V}O_2$**max**). As described above, the maximal oxygen intake is measured during an incremental maximal exercise test. As described in Chapter 11, $\dot{V}O_2$max can be defined by rearranging the Fick equation (see Equation 11.9) to the following equation:

$$\dot{V}O_2\text{max} = (\dot{Q}\text{max}) \times (a - vO_2\text{diff max})$$

The rectilinear increase in cardiac output during a maximal incremental exercise test is described above. The changes in the a-vO_2diff (discussed in Chapter 10) are an increase with a plateau at approximately 60% of $\dot{V}O_2$max. The result of these changes is the rectilinear rise in oxygen up to maximum, which has been discussed.

Maximal exercise tests that include the measurement of oxygen consumption for the determination of $\dot{V}O_2$max are routinely administered by coaches and trainers to determine an athlete's fitness or to track changes in fitness; by researchers to better understand the mechanisms that limit exercise or to probe questions related to physiological function under stressful conditions; and by medical personnel to assess cardiorespiratory function.

$\dot{V}O_2$max is commonly used as the criterion measure of cardiorespiratory (also called aerobic) fitness. In reality, $\dot{V}O_2$max is an integrated measure of fitness that encompasses the ability of the body to take in (respiratory

FIGURE 12.8 Changes in EDV and ESV That Account for Change in SV during Incremental Exercise.
Source: Based on data from Poliner, L. R., G. J. Dehmer, S. E. Lewis, R. W. Parkey, C. G. Blomqvist, & J. T. Willerson: Left ventricular performance in normal subjects: A comparison of the responses to exercise in the upright supine positions. *Circulation*. 62:528–534 (1980).

system), transport (cardiovascular system), and utilize (the metabolic system) oxygen. Thus, $\dot{V}O_2$max may be considered a cardiovascular, respiratory and metabolic variable and, indeed, for that reason it is also discussed in other chapters. However, $\dot{V}O_2$max has important implications for cardiovascular health and is normally thought to be limited by cardiovascular function; therefore, we will consider $\dot{V}O_2$max primarily as a cardiovascular variable and it is discussed in depth in this chapter.

CRITERIA FOR DETERMINING $\dot{V}O_2$max When the individual reaches volitional fatigue the highest oxygen consumption may or may not represent an actual maximal value. Before labeling the highest value as $\dot{V}O_2$max, the exercise tester has to decide whether any given test truly is a maximal one. The term $\dot{V}O_2peak$ is used to represent the highest value obtained during the test if the tester is not certain that a true maximal value was achieved. Criteria used to determine whether the test is a maximal test include:

1. A lactate value greater than 8–9 mmol·L^{-1} (Åstrand, 1956; Åstrand et al., 2003);
2. A heart rate ± 12 b·min^{-1} of predicted maximal heart rate (220 minus age) (Durstine and Pate, 1988);
3. A respiratory exchange ratio (RER, see Chapter 4) of 1.0 or 1.1, primarily depending on the age of the subject (Holly, 1988; MacDougall et al., 1982); and
4. A plateau in oxygen consumption. The classic definition of a plateau is a rise of 2.1 mL·kg^{-1}·min^{-1} or less, or a rise of 0.15 L·min^{-1} or less, in oxygen consumption ($\dot{V}O_2$) with an increase in workload that represents a change in grade of 2.5% while running at 7 mi·hr^{-1} (11.2 km·hr^{-1}) with 3-minute stages (Taylor et al., 1955). An alternative is to define a plateau as an increase of less than half the expected theoretical rise based on the change in speed, grade, or speed and grade (Plowman and Liu, 1999). The expected increase can be calculated using the American College of Sports Medicine (2006) equations provided in Appendix B.

FACTORS LIMITING $\dot{V}O_2$max At some point an individual cannot continue to increase the intensity of the exercise load or to work at maximum effort because the body cannot provide and utilize more oxygen to support an additional workload. But what specifically limits $\dot{V}O_2$max? **Figure 12.9** summarizes possible limitations to oxygen consumption within the major systems involved in oxygen delivery and use during exercise.

> **Maximal Oxygen Consumption ($\dot{V}O_2$max)** The highest amount of oxygen an individual can take in transport, and utilize to produce ATP aerobically while breathing air during heavy exercise.

Theoretically, maximal oxygen uptake could be limited by any system (or step) along the pathway of bringing oxygen into the body and delivering it to the mitochondria for the production of ATP. Thus, any of the following systems may limit $\dot{V}O_2$max:

1. The respiratory system, because of inadequate ventilation, oxygen diffusion limitations, or an inability to maintain the gradient for the diffusion of O_2 (a-vO_2diff)
2. the cardiovascular system, because of inadequate blood flow ($\dot{Q}$) or oxygen-carrying capacity (Hb)
3. the metabolic functions within skeletal muscle, such as an inability to produce additional ATP because of limited number of mitochondria, limited enzyme levels or activity, or limited substrates

Evidence suggests that each of these systems may limit $\dot{V}O_2$max in certain conditions (Bergh et al., 2000). For example, a reduction in the partial pressure of oxygen (PO_2) at altitude or with asthma causes a reduction in $\dot{V}O_2$max. Medications (such as beta-blockers) that limit cardiac output also cause a decrease in $\dot{V}O_2$max, as does a reduction in hemoglobin associated with anemia. Certain diseases in which muscle enzymes involved in metabolism are deficient can also result in reduced $\dot{V}O_2$max.

Although factors in each of these systems may limit $\dot{V}O_2$max, the question remains: What limits $\dot{V}O_2$max in healthy humans performing maximal exercise? This question has energized exercise physiologists for decades, beginning with the work of A. V. Hill in the 1920s, and it continues to engender lively debate among physiologists today (Bassett and Howley, 2000; Bergh et al., 2000; Grassi, 2000; Hale, 2008; Saltin, 1985).

Current research suggests that maximal oxygen uptake is limited by the ability of the cardiorespiratory system to deliver oxygen to the muscle, rather than the ability of the muscle mitochondria to utilize oxygen (Bergh et al., 2000; Hale, 2008; Rowell, 1993; Saltin, 1985). Specifically, cardiac output appears to be the limiting factor in $\dot{V}O_2$max (Bergh et al., 2000; di Prampero, 2003; Saltin, 1985).

Research evidence suggests that oxygen uptake is not limited by pulmonary ventilation in normal, healthy athletes without exercise-induced arterial hypoxemia (Chapter 10). Generally, the functional capacity of the respiratory system is believed to exceed the demands of maximal exercise (Rowell, 1993). The only respiratory or cardiovascular variable likely to impose a limitation on oxygen transport is a-vO_2diff.

Many researchers report that skeletal muscles have the ability to use more oxygen than can be supplied by the respiratory and cardiovascular systems (Richardson, 2000; Rowell, 1993; Saltin, 1985). Not all researchers agree with this view, though, and some have proposed that failure of muscle performance may explain exhaustion during maximal exercise (Noakes, 1988).

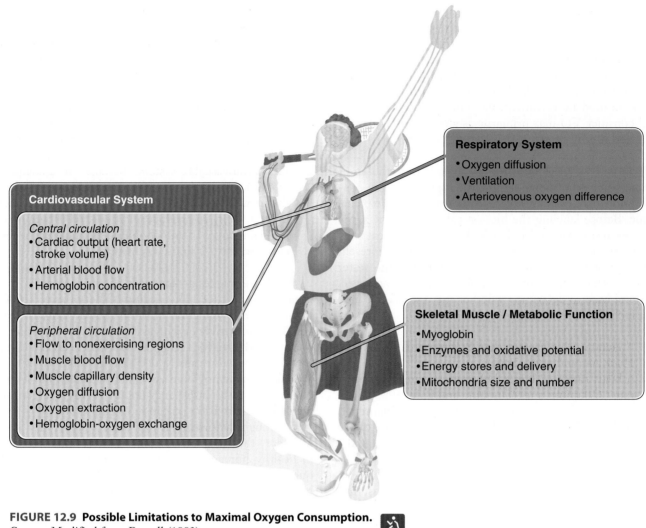

Cardiovascular System

Central circulation
- Cardiac output (heart rate, stroke volume)
- Arterial blood flow
- Hemoglobin concentration

Peripheral circulation
- Flow to nonexercising regions
- Muscle blood flow
- Muscle capillary density
- Oxygen diffusion
- Oxygen extraction
- Hemoglobin-oxygen exchange

Respiratory System
- Oxygen diffusion
- Ventilation
- Arteriovenous oxygen difference

Skeletal Muscle / Metabolic Function
- Myoglobin
- Enzymes and oxidative potential
- Energy stores and delivery
- Mitochondria size and number

FIGURE 12.9 Possible Limitations to Maximal Oxygen Consumption.
Source: Modified from Rowell (1993).

Possibly, the factors limiting $\dot{V}O_2$max vary with the fitness level of the individual. According to this hypothesis, in an untrained individual the respiratory capacity for gas exchange exceeds the cardiovascular system's capacity to deliver oxygen. A training program results in little change in the respiratory capacity but large changes in the cardiovascular capacity. Thus, in some highly trained individuals who have exercise-induced arterial hypoxemia (Chapter 10), the increased cardiovascular capacity may exceed the respiratory capacity (Dempsey, 1986; Legrand et al., 2005; Powers et al., 1989). In this case the respiratory system becomes the factor limiting $\dot{V}O_2$max. One final point to remember, although it is interesting to probe the question, "what limits $\dot{V}O_2$max?" we must resist the temptation to allow the search for an answer to obscure the fact that a close interaction exists among the various systems ensuring a continuous supply of oxygen to the working tissue during exercise (Mitchell and Saltin, 2003).

The reduction in plasma volume during submaximal exercise also occurs in incremental exercise to maximum. Because the magnitude of the reduction depends on the intensity of exercise, the reduction is greatest at maximal exercise. A decrease of 10–20% can be seen during incremental exercise to maximum (Wade and Freund, 1990).

Considerable changes in cardiac output occur during maximal incremental exercise. **Figure 12.10** illustrates the distribution of cardiac output at rest and at maximal aerobic exercise. Maximum cardiac output in this example is 25 L·min⁻¹. Again, the most striking change is the tremendous amount of cardiac output that is directed to the working muscles (88%). At maximal exercise, skin blood flow is reduced to direct the necessary blood to the muscles. Renal and splanchnic blood flows also decrease considerably. Blood flow to the brain and cardiac muscle is maintained.

Table 12.1 summarizes the cardiovascular responses to exercise.

TABLE 12.1 Cardiovascular Responses to Exercise*

	Short-Term, Light to Moderate Submaximal Aerobic Exercise	Long-Term, Moderate to Heavy Submaximal Aerobic Exercise[†]	Incremental Aerobic Exercise to Maximum	Static[‡] Exercise	Resistance[‡] Exercise
$\dot{Q}$	Increases rapidly; plateaus at steady state within 2 min	Increases rapidly; plateaus	Rectilinear increase with plateau at max	Modest gradual increase	Modest gradual increase
SV	Increases rapidly; plateaus at steady state within 2 min	Increases rapidly; plateaus; negative drift	Increases initially; plateaus at 40–50% $\dot{V}O_2$max	Relatively constant at low workloads; decreases at high workloads; rebound rise in recovery	Little change, slight decrease
HR	Increases rapidly; plateaus at steady state within 2 min	Increases rapidly; plateaus; positive drift	Rectilinear increase with plateau at max	Modest gradual increase	Increases gradually with numbers of reps
SBP	Increases rapidly; plateaus at steady state within 2 min	Increases rapidly; plateaus; slight negative drift	Rectilinear increase with plateau at max	Marked steady increase	Increases gradually with numbers of reps
DBP	Shows little or no change	Shows little or no change	Shows little or no change	Marked steady increase	No change or increase
MAP	Increases rapidly; plateaus at steady state within 2 min	Increases initially; little if any drift	Small rectilinear increase	Marked steady increase	Increases gradually with numbers of reps
TPR	Decreases rapidly; plateaus	Decreases rapidly; plateaus; slight negative drift	Curvilinear decrease	Decreases	Slight increase
RPP	Increases rapidly; plateaus at steady state within 2 min	Increases rapidly; plateaus; positive drift	Rectilinear increase with plateau at max	Marked steady increase	Increases gradually with numbers of reps

*Resting values are taken as baseline.

[†]The difference between a plateau during the short-term, light to moderate and long-term, moderate to heavy submaximal exercise response is one of magnitude; that is, a plateau occurs at a higher value with higher intensities.

[‡]The magnitude of a plateau change depends on the %MVC/load.

Upper-Body versus Lower-Body Aerobic Exercise

Upper-body exercise is routinely performed in a variety of industrial, agricultural, military, recreational, and sporting activities. The cardiovascular responses to exercise using muscles of the upper body are different in some important ways from exercise performed using muscles of the lower body. **Figure 12.11** presents data about cardiovascular responses to incremental exercise to maximum in able-bodied individuals using the upper body (arm cranking on an arm ergometer) versus lower body (cycling on a cycle ergometer). Notice that a higher peak $\dot{V}O_2$ was achieved during lower-body exercise. Comparisons at any given level of oxygen consumption also show differences in cardiovascular responses to submaximal upper- and lower-body exercise. When the oxygen consumption required to perform a submaximal workload is the same, cardiac output is similar for upper- and lower-body exercise (**Figure 12.11A**). However, the mechanism to achieve the required increase in cardiac output is not the same. As shown in **Figure 12.11B** and **C**, upper-body exercise results in a lower SV and a higher HR at any given submaximal workload (Clausen, 1976; Miles et al., 1989; Pendergast, 1989). SBP, DBP, MAP (**Figure 12.11D**), total peripheral resistance (**Figure 12.11E**), and rate-pressure product (**Figure 12.11F**) are significantly higher in upper-body exercise than in lower-body exercise performed at the same oxygen consumption.

There are several likely reasons for the differences. The higher HR observed during upper-body exercise is thought to reflect a greater sympathetic stimulation (Åstrand et al., 2003; Davies et al., 1974; Miles et al., 1989). SV is lower during upper-body exercise because of the absence of the skeletal muscle pump augmenting

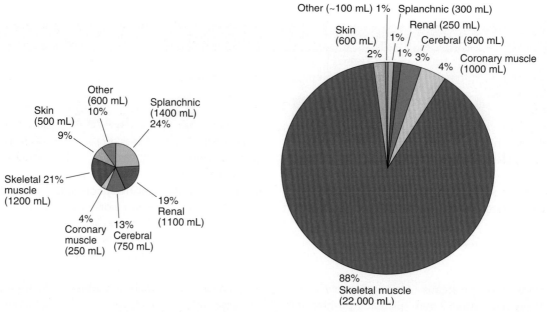

A Rest ($\dot{Q}$ = 5.8 L·min⁻¹)

Other (600 mL) 10%
Skin (500 mL) 9%
Splanchnic (1400 mL) 24%
Skeletal muscle 21% (1200 mL)
Coronary muscle 4% (250 mL)
Cerebral 13% (750 mL)
Renal 19% (1100 mL)

B Maximal Aerobic Exercise ($\dot{Q}$ = 25 L·min⁻¹)

Other (~100 mL) 1%
Splanchnic (300 mL) 1%
Skin (600 mL) 2%
Renal (250 mL) 1%
Cerebral (900 mL) 3%
Coronary muscle (1000 mL) 4%
88% Skeletal muscle (22,000 mL)

FIGURE 12.10 Distribution of Cardiac Output at Rest and during Maximal Aerobic Exercise.
Source: Data from Anderson, K. L.: The cardiovascular system in exercise. In Falls, H. B. (ed.): *Exercise Physiology*. New York, NY: Academic Press (1968).

FIGURE 12.11 Cardiovascular Response to Incremental Aerobic Maximal Upper-Body and Lower-Body Exercise.
A. Cardiac output ($\dot{Q}$). **B.** Stroke volume (SV). **C.** Heart rate (HR). **D.** Blood pressure (SBP, MAP, and DBP). **E.** Total peripheral resistance (TPR). **F.** Rate-pressure product (RPP).

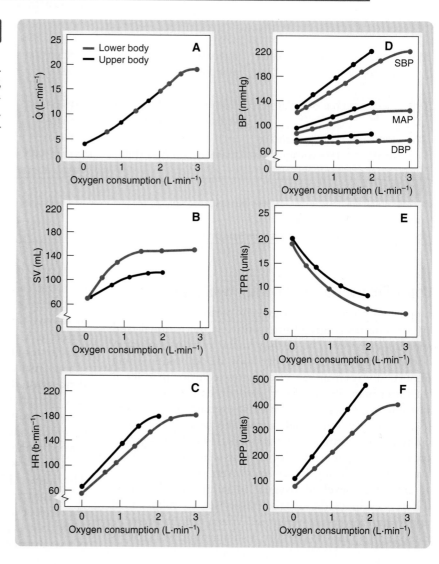

FOCUS ON APPLICATION: *Clinically Relevant*
Cardiovascular Demands of Shoveling Wet, Heavy Snow

As the text has described, upper-body exercise is associated with greater cardiovascular strain (exemplified by higher HRs and higher BPs at any given submaximal level of oxygen consumption) than lower-body exercise. Similarly, both static and dynamic resistance exercise are characterized by modest increases in HR but exaggerated increases in BP. Snow shoveling involves a unique combination of a predominantly upper-body activity with both static and dynamic components. In addition, snow shoveling is always done in cold and sometimes frigid conditions and often when the individual is under the added stress of digging out to get somewhere on time. It is not unusual to hear about individuals collapsing and dying of heart attacks while clearing snow.

In a classic study, Franklin et al. performed an experiment to determine the specific demands of snow shoveling on the heart. Ten sedentary, healthy, young adult males cleared two 15-m paths of wet, heavy snow 5–13 cm deep outside in the cold (2°C) for 10 minutes. In one trial, they used a 1.4-kg plastic shovel. They were told to repeatedly lift and throw the snow to the side at a self-selected rate. The group mean was 12 ± 2 loads per minute at approximately 7.3 kg per load for a total of 872.7 kg (1920 lb) over the 10-minute time span. In the second trial, they used a motorized snow blower. Ten to fifteen minutes of rest was permitted between the randomly assigned trials. On another day, each participant underwent a treadmill maximal oxygen consumption test in the laboratory. The results are presented in the accompanying table.

After only 2 minutes of snow shoveling, the participants' average HR was 85% of the treadmill HRmax. The HR continued to increase until it reached 98% HRmax. The SBP during the snow shoveling exceeded the treadmill maximum by 9.3%. The total body oxygen consumption was only 61.3% $\dot{V}O_2$max, but the myocardial oxygen consumption, as indicated by the rate-pressure product, was 107% of that required during maximal treadmill work. The disproportionate increase in myocardial oxygen demand relative to total body oxygen demand during shoveling was attributed to several factors: a reduced myocardial efficiency of arm exercise, a large static exercise component, the Valsalva maneuver, and the inhalation of cold air that could cause a spasm or constriction in the coronary arteries. These results clearly indicate that shoveling wet, heavy snow even for a short time period (10 minutes) places a tremendous physiological demand on the heart.

In contrast, using the snow blower resulted in elevations to only 69% HRmax, 89% maximal SBP, 25% $\dot{V}O_2$max, and 61% maximal myocardial oxygen consumption, as reflected by the rate-pressure product. Whereas the manual shoveling was perceived as "very heavy" work, using the snow blower resulted in a "fairly light" rating.

The healthy but untrained participants in this study completed the shoveling without any adverse cardiac or musculoskeletal complications. Such work, especially if continued for 20–60 minutes, would provide a heavy but acceptable workout. However, these results suggest that individuals with a history of heart disease, symptoms suggestive of cardiac disorder (dizziness, chest pain, and abnormal electrocardiograms), or one or more major coronary risk factors (see Chapter 15) should avoid this work or take precautions when faced with the task of clearing wet, heavy snow. These precautions include:

1. Take frequent breaks or use a work-rest approach.

2. Use both arms and legs in the lift-throw action.

3. Regulate body temperature with a hat, scarf over the mouth, and layers that can easily be added or removed.

4. Avoid large meals, alcohol consumption, and smoking immediately before and after shoveling.

5. Consider using a motorized snow blower.

Sources: Franklin (1997), Franklin et al. (1995).

Variable	Snow Shoveling	Snow Blower	Treadmill (Max)
HR (b·min⁻¹)	175 ± 15	124 ± 18	179 ± 17
SBP (mmHg)	198 ± 17	161 ± 14	181 ± 25
Rate-pressure product	347	199.6	324
$\dot{V}O_2$ (mL·kg⁻¹·min⁻¹)	19.95 ± 2.8	8.4 ± 2.5	32.55 ± 6.3
Rating of perceived exertion	16.70 ± 1.7	9.9 ± 1.0	17.90 ± 1.5

venous return from the legs. The greater sympathetic stimulation that occurs during upper-body exercise may also be partially responsible for the increased BP and total peripheral resistance. Upper-body exercise often involves a static component that causes an exaggerated BP response. For instance, using an arm-cranking ergometer has a static component because the individual must grasp the hand crank.

When maximal exercise is performed using upper-body muscles, $\dot{V}O_2$max values are approximately 30% lower than when maximal exercise is performed using lower-body muscles (Miles et al., 1989; Pendergast, 1989). Maximal HR values for upper-body exercise are 90–95% of those for lower-body exercise, and SV is 30–40% less during maximal upper-body exercise. Maximal SBP and the rate-pressure product are usually similar, but DBP is typically 10–15% higher during upper-body exercise (Miles et al., 1989).

The different cardiovascular responses to an absolute workload performed with the upper body versus the lower body dictate that exercise prescriptions for arm work cannot be based on data obtained from testing with leg exercises. Furthermore, the greater cardiovascular strain associated with upper-body work must be kept in mind when one prescribes exercise for individuals with cardiovascular disease.

CHECK YOUR COMPREHENSION 2

Kara has been working out at the YMCA for over a year. Her typical work includes 15 minutes of stair-climbing and 15 minutes of treadmill walking at an estimated 60% of HRmax (or 100 b·min⁻¹). Kara is interested in adding additional modalities to her workout routine and is considering using the newly purchased arm-crank ergometer. Is it appropriate for Kara to work out on the arm ergometer at an intensity that elicits a HR of 100 b·min⁻¹? Why or why not?

Check your answer in Appendix C.

Cardiovascular Responses to Static Exercise

Static work occurs repeatedly during daily activities, such as lifting and carrying heavy objects. It is also a common form of activity encountered in many occupational settings, particularly manufacturing jobs where lifting is common. Additionally, many sports and recreational activities have a static component associated with their performance. For example, weight lifting, rowing, and racquet sports all involve static exercise. The magnitude of the cardiovascular response to static exercise is affected by several factors, but most noticeably by the intensity of muscle contraction.

Intensity of Muscle Contraction

The cardiovascular response to static exercise depends on the intensity of contraction, provided the contraction is held for a specified time period. The intensity of a static contraction is expressed as a percentage of maximal voluntary contraction (%MVC). **Figure 12.12** illustrates the cardiovascular response to static contractions of the forearm (handgrip) muscles at 10%, 20%, and 50% MVC. Notice that at 10% and 20% MVC the contraction could be held for 5 minutes, but at 50% MVC the contraction could be held for only 2 minutes. Thus, as in aerobic exercise, intensity and duration are inversely related. Also note that the data presented in this figure are from handgrip exercises. Although the pattern of response appears to be similar for different muscle groups, the actual values may vary considerably depending on the amount of active muscle involved.

Cardiac output increases during static contractions due to an increase in HR, with the magnitude of the increase dependent on the intensity of exercise. SV (**Figure 12.12B**) remains relatively constant or decreases slightly during low-intensity contractions and decreases during high-intensity contractions. There is a marked increase in SV immediately following the cessation of high-intensity contractions (Lind et al., 1964; Smith et al., 1993). This is the same rebound rise in recovery as seen in a-vO₂diff, $\dot{V}_E$, and $\dot{V}O_2$ (see **Figure 4.5**). The reduction in SV during high-intensity contractions probably results from both a decreased preload and an increased afterload. Preload is decreased because of high intrathoracic pressure, which compresses the vena cava and thus decreases the return of venous blood to the heart. Because arterial BP is markedly elevated during static contractions (increased afterload), less blood is ejected at a given force of contraction. HR (**Figure 12.12C**) increases during static exercise. The magnitude and the rate of the increase in HR depend on the intensity of contraction. The greater the intensity, the greater the HR response.

Static exercise is characterized by a rapid increase in both systolic pressure and diastolic pressure, termed the **pressor response**, which appears to be inappropriate for the amount of work produced by the contracting muscle (Lind et al., 1964). Since both systolic and diastolic pressures increase, there is a marked increase in MAP (**Figure 12.12D**) (Donald et al., 1967; Lind et al., 1964; Seals et al., 1985; Tuttle and Horvath, 1957). As in any muscular work, static exercise increases metabolic demands of the active muscle. However, in static work, high intramuscular tension results in mechanical constriction of the blood vessels, which impedes blood flow to the muscle. The reduction in muscle blood flow during static exercise results in a buildup of local by-products of metabolism. These chemical by-products [H⁺, adenosine diphosphate, and others] stimulate sensory nerve endings, which leads to a pressor reflex, causing a rise in MAP (pressor response). This rise is substantially larger than the increase during aerobic exercise requiring similar energy expenditure (Asmussen, 1981; Hanson and Nagle, 1985). Notice in **Figure 12.12D** that holding a handgrip dynamometer at 20% MVC for 5 minutes resulted in an increase of 20–30 mmHg in MAP, and holding 50% MVC for 2 minutes caused a 50 mmHg increase in MAP!

Total peripheral resistance, indicated by TPR in **Figure 12.12E**, decreases during static exercise, although not to the extent seen in dynamic aerobic exercise. The smaller decrease in resistance helps to explain the higher BP response to static contractions. The high BP generated during static contractions helps overcome resistance to blood flow from mechanical occlusion. Because the SBP and the HR both increase during static exercise,

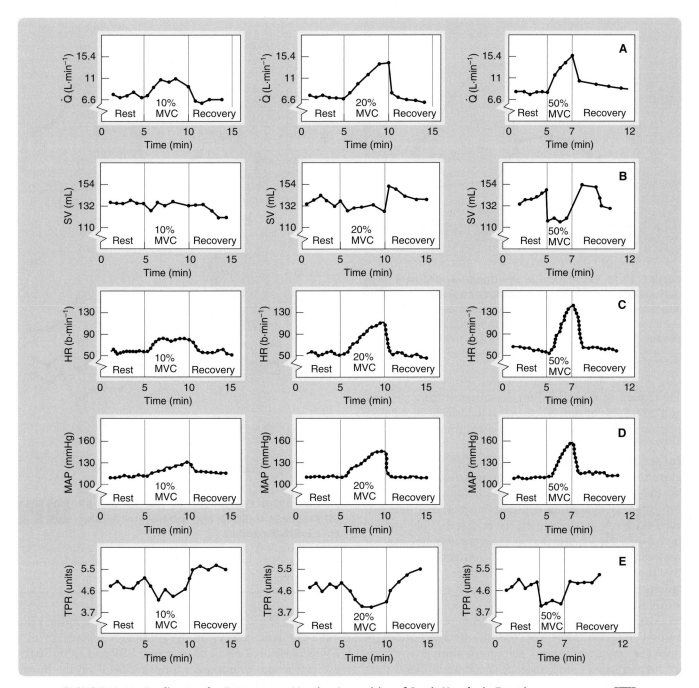

FIGURE 12.12 Cardiovascular Response to Varying Intensities of Static Handgrip Exercise.
A. Cardiac output ($\dot{Q}$). **B.** Stroke volume (SV). **C.** Heart rate (HR). **D.** Mean arterial pressure (MAP).
E. Total peripheral resistance (TPR).
Source: Modified from Lind, A. R., S. H. Taylor, P. W. Humphreys, B. M. Kennelly, & K. W. Donald: The circulatory effects of sustained voluntary muscle contraction. *Clinical Science*. 27:229–244 (1964). Reprinted with permission of the Biochemical Society and Portland Press.

there is a large increase in myocardial oxygen consumption and thus rate-pressure product.

Table 12.1 summarizes cardiovascular responses to static exercise.

> **Pressor Response** The rapid increase in both systolic pressure and diastolic pressure during static exercise.

Blood Flow during Static Contractions

Blood flow to the working muscle is impeded during static contractions because of the mechanical constriction of the blood vessel supplying the contracting muscle (Freund et al., 1979; Sjogaard et al., 1988). **Figure 12.13** depicts blood flow in the quadriceps muscle when a 5% and 25% MVC contraction were held to fatigue. The 5%

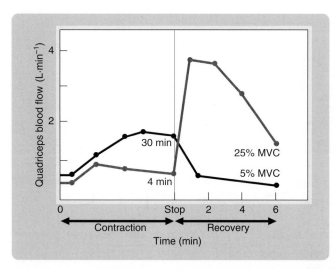

FIGURE 12.13 Blood Flow in the Quadriceps Muscle during Different Intensities of Static Contraction.
Source: Sjogaard, G., G. Savard, & C. Juel: Muscle blood flow during isometric activity and its relation to muscle fatigue. *European Journal of Physiology*. 57:327–335 (1988). Reprinted by permission.

MVC load could be held for 30 minutes; the 25% load could be held for only 4 minutes. Quadriceps blood flow is greater during the 5% MVC, suggesting that at 25% MVC there is considerable impedance to blood flow. In fact, blood flow during the 25% MVC load was very close to resting levels despite the metabolic work done by the muscle. The response occurring during recovery suggests that when contraction ceases, a mechanical occlusion to the muscle is released. The marked increase in blood flow during recovery compensates for the reduced flow during sustained contraction. The relative force at which blood flow is impeded varies greatly among different muscle groups (Lind and McNichol, 1967; Rowell, 1993).

Mechanical constriction also occurs during dynamic aerobic exercise. However, the alternating periods of muscular contraction and relaxation during rhythmical activity allow—and, indeed, encourage—blood flow, especially through the venous system.

Comparison of Aerobic and Static Exercise

Figure 12.14 compares the HR and the BP responses to fatiguing handgrip (static) exercise (30% MVC held to fatigue) and a maximal treadmill (incremental aerobic) test to fatigue. The incremental aerobic exercise is characterized by a large increase in the HR, which contributes to an increased cardiac output. The treadmill exercise response also shows a modest increase in the SBP and a relatively stable or decreasing DBP. Aerobic exercise is said to impose a "volume load" on the heart. Increased venous return leads to increased SV, which contributes to an increased cardiac output. In contrast, fatiguing static

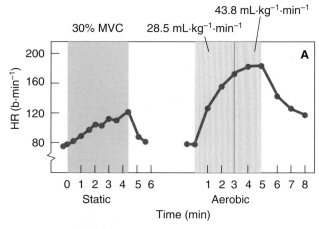

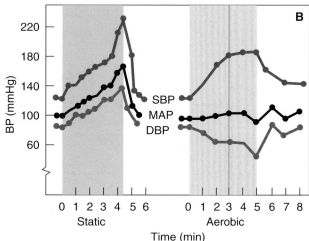

FIGURE 12.14 Comparison of HR (A) and BP (B) Response to Static and Incremental Aerobic Exercise to Maximum.
Source: Lind, A. Cardiovascular responses to static exercise. *Circulation*. XLI(2): 173–176 (1970). Reproduced with permission. Copyright 1970 American Heart Association.

exercise is characterized by a modest increase in the HR, but a dramatic increase in the BP (*pressor response*). Mean BP increases as a result of increased SBP and DBP. Static exercise is said to impose a "pressure load" on the heart. Increased MAP means that the heart must pump harder to overcome the pressure in the aorta.

Cardiovascular Responses to Dynamic Resistance Exercise

Weight-lifting or resistance exercise includes a combination of dynamic and static contractions (Hill and Butler, 1991; MacDougall et al., 1985). At the beginning of the lift, a static contraction exists until muscle force exceeds the load to be lifted and movement occurs, leading to a dynamic concentric (shortening) contraction as the lift continues. This is then followed by a dynamic eccentric (lengthening) contraction during the lowering phase (McCartney, 1999). A static component is always associated with gripping the barbell. During dynamic resistance exercise, cardiorespiratory system responses are dissociated from the energy demand. In contrast, during dynamic endurance activity, responses in the cardiorespiratory system are directly related to the use of oxygen for energy production. In part, the reason for this dissociation between oxygen use and cardiovascular response to resistance exercise is that much of the energy required for resistance exercise comes from anaerobic (without oxygen) sources. Another important difference between resistance exercise and aerobic exercise is the mechanical constriction of blood flow during resistance exercise because of the static nature of the contraction.

The magnitude of the cardiovascular response to resistance exercise depends on the intensity of the load (the weight lifted) and the number of repetitions performed. Cardiovascular responses also depend on how the load and repetitions are combined.

Varying Load/Constant Repetitions

As expected, cardiovascular responses are greater when heavier loads are lifted, assuming the number of repetitions is constant (Fleck, 1988; Fleck and Dean, 1987). For example, as shown in **Figure 12.15**, when participants performed 10 repetitions of arm curling exercises with dumbbells of three different weights (identified as light, moderate, and heavy), the SBP was highest at the completion of the heaviest set (Wescott and Howes, 1983). The SBP increased 16%, 22%, and 34% during the light, moderate, and heavy sets, respectively. The DBP, measured by auscultation, did not change significantly with any of the sets. There is disagreement about the DBP response to resistance exercise; some authors report an increase, while others report no change (Fleck, 1988; Fleck and Dean, 1987; Wescott and Howes, 1983).

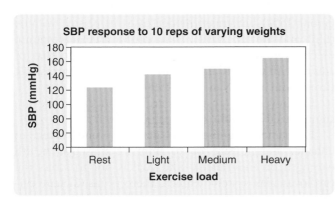

FIGURE 12.15 Systolic Blood Pressure (SBP) Response at the Completion of 10 Reps of Arm Curls Using Different Weights.
Source: Based on data from Wescott and Howes (1983).

These discrepancies may reflect differences in measurement techniques (auscultation versus intra-arterial assessment) and timing of the measurement.

Varying Load/Repetitions to Failure

A different pattern of response is seen when a given load is performed to fatigue, which lifters typically call failure. In this case, the individual performs maximal work regardless of the load. **Figure 12.16** shows the cardiovascular response at the completion of leg extension exercise performed to failure. Participants performed 50%, 80%, and 100% of their one repetition maximum (1-RM) as many times as they could, and cardiovascular variables were recorded at the end of each set (Falkel et al., 1992). Participants could perform the 100% load only one time, of course, but they could perform the 80% and 50% loads an average of 8 and 15 times, respectively. Thus, the greatest amount (volume) of work was performed when the lightest load was lifted the greatest number of times. Cardiac output at the completion of the set was highest when the lightest load was lifted for the most repetitions—that is, when the total work was greatest (**Figure 12.16A**).

The SV at the end of a set was similar for each condition (**Figure 12.16B**) and was slightly below resting levels. This is in contrast to significant increases in the SV that occur during aerobic exercise. Thus, dynamic resistance exercise does not produce the SV overload of dynamic aerobic exercise (Hill and Butler, 1991; McCartney, 1999). The HR was highest after completion of the set using the lightest load and lifting it the most times (**Figure 12.16C**). The HR was lowest when a single repetition using the heaviest weight was performed, and hence when the least amount of work was done. HRs between 130 and 160 b·min⁻¹ have been reported during resistance exercise (Hill and Butler, 1991). There is some evidence that the HR and the BP attained at fatigue are the same when loads between 60% and 100% of 1-RM are used, regardless of the number of times the load can be performed (Nau et al., 1990).

Constant Load/Repetitions to Failure

When the load is heavy, MAP and HR increase with succeeding repetitions in a set to failure (Fleck and Dean, 1987; MacDougall et al., 1985). **Figure 12.17A** shows the MAP, measured intra-arterially, during a set of leg press exercises that represented 95% of 1-RM; **Figure 12.17B** shows the HR during these exercises. In this study, peak SBP averaged 320 mmHg, and peak DBP averaged 250 mmHg! The dramatic increase in BP during dynamic resistance exercise results from the mechanical compression of blood vessels and performance of the Valsalva maneuver (as explained in Chapter 10). The TPR is higher during dynamic resistance exercise than during

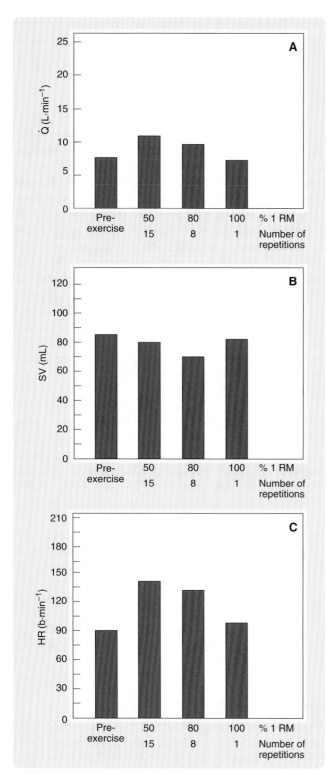

FIGURE 12.16 Cardiovascular Response at the Completion of Dynamic Resistance Exercise (Concentric Knee Extension Exercise) to Failure with Varying loads.
A. Cardiac output($\dot{\text{Q}}$). **B.** Stroke volume (SV). **C.** Heart rate (HR).
Source: Based on data from Falkel, J. E., S. J. Fleck, & T. F. Murray: Comparison of central hemodynamics between powerlifters and bodybuilders during resistance exercise. *Journal of Applied Sport Science Research*. 6(1):24–35 (1992).

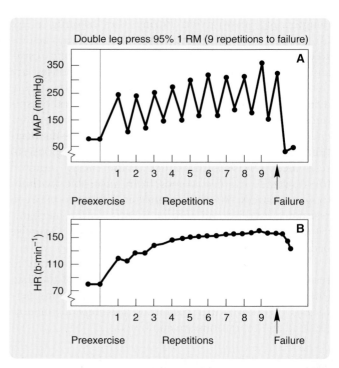

FIGURE 12.17 Mean arterial pressure (MAP; panel A) and heart rate (HR; panel B) Response during a Set of Dynamic Resistance Exercise to Failure.
Source: MacDougall, J. D., D. Tuxen, D. G. Sale, J. R. Moroz, & J. R. Sutton: Arterial blood pressure response to heavy resistance exercise. *Journal of Applied Physiology*. 58(3):785–790 (1985). Reprinted with permission.

dynamic aerobic exercise because of the vasoconstriction caused by the pressor reflex. In fact, some studies have reported a slight increase in the TPR during resistance exercise, rather than the decrease observed with aerobic exercise (Lentini et al., 1993; McCartney, 1999; Miles et al., 1987). Myocardial oxygen consumption and thus the rate-pressure product can reach extremely high levels because of the tachycardia and the exaggerated SBP response. Dynamic resistance exercise also causes large (about 15%) but transient decreases in plasma volume (Hill and Butler, 1991). The cardiovascular response of children to resistance exercise is similar to that of adults, with the HR and the BP increasing progressively throughout a set (Nau et al., 1990).

Cardiovascular responses to resistance exercise are summarized in **Table 12.1**.

Resistance exercises are generally undertaken to enhance muscle size or to improve muscular health (strength or endurance). The goal is not to stress the cardiovascular system. Hence, there is insufficient evidence to adequately compare cardiovascular responses to resistance exercise among different populations (male versus female, children versus adult, and young versus older adults). Therefore, this exercise category is not included in the following sections.

Male-Female Cardiovascular Differences during Exercise

The pattern of cardiovascular responses to aerobic exercise is similar for both sexes, although the magnitude of the response may vary for some variables. Many of the differences in cardiovascular responses between the sexes are related to differences in body size and structure.

Short-Term, Light to Moderate and Long-Term, Moderate to Heavy Submaximal Exercise

Females have a higher cardiac output and HR, but a lower SV, than males during submaximal exercise when work is performed at the same absolute workload (Åstrand et al., 1964; Becklake et al., 1965; Freedson et al., 1979). The higher HR more than compensates for the lower SV in females, resulting in the higher cardiac output seen at the same absolute workload. Thus, if a male and a female perform the same exercise, the female will typically be stressing the cardiovascular system to a greater extent (**Figure 12.18**). This relative disadvantage to women results from several factors. First, females typically are smaller than males; they have a smaller heart and less

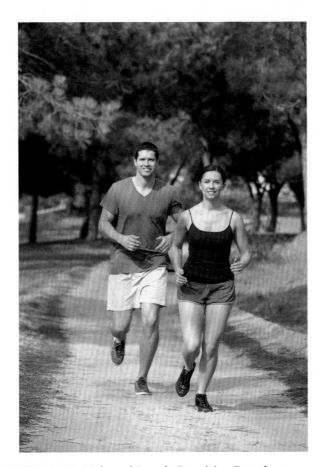

FIGURE 12.18 Male and Female Exercising Together.

muscle mass. Second, they have a lower oxygen-carrying capacity than males. Finally, they typically have lower aerobic capacity ($\dot{V}O_2$max).

When males and females perform the same relative workload (both working at the same percentage of their $\dot{V}O_2$max), a different pattern emerges. The importance of distinguishing between relative and absolute workloads is shown in **Figure 12.19**. This figure shows results from a study that compared the cardiovascular response of men and women to the same absolute work rate (600 kg·min⁻¹) and the same relative work rate (50% of $\dot{V}O_2$max). Although cardiac output was higher in women during the same absolute work rate, it is lower for women when the same relative work rate was performed (**Figure 12.19A**). The SV (**Figure 12.19B**) was lower in women than in men whether the work was expressed on an absolute or relative basis. Notice that the values are very similar for both conditions, suggesting that the SV has plateaued as would be expected at 50% of $\dot{V}O_2$max in both conditions. The difference in HR between the sexes (**Figure 12.19C**) was smaller when exercise was performed at the same relative work rate.

Males and females display the same pattern of response for BP; however, males tend to have a higher SBP at the same relative workloads (Deschenes et al., 2006; Malina and Bouchard, 1991; Ogawa et al., 1992). Much of the difference in the magnitude of the BP response is attributable to differences in resting SBP. The DBP response to submaximal exercise is very similar for both sexes. Thus, MAP is slightly greater in males during submaximal work at the same relative workload. The pattern of response for resistance is similar for males and females, although males typically have a lower resistance because of their greater cardiac output. Males and females both exhibit cardiovascular drift during heavy, prolonged submaximal exercise. Changes in plasma volume appear to be greater in men than in women at the same absolute submaximal exercise intensity (Deschenes et al., 2006).

Incremental Aerobic Exercise to Maximum

The cardiovascular response to incremental exercise is similar for both sexes, although again there are differences in the maximal values attained. Maximal oxygen consumption ($\dot{V}O_2$max) is higher for males than for females. When $\dot{V}O_2$max is expressed in absolute values (L·min⁻¹), males typically have values that are 40–60% higher than in females (Åstrand, 1952; Sparling, 1980). When differences in body size are considered and $\dot{V}O_2$max values are expressed relative to body weight (in mL·kg⁻¹·min⁻¹), the differences between the sexes decrease to 20–30%. If differences in body composition are considered and $\dot{V}O_2$max is expressed relative to fat-free mass (in mL·kg⁻¹ of fat-free mass per minute), the difference between the sexes is reduced to 0–15% (Sparling, 1980). Reporting $\dot{V}O_2$max relative to fat-free mass is important in terms of understanding the influence of adiposity and fat-free mass on

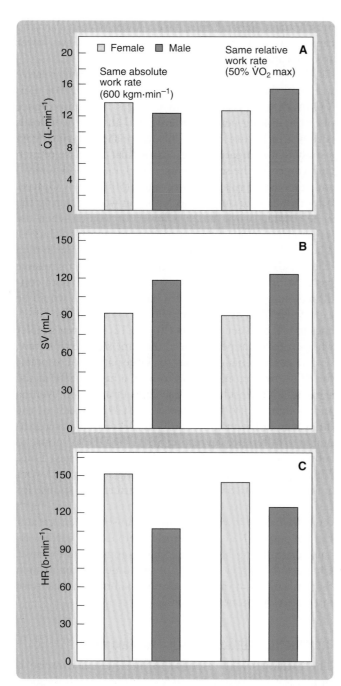

FIGURE 12.19 Comparison of Cardiovascular Responses of Men and Women to Submaximal Aerobic Exercise.
A. Cardiac output (Q̇). **B.** Stroke volume (SV). **C.** Heart rate (HR).
Source: Data from Astrand, P.: *Experimental Studies of Physical Working Capacity in Relation to Sex and Age.* Copenhagen, Munksgaard: University Microfilms International (1952).

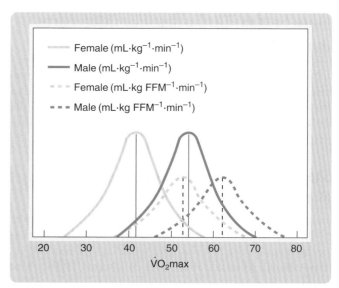

FIGURE 12.20 Distribution of V̇O$_2$max for Males and Females.
Source: Wells, C. L., & S. A. Plowman: Sexual differences in athletic performance: Biological or behavioral? *Physician and Sports Medicine.* 11(8):52–63 (1983). Reprinted by permission.

V̇O$_2$max. However, it is not a very practical way to express V̇O$_2$max because, in reality, consuming oxygen only in relation to fat-free mass is not an option. Individuals cannot leave their fat mass behind when exercising.

Figure 12.20 represents the distribution of V̇O$_2$max values for males and females expressed per kilogram of

weight and per kilogram of fat-free mass. This figure demonstrates the important point that there is considerable variability in V̇O$_2$max for both sexes. Thus, although males generally have a higher V̇O$_2$max, some females will have a higher V̇O$_2$max than the average male.

Figure 12.21 shows the differences in V̇O$_2$max, expressed in relative terms (**Figure 12.21A**) and absolute terms (**Figure 12.21B**), and average body weight (**Figure 12.21C**) between the sexes across the age span. Differences in V̇O$_2$max are largely explained by the differences in the size of the heart (and thus maximal cardiac output) and the differences in the oxygen-carrying capacity of the blood. Males have approximately 6% more red blood cells and 10–15% more hemoglobin than females; thus, males have a greater oxygen-carrying capacity (Åstrand et al., 2003).

Males typically have a maximal cardiac output that is 30% higher than that of females (Wells and Plowman, 1983). Maximal SV is higher for men, but the increase in SV during maximal exercise is achieved by the same mechanisms in both sexes (Sullivan et al., 1991). Furthermore, if maximal SV is expressed relative to body weight, there is no difference between the sexes. The maximal HR is similar for both sexes.

Males and females display the same pattern of BP response; however, males attain a higher SBP than females at maximal exercise (Malina and Bouchard, 1991; Ogawa et al., 1992; Wanne and Haapoja, 1988). The DBP response to maximal exercise is similar for both sexes. Thus, MAP is slightly greater in males at the completion of maximal work. The pattern of response for resistance and rate-pressure product is the same for both sexes. Resistance is greatly reduced during maximal exercise

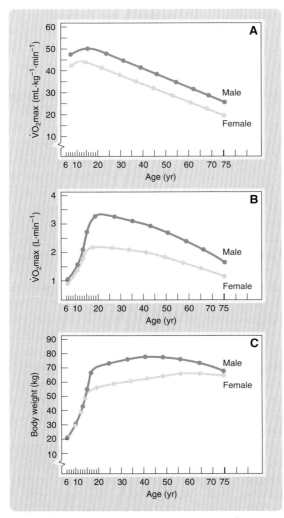

FIGURE 12.21 Maximal Oxygen Consumption (V̇O₂max) expressed in relative (A) and absolute terms (B) and Body Weight for Males and Females from 6 to 75 Years.
Source: Shvartz, E. & R. C. Reibold: Aerobic fitness norms for males and females aged 6 to 75 years: A review. *Aviation, Space, and Environmental Physiology*. 61:3–11 (1990). Reprinted by permission.

Table 12.2 summarizes the differences between the sexes in cardiovascular variables at various exercise levels.

Static Exercise

The HR response to static exercise (**Figure 12.22A**) is similar in males and females (Misner et al., 1990). However, as shown in **Figure 12.22B**, when a group of young adult, healthy participants held maximal contractions of the handgrip muscles for 2 minutes, the BPs reported for women were significantly lower than those reported for men (Misner et al., 1990). The SV and cardiac output responses in women during maximal static contraction of the finger flexors were similar to the responses previously reported in men, but no direct comparisons between men and women were made in this study (Smith et al., 1993).

Cardiovascular Responses of Children and Adolescents to Exercise

The pattern of responses in the cardiovascular variables in children and adolescents to aerobic exercise is similar to the pattern in adults. This is not meant to imply that children are simply "little adults." Often, the actual values are higher or lower than those for adults, but overall, the direction and the relative degree of change are very similar across the age range. Differences can frequently be attributed to differences in body size, structure, and maturity (Rowland, 2005a,b).

Short-Term, Light to Moderate and Long-Term, Moderate to Heavy Submaximal Exercise

The pattern of cardiac output response to submaximal aerobic exercise is similar in children and adolescents to adults, with cardiac output increasing rapidly at the onset of exercise and plateauing at a *steady state*. However, children have a lower cardiac output than adults at all levels of exercise, primarily because children have a lower SV at any level of exercise (Bar-Or, 1983; Rowland, 1990). As children grow and mature, cardiac output and SV increase

in both sexes. Because the HR response is similar and the SBP is greater in males, males tend to have a higher rate-pressure product at maximal exercise levels than do females.

TABLE 12.2 Cardiovascular Variables for Females Compared to Males				
Variable	**Rest**	**Exercise Condition**		
		Absolute, Submaximal	**Relative, Submaximal**	**Incremental, Maximal**
V̇O₂max	—	—	—	Lower
Q̇	Lower	Higher	?	Lower
SV	Lower	Lower	Lower	Lower
HR	Higher	Higher	Higher	Similar
Source: Wells, C. L.: *Women, Sport and Performance* (2nd edition). Champaign, IL: Human Kinetics (1991).				

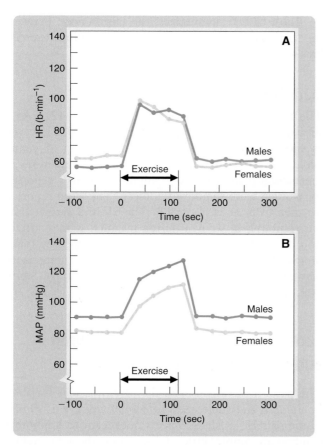

FIGURE 12.22 Heart rate (HR; panel A) and Mean arterial pressure (MAP; panel B) Response of Males and Females to Static Exercise.
Source: Misner, J. E., S. B. Going, B. H. Massey, T. E. Ball, M. G. Bemben, & L. K. Essandoh: Cardiovascular response in males and females to sustained maximal voluntary static muscle contraction. *Medicine and Science in Sports and Exercise.* 22(2):194–199 (1990). Reprinted by permission of Williams & Wilkins.

progressive rise in HR, simultaneous decreases in SV and MAP, and no change in cardiac output with prolonged exercise (Asano and Hirakoba, 1984; Rowland, 2005a). SV in girls is less than that in boys at all levels of exercise (Bar-Or, 1983).

As always, the magnitude of the cardiovascular response depends on the intensity of the exercise. **Table 12.3** reports the cardiac output, SV, and HR values of children 8–12 years old during treadmill exercise at 40%, 53%, and 68% of $\dot{V}O_2$max (Lussier and Buskirk, 1977). Both cardiac output and HR increase in response to increasing intensities of exercise. SV peaks at 40% of $\dot{V}O_2$max and changes little with increasing exercise intensity. This is consistent with the finding that SV plateaus at 40–50% of $\dot{V}O_2$max in adults (Åstrand et al., 1964).

The SBP in children increases during exercise, as it does in adults, and depends on the intensity of the exercise. Boys tend to have a higher SBP than girls (Malina and Bouchard, 1991). The magnitude of the increase in systolic pressure at submaximal exercise is less in children than in adults (James et al., 1980; Wanne and Haapoja, 1988). The failure of SBP to reach adult levels is probably the result of lower cardiac output in children. As children mature, the increases in the SBP during exercise become greater. Diastolic pressure changes little during exercise but is lower in children than adults (James et al., 1980; Wanne and Haapoja, 1988).

Similar decreases in resistance occur in children as in adults, a result of vasodilation in working muscles. Rate-pressure product increases in children and adolescents during exercise. However, the work of the heart reflects the higher HR and lower SBP for these age groups than for adults. Blood flow through the exercising muscle appears to be greater in children than in adults, resulting in a higher a-vO_2diff and thereby compensating partially for the lower cardiac output (Rowland, 1990; Rowland and Green, 1988).

Incremental Aerobic Exercise to Maximum

The cardiovascular responses to incremental exercise to maximum are similar for children, adolescents, and adults; however, children and adolescents achieve a lower maximal cardiac output and a lower maximal SV. HR rises in a rectilinear fashion with incremental exercise

at rest and during exercise. The lower SV in children is compensated for, to some extent, by a higher HR. The HR response to any given exercise intensity is highest in young children (Bar-Or, 1983; Cunningham et al., 1984) and declines as children grow into adolescents (Rowland, 2005a,b). Children, adolescents, and adults all exhibit the cardiovascular drift phenomenon of a slight (~15%)

TABLE 12.3	Cardiovascular Responses in Children to Submaximal Exercise of Various Intensities		
Variable	**Intensity of Exercise (%$\dot{V}O_2$max)**		
	40%	**53%**	**68%**
$\dot{Q}$ (L·min^{-1})	6.7	7.6	8.5
SV (mL·b^{-1})	53	51	49
HR (b·min^{-1})	126	149	173

Source: Lussier, L. & E. R. Buskirk: Effects of an endurance training regimen on assessment of work capacity in prepubertal children. *Annals of the New York Academy of Sciences.* 30:734–777 (1977).

in children as in adults. However, at approximately 60% $\dot{V}O_2$max, it begins to taper. Maximal HR is higher in children than in adults and is not age dependent until the late teens (Cunningham et al., 1984; Rowland, 1996, 2005a).

The maximal oxygen consumption typically attained by youths between the ages of 6 and 18 is shown in **Figure 12.23**. As children grow, their ability to take in, transport, and utilize oxygen improves. This improvement represents dimensional and maturational changes—specifically, heart volume, maximal SV, maximal cardiac output, blood volume and hemoglobin concentration, and a-vO_2diff increase.

The rate of improvement in absolute $\dot{V}O_2$max (expressed in L·min^{-1}) is similar for boys and girls until approximately 12 years of age (**Figure 12.23A**). Maximal oxygen uptake continues to increase in boys until the age of 18; it remains relatively constant in girls between the ages of 14 and 18 years.

When $\dot{V}O_2$max is expressed relative to body weight (expressed as mL·kg^{-1}·min^{-1}), it remains relatively constant throughout the years between 8 and 16 for boys (**Figure 12.23B**). However, $\dot{V}O_2$max (expressed as mL·kg^{-1}·min^{-1}) tends to decrease in girls as they enter puberty and their adiposity increases (**Figure 12.23B**). As children mature, they also grow, and the developmental changes indicated previously are largely offset if $\dot{V}O_2$max is described per kilogram of body weight. The large area of overlap for reported values of $\dot{V}O_2$max for boys and girls in **Figure 12.23** reflects the large variability in $\dot{V}O_2$max among children and adolescents.

There appears to be a major difference between children/adolescents and adults in terms of the meaning of $\dot{V}O_2$max. In adults, $\dot{V}O_2$max reflects both physiological function (cardiorespiratory power) and cardiovascular endurance (the ability to perform strenuous, large-muscle exercise for a prolonged period of time) (Taylor et al., 1955). In children and adolescents, $\dot{V}O_2$max is not as directly related to cardiorespiratory endurance as in adults (Bar-Or, 1983; Krahenbuhl et al., 1985; Rowland, 1990). **Figure 12.24B** shows performance as determined by the number of stages or minutes completed in the PACER test (Léger et al., 1988). This progressive aerobic cardiovascular endurance run (PACER) was described in Chapter 11. Recall that a higher number of laps completed is positively associated with a higher $\dot{V}O_2$max. **Figure 12.24A** shows that for boys, the mean estimated value of $\dot{V}O_2$max, expressed in mL·kg^{-1}·min^{-1}, changes very little from age 6 to 18. However, mean performance on the PACER test (**Figure 12.24B**) shows a definite linear improvement with age. The girls show the same trend as the boys before puberty, but thereafter, $\dot{V}O_2$max declines steadily and PACER performance plateaus. Similar results have been reported for treadmill endurance times and other distance runs (Cumming et al., 1978) and measured $\dot{V}O_2$max as well as estimated (Rowland, 2005a). Thus, in general, endurance performance improves

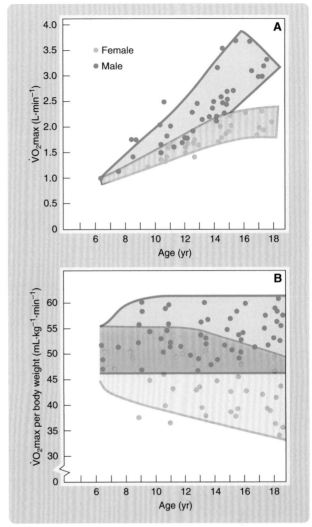

FIGURE 12.23 Maximal Oxygen Consumption ($\dot{V}O_2$max) of Children and Adolescents.
A. Changes in $\dot{V}O_2$max in children and adolescents during the ages of 6–18 years are expressed in absolute terms. The dots represent means from various studies. The outer lines indicate normal variability in values. **B.** Changes in $\dot{V}O_2$max in children and adolescents during the ages of 6–18 years are expressed relative to body weight. The dots represent means from various studies. The outer lines indicate normal variability in reported values.
Source: Bar-Or, O.: Physiologic principles to clinical applications. *Pediatric Sports Medicine for the Practitioner*. New York, NY: Springer-Verlag (1983). Reprinted by permission.

progressively throughout childhood, at least until puberty, but $\dot{V}O_2$max, expressed relative to body size, does not.

The reason for the weak association between $\dot{V}O_2$max and endurance performance in young people is unknown. The most frequent suggestion is that children use more aerobic energy (require greater oxygen) than adults at any submaximal pace. This phenomenon is called running economy and is fully discussed in the unit on metabolism (Chapter 4). More important than the actual oxygen consumption at a set pace, however, may be the percentage

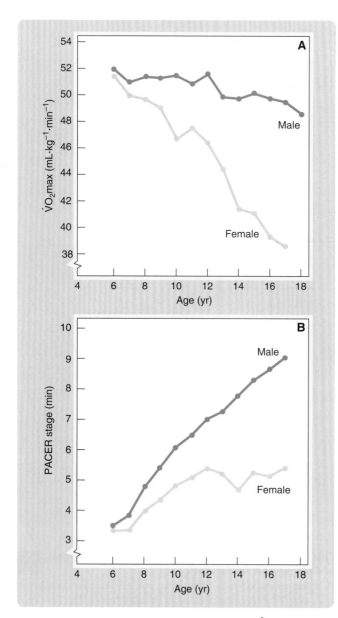

motivated to perform exercise tests and therefore do not perform well despite high $\dot{V}O_2$max capabilities.

The BP response is similar for children and adults; however, there are again age- or size-related quantitative differences. For a given level of exercise, a small child responds with a lower SBP and DBP than an adolescent, and an adolescent responds with lower BP than an adult. The lower BP response in young children is consistent with their lower SV response. Typically, boys have a higher peak SBP than girls (Riopel et al., 1979; Wade and Freund, 1990). This difference too is most likely attributable to differences in SV. Myocardial oxygen consumption at maximal exercise increases as children grow—predominantly through the influence of higher maximal SBP since maximal HR is stable until late adolescence.

Table 12.4 reports typical cardiovascular responses to maximal exercise in prepubescent and postpubescent children.

Static Exercise

Children's and adolescents' cardiovascular responses to static exercise appear to be similar to adults' (Rowland, 2005a,b). Table 12.5 presents data from two studies that investigated cardiovascular responses to 3 minutes of leg extension exercise at 30% of MVC. One study tested young men between the ages of 25 and 34 (Bezucha et al., 1982), and the other young boys aged 7–12 (Rowland et al., 2006). In both studies, static exercise resulted in typical responses: an increased MAP, an elevated HR, a decreased SV, and a small rise in cardiac output. Similarly, a study that compared premenarcheal girls and young women found no differences in cardiovascular responses to 3 minutes of 30% MVC of the handgrip muscles (Smith et al., 2000).

FIGURE 12.24 **Maximal Oxygen Consumption ($\dot{V}O_2$max; panel A) and Endurance Performance (panel B) in Children and Adolescents.**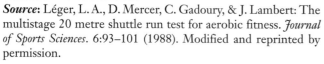
Source: Léger, L. A., D. Mercer, C. Gadoury, & J. Lambert: The multistage 20 metre shuttle run test for aerobic fitness. *Journal of Sports Sciences*. 6:93–101 (1988). Modified and reprinted by permission.

Cardiovascular Responses of Older Adults to Exercise

Aging is associated with diminishing function in many systems of the body. Thus, aging is characterized by a decreased ability to respond to physiological stress (Skinner, 1993). There is considerable debate, though, about how much loss of function is inevitably related to age, how much is related to disease, and how much can be attributed to a sedentary lifestyle often accompanying aging. Each of these factors causes decrements in function, but for an individual, it is often difficult to know which one or which combination may cause an observed change.

Many older adults remain active into their later years and perform amazing athletic feats. For example, Mavis Lindgren began an exercise program of walking in her early 60s. She slowly increased her training volume and began jogging. At age 70, she completed her first

of $\dot{V}O_2$max that value represents, and more so in children than adolescents (McCormack et al., 1991). Other factors that may affect endurance running performance in children and adolescents include body composition, particularly the percentage of body fat; sprint speed, possibly as a reflection of a high percentage of muscle fibers differentiated for speed and power; and various aspects of body size (Cureton et al., 1991, 1977; Mayhew and Gifford, 1975; McVeigh et al., 1995). There is also the possibility that many children and adolescents are not

TABLE 12.4 Cardiovascular Responses to Maximal Exercise in Prepubescent and Postpubescent Children

Variable	Boys		Girls	
	10 yr	15 yr	10 yr	15 yr
$\dot{Q}$ (L·min^{-1})	12	18	11	14
SV (mL·b^{-1})	60	90	55	70
HR (b·min^{-1})	200	200	200	200
$\dot{V}O_2$ (L·min^{-1})	1.7	3.5	1.5	2.0
SBP (mmHg)	144	174	140	170
DBP (mmHg)	64	64	64	64
MAP (mmHg)	105	110	103	117.5
TPR (units)	7.0	6.1	9.4	8.4
RPP (units)	290	350	280	340

Sources: Astrand, P.: *Experimental Studies of Physical Working Capacity in Relation to Sex and Age.* Copenhagent, Munksgaard: University Microfilms International (1952); Rowland, T. W.: *Exercise and Children's Health.* Champaign, IL: Human Kinetics (1990).

marathon. In the next 12 years, she raced in over 50 marathons (Nieman, 1990). Many studies of physical activity suggest that by remaining active in the older years, individuals can markedly reduce loss of cardiovascular function, even if they do not run a marathon.

Short-Term, Light to Moderate and Long-Term, Moderate to Heavy Submaximal Exercise

At the same absolute submaximal workload, cardiac output and SV are lower in older adults, but HR is higher than in younger adults. The pattern of systolic and diastolic pressure is the same for younger and older individuals. The difference in resting BP is maintained throughout the exercise, so that older individuals have a higher SBP, DBP, and MAP at any given level of exercise (Ogawa et al., 1992). The higher BP response is related to a higher TPR in older individuals, resulting from a loss of elasticity in the blood vessels. Because HR and SBP are higher for any given level of exercise in older adults, myocardial oxygen consumption and thus rate-pressure product are also higher in older individuals than in younger adults.

Incremental Aerobic Exercise to Maximum

Maximal cardiac output is lower in older individuals than in younger adults. This results from a lower maximal HR and a lower maximal SV. Maximal SV decreases with advancing age, and the decline is of similar magnitude for both men and women, although women have a much smaller maximal SV initially. Maximal HR decreases with age but does not vary significantly between the sexes. A decrease of approximately 10% per decade, starting at approximately age 30, has been reported for $\dot{V}O_2$max in sedentary and active adults (Åstrand, 1960; Heath et al., 1981; Wilson and Tanka, 2000). There is some indication that the rate of decline in $\dot{V}O_2$max is greater in men than in women (Stathokostas et al., 2004; Weiss et al., 2006). **Figure 12.21A** and **B** depict the change in $\dot{V}O_2$max from childhood to 75 years of age.

Like resting BP, SBP and DBP responses to maximal aerobic exercise are typically higher in older individuals than in younger individuals of similar fitness (Ogawa et al., 1992). Maximal SBP may be 20–50 mmHg higher in older individuals, and maximal DBP 15–20 mmHg higher. As a result of an elevated SBP and DBP, MAP is

TABLE 12.5 Cardiovascular Responses of Boys and Men to Static Exercise

	Men		Boys	
	Rest	Exercise	Rest	Exercise
HR (b·min^{-1})	70	110	77	106
SV (mL·b^{-1})	85	62	59	52
$\dot{Q}$ (L·min^{-1})	5.7	6.8	4.8	5.6
MAP (mmHg)			86	109

Sources: Based on the data from Bezucha, G. R., M. C. Lenser, P. G. Hanson, & F. J. Nagle: Comparison of hemodynamic responses to static and dynamic exercise. *Journal of Applied Physiology.* 31:1589–1593 (1982) and Rowland, T.W., K. Heffernan, S. Y. Jae, G. Echols, G. Krull, & B. Fernhall: Cardiovascular responses to static exercise in boys: Insights from tissue Doppler Imaging. *European Journal of Applied Physiology.* 97(5):637–642 (2006).

TABLE 12.6 Cardiovascular Responses to Maximal Exercise in Young and Older Adults

Variable	Men		Women	
	25 yr	65 yr	25 yr	65 yr
$\dot{Q}$ (L·min^{-1})	25	16	18	12
SV (mL·b^{-1})	128	100	92	75
HR (b·min^{-1})	195	155	195	155
$\dot{V}O_2$ (L·min^{-1})	3.5	2.5	2.5	1.5
SBP (mmHg)	190	200	190	200
DBP (mmHg)	70	84	64	84
MAP (mmHg)	130	143	128	143
TPR (units)	5.2	8.9	7.1	11.9
RPP (units)	371	310	371	310

Source: Ogawa, T., R. J. Spina, W. H. Martin, W. M. Kohrt, K. B. Schechtman, J. O. Holloszy, & A. A. Ehsani: Effects of aging, sex, and physical training on cardiovascular responses to exercise. *Circulation.* 86:494–503 (1992).

FIGURE   12.25 Cardiovascular Response of Males by Age to Static Exercise.
A. Cardiac output ($\dot{Q}$). **B.** Stroke volume (SV). **C.** Heart rate (HR). **D.** Systolic blood pressure (SBP). **E.** Diastolic blood pressure (DBP). **F.** Rate-pressure product (RPP).
Source: VanLoan, M. D., B. H. Massey, R. A. Boileau, T. G. Lohman, J. E. Misner, & P. L. Best: Age as a factor in the hemodynamic responses to isometric exercise. *Journal of Sports Medicine and Physical Fitness.* 29(3): 262–268 (1989). Reprinted with permission.

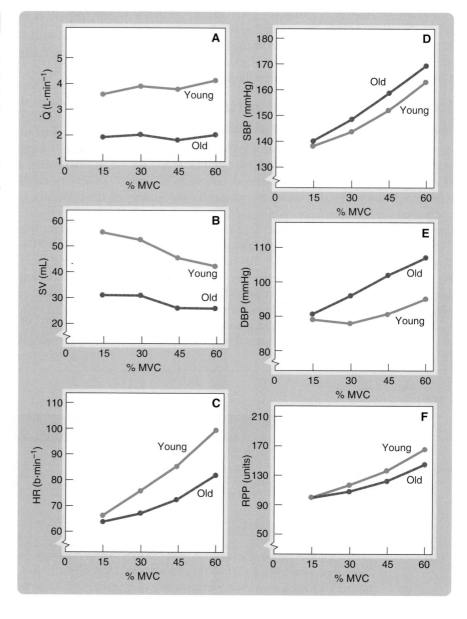

considerably higher at maximal exercise in older than in younger adults.

TPR decreases during aerobic exercise in older adults but not to the same extent as in younger individuals. This difference is a consequence of the loss of elasticity of the connective tissue in the vasculature that accompanies aging. Since the decrease in maximal HR for older individuals is greater than the increase in maximal SBP when compared to younger adults, older individuals have a lower rate-pressure product at maximal exercise. **Table 12.6** presents typical cardiovascular values at maximal exercise in young and old adults of both sexes.

Static Exercise

Many studies have described the cardiovascular responses to static exercise in older adults (Goldstraw and Warren, 1985; Petrofsky and Lind, 1975; Sagiv et al., 1988; VanLoan et al., 1989). As an example, **Figure 12.25** depicts the cardiovascular responses of young and old men to sustained handgrip and leg extension exercise over a range of submaximal static workloads (VanLoan et al., 1989). Note that cardiac output (**Figure 12.25A**) and SV (**Figure 12.25B**) values are lower than normally reported, because of the measurement technique. However, the relative differences between the responses of the young and the older participants show that cardiac output, SV, and HR (**Figure 12.25C**) were lower for the older men than for the younger men at each intensity. In contrast, BP responses (**Figure 12.25D** and **E**) were higher for the older men at each intensity. As with dynamic aerobic exercise, the differences in the cardiovascular responses between the two age groups are probably due to an age-related increase in resistance due to a loss of elasticity in the vasculature and a decreased ability of the myocardium to stretch and contract forcibly (VanLoan et al., 1989). The rate-pressure product (**Figure 12.25F**) was higher for the younger participants than for the older participants at 30%, 45%, and 60% MVC. The small difference in rate-pressure product reflected a higher HR in younger participants at each intensity of contraction, which was not completely offset by a lower SBP in the younger participants.

SUMMARY

1. During short-term, light to moderate aerobic exercise, cardiac output (Q), stroke volume (SV), heart rate (HR), systolic blood pressure (SBP), and rate-pressure product (RPP) increase rapidly at the onset of exercise and reach steady state within approximately 2 minutes. Diastolic blood pressure (DBP) remains relatively unchanged, and resistance decreases rapidly and then plateaus.

2. During long-term, moderate to heavy aerobic exercise, Q, SV, HR, SBP, and RPP increase rapidly. Once steady state is achieved, cardiac output remains relatively constant owing to the downward drift of SV and the upward drift of HR. SBP and resistance may also drift downward during prolonged, heavy work. This cardiovascular drift is associated with rising body temperature.

3. During incremental exercise to maximum, Q, HR, SBP, and RPP increase in a rectilinear fashion with increasing workload. SV increases initially and then plateaus at a workload corresponding to approximately 40–50% of $\dot{V}O_2$max in normally active adults and children. DBP remains relatively constant throughout an incremental exercise test. Resistance decreases rapidly with the onset of exercise and reaches its lowest value at maximal exercise.

4. The decrease in resistance during aerobic exercise has two important implications. It allows greater blood flow to the working muscles and keeps blood pressure from rising excessively. The increase in cardiac output would produce a much greater rise in blood pressure if it were not for the fact that there is a simultaneous decrease in resistance.

5. The highest oxygen consumption during an incremental test may or may not represent an actual maximal value. The term $\dot{V}O_2$peak is used to represent the highest value obtained during the test if the tester is not certain that a true maximal value was achieved. Specific criteria should be used to determine whether the test is truly a maximal test.

6. Maximal oxygen uptake may be limited by any system (or step) along the pathway of bringing oxygen into the body and delivering it to the mitochondria for the production of ATP. Although factors in each of these systems may limit the $\dot{V}O_2$max, research suggests that cardiac output is the limiting factor in $\dot{V}O_2$max.

7. Blood volume decreases during aerobic exercise. Most of the decrease occurs within the first 10 minutes of activity and depends on exercise intensity. A decrease of 10% of blood volume is not uncommon.

8. SV initially increases during dynamic aerobic exercise and then plateaus at a level that corresponds to 40–50% of $\dot{V}O_2$max. The increase in SV results from changes in end-diastolic volume (EDV) and end-systolic volume (ESV). EDV increases primarily because the active muscle pump returns blood to the heart. ESV decreases owing to augmented contractility of the heart, thus ejecting more blood and leaving less blood in the ventricle.

9. The pattern of cardiovascular response is the same for both sexes. However, males have a higher cardiac output, SV, and SBP at maximal exercise. Additionally, males have a higher $\dot{V}O_2$max. Most of these differences are attributable to differences in body size and heart size between the sexes and to the greater hemoglobin concentration of males.

10. The pattern of cardiovascular response in children and adolescents is similar to the adult response.

However, children have a lower $\dot{Q}$, SV, and SBP at an absolute workload and at maximal exercise. Most of these differences are attributable to differences in body size and heart size.

11. As adults age, their cardiovascular responses change. Maximal $\dot{Q}$, SV, HR, and $\dot{V}O_2$max decrease. Maximal SBP, DBP, and mean arterial pressure (MAP) increase.

12. Static exercise is characterized by modest increases in HR and $\dot{Q}$ and exaggerated increases in SBP, DBP, and MAP, known as the pressor response.

13. Dynamic resistance exercise results in a modest increase in $\dot{Q}$, an increase in HR, little change or a decrease in SV, and a large increase in blood pressure.

REVIEW QUESTIONS

1. Graph and explain the pattern of response for each of the major cardiovascular variables during short-term, light to moderate aerobic exercise. Explain the mechanisms responsible for each response.

2. Graph and explain the pattern of response for each of the major cardiovascular variables during long-term, moderate to heavy aerobic exercise. Explain the mechanisms responsible for each response.

3. Graph and explain the pattern of response for each of the major cardiovascular variables during incremental aerobic exercise to maximum. Explain the mechanisms responsible for each response.

4. List the criteria used to determine if an individual reached maximal oxygen consumption during an incremental test.

5. Discuss the factors that may limit $\dot{V}O_2$max and indicate which factor is mostly likely to limit $\dot{V}O_2$max in normal healthy individuals. Graph and explain the pattern of response for each of the major cardiovascular variables during static exercise. Explain the mechanisms responsible for each response.

6. Graph and explain the pattern of response for each of the major cardiovascular variables during dynamic resistance exercise. Explain the mechanisms responsible for each response.

7. Discuss the change that occurs in TPR during exercise, and explain its importance for blood flow and BP. Why is resistance altered in older adults?

8. Describe the pressor response to static exercise, and explain the mechanisms by which BP is elevated.

9. Describe the differences in male and female response to incremental maximal exercise.

10. Explain why the $\dot{V}O_2$max, expressed in relative terms, of females decrease as children age.

11. Compare the cardiovascular responses to incremental exercise in young and older adults.

For further review and additional study tools, visit the website at http://thePoint.lww.com/Plowman4e ✳ ▶

REFERENCES

American College of Sports Medicine: Position stand: Physical activity, physical fitness, and hypertension. *Medicine and Science in Sports and Exercise*. 25(10):I–X (1993).

American College of Sports Medicine: *Guidelines for Exercise Testing and Prescription* (7th edition). Philadelphia, PA: Lippincott Williams & Wilkins (2006).

Anderson, K. L.: The cardiovascular system in exercise. In H. B. Falls (ed.): *Exercise Physiology*. New York, NY: Academic Press (1968).

Asano, K. & K. Hirakoba: Respiratory and circulatory adaptation during prolonged exercise in 10–12 year-old children and adults. In J. Ilmarinen & I. Valimaki (eds.): *Children and Sports*. Berlin: Springer-Verlag (1984).

Asmussen, E.: Similarities and dissimilarities between static and dynamic exercise. *Circulation Research*. 48(6 Suppl. I):3–10 (1981).

Åstrand, P.: *Experimental Studies of Physical Working Capacity in Relation to Sex and Age*. Copenhagen, Munksgaard: University Microfilms International (1952).

Åstrand, I.: Human physical fitness with special reference to sex and age. *Physiological Reviews*. 36:307 (1956).

Åstrand, I.: Aerobic work capacity in men and women with special reference to age. *Acta Physiologica Scandinavica*. 49(Suppl. 169):1–92 (1960).

Åstrand, P., T. E. Cuddy, B. Saltin, & J. Stenberg: Cardiac output during submaximal and maximal work. *Journal of Applied Physiology*. 19(2):268–274 (1964).

Åstrand, P.-O. & I. Rhyming: A nomogram for calculation of aerobic capacity (physical fitness) from pulse rate during submaximal work. *Journal of Applied Physiology*. 7:218–221 (1954).

Åstrand, P. O., K. Rodahl, H. A. Dahl, S. B. Stromme: *Textbook of Work Physiology* (4th edition). Champaign, IL: Human Kinetics (2003).

Bar-Or, O.: *Physiologic Principles to Clinical Applications*. Pediatric Sports Medicine, for the Practitioner. New York, NY: Springer-Verlag (1983).

Bassett, D. R., & E. T. Howley: Limiting factors for maximum oxygen uptake and determinants of endurance performance. *Medicine & Science in Sports & Exercise*. 32:85–88 (2000).

Becklake, M. R., H. Frank, G. R. Dagenais, G. L. Ostiguy, & C. A. Guzman: Influence of age and sex on exercise cardiac output. *Journal of Applied Physiology*. 20(5):938–947 (1965).

Bergh, U., B. Ekblom, & P.-O. Åstrand: Maximal oxygen uptake: "Classical" versus "contemporary" viewpoints. *Medicine & Science in Sports & Exercise*. 32:70-84 (2000).

Bezucha, G. R., M. C. Lenser, P. G. Hanson, & F. J. Nagle. Comparison of hemodynamic responses to static and dynamic exercise. *Journal of Applied Physiology*. 31:1589–1593 (1982).

Clausen, J. P.: Circulatory adjustments to dynamic exercise and effect of physical training in normal subjects and in patients with coronary artery disease. *Progressive Cardiovascular Disease*. 18:459–495 (1976).

Cumming, G. R., D. Everatt, & L. Hastman: Bruce treadmill test in children: Normal values in a clinic population. *American Journal of Cardiology*. 41:69–75 (1978).

Cunningham, D. A., D. H. Paterson, C. J. R. Blimkie, & A. P. Donner: Development of cardiorespiratory function in circumpubertal boys: A longitudinal study. *Journal of Applied*

Physiology: Respiratory Environment Exercise Physiology. 56(2): 302–307 (1984).

Cureton, K. J., T. A. Baumgartner, & B. McManis: Adjustment of 1-mile run/walk test scores for skinfold thickness in youth. *Pediatric Exercise Science*. 3:152–167 (1991).

Cureton, K. J., R. A. Boileau, T. G. Lohman, & J. E. Misner: Determinants of distance running performance in children: Analysis of a path model. *Research Quarterly*. 48(2):270–279 (1977).

Davies, C. T. M., J. Few, K. G. Foster, & A. J. Sargeant: Plasma catecholamine concentration during dynamic exercise involving different muscle groups. *European Journal of Applied Physiology*. 32:195–206 (1974).

Dempsey, J. A.: Is the lung built for exercise? *Medicine and Science in Sports and Exercise*. 18(2):143–155 (1986).

Deschenes, M. R., M. N. Hillard, J. A. Wilson, M. I. Dubina, & M. K. Eason: Effects of gender on physiological responses during submaximal exercise and recovery. *Medicine & Science in Sports & Exercise*. 38(7):1304–1310 (2006).

di Prampero, P. E.: Factors limiting maximal performance in humans. *European Journal of Applied Physiology*. 90:420–429 (2003).

Donald, K. W., S. R. Lind, G. W. McNichol, P. W. Humphreys, S. H. Taylor, & H. P. Stauton: Cardiovascular responses to sustained (static) contractions. *Circulation Research*. 20(Suppl. I):15–32 (1967).

Durstine, J. L. & R. R. Pate: Cardiorespiratory responses to acute exercise. In S. N. Blair (ed.) et al., *Resource manual for guidelines for exercise testing and prescription*, Philadelphia: Lea & Febiger, 48–54 (1988).

Ekelund, L. G. & A. Holmgren: Central hemodynamics during exercise. *Circulation Research*. 22(Suppl. I):33–43 (1967).

Falkel, J. E., S. J. Fleck, & T. F. Murray: Comparison of central hemodynamics between powerlifters and bodybuilders during resistance exercise. *Journal of Applied Sport Science Research*. 6(1):24–35 (1992).

Ferguson, S., N. Gledhill, V. K. Jamnik, C. Wiebe, & N. Payne: Cardiac performance in endurance-trained and moderately active young women. *Medicine & Science in Sports & Exercise*. 33:1114–1119 (2001).

Fleck, S. J.: Cardiovascular adaptations to resistance training. *Medicine and Science in Sports and Exercise*. 20:S146–S151 (1988).

Fleck, S. J. & L. S. Dean: Resistance-training experience and the pressor response during resistance exercise. *Journal of Applied Physiology*. 63:116–120 (1987).

Fortney, S. M., C. B. Wenger, J. R. Bove, & E. R. Nadel: Effect of blood volume on sweating rate and body fluids in exercising humans. *Journal of Applied Physiology*. 51(6):1594–1600 (1981).

Foster, C., K. Meyer, N. Georgakopoulos, et al.: Left ventricular function during interval and steady state exercise. *Medicine & Science in Sports & Exercise*. 31(8):1157–1162 (1999).

Franklin, B. A.: Prevention of heart attacks during snow shoveling. *ACSM's Health & Fitness Journal*. 1(6):20–23 (1997).

Franklin, B. A., P. Hogan, K. Bonzheim, D. Bakalyar, E. Terrien, S. Gordon, & G. C. Timmis: Cardiac demands of heavy snow shoveling. *Journal of the American Medical Association*. 273:880–882 (1995).

Freedson, P., V. L. Katch, S. Sady, & A. Weltman: Cardiac output differences in males and females during mild cycle ergometer exercise. *Medicine and Science in Sports*. 11(1):16–19 (1979).

Freund, P. R., S. F. Gobbs, & L. B. Rowell: Cardiovascular responses to muscle ischemia in man, dependency on muscle mass. *Journal of Applied Physiology*. 45:762–767 (1979).

Grassi, B.: Skeletal muscle $\dot{V}O_2$ on kinetics: Set by O_2 delivery or by O_2 utilization? New insights into an old issue. *Medicine & Science in Sports & Exercise*. 32:108–116 (2000).

Gledhill, N., D. Cox, & R. Jamnik: Endurance athletes' stroke volume does not plateau: Major advantage is diastolic function. *Medicine and Science in Sports and Exercise*. 26:1116–1121 (1994).

Goldstraw, P. W. & D. J. Warren: The effect of age on the cardiovascular responses to isometric exercise: A test of autonomic function. *Gerontology*. 31:54–58 (1985).

González-Alonso, J.: Point: Counterpoint: Stroke volume does/does not decline during exercise at maximal effort in healthy individuals. *Journal of Applied Physiology*. 104:275–276 (2008).

Hale, T.: History of developments in sport and exercise physiology: A.V. Hill, maximal oxygen uptake, and oxygen debt. *Journal of Sports Sciences*. 26(4):365–400 (2008).

Hamilton, M. T., J. G. Alonso, S. J. Montain, & E. F. Coyle: Fluid replacement and glucose infusion during exercise prevents cardiovascular drift. *Journal of Applied Physiology*. 71:871–877 (1991).

Hanson, P. & F. Nagle: Isometric exercise: Cardiovascular responses in normal and cardiac populations. *Cardiology Clinics*. 5(2):157–170 (1985).

Heath, G. W., J. M. Hagberg, A. A. Ehsani, & J. O. Holloszy: A physiological comparison of young and older endurance athletes. *Journal of Applied Physiology*. 51:634–640 (1981).

Higginbotham, M. B., K. G. Morris, R. S. Williams, P. A. McHale, R. E. Coleman, & F. R. Cobb: Regulation of stroke volume during submaximal and maximal upright exercise in normal man. *Circulation Research*. 58:281–291 (1986).

Hill, D. W. & S. D. Butler: Haemodynamic responses to weight-lifting exercise. *Sports Medicine*. 12(1):1–7 (1991).

Holly, R. G.: Measurement of the maximal rate of oxygen uptake. In American college of Sports Medicine (ed.), *Resource manual for guidelines for exercise testing and prescription*. Philadelphia: Lea & Febiger (1988).

Jae, S. Y., B. Fernhall, K. S. Heffernan, et al.: Exaggerated blood pressure response to exercise is associated with carotid atherosclerosis in apparently healthy men. *Journal of Hypertension*. 24:881–887 (2006).

James, F. W., S. Kaplan, C. J. Glueck, J. Y. Tsay, M. J. S. Knight, & C. J. Sarwar: Responses of normal children and young adults to controlled bicycle exercise. *Circulation*. 61:902–912 (1980).

Krahenbuhl, G. S., J. S. Skinner, & W. M. Kohrt: Developmental aspects of maximal aerobic power in children. In Terjung, R. L. (ed.): *Exercise and Sport Science Reviews*. New York, NY: Macmillan, 13:503–538, (1985).

Kurl, S., J. A. Laukkanen, R. Rauramaa, T. A. Lakka, J. Sivenius, & J. T. Salonen: Systolic blood pressure response to exercise stress test and risk of stroke. *Stroke*. 32:2036–2041 (2001).

Léger, L. A., D. Mercer, C. Gadoury, & J. Lambert: The multistage 20 metre shuttle run test for aerobic fitness. *Journal of Sports Sciences*. 6:93–101 (1988).

Lentini, A. C., R. S. McKelvie, N. McCartney, C. W. Tomlinson, & J. D. MacDougall. Left ventricular responses in healthy young men during heavy-intensity weight-lifting exercise. *Journal of Applied Physiology*. 75:2703–2710 (1993).

Legrand, R., Ahmaidi, S., Moalla, W., Chocquet, D., Marles, A., Prieur, F., & P. Mucci: O_2 arterial desaturation in endurance athletes increases muscle deoxygenation. *Medicine & Science in Sports & Exercise.* 37(5):782–788 (2005).

Lind, A.: Cardiovascular responses to static exercise. *Circulation.* XLI(2, Suppl II):173–176 (1970).

Lind, A. R. & G. W. McNichol: Circulatory responses to sustained handgrip contractions performed during other exercise. *Journal of Physiology.* 192:595–607 (1967).

Lind, A. R., S. H. Taylor, P. W. Humphreys, B. M. Kennelly, & K. W. Donald: The circulatory effects of sustained voluntary muscle contraction. *Clinical Science.* 27:229–244 (1964).

Lussier, L. & E. R. Buskirk: Effects of an endurance training regimen on assessment of work capacity in prepubertal children. *Annals of the New York Academy of Sciences.* 30:734–777 (1977).

MacDougall, J. D., D. Tuxen, D. G. Sale, J. R. Moroz, & J. R. Sutton: Arterial blood pressure response to heavy resistance exercise. *Journal of Applied Physiology.* 58(3):785–790 (1985).

Malina, R. M. & C. Bouchard: *Growth, Maturation and Physical Activity.* Champaign, IL: Human Kinetics (1991).

Mayhew, J. L. & P. B. Gifford: Prediction of maximal oxygen intake in preadolescent boys from anthropometric parameters. *Research Quarterly.* 46(3):302–311 (1975).

McCartney, N.: Acute responses to resistance training and safety. *Medicine & Science in Sports & Exercise.* 31(1):31–37 (1999).

McCormack, W. P., K. J. Cureton, T. A. Bullock, & P. G. Weyand: Metabolic determinants of 1-mile run/walk performance in children. *Medicine and Science in Sport and Exercise.* 23(5):611–617 (1991).

MacDougall, J. D., H. A. Wenger, & H. J. Green: *Physiological testing of the elite athlete.* Ottawa, Canada: Canadian Association of Sport Sciences: Sports Medicine Council of Canada (1982).

McVeigh, S. K., A. C. Payne, & S. Scott: The reliability and validity of the 20-meter shuttle test as a predictor of peak oxygen uptake in Edinburgh school children, ages 13 to 14 years. *Pediatric Exercise Science.* 7:69–79 (1995).

Miles, D. S., M. H. Cox, & J. P. Bomze: Cardiovascular responses to upper body exercise in normal and cardiac patients. *Medicine and Science in Sport and Exercise.* 21(5):s126–s131 (1989).

Miles, D. S., J. J. Owens, J. C. Golden, & R. W. Gotshall: Central and peripheral hemodynamics during maximal leg extension exercise. *European Journal of Applied Physiology.* 56:12–17 (1987).

Misner, J. E., S. B. Going, B. H. Massey, T. E. Ball, M. G. Bemben, & L. K. Essandoh: Cardiovascular response in males and females to sustained maximal voluntary static muscle contraction. *Medicine and Science in Sports and Exercise.* 22(2):194–199 (1990).

Mitchell, J. H. & B. Saltin: The oxygen transport system and maximal oxygen uptake. In Tipton, C. M. (ed): *Exercise Physiology: People and Ideas.* Oxford: Oxford University Press (2003).

Miyai, N., M. Arita, K. Miyashita, I. Moriokia, T. Shiraishi, & I. Nishio: Blood pressure response to heart rate during exercise test and risk of future hypertension. *Hypertension.* 39:761–766 (2002).

Mortensen, S. P., E. A. Dawson, C. C. Yoshiga, M. K. Dalsgaard, R. Damsgaard, N. H. Secher, & J. González-Alonso: Limitations to systemic and locomotor limb muscle oxygen delivery and uptake during maximal exercise in humans. *Journal of Physiology.* 566:273–285 (2005).

Mundal, R., S. E. Kjeldsen, L. Sandvik, G. Erikssen, E. Thaulow, & J. Erikssen: Exercise blood pressure predicts cardiovascular mortality in middle-aged men. *Hypertension.* 24:56–62 (1994).

Nau, K. L., V. L. Katch, R. H. Beekman, & M. Dick II: Acute intra-arterial blood pressure response to bench press weight lifting in children. *Pediatric Exercise Science.* 2:37–45 (1990).

Nieman, D.: *Fitness and Sports Medicine.* Palo Alto, CA: Bull Publishing (1990).

Noakes, T.D.: Implications of exercise testing for prediction of athletic performance: A contemporary perspective. *Medicine and Science in Sports and Exercise.* 20(4):319–330 (1988).

Ogawa, T., R. J. Spina, W. H. Martin, W. M. Kohrt, K. B. Schechtman, J. O. Holloszy, & A. A. Ehsani: Effects of aging, sex, and physical training on cardiovascular responses to exercise. *Circulation.* 86:494–503 (1992).

Pendergast, D. R.: Cardiovascular, respiratory, and metabolic responses to upper body exercise. *Medicine and Science in Sport and Exercise.* 21(5):s122–s125 (1989).

Petrofsky, J. S. & A. R. Lind: Aging, isometric strength and endurance, and cardiovascular responses to static effort. *Journal of Applied Physiology.* 38(1):91–95 (1975).

Plowman, S.A., & N. Y-S. Liu: Norm-referenced and criterion-referenced validity of the one-mile run and PACER in college age individuals. *Measurement in Physical Education and Exercise Science.* 3:63–84 (1999).

Poliner, L. R., G. J. Dehmer, S. E. Lewis, R. W. Parkey, C. G. Blomqvist, & J. T. Willerson: Left ventricular performance in normal subjects: A comparison of the responses to exercise in the upright supine positions. *Circulation.* 62:528–534 (1980).

Powers, S. K., J. Lawler, J. A. Dempsey, S. Dodd, & G. Landry: Effects of incomplete pulmonary gas exchange on $\dot{V}O_2max$. *Journal of Applied Physiology.* 66:2491–2495 (1989).

Richardson, R. S.: What governs skeletal muscle $\dot{V}O_2max$? New Evidence. *Medicine & Science in Sports & Exercise.* 32(1):100–107 (2000).

Riopel, D. A., A. B. Taylor, & A. R. Hohn: Blood pressure, heart rate, pressure-rate product and electrocardiographic changes in healthy children during treadmill exercise. *American Journal of Cardiology.* 44:697–704 (1979).

Rowell, L.: Human cardiovascular adjustments to exercise and thermal stress. *Physiological Reviews.* 54:75–159 (1974).

Rowell, L. B.: *Human Circulation: Regulation during Physical Stress.* New York, NY: Oxford University Press (1986).

Rowell, L. B.: *Human Cardiovascular Control.* New York, NY: Oxford University Press (1993).

Rowland, T. W.: *Exercise and Children's Health.* Champaign, IL: Human Kinetics (1990).

Rowland, T. W.: *Developmental Exercise Physiology.* Champaign, IL: Human Kinetics (1996).

Rowland, T. W.: *Children's Exercise Physiology* (2nd edition). Champaign, IL: Human Kinetics (2005a).

Rowland, T. W.: Circulatory responses to exercise: Are we misreading Fick? *Chest.* 127(3):1023–1030 (2005b).

Rowland, T. W. & G. M. Green: Physiological responses to treadmill exercise in females: Adult-child differences. *Medicine and Science in Sports and Exercise.* 20(5):474–478 (1988).

Rowland, T. W., K. Heffernan, S. Y. Jae, G. Echols, G. Krull, & B. Fernhall: Cardiovascular responses to static exercise in boys: Insights from tissue Doppler Imaging. *European Journal of Applied Physiology*. 97(5):637–642 (2006).

Sagiv, M., E. Goldhammer, E. G. Abinader, & J. Rudoy: Aging and the effect of increased after-load on left ventricular contractile state. *Medicine and Science in Sports and Exercise*. 20(3):281–284 (1988).

Saltin, B.: Hemodynamic adaptations to exercise. *American Journal of Cardiology*. 55:42D–47D (1985).

Seals, D. R., R. A. Washburn, & P. G. Hanson: Increased cardiovascular response to static contraction of larger muscle groups. *Journal of Applied Physiology*. 54(2):434–437 (1985).

Secher, N. H., J. P. Clausen, K. Klausen, I. Noer, & J. Trap-Jensen: Central and regional circulatory effects of adding arm exercise to leg exercise. *Acta Physiologica Scandinavica*. 100:288–297 (1977).

Shvartz, E. & R. C. Reibold: Aerobic fitness norms for males and females aged 6 to 75 years: A review. *Aviation, Space, and Environmental Physiology*. 61:3–11 (1990).

Sjogaard, G., G. Savard, & C. Juel: Muscle blood flow during isometric activity and its relation to muscle fatigue. *European Journal of Physiology*. 57:327–335 (1988).

Skinner, J. S.: *Exercise Testing and Exercise Prescription for Special Cases* (2nd edition). Philadelphia, PA: Lea & Febiger (1993).

Smith, D. L., B. Kocher, A. Kolesnikoff, & T. Rowland: Cardiovascular responses to isometric contractions in girls and young women [abstract]. *Medicine & Science in Sports & Exercise*. 32:S95 (2000).

Smith, D. L., J. E. Misner, D. K. Bloomfield, & L. K. Essandoh: Cardiovascular responses to sustained maximal isometric contractions of the finger flexors. *European Journal of Applied Physiology*. 67:48–52 (1993).

Sparling, P. B.: A meta-analysis of studies comparing maximal oxygen uptake in men and women. *Research Quarterly for Exercise and Sport*. 51(3):542–552 (1980).

Stathokostas, L., S. Jacob-Johnson, R. J. Petrella, & D. H. Paterson: Longitudinal changes in aerobic power in older men and women. *Journal of Applied Physiology*. 97:781–789 (2004).

Stringer, W. W., J. E. Hansen, & K. Wasserman: Cardiac output estimated noninvasively from oxygen uptake during exercise. *Journal of Applied Physiology*. 82:908–912 (1997).

Sullivan, M. J., F. R. Cobb, & M. B. Higginbotham: Stroke volume increases by similar mechanisms during upright exercise in normal men and women. *American Journal of Cardiology*. 67:1405–1412 (1991).

Taylor, H. L., E. Buskirk, & A. Henshel: Maximal oxygen intake as an objective measure of cardio-respiratory performance. *Journal of Applied Physiology*. 8:73–80 (1955).

Tuttle, W. W. & S. M. Horvath: Comparison of effects of static and dynamic work on blood pressure and heart rate. *Journal of Applied Physiology*. 10(2):294–296 (1957).

VanLoan, M. D., B. H. Massey, R. A. Boileau, T. G. Lohman, J. E. Misner, & P. L. Best: Age as a factor in the hemodynamic responses to isometric exercise. *Journal of Sports Medicine and Physical Fitness*. 29(3):262–268 (1989).

Wade, C. E. & B. J. Freund: Hormonal control of blood volume during and following exercise. In Gisolfi, C. V. & D. R. Lamb (eds.): *Perspectives in Exercise Science and Sports Medicine*. 3:1405–1412 (1990).

Wanne, O. P. S. & E. Haapoja: Blood pressure during exercise in healthy children. *European Journal of Applied Physiology*. 58:62–67 (1988).

Warburton, D. E. & N. Gledhill: Counterpoint: Stroke volume does not decline during exercise at maximal effort in healthy individuals. *Journal of Applied Physiology*. 104(1):276–278 (2008).

Warburton, D. E., M. J. Haykowsky, H. A. Quinney, D. P. Humen, & K. K. Teo: Reliability and validity of measures of cardiac output during incremental to maximal aerobic exercise. Part II: Novel techniques and new advances. *Sports Medicine*. 27:241–260 (1999).

Weiss, E. P., R. J. Spina, J. O. Holloszy, & A. A. Ehsani: Gender differences in the decline in aerobic capacity and its physiological determinants during the later decades of life. *Journal of Applied Physiology*. 101:938–944 (2006).

Wells, C. L.: *Women, Sport and Performance* (2nd edition). Champaign, IL: Human Kinetics (1991).

Wells, C. L. & S. A. Plowman: Sexual differences in athletic performance: Biological or behavioral? *Physician and Sports Medicine*. 11(8):52–63 (1983).

Wescott, W. & B. Howes: Blood pressure response during weight training exercise. *National Strength and Conditioning Association Journal*. 5:67–71 (1983).

Wilson, T. & H. Tanka: Meta-analysis of the age-associated decline in maximal aerobic capacity in men: Relation to training status. *American Journal of Applied Physiology*. 278:H829–H834 (2000).

13 Cardiorespiratory Training Principles and Adaptations

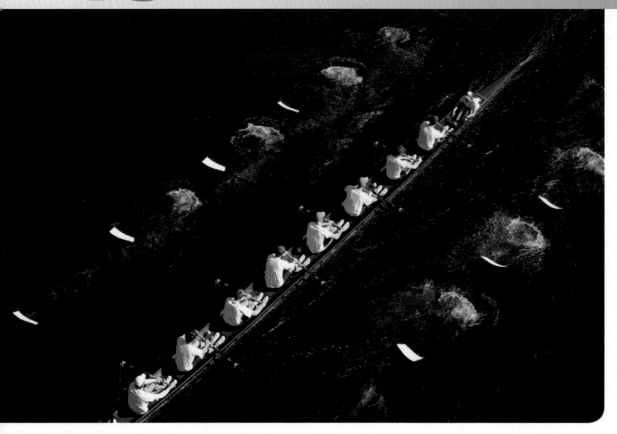

OBJECTIVES

After studying the chapter, you should be able to:

> Describe the exercise/physical activity recommendations of the American College of Sports Medicine, the Canadian Society for Exercise Physiology, the National Association for Sport and Physical Education, and the CDC Expert Panel. Discuss the commonalities and differences of these reports.

> Discuss the application of each of the training principles in a cardiorespiratory training program.

> Explain how the FIT principle is related to the overload principle.

> Differentiate among the methods used to classify exercise intensity.

> Calculate training intensity ranges by using different methods including the percentage of maximal heart rate, the percentage of heart rate reserve, and the percentage of oxygen consumption reserve.

> Discuss the merits of specificity of modality and cross-training in bringing about cardiovascular adaptations.

> Identify central and peripheral cardiovascular adaptations that occur at rest, during submaximal exercise, and at maximal exercise following an aerobic endurance or dynamic resistance training program.

Introduction

In the last decade, *physical fitness*–centered exercise prescriptions, which emphasize continuous bouts of relatively vigorous exercise, have evolved (for the nonathlete) into public health recommendations for daily moderate-intensity *physical activity*. Early scientific investigations that led to the development of training principles for the cardiovascular system almost always focused on the improvement of physical fitness, operationally defined as an improvement of maximal oxygen consumption ($\dot{V}O_2$max). Such studies formed the basis for the guidelines developed by the American College of Sports Medicine (ACSM) and first published in 1978 as "the recommended quantity and quality of exercise for developing and maintaining fitness in healthy adults." These guidelines were revised in 1998 and again in 2011 to "Quantity and quality of exercise for developing and maintaining cardiorespiratory, musculoskeletal, and neuromotor fitness in apparently healthy adults: Guidance for prescribing exercise." After 1978, these guidelines were increasingly applied not only to healthy adults intent on becoming more *fit* but also to individuals seeking only *health benefits* from exercise training.

Although evidence shows that health benefits accrue when fitness is improved, health and fitness are different goals, and exercise training and physical activity are different processes (Plowman, 2005). The quantity and quality of exercise required to develop or maintain cardiorespiratory fitness may not be (and probably is not) the same as the amount of physical activity required to improve and maintain cardiorespiratory health (American College of Sports Medicine, 2011; Haskell, 1994; Haskell, 2005; Haskell et al., 2007; Nelson et al., 2007). Furthermore, most exercise science or physical education majors and competitive athletes who want or need high levels of fitness can handle physically rigorous and time-consuming training programs. Such programs, however, carry a risk of injury and are often intimidating to those who are sedentary, elderly, or obese.

Studies also suggest that different physical activity recommendations are warranted for children and adolescents. Thus, an optimal cardiovascular training program—maximizing the benefit while minimizing the time, effort, and risk—varies with both the population and the goal. **Table 13.1** summarizes recommendations for cardiorespiratory health and fitness from leading authorities.

Application of the Training Principles

This chapter focuses on cardiovascular fitness and cardiorespiratory function that can impact health. Thus, only the cardiovascular portion of the exercise prescription recommendations of the ACSM and the Canadian Society for Exercise Physiology (CSEP) are discussed here for adults and children/adolescents. The emphasis will be on changes that accompany a change in $\dot{V}O_2$max. Additional information about physical fitness and physical activity in relation to cardiovascular disease is presented in Chapter 15, Cardiovascular Disease Risk Factors and Physical Activity.

Obviously, there are other goals for exercise prescription and physical activity guidelines in addition to cardiovascular ones. There is also some overlap in the cardiovascular benefits of physical activity/exercise with other health and fitness areas, especially those pertaining to body weight/composition and metabolic function. Body weight aspects are discussed in the metabolic unit, and the recommendations for and benefits of resistance training, flexibility, and balance are discussed in the neuromuscular unit.

This first section of the chapter, focusing on how the training principles are applied for cardiovascular fitness, relies heavily on the cardiorespiratory portion of the 2011 ACSM guidelines for healthy adults. **Cardiovascular fitness** (also known as cardiorespiratory fitness) is defined as the ability to deliver and use oxygen during intense and prolonged exercise or work. Cardiovascular fitness is evaluated by measures of maximal oxygen consumption ($\dot{V}O_2$max). Sustained exercise training programs using these principles to improve $\dot{V}O_2$max are rarely included in the daily activities of children and adolescents. However, in the absence of more specific exercise prescription guidelines for younger individuals, these guidelines are often applied to adolescent athletes and youngsters in scientific training studies (Rowland, 2005).

Specificity

Any activity that involves large muscle groups and is sustained for prolonged periods of time has the potential to increase cardiorespiratory fitness. This includes such exercise modes as aerobics, bicycling, cross-country skiing, various forms of dancing, jogging, rollerblading, rowing, speed skating, stair-climbing or stepping, swimming, and walking. Sports involving high-energy, nonstop action, such as field hockey, lacrosse, and soccer, can also positively benefit the cardiovascular system (American College of Sports Medicine, 2011; Pollock, 1973).

Exercise is beneficial only if an individual participates in it. Therefore, for fitness participants, the choice of exercise modalities should be based on interest, availability, and minimal risk of injury. An individual who enjoys the activity is more likely to adhere to the program. Although jogging or running may be the most time-efficient way to achieve cardiorespiratory fitness, these activities are not enjoyable for many individuals. They also have a relatively high incidence of overuse injuries. Therefore, other options should be available in fitness programs.

Cardiovascular Fitness The ability to deliver and use oxygen under the demands of intensive, prolonged exercise or work.

TABLE 13.1   Physical Activity and Exercise Prescription for Health and Physical Fitness

Source	Frequency	Intensity	Duration	Modality Cardiorespiratory	Neuromuscular
American College of Sports Medicine (ACSM) (2011): Adults	5 d·wk^{-1} or 3 d·wk^{-1} or combination	Moderate Vigorous Moderate + Vigorous	≥30 min·d^{-1} ≥20 min·d^{-1} ≥500–1000 MET·min·wk^{-1}*	Rhythmical, aerobic, large muscles	Dynamic resistance: 2–4 sets of 8–12 reps; major muscle groups; 2–3 d·wk^{-1} Flexibility: Major muscle groups 60s total each; 2–3 d·wk^{-1} balance, agility, coordination and gait ≥20–30 min·d^{-1} 2–3 d·wk^{-1}
Canadian Society for Exercise Physiology (CSEP) (2011): Adults 18–65 yr		Moderate to Vigorous	150 min·wk^{-1}		Muscle and bone strength training exercises: ≥2 d·wk^{-1}
Canadian Society for Exercise Physiology (CSEP) (2011): Children/Adolescents 5–18 yr	Daily	Moderate to Vigorous; Vigorous ≥3 d·wk^{-1}	60 min·d^{-1}		Muscle and bone strength training exercises: ≥3 d·wk^{-1}
National Association for Sport and Physical Education (NASPE) (2004): Children 5–12 yr	All, or most days	Moderate to Vigorous	≥60 min·d^{-1} Intermittent, but several bouts >15 min	Age-appropriate aerobic sports	
Centers for Disease Control and Prevention (CDC) Expert Panel (Strong et al., 2005): Children/Adolescents 6–18 yr	Daily	Moderate to Vigorous	≥60 min·d^{-1}	Age-appropriate, enjoyable, varied	

*MET·min = (Energy expenditure of selected activity ÷ Resting energy expenditure) × minutes of activity per day or week. For example, jogging at an energy expenditure of 24.5 mL·kg·min^{-1} ÷ 3.5 mL·kg·min^{-1} resting energy expenditure = 7 METs; 7 METs × 30 min × 4 d·wk^{-1} = 840 MET·min·wk^{-1}.

Although many different modalities can improve cardiovascular function, the greatest improvements in performance occur in the modality used for training, that is, there is modality specificity. For example, individuals who train by swimming improve more in swimming than in running (Magel et al., 1975), and individuals who train by bicycling improve more in cycling than running (Pechar et al., 1974; Roberts and Alspaugh, 1972). Modality specificity has two important practical applications. First, to determine whether improvement is occurring, the individual should be tested in the modality used for training. Second, the more the individual is concerned with sports competition rather than fitness or rehabilitation, the more important the mode of exercise becomes. A competitive rower, for example, whether competing on open water or an indoor ergometer, should train mostly in that modality. Running, however, seems to be less specific than most other modalities; running forms the basis of many sports other than track or road races (Pechar et al., 1974; Roberts and Alspaugh, 1972; Wilmore et al., 1980).

Although modality specificity is important for competitive athletes, cross-training also has value. Originally, the term cross-training referred to the development or maintenance of muscle function in one limb by exercising the contralateral limb or upper limbs as opposed to lower limbs (American College of Sports Medicine, 2011; Housh and Housh, 1993; Kilmer et al., 1994; Pate et al., 1978). Such training remains important, especially in situations where one limb has been injured or placed in a cast. As used here, however, the term **cross-training** means the development or maintenance of cardiovascular fitness by training in two or more modalities either alternatively or concurrently. Two sets of athletes in particular are interested in cross-training. First, injured athletes, especially those with injuries associated with high-mileage running, who wish to prevent detraining. Second, an increasing number of athletes who participate in multisport competitions such as biathlons and triathlons and need to be conditioned in each.

Theoretically, both specificity and cross-training have value for a training program. Any form of aerobic endurance exercise affects both central and peripheral cardiovascular functioning. **Central cardiovascular adaptations** occur in the heart and contribute to an increased ability to deliver oxygen. Central cardiovascular adaptations are the same in all modalities when the heart is stressed to the same extent. Thus, many modalities can

TABLE 13.2 Situations in Which Cross-Training is Beneficial

Reason	Fitness Participant	Competitive Athlete
Multisport participation		General preparation phase, specific preparation phase, competitive phase
Injury or rehabilitation; fitness maintenance	As needed	As needed
Inclement weather	As needed	As needed
Baseline or general conditioning	Always	General preparation phase
Recovery	After intense workout	After intense workout or competition
Prevention of boredom and burnout	Always	Transition phase

Source: Kibler, W. B. & T. J. Chandler: Sport-specific conditioning. *The American Journal of Sports Medicine.* 22(3):424–432 (1994).

have the same overall training benefit by leading to central cardiovascular adaptations.

Peripheral cardiovascular adaptations occur in the vasculature or the muscles and contribute to an increased ability to extract oxygen. Peripheral cardiovascular adaptations are specific to the modality and the specific muscles used in that exercise. For example, additional capillaries will form to carry oxygen to habitually active muscles but not to habitually inactive ones. Other factors within exercising muscles such as mitochondrial density and enzyme activity also affect the body's ability to reach a high $\dot{V}O_2max$. Specificity of modality operates because peripheral adaptations occur in the muscles that are used in the training. Thus, the specific activity—or closely related activities that mimic the muscle action of the primary sport—are needed to maximize peripheral adaptations. Examples of mimicking muscle action include side sliding or cycling for speed skating and water running in a flotation vest for jogging or running.

Table 13.2 lists several situations, in addition to the maintenance of fitness when injured, in which cross-training may be beneficial (Kibler and Chandler, 1994; O'Toole, 1992). Note that multisport athletes may or may not be limited to the sports in which they are competing. For example, although a duathlete needs to train for both running and cycling, this training will have the benefits of both specificity and cross-training. In addition, this athlete may also cross-train by doing other activities such as rollerblading or speed skating. Note also that cross-training can be recommended at any time for a fitness participant to help avoid physiological monotony and mental boredom. For a healthy competitive athlete the value of cross-training is modest during the season. Cross-training is most valuable for single-sport competitive athletes during the transition (active rest) phase but may also be beneficial during the general preparation phase of periodization.

Overload

Overload of the cardiovascular system is achieved by manipulating the intensity, duration, and frequency of the training bouts. These variables are easily remembered by the acronym FIT (F = frequency, I = intensity, and T = time or duration). **Figure 13.1** presents the results of a study in which the components of overload were investigated relative to their effect on changes in $\dot{V}O_2max$. As the most critical component, intensity will be discussed first.

Intensity

Figure 13.1A shows the relationship between change (Δ) in $\dot{V}O_2max$ and exercise intensity. In general, as exercise intensity increases, so do improvements in $\dot{V}O_2max$. The greatest amount of improvement in $\dot{V}O_2max$ is seen following training programs that utilize exercise intensities of 90–100% of $\dot{V}O_2max$. In order to achieve such high-intensity training individuals may alternate work and rest intervals (interval training). At exercise levels greater than 100% (supramaximal exercise), in which the total amount of training that can be performed decreases, improvement in $\dot{V}O_2max$ is somewhat less than is seen at 90–100% $\dot{V}O_2max$.

Intensity, both alone and in conjunction with duration, is very important for improving $\dot{V}O_2max$. Intensity may be described in relation to heart rate, oxygen consumption, or rating of perceived exertion (RPE). Laboratory studies typically use $\dot{V}O_2$ for determining intensity, but heart rate and RPE are more practical for individuals outside the laboratory. **Table 13.3** includes techniques used to classify intensity and suggested percentages for very light to near maximal activity (American College of Sports Medicine, 2011). Note that these percentages and classifications are intended to be used when the exercise duration is 20–60 minutes and the frequency is 3–5 d·wk⁻¹.

Cross-Training The development or maintenance of cardiovascular fitness by alternating between or concurrently training in two or more modalities.

Central Cardiovascular Adaptations Adaptations that occur in the heart that increase the ability to deliver oxygen.

Peripheral Cardiovascular Adaptations Adaptations that occur in the vasculature or muscles that increase the ability to extract oxygen.

FIGURE 13.1 Changes in $\dot{V}O_2$max Based on Intensity (A), Duration (B), Frequency (C) and Initial Fitness Level (D). *Source*: Wenger, H. A. & G. J. Bell. The interactions of intensity, frequency and duration of exercise training in altering cardiorespiratory fitness. *Sports Medicine*. 3:346–356 (1986). Reprinted by permission of Adis International, Inc.

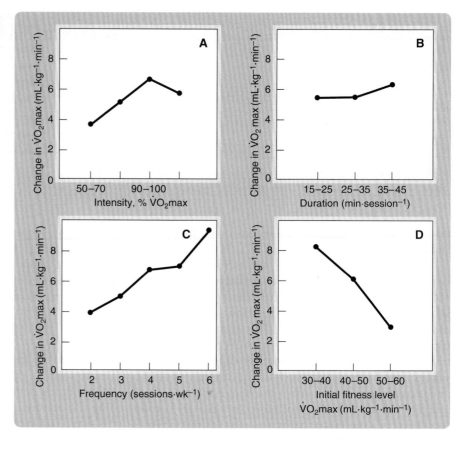

HEART RATE METHODS Exercise intensity can be expressed as a percentage of either maximal heart rate (%HRmax) or heart rate reserve (% HRR). The %HRR method may be preferable because it reflects the rate of energy expenditure during exercise well, and because exercise intensity can be underestimated or overestimated when using %HRmax (American College of Sports Medicine, 2011). Both techniques, explained below, require maximal heart rate to be known or estimated. The methods are most accurate if the maximal heart rate is actually measured during an incremental exercise test to maximum. If such a test cannot be performed, maximal heart rate can be estimated. ACSM recommends the following traditional, empirically based, easy formula using age despite the equation's large (±12–15 b·min⁻¹) standard deviation (American College of Sports

Medicine, 2011; Wallace, 2006). This large standard deviation, based on population averages, means that the calculated value may either overestimate (in individuals over 40 years) or underestimate (in individuals under 40 years) the true HRmax by as much as 12–15 b·min⁻¹ (American College of Sports Medicine, 2010; Miller et al., 1993; Wallace, 2006).

13.1a maximal heart rate (b·min⁻¹) = 220 − age (yr)

For obese individuals, the following equation is more accurate (Miller et al., 1993):

13.1b maximal heart rate (b·min⁻¹) = 200 − [0.5 × age (yr)]

TABLE 13.3 Classification of Intensity of Exercise Based on 20–60 min of Endurance Training

Classification of Intensity	Relative Intensity		
	%HRmax	**%HRR/%$\dot{V}O_2$R**	**Borg's Rating of Perceived Exertion**
Very light	<57	<30	<9
Light	57–63	30–39	9–11
Moderate	64–76	40–59	12–13
Vigorous	77–95	60–89	14–17
Near-maximal to maximal	≥96	≥90	≥18

Source: American College of Sports Medicine: Position stand: Quantity and quality of exercise for developing and maintaining cardiorespiratory, musculoskeletal, and neuromotor fitness in apparently healthy adults: Guidance for prescribing exercise. *Medicine & Science in Sports & Exercise*. 43(7):1334–1359 (2011).

For older adults, the following equation is more accurate (Tanaka et al., 2001).

13.1c maximal heart rate $(b \cdot min^{-1}) = 208 - [0.7 \times$ age (yr)]

As indicated in Chapter 12, maximal heart rate is independent of age between the growing years of 6 and 16. This means that the 220 – age formula cannot be used for youngsters at this age (Rowland, 2005). During this age span for both boys and girls, the average HRmax resulting from treadmill running is 200–205 $b \cdot min^{-1}$. Values obtained during walking and cycling are typically 5–10 $b \cdot min^{-1}$ lower at maximum. As with adults, measured values are always preferable but may not be practical. Therefore, the value estimated for HRmax for children and young adolescents should depend on modality rather than age.

EXAMPLE

Calculate the predicted or estimated HRmax for a 28-year-old female with a normal body composition.

$$HRmax = 220 - age = 220 - (28\,yr) = 192\,b \cdot min^{-1}$$

If the female is obese, her estimated maximal heart rate is

$$HRmax = 200 - (0.5 \times age) = 200 - (0.5 \times 28\,yr)$$
$$= 186\,b \cdot min^{-1}$$

Once the maximal heart rate is known or estimated, the %HRmax is calculated as follows:

13.2 Target exercise heart rate (TExHR) = maximal heart rate $(b \cdot min^{-1}) \times$ percentage of maximal heart rate (expressed as a decimal)

or

TExHR = HRmax × %HRmax

1. Determine the desired intensity of the workout.
2. Use **Table 13.3** to find the %HRmax associated with the desired exercise intensity.
3. Multiply the percentages (as decimals) times the HRmax.

EXAMPLE

Determine the appropriate HR training range for a moderate workout for a nonobese 28-year-old using the HRmax.

1. Determine the HRmax:

$$220 - 28 = 192\,b \cdot min^{-1}$$

2. Determine the desired intensity of the workout. **Table 13.3** shows 64–76% of HRmax corresponds to a moderate workout.

EXAMPLE (continued)

3. Multiply the percentages (as decimals) times the HRmax for the upper and lower exercise limits. Thus:

HRmax	192	192
desired intensity (decimal)	× 0.64	× 0.76
Target HR Range (rounded)	123	146

Thus, a HR of 122 $b \cdot min^{-1}$ represents 64% of HRmax and a HR of 146 $b \cdot min^{-1}$ represents 76% of HRmax. To exercise between 64% and 76% of HRmax, a moderate workload, this individual should keep the heart rate between 122 and 146 $b \cdot min^{-1}$.

It is always best to provide the potential exerciser with a target heart rate range rather than a threshold heart rate. In fact, the term threshold may be a misnomer since no particular percentage has been shown to be a minimally necessary threshold for all individuals in all situations (Haskell, 1994). Evidence of a minimum threshold is supported in some, but not all, studies and may be related to the initial fitness level of the individual, the precise program followed, and individual variability of response (American College of Sports Medicine, 2011). Additionally, a range allows for the heart rate drift that occurs in moderate to heavy exercise after about 30 minutes and for variations in weather, terrain, fluid replacement, and other influences. The upper limit serves as a boundary against overexertion.

Alternatively, a target heart rate range can be calculated as a percentage of heart rate reserve (%HRR), a technique also called the *Karvonen* method. It involves additional information and calculations but has the advantage of considering resting heart rate. The steps are as follows:

1. Determine the heart rate reserve (HRR) by subtracting the resting heart rate from the maximal heart rate:

13.3 Heart rate reserve $(b \cdot min^{-1})$ = maximal heart rate $(b \cdot min^{-1})$ – resting heart rate $(b \cdot min^{-1})$

or

HRR = HRmax – RHR

The resting heart rate is best determined when the individual is truly resting, such as immediately on awakening in the morning. However, for purposes of exercise prescription, this can be a seated or standing resting heart rate, depending on the exercise posture. Heart rates taken before an exercise test are anticipatory, not resting, and are higher than actual resting heart rate.

2. Choose the desired intensity of the workout.
3. Use **Table 13.3** to find the %HRR associated with the desired exercise intensity.

4. Multiply the percentages (as decimals) for the upper and lower exercise limits by the HRR and add RHR using Equation 13.4.

13.4 Target exercise heart rate $(b \cdot min^{-1})$ = [heart rate reserve $(b \cdot min^{-1}) \times$ percentage of heart rate reserve (expressed as a decimal)] + resting heart rate $(b \cdot min^{-1})$

or

$$TExHR = (HRR \times \%HRR) + RHR$$

EXAMPLE

Determine the appropriate HR range for a moderate workout for a normal weight 28-year-old using the HRR method, assuming a RHR of 80 b·min⁻¹.

1. Determine the HRR:

$$192b \cdot min^{-1} - 80b \cdot min^{-1} = 112b \cdot min^{-1}$$

2. Determine the desired intensity of the workout. Again, using **Table 13.3**, 40–59% of HRR corresponds to a moderate workout. This reinforces the point that the %HRmax does not equal %HRR.
3. Multiply the percentages (as decimals) for the upper and lower exercise limits by the HRR. Thus:

HRR	112	112
desired intensity (decimal)	$\times \underline{0.4}$	$\times \underline{0.59}$
	45	66

4. Add RHR as follows:

	45	66
resting HR	+80	+80
target HR training range $(b \cdot min^{-1})$	125	146

Thus, a HR of 125 b·min⁻¹ represents 40% of HRR and a HR of 146 b·min⁻¹ represents 59% of HRR. So, in order to be exercising between 40% and 59% of HRR, a moderate workload, this individual should keep the heart rate between 125 and 146 b·min⁻¹.

This heart rate range (125–146 b·min⁻¹), is only slightly different from the one calculated by using %HRmax (122–146 b·min⁻¹) but the %HRR technique has the advantage of taking into account any training adaptations that occur in resting heart rate for future adjustments and is more closely tied with energy expenditure.

Work through the problem presented in the Check Your Comprehension 1 box, paying careful attention to the influence of resting heart rate when determining the training heart rate range using the heart rate reserve (Karvonen) method. Check your answer in Appendix C.

CHECK YOUR COMPREHENSION 1

Calculate the target HR range for a light workout for two normal-weight individuals, using the %HRmax and %HRR methods and the following information.

	Age	RHR
Mei	50	62
Serena	60	82

Maximal heart rate declines in a rectilinear fashion with advancing age in adults. Thus, the heart rate needed to achieve a given intensity level, calculated by either the maximal heart rate or heart rate reserve method, decreases with age.

OXYGEN CONSUMPTION/%V̇O₂R METHODS In a laboratory setting where an individual has been tested for $\dot{V}O_2max$ and equipment is available for monitoring $\dot{V}O_2$ during training, $\%\dot{V}O_2R$ may be used to prescribe exercise intensity. Oxygen reserve is parallel to heart rate reserve in that it is the difference between a resting and maximal value. It is calculated according to the formula:

13.5 Oxygen consumption reserve $(mL \cdot kg^{-1} \cdot min^{-1})$ = maximal oxygen consumption $(mL \cdot kg^{-1} \cdot min^{-1})$ − resting oxygen consumption $(mL \cdot kg^{-1} \cdot min^{-1})$

or

$$\dot{V}O_2R = \dot{V}O_2max - \dot{V}O_2rest$$

Target exercise oxygen consumption is then determined by the equation:

13.6 Target exercise oxygen consumption $(mL \cdot kg^{-1} \cdot min^{-1})$ = [oxygen consumption reserve $(mL \cdot kg^{-1} \cdot min^{-1} \times$ percentage of oxygen consumption reserve (expressed as a decimal)] + resting oxygen consumption $(mL \cdot kg^{-1} \cdot min^{-1})$

or

$$TEx\dot{V}O_2 = (\dot{V}O_2R \times \%\dot{V}O_2R) + \dot{V}O_2rest$$

Use these steps to calculate training intensity with this method:

1. Choose the desired intensity of the workout.
2. Use **Table 13.3** to find the $\%\dot{V}O_2R$ for the desired exercise intensity.
3. Multiply the percentage (as a decimal) of the desired intensity times the $\dot{V}O_2max$.
4. Add the resting oxygen consumption to the obtained values. Note that this may be an individually measured value or the estimated 3.5 mL·kg⁻¹·min⁻¹ that represents 1 MET.
5. Because oxygen drifts, as does heart rate, it is best to use a target range.

Basing the intensity of a workout on $\%\dot{V}O_2R$ is not very practical because most people do not have access to the needed equipment. However, the technique can be modified for individuals who wish to use it. First, one can use the formula in Appendix B (The Calculation of Oxygen Consumed Using Mechanical Work or Speed of Movement) to solve for the workload (velocity of level or inclined walking or running; resistance for arm or leg cycling; height or cadence for bench stepping). Then the prescription can be based on minutes per mile, cadence of stepping at a particular height, or load setting at a specific revolutions per minute pace. Because the oxygen cost of submaximal exercise is higher for children and changes as they age and grow, this technique is rarely used for children (Strong et al., 2005).

A second practical use of the $\dot{V}O_2R$ approach is based on the direct relationship between heart rate and oxygen consumption. Look closely again at **Table 13.3**. Note that the column for $\%\dot{V}O_2R$ is also the column for $\%HRR$; that is, any given $\%HRR$ has an equivalent $\%\dot{V}O_2R$ in adults. For example, an adult who is working at 50% HRR is also working at 50% $\dot{V}O_2R$. Therefore, heart rate can be used to estimate oxygen consumption when an individual is training or competing. The equivalency between $\%\dot{V}O_2R$ and $\%HRR$ has been demonstrated experimentally in both young and elderly adult males and females, and for the modalities of cycle ergometry and treadmill walking and running (Swain, 2000).

Although there is also a rectilinear relationship between $\%HRR$ and $\%\dot{V}O_2R$ in children and adolescents, this relationship in not the same as for adults. In children and adolescents, the two percentages are not equal. In a recent study, 50–85% $\dot{V}O_2R$ was found to equate with 60–89% HRR in boy and girls 10–17 years of age (Hui and Chan, 2006). Therefore, it is probably best to simply use either $\%HRmax$ or $\%HRR$ when prescribing exercise intensity for children and adolescents, and not make any equivalency assumption with $\%\dot{V}O_2R$.

Table 13.4 shows how long one can run at a specific percentage of maximal oxygen consumption. The Check Your Comprehension 2 box provides an example of how this information can be used in training and competition. Take the time now to work through the situation described in the box.

CHECK YOUR COMPREHENSION 2

Four friends meet at the track for a noontime workout. Their physiological characteristics are as follows. (The estimated $\dot{V}O_2$max values have been calculated from a 1-mi running test.)

Individual	Age (yr)	Estimated $\dot{V}O_2$max (mL·kg^{-1}·min^{-1})	Resting HR (b·min^{-1})
Janet	23	52	60
Juan	35	64	48
Mark	22	49	64
Gail	28	56	58

The following oxygen requirements have been calculated for a given speed based on the equations that are presented in Appendix B.

Speed (mph)	Oxygen Requirement (mL·kg^{-1}·min^{-1})
4	27.6
5	30.3
6	35.7
7	41.0
8	46.4
9	51.7

The friends wish to run together in a moderate workout. Assume temperate weather conditions.

1. At what speed should they be running?

2. What heart rate should be achieved by each runner at that pace?

Check your answers with the ones provided in Appendix C.

TABLE 13.4	Time Period of a Selected $\%\dot{V}O_2$max Can Be Sustained during Running
$\%\dot{V}O_2$max	**Time (min)**
100.00	8–10
97.5	15
90	30
87.5	45
85	60
82.5	90
80	120–210

Source: Daniels, J. & J. Gilbert: *Oxygen Power: Performance Tables for Distance Runners.* Tempe, AZ: Author (1979).

Rating of Perceived Exertion A subjective impression of overall physical effort, strain, and fatigue during acute exercise.

RATING OF PERCEIVED EXERTION METHODS The third way exercise intensity can be prescribed is by a subjective impression of overall effort, strain, and fatigue during the activity. This impression is known as a **rating of perceived exertion** (RPE). Although RPE can be used alone as a prescriptive method (American College of Sports Medicine, 2010), it is best used to fine-tune an exercise prescription (American College of Sports Medicine, 2011). Perceived exertion is typically measured using either Borg's 6–20 RPE scale or the revised 0–10+ Category Ratio Scale (Borg,

TABLE 13.5 Scales for Ratings of Perceived Exertion

RPE Scale	CR-10 Scale
6	0.0
7 Very, very light	0.0
8	0.5 Just noticeable
9 Very light	1.0 Very weak
10	1.5
11 Fairly light	2.0 Light/weak
12	3.0 Moderate
13 Somewhat hard	3.5
	4.0 Somewhat strong
14	4.5
	5.0
15 Hard	5.5
	6.0
16	6.5 Very strong
	7.0
17 Very hard	7.5
	8.0
18	9.0
19 Very, very hard	10.0 Extremely strong
20	10+(~12) Highest possible

1998). **Table 13.5** presents and compares both scales. The RPE scale is designed so that these perceptual ratings rise in a rectilinear fashion with heart rate, oxygen consumption, and mechanical workload during incremental exercise; thus, it is the primary scale used for cardiovascular exercise prescription (**Table 13.3**). The CR-10 scale

increases in a positively accelerating curvilinear fashion and closely parallels the physiological responses of pulmonary ventilation and blood lactate. Chapter 5 describes the use of these scales for metabolic exercise prescription.

Both the Borg RPE and CR-10 scales are intended for use with postpubertal adolescents and adults. Because children (~6–12 years) have difficulty consistently assigning numbers to words or phrases to describe their exercise-related feelings, Robertson et al. (2002) developed the Children's OMNI Scale of Perceived Exertion. The OMNI Scale uses numerical, pictorial, and verbal descriptors. The original scale, depicted in **Figure 13.2**, was validated for cycling activity. Since then, variations have been developed for walking/running (Utter et al., 2002) and stepping (Robertson et al., 2005). Children have been shown to be able to self-regulate their cycling exercise intensity using the OMNI Scale (Robertson et al., 2002). In addition, observers can determine children's exercise intensity using the OMNI Scale (Robertson et al., 2006). This could be very helpful for teachers.

The classification of exercise intensity and the corresponding relationships among %HRmax, %$\dot{V}O_2$R, % HRR, and RPE presented in **Table 13.3** have been derived from and are intended for use with land-based activities in moderate environments.

Whether a water activity is performed horizontally, as in swimming, or vertically, as in running or water aerobics, postural and pressure changes shift the blood volume centrally and cause changes in blood pressure, cardiac output, resistance, and respiration. Although the magnitude of changes in the cardiovascular system vary considerably among individuals, the most consistent changes are lower submaximal HR (8–12 b·min⁻¹) at any given $\dot{V}O_2$, a lower

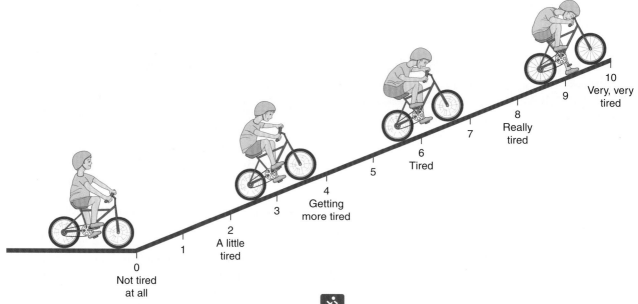

FIGURE 13.2 Children's OMNI Scale of Perceived Exertion.
Source: Robertson, R. J., F. L. Goss, N. F. Boer, et al.: Children's OMNI Scale of Perceived Exertion: Mixed gender and race validation. *Medicine & Science in Sports & Exercise*. 32(3):452–458 (2000). Reprinted with Permission.

Ratings of Perceived Exertion and Environmental Conditions

Rating of Perceived Exertion (RPE) is a useful, common way to assist in exercise intensity prescription. Note, however, that the estimation of RPE (when exercisers are asked how hard they feel they are exercising) and actual physiological responses to exercise are affected by environmental conditions. Both HR and RPE are higher when exercise is performed in a hot environment (or while wearing clothing that interferes with heat dissipation) compared to a thermoneutral environment. The relationship between HR and RPE is also affected by environmental conditions. At any given RPE, HR is 10–15 b·min^{-1} higher in the heat (Maw et al., 1993). When exercisers are instructed to produce a given exercise intensity based on a specific RPE, they usually automatically adjust the exercise intensity to environmental conditions. For example, running at 8 min·mi^{-1} in thermal neutral conditions may elicit an RPE estimation of 13. However, in hot humid conditions, an individual may only run at 9 min·mi^{-1} at an RPE of 13.

HRmax (~15 b·min^{-1}), and a lower $\dot{V}O_2$max when exercise is performed in the water. A greater reliance on anaerobic metabolism is evident, and the RPE is higher in water than at the same workload on land (Svedenhag and Seger, 1992). The lower HR is probably a compensation for the increased stroke volume when blood is shifted centrally. As a result, the HR prescription should be about 10% lower for water workouts than for land-based workouts. For example, if an individual normally works out at 75% HRmax on land, the prescription for an equivalent workout in the water should be 65% HRmax. Another way to achieve the adjustment, if an estimated HRmax is used, is to start with 205 b·min^{-1} minus age rather than 220 b·min^{-1} minus age. Either of these changes should effectively reduce the RPE as well.

Regardless of the method chosen to prescribe exercise intensity, always consider three factors:

1. Exercise intensity should generally be prescribed within a range. Many activities require different levels of exertion throughout the activity. This is particularly true of games and athletic activities, but it also applies to activities like jogging and bicycling, in which changes in terrain can greatly affect exertion. In addition, a range allows for cardiovascular and oxygen consumption drifts during prolonged exercise.
2. Exercise intensity must be considered in conjunction with duration and frequency.
   a. Intensity cannot be prescribed without regard to duration. These two variables are inversely related: In general, the more intense an activity is, the shorter it should be.
   b. The appropriate intensity of exercise also depends on the individual's fitness level and, to some extent, the point within his or her fitness program. Individuals should begin an exercise program at a low exercise intensity and gradually increase intensity in a steploading progression until the desired level is achieved.
3. Using heart rate or perceived exertion to monitor training sessions, rather than merely time over distance, allows the influence of weather, terrain, surfaces, and the way the individual is responding to be taken into account when assessing the person's adaptation to a training program.

Duration

As shown in **Figure 13.1B**, improvements in $\dot{V}O_2$max can be achieved when exercise is sustained for durations of 15–45 minutes (Wenger and Bell, 1986). Slightly greater improvements are achieved from longer sessions (35–45 minutes) than from shorter sessions (either 15–25 or 25–35 minutes). Indeed, greater improvements in $\dot{V}O_2$max can be achieved if the sessions are long (35–45 minutes) and the intensity moderate to heavy (50–90%) than if the sessions are short (25–35 minutes) and the intensity very hard to maximal (90–100%). Apparently, the total volume of work is more important in determining cardiorespiratory adaptations than either intensity or duration considered individually. This is good news, because the risk of injury is lower in moderate-intensity, long-duration activity than in high, near-maximal, short-duration activity; and the compliance rate is higher. Although a program of all moderate or all vigorous exercise will result in fitness improvements, most adult fitness programs should emphasize a combination of moderate and vigorous-intensity workouts for a duration of 20–60 minutes for optimal improvements (American College of Sports Medicine, 2006, 2010, 2011). Light to moderate intensity may be necessary and beneficial in severely deconditioned individuals. The recommended duration of exercise is approximately equal to 150 min·wk^{-1} for moderate activity and 75 min·wk^{-1} for vigorous activity.

The 20–60 minute recommendation does not mean that exercise sessions less than 20 minutes are not valuable for $\dot{V}O_2$max or health benefits or that at least 20 minutes must be accumulated during one exercise session. Similarly, although it is most often the case in practice, it does not mean that the exercise must be continuous within any single session. The technique of interval training (alternating predetermined periods of exercise and rest) often used by athletes can be very effective in improving cardiorespiratory fitness (American College of Sports Medicine, 2011). Exercise bouts of 10 minutes are acceptable if the individual accumulates at least 20–60 minutes for the day, 3–5 d·wk^{-1}. For example, two groups of adult males participated in a walk-jog program at 65–75% HRmax, for 5 d·wk^{-1} for 8 weeks (De Busk et al., 1990). The only variation was that one group did the 30-minute workout continuously while the other had 10-minute sessions at three different times during the day. Both groups increased the primary fitness variable $\dot{V}O_2$max significantly (although the 30-minute consecutive group did so to a greater extent) and lost equal amounts of weight—an important health benefit.

Thus, for individuals who claim they do not have time to exercise, suggesting a 10-minute brisk walk in the morning (perhaps to work or walking the kids to school), at noon (to a favorite restaurant and back), and in the evening (perhaps walking to the movie or taking the dog for a walk) might make it easier to achieve a total of 30 minutes of activity. The benefit of split sessions is particularly important for those in rehabilitation programs. An injured person may simply not be able to exercise for a long period, while short bouts may be possible spread throughout the day.

Pedometer step counts are another way of assessing the quantity of exercise. Attainment of 10,000 or more steps per day has been recommended as an exercise prescription, but this recommendation needs further study in different populations and with a variety of health outcomes taking into account the intensity of the steps (American College of Sports Medicine, 2010). Recent studies suggest that fewer than 10,000 steps per day may provide health benefits. Moderate-intensity walking (at ~100 steps·min^{-1}) for 30 minutes equates to 3000–4000 steps and can be used as a realistic minimal daily goal. Increasing pedometer steps counts to reach ≥7000 steps per day is beneficial (American College of Sports Medicine, 2011).

Frequency

If the total work done or the number of exercise sessions is held constant, there is basically no difference in the improvement of $\dot{V}O_2$max over 2, 3, 4, or 5 days (Pollock, 1973). However, when these conditions are not adhered to, there does seem to be an advantage to more frequent training. As **Figure 13.1C** shows, the improvement in $\dot{V}O_2$max is proportional to the number of training sessions per week (Wenger and Bell, 1986). In general, training fewer than 2 d·wk^{-1} did not result in improvements in $\dot{V}O_2$max. Likewise, further improvement in $\dot{V}O_2$max was not meaningful when exercise participation was increased from 4 to 5 days a week. Although the graph in **Figure 13.1C** reveals that there is the potential for further improvement in $\dot{V}O_2$max if a sixth day of training is added, it is not generally recommended for those pursuing fitness goals because of a higher incidence of

injury and fatigue. The optimal frequency for improving $\dot{V}O_2$max for all intensities appears to be 4 d·wk^{-1}.

The American College of Sports Medicine (2010, 2011) recommendation for healthy individuals is a frequency of 3–5 with moderated intensity being done 5 d·wk^{-1} or vigorous done 3 d·wk^{-1} with the assumption that these days are nonconsecutive. However, individuals at very low fitness levels may start a program of only 2 d·wk^{-1} if they are attempting to meet the ACSM intensity and duration guidelines. Athletes in training may train 6 d·wk^{-1} as a way of increasing their total training volume. In this case "easy" and "hard" days should be interspersed within most microcycles. Cross-training may also be employed. A special case is the "weekend warrior," that is, the individual who accumulates a large volume of physical activity in a 2-day weekend. Existing evidence supports the possibility of benefit, although the injury risks are unknown (American College of Sports Medicine, 2011).

Individualization

Fitness programs should be individualized for participants. Not only do individual goals vary, but individuals also respond to and adapt to exercise differently. One of the major determinants of the individual's response is genetics. Another major determinant is initial fitness level. **Figure 13.1D** clearly shows that independent of frequency, intensity, or duration, the greatest improvements in $\dot{V}O_2$max occur in individuals with the lowest initial-fitness level. Thus, both absolute and relative increases in $\dot{V}O_2$max are inversely related to one's initial fitness level. Although improvements in $\dot{V}O_2$max are smallest in highly fit individuals; at this level small changes may have a significant influence on performance, because many athletic events are won by fractions of a second.

The initial fitness-level generalization also applies to health benefits. Health benefits are greatest when a person moves from a low-fitness to a moderately fit category. Most sedentary individuals can accomplish this if they participate in a regular, low-to-moderate–endurance exercise program (Haskell, 1994).

Rest/Recovery/Adaptation

Training programs can be divided into initial, improvement, and maintenance stages. The initial stage usually lasts 1–6 weeks, although this varies considerably among individuals. This stage should include low-level aerobic activities that cause a minimum of muscle soreness or discomfort. It is often prudent to begin an exercise program at an intensity lower than the desired exercise range (40–59% HRR). The aerobic exercise session should last at least 10 minutes and gradually become longer by 5–10 minutes every 1–2 weeks over the first 4–6 weeks (American College of Sports Medicine, 2010). For individuals at very low levels of fitness, a discontinuous or interval format training program may be warranted, using several repetitions of exercise, each lasting 2–5 minutes. Rest periods between the intervals reduce the overall stress on the individual by allowing intermittent recovery. Frequency may vary from short, light daily activity to longer exercise sessions two or three times per week. Adaptation occurs during the off days. An important part of this stage is helping the individual achieve the "habit" of exercise and orthopedically adapt to workouts. Soreness, discomfort, and injury should be avoided to encourage the individual to continue.

During the improvement stage, significant changes in physiological function indicate that the body is adapting to the stress of the training program. Again, the individual adapts during rest days when the body is allowed to recover. Adaptation has occurred when the same amount of work is accomplished in less time, when the same amount of work is accomplished with less physiological (homeostatic) disruption, when the same amount of work is accomplished with a lower perception of fatigue or exertion, or when more work is accomplished. Once the body has adapted to the stress of exercise, progression is necessary to induce additional adaptations, or maintenance is required to preserve the adaptations.

Progression

Once adaptation occurs, the workload must be increased for further improvement to occur. The workload can be increased by manipulating the frequency, intensity, and duration of the exercise. Increasing any of these variables effectively increases the volume of exercise and thus provides the overload necessary for further adaptation. The rate of progression depends on the individual's needs or goals, fitness level, health status, exercise tolerance, and age but should always be done in a steploading fashion of 2–3 weeks of increase followed by a decrease for recovery and regeneration before increasing training volume again.

The improvement stage of a training program typically lasts 4–8 months and is characterized by relatively rapid progression. For an individual with a low fitness level, the progression from a discontinuous activity to a continuous activity should occur first. Then the duration of the activity should be increased. This increase in duration should not exceed 20% per week until 20–30 minutes of moderate to vigorous intensity activity can be completed, and 10% per week thereafter. Frequency can then be increased. Intensity should be the last variable to be increased. Adjustments of no more than 5% HRR every six exercise sessions (1.5–2 weeks) are well tolerated.

The principles of adaptation and progression are intertwined. Adaptation and progression may be repeated several times until the desired level of fitness or performance is achieved. Each time an exercise program is modified, there will be a period of adaptation that may be followed by further progression if desired.

Maintenance

Athletes often vary their training levels according to a general preparation phase (off-season), specific preparation phase (preseason), competitive phase (in-season), and transition phase (active rest). In transition and competitive phases they can shift to a maintenance schedule. For rehabilitation and fitness participants, maintenance typically begins after the first 4–8 months of training. Reaching the maintenance stage indicates that the individual has achieved a personally acceptable level of cardiorespiratory fitness and is no longer interested in increasing the conditioning load (American College of Sports Medicine, 2006).

After attaining a desired level of aerobic fitness, this level can be maintained either by continuing the same volume of exercise or by decreasing the volume of training, as long as intensity is maintained. **Figure 13.3** shows the results of research that investigated changes in $\dot{V}O_2max$ with 10 weeks of relatively intense interval training and a subsequent 15-week reduction in training frequency (13.3A), duration (13.3B), or intensity (13.3C) (Hickson and Rosenkoetter, 1981; Hickson et al., 1982, 1985). When training frequency was reduced from 6 $d \cdot wk^{-1}$ to 4 or 2 $d \cdot wk^{-1}$ and intensity and duration were held constant, training-induced improvements in $\dot{V}O_2max$ were maintained. Similarly, when training duration was reduced from 40 to 26 or 13 minutes, improvements in $\dot{V}O_2max$ were maintained or continued to improve. However, when intensity was reduced by two thirds, improvements in $\dot{V}O_2max$ were not maintained. These results indicate that intensity plays a primary role in maintaining cardiovascular fitness. Thus, although the total volume of exercise is most important for attaining a given fitness level, intensity is most important for maintaining the achieved fitness level. That is, in general, more exercise is required to improve cardiorespiratory fitness and health than is required to maintain the resultant improvements (American College of Sports Medicine, 2011).

During the maintenance phase of a training program, cross-training is particularly beneficial, especially on days when a high-intensity workout is not called for. For example, one study divided endurance-trained runners into three groups. One third continued to train by running, one third trained on a cycle ergometer, and one third trained by deep water running. The intensity, frequency, and duration of workouts in each modality were equal. After 6 weeks, performance in a 2-mi run had improved slightly (~1%) in all three groups (Eyestone et al., 1993). Thus, running performance was maintained by each of the modalities. On the other hand, arm ergometer training has not been shown to maintain training benefits derived from leg ergometer activity (Pate et al., 1978). Apparently, the closer the activities are in terms of muscle action, the greater the potential maintenance benefit of cross-training.

Retrogression/Plateau/Reversibility

Sometimes, an individual in training may fail to improve (plateau) or exhibit a performance or physiological decrement (retrogression), despite progression of the training program. When such a pattern occurs, it is important to

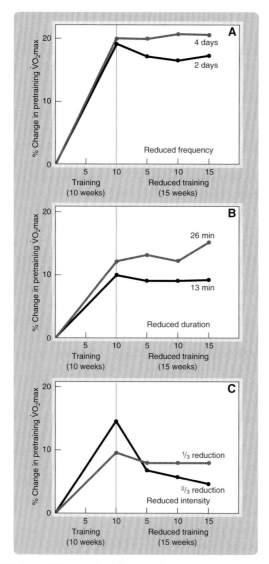

FIGURE 13.3 Effects of Reducing Exercise Frequency, Intensity, and Duration on Maintenance of V̇O₂max.

A. Improvements in V̇O₂max during 10 weeks of training (bicycling and running) for 40 minutes a day, 6 days a week were maintained when training intensity and duration were maintained with a reduction in frequency from 6 days a week to 4 or even 2 d·wk⁻¹. **B.** V̇O₂max was maintained when frequency of training and intensity were maintained with a reduction of training duration to 13 minutes. V̇O₂max continued to improve when training duration was reduced to 26 minutes. **C.** V̇O₂max was maintained when frequency and duration were maintained and intensity was reduced by one third. V̇O₂max was not maintained when training was reduced by two thirds.

Sources: Hickson, R. C. & M. A. Rosenkoetter: Reduced training frequencies and maintenance of increased aerobic power. *Medicine and Science in Sports and Exercise*. 13:13–16 (1981); Hickson, R. C., C. Kanakis, J. R. Davis, A. M. Moore, & S. Rich: Reduced training duration effects on aerobic power, endurance, and cardiac growth. *Journal of Applied Physiology*. 53(1):225–229 (1982); Hickson, R. C., C. Foster, M. L. Pollock, T. M. Galassi, & S. Rich: Reduced training intensities and loss of aerobic power, endurance, and cardiac growth. *Journal of Applied Physiology*. 58:492–499 (1985).

check for other signs of overtraining (see Chapters 1 and 22). A shift in training emphasis or the inclusion of more easy days is warranted. Remember that a reduction in the frequency of training does not necessarily lead to detraining and may actually enhance performance.

If training is discontinued for a significant period of time, detraining will occur. This principle, often referred to as the reversibility concept, holds that when a training program is stopped or reduced, body systems readjust in accordance with the decreased physiological stimuli. Increases in V̇O₂max with low to moderate exercise programs are completely reversed after training is stopped. Values of V̇O₂max decrease rapidly during a month of detraining, followed by a slower rate of decline during the second and third month (Bloomfield and Coyle, 1993).

Warm-Up and Cooldown

A warm-up period allows the body to adjust to the cardiovascular demands of exercise. At rest the skeletal muscles receive about 15–20% of the blood pumped from the heart; during moderate exercise they receive approximately 70%. This increased blood flow is important for warming the body since the blood carries heat from the metabolically active muscle to the rest of the body.

A warm-up period of 5–15 minutes at low to moderate intensity should precede the conditioning portion of an exercise session (American College of Sports Medicine, 2010). The warm-up should gradually increase in intensity until the desired intensity of training is reached. For many activities the warm-up period simply continues into the aerobic portion of the exercise session. For example, if an individual is going for a noontime run and wants to run at an 8 min·mi⁻¹ pace, he or she may begin with a slow jog for the first few minutes (say a 10 min·mi⁻¹ pace), increase to a faster pace (say a 9 min·mi⁻¹ pace), and then proceed into the desired pace (the 8 min·mi⁻¹ pace).

A warm-up period has the following beneficial effects on cardiovascular function.

- It increases blood flow to the active skeletal muscles.
- It increases blood flow to the myocardium.
- It increases the dissociation of oxyhemoglobin.
- It causes sweating, which plays a role in temperature regulation.
- It may reduce the incidence of abnormal rhythms in the heart's conduction system (dysrhythmias), which can lead to abnormal heart function (Barnard et al., 1973).

A cooldown period of 5–15 minutes of moderate- to low-intensity activity should follow the conditioning period of the exercise session (American College of Sports Medicine, 2010). The cooldown period prevents venous pooling by keeping the muscle pump active and thus may reduce the risk of postexercise hypotension (and possible fainting) and dysrhythmias. A cooldown also facilitates

FOCUS ON APPLICATION

Manipulation of Training Overload in a Taper

Peaking for performance often involves manipulating the training principles of specificity, overload, and maintenance within a periodization plan. This is exemplified by a study in which 18 male and 6 female distance runners were pretested, matched, and then divided into three groups. The run taper group systematically reduced its weekly training volume to 15% of their previous training volume over a 7-day period, performing 30% of the calculated reduced training distance on day 1, and then 20%, 15%, 12%, 10%, 8%, and 5% on each succeeding day. Training consisted of 400-m intervals at close to 5-km pace (~100% $\dot{V}O_2$peak) resulting in a HR of 170–190 b·min^{-1} with recovery to 100–110 b·min^{-1} before the next interval. The cycle taper group performed approximately the same number of intervals for the same duration as paired athletes in the run taper group, at the same work and recovery heart rates. The control group continued normal training, of which 6–10% of the weekly training

distance was interval/fartlek work. All subjects participated in a 10-minute submaximal treadmill run, an incremental treadmill test to volitional fatigue in which the grade remained constant at 0% and the speed increased, and a 5-km time trial on the treadmill.

At the same absolute speed during the submaximal run, the run taper group (and seven of the eight individual runners) exhibited a 5% reduction (2.4 mL·kg^{-1}·min^{-1}) in oxygen consumption and a decrease of 7% (0.9 kcal·min^{-1}) in calculated energy expenditure. No changes were evident in either the cycle taper or control group. Both maximal treadmill speed (2%) and total exercise time (4%) increased for the run taper group without a concomitant increase in $\dot{V}O_2$max or HRmax. No changes occurred in any maximal value for the cycle taper or control groups. The run taper group (all eight individuals) significantly improved 5-km performance by a mean of 2.8 ± 0.4%, or an average of almost 30 seconds. No improvement in

performance was seen in either the cycle taper or control groups.

These results clearly demonstrate the benefits of a 7-day taper in which intensity is maintained, training volume drastically reduced, and specificity of training utilized. Of the variables measured, the most likely explanation for the improved 5-km performance was the increase in submaximal running economy (decreased submaximal oxygen and energy cost). Note, however, that all three groups maintained their $\dot{V}O_2$max values. This cross-training benefit exhibited by the cycle taper group is particularly important. Distance runners often have nagging injuries. These results imply that a non–weight-bearing taper may be used in such cases and allow the runner to possibly heal (or at least not aggravate an injury) while maintaining cardiovascular fitness. Performance enhancement, however, appears to require mode specificity during the taper.

Source: Houmard et al. (1994).

heat dissipation and promotes a more rapid removal of lactic acid and catecholamines from the blood.

Training Principles and Physical Activity Recommendations

Much evidence has been compiled that demonstrates the health-related benefits of moderate physical activity, including reduced incidence of cardiac events, stroke, hypertension, type 2 diabetes, some types of cancer, obesity, the metabolic syndrome, depression, and anxiety. This evidence summarized in The Surgeon General's Report (SGR) on Physical Activity and Health recomendation (U.S. Department of Health and Human Services, 1996) have been updated in the American College of Sports Medicine position stand (2011). The SGR was an important public health statement that recognized the health benefits associated with moderate levels of physical activity and encouraged increased activity among Americans by widely publicizing those health benefits and recommending levels of activity (an accumulation of 30 minutes of moderate-intensity physical activity on most, if not all, days of the week) that were intended to

be nonintimidating for currently sedentary individuals. Both joint statements by the American Heart Association and ACSM (Haskell et al., 2007; Nelson et al., 2007) and the "2008 Physical Activity Guidelines for Americans" (U.S. Department of Health and Human Services, 2008) clarified that moderate activity should be done 5 days a week or vigorous activity 3 d·wk^{-1} instead of the generic "on most days" for moderate activity. Such moderate- and vigorous-intensity activities were to be in addition to routine activities of daily living, which are of light intensity such as casual walking or grocery shopping. However, moderate or vigorous activities performed as part of daily life such as brisk walking to work or other manual labor performed in bouts of 10 minutes or more could be counted toward the time recommendation. In addition, the dose-response relationship between physical activity and health benefit was now emphasized. This continues to be the case. That is, while some activity of moderate intensity is better than no activity, more activity and more vigorous activity is better than less activity, within reasonable limits. All of these previous recommendations for adults have been incorporated into the current ACSM guidelines (2011). Canadian guidelines for adults (Canadian Society for Exercise Physiology, 2011) are similar but stated in terms of time (150 min·wk^{-1})

indicating that it is unclear which frequency of activity is best for maximal benefit. The 150 minutes is exclusive of any neuromuscular training (Tremblay et al., 2011).

Table 13.1 contains three sets of recommendations for physical activity for children and adolescents (Canadian Society for Exercise Physiology (CSEP); National Association for Sport and Physical Education (NASPE); Centers for Disease Control and Prevention (CDC)). Recent evidence has indicated that 30 min·d^{-1} is not sufficient exercise for school-age individuals. This is reflected in the recommendations of 60+ min·d^{-1} of moderate to vigorous physical activity (CSEP, 2011; NASPE, 2004; Strong et al., 2005) for this age group. CSEP specifies that children/adolescents should participate in vigorous-intensity activity at least 3 d·wk^{-1}. The 60-minute recommendation is inclusive of both the aerobic activity and the bone/muscle strengthening activity.

As with adults, children/adolescents can accumulate the recommended duration of activity throughout the day rather than in a single more structured training session. Children by nature tend to be sporadic exercisers, and getting them to exercise continuously is both unrealistic and unnecessary (Corbin et al., 2004). However, the NASPE guidelines do recommend that children should participate in several bouts of physical activity each day each lasting 15 minutes or more. Note that the 60-minute recommendation for those between 5 and 18 years of age is considered a minimum. Also, although not presented in Table 13.1, NASPE and CSEP recommend that extended periods of inactivity (2 or more hours at one time) be discouraged for children during waking hours. This includes screen time, motorized transport, extended sitting, and nonactive indoor time.

In contrast to the more formal exercise prescription recommendations of a frequency of 3–5 d·wk^{-1} for adults (to allow for the necessary rest and recovery to achieve adaptation to high-intensity exertion) the physical activity recommendations for children call for daily participation. This is actually easier for many youngsters because the activity behavior becomes a habit. Of course, older adolescents involved in specific sport training may modify this guideline according to their increased training needs. Unfortunately for nonathletes, a decline in physical activity commonly occurs through adolescence (Strong et al., 2005).

With few exceptions, children and adolescents ideally should be involved in a wide variety of age-appropriate activities. As with adults, large muscle activities involving rhythmical dynamic muscle contractions are best for the development of cardiovascular fitness, but children and adolescents should try as many different activities as possible to develop their skills and learn which they enjoy most. Enjoyable activities are more likely to be continued throughout life.

All guidelines presented in Table 13.1 are intended for "apparently healthy" individuals of the appropriate age irrespective of gender, race, ethnicity, or socioeconomic status. Additionally, with appropriate evaluation, medical advisement, and initial modification to gradually progress to achieving the recommendations they may be used for individuals with certain chronic diseases or disabilities.

Physical activity recommendations are the manifestation of the cardiorespiratory training principles for public health. In addition to documented health benefits, moderate-intensity physical activity was and is promoted as a way to increase the palatability of exercise so that more people would participate. Unfortunately, there is still a large segment of the adult US population who report no leisure-time physical activity (Figure 13.4). The Centers for Disease Control and Prevention (CDC) periodically polls the US population on a variety of issues. Their latest published results indicate that the proportion of the population reporting no physical activity has decreased from about 31% in 1989 to about 25% in 2003 and has remained there through 2008 (CDC, 2011b). While this improvement is obviously a good thing, it does not mean that the remaining 75% are meeting the recommended levels. Data from 2005 indicated that 49.7% of adult males and 46.7% of adult females participated in at least minimal recommended levels of physical activity (CDC, 2007). For high school students in 2010 the percentages are considerably lower: 21.9% for males and 8.4% for females (CDC, 2011a). There is much room for improvement.

Cardiovascular Adaptations to Aerobic Endurance Training

As has been discussed, regular physical activity results in improvements in cardiovascular health and function. Although the primary goal and most obvious adaptation is an increase in $\dot{V}O_2$max, this adaptation is supported and accompanied by changes in numerous other physiological variables. The magnitude of the improvement depends on the training program—specifically on the frequency, intensity, and duration of the exercise and the individual's initial level of fitness. Figure 13.5 presents cardiovascular responses to incremental exercise to maximum following aerobic exercise training. Changes in cardiovascular variables may be evident at rest, during submaximal exercise, and during maximal exercise. Many of these changes have health implications.

Cardiac Dimensions

Cardiac dimensions and mass increase with endurance training (Huston et al., 1985; Keul et al., 1981; Longhurst et al., 1981). These changes are associated with high cardiac output during sustained aerobic exercise. Endurance training exposes the heart to conditions of increased ventricular filling, with subsequent high stroke volume and cardiac output. This chronic exposure to high levels of ventricular filling (large end-diastolic volume) is known as volume overload (Morganroth et al., 1975).

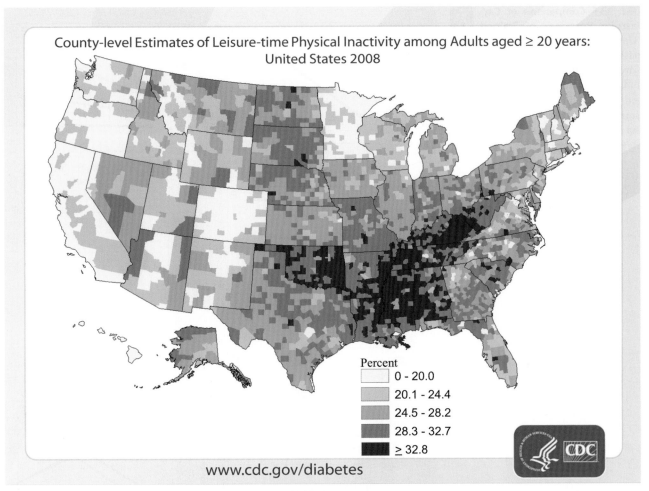

County-level Estimates of Leisure-time Physical Inactivity among Adults aged ≥ 20 years: United States 2008

Percent

	0 - 20.0
	20.1 - 24.4
	24.5 - 28.2
	28.3 - 32.7
	≥ 32.8

www.cdc.gov/diabetes

FIGURE 13.4 County Level Estimates of Leisure-time Physical Inactivity.
2008 Age-adjusted estimates of the percentage of adults who are physically inactive.
Source: Centers for Disease Control and Prevention: National Diabetes Surveillance System. Available online at: http://apps. nccd.cdc.gov/DDTSTRS/default.aspx. Retrieved 7/11/2011.

Chronic volume overload results in an increased left ventricular end-diastolic diameter (Huston et al., 1985; Keul et al., 1981) and left ventricular mass (Cohen and Segal, 1985; Longhurst et al., 1981). To better characterize the effect of aerobic training on both left and right ventricular mass and volume, Scharhag et al. (2002) used magnetic resonance imaging (MRI) to measure heart size and volume in a group of endurance-trained male athletes and a group of age- and size-matched controls. As shown in **Figure 13.6**, the aerobically trained athletes had greater right and left ventricular mass (**Figure 13.6A**) and greater right and left end-diastolic volume (**Figure 13.6B**).

Vascular Structure and Function

As described in Chapter 11, blood vessel walls contain a layer of smooth muscle, the tunica media. Blood flow to a given region is determined by the pressure gradient and the resistance ($F = \Delta P/R$). By far the greatest influence on resistance is the diameter of the vessel. Vessel diameter is determined by the actual size of the vessel and the relative degree of contraction of the smooth muscle in the tunica media. The greater the size of the vessel or the greater its ability to dilate, the greater the ability of the vasculature to provide increased blood flow to meet the needs of active tissue. Evidence shows that aerobic training can increase both the size of vessels and their ability to dilate.

Arterial Remodeling

Strong evidence suggests that endurance athletes have enlarged arteries, thus demonstrating that aerobic exercise leads to structural changes in arteries that increase resting lumen diameter (Dinenno et al., 2001; Prior et al., 2003; Schmidt-Trucksass et al., 2000). This is called arterial remodeling. Naylor et al. (2006) reported that the resting brachial artery diameter of elite rowers was significantly greater than that of untrained volunteers. Certainly, an increased arterial diameter to working muscle represents a positive adaptation to exercise, but evidence also

FIGURE 13.5 Comparison of Cardiovascular Response of Trained and Untrained Individuals to Incremental Exercise to Maximum.
A: Cardiac output (Q̇). **B:** Stroke volume (SV). **C:** Heart rate (HR). **D:** Maximal oxygen consumption (V̇O₂max). **E:** Blood pressure (BP). **F:** Resistance (R). **G:** Rate-pressure product (RPP).

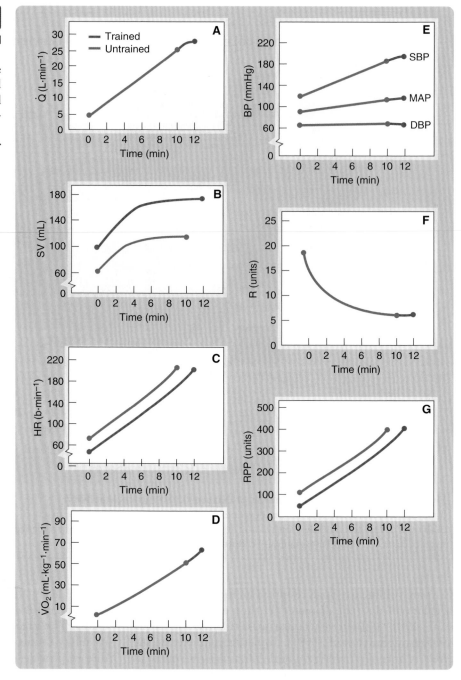

suggests that the coronary arteries, supplying blood to the working myocardium, are enlarged in highly trained athletes. Several studies (including the classic autopsy report of Clarence DeMar, winner of seven Boston marathons) have shown that habitual exercise is related to a larger cross-sectional arterial size. DeMar's arteries were reportedly two to three times the normal size (Currens and White, 1961).

Improved Endothelial Function

Exercise training leads to an improved ability of arterial vessels to vasodilate; the increased vasodilatory potential is directly related to endothelium nitric oxide production.

Aerobic training is therefore said to improve endothelial function. Improvements in endothelial function following aerobic exercise programs have been reported in healthy individuals with low risk for cardiac disease and in individuals with several risk factors as well as those with known cardiovascular disease (Green et al., 2003; Hambrecht et al., 1998; Niebauer and Cooke, 1996). Increasing evidence from animal studies shows that aerobic exercise leads to increased vasodilatory potential at several sites along the vascular tree, including the aorta, coronary arteries, and the brachial and femoral arteries (Jasperse and Laughlin, 2006).

Coronary vessels apparently have an increased vasodilatory response to exercise following exercise training.

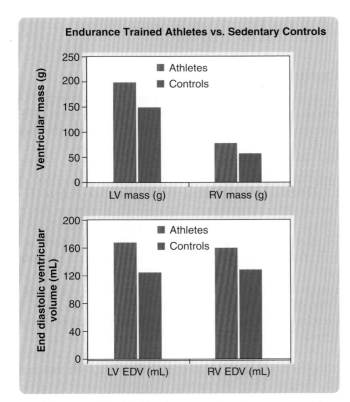

FIGURE 13.6 Comparison of Ventricular Mass (A) and End-Diastolic Ventricular Volumes (B) in a Group of Endurance Trained Athletes and Sedentary Controls.
Source: Based on Data in Scharhag, J., G. Schneider, A. Urhausen, V. Rochette, B. Kramann, & W. Kindermann: Athlete's heart: Right and left ventricular mass and function in male endurance athletes and untrained individuals determined by magnetic resonance imaging. *Journal of American College of Cardiology*. 40(10):1856–1863 (2002).

In a study that compared ultra marathoners to sedentary individuals, investigators found no difference in the internal diameter of the coronary arteries in the two groups at rest, but the capacity of the coronary arteries to dilate was two times greater in the marathoners than in the sedentary individuals (13.2 mm² versus 6 mm²) (Haskell et al., 1993). The ability of arteries to dilate during exercise may be even more important than the resting diameter, because the myocardial demand for oxygen is low during rest and high during exercise, as evidenced by the low rate-pressure product (RPP) at rest and the high RPP during exercise.

It is not yet possible to definitively describe the effect of aerobic training on endothelial function because the adaptation appears to depend on several factors, including the exercise stimulus, the species studied, the vessel size, the organ supplied, and the health status.

Clot Formation and Breakdown

As discussed in Chapter 11, a blood clot forms when needed to prevent blood loss from a damaged vessel. The body also breaks down clots (fibrinolysis) when they are no longer needed. Although blood clots are very useful when a vessel is damaged, unnecessary clots greatly increase the risk of heart attack and stroke.

Aerobic exercise training decreases the blood's tendency to clot and enhances the process of dissolving unnecessary clots (enhanced fibrinolytic activity), thus decreasing the risk for vascular clot formation. These are important mechanisms by which regular exercise decreases the risk of cardiovascular death. Moderate-intensity aerobic exercise alters coagulatory potential in part by depressing platelet aggregation (first step in clot formation) in healthy men and women (Wang et al., 1997, 1995). Since the endothelium releases factors that inhibit platelet aggregation, improved endothelial function with exercise may be related to the beneficial changes observed in platelets following a training program. In addition to suppressing platelet aggregation, some inconclusive evidence suggests that moderate levels of aerobic training decrease coagulatory potential in healthy adults, as evidenced by a decrease in clotting factors (Womack et al., 2003). While evidence shows that moderate exercise training decreases clotting potential, thus decreasing the risk of coronary thrombus formation, evidence also shows that the ability to break down clots is enhanced following a moderate training program (Womack et al., 2003). Furthermore, it has been reported that fibrinolytic activity is greater after exercise in active individuals than in sedentary individuals (Szymanski and Pate, 1994).

Blood Volume

Blood volume increases as a result of endurance training. Highly trained endurance athletes have a 20–25% larger blood volume than untrained subjects. The increase in blood volume is primarily due to an expansion of plasma volume. This increase has been reported for both males and females and appears to be independent of age (Convertino, 1991). Increases in plasma volume occur soon after beginning an endurance training program, with changes between 8% and 10% occurring within the first week of training (Convertino et al., 1980) followed by a plateauing of plasma volume. For up to 10 days of training an expansion of plasma volume accounts for increases in blood volume, with little or no change in red blood cell mass (Convertino, 1991; Convertino et al., 1980).

Hematocrit and hemoglobin concentration during this period are often lower, because the red blood cells and hemoglobin are diluted by the larger plasma volume. This condition has sometimes been called *sports anemia*, but this term is a misnomer because the number of red blood cells is almost the same or may actually be increased above pretraining levels. Thus, there is no reason for alarm about this condition; in fact, it may actually be beneficial. The lower hematocrit as a result of elevated plasma volume and normal or slightly elevated number of red blood cells means that the blood is less viscous, which decreases resistance to flow and facilitates the transportation of oxygen.

After approximately 1 month of training, the increase in blood volume is distributed more equally between increases in plasma volume and red blood cell mass (Convertino, 1991; Convertino et al., 1991). Blood volume and plasma volume return to pretraining levels when exercise is discontinued. **Figure 13.7** depicts these changes in blood volume, plasma volume, and red blood cell volume during 8 days of exercise training and after 7 days of cessation of exercise.

Cardiac Output

As seen in **Figure 13.5A** cardiac output is unchanged at rest and during submaximal exercise following an aerobic exercise training program. However, following a training program, more work can be done, meaning that the exercise test to maximum can continue longer, and a higher maximal cardiac output can be achieved.

Although resting cardiac output does not change following a training program, it is achieved by a larger stroke volume and a lower heart rate than in the untrained (Saltin, 1969). Cardiac output at an absolute submaximal workload is decreased or unchanged with training but, as at rest, the relative contribution of stroke volume and heart rate is changed (Åstrand and Rodahl, 1986; Mitchell and Raven, 1994). Maximal cardiac output increases at maximal levels of exercise following an endurance exercise training program (**Figure 13.5A**). This increase results from an increase in stroke volume, since maximal heart rate does not change to a degree that has any physiological meaning with training. The magnitude of the increase in cardiac output depends on the level of training. Elite endurance athletes may have cardiac output values in excess of 35 L·min^{-1}.

Stroke Volume

As shown in **Figure 13.5B**, endurance training results in an increased stroke volume at rest, during submaximal exercise, and during maximal exercise. This increase results from increased plasma volume, increased cardiac dimensions, increased venous return, and an enhanced ability of the ventricle to stretch and accommodate increased venous return (Mitchell and Raven, 1994; Smith and Mitchell, 1993). Since several of these are structural changes, they exert their influence both at rest and during exercise.

It has traditionally been reported that the pattern of stroke volume response during incremental work to maximum is best described as an initial rectilinear rise that plateaus at about 40–50% of $\dot{V}O_2max$. This is seen in **Figure 13.5B**. However, as shown in **Figure 13.8**, some evidence suggests that stroke volume does not plateau in highly trained endurance athletes (Gledhill et al., 1994; Wiebe et al., 1999), although most studies suggest that it does in untrained individuals (**Figures 13.5B** and **13.8**). The question of whether endurance trained athletes have a qualitatively different stroke volume response to incremental exercise remains unanswered (Rowland, 2009a).

Heart Rate

Resting heart rate is lower following endurance training (**Figure 13.5C**). Although bradycardia is technically defined as a resting heart rate less than 60 b·min^{-1}, the term

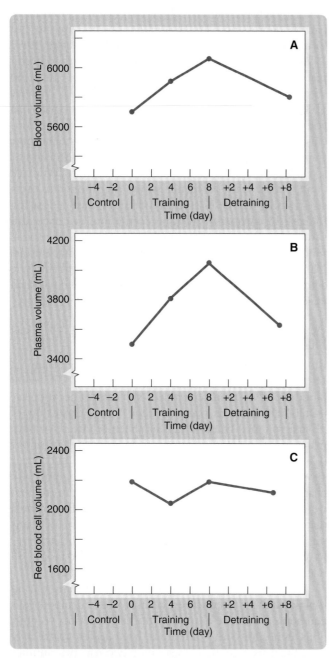

FIGURE 13.7 Changes in Blood Volume as a Result of Training and Detraining.
A: Blood volume. **B:** Plasma volume. **C:** Red blood cell volume. *Source*: V. A. Convertino, P. J. Brock, L. C. Keil, E. M. Bernauer, & J. E. Greenleaf. Exercise training-induced hypervolemia: Role of plasma albumin, renin, and vasopressin. *Journal of Applied Physiology*. 48:665–669 (1980). Reprinted by permission.

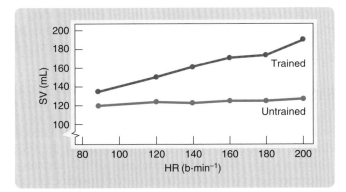

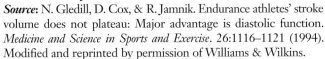

FIGURE 13.8 Stroke Volume Response in Trained and Untrained Subjects.
Source: N. Gledill, D. Cox, & R. Jamnik. Endurance athletes' stroke volume does not plateau: Major advantage is diastolic function. *Medicine and Science in Sports and Exercise*. 26:1116–1121 (1994). Modified and reprinted by permission of Williams & Wilkins.

is sometimes used to refer to the lower resting heart rate resulting from exercise training. Bradycardia is one of the classic and most easily assessed indicators of training adaptation. A reduced heart rate reflects a more efficient heart as the same amount of blood can be pumped each minute (cardiac output) with fewer beats. Fewer heart beats are needed to achieve the same cardiac output because stroke volume is increased following training. The heart rate response to an absolute submaximal amount of work is significantly reduced following endurance training. Maximal heart rate is unchanged or slightly decreased (2–3 b·min⁻¹) with endurance training (Ekblom et al., 1968; Saltin, 1969).

Maximal Oxygen Consumption

Maximal oxygen consumption ($\dot{V}O_2max$) increases as a result of endurance training (**Figure 13.5D**). The magnitude of the increase depends on the type of training program. Improvements of 5–30% are commonly reported, with improvements of 15% routinely found for training programs that meet the recommendations of the American College of Sports Medicine (1998). $\dot{V}O_2max$ rapidly improves during the first 2 months of an endurance training program. Then improvements continue to occur, but at a slower rate. This pattern appears to be independent of sex and is consistent over a wide age range, although elderly individuals may take longer to adapt to endurance training (American College of Sports Medicine, 1998; Cunningham and Hill, 1975; Seals et al., 1984).

The improvement in $\dot{V}O_2max$ results from central and peripheral cardiovascular adaptations. Recall that $\dot{V}O_2max$ can be calculated as the product of cardiac output and arteriovenous oxygen difference (a-vO_2diff) (Equation 11.13). As previously discussed, maximal cardiac output increases as a result of endurance training, representing a central adaptation that supports the training-induced improvement in $\dot{V}O_2max$. The a-vO_2diff reflects

oxygen extraction by the working tissue and thus represents a peripheral adaptation that supports the improvement in $\dot{V}O_2max$ (see Chapter 10). Changes in cardiac output are a more consistent training adaptation than changes in a-vO_2diff, and stroke volume appears to be the principal factor responsible for the increase in cardiac output.

Figure 13.9 uses compiled data to compare $\dot{V}O_2max$ of various athletic groups (Wilmore and Costill, 1988). Several conclusions can be drawn from this graph. First,

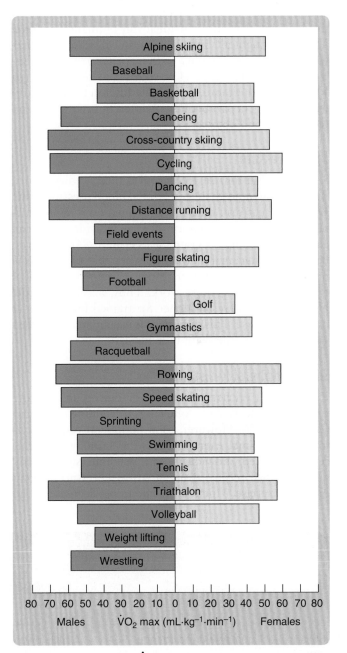

FIGURE 13.9 Average $\dot{V}O_2$max of Male and Female Athletes in Selected Sports.
Source: Based on data from Wilmore, J. H. & D. L. Costill: *Training for Sport and Activity: The Physiological Basis of the Conditioning Process* (3rd edition). Dubuque, IA: Brown (1988).

even among athletes a male-female difference occurs, with males generally having a greater $\dot{V}O_2$max than females. Second, $\dot{V}O_2$max varies considerably among athletes. Third, $\dot{V}O_2$max is related to the demands of the sport. Athletes whose performance depends on the ability of the cardiovascular system to sustain dynamic exercise consistently have higher $\dot{V}O_2$max values than athletes whose sport performance is based primarily on motor skills, such as baseball. **Figure 13.9** does not show, however, the relative influence of genetics and training in determining an individual's $\dot{V}O_2$max. Genetics set the upper limit on the $\dot{V}O_2$max that any individual can ultimately achieve. Thus, although all individuals can increase $\dot{V}O_2$max with training, an individual with a greater genetic potential is more likely to excel at sports that require a high $\dot{V}O_2$max. Furthermore, individuals differ in their sensitivity to training, in part because of different genetic makeup (Bouchard and Persusse, 1994).

Blood Pressure

As indicated in **Figure 13.5E** and as most studies report, there is little or no change in arterial blood pressure (SBP, DBP, MAP) at rest, during submaximal exercise, or during maximal exercise in normotensive individuals after an endurance training program (Seals et al., 1984). However, because the maximal amount of work that can be done increases with exercise training, a trained individual is capable of doing more work. Thus, maximal systolic blood pressure may be higher for trained individuals at maximal exercise. This difference is usually small between sedentary and normally fit individuals.

Total Peripheral Resistance

Resistance is unchanged at rest or during an absolute submaximal workload following a training program (**Figure 13.5F**). However, total peripheral resistance is lower at maximal exercise following training. For this reason, trained individuals can generate significantly higher cardiac outputs at similar arterial pressures during maximal exercise. Much of the additional decrease in the

total peripheral resistance at maximal exercise in trained individuals results from the increased capillarization of the skeletal muscle in these individuals (Blomqvist and Saltin, 1983).

Rate-Pressure Product

Myocardial oxygen consumption, indicated by the rate-pressure product, is lower at rest and during submaximal exercise following endurance training (**Figure 13.5G**). This result reflects the greater efficiency of the heart, since fewer contractions are necessary to eject the same amount of blood during submaximal exercise (Mitchell and Raven, 1994). Because maximal heart rate is unchanged and systolic blood pressure is either unchanged or increases slightly with exercise training, it follows that the maximal rate-pressure product is unchanged or increases slightly.

Table 13.6 summarizes the training adaptations that occur within the cardiovascular system as a result of a dynamic aerobic exercise program.

Cardiovascular Adaptations to Dynamic Resistance Training

Low-volume dynamic resistance training (few repetitions and low weight) has not been shown to lead to any consistent or significant changes in cardiovascular variables. Thus, the changes described in the following sections depend on high-volume (high total workload) dynamic resistance training programs (Stone et al., 1991).

Cardiac Dimensions

Dynamic resistance–trained athletes often have increased left ventricular wall and septal thicknesses, although this is not consistently seen in short-term training studies (Keul et al., 1981; Longhurst et al., 1981; Morganroth et al., 1975). When the increase in wall thickness is reported relative to body surface area or lean body mass, the increase is greatly reduced or even nonexistent (Fleck, 1988a). The increase in wall thickness results from the work the heart must do

TABLE 13.6	Cardiovascular Adaptations to Dynamic Aerobic Exercise		
	Rest	**Absolute Submaximal Exercise**	**Maximal Exercise**
$\dot{Q}$	Unchanged	Decreased or unchanged	Increased
SV	Increased	Increased	Increased
HR	Decreased	Decreased	Unchanged or slight decrease
SBP	Little or no change	Little or no change	Little increase or no change
DBP	Little or no change	Little or no change	Little decrease or no change
MAP	Little or no change	Little or no change	Little increase or no change
$\dot{V}O_2$	—	—	Increased
TPR	Unchanged	Unchanged	Decreased
RPP	Decreased	Decreased	Unchanged or slight increase

Benefits of Lifestyle versus Structured Exercise Training

Preprofessional students involved in athletics or high-intensity personal exercise training programs often find it difficult to accept that the level of activity recommended in the Surgeon General's Report (30 min · day⁻¹, most days) can have any meaningful impact on measures of cardiorespiratory fitness or physiological variables. A study conducted at the Cooper Institute for Aerobics Research (and reported in these two articles) provides evidence for the effectiveness of this approach. Subjects were randomized into either a structured intervention program or lifestyle activity intervention program. Individuals in the structured group were given free memberships to the Cooper Fitness Center and trained with a designated exercise leader. Their program began with 30 minutes of walking 3 d·wk⁻¹, but after 3 weeks they were allowed to select any available aerobic program and eventually progressed to 5 d·wk⁻¹. The lifestyle group received curricular material at weekly meetings centered around individual motivational readiness and behavioral motivation techniques. They were asked to accumulate no fewer than 30 minutes of at least moderate-intensity activity most days in any way that could be adapted to their individual lifestyle and to progress at their own rate. After 6 months both groups were put on maintenance programs, during which they were requested simply to continue their respective activities. Direct leadership and the number of group meetings were reduced. Selected cardiovascular results are presented in the accompanying table.

As anticipated, the greatest changes were made in the initial 6 months in both groups. Both interventions were effective in increasing physical activity, as indicated by the increases in energy expenditure

and walking and the decreases in sitting. However, the structured group increased hard activity more than the lifestyle group and hence improved more than the lifestyle group in physical fitness. The improvement was measured by a greater decrease in HR during submaximal treadmill walking and a greater increase in VO₂peak. In the ensuing 18 months, both groups decreased physical activity (energy expenditure) and physical fitness (VO₂peak) from the 6-month level but maintained significant improvements over their initial values. Although the absolute magnitude of the changes is not great, it is important to realize that during the first 6 months only 32% and 27% of the lifestyle and structure groups attained the level of activity suggested by the Surgeon General's Report. During the maintenance phase, these numbers were reduced to 20% in each group. Those in both groups who reported that they were active 70% or more of the weeks had

at least twice as much improvement as those who did not.

The "take home" messages from this study are that even under the conditions of well-designed and well-delivered external intervention, getting all individuals to include minimal but meaningful levels of activity into their lives is difficult. However, in previously sedentary healthy adult males and females, lifestyle intervention can be as effective as a structured exercise program in improving physical activity and cardiorespiratory fitness.

Sources: Dunn, A. L., M. E. Garcia, B. H. Marcus, J. B. Kampert, H. D. Kohl, III, & S. N. Blair: Six-month physical activity and fitness changes in Project Active, a randomized trial. *Medicine & Science in Sports & Exercise.* 30(7):1076–1083 (1998); Dunn, A. L., B. H. Marcus, J. B. Kampert, M. E. Garcia, H. W. Kohl, III, & S. N. Blair: Comparison of lifestyle and structured interventions to increase physical activity and cardiorespiratory fitness: A randomized trial. *Journal of the American Medical Association.* 281(4):327–334 (1999).

	Lifestyle 6 mo	Lifestyle 24 mo	Structured 6 mo	Structured 24 mo
Activity energy expenditure (kcal·kg⁻¹·d⁻¹)	+1.53*	+0.84*	+1.34*	+0.69*
Achieved SG goal (2 kcal·kg⁻¹·d⁻¹)	32%	20%	27%	20%
Walking (min·d⁻¹)	+19.80*	+13.07	+16.52*	+26.75*
Sitting (hr·wk⁻¹)	−5.27*	−1.18	−6.88*	−6.85*,†
Treadmill time (min)	+0.46*	+0.23*	+0.92*	+0.37*,†
Submaximal HR (b·min⁻¹)	−4.75*	−2.62*	−10.22*,†	−4.88*
V̇O₂peak (mL·kg⁻¹·min⁻¹)	−1.58*	+0.77*	+3.64*,†	+1.34*
SBP (mmHg)		−3.63*		−3.26*
DBP (mmHg)		−5.38*		−5.14*
Body fat (%)		−2.39*		−1.85*

*Significant difference in each group compared to its own baseline.
†Significant difference between groups at 6 or 24 mo.

to overcome the high arterial pressures (increased pressure afterload) encountered during resistance training; this depends on training intensity and volume.

Stroke Volume and Heart Rate

Resting stroke volume in highly trained dynamic resistance athletes has been reported to be both greater than

normal and not different from normal (Effron, 1989; Fleck, 1988b). Because stroke volume is so seldom measured during resistance activities, changes that may occur in stroke volume from this type of training are not known (Sjogaard et al., 1988).

Highly trained dynamic resistance athletes have average or below-average resting heart rates (Stone et al., 1991). Heart rate at a specified submaximal dynamic

Resistance Training Improves Vascular Function in Overweight Women

Aerobic exercise is known to improve endothelial function. Aerobic exercise significantly elevates blood flow under moderately high pressure for a prolonged period of time. This increase in shear stress on the endothelium is thought to increase nitric oxide production leading to enhanced vasodilation. A recent study, however, hypothesized that resistance training, which elevates blood flow for shorter periods but under higher pressure, would also provide a stress stimulus on the endothelium resulting in improved vascular function.

The study included 30 overweight women, 15 of whom engaged in a 1-year resistance training program and 15 who served as controls. The researchers measured the resting diameter of the brachial artery before and after training. They also measured the artery's ability to vasodilate after 3 minutes of occlusion, which is known to cause an increase in blood flow; this phenomenon is known as reactive hyperemia. The brachial diameter during the reactive hyperemia was reported as peak flow-mediated dilation and expressed as a percent.

This study found that resistance training positively affects vascular function in overweight women. This finding suggests that resistance training has

important cardiovascular benefits and provides further support for the recommendation of including resistance training in an overall fitness program. However, given the small sample size and the narrow population studied, additional research into the effects of

resistance training on vascular structure and function are warranted.

Source: Olson, T. P., D. R. Dengel, A. S. Leon, & K. H. Schmitz: Moderate resistance training and vascular health in overweight women. *Medicine & Science in Sports & Exercise.* 38: 1558–1564 (2006).

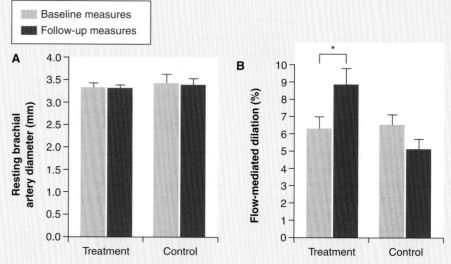

A. Resting baseline diameter of the brachial artery in the resistance-trained and control groups. **B.** Peak flow-mediated dilation of the brachial artery in the resistance-trained and control groups. Data are presented as mean ± SEM. *$p < 0.05$ for within-group analysis.

resistance workload is lower following resistance training (Fleck and Dean, 1987).

Blood Pressure

Dynamic resistance–trained athletes do not have elevated resting blood pressures, provided that they are not chronically overtrained, do not have greatly increased muscle mass, and are not using anabolic steroids. This information contradicts the popular misconception that resistance-trained individuals have a higher resting blood pressure than endurance-trained or untrained individuals. Indeed, most scientific investigations report that highly trained resistance athletes have average or lower-than-average systolic and diastolic blood pressures (Fleck, 1988b). Resistance-trained individuals also exhibit a lower blood pressure response to the same relative workload of resistance exercise than untrained individuals,

even though the trained individuals are lifting a greater absolute load.

Dynamic resistance training has not been shown to consistently lower blood pressure in hypertensive individuals and therefore is not recommended as the only exercise modality for hypertensives except in the form of circuit training. Circuit training relies on high repetitions, low loads, and short rest periods in a series of stations. A supercircuit integrates aerobic endurance activities between the stations.

The rate-pressure product, which reflects myocardial oxygen consumption, is decreased at rest following strength training, during weight lifting or circuit training, and during aerobic exercise that includes a resistance component (such as holding hand weights while walking) (Fleck, 1988b; Stone et al., 1991). Researchers have suggested that these results occur because of a reduction in peripheral resistance.

Maximal Oxygen Consumption

Small increases (4–9%) in $\dot{V}O_2$max have been reported following circuit training and Olympic-style weightlifting programs (Gettman, 1981; Stone et al., 1991). However, other studies have failed to identify any increase in $\dot{V}O_2$max with resistance training (Hurley et al., 1984). $\dot{V}O_2$max probably does not change much because of the low percentage of $\dot{V}O_2$max achieved during resistance training. Weight training may impact the central cardiovascular variables as described earlier (i.e., resulting in a reduced resting heart rate), but it does not enhance peripheral cardiovascular adaptations (i.e., a-vO_2diff). Thus, to improve cardiorespiratory fitness, individuals should not rely on resistance training programs but instead use dynamic resistance training in conjunction with aerobic endurance training.

The Influence of Age and Sex on Cardiovascular Training Adaptations

Few data are available regarding the influence of age and sex on cardiovascular adaptations to dynamic resistance exercise. Therefore, this section addresses only cardiovascular adaptations to aerobic endurance exercise.

Male-Female Differences in Adaptations

Research evidence suggests no differences between the sexes in central or peripheral adaptations to aerobic endurance training. Both sexes exhibit similar cardiovascular adaptations at rest, during submaximal exercise, and at maximal exercise (Drinkwater, 1984; Mitchell et al., 1992). Maximal cardiac output is higher in both sexes because of the increased stroke volume following training; however, the absolute value achieved by a woman is less than that attained by a similarly trained man.

When males and females of similar fitness level train at the same frequency, intensity, and duration, they show no differences in the relative increase in $\dot{V}O_2$max (Lewis et al., 1986; Mitchell et al., 1992). As shown earlier in **Figure 12.12**, $\dot{V}O_2$max overlaps considerably between the sexes. Thus, a well-trained female may have a higher $\dot{V}O_2$max than a sedentary or even normally active male; however, a female will always have a lower $\dot{V}O_2$max than a similarly trained and similarly genetically endowed male.

The blood pressure (SBP, DBP, MAP) response to exercise is unchanged in both sexes following endurance training. Males and females show the same adaptations in total peripheral resistance and rate-pressure product. The effects of endurance training on cardiovascular variables at maximal exercise are reported in **Table 13.7** for both sexes. In summary, the trainability of females does not differ from that of males, and similar benefits can and should be gained from regular activity by both sexes (Hanson and Nedde, 1974). However, the absolute values achieved for maximal oxygen consumption, cardiac output, and stroke volume are generally lower in females because of their smaller body and heart size.

Adaptations in Children and Adolescents

Endurance training has been documented to result in increased left ventricular mass and heart volume in children, as it does in adults (Bar-Or, 1983; Greenen et al., 1982). The increase in heart size is associated with an increased resting stroke volume (Gutin et al., 1988) and a decreased resting heart rate but not with any change in cardiac output (Eriksson and Koch, 1973). Research also suggests an increased blood volume and hemoglobin level in young endurance athletes compared with sedentary children (Eriksson and Koch, 1973; Koch and Rocher, 1980; Zauner et al., 1989), but possibly not as much as in adults. Information about changes in capillary density with training in children is not available (Rowland, 2005).

At submaximal levels of exercise, cardiac output is unchanged or slightly decreased in youngsters after endurance training (Bar-Or, 1983; Soto et al., 1983) as a result of increased submaximal stroke volume and

TABLE 13.7 Comparison of Cardiovascular Responses to Maximal Exercise in Sedentary and Trained Young Adults (20–30 yr)				
	Men		**Women**	
Variable	**Sedentary**	**Trained**	**Sedentary**	**Trained**
$\dot{Q}$max (L·min⁻¹)	22	30	16	20
SVmax (mL·b⁻¹)	115	155	80	105
HRmax (b·min⁻¹)	195	195	195	195
$\dot{V}O_2$max (mL·kg⁻¹·min⁻¹)	50	65	37	52
SBP (mmHg)	200	200	190	190
DBP (mmHg)	70	70	66	66
MAP (mmHg)	135	135	128	128
TPR (units)	6.1	4.5	8.0	6.4
RPP (units)	390	390	370	370

decreased heart rate (Bar-Or, 1983; Lussier and Buskirk, 1977). Neither systolic nor diastolic blood pressure changes significantly as a result of endurance training during submaximal work (Lussier and Buskirk, 1977).

At maximal work, cardiac output increases in children and adolescents as a result of endurance training. This is caused by an increased maximal stroke volume and stable maximal heart rate (Eriksson and Koch, 1973; Lussier and Buskirk, 1977).

Children and adolescents can participate in a wide variety of training programs in school or community settings (**Figure 13.10**). Research has consistently shown improvements in endurance performance as a result of exercise training. Such improvements have occurred when endurance performance was measured as an increase in the workload performed (longer treadmill times or distances run, more distance covered in a set time, higher work output on a cycle ergometer, or longer rides at the same load) or as a faster time for a given distance (Cooper et al., 1975; Daniels and Oldridge, 1971; Daniels et al., 1978; Duncan et al., 1983; Dwyer et al., 1983; Goode et al., 1976; Graunke

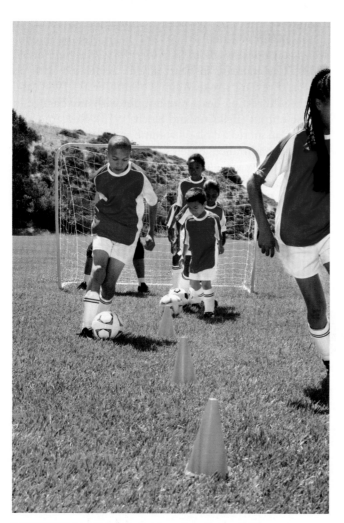

FIGURE 13.10 Children Performing Soccer Drills.

et al., 1990; Mosellin and Wasmund, 1973; Siegel and Manfredi, 1984). Given the lack of association between endurance performance and $\dot{V}O_2$max in children, it is not surprising that endurance performance improvements are not always accompanied by a comparable improvement in $\dot{V}O_2$max (Daniels and Oldridge, 1971; Daniels et al., 1978). Although children and adolescents who participate in organized athletic activities have higher $\dot{V}O_2$max values than those who do not, the relationship between measures of physical activity (such as self-report questionnaires, heart rate monitoring, and motion detection devices) and measures of $\dot{V}O_2$max is generally only low to moderate (Morrow and Freedson, 1994; Vaccaro and Mahon, 1987; Rowland, 2005). The most consistent finding of cardiovascular adaptations in prepubertal children is a diminished level of aerobic trainability compared to adults (Rowland, 2005). This occurs even in those studies in which the training meets the standards of intensity, duration, and frequency that result in substantial improvements in adults. Thus, where an adult (or postpubertal adolescent) might show a 25–30% increase, this is more likely to be 10–15% in prepubertal children. It has been suggested (Rowland, 2009b) that this difference may be the result of metabolic differences between children and adults (as discussed in Chapter 5). Clarification requires further research.

Adaptations in Children and Older Adults

Older men and women respond to endurance exercise training with adaptations similar to those in younger adults (Hagberg et al., 1989; Heath et al., 1981; Ogawa et al., 1992). Left ventricular wall thickness and myocardial mass are greater in elderly athletes than in elderly sedentary individuals, although these training adaptations may not be as pronounced or as quickly achieved as in younger adults (Green and Crouse, 1993; Heath et al., 1981; Ogawa et al., 1992).

Left ventricular end-diastolic volume and ejection fraction increase as a result of endurance training in older individuals. These changes enhance myocardial contractile function, especially the Frank-Starling mechanism, and help maintain cardiac output in the active elderly (Green and Crouse, 1993).

Resting cardiac output is unchanged as a result of endurance training in the elderly. Elderly athletes with an extensive history of endurance training consistently show lower resting heart rates than sedentary older adults. However, short-term training programs sometimes cause the expected decrease in resting heart rates and sometimes do not. Resting stroke volume typically increases, but the increase is generally small (Green and Crouse, 1993).

As in normotensive individuals of other ages, endurance training does not affect systolic blood pressure, diastolic blood pressure, or mean arterial blood pressure at rest in elderly people. Both hemoglobin levels and blood volume increase in the elderly as a result of endurance training, as does the density of capillaries supplying blood to the active musculature (Green and Crouse, 1993).

Most training studies show no change in cardiac output during any given submaximal workload. The components of cardiac output, however, often change reciprocally, with the expected decrease in heart rate and increase in stroke volume. Again, the stroke volume changes tend to be small and do not always reach statistical significance. Submaximal values for systolic blood pressure, mean arterial blood pressure, and total peripheral resistance are lower in elderly athletes than in nonathletes and decrease with endurance training (Green and Crouse, 1993).

Maximal cardiac output may be increased by exercise training in elderly individuals. This increase is completely accounted for by the increased maximal stroke volume, since maximal heart rate is unchanged. The reported effects of endurance training on blood pressures and systematic vascular resistance are inconsistent, although most evidence suggests no change in these variables (Green and Crouse, 1993).

The results of training status on cardiovascular responses to maximal exercise in the elderly, including $\dot{V}O_2$max, are shown in **Table 13.8** for both men and women. $\dot{V}O_2$max is higher in trained than in untrained elderly. Thus, training programs can result in increases in $\dot{V}O_2$max in the elderly. The magnitude of this increase depends on the individual's initial fitness level and the training program. Research suggests, however, that healthy, elderly untrained males and females can improve their $\dot{V}O_2$max by 15–30% with training (Hagberg et al., 1989; Ogawa et al., 1992; Seals et al., 1984).

One study using a short-duration exercise program (9 weeks) of endurance training reported that a low-intensity exercise prescription (30–45% HRR) was as effective as a high-intensity exercise prescription (60–75% HRR) in eliciting improvements in $\dot{V}O_2$max (Badenhop, 1983). However, a 1-year training program found that 6 months of training at low intensities (40% HRR) resulted in only a 10.5% improvement in $\dot{V}O_2$max in elderly subjects. When the training program was progressively changed to a high-intensity program (85% HRR) and the duration extended, their $\dot{V}O_2$max increased by another 16.5%. This research suggests that elderly individuals respond to exercise training in much the same way as younger individuals.

When starting a training program for elderly people, it is important to begin at low intensities to avoid injury. Significant improvements in function can be gained from low-intensity programs. After individuals become accustomed to the program, the training can be upgraded to a more intense level if desired. Note that the rate of adaptation may be slower in older individuals (American College of Sports Medicine, 1998).

Although elderly athletes are more similar to younger individuals than to their sedentary counterparts, and training programs tend to show the same beneficial changes in the elderly as in younger subjects, exercise training does not stop the effects of aging on the cardiovascular system. At best, exercise training can only lessen normal age-related losses in cardiovascular function. This conclusion is exemplified in **Figure 13.11**, where the average rate of decline in $\dot{V}O_2$max is shown for both an active, highly fit (HF) group of females and a relatively sedentary, low-fitness (LF) comparison group (Plowman et al., 1979). The first thing to notice is that the HF group had higher $\dot{V}O_2$max values than the LF group in every decade. Indeed, the $\dot{V}O_2$max values of active 45-year-olds equaled those of inactive 20-year-olds. Second, $\dot{V}O_2$max expressed per kilogram of body weight declined with age, and the rate of decline was similar in the two groups. More recent data suggest that the rate of decline in peak $\dot{V}O_2$ in healthy adults is not constant across the age span but accelerates markedly with each successive decade, regardless of physical activity habits (Fleg et al., 2005). It appears that declining FEV_1 and maximal exercise heart rates account for much of the "aging effect" on aerobic capacity (Hollenberg et al., 2006). The decline of peak aerobic capacity has substantial implications with regard to functional independence and quality of life for older adults.

TABLE 13.8 Comparison of Cardiovascular Responses to Maximal Exercise in Sedentary and Trained Elderly Individuals (60–70 yr)				
	Men		**Women**	
Variable	**Sedentary**	**Trained**	**Sedentary**	**Trained**
$\dot{Q}$max (L·min^{-1})	16	19.4	12	15
SVmax (mL·b^{-1})	100	125	75	90
HRmax (b·min^{-1})	155	155	155	155
$\dot{V}O_2$max (mL·kg^{-1}·min^{-1})	28	48	22	35
SBP (mmHg)	190	190	190	190
DBP (mmHg)	84	84	84	84
MAP (mmHg)	138	138	138	138
TPR (units)	8.6	7.3	11.5	9.2
RPP (units)	290	290	290	290

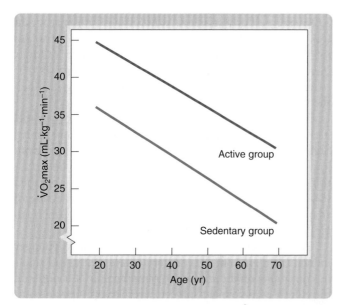

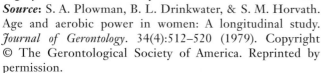

FIGURE 13.11 Age-Related Decline in $\dot{V}O_2$max in Highly Active and Sedentary Women.
Source: S. A. Plowman, B. L. Drinkwater, & S. M. Horvath. Age and aerobic power in women: A longitudinal study. *Journal of Gerontology*. 34(4):512–520 (1979). Copyright © The Gerontological Society of America. Reprinted by permission.

Detraining in the Cardiorespiratory System

It is clear that athletes and physically active individuals enjoy fitness and health benefits from the physiological adaptations resulting from their lifestyle. It is also clear, as expressed in the reversibility training principle, that individuals lose the benefits of physical activity when they cease being active or detrain.

The consequences of detraining depend on many factors, including the individual's training status and the extent of the inactivity (decreased or ceased completely). The extent of these physiological reversals also depends on how long detraining continues. Further complicating the impact of detraining is normal aging. In fact, it is often not possible to distinguish between the effects of aging and detraining in an elderly population.

All available research evidence suggests that all physiological variables that are responsive to exercise training also respond to detraining, and adaptations in the cardiovascular system are no exception. In general, detraining leads to lower maximal oxygen consumption ($\dot{V}O_2$max). Brief periods of detraining (10–14 days) appear not to result in a decrease in $\dot{V}O_2$max in highly trained individuals (Cullinane et al., 1986; Houston et al., 1979). On the other hand, a training cessation of 2–4 weeks results in decreases in $\dot{V}O_2$max of approximately 4–15% (Mujika and Padilla, 2000; Coyle et al., 1984; 1986). This reduction

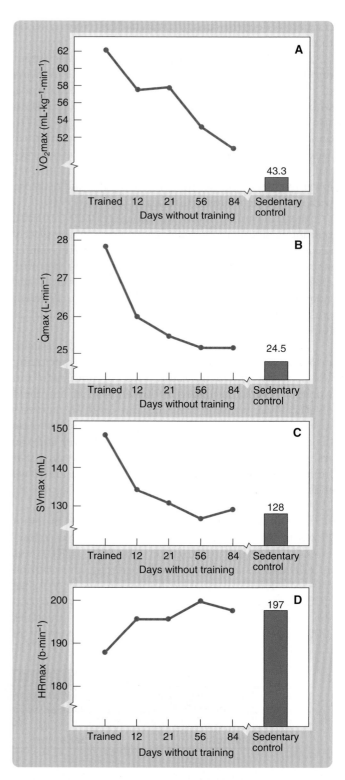

FIGURE 13.12 Effects of Detraining on Highly Conditioned Athletes.
A: Maximal oxygen consumption ($\dot{V}O_2$max). **B:** Maximal cardiac output ($\dot{Q}$ max). **C:** Maximal stroke volume (SVmax). **D:** Maximal heart rate (HRmax).
Source: E. F. Coyle, W. H. Martin, D. R. Sinacore, M. J. Joymer, J. M. Hagberg, & J. O. Holloszy. Time course of loss of adaptations after stopping prolonged intense endurance training. *Journal of Applied Physiology*. 57:1857–1864 (1984). Reprinted by permission.

is greater in highly trained than in recently trained individuals (Mujika and Padilla, 2000). In 1993 a study by Madsen et al. in which exercise training was severely reduced in highly trained athletes reported that $\dot{V}O_2$max was maintained during the 4 weeks of detraining (Madsen et al., 1993). This finding can be attributed to the fact that in the Madsen study athletes severely reduced their training but did not cease to train (the athletes performed one 35-minute bout of intense training rather than their normal training of 6–10 hours a week).

Figure 13.12 presents changes in $\dot{V}O_2$max over an 84-day period in a group of endurance-trained subjects (Coyle et al., 1984). These data suggest that in highly trained individuals, $\dot{V}O_2$max may decline as much as 20% with detraining but still remain above levels of sedentary individuals. Other studies report the complete reversal of $\dot{V}O_2$max to pretraining levels in individuals who are recently trained (Mujika and Padilla, 2000). Changes in $\dot{V}O_2$max during detraining are accompanied by reductions in maximal stroke volume and cardiac output and increased maximal heart rate (Figure 13.12). The decrease in stroke volume and thus cardiac output can most likely be attributed to changes in blood volume. Detraining leads to 5–10% decreases in blood volume, and these reductions may occur within 2 days of inactivity (Mujika and Padilla, 2001; Cullinane et al., 1986). Coyle et al. (1986) investigated the effects of 2–4 weeks of inactivity on endurance-trained men and reported a 9% decline in blood volume and a 12% reduction in stroke volume. When blood volume was expanded (by infusing a dextran solution in saline) to a level equal to the trained state, both stroke volume and $\dot{V}O_2$max increased to within 2–4% of the trained state.

Collectively, these findings suggest that cardiovascular training adaptations are lost relatively quickly when training ceases.

SUMMARY

1. A cardiovascular training program depends on the individual's age and health status and the program's goals.

2. Any activity involving large muscle groups for a prolonged time has the potential to increase cardiovascular fitness. The choice of exercise modalities should be based on interest, availability, and a low risk of injury.

3. Training using different exercise modalities causes the same overall benefits with central cardiovascular adaptations, but peripheral cardiovascular adaptations are specific to the muscles being exercised.

4. Intensity is very important for improving maximal oxygen consumption ($\dot{V}O_2$max) primarily in conjunction with duration, which determines training volume. Intensity can be prescribed in relation to heart rate,

oxygen consumption, or rating of perceived exertion (RPE). Training intensity is the most important factor for maintaining cardiovascular fitness.

5. The ACSM recommends the following training goals to develop and maintain cardiorespiratory fitness in healthy adults: frequency of 3–5 d·wk⁻¹, intensity of 64–95% HRmax, 40–89% $\dot{V}O_2$R or %HRR, and duration of 20–60 minutes of continuous aerobic activity.

6. The Canadian Society for Exercise Science recommends a total of 150 min·wk⁻¹ of moderate to vigorous physical activity at a frequency determined by the individual.

7. Children and adolescents should participate in at least 60 min·d⁻¹ of moderate to vigorous physical activity that is age appropriate while minimizing sedentary activity the rest of the day.

8. The absolute and relative increases in $\dot{V}O_2$max and the health benefits thereof are inversely related to the individual's initial fitness level. The greatest improvements in fitness and health occur when very sedentary individuals begin a regular, low- to moderate-endurance exercise program. Meaningful health benefits can be achieved with minimal increases in activity or fitness by those who need it most.

9. Endurance training results in increased cardiac dimensions and mass and leads to positive adaptations in the vasculature because of vascular remodeling and improved endothelial function.

10. Endurance training results in changes in blood formation and clot breakdown that decrease the likelihood of unnecessary clot formation.

11. Endurance training results in increased blood volume, with highly trained endurance athletes having 20–25% greater volume than untrained subjects. Changes in plasma volume occur early in a training program, with an 8–10% change occurring within the first week. Early changes (at 1 month) are due almost entirely to increases in plasma volume, whereas increases in red blood cells and hemoglobin occur later.

12. Cardiac output at rest and at an absolute submaximal workload is not changed by an endurance training program. However, cardiac output at the same relative workload and at maximal exercise is greater with endurance training.

13. Stroke volume is greater at rest, at submaximal exercise (absolute and relative workloads), and at maximal exercise with endurance training.

14. Heart rate is lower at rest and during an absolute submaximal workload with endurance training. It is unchanged at the same relative submaximal workload and at maximal exercise.

15. Blood pressure changes little or not at all at rest, during submaximal exercise, or during maximal exercise in normotensive individuals with endurance training.

16. $\dot{V}O_2$max increases with endurance training; improvements of 15% are routinely reported with training programs that meet the recommendations of ACSM.

REVIEW QUESTIONS

1. How is overload manipulated to bring about cardiorespiratory adaptation? Consider exercise recommendations for fitness and physical activity guidelines for health benefit in your response.

2. Differentiate between central and peripheral cardiovascular adaptations.

3. Compare and contrast adaptations in cardiac output, stroke volume, heart rate, and blood pressure with endurance training at rest and during submaximal and maximal exercise.

4. Discuss the relevance of an individual's initial fitness level for expected improvements in fitness and health-related benefits.

5. Describe the physiological benefits of a warm-up and a cooldown period.

6. Explain the changes in blood volume that result from endurance training.

7. Describe changes in cardiac dimensions that result from endurance training, and explain how these structural changes support improved cardiac function.

8. Describe changes in blood clotting and breakdown that result from endurance training, and explain how these physiological changes support improved cardiovascular health.

9. Compare and contrast cardiovascular adaptations to dynamic endurance and dynamic resistance training.

For further review and additional study tools go to the Student Study Guide for Exercise Physiology for Health, Fitness, and Performance by Sharon A. Plowman and Denise L. Smith.

REFERENCES

American College of Sports Medicine: Position stand on the recommended quantity and quality of exercise for developing and maintaining fitness in healthy adults. *Medicine and Science in Sports and Exercise.* 10(3):vii–x (1978).

American College of Sports Medicine: Position stand on the recommended quantity and quality of exercise for developing and maintaining cardiorespiratory and muscular fitness and flexibility in healthy adults. *Medicine & Science in Sports & Exercise.* 30(6):975–985 (1998).

American College of Sports Medicine: Position stand: Quantity and quality of exercise for developing and maintaining cardiorespiratory, musculoskeletal, and neuromotor fitness in apparently healthy adults: Guidance for prescribing exercise. *Medicine & Science in Sports & Exercise.* 43(7):1334–1359 (2011).

American College of Sports Medicine: *ACSM's Guidelines for Exercise Testing and Prescription.* (8th edition). Philadelphia, PA: Lippincott Williams & Wilkins (2010).

Åstrand, P. O. & K. Rodahl: *Textbook of Work Physiology.* New York, NY: McGraw-Hill (1986).

Badenhop, D. T., P. A. Cleary, S. F. Schaal, E. L. Fox, & R. L. Bartels: Physiological adjustments to higher- or lower-intensity exercise in elders. *Medicine and Science in Sports and Exercise.* 15(6):496–502 (1983).

Barnard, R. J., G. W. Gardner, N. V. Diasco, R. N. MacAlpin, & A. A. Kattus: Cardiovascular responses to sudden strenuous exercise—Heart rate, blood pressure and ECG. *Journal of Applied Physiology.* 34:833–837 (1973).

Bar-Or, O.: *Pediatric Sports Medicine for the Practitioner.* New York, NY: Springer-Verlag (1983).

Blomqvist, C. G. & B. Saltin: Cardiovascular adaptations to physical training. *Annual Review of Physiology.* 45:169 (1983).

Bloomfield, S. & E. F. Coyle: Bedrest, detraining, and retention of training-induced adaptations. In American College of Sports Medicine (ed.): *Resource Manual for Guidelines for Exercise Testing and Prescription.* Philadelphia, PA: Lea & Febiger (1993).

Borg, G.: *Borg's Perceived Exertion and Pain Scales.* Champaign, IL: Human Kinetics (1998).

Bouchard, C. & L. Persusse: Heredity, activity level, fitness, and health. In Bouchard, C., R. J. Shephard, & T. Stephens (eds.): *Physical Activity, Fitness, and Health, International Proceedings and Consensus statement.* Champaign, IL: Human Kinetics (1994).

Canadian Society for Exercise Physiology: Canadian Physical Activity Guidelines. www.csep.ca/guidelines. (2011)

Centers for Disease Control and Prevention: National Diabetes Surveillance System. Available online at: http://apps.nccd.cdc.gov/DDTSTRS/default.aspx. Retrieved 7/11/2011

Centers for disease control and prevention: Physical activity levels of high school students—United States, 2010. *MMWR Weekly.* 60(23):773–777 (2011a).

Centers for disease control and prevention: Prevalence of regular physical activity among adults—United States 2001 and 2005. *MMWR Weekly.* 56(46):1209–1212 (2007).

Centers for disease control and prevention: 1988–2008 no leisure-time physical activity trend chart. www.cdc.gov. (2011b)

Cohen, J. L. & K. R. Segal: Left ventricular hypertrophy in athletes: An exercise-echocardiographic study. *Medicine and Science in Sports and Exercise.* 17:695–700 (1985).

Convertino, V. A.: Blood volume: Its adaptation to endurance training. *Medicine and Science in Sports and Exercise.* 23:1338–1348 (1991).

Convertino, V. A., P. J. Brock, L. C. Keil, E. M. Bernauer, & J. E. Greenleaf: Exercise training–induced hypervolemia: Role of plasma albumin, renin, and vasopressin. *Journal of Applied Physiology.* 48:665–669 (1980).

Convertino, V. A., G. W. Mack, & E. R. Nadel: Elevated central venous pressure: A consequence of exercise training–induced hypervolemia? *American Journal of Physiology.* 29:R273–R277 (1991).

Cooper, K. H., J. G. Purdy, A. Friedman, R. L. Bohannon, R. A. Harris, & J. A. Arends: An aerobics conditioning program for the Fort Worth, Texas, School District. *Research Quarterly.* 46:345–380 (1975).

Corbin, C. B., R. P. Pangrazi, & G. C. LeMasurier: Physical Activity for children: Current patterns and guidelines. *President's Council on Physical Fitness and Sports Research Digest.* 5(2):1–8 (2004).

Coyle, E. F., M. K. Hemmert, & A. R. Coggan: Effects of detraining on cardiovascular responses to exercise: Role of blood volume. *Journal of Applied Physiology*. 60:95–99 (1986).

Coyle, E. F., W. H. Martin, D. R. Sinacore, M. J. Joymer, J. M. Hagberg, & J. O. Holloszy: Time course of loss of adaptations after stopping prolonged intense endurance training. *Journal of Applied Physiology*. 57:1857–1864 (1984).

Cullinane, E. M., S. P. Sady, L. Vadeboncoeur, M. Burke, & P. D. Thompson: Cardiac size and VO_2max do not decrease after short-term exercise cessation. *Medicine and Science in Sports and Exercise*. 18:420–424 (1986).

Cunningham, D. A. & J. S. Hill: Effect of training on cardiovascular response to exercise in women. *Journal of Applied Physiology*. 39:891–895 (1975).

Currens, J. G. & P. D. White: Half century of running: Clinical, physiologic and autopsy findings in the case of Clarence De Mar, "Mr. Marathoner." *The New England Journal of Medicine*. 265:988–993 (1961).

Daniels, J. & J. Gilbert: *Oxygen Power: Performance Tables for Distance Runners*. Tempe, AZ: Author (1979).

Daniels, J. & N. Oldridge: Changes in oxygen consumption of young boys during growth and running training. *Medicine and Science in Sports and Exercise*. 3:161–165 (1971).

Daniels, J., N. Oldridge, F. Nagle, & B. White: Differences and changes in VO_2 among young runners 10 to 18 years of age. *Medicine and Science in Sports and Exercise*. 10:200–203 (1978).

De Busk, R. F., U. Hakanssan, M. Sheehan, & W. L. Haskell: Training effects of long versus short bouts of exercise. *The American Journal of Cardiology*. 65:1010–1013 (1990).

Dinenno, F. A., D. R. Seals, C. A. DeSouza, & H. Tanaka: Age-related decreases in basal limb blood flow in humans: Time course, determinants and habitual exercise effects. *The Journal of Physiology*. 531(2):573–579 (2001).

Drinkwater, B. L.: Women and exercise: Physiological aspects. *Exercise and Sport Sciences Reviews*. 12:21–52 (1984).

Duncan, B., W. T. Boyce, R. Itami, & N. Puffengarger: A controlled trial of a physical fitness program for fifth grade students. *The Journal of School Health*. 53:467–471 (1983).

Dunn, A. L., M. E. Garcia, B. H. Marcus, J. B. Kampert, H. D. Kohl, III, & S. N. Blair: Six-month physical activity and fitness changes in Project Active, a randomized trial. *Medicine & Science in Sports & Exercise*. 30(7):1076–1083 (1998).

Dunn, A. L., B. H. Marcus, J. B. Kampert, M. E. Garcia, H. W. Kohl, III, & S. N. Blair: Comparison of lifestyle and structured interventions to increase physical activity and cardiorespiratory fitness: A randomized trial. *Journal of the American Medical Association*. 281(4):327–334 (1999).

Dwyer, T., W. E. Coonan, D. R. Leitch, B. S. Hetzel, & R. A. Boghurst: An investigation of the effects of daily physical activity on the health of primary school students in South Australia. *International Journal of Epidemiology*. 12:308–313 (1983).

Effron, M. B.: Effects of resistance training on left ventricular function. *Medicine and Science in Sports and Exercise*. 21:694–697 (1989).

Ekblom, B., P. O. Åstrand, B. Saltin, J. Stenberg, & B. Wallstrom: Effect of training on circulatory response to exercise. *European Journal of Applied Physiology*. 24:518–528 (1968).

Eriksson, B. O. & G. Koch: Effects of physical training on hemodynamic response during submaximal and maximal exercise in 11 to 13 year old boys. *Acta Physiologica Scandinavia*. 87:27–39 (1973).

Eyestone, E. D., G. Fellingham, J. George, & A. G. Fisher: Effect of water running and cycling on maximum oxygen consumption and 2-mile run performance. *The American Journal of Sports Medicine*. 21(1):41–44 (1993).

Fleck, S. J.: Cardiovascular adaptations to resistance training. *Medicine and Science in Sports and Exercise*. 20:S146–S151 (1988a).

Fleck, S. J.: Cardiovascular responses to strength training. In Komi, P. V. (ed.): *Strength and Power in Sport*. Champaign, IL: Human Kinetics, 305–319 (1988b).

Fleck, S. J. & L. S. Dean: Resistance-training experience and the pressor response during resistance exercise. *Journal of Applied Physiology*. 63:116–120 (1987).

Fleg, J. L., C. H. Morrell, A. G. Bos, J. Brant, L. A. Talbot, J. G. Wright, & E. G. Lakatta: Accelerated longitudinal decline of aerobic capacity in healthy older adults. *Circulation*. 112:674–682 (2005).

Gettman, L. R.: Circuit weight-training: A critical review of its physiological benefits. *The Physician and Sports Medicine*. 9(1):44–59 (1981).

Gledhill, N., D. Cox, & R. Jamnik: Endurance athletes' stroke volume does not plateau: Major advantage is diastolic function. *Medicine and Science in Sports and Exercise*. 26:1116–1121 (1994).

Goode, R. C., A. Virgin, T. T. Romet, P. Crawford, J. Duffin, T. Palland, & Z. Woch: Effects of a short period of physical activity in adolescent boys and girls. *Canadian Journal of Applied Sport Sciences*. 1:241–250 (1976).

Graunke, J. M., S. A. Plowman, & J. R. Marett: Evaluation of a fitness based physical education curriculum for the high school freshman. *Illinois Journal of Health, Physical Education, Recreation and Dance*. 27:24–27 (1990).

Green, D. J., J. H. Walsh, A. Maiorana, M. J. Best, R. R. Taylor, & J. G. O'Driscoll: Exercise-induced improvements in endothelial dysfunction is not mediated by changes in CV risk factors: Pooled analysis of diverse patient populations. *American Journal of Physiology: Heart and Circulation Physiology*. 285:H2679–2687 (2003).

Green, J. S. & S. F. Crouse: Endurance training, cardiovascular function and the aged. *Sports Medicine*. 16(5):331–341 (1993).

Greenen, D. L., T. B. Gilliam, D. Crowley, C. Moorehead-Steffens, & A. Rosenthal: Echocardiographic measures in 6 to 7 year old children after an 8 month exercise program. *The American Journal of Cardiology*. 49:1990–1995 (1982).

Gutin, B., N. Mayers, J. A. Levy, & M. V. Herman: Physiologic and echocardiographic studies of age-group runners. In Brown. E. W. & C. F. Branta (eds.): *Competitive Sports for Children and Youth*. Champaign, IL: Human Kinetics, 115–128 (1988).

Hagberg, J. M., J. E. Graves, M. Limacher, D. R. Woods, S. H. Leggett, C. Cononie, J. J. Gruber, & M. L. Pollock: Cardiovascular responses of 70- to 79-yr-old men and women to exercise training. *Journal of Applied Physiology*. 66:2589–2594 (1989).

Hambrecht, R., E. Fiehn, C. Weigl, S. Gielen, C. Hamann, R. Kaiser, J. Yu, V. Adams, J. Niebauer, & G. Schuler: Regular physical exercise corrects endothelial dysfunction and improves exercise capacity in individuals with chronic heart failure. *Circulation*. 98:2709–2715 (1998).

Hanson, J. S. & W. H. Nedde: Long-term physical training effect in sedentary females. *Journal of Applied Physiology*. 37:112–116 (1974).

Haskell, W. L.: Dose-response issues in physical activity, fitness, and health. pp. 303–317. In Bouchard, C., S. N. Blair, & W. L. Haskell (eds.): *Physical Activity and Health*. Champaign, IL: Human Kinetics (2005).

Haskell, W. L.: Health consequences of physical activity: Understanding and challenges regarding dose response. *Medicine and Science in Sports and Exercise.* 26(6):649–660 (1994).

Haskell, W. L., I. Lee, R. R. Pate, K. E. Powell, S. N. Blair, B. A. Franklin, C. A. Macera, G. W. Heath, P. D. Thompson, & A. Bauman: Physical activity and public health: Updated recommendation for adults from the American College of Sports Medicine and the American Heart Association. *Medicine & Science in Sports & Exercise.* 39(8):1423–1434 (2007).

Haskell, W. L., C. Sims, J. Myll, W. M. Bortz, F. G. St. Goar, & E. L. Alderman: Coronary artery size and dilating capacity in ultra distance runners. *Circulation.* 87(4):1076–1082 (1993).

Heath, G. W., J. M. Hagberg, A. A. Ehsani, & J. O. Holloszy: A physiological comparison of young and older endurance athletes. *American Physiological Society.* 51(3):634–640 (1981).

Hickson, R. C., C. Foster, M. L. Pollock, T. M. Galassi, & S. Rich: Reduced training intensities and loss of aerobic power, endurance, and cardiac growth. *Journal of Applied Physiology.* 58:492–499 (1985).

Hickson, R. C., C. Kanakis, J. R. Davis, A. M. Moore, & S. Rich: Reduced training duration effects on aerobic power, endurance, and cardiac growth. *Journal of Applied Physiology.* 53(1):225–229 (1982).

Hickson, R. C. & M. A. Rosenkoetter: Reduced training frequencies and maintenance of increased aerobic power. *Medicine and Science in Sports and Exercise.* 13:13–16 (1981).

Hollenberg, M., J. Yang, T. J. Haight, & I. B. Tager: Longitudinal changes in aerobic capacity: Implications for concepts of aging. *The Journals of Gerontology Series A: Biological Sciences and Medical Sciences* 61:851–858 (2006).

Houmard, J. A., B. K. Scott, C. L. Justice, & T. C. Chenier: The effects of taper on performance in distance runners. *Medicine and Science in Sports and Exercise.* 26(5):624–631 (1994).

Housh, D. J. & T. J. Housh: The effects of unilateral velocity—Specific concentric strength training. *The Journal of Orthopaedic and Sports Physical Therapy.* 17(5):252–260 (1993).

Houston M. E., H. Bentzen, & H. Larsen: Interrelationships between skeletal muscle adaptations and performance as studied by detraining and retraining. *Acta Physiologica Scandinavica.* 105:163–170 (1979).

Hui, S. S. & J. W. Chan: The relationship between heart rate reserve and oxygen uptake reserve in children and adolescents. *Research Quarterly for Exercise and Sport.* 77(1):41–49 (2006).

Hurley, B. F., D. R. Seals, A. A. Ehsani, L. J. Cartier, G. P. Dalsky, J. M. Hagberg, & J. O. Holloszy: Effects of high-intensity strength training on cardiovascular function. *Medicine and Science in Sports and Exercise.* 16(5):483–488 (1984).

Huston, T. P., J. C. Puffer, & W. MacMillan: The athletic heart syndrome. *The New England Journal of Medicine.* 313:24–32 (1985).

Jasperse, J. L. & M. H. Laughlin: Endothelial function and exercise training: Evidence from studies using animal models. *Medicine & Science in Sports & Exercise.* 38:445–454 (2006).

Keul, J., H. H. Dickhuth, G. Simon, & M. Lehmann: Effect of static and dynamic exercise on heart volume, contractility, and left ventricular dimensions. *Circulation Research.* 48:I162–I170 (1981).

Kibler, W. B. & T. J. Chandler: Sport-specific conditioning. *The American Journal of Sports Medicine.* 22(3):424–432 (1994).

Kilmer, D. D., M. A. McCrory, N. C. Wright, S. G. Aitkens, & E. M. Bernaver: The effect of a high resistance exercise program in slowly progressive neuro-muscular disease. *Archives of Physical Medicine and Rehabilitation.* 75(5):560–563 (1994).

Koch, G. & L. Rocher: Total amount of hemoglobin, plasma and blood volumes, and intravascular protein masses in trained boys. In Berg, K. & B. O. Erickson (eds.): *Children and Exercise IX*. Baltimore, MD: University Park Press, 109–115 (1980).

Lewis, D. A., E. Kamon, & J. L. Hodgson: Physiological differences between genders. Implications for sports conditioning. *Sports Medicine.* 3:357–369 (1986).

Longhurst, J. C., A. R. Kelly, W. J. Gonyea, & J. H. Mitchell: Chronic training with static and dynamic exercise: Cardiovascular adaptation and response to exercise. *Circulation Research.* 48:I171–I178 (1981).

Lussier, L. & E. R. Buskirk: Effects of an endurance training regimen on assessment of work capacity in prepubertal children. *Annals of the New York Academy of Sciences.* 301:734–747 (1977).

Madsen, K., P. K. Pedersen, M. S. Djurhuus, & N. A. Klitgaard: Effects of detraining on endurance capacity and metabolic changes during prolonged exhaustive exercise. *Journal of Applied Physiology.* 75:1444–1451 (1993).

Magel, J. R., G. F. Foglia, W. D. McArdle, B. Gutin, G. S. Pechar, & F. I. Katch: Specificity of swim training on maximum oxygen uptake. *Journal of Applied Physiology.* 38(1):151–155 (1975).

Maw, G. J., S. H. Boutcher, & N. A. S. Taylor: Ratings of perceived exertion and affect in hot and cool environments. *European Journal of Applied Physiology.* 67:174–179 (1993).

Miller, W. C., J. P. Wallace, & K. E. Eggert: Predicting max HR and the HR-VO_2 relationship for exercise prescription in obesity. *Medicine and Science in Sports and Exercise.* 25:1077–1081 (1993).

Mitchell, J. H. & P. Raven: Cardiovascular adaptation to physical activity. In Bouchard, C. R., R. J. Shepard, & T. Stephens (eds.): *Physical Activity, Fitness, and Health: International Proceedings and Consensus Statement*. Champaign, IL: Human Kinetics, 286–301 (1994).

Mitchell, J. H., C. Tate, P. Raven, F. Cobb, W. Kraus, R. Moreadith, M. O'Toole, B. Saltin, & N. Wenger: Acute response and chronic adaptation to exercise in women. *Medicine and Science in Sports and Exercise* (Suppl.). 24(6):258–265 (1992).

Morganroth, J., B. J. Maron, W. L. Henry, & S. E. Epstein: Comparative left ventricular dimensions in trained athletes. *Annals of Internal Medicine.* 82:521 (1975).

Morrow, J. R. & P. S. Freedson: Relationship between habitual physical activity and aerobic fitness in adolescents. *Pediatric Exercise Science.* 6:315–329 (1994).

Mosellin, R. & U. Wasmund: Investigations on the influence of a running-training program on the cardiovascular and motor performance capacity in 53 boys and girls of a second and third primary school class. In Bar-Or, O. (ed.): *Pediatric Work Physiology: Proceedings of the Fourth International Symposium*. Natanya, Israel: Wingate Institute (1973).

Mujika, I. & S. Padilla: Detraining: loss of training-induced physiological and performance adaptations. Part I. *Sports Medicine.* 30(2):79–87 (2000).

National Association for Sport and Physical Education: *Physical activity for children: A statement of guidelines for children ages 5-12* (2nd edition). Reston, VA: Author (2004).

Naylor, L. H., G. O'Driscoll, M. Fitzsimons, L. F. Arnolda, and D. J. Green: Effects of training resumption on conduit arterial diameter of elite rowers. *Medicine & Science in Sports & Exercise.* 38(1):86–92 (2006).

Nelson, M. E., W. J. Rejeski, S. N. Blair, P. W. Duncan, J. O. Judge. A. C. King, C. A. Macera, & C. Castaneda-Sceppa: Physical activity and public health in older adults: recommendation from the American College of Sports Medicine and the American Heart Association. *Medicine & Science in Sports & Exercise.* 39(8):1435–1445 (2007).

Niebauer, J. J. & P. Cooke: Cardiovascular effects of exercise: Role of endothelial shear stress. *Journal of American College of Cardiology.* 28:1652–1660 (1996).

Ogawa, T., R. J. Spina, W. H. Martin, W. M. Kohrt, K. B. Schechtman, J. O. Holloszy, & A. A. Ehsani: Effects of aging, sex, and physical training on cardiovascular responses to exercise. *Circulation.* 86:494–503 (1992).

Olson, T. P., D. R. Dengel, A. S. Leon, & K. H. Schmitz: Moderate resistance training and vascular health in overweight women. *Medicine & Science in Sports & Exercise.* 38:1558–1564 (2006).

O'Toole, M.: Prevention and treatment of injuries to runners. *Medicine and Science in Sports and Exercise.* 24(9 Suppl.):5360–5363 (1992).

Pate, R. R., R. D. Hughes, J. V. Chandler, & J. L. Ratliffe: Effects of arm training on retention of training effects derived from leg training. *Medicine and Science in Sports.* 10(2):71–74 (1978).

Pechar, G. S., W. D. McArdle, F. I. Katch, J. R. Magel, & J. Deluca: Specificity of cardiorespiratory adaptation to bicycle and treadmill training. *Journal of Applied Physiology.* 36(6):753–756 (1974).

Plowman, S. A.: Physical activity and physical fitness: Weighing the relative importance of each. *Journal of Physical Activity and Health.* 2(2):143–158 (2005).

Plowman, S. A., B. L. Drinkwater, & S. M. Horvath: Age and aerobic power in women: A longitudinal study. *Journal of Gerontology.* 34(4):512–520 (1979).

Pollock, M. L.: The quantification of endurance training programs. In Wilmore, J. H. (ed.): *Exercise and Sport Sciences Reviews.* 1:155–188 (1973).

Prior, B. M., P. G. Lloyd, H. T. Yang & R. L. Terjung: Exercise-induced vascular remodeling. *Exercise and Sport Science Reviews.* 31:26–33 (2003).

Roberts, J. A. & J. W. Alspaugh: Specificity of training effects resulting from programs of treadmill running and bicycle ergometer riding. *Medicine and Science in Sports.* 4(1):6–10 (1972).

Robertson, R. J., F. L. Goss, J. L. Andreacci, J. J. Dubé, J. J. Rutkowski, B. M. Snee, R. A. Kowallis, K. Crawford, D. J. Aaron, K. F. Metz: Validation of the children's OMNI RPE scale for stepping exercise. *Medicine & Science in Sports & Exercise.* 37(2):290–298 (2005).

Robertson, R. J., F. L. Goss, D. J. Aaron, K. A. Tessmer, A. Gairola, J. J. Ghigiarelli, R. A. Kowallis, S. Thekkada, Y. Liu, C. R. Randall, & K. A. Weary: Observation of perceived exertion in children using the OMNI pictorial scale. *Medicine & Science in Sports & Exercise.* 38(1):158–166 (2006).

Robertson, R. J., F. L. Goss, J. A. Bell, C. B. Dixon, K. I. Gallagher, K. M. Lagally, J. M. Timmer, K. L. Abt, J. D. Gallagher, & T. Thompkins: Self-regulated cycling using the children's OMNI scale of perceived exertion. *Medicine & Science in Sports & Exercise.* 34(7):1168–1175 (2002).

Robertson, R. J., F. L. Goss, N. F. Boer, J. A. Peoples, A. J. Foreman, I. M. Dabayebeh, N. B. Millich, G. Balasekaran, S. E. Riechman, J. D. Gallagher, & T. Thompkins: Children's OMNI scale of perceived exertion: Mixed gender and race validation. *Medicine & Science in Sports & Exercise.* 32(3):452–458 (2000).

Rowland, T. W.: *Children's Exercise Physiology.* Champaign, IL: Human Kinetics (2005).

Rowland, T.W.: Endurance Athletes' Stroke Volume Response to Progressive Exercise: A Critical Review. *Sports Medicine,* 39(8):687–695 (2009a).

Rowland, T.W.: Aerobic (un)trainability of children: Mitochondrial biogenesis and the "crowded cell" hypothesis. *Pediatric Exercise Science.* 21:1–9 (2009b)

Saltin, B.: Physiological effects of physical conditioning. *Medicine and Science in Sports.* 1:50–56 (1969).

Scharhag, J., G. Schneider, A. Urhausen, V. Rochette, B. Kramann, & W. Kindermann: Athlete's Heart: Right and left ventricular mass and function in male endurance athletes and untrained individuals determined by magnetic resonance imaging. *Journal of American College of Cardiology.* 40(10):1856–1863 (2002).

Schmidt-Trucksass, A., A. Schmid, C. Brunner, N. Scherer, G. Zack, J. Keul, & M. Hounker: Arterial properties of carotid and femoral artery in endurance-trained and paraplegic subjects. *Journal of Applied Physiology.* 89:1959–1963 (2000).

Seals, D. R., J. M. Hagberg, B. F. Hurley, A. A. Ehsani, & J. O. Holloszy: Endurance training in older men and women. *Journal of Applied Physiology.* 57(4):1024–1029 (1984).

Siegel, J. A. & T. G. Manfredi: Effects of a ten month fitness program on children. *The Physician and Sports Medicine.* 12:91–97 (1984).

Sjogaard, G., G. Savard, & C. Juel: Muscle blood flow during isometric activity and its relation to muscle fatigue. *European Journal of Applied Physiology.* 57:327–335 (1988).

Smith, M. L. & J. H. Mitchell: Cardiorespiratory adaptations to exercise training. In American College of Sports Medicine (ed.): *Resource Manual for Guidelines for Exercise Testing and Prescription.* Philadelphia, PA: Lea & Febiger (1993).

Soto, K. I., C. W. Zauner, & A. B. Otis: Cardiac output in preadolescent competitive swimmers and in untrained normal children. *Journal of Sports Medicine.* 23:291–299 (1983).

Stone, M. H., S. J. Fleck, N. T. Triplett, & W. J. Kraemer: Health- and performance-related potential of resistance training. *Sports Medicine.* 11(4):210–231 (1991).

Strong, W. B., R. M. Malina, C. J. Blimkie, S. R. Daniels, R. K. Dishman, B. Gutin, A. C. Hergenroeder, A. Must, P. A. Nixon, J. M. Pivarnik, T. Rowland, S. Trost, & F. Trudeau: Evidence based physical activity for school-age youth. *The Journal of Pediatrics.* 146:732–737 (2005).

Svedenhag, J. & J. Seger: Running on land and in water: Comparative exercise physiology. *Medicine and Science in Sports and Exercise.* 24(10):1155–1160 (1992).

Swain, D. P.: Energy cost calculations for exercise prescription: An update. *Sports Medicine.* 30(1):17–22 (2000).

Szymanski, L. M. & R. R. Pate: Effects of exercise intensity, duration, and time of day on fibrinolytic activity in physically active men. *Medicine and Science in Sports and Exercise*. 26: 1102–1108 (1994).

Tanaka, H., K. D. Monahan, & D. R. Seals: Age-predicted maximal heart rate revisited. *Journal of the American College of Cardiology*. 37(1):153–156 (2001).

Tremblay, M. S., Warburton, D. E. R., Janssen, I., Paterson, D. H., Latimer, A. E., Rhodes, R. E., et al.: New Canadian physical activity guidelines. *Applied Physiology, Nutrition, and Metabolism*. 36:36–46 (2011).

U.S. Department of Health and Human Services: *Physical Activity and Health: A Report of the Surgeon General*. Atlanta, GA: U.S. Department of Health and Human Services, Centers for Disease Control and Prevention, National Center for Chronic Disease Prevention and Health Promotion (1996).

U.S. Department of Health and Human Services: Physical Activity and Health: 2008 Physical Activity Guidelines for Americans: U.S. Department of Health and Human Services, Centers for Disease Control and Prevention, National Center for Chronic Disease Prevention and Health Promotion (2008). www.health.gov/paguidelines

Utter, A. C., R. J. Robertson, D. C. Nieman, & J. Kang: Children's OMNI Scale of perceived exertion: walking/running evaluation. *Medicine & Science in Sports & Exercise*. 34(1):139–144 (2002).

Vaccaro, P. & A. Mahon: Cardiorespiratory responses to endurance training in children. *Sports Medicine*. 4:352–363 (1987).

Wallace, J.: "Principles of cardiorespiratory endurance programming" In: Kaminsky, A. (ed.): *ACSM's Resource Manual for Guidelines for Exercise Testing and Prescription* (5 edition).

pp. 336–349. Philadelphia, PA: Lippincott Williams & Wilkins (2006).

Wang, J. S., C. J. Jen, & H. I. Chen: Effects of chronic exercise and deconditioning on platelet function in women. *Journal of Applied Physiology*. 83:2080–2085 (1997).

Wang, J. S., C. J. Jen, & H. I. Chen: Effects of exercise and deconditioning on platelet function in men. *Atherosclerosis, Thrombosis, and Vascular Biology*. 15:1668–1674 (1995).

Wenger, H. A. & G. J. Bell: The interactions of intensity, frequency and duration of exercise training in altering cardiorespiratory fitness. *Sports Medicine*. 3:346–356 (1986).

Wiebe, C. G., N. Gledhill, V. K. Jamnik, & S. Ferguson: Exercise cardiac function in young through elderly endurance trained women. *Medicine & Science in Sports & Exercise*. 31(5):684–691 (1999).

Wilmore, J. H. & D. L. Costill: *Training for Sport and Activity: The Physiological Basis of the Conditioning Process* (3rd edition). Dubuque, IA: Brown (1988).

Wilmore, J. H., J. A. Davis, R. S. O'Brien, P. A. Vodak, G. R. Walder, & E. A. Amsterdam: Physiological alterations consequent to 20-week conditioning programs of bicycling, tennis, and jogging. *Medicine and Science in Sports and Exercise*. 12(1):1–8 (1980).

Womack, C. J., P. R. Nagelkirk, & A. M. Coughlin: Exercise-induced changes in coagulation and fibrinolysis in healthy populations and patients with cardiovascular disease. *Sports Medicine*. 33:795–807 (2003).

Zauner, C. W., M. G. Maksud, & J. Melichna: Physiological considerations in training young athletes. *Sports Medicine*. 8:15–31 (1989).

Thermoregulation

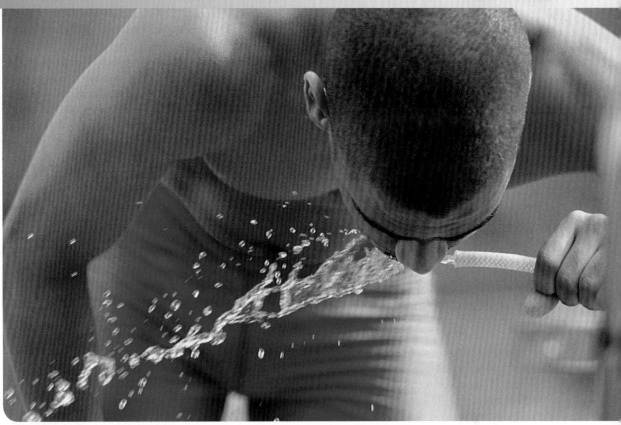

OBJECTIVES

After studying the chapter, you should be able to:

> Identify environmental factors that affect thermoregulation and be able to use indices of heat stress and windchill to assess the risks associated with exercise under various conditions.

> Describe thermal balance and discuss factors that contribute to heat gain and heat loss.

> Define the mechanisms by which heat is lost from the body, and describe how they differ under exercise conditions.

> Describe the body's regulatory system for temperature control in terms of the sensory input, neural integration, and effector responses to increase or decrease heat loss.

> Identify the factors that influence heat exchange between an individual and the environment.

> Describe the challenges to the cardiovascular system during exercise in a hot environment and in a cold environment.

> Describe the goals for fluid ingestion before, during, and after exercise.

> Differentiate among the types of heat illness in terms of severity and symptoms.

> Identify ways in which an exercise leader can prevent heat and cold injuries and illness.

Introduction

Many athletic competitions and recreational activities occur in settings in which hot or cold environmental conditions affect or may threaten physical performance, health, and even life. **Thermoregulation** is the process whereby body temperature is maintained or controlled under a wide range of such environmental conditions. In human beings, body temperature is maintained within a fairly narrow range by mechanisms that match heat production to heat loss. Human thermoregulatory responses rely heavily on the cardiovascular system to maintain body temperature. This chapter addresses issues related to exercise in environmental extremes, emphasizing the role of the cardiovascular system in mediating the body's responses to exercise under such conditions.

Exercise in Environmental Extremes

Exercise in conditions of environmental extremes can present a serious challenge to the thermoregulatory and cardiovascular systems of the body. If the cardiovascular system cannot meet the concurrent demands of supplying adequate blood to the muscles and maintaining thermal balance, *exertional heat illness (EHI)* may ensue. Heat illness includes a spectrum of disorders from heat cramps to life-threatening heatstroke. Cold conditions can also pose problems. If an exerciser is unprepared or inadequately clothed for exercise in a cold environment, heat loss can exceed heat production, leading to cold-induced injury.

Exercise professionals have a responsibility to understand the problems associated with exercise in extreme environmental conditions because they may affect an individual's performance or place an exerciser at risk for injury or even death. Understanding the body's responses to extreme environmental conditions is necessary for minimizing performance decrements and avoiding injury or illness in those who train and compete in adverse conditions.

Basic Concepts

Understanding the body's responses to exercise in different environments begins with basic environmental measures and the measurement of body temperature.

Measurement of Environmental Conditions

Human thermoregulation is affected by several environmental conditions: ambient temperature (T_{amb}), relative humidity, and wind speed. Ambient temperatures are often measured with a mercury or digital thermometer and can vary greatly in areas that are in shade or direct sunlight. **Relative humidity** is a measure of the moisture in the air relative to how much moisture, or water vapor,

can be held by the air at a given ambient temperature. Thus, 70% humidity means that the air contains 70% of the moisture that it can hold at that temperature.

Specific scales are used to assess thermal heat load imposed by the environment. Wet bulb globe temperature (WBGT), developed by the military, is often used in industrial settings and athletic situations. The WBGT is calculated based on a formula that includes measures of air temperature, radiant heat load (measured by a thermometer in a small black globe that absorbs radiant heat), and relative humidity (measured by a thermometer covered with a wet cotton wick). Recommendations about the risk of heat stress at various WBGT levels are available in the American College of Sports Medicine (ACSM) Position Stand on exertional heat illness (American College of Sports Medicine, 2007a). Included in this publication are guidelines for modifying or canceling high-intensity or long-duration exercise when WBGT conditions are a risk for adults and children. In many cases, however, WBGT measurements are not available, and a simpler measure of environmental heat stress—the heat stress index—can be used to assess the risk. The **heat stress index** is used to estimate the risk of heat stress based on the ambient temperature and relative humidity (**Figure 14.1**).

Wind speed affects the amount of heat lost from the body and is used to calculate the windchill factor. **Table 14.1** presents the most recent windchill chart

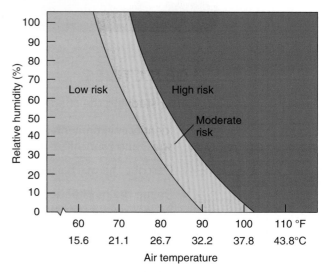

FIGURE 14.1 Heat Stress Index.
Low risk: Use discretion, especially if unconditioned or unacclimatized; little danger of heat stress for acclimatized individuals who hydrate adequately. Moderate risk: Heat-sensitive and unacclimatized individuals may suffer; avoid strenuous activity in the sun; take adequate rest periods and replace fluids. High risk: Extreme heat stress conditions exist; consider canceling all exercise.
Source: Modified from Armstrong, L. E. & R. W. Hubbard: High and dry. *Runners World.* June:38–45 (1985).

TABLE 14.1 Windchill Index

Wind Speed (mi·hr⁻¹)	Thermometer Reading (°F)*																
	40	35	30	25	20	15	10	5	0	−5	−10	−15	−20	−25	−30	−35	−40
5	36	31	25	19	13	7	1	−5	−11	−16	−22	−28	−34	−40	−46	−52	−57
10	34	27	21	15	9	3	−4	−10	−16	−22	−28	−35	−41	−47	−53	−59	−66
15	32	25	19	13	6	0	−7	−13	−19	−26	−32	−39	−45	−51	−58	−64	−71
20	30	24	17	11	4	−2	−9	−15	−22	−29	−35	−42	−48	−55	−61	−68	−74
25	29	23	16	9	3	−4	−11	−17	−24	−31	−37	−44	−51	−58	−64	−71	−78
30	28	22	15	8	1	−5	−12	−19	−26	−33	−39	−46	−53	−60	−67	−73	−80
35	28	21	14	7	0	−7	−14	−21	−27	−34	−41	−48	−55	−62	−69	−76	−82
40	27	20	13	6	−1	−8	−15	−22	−29	−36	−43	−50	−57	−64	−71	−78	−84
45	26	29	12	5	−2	−9	−16	−23	−30	−37	−44	−51	−58	−65	−72	−79	−86
	Low risk						Moderate risk			High risk							

Low Risk: Use discretion; little danger, if properly clothed.

Moderate Risk: Postpone exercise, if possible. Proper clothing is essential. Individuals at risk should take added precautions against overexposure.

High Risk: There is great danger from cold exposure; consider canceling all exercise.

*Note that this table uses °F; see Appendix A for conversion.

Source: U.S. Weather Service.

adopted by the U.S. National Weather Service in 2001. This chart uses the wind velocity measured at a height of 1.3 m (5 ft), as opposed to a height of 8.7 m (33 ft) as in the original windchill chart from the 1940s. The windchill chart was developed as a public health tool to help prevent frostbite and cold-induced injuries by providing information for choosing appropriate clothing and activities based on available environmental data.

Measurement of Body Temperature

Exercise physiologists differentiate among temperatures in different body sites; most commonly used are core temperature (T_{co}) and skin temperature (T_{sk}). Even this distinction is simplistic, however, because core and skin temperature both vary among different specific sites. Core temperature is normally maintained within fairly narrow limits of approximately 36.1–37.8°C (97–100°F) in the resting individual (Marieb and Hoehn, 2010). Skin temperature is considerably cooler, averaging approximately 33.3°C (91.4°F). Skin temperature is more variable than core temperature because it is greatly influenced by environmental conditions.

Body temperature is commonly measured with a thermometer placed in the mouth. However, this method is affected by many factors, including breathing rate and recent fluid ingestion. Heavy breathing through the mouth and the ingestion of cold fluids result in artificially low oral temperatures, whereas the ingestion of hot liquids can artificially raise oral temperatures. For these reasons, oral measurement is not the method of choice among physiologists.

Core temperature is most accurately assessed by measuring the temperature of the blood as it enters the right atrium or measuring esophageal temperature. These measurements are invasive procedures, however, and are not practical for routinely measuring core temperature. Therefore, rectal temperature (T_{re}) or gastrointestinal (T_{GI}) temperature (via an ingested radio transmitter—see "Focus on Research") is often used in laboratory and research settings to measure core body temperature.

Although rectal and GI temperature measurements are accurate and reliable, they are not feasible for mass testing, nor are they routinely used to assess temperatures in exercise participants or athletes. Despite the importance of assessing body temperature for preventing and

Thermoregulation The process whereby body temperature is maintained or controlled under a wide range of environmental conditions.

Relative Humidity The moisture in the air relative to how much moisture (water vapor) can be held by the air at any given ambient temperature.

Heat Stress Index A scale used to determine the risk of heat stress from measures of ambient temperature and relative humidity.

Core Temperature during a Half Marathon

Advances in technology now permit temperature to be measured relatively noninvasively by swallowing a vitamin-sized telemetric temperature sensor. Core body temperature in the lower GI tract is then transmitted to a small recorder (see Photo).

This technology was used to continuously measure core temperature of male soldiers participating in a half marathon (21 km or 13.1 mi) in a tropical environment. The soldiers were heat acclimatized and regularly participated in fitness training. The soldiers consumed an average of 1.18 L of fluid before and during the race and lost an average of 2.89 L of sweat—meaning on average they replaced only about 42% of sweat loss. The figure below shows their individual core temperatures by race finish time (panel A, 105–111 minutes; panel B, 111–117 minutes; panel C, 122–146 minutes).

These measurements highlight the considerable variability in core temperature response even in a relatively homogeneous group of young, trained, acclimatized soldiers. Also seen here is the magnitude of core temperature rise that these runners voluntarily achieved during a distance run in a hot, humid environment without medical consequence.

It is important to recognize that the core temperatures reported in this study do not indicate "safe" levels of core temperature for all individuals. Indeed, many unfit or unacclimatized individuals would suffer from heat illness at much lower core temperatures.

Source: Byrne, C., J. K. Lee, S. A. Chew, C. L. Lim, & E. Y. Tan: Continuous thermoregulatory responses to mass-participation distance running in the heat. *Medicine & Science in Sports & Exercise.* 38(5):803–810 (2006).

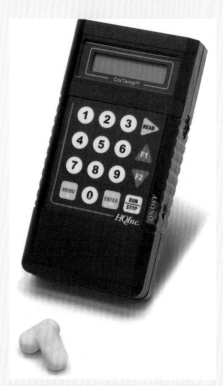

CorTemp Data Recorder and CorTemp Ingestible Core Body Temperature Sensor (photos courtesy of HQ, Inc.).

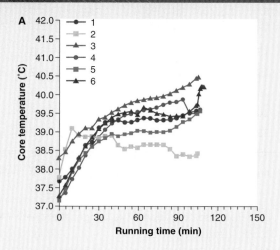

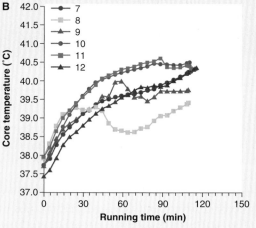

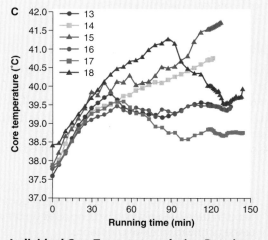

Individual Core Temperature during Running.
Individual core temperature responses of 18 runners during the half marathon, presented in order of finishing time: 105–111 min, N = 6 (top); 111–117 min, N = 6 (middle); 122–146 min, N = 6 (bottom).

treating heat illness, there is no readily available, accurate, and convenient way of assessing core temperature in many situations such as athletic events. Often practitioners must rely on oral temperature measurements despite problems associated with this method. When appropriate, medical personnel often obtain rectal temperatures. Tympanic membrane (ear) temperatures (T_{tym}) are sometimes used to measure body temperature, but these instruments do not accurately detect exercise-induced changes in body temperature and thus should not be used to assess exertional heat stress (Casa and Armstrong, 2003).

Skin temperature is not routinely measured in field settings, but it is important because it affects the amount of heat that can be exchanged with the environment. Heat moves down a thermal gradient (both between the core and the skin and between the skin and the environment). Therefore, more heat is lost from the body when the skin is considerably hotter than the environment (larger gradient) than when the two temperatures are similar (smaller gradient). In the same way, more heat is gained by the body when the environment is considerably hotter than the skin. Skin temperatures are measured with thermocouples attached to the skin.

Thermal Balance

Body temperature results from a balance between heat gain and heat loss (**Figure 14.2**). Although heat can be gained from the environment, most heat is typically produced in the body by metabolic activity. Heat is a by-product of cellular respiration; at rest the body liberates approximately 60–80% of the energy from aerobic metabolism as heat (**Figure 2.1**). The minimum energy required to meet the metabolic demands of the body at rest is called basal metabolic rate or resting metabolic rate; this accounts for a large proportion of the body's heat production.

The ingestion of food increases the body's production of heat. This is known as *thermogenesis* (see Chapter 8). Muscular activity also increases heat production, including activity related to muscle tone and posture; activities of daily living, such as bathing, dressing, and meal preparation; and planned exercise. Because metabolism increases greatly during physical activity, heat production also increases dramatically.

Heat can be exchanged (gained or lost) from the body through four processes: radiation, conduction, convection, and evaporation. The extent of heat gain or loss through these processes depends on environmental conditions: ambient temperature, relative humidity, and wind speed.

Radiant heat loss occurs through the emission of electromagnetic heat waves to the environment. It depends on the thermal gradient between the body and the environment. When the environmental temperature equals the skin temperature, no heat is lost through radiation. If the environmental temperature exceeds the skin temperature, radiation adds to the heat load of the body.

FIGURE 14.2 Thermal Balance.
Body temperature is maintained within a narrow range by a balance of heat gain and heat loss mechanisms.

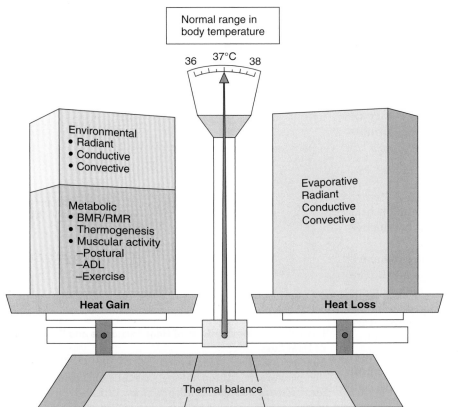

Conduction involves the direct transfer of heat from one molecule in contact with another. Conduction in humans primarily involves contact between the skin and the molecules of air and other substances in contact with the skin. The extent of conductive heat loss depends on the thermal gradient between the skin and the molecules in contact with the skin and on the thermal properties of the molecules in contact with the skin. Because water absorbs and conducts heat much better than air, submersion in cool water can more rapidly lower body temperature.

Convective heat loss depends on the movement of the molecules in contact with the skin. When there is a breeze, heat loss is greater because the warmer molecules are moved away from the skin. Thus, the thermal gradient is maintained and more heat is lost through conduction.

Evaporation is the conversion of liquid into vapor. The evaporation of unnoticed water from the skin, called *insensible perspiration*, contributes to heat dissipation under resting and exercise conditions. However, the evaporation of sweat is the major mechanism for cooling the body under exercise conditions. Sweat is 99% water derived from plasma and released from eccrine glands. These glands are located throughout the body but are more concentrated on the forehead, hands, and feet (Marieb and Hoehn, 2010). The remaining 1% includes the electrolytes sodium (Na^+), chloride (Cl^-), and potassium (K^+) and traces of amino acids, bicarbonate (HCO_3^-), carbon dioxide (CO_2), copper, glucose, hormones, iron, lactic acid, magnesium (Mg^{2+}), nitrogen (N), phosphates (PO_4^-), urea, vitamins, and zinc (Murray, 1987). The exact proportion of these elements in sweat varies among individuals and within the same individual under different conditions; it is also influenced by the individual's fitness level (Haymes and Wells, 1986).

When the body is in *thermal balance*, the amount of heat lost equals the amount of heat produced, and body temperature remains constant. In this situation, when all heat exchange processes are added, the sum is equal to zero. This can be shown by the following formula (Winslow et al., 1939):

14.1 $\quad M \pm R \pm C \pm K - E = 0$

where M is metabolic heat production, R is radiant heat exchange, C is convective heat exchange, K is conductive heat exchange, and E is evaporative heat loss.

The ± sign for radiant, convective, and conductive processes indicates that heat can be lost or gained by the body through these mechanisms. When the environment is hotter than the skin temperature, heat is gained by the body (a + sign in the equation). When skin temperature is higher than the environment temperature, heat is lost from the body (a − sign in the equation). Evaporation cannot add to the heat load of the body. This mechanism can only dissipate heat; thus, there is only a negative sign in the equation for evaporation.

Heat Exchange

The exchange (transfer) of heat between the body and the environment occurs by the mechanisms just described: conduction, convection, radiation, and evaporation. Heat exchange is represented schematically in **Figure 14.3**. These four mechanisms are important for dissipating heat to the environment under most conditions. However, when ambient temperatures are high, conduction, convection, and radiation may actually add heat to the body.

The effectiveness of heat exchange between an individual and the environment is affected by five factors:

1. The thermal gradient
2. The relative humidity
3. Air movement
4. The degree of direct sunlight
5. The clothing worn

The greater the difference between two temperatures—called the thermal gradient—the greater the heat loss is from the warmer of the two. Typically, the body is warmer than the environment, so heat moves down its thermal gradient to the environment. More heat is lost in cooler environments because the thermal gradient is greater.

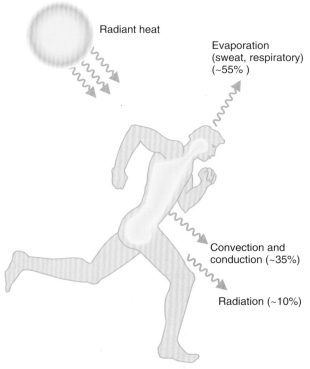

Radiant heat

Evaporation (sweat, respiratory) (~55%)

Convection and conduction (~35%)

Radiation (~10%)

FIGURE 14.3 Mechanisms of Heat Exchange and Percentage of Heat Loss.
Source: Modified from Gisolfi, C. V. & C. B. Wenger: Temperature regulation during exercise: Old concepts, new ideas. *Exercise and Sport Sciences Reviews*. 12:339–372 (1984).

High humidity decreases evaporative heat loss from the body because the air is already largely saturated with water vapor. Relative humidity is the primary determinant of the extent of evaporative cooling; on humid days, evaporative cooling is limited. Although an exerciser may sweat profusely when humidity is high, the sweat does not evaporate as effectively.

Air movement increases convective heat loss from the skin to the environment. Thus, on windy days more heat is lost from the body.

Direct sunlight can add considerably to the radiant heat load of an individual. Conversely, shade or cloud cover can often provide significant relief from heat.

Clothing also influences the extent of heat transfer with the environment. In cold weather, clothing protects against excessive heat loss. For example, long sleeve undershirts and tights are often added to football uniforms to help retain heat in cold weather outdoor games. Conversely, clothing can interfere with heat dissipation in hot weather by decreasing convective heat loss. Clothing that is lightweight, nonrestrictive, and light-colored promotes heat loss; heavy, dark clothing interferes with the dissipation of heat. Football uniforms, especially the protective padding, are an example of heavy, restrictive clothing that has been shown to increase physiological strain (Armstrong et al., 2010). Helmets, in particular, limit heat loss by encapsulating the head. The color of the clothing is also a consideration. Dark colors absorb light and thereby add to the radiant heat load; light colors reflect light. Thus, dark-colored uniforms can contribute to the heat stress of athletes as they play on a synthetic field that radiates heat in the hot sun. Short shirts and the use of mesh materials are attempts to aid in heat dissipation under these conditions.

Thermoregulation

The body regulates its internal body temperature within a narrow range despite wide variations in environmental temperatures. The process by which the body regulates body temperature is termed thermoregulation.

Normal Body Temperature

The human body typically regulates its temperature within approximately 1°C near 37°C (98.6°F) (**Figure 14.4**). Maintaining temperature within this range is important because changes in body temperature dramatically

Heat Stress The physical work and environmental components that combine to create heat load on an individual.

Heat Strain The physiological responses and resulting thermoregulatory processes to combat heat stress.

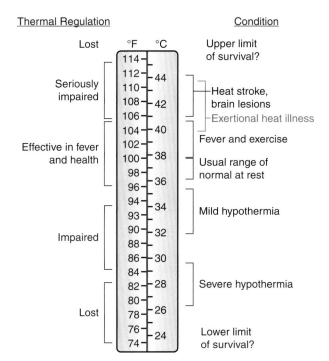

FIGURE 14.4 Range of Core Temperature and Associated Conditions.
A range of temperatures is associated with each condition. A given temperature may fall into more than one category depending on individual characteristics.
Source: Modified from Wenger, C. B. & J. D. Hardy: Temperature regulation and exposure to heat and cold. In Lehmann, J. F. (ed.): *Therapeutic Heat and Cold* (4th edition). Baltimore, MD: Williams & Wilkins, 150–178 (1990).

affect biological function by altering chemical reactions and ultimately directly damaging body tissue. Although body temperature is carefully regulated, it is not consistent throughout the body. The core is tightly regulated to maintain a temperature near 37°C. The shell (skin), on the other hand, varies greatly in temperature because it is strongly influenced by environmental conditions.

Core body temperature fluctuates throughout the day (circadian rhythm) and is typically 0.7–0.8°C higher in the late afternoon than in the early morning hours. Core temperature can also vary throughout the menstrual cycle, increasing by 0.5–0.75°C at ovulation (Stitt, 1993).

Physiological Thermoregulation

Heat stress refers to physical work and environmental components that combine to create heat load on an individual. The physiological responses and resulting thermoregulatory processes that combat this heat stress are known as **heat strain**. A relatively stable core temperature is achieved through the interaction of behavioral and physiological reactions to thermal stimuli. Core body temperature is controlled by regulatory centers in the hypothalamus. These regulatory centers can modify

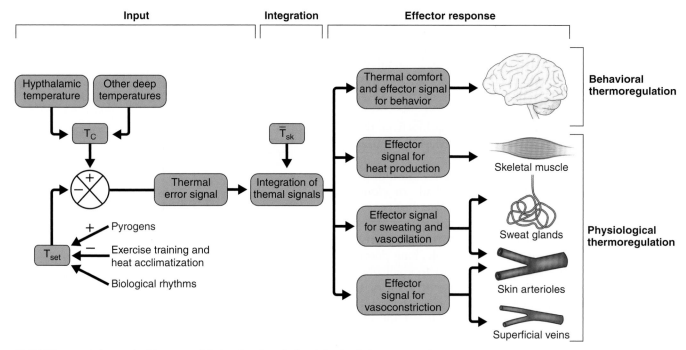

FIGURE 14.5 Schematic Diagram of Behavioral and Physiological Thermoregulation.
Several factors (biological rhythms, training and acclimatization, and circulating pyrogens) influence the core temperature set point (T_{set}). Core temperature is compared to the T_{set}, which is integrated with thermal input from the skin to produce effector signals for behaviors and physiological thermoregulatory responses.
Sources: Modified from Sawka, M. N. & C. B. Wenger: Physiological responses to acute exercise-heat stress. In Pandolf, K. B., M. N. Sawka, & R. R. Gonzalez (eds.): *Human Performance Physiology and Environmental Medicine at Terrestrial Extremes*. Dubuque, IA: Brown & Benchmark, 97–151 (1988), and Guyton, A. C. & J. E. Hall: *Textbook of Medical Physiology* (12th edition). Philadelphia, PA: Elsevier Saunders (2011).

heat production by affecting muscular activity and can modify heat loss by changing skin blood flow and sweating. Two systems regulate body temperature: behavioral thermoregulation and physiological thermoregulation. Behavioral thermoregulation involves conscious efforts to regulate body temperature such as adding clothing or increasing activity to stay warm. Physiological thermoregulation involves the reflex control of effector organs (blood vessels, sweat glands, and skeletal muscle) to maintain temperature within homeostatic limits. **Figure 14.5** summarizes the thermoregulatory system that maintains core body temperature (Guyton and Hall, 2011; Sawka and Wenger, 1988).

The hypothalamus is the primary integration center for the control of body temperature. The hypothalamus receives input from sensors that detect core body temperature and skin (shell) body temperature. These signals are compared to the body's "set point" for temperature, and if necessary, effector responses are initiated to increase heat production or facilitate heat loss. Importantly, during exercise, increased skeletal muscle activity is the primary factor that increases core temperature, which causes the hypothalamus to provide effector signals to increase heat dissipation through sweating and vasodilation. **Figure 14.6** reveals how the primary

heat dissipation mechanisms, sweating (**Figure 14.6A**) and vasodilation, shown in terms of blood flow (**Figure 14.6B**), are affected by changes in core temperature.

Exercise in the Heat

Many sporting events and recreational activities occur in hot environments. As just described, the body's thermoregulatory system dissipates excess body heat resulting from muscle activity and environmental heat. However, strenuous exercise and environmental extremes can combine to overwhelm the thermoregulatory capacity of the body.

Body Temperature during Exercise in the Heat

Body temperature increases during prolonged exercise because heat production exceeds heat dissipation. As shown in **Figure 14.7**, the increase in core temperature is proportional to the metabolic power output performed (measured in watts), and is largely independent of environmental temperature over a fairly wide range of temperatures. This suggests that the heat-dissipating mechanisms of the body can compensate for the increased metabolic

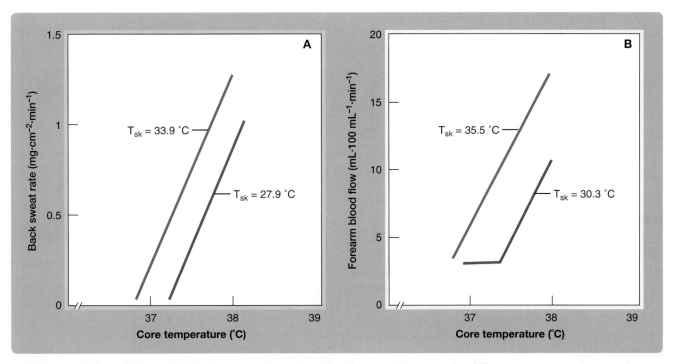

FIGURE 14.6 Effect of Core and Skin Temperature on Sweating Rate and Forearm Blood Flow.
At any given core temperature, sweating **(A)** is greater when the skin is warmer. Forearm blood flow **(B)** is constant with an increase of core temperature to approximately 37.5°C, after which blood flow increases with rising core temperature when skin temperature is approximately 30°C. When the skin is warm (35.5°C), any increase in core temperature is associated with increased blood flow.
Sources: Modified from Sawka, M. N., R. R. Gonzalez, L. L. Drolet, & K. B. Pandolf: Heat exchange during upper- and lower-body exercise. *Journal of Applied Physiology*. 57(4):1050–1054 (1984), and Wenger, C. B., M. F. Roberts, J. A. J. Stolwijk, & E. R. Nadel: Forearm blood flow during body temperature transients produced by leg exercise. *Journal of Applied Physiology*. 38(1):58–63 (1975).

heat production and stabilize body temperature. The term "prescriptive zone" is used to describe the combination of environmental conditions and work intensities at which thermoregulatory mechanisms are effective in preventing dangerous rises in body temperature during prolonged work (Lind, 1963). More generally, this zone might also be described as a compensable zone, in which

the thermoregulatory system can effectively compensate for increased metabolic heat production by increasing heat dissipation so that body temperature does not continue to rise, even though it reaches a steady state that is greater than resting body temperature.

When the body cannot dissipate the metabolic heat generated during exercise, body temperature continues

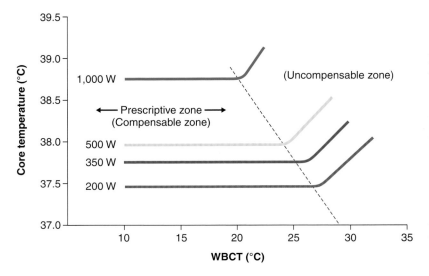

FIGURE 14.7 Core Temperature Responses during Exercise of Various Intensities (200–1000 W) in Different Environmental Conditions.
In the compensable zone, core temperature is elevated due to increased metabolic heat production but reaches a steady state because the body is able to dissipate the heat that is being generated. In the uncompensable zone, the heat-dissipating mechanism of the body cannot fully compensate for the increased heat production and body temperature continues to rise—sometimes dangerously.
Source: Modified from Lind, R. A.: A physiological criterion for setting thermal environmental limits for everyday work. *Journal of Applied Physiology*. 18:51–56 (1963).

to rise (see **Figure 14.7**, area to the right of dashed line). **Uncompensable heat stress** is a condition in which the evaporative cooling that is needed is greater than the evaporative cooling permitted by the environment (Montain et al., 1994; Sawka and Pandolf, 2001). During uncompensable heat stress, steady-state core temperature cannot be achieved and body temperature continues to rise until exhaustion occurs. Uncompensable heat stress is associated with exhaustion from heat strain at relatively low core temperatures (Montain et al., 1994; Sawka and Pandolf, 2001).

Heat Exchange during Exercise

Heat production and heat transfer occur by the same mechanisms during exercise as they do at rest. However, during exercise the total body metabolism may increase to 15–20 times the resting rate (Sawka and Pandolf, 1990). In this situation, metabolic heat production may increase to a greater extent than heat dissipation; thus, the body stores heat and body temperature increases. The increase in body temperature with exercise is termed **hyperthermia**.

Metabolic heat produced in the muscles is transported to the core of the body and skin by the blood. Heat is also transferred to the skin and exchanged with the environment by conduction, convection, radiation, and evaporation. Two physiological mechanisms allow the body to dissipate heat in an attempt to maintain thermal balance during exercise: an increase in sweating rate and vasodilation of the cutaneous (skin) vessels. Evaporative cooling of sweat is the primary mechanism by which the body cools itself during exercise in warm temperatures. Vasodilation of cutaneous vessels brings the more warm blood close to the body's surface so that heat can be dissipated to the environment via conduction, radiation, and convection, assuming that the ambient temperature is cooler than the body.

Figure 14.8 depicts the relative importance of heat exchange mechanisms during 60 minutes of cycling exercise (900 kpm·min⁻¹) at various ambient temperatures. Total heat loss (THL) remains relatively constant across a wide range of ambient temperatures. The fact that the metabolic heat production (M) exceeds the THL accounts for the increased temperature that occurs with exercise. **Figure 14.8** reinforces the earlier observation that the increase in body temperature (heat storage) is relatively constant over a wide range of ambient temperatures as long as the work rate is constant. This is true because the metabolic heat production depends on the amount of work being done, regardless of temperature. The THL also remains the same. Thus, the difference between metabolic heat production and THL—that is, heat storage—is constant. Although THL remains relatively constant, it occurs through different processes at different ambient temperatures. At high temperatures, evaporative

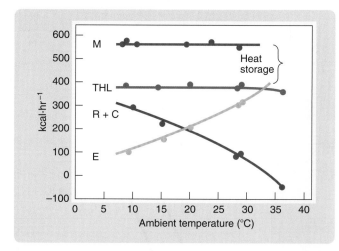

FIGURE 14.8 Mechanisms of Heat Loss during Exercise at Different Ambient Temperatures.
M, metabolic heat production; THL, total heat loss; R + C, heat loss by radiation and conduction; E, heat loss by evaporation. Exercise was performed for 60 minutes at the work rate of 900 kpm·min⁻¹ at each ambient temperature. Notice that the metabolic heat produced and the THL (and thus the heat storage) are constant over a wide range of temperatures (~10–36°C; 50–97°F) although they are achieved via different mechanisms. Evaporative heat loss becomes increasingly important as ambient temperature increases.
Source: Gisolfi, C. V. & C. B. Wenger: Temperature regulation during exercise: Old concepts, new ideas. *Exercise and Sport Sciences Reviews*. 12:339–372 (1984). Reprinted by permission of Williams & Wilkins.

heat loss is primary, and radiant and convective heat losses are less effective. This combination is effective, however, only when the humidity is low enough to allow sweat to evaporate. In high humidity, evaporative heat loss is less effective, and heat storage (body temperature) increases. This explains why temperature and humidity must be considered together (using the heat index in **Figure 14.1**, or the WBGT) for determining when activity is safe.

During heavy exercise, the sweat rate can increase dramatically. Sweat rates vary considerably among individuals, depending on genetics and fitness level. A fit person begins sweating at a lower body temperature and sweats more profusely. For any one individual, sweat rate depends on environmental conditions, exercise intensity, fitness level, degree of acclimatization, and hydration status. **Figure 14.9** estimates hourly sweating rates for running at various speeds in different environmental conditions (Sawka and Pandolf, 1990). Notice how common it is for sweating rates to exceed 1 L·hr⁻¹ of sweat. Clearly, such a water loss will lead to a decrease in total body water and plasma volume and will have deleterious effects on cardiovascular function if fluid is not replaced. The evaporation of sweat is the primary defense against heat stress. Sweating itself does not cool

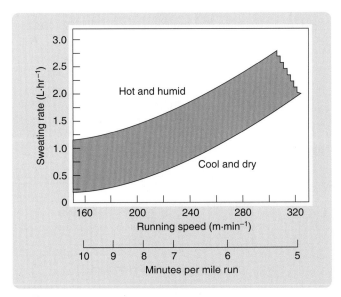

FIGURE 14.9 Estimated Sweating Rate at Various Running Speeds.
Source: Sawka, M. N. & K. B. Pandolf: Effects of body water loss on physiological function and exercise performance. In Gisolfi, C. V. & D. R. Lamb (eds.): *Perspectives in Exercise Science and Sports Medicine. Vol. 3: Fluid Homeostasis during Exercise.* Carmel, IN: Cooper Publishing Group, 97–151 (1993). Reprinted by permission.

the body; the sweat must evaporate. The evaporation of sweat produces a cooling of the body because energy is needed to convert the liquid sweat into a vapor, and this energy is extracted from the immediate surroundings. The amount of energy needed for the evaporation of sweat can be quantified: 580 kcal of heat energy is released for each liter of water that is vaporized (Guyton and Hall, 2011).

Cardiovascular Demands of Exercise in the Heat

As discussed fully in previous chapters, the cardiovascular system responds to exercise by increasing blood flow to the active tissue to support energy production. The cardiovascular system is also directly involved in thermoregulation, and heat dissipation in particular. The cardiovascular system faces several interrelated problems when exercise is performed in hyperthermic conditions:

> **Uncompensable Heat Stress** A condition in which the evaporative cooling that is needed is greater than the evaporative cooling permitted by the environment.
>
> **Hyperthermia** The increase in body temperature with exercise.

1. The skin and the muscles compete for blood flow. The muscles need increased blood flow to meet the demands of metabolic activity, and the skin needs increased blood flow to dissipate heat from the body's core.
2. Vasodilation in cutaneous vessels effectively decreases venous return, thus decreasing stroke volume. Therefore, cardiac output may be reduced at a time when the demands for flow are greatest (Rowell, 1986).
3. Sweating results in a reduced plasma volume, contributing to the reduction in stroke volume and, therefore, cardiac output.
4. Adequate blood pressure must be maintained to perfuse the vital organs, including the brain, kidney, and liver. The ability to maintain blood pressure is challenged by widespread vasodilation in the skeletal muscle beds and cutaneous vessels, which decreases total peripheral resistance.

Figure 14.10 presents cardiovascular responses to various intensities of exercise (light, moderate, and heavy) under hot and thermoneutral conditions. As seen in **Figure 14.10A**, during short-term, light submaximal exercise, cardiac output increases to a similar degree in both hot and thermoneutral environments (Rowell, 1974). However, cardiac output in a hot environment is achieved by a higher heart rate (**Figure 14.10C**) and a lower stroke volume (**Figure 14.10B**) than in a thermoneutral environment. This reduced stroke volume occurs during hot conditions because of sweating and vasodilation in the cutaneous vessels, which decreases central venous volume. Mean arterial pressure is similar to or only slightly lower in hot environments than in thermoneutral environments because of vasoconstriction in the kidneys and digestive tract.

During prolonged, heavy submaximal exercise in the heat, cardiac output increases less than in a thermoneutral environment (**Figure 14.10**). Cardiac output in hot environments fails to reach levels attained under thermoneutral conditions during heavy exercise because stroke volume declines progressively as the intensity of exercise increases. Although the heart rate is higher, it cannot compensate fully for the reduced stroke volume during heavy exercise in hot conditions. Thus, cardiac output is lower in hot conditions than in thermoneutral conditions.

During long-term, heavy submaximal exercise in the heat, vasoconstriction occurs in the digestive and renal areas in an attempt to maintain mean arterial blood pressure. Vasoconstriction may result in ischemia and even tissue damage in extreme conditions (Rowell, 1986). The regulatory mechanisms that maintain blood pressure are stressed by the excessive water loss that occurs with profuse sweating. If this fluid is not replaced, stroke volume, cardiac output, and blood pressure will decrease. Additionally, performance will suffer, and heat illness becomes increasingly likely.

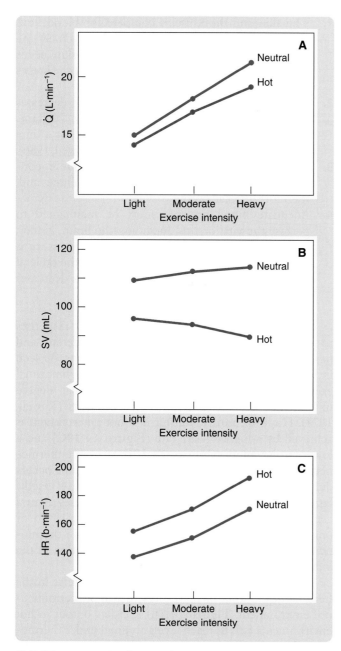

FIGURE 14.10 Cardiovascular Responses to Hot or Thermoneutral Conditions.
A. Cardiac output ($\dot{Q}$). **B.** Stroke volume (SV). **C.** Heart rate (HR).
Source: Rowell, L. B.: Human cardiovascular adjustments to exercise and thermal stress. *Physiological Reviews.* 54:75–159 (1974). Reprinted by permission.

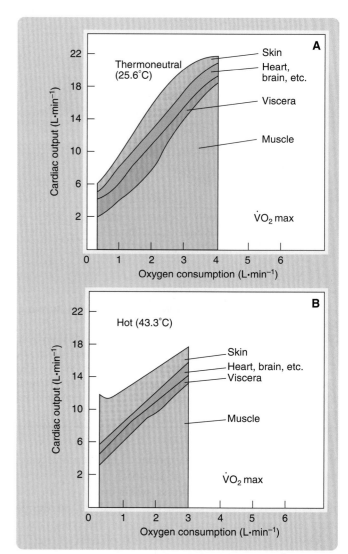

FIGURE 14.11 Distribution of Cardiac Output during Incremental Exercise in (A) Thermoneutral (25.6°C; 78°F) and (B) Hot (43.3°C; 110°F) Conditions.
Source: Modified from Rowell, L. B.: *Human Circulation Regulation During Physical Stress.* New York, NY: Oxford University Press (1986).

Maximal cardiac output during incremental exercise to maximum is lower when performed in hot conditions than in thermoneutral conditions. This decreased cardiac output results from a lower stroke volume, because maximal heart rate is unchanged, although maximal heart rate may occur earlier in the heat. The estimated distribution of cardiac output during an incremental exercise test performed under neutral and hot conditions is presented in **Figure 14.11**.

When exercise is performed in a hot environment, it cannot be performed as long as in cooler conditions. Consequently, $\dot{V}O_2$max is lower in a hot environment (**Figure 14.11B**). Cardiac output increases during exercise in both conditions. However, cardiac output at $\dot{V}O_2$max is less in the hot environment, presumably because blood is displaced in cutaneous veins, thus decreasing venous return and stroke volume. Blood flow to the active skeletal muscles increases throughout exercise in both conditions. However, blood flow to skeletal muscle is a smaller proportion of total blood flow in a hot environment than in a thermoneutral environment, because skin blood flow accounts for a larger portion of the blood flow in the hot environment. At $\dot{V}O_2$max in the hot condition, visceral blood flow is severely reduced in an effort to support the muscles with adequate blood flow and maintain blood pressure. The lower cardiac output and the decrease in blood flow when maximal exercise is performed in a hot environment both contribute to a lower $\dot{V}O_2$max and an earlier onset of fatigue.

Factors Affecting Cardiovascular Response to Exercise in the Heat

Several factors affect an individual's response to exercise in the heat. The following sections discuss four key factors: acclimatization, cardiovascular fitness, body composition, and hydration level.

Acclimatization

Acclimatization refers to adaptive changes in an individual who undergoes prolonged or repeated exposure to a stressful environment; these changes reduce the physiological strain produced by such an environment. Although acclimatization and acclimation are often used interchangeably, scientists distinguish between *acclimation*—which is a short-term adaptation (i.e., one that occurs in days or weeks) that is induced in a laboratory—and acclimatization—which is an adaptation that occurs over a longer time period and occurs in a natural climate. Acclimatization to heat results from repeated exposure to heat sufficient to increase core body temperature and elicit moderate to profuse sweating (Werner, 1993). Repeated exercise in hot climatic conditions results in improved efficiency of the thermoregulatory responses, augmented cardiovascular function, and enhanced endurance performance (Tipton et al., 2008). Light to moderate exercise in the heat for 1–2 hours a day can lead to positive adaptations within a few days.

Acclimatization to heat involves several underlying mechanisms:

1. There is an expansion of plasma volume that leads to an enhanced cardiac output during exercise and a decrease in heart rate and cardiovascular strain at a given level of exercise in the heat (Lorenzo et al., 2010; Nielsen et al., 1993).
2. Sweating begins earlier and at a lower body temperature.
3. The sweating rate for a given core temperature is higher and can be maintained longer (Tipton et al., 2008; Wenger, 1988).

> **Acclimatization** The adaptive changes that occur when an individual undergoes prolonged or repeated exposure to a stressful environment; these changes reduce the physiological strain produced by such an environment.

Figure 14.12 compares changes in rectal temperature, heart rate, and sweating rate during 4 hours of aerobic exercise before and after acclimatization (Wyndham et al., 1964). These data support the benefits of heat acclimatization as lowered thermal and cardiovascular strain. Proper acclimatization ensures that individuals can perform longer and more safely in the heat.

Fitness Level

Aerobic fitness improves an individual's thermoregulatory function and heat tolerance (Wenger, 1988). Endurance training results in a lower resting core temperature, a larger plasma volume, an earlier onset of sweating, and a smaller decrease in plasma volume during exercise (Drinkwater, 1984; Werner, 1993). Therefore, individuals who are aerobically fit are better able to handle the cardiovascular demands of exercise in hot conditions than sedentary individuals. High-intensity interval training in thermoneutral conditions also decreases the time required for acclimatization to exercise in a hot environment (Cohen and Gisolfi, 1982). In fact, exercise training results in an expansion of the plasma volume. Thus, many of the changes in cardiovascular function that are seen when repeated bouts of exercise are used to induce acclimatization may primarily reflect a training adaptation (Tschakovasky and Pyke, 2008).

Body Composition

Excessive body fat is a liability for thermoregulation during exercise in the heat. Greater adiposity contributes to heat stress by two primary mechanisms. First, adipose tissue interferes with the dissipation of heat; body fat acts to insulate the core. Second, body fat adds to the metabolic cost of activity by adding weight to the body that must be moved. Heat illness is more common in overweight individuals and is more likely to be fatal to these individuals (Bedno et al., 2010; Henshell, 1967).

Hydration Level

An individual's level of hydration has a large impact on exercise tolerance and on the cardiovascular responses to long-term exercise in the heat. Dehydration increases physiological strain and perceived effort for the same absolute amount of exercise and this effect is exacerbated when exercise is performed in the heat (American College of Sports Medicine, 2007a). Body water accounts for 65–70% of the total body mass of an average adult. Water balance is generally well regulated on a daily basis as long as water and food are readily available (Sawka et al., 2005). However, during long-term exercise in the heat, if fluid is not replaced profuse sweating leads to large acute losses of total body water and a reduction in plasma volume (Wade and Freund, 1990). The reduced plasma volume, in turn, leads to decreased stroke

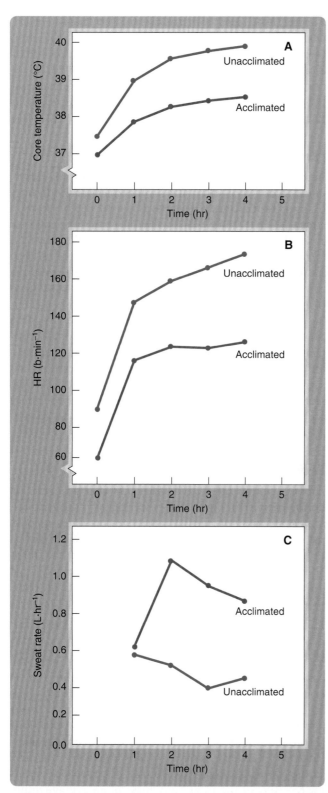

FIGURE 14.12 Comparison of Core (Rectal) Temperature (A), Heart Rate (B), and Sweat Rate (C) in Acclimated and Unacclimated Individuals during Long-Term, Moderate to Heavy Submaximal Exercise.
Source: Based on data in Wyndham, C. H., N. B. Strydom, J. F. Morrison, et al.: Heat reactions of Caucasians and Bantu in South Africa. *Journal of Applied Physiology.* 19:598–606 (1964).

volume and an increased heart rate during prolonged exercise. Therefore, it is recommended that fluid ingestion during exercise be sufficient to prevent excessive dehydration (>2% of body weight) and excessive loss of electrolytes to prevent compromised performance and health risks. Individuals vary considerably in the amount of sweat lost during activity, because of both external factors (such as the exercise intensity and duration, environmental conditions, clothing) and individual factors (such as genetic makeup, heat acclimatization, initial hydration status, and training and health status). Thus, unfortunately, general recommendations about fluid ingestion are not feasible. Instead, it is recommended that individuals develop a personalized fluid replacement plan to ensure that dehydration does not account for more than 2% of their body weight during exercise (American College of Sports Medicine, 2007a). Careful monitoring of body weight following an exercise bout is necessary to determine an individual's typical sweat loss with exercise and the required fluid intake to offset this loss.

Thirst is an inadequate stimulus for adequately replacing the fluid lost during exercise. Even with unlimited access to water, most individuals do not voluntarily consume enough water to replace the water lost during physical activity, resulting in a relative state of dehydration. **Voluntary dehydration** refers to exercise-induced dehydration that develops despite an individual's unlimited access to water. **Figure 14.13** shows the sweat loss and voluntary fluid intake of men and women in various sports. Clearly, voluntary fluid intake does not fully replace sweat loss. Thus, the coach or exercise leader needs to encourage participants to consume fluid beyond what thirst dictates. Experts recommend that proper hydration be achieved by paying attention to prehydration, fluid ingestion during exercise, and rehydration following exercise (American College of Sports Medicine, 2007a). See the Focus on Application box for additional details.

Fluid Ingestion during and after Exercise

During heavy exercise, metabolic heat production in active muscles increases up to 100 times that of inactive muscle. If this heat were not dissipated, the internal temperature would rise 1°C every 5–8 minutes, resulting in overheating (hyperthermia) and collapse of the individual within 15–20 minutes. Thus, sweating under these conditions is absolutely essential (Nadel, 1988). However, sweating does not occur without a price—the removal of fluid from the body (Maughan, 1991). A 70-kg, 2:30 marathoner can lose 5 L of body water, or 1–2 L·hr^{-1}. As previously described, sweat is not pure water but contains a variety of substances. The most important electrolytes are sodium (Na$^+$), chloride (Cl$^-$), and potassium (K$^+$).

FOCUS ON APPLICATION
Exercise and Fluid Replacement

The ACSM publishes a wide variety of Position Stands on issues related to Exercise, Physical Activity, and Health (go to thepoint.lww.com/Plowman4e for a complete list). These pronouncements written by members of the ACSM represent research-based consensus views from leading experts in the area. The Position Stand titled "Exercise and Fluid Replacement" provides important recommendations about fluid and electrolyte requirements during physical activity and a review of research documenting the effect of hydration status on performance, physiology, and health. The accompanying tables summarize the goals and recommendations for prehydration, fluid intake during physical activity, and postexercise rehydration and estimate the approximate fluid intake needed to compensate for the sweating rate of individuals of different body sizes who are running at different speeds in different environmental conditions. It is recommended that changes in body weight be directly measured by individuals to personalize their fluid replacement regimes.

Please see the Position Stand in its entirety for additional recommendations on fluid and electrolyte replacement.

Source: American College of Sports Medicine (2007a).

Approximate Fluid Intake (L) Needs Based on Body Weight and Running Speed in Cool and Hot Conditions			
Cool Temperature (18°C; 64.4°F)			
Body Weight (kg)	**10 km·hr⁻¹ (~5.3 mi·hr⁻¹)**	**12.5 km·hr⁻¹ (~6.3 mi·hr⁻¹)**	**15 km·hr⁻¹ (~9.5 mi·hr⁻¹)**
50	0.53	0.69	0.86
70	0.79	1.02	1.25
90	1.04	1.34	1.64
Warm Temperature (28°C; 82.4°F)			
Body Weight (kg)	**10 km·hr⁻¹ (~5.3 mi·hr⁻¹)**	**12.5 km·hr⁻¹ (~6.3 mi·hr⁻¹)**	**15 km·hr⁻¹ (~9.5 mi·hr⁻¹)**
50	0.62	0.79	0.96
70	0.89	1.12	1.36
90	1.15	1.46	1.76

Fluid Intake Goals and Recommendations		
Time Period	**Goal**	**Recommended Intake**
Prephysical activity (prehydration)	Begin activity euhydrated—with normal electrolytes	If not already adequately, hydrated drink ~5–7 mL·kg⁻¹ BW 4 hr prior and, if still not hydrated, drink ~3–5 mL·kg⁻¹ BW 2 hr prior to the event
During activity	Prevent excessive (>2% loss of body weight) dehydration and excessive change in electrolyte balance to avert compromised performance	Customize based on type of exercise, clothing, weather, and individual factors (genetics, acclimatization, training, and health status) (Use the table above to approximate necessary fluid intake)
Postphysical activity (rehydration)	Replace any fluid and electrolyte deficit	• If recovery time permits, this can be achieved with increased water and food containing enough Na⁺ to replace Na⁺ sweat loss • If recovery time is short, exercisers should ingest 1.5 L of fluid that includes electrolytes for each kg of body weight lost

Although shifts in internal water compartments provide the liquid portion of sweat, ultimately some of the water lost through sweating comes from blood plasma. If this water is not replaced, the individual may perform poorly and suffer from heat injuries.

Voluntary Dehydration Exercise-induced dehydration that develops despite an individual's access to unlimited water.

Type of Fluid Ingested

Whether to supplement with plain water or a carbohydrate and/or electrolyte beverage (sports drink) has been much debated. For the vast majority of sports or fitness workouts, plain water is the beverage of choice (**Figure 14.14**), but endurance events may be the exception (American Dietetic Association, 1987; Coyle, 2004).

The rate at which an ingested fluid enters the body's water supply depends on the rate at which it leaves the stomach (*gastric emptying*) and the rate at which it is

FIGURE 14.13 Sweating Rate and Voluntary Fluid Intake for Males and Females in Various Sports.
Source: Based on data in American College of Sports Medicine: Position stand: Exercise and fluid replacement. *Medicine & Science in Sports & Exercise.* 39:377–390 (2007a).

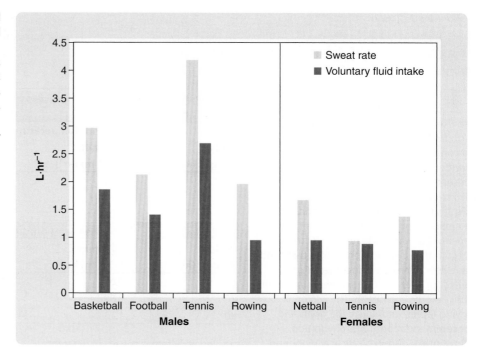

absorbed across the intestinal membrane (*intestinal absorption*). Both gastric emptying and intestinal absorption are influenced by the composition of the ingested fluid.

Three factors affect gastric emptying. First, the gastric-emptying rate decreases as the caloric content of the ingested fluid increases. However, the differences in the gastric-emptying rate of solutions of 2.5–10% carbohydrate are negligible and are similar to that of plain water (Coleman, 1988; Maughan, 1991). Second, the rate of gastric emptying is exponentially related to the volume of fluid in the stomach (Maughan, 1991; Murray, 1987). That is, the amount of fluid emptied from the stomach is relatively large in the first minutes and then the

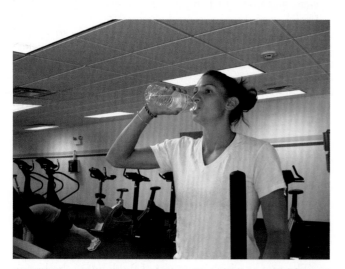

FIGURE 14.14 Water is an Appropriate Way to Replace Fluid Loss during Most Types of Physical Activity.

rate slows down. Therefore, frequent ingestion of small amounts of fluid is preferable to infrequent ingestion of large amounts; 200–400 mL of fluid should be ingested every 15–30 minutes, because approximately 400 mL can be cleared in 15 minutes (American Dietetic Association, 1987; Nieman, 1990). Third, the temperature of the fluid may be relevant. Although it has been suggested that cold sports drinks enhance gastric emptying, the evidence suggests that the gastric-emptying rates of hot and cold beverages are the same (Maughan, 1991). The real advantage of a cold drink may simply be that it tastes better to a hot, sweaty athlete, thereby encouraging more drinking. In addition, a cold fluid does not add heat to the body, as a hot fluid would. Fluid temperatures of 15–22°C (59–72°F) are recommended (American College of Sports Medicine, 2007a).

Intestinal absorption is not influenced by as many factors as gastric emptying. However, research has shown that glucose combined with sodium greatly increases intestinal fluid absorption compared to plain water. Thus, small percentages of glucose do not inhibit gastric emptying but enhance intestinal absorption if accompanied by sodium.

Although it has been claimed that electrolytes make sports drinks more palatable and hence encourage drinking, evidence indicates that sodium is the only physiologically beneficial electrolyte consumed during exercise (Maughan, 1991; Murray, 1987). Evidence does not indicate that matching the content of sweat—even if this were possible, considering its extreme variability—is necessary in replacement fluid (Haymes and Wells, 1986). Despite considerable attention given to potassium loss, its loss in sweat is low and of little consequence during exercise.

The general consensus is that electrolyte losses will be replaced through normal food intake after exercise, with the possible exception of sodium. Sodium appears to be important in postexercise beverages for reasons other than intestinal absorption. After exercise, if drinks with little or no sodium are ingested, the plasma becomes diluted, stimulating urine production and fluid excretion. This also shuts off the thirst drive, delaying rehydration (American College of Sports Medicine, 2007a; Maughan, 1991; Nose et al., 1988). Once again, however, if some is good, more is not better. Salt tablets should never be ingested because highly concentrated amounts of salt can lead to GI discomfort, dehydration, and electrolyte loss (Steen, 1994).

Because most commercially available sports drinks (see **Table 6.4** in Chapter 6) contain varying amounts of electrolytes other than sodium, some have wondered whether these other electrolytes may be harmful. Studies have not provided evidence one way or the other. However, no cases of problems arising from the ingestion of commercial sports drinks have been reported in the literature (Nose et al., 1988). One would assume, given the ongoing debate about such products, that such incidences would have been publicized had they occurred.

In situations where fluid replacement is more important than energy substrate supplementation (such as in a relatively short endurance event of 1–2 hours or an activity in high heat and humidity), the carbohydrate concentration should be low (2.5–8%) and the sodium content moderately high (30–110 mg). To put this amount of sodium in context, an 8 oz glass of 2% milk or tomato juice contains over 100 mg of sodium. Conversely, in those situations where substrate provision is needed (a long endurance event of over 2 hours in temperate environmental conditions), a more concentrated carbohydrate solution (6–10%) with sodium should be ingested (Maughan, 1991; Murray, 1987).

Exercise-Associated Hyponatremia (EAH)

While it is clear that dehydration can lead to impaired performance and serious health problems, it is also clear that excessive fluid ingestion can also be dangerous—even fatal. If large quantities of fluids are ingested in events lasting longer than 4 hours, hyponatremia (low sodium, sometimes called "water intoxication") may occur. **Exercise-associated hyponatremia (EAH)** is the occurrence of hyponatremia during or up to 24 hours after prolonged physical activity; it is diagnosed by a plasma

> **Exercise-Associated Hyponatremia (EAH)** The occurrence of hyponatremia during or up to 24 hours after prolonged physical activity; it is diagnosed by a plasma sodium concentration below normal values (usually 135 mmol·L⁻¹).

sodium concentration below normal values (usually 135 mmol·L⁻¹) (Hew-Butler et al., 2008). Hyponatremia not only affects performance but can lead to brain damage and death. Death due to hyponatremia has been reported following marathons, ultraendurance events, and military training. The primary cause of hyponatremia during exercise is sustained overdrinking, in which fluid ingestion exceeds fluid loss through sweating and urination. Risk factors associated with the development of EAH include excessive drinking behavior, weight gain during exercise, low body weight, female sex, slow running or performance pace, and event inexperience (Hew-Butler et al., 2008). Recent research also indicates that the use of nonsteroidal anti-inflammatory drugs increases the risk of developing EAH (American College of Sports Medicine, 2007a; Wharam et al., 2006). Thus, in ultraendurance events athletes are urged to drink electrolyte beverages in addition to water and to avoid fluid consumption in excess of fluid loss.

Influence of Sex and Age on the Exercise Response in Heat

Male-Female Differences in Exercise Response in Heat

Most scientific evidence suggests that the response of individuals to exercise in a hot environment depends more on the state of their cardiovascular system and their hydration status than on their sex (Drinkwater, 1984; Stephenson and Kolka, 1988, 1993). A confounding factor, however, is the phase of the menstrual cycle. Core temperature is greater, at rest and during exercise, in the luteal phase (days 14–28) than in the follicular phase (days 1–13) of the menstrual cycle (Pivarnik et al., 1992; Stephenson and Kolka, 1993). Although early studies reported that women experienced more heat strain than men when both performed the same absolute work, the women in these studies were working at a higher percentage of maximal effort, and core temperature response to exercise is related more to relative exercise intensity than absolute intensity (Drinkwater, 1984). Studies that have matched subjects for fitness level, body size, body fat, and degree of heat acclimatization have found few thermoregulatory differences between the sexes, particularly if the phase of the menstrual cycle was controlled for (Stephenson and Kolka, 1988).

There does appear to be a difference between the sexes in sweating response. Females generally sweat less and rely more on convection and conduction to dissipate heat than men. Males begin sweating at a lower core temperature and have a greater sweat rate and loss of electrolytes in humid conditions than similarly trained females (American College of Sports Medicine, 2007a; Avellini et al., 1980a; Drinkwater, 1984). Whether this difference is an asset or a liability to males is unknown. Some researchers have suggested that the higher sweat production of males is inefficient and wasteful and that females have the advantage of sweating less and thus decreasing blood volume to a lesser extent (Avellini et al., 1980b; Wyndham et al., 1965). Others counter that higher sweat rates might be advantageous in situations where evaporative heat loss is important, such as in a drier environment (Frye and Kamon, 1981). Although the sweating response is slightly different in males and females, heart rate and core temperature responses to exercise in the heat are similar (Frye and Kamon, 1983). Heat acclimatization also produces similar results in both sexes (Frye and Kamon, 1983).

Exercise Response of Children and Adolescents in the Heat

Thermoregulatory responses are different between adults and children. Heat is produced by active muscle mass but dissipated by exposed surface area. Despite a lower muscle mass, children produce more metabolic heat during the same amount of weight-bearing exercise (walking, running) than adults. On the other hand, the surface area-to-mass ratio is greater in children than in adults. This progressively decreases during growth and maturation until the adolescent reaches adult size. Therefore, in thermoneutral or moderate heat situations, the higher metabolic heat production of children is compensated for, to a large extent, by a relatively larger body surface area over which to dissipate this heat by dry heat exchange (radiation, convection, conduction). Thus, children rely less on evaporative cooling than adults. However, in high heat situations this variation becomes a liability. Not only does the higher metabolic heat production continue, but the body absorbs heat from the surroundings over this larger surface area and evaporative cooling may not be able to sufficiently compensate (Falk, 1998).

With high ambient temperatures, sweat evaporation is the main process for heat dissipation, and this requires the involvement of sweat glands. Children have the same total number of sweat glands as adults by the age of 2 or 3 years, and thus children have a higher number of sweat glands per unit of area than adolescents or adults. However, sweat gland size and sensitivity appear directly related to age. Sensitivity is lower in children, meaning that the threshold at which sweating begins is higher; it takes longer for sweating to start and the rate of sweating may be different in children and adolescents than in adults. Sweat rate is the best indicator for evaporative heat loss. Sweat rates are lower (by as much as 40%) in boys than in young adult males. The sweat rate increases progressively in young males both per gland and per surface area as they progress from prepubertal to midpubertal and late pubertal stages of maturation. Girls appear to sweat less than boys, but most studies have not found any difference between prepubertal girls and adult females in sweat rate (Falk, 1998; Meyer et al., 1992; Rowland, 2005).

The effectiveness of thermoregulation is judged by the stability of core temperature. In children, the body can prevent a detrimental rise in core temperature with exercise in the heat as well as adults under moderate conditions. However, when the ambient temperature is very high or exceeds skin temperature by 5–10°C, symptoms of fatigue and intolerance are more common in children than in adults (Rowland, 2005).

There is no clear evidence that exercise affects the level of dehydration or circulatory function more in children than in adults. The size of voluntary dehydration does not appear to differ across the age span (Rowland, 2005), although voluntary dehydration is typically not a problem in activities lasting less than 45 minutes for children. However, the same degree of dehydration, corrected for body weight, results in a greater core temperature rise in children than adults during exercise in the heat. The levels of sodium and chloride in children's sweat during exercise in a hot environment are lower, and the level of potassium is higher, compared with adults. However, these differences do not require most currently available sports drinks to be diluted for children. Evidence suggests that adding flavoring and enriching water with sodium chloride (NaCl) and carbohydrates (as in sports drinks) increases voluntary ingestion in children and adolescents and, when freely available, can prevent dehydration (Falk, 1998; Kenney and Chiu, 2001).

Aerobic training improves heat tolerance and thermoregulatory effectiveness in adults but has only a minor effect in children (Bar-Or and Rowland, 2004). However, children, adolescents, and adults all appear to successfully acclimatize to heat. The main difference is the rate of acclimatization, although the time period needed for acclimatization may not vary. For example, at the end of 2 weeks, both children and adults may have acclimatized, but throughout the process adult adaptations (sweat rate, core temperatures, etc.) are ahead of the children's (Falk, 1998). Children should undergo a long and gradual acclimatization program to ensure that they are physiologically prepared for exercise in the heat (Rowland, 1990). Children subjectively feel acclimatized before physiological acclimatization has occurred, and thus they are likely to try to do too much too soon (Falk, 1998).

Exercise Response of Older Adults in the Heat

Cardiac output increases above resting levels during exercise in the heat for both young and older individuals. However, at higher workloads the increase in cardiac output is not as great when exercise is performed in the heat as when it is performed under thermoneutral conditions (see **Figure 14.10**). The increase in cardiac output during exercise in a hot environment is less in older persons than in younger individuals of similar fitness levels (Kenney

FOCUS ON RESEARCH
Heat Dissipation and Age

The two primary physiological mechanisms to dissipate heat are an increased sweat rate and an increased skin blood flow. It has long been known that the ability to dissipate heat during exercise in hot environments declines with increasing age. However, for many years it was unclear what physiological mechanisms caused the alterations in sweat rate and skin blood flow that occur as a person ages. The obvious way to explore an answer to this question is to design a study that compares younger adults with their older counterparts. However, one inherent difficulty in such studies is that older adults typically have a lower $\dot{V}O_2$max. It is known that an increase in $\dot{V}O_2$max is associated with an earlier onset of sweating, presumably because in a trained individual the body has adapted to maintain thermal balance more effectively. Thus, it has been unclear whether aging itself or the age-related decline in $\dot{V}O_2$max is responsible for the decreased sweating and reduced heat loss in older exercisers.

To overcome these difficulties, Tankersley et al. designed a study that compared young normally fit individuals to a group of older normally fit individuals and to a group of older highly fit individuals during 20 minutes of submaximal exercise (67.5% of $\dot{V}O_2$max). Thus, the younger group could be compared to an older group with a lower $\dot{V}O_2$max (the normally fit older group) and an older group with a similar $\dot{V}O_2$max (the highly fit older group). The accompanying graphs present the esophageal temperature, chest sweating rate, and forearm blood flow in the three groups.

The graphs indicate the following:

1. Esophageal temperature during the exercise was not different among the three groups working at the same relative workload. However, because the normally fit older group had the lowest $\dot{V}O_2$max, they were working at a lower absolute workload and thus should be producing less metabolic heat. Therefore, the fact that the increased temperature among the three groups was similar may indicate an impaired ability to dissipate heat in the normally fit older group compared to the two groups with a higher $\dot{V}O_2$max.

2. In general, the average forearm blood flow and chest sweating rates for the highly fit older individuals were intermediate to those in the normally fit older group and the normally fit younger group.

3. The normally fit older individuals had a lower forearm blood flow and lower sweating response during most of the exercise protocol compared to the normally fit younger individuals.

These results suggest that younger and older subjects matched for similar $\dot{V}O_2$max have similar heat loss responses to submaximal exercise. Therefore, it appears that the decreased $\dot{V}O_2$max that typically accompanies aging is primarily responsible for the changes in sweating and blood flow reported in older adults. A person who maintains a high fitness level as he or she ages is not likely to experience these detrimental changes in the thermoregulatory response to aging.

Source: Tankersley, C. G., J. Smolander, W. L. Kenney, & S. M. Fortney: Sweating and skin blood flow during exercise: The effects of age and maximal oxygen uptake. *Journal of Applied Physiology.* 71(1):236–242 (1991).

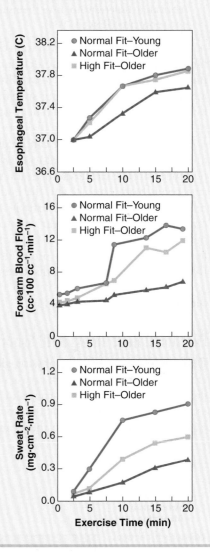

and Anderson, 1988). Furthermore, it appears that young adults increase cardiac output by augmenting heart rate, but older individuals increase cardiac output by increasing stroke volume (Kenney and Anderson, 1988). This helps explain why differences exist in cardiac output at higher workloads; apparently, there is a limit to the extent to which older individuals can increase stroke volume.

Exercise-induced reductions in plasma volume are greater in older individuals than in young individuals when they exercise in hot and humid conditions. When exercising at the same relative workload, young and older individuals demonstrate similar changes in systolic, diastolic, and mean arterial blood pressure. The accompanying Focus on Research box explores the influence of age and fitness level on thermoregulatory (temperature, forearm blood flow, and sweating) responses to exercise. As noted in the Focus on Research box, there is no difference in core temperature between young and older individuals when they exercise in the heat when the individuals are matched for fitness level. Furthermore, acclimatization to heat results in similar changes in older individuals and in young people (Pandolf et al., 1988).

Heat Illness

The magnitude of cardiovascular stress placed on the body by exercise in the heat was addressed in compelling language by Loring Rowell over 35 years ago:

> Probably the greatest stress ever imposed on the human cardiovascular system (except for hemorrhage) is the combination of exercise and hyperthermia. Together these stresses can present life-threatening challenges, especially in highly motivated athletes who drive themselves to extremes in hot environments (Rowell 1986).

When the cardiovascular system cannot meet the thermoregulatory and metabolic demands of the body, heat illness ensues. **Exertional heat illness (EHI)** involves a range of disorders resulting specifically from the combined stresses of exertion and heat stress. This is the type of heat illness that is most likely to be encountered by exercise professionals. EHI can be defined as a range of multisystem illnesses related to elevated body core temperature and the cardiovascular and metabolic responses that result from exercise and the body's attempts at thermoregulation. EHI varies greatly in severity and includes exertional dehydration, heat cramps, heat exhaustion, heat injury, and heatstroke. One of the greatest challenges of EHI is that it is often difficult or impossible to distinguish among these disorders because they often overlap and frequently evolve into a different form over time (Gardner and Kark, 2001).

Exertional Heat Illness (EHI) Syndromes

EHI syndromes involve the physiological disruption of several organs or systems and can vary in severity. **Figure 14.15** depicts the major EHI syndromes in terms of physiological disruption and severity. Within each category along the EHI range (minor to serious), there can be different levels of

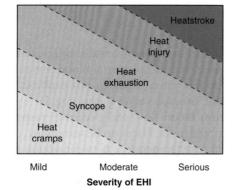

FIGURE 14.15 Spectrum of EHIs.

physiological disruption, and each illness may differ in severity and consequence. Furthermore, the shading within the figure reinforces the considerable overlap among the EHS syndromes and suggests that clear distinctions among them are not always possible (Gardner and Kark, 2001). Although clinicians have long sought to categorize heat illnesses in discrete categories, and have attempted to use core temperature as a way to define thresholds for defining categories, current thought is that such categorization is not possible and that body temperature alone does not accurately reveal the severity of heat illness.

Minor Exertional Heat Illness

Minor EHI includes mild dehydration, heat cramps, and heat syncope (Carter et al., 2006; Gardner and Kark, 2001). Symptoms of heat stress may be nonspecific, particularly in the early stages of heat illness. As heat illness progresses, so does the severity of orthostatic signs and symptoms (**Table 14.2**).

Heat cramps are an acute disorder consisting of brief, recurrent, and excruciating pain in the voluntary muscles of the legs, arms, or abdomen. Typically, the muscles have recently been engaged in intense physical activity and are fatigued. Heat cramps may result from a fluid-electrolyte imbalance. Profuse sweaters who lose large quantities of sodium may be more susceptible than others. Skeletal muscle heat cramps frequently occur in football and tennis players competing in late summer or early fall heat and humidity (American College of Sports Medicine, 2007a,b), but other athletes are not immune. A combination of rest, stretching, and ingestion of fluids or foods containing NaCl typically leads to recovery. *Heat syncope* (fainting) is characterized by vertigo (dizziness) and weakness during or following standing or with a rapid change to the upright posture during heat stress (Carter et al., 2006).

Serious Exertional Heat Illnesses

Serious EHIs include heat exhaustion, heat injury, and heatstroke (Carter et al., 2006). **Exertional heat exhaustion** is characterized by an inability to maintain adequate cardiac output and moderate (38.5°C; 101.3°F) to high (>40°C; 104°F) body temperatures. The person experiences a rapid and weak pulse, fatigue, weakness, profuse sweating, psychological disorientation, and fainting. Heat exhaustion is caused by an acute fluid loss and the inability of the cardiovascular system to adequately compensate for the concurrent demands of muscle and skin blood flow.

Children may be more susceptible to heat exhaustion because they have a smaller plasma pool from which to draw fluid. Thus, they have a potential greater deficiency of peripheral blood supply during strenuous activity in the heat than adults (Zwiren, 1992).

Individuals suffering from heat exhaustion should be moved to a cool place, given fluids, and encouraged to lie

TABLE 14.2 Symptoms of Exertional Heat Illness (EHI)

Nonspecific Symptoms			
Thirst	Weakness	Headache	Nausea
Hyperventilation	Fatigue	Poor concentration	Vomiting
Tachycardia	Cramps	Impaired judgment	Diarrhea
		Anxiety	
		Hysteria	

Progressive Orthostatic Signs and Symptoms		
Severity	**Sign or Symptom**	**Action**
Mild	Faintness	Cool body, rehydrate
	Dizziness	
	Wobbly legs	
	Stumbling gait	
Moderate	Blurred vision, tunnel vision, blackout	Seek medical help
	Collapse (without loss of consciousness)	
Severe	Collapse—brief (<3 min), loss of consciousness	Seek medical help
	Sustained hypotension	Medical emergency
	Shock, cardiovascular collapse	

down. In severe cases of heat exhaustion, a person may require medical intervention including the intravenous administration of fluids and electrolytes.

Exertional heat injury is a moderate to severe progressive multisystem disorder, with hyperthermia accompanied by organ damage or severe dysfunction. Muscle cell breakdown (rhabdomyolysis) occurs when heat decomposes the muscle cell membrane, which in turn may cause liver and kidney damages (Carter et al., 2006; Gardner and Kark, 2001). Exertional heat injury is more severe than heat exhaustion but less severe than heatstroke. Exertional heat injury may progress into heatstroke, however.

Exertional heatstroke is a life-threatening illness characterized by central nervous system dysfunction (Carter et al., 2006; Leon and Helwig, 2010). Heatstroke is a progressive multisystem disease that can lead to death due to multiorgan failure (Leon and Helwig, 2010). It often involves severe muscle and liver cell deaths, cardiovascular

collapse, and seizures (Gardner and Kark, 2001). It can be accompanied by elevated skin and core temperatures in excess of 40.5°C, tachycardia (rapid heart rate), vomiting, diarrhea, hallucinations, and coma. Heatstroke involves a failure of the thermoregulatory mechanisms. If heatstroke is suspected, the individual should be cooled as quickly as possible (preferably by cold water immersion) and medical personnel notified immediately. Unfortunately, a recent study found that although athletic trainers know that cold water immersion is the most effective way to treat this condition, only about half (49.7%) of those surveyed have adopted this method of cooling for their cooling treatment in cases of suspected heatstroke (Mazerolle et al., 2010).

Prevention of Exertional Heat Illness

Although exercise professionals must be able to recognize and respond to heat illness, preferably they should prevent heat injuries by using sound judgment and observing basic recommendations. The ACSM position stand entitled "The Prevention of Thermal Injuries During Distance Running" (1987) outlines strategies to decrease thermal injuries during road races. Following are basic recommendations for people who exercise in hot environments:

1. Allow adequate time for acclimatization (10–14 days).
2. Exercise during cooler parts of the day (early morning or evening).
3. Limit or defer exercise if the heat stress index is in the high-risk zone (see **Figure 14.1**).
4. Adequately hydrate before exercise and replace fluid loss during exercise. Monitor daily body weight changes closely, because they reflect acute water loss.
5. Wear light-colored, loose-fitting clothing that exposes large areas of skin to the air to enhance evaporation.

Exertional Heat Illness (EHI) A range of multisystem illnesses related to elevated body core temperature and the cardiovascular and metabolic processes that result from exercise and the body's thermoregulatory response.

Exertional Heat Exhaustion A moderate illness characterized by an inability to maintain adequate cardiac output at moderate (38.5°C) to high (>40°C) body temperatures.

Exertional Heat Injury A moderate to severe progressive multisystem disorder, with hyperthermia accompanied by organ damage or severe dysfunction.

Exertional Heatstroke A life-threatening illness characterized by high body temperature and central nervous system dysfunction.

FOCUS ON APPLICATION
Working under Environmental Extremes

Many occupational workers, such as construction workers, miners, and hazardous material crews, are routinely required to perform muscular work under extreme environmental conditions. Probably no workers are exposed to higher thermal environments than are firefighters. Firefighters produce large amounts of metabolic heat and are often exposed to very high temperatures. Firefighters wear vapor-impermeable gear weighing approximately 20 kg and perform heavy muscular work, often in temperatures ranging from 100 to 400°C. Thus, it is not surprising that firefighters experience severe cardiac strain. In fact, the leading cause of death in the line of duty among firefighters is myocardial infarction. It accounts for approximately 50% of the line-of-duty deaths each year—far more than deaths due to burn injuries (<10% in most years).

To better understand the magnitude of the cardiovascular stress, Smith et al. (2001) had firefighters perform three trials of a standardized set of firefighting tasks in a training building that contained live fires. Each set of drills took approximately 7 minutes to complete. A 10-minute rest period was provided between the second and third trials, during which firefighters removed their helmets, face masks, and coats in an attempt to cool the body and were strongly encouraged to consume cold water. As seen in the accompanying graphs, their heart rates increased quickly during the first trial and reached age-predicted maximal values by the end of the third trial. Stroke volume increased following the first trial but was significantly below resting values by the end of the third trial. Stroke volume was lower following several minutes of firefighting due to profuse sweating and vasodilation of cutaneous vessels. This occurred despite the attempt to cool the body and replace fluid during the 10-minute rest period.

Because of the severe cardiovascular strain associated with firefighting and the risk of myocardial infarction, many fire departments are initiating fitness programs for their personnel. Aerobic fitness programs help lessen the cardiovascular strain associated with firefighting by increasing plasma volume and improving heart function.

Source: Smith et al. (2001).

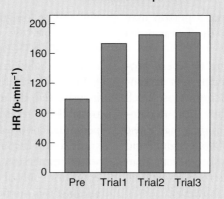

Heart Rate Response

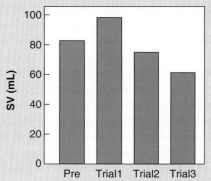

Stroke Volume Response

CHECK YOUR COMPREHENSION

Coach Brown, a high school lacrosse coach, is preparing for the start of the fall season in Charleston, SC. When practice begins in late August, the coach expects a mix of returning players and new players trying out for the team.

What environmental and physical factors should he consider in relation to heat stress on his players?

What individual characteristics should he consider in relation to heat stress on his players?

What can he do to lessen the risk of heat stress among his players?

Check your answer in Appendix C.

Exercise in the Cold

Cold weather can cause significant injuries to individuals who are unprepared or inadequately equipped for exercise training or competition. Although cold-related injuries are less common than heat-related injuries, they can be serious and even life threatening. Most commonly, exercise in the cold involves sporting events or wilderness experiences. Sporting events include winter sports, such as skiing and ice skating, and athletic contests, such as football. In these activities, hypothermia (low body temperature) is typically not a threat because individuals usually wear proper clothing, produce much metabolic heat, and have access to shelter when necessary. Wilderness activities, such as hiking and backpacking, present more risk because exposure can be prolonged (**Figure 14.16**).

Exposure to cold results in several physiological responses that alter thermal balance. Heat production increases, and heat loss is minimized by vasoconstriction. Heat production increases through nonshivering thermogenesis, shivering thermogenesis, and exercise metabolism. Nonshivering thermogenesis refers to increased metabolic heat production other than through muscular contraction. Circulating hormones—catecholamines, glucocorticoids, and thyroxine—increase metabolic rate during cold exposure (Toner and McArdle, 1988). Muscular

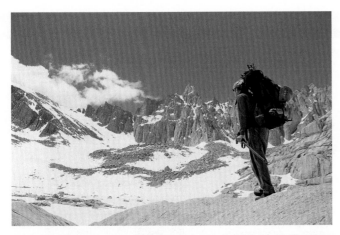

FIGURE 14.16 Prolonged Activities in Cold Environments Can Pose a Risk of Hypothermia or Frost Bite.

tensing without noticeable shivering accounts for over 30% of the increase in heat production in response to cold exposure (Toner and McArdle, 1988). This response is sometimes called preshivering. Shivering can also contribute significantly to heat production. Finally, although it varies with intensity and duration, exercise can be the greatest contributor to increased metabolic heat in the cold. Conversely, cool temperatures are often useful for dissipating the large amount of heat produced by exercise.

Very often, individuals who are exposed to the cold will voluntarily increase muscular activity as a means to increase heat production and thus feel more comfortable. Heat loss is minimized by widespread vasoconstriction, which decreases blood flow to the periphery in an attempt to maintain core temperature.

Despite the compensatory mechanisms, in some situations, being in a cold environment leads to heat loss that exceeds heat production, and body temperature drops. When an individual is exposed to the cold and heat loss is greater than heat production, serious injuries can result. The two most common cold-induced injuries of concern to exercise professionals are hypothermia and frostbite.

Cold-Induced Injuries

Hypothermia, defined as a core temperature less than 35°C (95°F) is a lowering of the body temperature to the point that it affects normal function (Bar-Or and Baranowski, 1994). This condition is potentially fatal. Body temperature drops when heat loss exceeds heat production. The magnitude of heat loss is affected by temperature, wind speed, and whether the individual becomes wet. The windchill chart (**Table 14.1**) takes into account the combined effects of temperature and wind speed and should be consulted before activity in the cold.

> **Hypothermia** A core temperature less than 35°C (95°F), resulting in the loss of normal function.

Because heat production increases greatly during exercise, hypothermia is seldom a concern for an exerciser who is properly clothed and not exposed to the environment for a prolonged time. However, during long-term events, such as a marathon, hypothermia may occur as a result of reduced heat production and increased heat loss. For instance, many runners run the second half of a race at a slower pace, resulting in less heat production. At this time, the runner may also have removed some clothing because of greater heat production earlier in the run and may be wet due to accumulated sweat, thus increasing the rate of conductive and evaporative heat loss.

As body temperature decreases, physical signs of hypothermia can be observed. Early signs include depressed heart rate, respiration, and reflexes. Mild hypothermia is marked by a loss of judgment and reduced ability to reason. The person often complains of being cold and is focused on getting warm. As hypothermia progresses, fine motor skills are affected and speech may become slurred. Severe hypothermia is characterized by agitation and inappropriate behavior and may progress to unconsciousness and coma. Mild hypothermia can be managed by warming the individual with blankets and warm beverages. However, moderate and severe cases of hypothermia should be treated by medical personnel. It is important to replace wet clothing and to protect a person with hypothermia from wind so that additional heat from the body is not lost. Because a person suffering from hypothermia often has an impaired ability to reason, the person should not be left alone.

Frostbite results from water crystallization within tissues that causes cellular dehydration and leads to tissue destruction. Frostbite usually occurs in insufficiently insulated skin. Severe frostbite can cause permanent circulatory damage, potentially leading to a need for amputation. Moving quickly (such as when running, skiing, and cycling) can create a windchill condition that increases the likelihood of frostbite.

Prevention of Cold-Induced Injuries

Injury prevention is preferable to injury treatment. To avoid cold injuries, individuals should exercise in appropriate clothing. Windproof and water-repellent outer garments are necessary. Layering loose-fitting clothing is more advantageous than wearing a single layer of heavy, bulky clothes. Clothing next to the skin should be composed of a material that wicks moisture away from the skin. Cotton should not be worn next to the skin because it holds moisture, which will draw heat away from the body.

Exercisers should consider warming up indoors, but only to the point at which they begin to sweat, so that they are not wet when they go outside. If possible, runners should run against the wind first and return with the wind at their back. Exercisers should also avoid periods of decreased

Preventing Cold Injuries during Exercise

The American College of Sports Medicine has published a Position Statement titled "Prevention of Cold Injuries during Exercise" to increase the safety of individuals performing work or exercise in cold environments. The adjacent flowchart provides an overall strategy for identifying and managing potential threats to performance and safety in cold conditions.

Please see the Position Stand in its entirety for additional recommendations for preventing cold injuries during exercise.

Source: American College of Sports Medicine (2006).

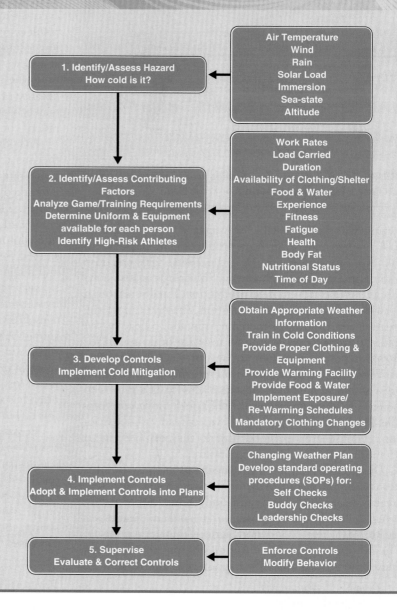

metabolic heat production unless they can compensate by adding clothing or leaving the cold environment. The cooldown period at the end of exercise is potentially dangerous because heat production has decreased although heat loss remains high. Additionally, the exerciser may be fatigued, which further exacerbates the condition. The exerciser should ideally cool down inside also.

Influence of Sex and Age on Cold Tolerance

Male-Female Differences

Body size and composition are important influences on an individual's response to cold exposure. Body fat protects against heat loss and can thus be advantageous in the cold (Toner and McArdle, 1988). Because women on average have a greater percentage of body fat than men, they may tolerate cold better.

Children and Adolescents

Because children have a larger surface area per kilogram of body weight, they lose heat faster in the cold than adults (Falk, 1998). As compensation, however, peripheral vasoconstriction occurs to a greater extent in children to protect core temperature. This reduced blood flow lowers skin temperature, however, and increases the risk of frostbite in the extremities (Bar-Or and Baranowski, 1994).

Children also cool faster in water than adults because of their relatively larger surface area and smaller amount of subcutaneous fat. Special attention should be given, therefore, when children are swimming on cool days or when water temperatures are cool.

Older Adults

Older adults have a greater risk of hypothermia due to blunted physiological and behavioral responses to the cold. In older adults, vasoconstriction to conserve heat is reduced from that in young adults. Because older adults also have a lower exercise capacity, they will become fatigued earlier when performing the same absolute workload. An older person is more likely to produce less heat (due to fatigue and discontinuing exercise) and may be less able to limit heat loss (due to reduced vasoconstriction), placing them at greater risk for hypothermia. Evidence suggests that older adults often have a blunted sensitivity to cold, such that they may be slower to make appropriate behavioral changes in a cold environment (American College of Sports Medicine, 2006).

SUMMARY

1. Environmental conditions that affect human thermoregulation are ambient temperature (T_{amb}), relative humidity, and wind speed. The heat stress index assesses the risk of thermal injury from measures of ambient temperature and relative humidity. The windchill index assesses the risk of cold-induced injury from wind speed and ambient temperature.

2. Body temperature results from a balance of heat gain and heat loss. Most heat gain results from the body's metabolic heat production. Heat can be lost from the body through radiation, conduction, convection, and evaporation.

3. Sweat evaporation is the primary defense against heat stress. For each liter of sweat vaporized, 580 kcal of heat energy is released.

4. The extent of heat exchange depends on the thermal gradient, relative humidity, air movement, degree of direct sunlight, and clothing worn.

5. Several interrelated problems challenge the cardiovascular system under hyperthermic conditions.
   a. The skin and the muscles compete for blood flow.
   b. Vasodilation in the cutaneous vessels effectively decreases venous return and thus stroke volume.
   c. Adequate blood pressure must be maintained to perfuse the vital organs.
   d. Plasma volume is reduced, contributing to reduced cardiac output.

6. An individual's response to exercise is influenced by the degree of acclimatization, cardiovascular fitness, body composition, and hydration level.

7. Water balance is generally well maintained, but athletes need to pay particular attention to hydration before, during, and after exercise.

8. The response of males and females to exercise in a hot environment is similar, although males appear to have a greater sweat rate.

9. In children and adolescents, thermoregulation is slightly different from that in adults, and they may be at greater risk of heat stress when exercising in hot environments.

10. When the cardiovascular system cannot meet the body's thermoregulatory and metabolic demands, heat illness ensues. Heat illness is a range of disorders that vary in intensity, complexity, and severity. Exertional heat illnesses include heat exhaustion, heat injury, and heatstroke.

11. During exercise in the cold, heat loss may exceed heat production, potentially resulting in serious injuries: hypothermia and frostbite.

REVIEW QUESTIONS

1. Diagram the thermal balance that is typically maintained at rest. Indicate how this balance is altered during exercise in hot and cold environments.

2. Identify the factors that influence heat exchange, and discuss how each facilitates or impedes the transfer of heat to and from the body.

3. Describe the cardiovascular responses to incremental exercise in a hot environment compared to a thermoneutral environment, and explain why these occur.

4. What is the importance of acclimatization? How much time is needed for acclimatization to occur?

5. Explain the influence of hydration level on an individual's response to exercise in the heat. What is necessary to maintain adequate hydration?

6. Discuss the effects of fitness level and body composition on an individual's response to exercise in the heat.

7. Provide a definition, cause, and treatment for exertional heat cramps, heat syncope, heat exhaustion, heat injury, and heatstroke.

8. Identify ways to minimize the risk of heat illness.

9. Explain the underlying cause of hypothermia and frostbite. Suggest ways in which these conditions can be prevented.

For further review and additional study tools, visit the website at http://thepoint.lww.com/Plowman4e ✳ 🔘

REFERENCES

American College of Sports Medicine: Position stand: Prevention of cold injuries during exercise. *Medicine & Science in Sports & Exercise*. 38(11):2012–2029 (2006).

American College of Sports Medicine: Position stand: Exercise and fluid replacement. *Medicine & Science in Sports & Exercise*. 39:377–390 (2007a).

American College of Sports Medicine: Position stand: Exertional heat illness during training and competition. *Medicine & Science in Sports & Exercise*. 39(3):556–572 (2007b).

American Dietetic Association: Nutrition for physical fitness and athletic performance for adults: Technical support paper. *Journal of the American Dietetic Association*. 87(7):934–939 (1987).

Armstrong, L. E. & R. W. Hubbard: High and dry. *Runners World*. June:38–45 (1985).

Armstrong, L. E., E. C. Johnson, D. J. Casa, M. S. Ganio, B. P. McDermott, L. M. Yamamoto, R. M. Lopez, & H. Emmanuel: The American football uniform: Uncompensable heat stress and hyperthermic exhaustion. *Journal of Athletic Training*. 45(2):117–127 (2010).

Avellini, B. A., E. Kamon, & J. T. Krajewski: Physiological responses of physically fit men and women to acclimation to humid heat. *Journal of Applied Physiology*. 49:254–261 (1980a).

Avellini, B. A., Y. Shapiro, K. B. Pandolf, N. A. Pimental, & R. F. Goldman: Physiological responses of men and women to prolonged dry heat exposure. *Aviation Space Environmental Medicine*. 51:1081–1085 (1980b).

Bar-Or, O. & T. Baranowski: Physical activity, adiposity, and obesity among adolescents. *Pediatric Exercise Science*. 6(4):348–360 (1994).

Bar-Or, O. & T. W. Rowland: *Pediatric Exercise Medicine: From Physiological Principles to Health Care Application*. Champaign, IL: Human Kinetics (2004).

Bedno, S. A., Y. Li, W. Han, D. N. Cowan, C. T. Scott, M. A. Cavicchia, & D. W. Niebuhr: Exertional heat illness among overweight U.S. army recruits in basic training. *Aviation, Space, and Environmental Medicine*. 81(2):107–111 (2010).

Byrne, C., J. K. Lee, S. A. Chew, C. L. Lim, & E. Y. Tan: Continuous thermoregulatory responses to mass-participation distance running in the heat. *Medicine & Science in Sports & Exercise*. 38(5):803–810 (2006).

Carter, R., S. N. Cheuvront, & M. N. Sawka: Heat Related Illnesses. Gatorade Sport Science Institute. *Sports Science Exchange*. 19(3):1–12 (2006).

Casa, D. J. & L. E. Armstrong: Exertional heatstroke: A medical emergency. In Armstrong, L. E. (ed.): *Exertional Heat Illnesses*. Champaign, IL: Human Kinetics, 29–56 (2003).

Cohen, J. S. & C. V. Gisolfi: Effects of interval training on work-heat tolerance of young women. *Medicine and Science in Sports and Exercise*. 14:46–52 (1982).

Coleman, E.: Sports Drink Update. Gatorade Sports Science Institute. *Sports Science Exchange*. 1(5):1–4 (1988).

Coyle, E. F.: Fluid and fuel intake during exercise. *Journal of Sports Sciences*. 22:39–55 (2004).

Drinkwater, B. L.: Women and exercise: Physiological aspects. *Exercise and Sport Sciences Reviews*. 12:21–52 (1984).

Falk, B.: Effects of thermal stress during rest and exercise in pediatric population. *Sports Medicine*. 25(4):221–240 (1998).

Frye, A. J. & E. Kamon: Responses to dry heat of men and women with similar aerobic capacities. *Journal of Applied Physiology*. 50:65–70 (1981).

Frye, A. J. & E. Kamon: Sweating efficiency in acclimated men and women exercising in humid and dry heat. *Journal of Applied Physiology*. 54:972–977 (1983).

Gardner, J. W. & J. A. Kark: Clinical diagnosis, management, and surveillance of exertional heat illness. In Zajtchuk, R (ed.) *Textbook of Military Medicine: Medical Aspects of Harsh Environments* (Vol. 1). Bethesda, MD: Office of the Surgeon General, 231–280 (2001).

Gisolfi, C. V. & C. B. Wenger: Temperature regulation during exercise: Old concepts, new ideas. *Exercise and Sport Sciences Reviews*. 12:339–372 (1984).

Guyton, A. C. & J. E. Hall: *Textbook of Medical Physiology* (12th edition). Philadelphia, PA: Elsevier Saunders (2011).

Haymes, E. M. & C. L. Wells: *Environment and Human Performance*. Champaign, IL: Human Kinetics (1986).

Henshell, A.: Obesity as an occupational hazard. *Canadian Journal of Public Health*. 58:491–497 (1967).

Hew-Butler, T., J. C. Ayus, C. Kipps, R. J. Maughan, S. Mettler, W. H. Meeuwisse, A. J. Page, S. A. Reid, N. J. Rehrer, W. O. Roberts, I. R. Rogers, M. H. Rosner, A. J. Siegel, D. B. Speedy, K. J. Stuempfle, J. G. Verbalis, L. B. Weschler, & P. Wharam: Statement of the second international exercise-associated hyponatremia consensus development conference, New Zealand, 2007. *Clinical Journal of Sports Medicine*. 18:111–121 (2008).

Kenney, W. L. & R. K. Anderson: Responses of older and younger women to exercise in dry and humid heat without fluid replacement. *Medicine and Science in Sports and Exercise*. 20:155–160 (1988).

Kenney, W. L. & P. Chiu: Influence of age on thirst and fluid intake. *Medicine & Science in Sports & Exercise*. 33(9): 1524–1532 (2001).

Leon, L. R. & B. G. Helwig: Heat stroke: Role of the systemic inflammatory response. *Journal of Applied Physiology*. 109:1980–1988 (2010).

Lind, R. A.: A physiological criterion for setting thermal environmental limits for everyday work. *Journal of Applied Physiology*. 18:51–56 (1963).

Lorenzo, S., J. R. Halliwill, M. N. Sawka, & C. T. Minson: Heat acclimation improves exercise performance. *Journal of Applied Physiology*. 109(4):1140–1147 (2010).

Marieb, E. N. & K. Hoehn: *Human Anatomy and Physiology* (8th edition). Redwood City, CA: Benjamin Cummings (2010).

Maughan, R. J.: Fluid and electrolyte loss and replacement in exercise. *Journal of Sports Sciences*. 9:117–142 (1991).

Mazerolle, S. M., I. C. Scruggs, D. J. Casa, L. J. Burton, B. P. McDermott, L. E. Armstrong, & C. M. Maresh: Current knowledge, attitudes, and practices of certified athletic trainers regarding recognition and treatment of exertional heat stroke. *Journal of Athletic Training*. 45(2):170–180 (2010).

Meyer, F., O. Bar-Or, D. MacDougall, & G. J. F. Hiegenhauser: Sweat electrolyte loss during exercise in the heat: Effects of gender and maturation. *Medicine and Science in Sports and Exercise*. 24(7):776–781 (1992).

Montain, S. J., M. N. Sawka, B. S. Cadarette, M. D. Quigley, & J. M. McKay: Physiological tolerance to uncompensable heat stress: Effects of exercise intensity, protective clothing, and climate. *Journal of Applied Physiology*. 77:216–222 (1994).

Murray, R.: The effects of consuming carbohydrate-electrolyte beverages on gastric emptying and fluid absorption during and following exercise. *Sports Medicine*. 4:322–351 (1987).

Nadel, E. R.: Temperature regulation and prolonged exercise. In D. R. Lamb & R. Murray (eds.): *Perspectives in Exercise Science and Sports Medicine. Vol. 1: Prolonged Exercise*. Indianapolis: Benchmark Press, 125–152 (1988).

Nielsen, R., J. R. Hales, S. Strange, N. J. Christensen, J. Warberg, & B. Stalin: Human circulatory and thermoregulatory adaptations with heat acclimation and exercise in a hot, dry environment. *Journal of Physiology*. 460:467–486 (1993).

Nieman, D. C.: *Fitness and Sports Medicine: An Introduction*. Palo Alto, CA: Bull Publishing (1990).

Nose, H. M., G. W. Mack, X. Shi, & E. R. Nadel: Involvement of sodium retention hormones during rehydration in humans. *Journal of Applied Physiology*. 65(1):332–336 (1988).

Pandolf, K. B., B. S. Cadarette, M. N. Wawka, A. J. Young, R. P. Francesconi, & R. R. Gonzalez: Thermoregulatory responses of matched middle-aged and young men during dry-heat acclimation. *Journal of Applied Physiology*. 65(1):65–71 (1988).

Pivarnik, J. M., C. J. Marichal, T. Spillman, & J. R. Marrow, Jr.: Menstrual cycle phase affects temperature regulation during endurance exercise. *Journal of Applied Physiology*. 72:543–548 (1992).

Rowell, L. B.: Human cardiovascular adjustments to exercise and thermal stress. *Physiological Reviews*. 54:75–159 (1974).

Rowell, L. B.: *Human Circulation Regulation during Physical Stress*. New York, NY: Oxford University Press (1986).

Rowland, T. W.: *Exercise and Children's Health*. Champaign, IL: Human Kinetics (1990).

Rowland, T. W.: *Children's Exercise Physiology* (2nd edition). Champaign, IL: Human Kinetics (2005).

Sawka, M. N., S. N. Cheuvront, & R. Carter III: Human water needs. *Nutrition Reviews*. 63(6):S30–S39 (2005).

Sawka, M. N., R. R. Gonzalez, L. L. Drolet, & K. B. Pandolf: Heat exchange during upper- and lower-body exercise. *Journal of Applied Physiology*. 57(4):1050–1054 (1984).

Sawka, M. N. & K. B. Pandolf: Effects of body water loss on physiological function and exercise performance. In C. V. Gisolfi & D. R. Lamb (eds.): *Perspectives in Exercise Science and Sports Medicine. Vol. 3: Fluid Homeostasis During Exercise*. Indianapolis, IN: Benchmark Press, 1–38 (1990).

Sawka, M. N. & K. B. Pandolf: Physical exercise in hot climates: Physiology, performance, and biomedical issues. In Zajtchuk, R (ed.) *Textbook of Military Medicine: Medical Aspects of Harsh Environments* (*Vol. 1*). Bethesda, MD: Office of the Surgeon General, 87–133 (2001).

Sawka, M. N. & C. B. Wenger: Physiological responses to acute exercise-heat stress. In Pandolf, K. B., M. N. Sawka, & R. R. Gonzalez (eds.): *Human Performance Physiology and Environmental Medicine at Terrestrial Extremes*. Dubuque, IA: Brown & Benchmark, 97–151 (1988).

Smith, D. L., T. S. Manning, & S. J. Petruzzello: The effect of strenuous live-fire drills on cardiovascular and psychological responses of recruit firefighters. *Ergonomics*. 44(3):244–254 (2001).

Steen, S. N.: Nutrition for young athletes: Special considerations. *Sports Medicine*. 17(3):152–162 (1994).

Stephenson, L. A. & M. A. Kolka: Effect of gender, circadian period and sleep loss on thermal responses during exercise. In Pandolf, K. B., M. N. Sawka, & R. R. Gonzalez (eds.): *Human Performance Physiology and Environmental Medicine at Terrestrial Extremes*. Dubuque, IA: Brown & Benchmark, 267–304 (1988).

Stephenson, L. A. & M. A. Kolka: Thermoregulation in women. *Exercise and Sport Sciences Reviews*. 21:231–262 (1993).

Stitt, J. T.: Central regulation of body temperature. In Gisolfi, C. V., D. R. Lamb, & E. R. Nadel (eds.): *Perspectives in Exercise Science and Sports Medicine. Vol. 6: Exercise, Heat, and Thermoregulation*. Indianapolis, IN: Benchmark Press, 1–48 (1993).

Tankersley, C. G., J. Smolander, W. L. Kenney, & S. M. Fortney: Sweating and skin blood flow during exercise: The effects of age and maximal oxygen uptake. *Journal of Applied Physiology*. 71:236–242 (1991).

Tipton, M. J., K. B. Pandolf, M. N. Sawka, J. Werner, & N. Taylor: Physiological adaptations to hot and cold environments. In Taylor, N. & H. Groeller (eds.): *Physiological Bases of Human Performance During Work and Exercise*. Edinburgh, UK: Churchill Livingstone, 379–400 (2008).

Toner, M. M. & W. D. McArdle: Physiological adjustments of man to the cold. In Pandolf, K. B., M. N. Sawka, & R. R. Gonzalez (eds.): *Human Performance Physiology and Environmental Medicine at Terrestrial Extremes*. Dubuque, IA: Brown & Benchmark, 361–400 (1988).

Tschakovsky, M. E. & M. E. Pyke: Cardiovascular responses to exercise and limitations to human performance. In Tyalor, N. & Groeller, H. (eds.): *Physiological Bases of Human Performance During Work and Exercise*. Edinburgh, UK: Churchlivingstone, 5–27 (2008). U.S. Weather Service: http://www.weather.gov/os/windchill/index.shtml. Accessed 11/1/08.

Wade, C. E. & B. J. Freund: Hormonal control of blood volume during and following exercise. In Gisolfi, C. V. & D. R. Lamb (eds.): *Perspectives in Exercise Science and Sports Medicine. Vol. 3: Fluid Homeostasis during Exercise*. Indianapolis, IN: Benchmark Press, 201–246 (1990).

Wenger, C. B.: Human heat acclimatization. In Pandolf, K. B., M. N. Sawka, & R. R. Gonzalez (eds.): *Human Performance Physiology and Environmental Medicine at Terrestrial Extremes*. Dubuque, IA: Brown & Benchmark, 153–198 (1988).

Wenger, C. B. & J. D. Hardy: Temperature regulation and exposure to heat and cold. In Lehmann, J. F. (ed.): *Therapeutic Heat and Cold* (4th edition). Baltimore, MD: Williams and Wilkins, 150–178 (1990).

Wenger, C. B., M. F. Roberts, J. A. J. Stolwijk, & E. R. Nadel: Forearm blood flow during body temperature transients produced by leg exercise. *Journal of Applied Physiology*. 38(1):58–63 (1975).

Werner, J.: Temperature regulation during exercise: An overview. In Gisolfi, C. V., D. R. Lamb, & E. R. Nadel (eds.): *Perspectives in Exercise Science and Sports Medicine. Vol. 6: Exercise, Heat, and Thermoregulation*. Indianapolis, IN: Benchmark Press, 49–79 (1993).

Wharam, P. C., D. B. Speedy, T. D. Noakes, J. M. D. Thompson, S. A. Reid, & L. Holtzhausen: NSAID use increases the risk of developing hyponatremia during an Ironman Triathlon. *Medicine & Science in Sports & Exercise*. 38:618–622 (2006).

Winslow, C. E. A., A. P. Gagge, & L. P. Herrington: The influence of air movement upon heat losses from clothed human body. *American Journal of Physiology*. 127:505 (1939).

Wyndham, C. H., J. F. Morrison, & C. G. Williams: Heat reaction of male and female Caucasians. *Journal of Applied Physiology*. 20:357–364 (1965).

Wyndham, C. H., N. B. Strydom, J. F. Morrison, et al.: Heat reactions of Caucasians and Bantu in South Africa. *Journal of Applied Physiology*. 19:598–606 (1964).

Zwiren, L. D.: Children and exercise. In Shephard, R. J. & H. S. Miller (eds.): *Exercise and the Heart in Health and Disease*. New York, NY: Dekker, 105–163 (1992).

Cardiovascular Disease Risk Factors and Physical Activity

15

OBJECTIVES

After studying the chapter, you should be able to:

> Discuss the prevalence of cardiovascular disease and its impact in terms of mortality and economic costs.

> Describe the progression of atherosclerosis and indicate how atherosclerosis can lead to a heart attack.

> Identify the cardiovascular risk factors and classify them as risk factors that cannot be modified, major modifiable risk factors, or contributing (nontraditional) risk factors.

> Describe the relationship between each risk factor and cardiovascular disease in terms of the degree of risk and the underlying pathology.

> Identify how exercise/physical activity, exercise training, and physical fitness impact each of the risk factors.

> Track the cardiovascular risk factors from childhood to adulthood.

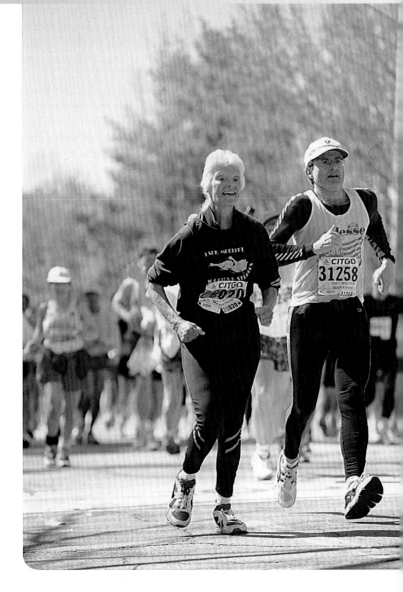

Introduction

Earlier in this unit a distinction was made between the application of the training principles for the achievement of health and for fitness. The health factor of primary concern is cardiovascular disease. Cardiovascular disease (CVD) affects nearly 80 million Americans (one in three) and has been the leading cause of death in the United States every year since 1900, except 1918. Cardiovascular disease is the underlying cause of nearly 34% of all deaths in the United States. Nearly 2200 Americans die from CVD every day, an average of one every 39 seconds (American Heart Association, 2011). Worldwide, cardiovascular disease is also increasing as a cause of death and disability. The proportion of worldwide deaths from cardiovascular disease is projected to increase from 28% in 1990 to 36% in 2020 (Gaziano, 2005).

Several terms have a very specific meaning in regard to statistics about disease. **Prevalence** refers to the number of cases of a disease in a specific population at a given time. **Incidence** is the rate of new cases of a disease in a specific population. **Mortality** is the number of deaths in a population. **Morbidity** refers to the number of people with a sickness or disease in a population.

Figure 15.1 depicts the number of CVD deaths in the United States from 1979 to 2008 in men and women (American Heart Association, 2011). Notice that more women than men have died of CVD every year since 1984. Furthermore, the patterns of CVD mortality are different between the sexes. For men, there is a pattern of gradual decline since 1980. Women, on the other hand, had a relatively stable CVD mortality rate through 2001, when the death rate began consistently declining.

In addition to the emotional tragedy of lives cut short, the economic cost of cardiovascular disease is staggering. In 1994, the estimated economic cost of CVD in the United States was $128 billion. Between 2010 and 2030, total direct medical costs of CVD are projected to climb from $272.5 billion to $818.1 billion (Heidenreich et al., 2011).

Cardiovascular disease (CVD) includes coronary heart disease (which can lead to heart attack, also called *myocardial infarction*), stroke, hypertension, heart failure, diseases of the arteries, congenital cardiovascular defects, rheumatic heart diseases, and other diseases. Coronary heart disease is the most common form of heart disease, accounting for approximately 50% of all CVD (American Heart Association, 2011).

Figure 15.2 presents the incidence of heart attack with advancing age. Advancing age increases the possibility of death from heart attack, but being young is not an automatic protection from impairment or death. This figure also reinforces the important point that the death rate from heart attack is not consistent across ethnic groups. In almost every age category, black men have the highest incidence of heart attacks, followed closely by white men. Black women have a higher incidence than white women. Note that although the number of females dying from CVD is higher than males (**Figure 15.1**), when heart attacks are prorated per 1000 population (**Figure 15.2**), more men die of heart attacks than women. The former is at least partially a reflection of a larger population of females than males. Additionally, females who have had heart attacks are more likely to die from them within a few weeks to a year or to suffer a second heart attack (American Heart Association, 2011).

Progression of Coronary Heart Disease

Coronary heart disease (CHD) (also called *coronary artery disease* or *ischemic heart disease*) results from damage to the coronary arteries supplying the heart muscle (myocardium). Coronary heart disease often leads to a heart attack, which may or may not be fatal. The damage

FIGURE 15.1 Cardiovascular Disease Mortality Trends for US Males and Females.
Source: Roger, V. L., A. S. Go, D. M. Lloyd-Jones, E. J. Benjamin, J. D. Berry, W. B. Borden, et al.: Heart Disease and Stroke Statistics—2012 Update: A Report from the American Heart Association. *Circulation*. 125:e02–e220 (2011). Reprinted with permission.

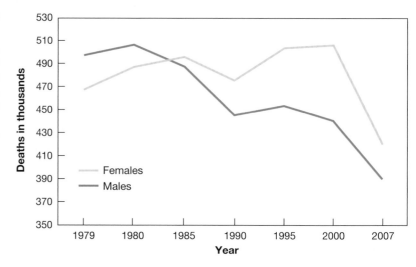

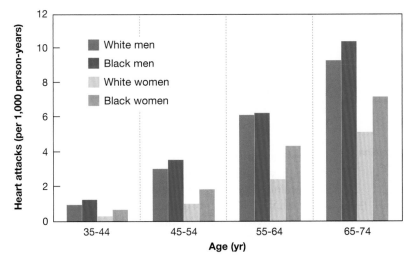

FIGURE 15.2 Incidence of Heart Attack by Age, Race, and Sex.
Source: Roger, V. L., A. S. Go, D. M. Lloyd-Jones, E. J. Benjamin, J. D. Berry, W. B. Borden, et al.: Heart Disease and Stroke Statistics—2012 Update: A Report from the American Heart Association. *Circulation*. 125:e02–e220 (2011). Reprinted with permission.

to the coronary artery is caused by **atherosclerosis**, an inflammatory disease arising in response to endothelial cell injury or dysfunction (Libby and Theroux, 2005) and characterized by lipid accumulation (plaque) in the arterial wall. In contrast to atherosclerosis, **arteriosclerosis** encompasses the natural aging changes that occur in blood vessels—namely, thickening of the wall, loss of elastic connective tissue, and hardening of the vessel wall.

While this text cannot fully describe the pathology of atherosclerosis, a basic understanding of the evolution of atherosclerotic plaque formation is needed to understand how cardiovascular risk factors are related to disease and how exercise training can effectively reduce cardiovascular disease.

The process of atherosclerosis begins with damage to the endothelium of the artery. The initial injury to the endothelial cells of the arterial wall may result from chemical irritants in tobacco smoke, the turbulent blood flow resulting from hypertension, hyperglycemia, high cholesterol (specifically low-density lipoprotein cholesterol—LDL-C) levels, immune complexes, vasoconstrictor substances, homocysteine (a proclotting factor), and viral or bacterial infection (Libby, 2006). Damaged endothelium allows LDL-C to enter the arterial wall and become oxidized (modified) by free radicals (see the Focus on Application box in Chapter 5). Oxidized LDL-C in the arterial wall initiates an inflammatory response that attracts immune cells (macrophages) into the arterial wall. An inflammatory response by the immune system is a normal reaction to such an injury (see **Figure 22.3**). Macrophages ingest (phagocytize) the LDL-C and release chemicals that stimulate smooth muscle cells in the tunica media of the vessel wall to divide and migrate into the intima. The result of this complex process is the formation of an atherosclerotic plaque (or lesion) inside the blood vessels composed of connective tissue, smooth muscle cells, cellular debris, cholesterol, and, in advanced cases, calcium. This leads to an increased thickness of the tunica intima layer and can seriously decrease the internal diameter of the coronary artery. **Figure 15.3** summarizes the process of atherosclerotic plaque development.

The growing plaque can interfere with arterial function in many ways. Early in the progression of atherosclerosis, there is evidence of endothelial dysfunction (an impaired ability to vasodilate in response to increased need for blood flow). As the plaque progresses, it can cause narrowing of the artery to the extent that blood flow cannot increase sufficiently during periods of increased cardiac work (causing pain called angina pectoris if in the chest or claudication if in the legs). Plaque can also cause turbulent blood flow that may lead to the rupture of an aneurism or further injury to the endothelium. Finally, advanced atherosclerotic plaque is highly thrombotic, meaning that if the plaque ruptures, the material in the plaque will lead to the formation of a blood clot that could occlude a coronary artery, leading to a heart attack (or a stroke if an artery to the brain is occluded).

Prevalence The number of cases of a disease in a specific population at a given time.

Incidence The rate of new cases of a disease in a specific population.

Mortality The number of deaths in a population.

Morbidity The number of people with a sickness or disease in a population.

Coronary Heart Disease (CHD) Also called coronary artery disease or ischemic heart disease, CHD results from damage to the coronary arteries supplying the heart muscle (myocardium).

Atherosclerosis A pathological process that results in the buildup of plaque inside blood vessels.

Arteriosclerosis The natural aging changes that occur in blood vessels, including thickening of the walls, loss of elastic connective tissue, and hardening of the vessel wall.

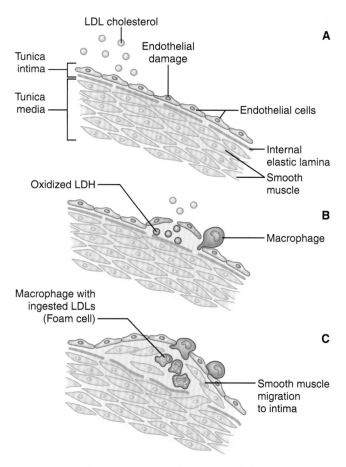

FIGURE 15.3 Progression of Atherosclerotic Plaque.
A. Atherosclerosis is initiated by damage to the endothelial lining of the vessel wall allowing LDL-C to enter the vessel wall.
B. LDL-C in the intimal layer of the arterial wall is oxidized, leading to an inflammatory response, which is evident by the entry of macrophages into the arterial wall. **C.** Macrophages ingest the oxidized lipids and release chemical signals that enhance the inflammatory response and signal smooth muscle division and migration into the tunica intima, resulting in an atherosclerotic plaque that increases intimal thickness.

If the affected area of the myocardium is small, the individual may recover from the heart attack. However, if the affected area of the myocardium is large, the heart can no longer pump blood, and the heart attack will be fatal. The process of atherosclerotic plaque development may begin in childhood and progress for years before any clinical symptoms of disease occur (Squires, 1998).

The Influence of Exercise Training on Atherosclerosis

While there is substantial evidence that regular physical exercise delays the development of atherosclerosis and decreases the risk of cardiovascular mortality, the direct impact of exercise training on the process of atherosclerosis has been difficult to document in humans.

In a 1992 study (Schuler et al., 1992), a group of patients were placed on a low-fat diet (<20% of total calories, <200 mg of cholesterol), and a high-intensity daily aerobic exercise program (75% HRmax). This study showed that 32% of the subjects experienced a regression in their coronary atherosclerotic lesion, 45% stayed the same, and only 23% exhibited a progression in their lesions. These changes were significantly better than the changes in the control group, who were advised to eat less fat and to exercise but were left to their own initiative. Other studies have supported this tendency (Froelicher, 1990; LaFontaine, 1994; Squires and Williams, 1993; Wood and Stefanik, 1990). Nordstrom et al. (2003) found that physical activity during leisure, although not workplace physical activity, was inversely related to the progression of carotid artery atherosclerosis.

Exercise training has been shown to improve endothelial function and myocardial perfusion in patients with coronary heart disease (Gielen and Hambrecht, 2001; Gielen et al., 2002). These beneficial effects appear to be mediated through increased nitric oxide (NO) availability (Linke et al., 2006). However, much of the influence of physical activity or exercise training on atherosclerosis is mediated through changes in cardiovascular risk factors, which is discussed in detail in the following section. Of course, it is also probable that changes in those risk factors lessen the risk of CVD by effecting positive changes in endothelial function, including the increased production of NO.

Physical Activity and Cardiovascular Risk Factors

Given the high prevalence of CVD and its morbidity (disease) and mortality (death) consequences, the ability to predict who is at greatest risk for developing CVD is valuable. A **risk factor** is an aspect of personal behavior or lifestyle, an environmental exposure, or an inherited characteristic that has been shown by epidemiological evidence to predispose an individual to the development of a specific disease (Caspersen and Heath, 1993). **Table 15.1** lists various classifications of risk factors for coronary heart disease. Age, race, sex, and heredity are risk factors that cannot be changed. Age becomes a risk factor for males at 45 years, and for females at 55 years. Heredity is interpreted as a family history (parent or sibling) with premature (<55 years of age if male; <65 years of age if female) cardiovascular disease or death from cardiovascular disease, especially heart attack or stroke. A family history of coronary revascularization (bypass surgery), diabetes mellitus, hypertension, and/or hyperlipidemia (high cholesterol levels) also increases the risk of coronary heart disease.

The major modifiable risk factors are, at least to some degree, changeable through diet, exercise, medication, or

TABLE 15.1 Coronary Heart Disease Risk Factors

Nonmodifiable Risk Factors	Major Modifiable Risk Factors	Contributing and Selected Nontraditional Risk Factors
Age	Cholesterol-lipid fractions	C-Reactive Protein (CRP)
Heredity	Cigarette smoking	Fibrinogen levels
Race	Diabetes mellitus	Fibrinolytic activity
Sex	Hypertension	Stress
	Obesity	Apolipoproteins
	Physical inactivity	

other lifestyle alterations. The following sections discuss these major modifiable risk factors and the role of physical activity or exercise training in modifying each. Each major risk factor acts independently, but many are also interrelated and act jointly. In general, the greater the number of risk factors, the greater the level of risk.

The contributing and nontraditional risk factors are a relatively new set of risk factors that may predict cardiovascular disease but that are not yet universally considered major risk factors because of a lack of evidence from large-scale studies, because of the infeasibility of measuring these factors in large numbers of people, or because they do not significantly increase the predictability of cardiovascular disease beyond the traditional risk factors. Additional contributing and nontraditional factors, beyond those discussed here, are under study.

Major Modifiable Risk Factors

Cholesterol-Lipid Fractions

Lipids, or fats, are by definition water-insoluble substances. They may be classified as simple (or neutral) fats, compound fats, and derived fats. The primary simple fat is triglyceride. Compound fats are combinations of a neutral fat and another substance such as phosphate (phospholipid), glucose (glucolipid), or protein (lipoprotein). Derived fats originate from simple and compound fats. Chief among them is **cholesterol**, a derived fat that is essential for the body but may be detrimental in excessive amounts.

Combining fats with another substance typically makes the compound water-soluble, and it is through such compounds—specifically **lipoproteins**—that fat is transported in the bloodstream. The protein portions of lipoproteins are called **apolipoproteins**. Five types of lipoproteins circulate in blood: chylomicrons, very low density lipoproteins, intermediate-density lipoproteins, low-density lipoproteins, and high-density lipoproteins. *Chylomicrons* are microscopic fat particles formed after digestion that enter the bloodstream via the lymphatic system. Triglycerides and some cholesterol are transported in the blood, from the small intestines or liver to adipose tissue or muscle for storage or use as fuel, by chylomicrons and *very low density lipoproteins (VLDLs)*. The VLDL from which the triglyceride has been removed is degraded into an *intermediate-density lipoprotein (IDL)*, which in turn is converted in the liver to a **low-density lipoprotein (LDL-C)**. LDL is composed of protein, a small portion of triglyceride, and a large portion of cholesterol. LDL transports 60–70% of the total cholesterol in the body to all cells except liver cells, hence the abbreviation LDL-C. The major apolipoprotein of LDL is called Apo-B. As mentioned earlier, LDL-C is involved in the formation of atherosclerotic plaque.

High-density lipoprotein (HDL-C) is a lipoprotein in blood plasma composed primarily of protein and a minimum of cholesterol or triglyceride. The purpose of HDL is to transport cholesterol from body tissues to the liver where the cholesterol can be broken down and eliminated in bile. Because HDL transports cholesterol it is abbreviated HDL-C. Some speculate that HDL-C may also block or in some way interfere with the deposition of cholesterol in the arterial wall lining. The major apolipoprotein of HDL-C is called Apo-A1 (Squires and Williams, 1993).

Triglycerides (but not the associated VLDLs) represent an independent risk factor (Summary of the Third

---

Risk Factor An aspect of personal behavior or lifestyle, an environmental exposure, or an inherited characteristic that has been shown by epidemiological evidence to predispose an individual to develop a specific disease.

Cholesterol A derived fat that is essential for the body but may be detrimental in excessive amounts.

Lipoprotein Water-soluble compound composed of apolipoprotein and lipid components that transport fat in the bloodstream.

Apolipoprotein The protein portion of lipoproteins.

Low-Density Lipoprotein (LDL-C) A lipoprotein in blood plasma composed of protein, a small portion of triglyceride, and a large portion of cholesterol whose purpose is to transport cholesterol to the cells.

High-Density Lipoprotein (HDL-C) A lipoprotein in blood plasma composed primarily of protein and a minimum of cholesterol or triglyceride whose purpose is to transport cholesterol from the tissues to the liver.

TABLE 15.2 Classification of Total, LDL-C, HDL-C Blood Levels, and Triglycerides

Lipid and Category	Level for Adults (mg·dL⁻¹)	Level for Children and Adolescents (mg·dL⁻¹)
Total cholesterol		
Desirable	<200	<170
Borderline high	200–239	170–199
High	≥240	≥200
LDL-cholesterol		
Optimal	<100	<110
Near optimal	100–129	
Borderline high	130–159	110–129
High	160–189	130
Very high	≥190	
HDL-cholesterol		
Low	<40	
High	≥60	
Triglyceride level		
Normal	<150	
Borderline high	150–199	
High	200–499	

Sources: Summary of the Third Report of the National Cholesterol Education Program (NCEP): Expert panel on detection, evaluation and treatment of high blood cholesterol in adults (adult treatment panel II). *Journal of the American Medical Association.* 285:2486–2497 (2001).

Report of the National Cholesterol Education Program, 2001). Chylomicrons are not thought to be atherosclerotic. Abundant evidence shows, however, that an elevated total cholesterol (TC) level is independently and directly related to CHD incidence. A classification system for TC is presented in **Table 15.2** (Summary of the Third Report of the National Cholesterol Education Program, 2001). In the United States, an adult level of 240 mg·dL⁻¹ carries twice the risk of a level of 200 mg·dL⁻¹. These values thus represent high-risk and desirable levels, respectively. They apply to all adults regardless of age or sex. (The risks in children are considered later.) The term *hyperlipidemia* (excessive fat in the blood) is commonly used to describe this risk factor. **Figure 15.4** shows the percentages of

Americans between the ages of 20 and 74 years with obesity/overweight, hypertension, or high blood cholesterol at different time points between 1971 and 2008. As seen in this figure, the percentage of Americans with high cholesterol declined through this 37-year period but still represents nearly 15% of the population.

Not only is the total amount of cholesterol important, but also the fractions of LDL-C and/or HDL-C are important. High levels of LDL-C and/or Apo-B are positively related to CHD. High levels of HDL-C and/or Apo-A1 are inversely related to CHD. Optimal levels of LDL-C are 100 mg·dL⁻¹ or less. Low levels of HDL-C are 40 mg·dL⁻¹ or less. An HDL-C level greater than or equal to 60 mg·dL⁻¹ is actually so good that it is said

FIGURE 15.4 Trends in the Prevalence of Health Conditions among US Adults, Aged 20–74 years. *Sources:* Data based on Briefel, R. R. & C. L. Johnson: Secular trends in dietary intake in the United States. *Annual Review of Nutrition.* 24:401–431 (2004); Roger, V. L., A. S. Go, D. M. Lloyd-Jones, E. J. Benjamin, J. D. Berry, W. B. Borden, et al.: Heart Disease and Stroke Statistics—2012 Update: A Report from the American Heart Association. *Circulation.* 125:e02–e220 (2011). Reprinted with permission.

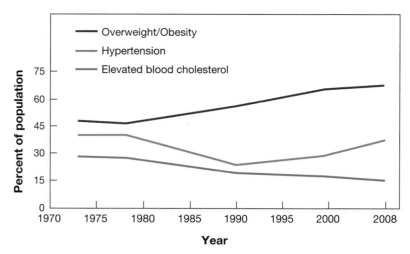

to be a negative risk factor, which means it lowers one's risk for disease (American College of Sports Medicine, 2010). Some researchers consider decreased Apo-A1 and increased Apo-B to be independent risk factors and believe they add considerably to risk prediction (Barter et al., 2006; Sacks, 2006; Wood and Stefanik, 1990). However, other researchers have found that these values add little to the predictive value of existing risk factors (van der Steeg et al., 2007) while still other authorities are cautious about the ability of any new risk factor to add substantially to the prediction of a chronic medical disease with many contributing causes (Berkwits and Guallar, 2007). For these reasons, and because specific levels have not been determined, the apolipoproteins are considered here to be nontraditional risk factors.

THE INFLUENCE OF EXERCISE AND EXERCISE TRAINING ON BLOOD LIPIDS The impact of exercise on lipid levels may be both transient (a last-bout effect from a single bout of exercise) and chronic (a consistent adaptation resulting from exercise training). Triglycerides, total cholesterol, and LDL-C all decease in the 24–48 hours following vigorous aerobic exercise, and HDL-C may increase. Many of these changes appear to require 9–12 months of training to become more or less permanent (Thomas and LaFontaine, 1998).

Cross-sectional studies in adults have generally shown that active individuals have lipid profiles with a reduced risk for CHD. This result is weak for TC (lower in more active individuals) but strong for HDL-C (higher in more active individuals) and TG (lower in more active individuals). However, there is little, if any, consistent difference in LDL-C levels between active and inactive individuals (Lippi et al., 2006). Cross-sectional studies, however, are by their very design difficult to interpret, because the element of self-selection may influence the results. Perhaps individuals who have a good cholesterol profile and healthy lifestyle habits are simply more likely to be active. This problem can be overcome by the use of training studies.

In general, exercise training studies have supported a reduction in TC levels, but often not to statistically significant levels. When present, TC changes are relatively small (3–5%) and short-term (24 hours) unless the energy expenditure is very high. Some individuals may be genetic "nonresponders" whose TC actually rises after exercise. Likewise, LDL-C levels are not consistently reduced significantly as a result of exercise training. On the other hand, the vast majority of studies that last longer than 12 weeks and have a training volume equivalent to at least 15 km·wk^{-1} (9.3 mi·wk^{-1}) of running or 1000–1200 kcal·wk^{-1} (4180–5016 kJ) of aerobic activity have shown a significant increase in HDL-C levels. Postexercise increases in HDL-C range from 3 to 34% and last from 24 to 72 hours (Grandjean and Crouse, 2004). These positive changes in HDL-C with high-intensity training appear to be similar for men and women, independent of age (Tambalis et al., 2009).

A high level of energy expenditure is apparently needed to positively alter blood lipids. For example, one study (Pfeiffer et al., 2006) investigated the impact of 30 minutes of moderate activity on lipid concentrations after a meal. Participants engaged in three bouts of 30 minutes of light to moderate cycling that expended 100, 150, or 200 kcal (420, 630, or 840 kJ) and a control trial. No significant differences occurred in any blood lipids during any exercise trial or the control trial. This indicates that if the objective is to modify one's lipid profile, more than 30 minutes of light to moderate activity is needed. A dose-response relationship seems to occur such that more vigorous activity and higher total calorie expenditure result in greater HDL-C increases. **Figure 15.5** presents data on HDL-C and triglycerides based on distance run per week in a group of over 8000 male recreational runners (Williams, 1997). As the figure shows, increased running mileage was associated with a proportional increase in HDL-C levels over most of the range. The lack of a proportional increase in the mean HDL-C value for those running more than 80 km·wk^{-1} (~50 mi·wk^{-1}) reflects more on the low number of individuals in that category than any ceiling effect for HDL-C change. The percentage of individuals with HDL-C values greater than 60 mg·dL^{-1} for each 15 km (~10 mi) category of running per week was 17, 20, 26, 31, 39, and 42, respectively. Remember that at 60 mg·dL^{-1} HDL-C becomes a negative risk factor. A meta-analysis (Kelley and Kelley, 2006) has shown consistent increases in HDL-C with aerobic training of at least 8 weeks, independent of decreases in body weight, body mass index (BMI), and percent body fat. Triglycerides are also consistently reduced (Wood and Stefanik, 1990) for up to 44 hours after activity (Grandjean and Crouse, 2004). Also, as indicated in **Figure 15.5**, TG show a dose-response relationship with greater reductions occurring as mileage run per week increases.

Favorable changes in blood lipids measured after eating are generally seen when aerobic exercise is completed in the period extending from 16 hours before to 1.5 hours after the meal, is of at least moderate intensity, and expends at least 500 kcal (2090 kJ) (Katsanos, 2006). Highly trained individuals may need a higher caloric expenditure to elicit HDL-C increases. In addition, to maintain the beneficial effects in lipid variables, the individual must consistently engage in aerobic exercise of sufficient intensity and duration, that is, at least every third day and preferably, every second day (Grandjean and Crouse, 2004). Note also that both the positive results in lipid profiles and the exercise recommendations pertain only to aerobic activities. Individuals who participate exclusively in anaerobic training programs, including dynamic resistance training, appear to have lipid profiles similar to those of untrained individuals (Grandjean and Crouse, 2004; Thomas and LaFontaine, 1998).

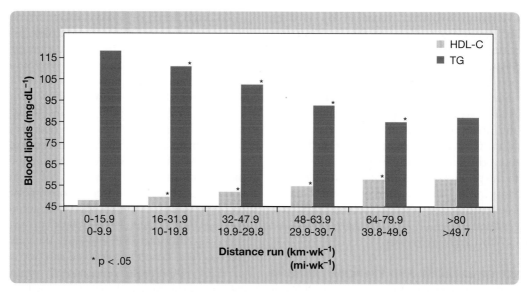

FIGURE 15.5 Dose-Response Relationship between Distance Run per Week and Levels of High-Density Lipoprotein (HDL-C) and Triglycerides (TG) in Males.
*Significantly different from next lower distance category.
***Source**: Based on data from Williams, P. T.: Relationship of distance run per week to coronary heart disease risk factors in 8283 male runners. *Archives of Internal Medicine*. 157:191–198 (1997).

Cigarette Smoking

From 2000 to 2004, an estimated 443,000 Americans died each year from smoking-related illnesses, 32.7% of those deaths being related to cardiovascular disease (American Heart Association, 2011). Of course, smoking also increases the risk of cancer and other respiratory diseases. For males, smoking one pack a day doubles the risk compared to not smoking, and smoking more than one pack a day triples the risk. For females, smoking as few as 1–4 cigarettes per day doubles the risk. The longer an individual smokes, the higher the risk (Gordon et al., 2006). Individuals who currently smoke and those who have quit within the last 6 months are considered to have the same risk (American College of Sports Medicine, 2010). On average, male smokers die 13.2 years earlier than nonsmokers, and female smokers 14.5 years earlier (American Heart Association, 2011). Breathing secondhand smoke also increases the risk of heart disease by at least 25% (Gordon et al., 2006). Cigar and pipe smokers have a higher risk for CVD than nonsmokers but lower than cigarette smokers. The percentage of Americans who smoke has declined from approximately 39% in 1960 to just over 20% in 2009 (American Heart Association, 2011).

The chemicals in cigarettes, particularly nicotine, stimulate the sympathetic nervous system, causing an acute increase in heart rate and blood pressure, thus making the heart work harder. Carbon monoxide in smoke binds with hemoglobin, thus reducing oxygen transport. The atherosclerotic process is accelerated because smoking injures the arterial wall lining (endothelium), increases the levels of circulating TC, LDL-C, and TG, and decreases the amount of HDL-C.

Smoking also causes blood platelets to adhere to each other, speeds up internal blood clotting, and makes what clots that do form tougher to dissolve. Prostacyclin, which is partially responsible for blood vessel dilation, is decreased. Capillaries and small arteries constrict and may spasm shut. Thus, smoking increases the possibility of a thrombus (clot) or an embolism (moving clot) blocking an artery already narrowed by atherosclerosis.

Narrowing of blood vessels to the arms and legs also makes smokers vulnerable to peripheral vascular disease, which may lead to gangrene and amputation. Smokers are 10 times more likely to develop peripheral vascular disease than nonsmokers (American Heart Association, 2007). Certain life-threatening dysrhythmias of the heartbeat are also more likely to occur. Thus, smoking both operates independently and contributes to other CHD risk factors (American Heart Association, 2011; Caspersen and Heath, 1993; Squires and Williams, 1993; Wood and Stefanik, 1990).

THE INFLUENCE OF EXERCISE AND EXERCISE TRAINING ON CIGARETTE SMOKING The relationship between exercise training and smoking is only indirect. One study of over 3000 individuals showed a consistent and statistically significant inverse relationship between the number of cigarettes smoked and the level of physical activity in both males and females (Dannenberg et al., 1989). Another study (a random sampling of Peachtree Road Race runners) indicated that 85% of both male and female runners had never smoked. In addition, 81% of the men and 75% of the women who had smoked when they began running had since stopped. Only 1% of the men and 2% of the women who had been nonsmokers started smoking after beginning to run (Koplan et al., 1982).

Brief bouts of aerobic exercise have been shown to result in an acute reduction in tobacco withdrawal symptoms and cravings to smoke (Elibero et al., 2011). Similar results were found with static exercise (pushing one hand against another) performed for a short period of time (Ussher et al., 2006). Although these results are encouraging, there is no direct cause-and-effect relationship between exercise training and smoking or not. You may know someone who is active or a good athlete who also smokes. Individuals must make a conscious decision to stop smoking. Then it takes 15 years of abstinence for the risk of former smokers to approach that of lifelong nonsmokers (Hahn et al., 1998).

Prediabetes and Diabetes Mellitus

Diabetes mellitus is a complex metabolic disease characterized by an inability to use carbohydrates effectively (glucose intolerance). There are four categories of diabetes based on etiology (cause): Type 1, Type 2, gestational (onset during pregnancy), and other (due to genetic abnormalities, medication, or other illnesses). Only Type 1 and Type 2 are considered here. Diabetes has become a widespread epidemic in the country, with Type 2 diabetes accounting for 90–95% of all cases of diabetes in the United States. Approximately 25.8 million Americans have diabetes, and about 7 million of these people are undiagnosed (Centers for Disease Control and Prevention, 2011). People with prediabetes have an increased risk for developing Type 2 diabetes, heart disease, stroke, blindness and kidney disease.

Type 1 diabetes begins most commonly in childhood and adolescence but is occurring more frequently in older individuals. In Type 1 diabetes, an environmentally triggered autoimmune process destroys the insulin-producing beta cells in the pancreas. Thus, an external source of insulin must be supplied.

Type 2 diabetes is a progressive disease whose diagnosis is often delayed for years. The underlying causes of Type 2 diabetes are insulin resistance (an inability to achieve normal rates of glucose uptake in response to insulin) and defective secretion of insulin by pancreatic beta cells. **Prediabetes**, also called *insulin resistance (IR)*, typically precedes the onset of Type 2 diabetes. Prediabetes is characterized by elevations in blood sugar level that get progressively higher until reaching the level of actual diabetes.

The normal fasting glucose level is less than 100 mg·dL^{-1}. Values between 100 and 125 mg·dL^{-1} confirmed by measurements on at least two separate occasions are designated as prediabetes. The threshold for the diagnosis of diabetes is a blood glucose of 126 mg·dL^{-1} (American College of Sports Medicine, 2007). Genetic and environmental factors affect the development of Type 2 diabetes, but the risk of developing prediabetes and Type 2 diabetes increases with age, obesity (predominantly abdominal visceral obesity), and a lack of physical activity (American College of Sports Medicine, 2010; Grundy et al., 1999). Type 2 diabetes used to occur predominantly in adults over the age of 40 years but in recent years has become increasingly prevalent in younger individuals, including children and adolescents.

Early in the progression of Type 2 diabetes, insulin may be produced in sufficient or even excessive amounts. Thus, individuals with Type 2 diabetes are initially not insulin dependent, but eventually approximately 40% of these individuals will require insulin injections. Among the many pathological complications resulting from prediabetes and diabetes is an acceleration of atherosclerosis, impaired myocardial contraction, poor peripheral perfusion, and alterations in blood coagulation mechanisms, including increased fibrinogen levels (Aronson and Rayfield, 2005).

Figure 15.6 illustrates the complex interactions between prediabetes/diabetes and increased cardiovascular risk. In the prediabetic state, cells of the body are insulin resistant; thus, the pancreas secretes more insulin in order to facilitate the transfer of glucose into the cell. At this stage, blood glucose levels are slightly elevated and the damage done to the cardiovascular system is mediated primarily through the negative consequences of hyperinsulinemia (elevated insulin) and insulin resistance. As seen in the large wedge at the bottom of **Figure 15.6**, insulin resistance is associated with several negative cardiovascular consequences, including dyslipidemia, hypertension, impaired fibrinolysis (clot breakdown), endothelial dysfunction, and inflammation. As the disease progresses, the beta cells of the pancreas become unable to continue secreting elevated insulin, and insulin levels fall. The falling levels of insulin, along with the increasing insulin resistance of cells, means that blood glucose levels rise (the defining characteristic of diabetes). At this stage in the disease, the cardiovascular system is negatively impacted by the high glucose levels (hyperglycemia). As depicted in the top wedge in the diagram, hyperglycemia is also associated with a number of negative cardiovascular consequences, including increased oxidative stress, endothelial dysfunction, and hypercoagulability (increased clotting potential). Thus, both hyperglycemia and insulin resistance contribute to increased cardiovascular complications. Importantly, **Figure 15.6** illustrates that the negative cardiovascular consequences associated with insulin resistance can precede the diagnosis of diabetes by many years. In other words, prediabetes is a very serious condition.

THE INFLUENCE OF EXERCISE AND EXERCISE TRAINING ON PREDIABETES AND DIABETES The evidence is solid and consistent that exercise training is important in both the prevention and treatment of Type 2 diabetes and a reduction in the progression of prediabetes to Type 2 diabetes. Evidence also consistently shows a reduction of CVD risk in individuals with prediabetes and diabetes as a result of exercise training (American College of Sports Medicine/American Diabetes Association, 2010; Alcazar et al., 2006; Sigal et al., 2006).

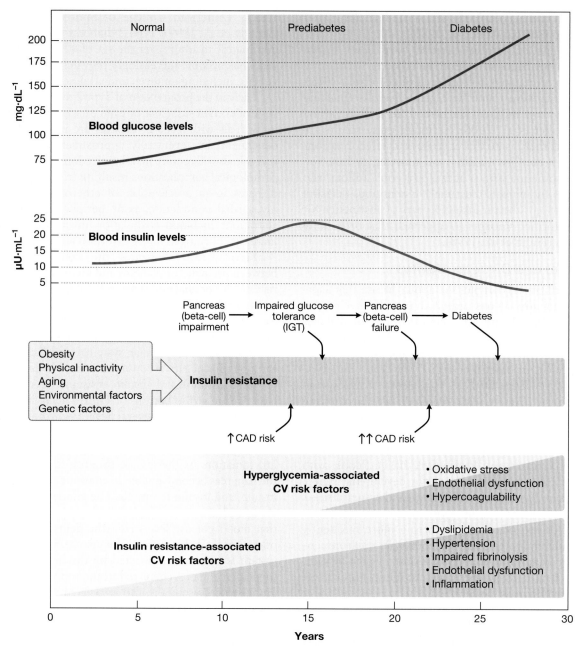

FIGURE 15.6 Relationship between Prediabetes/Diabetes and Increased Cardiovascular Risk.
CAD = Coronary artery disease; CV = Cardiovascular.
Source: Modified from Aronson, D. & E. J. Rayfield: Diabetes and obesity. In Fuster, V., R. Ross, E. J. Topol (eds.): *Atherosclerosis and Coronary Artery Disease* (2nd edition). Philadelphia, PA: Lippincott-Raven (2005).

One of the acute effects of exercise is an increase in non–insulin-dependent uptake of glucose into the active skeletal muscle. This effect continues after exercise while the depleted stores of glucose (as glycogen) are restored. Studies have shown increased insulin sensitivity and glucose tolerance as a result of exercise training. These changes are transient last-bout or augmented last-bout effects persisting from 12 to 72 hours from a single bout of aerobic exercise. The effect of a dynamic resistance exercise session may last somewhat longer. This means, of course, that a constant pattern of exercise (defined as no more than two consecutive days without exercise) must be established to maintain the benefits. The American College of Sports Medicine and American Diabetes Association recommend at least 2.5 hr·wk^{-1} of moderate to vigorous physical activity for the prevention of Type 2 diabetes. Persons with Type 2 diabetes should also undertake at least 2.5 hr·wk^{-1} of moderate to vigorous aerobic activity spread out during at least 3 d·wk^{-1}. Additionally, individuals with Type 2 diabetes should undertake moderate to vigorous resistance exercise at least

Understanding Short-Term Inactivity

Endurance training improves glucose tolerance and enhances insulin sensitivity. This means that if a trained individual ingests a given amount of glucose, that glucose is transported into the cells more readily, leaving less glucose in the blood than in an untrained individual. Insulin plays an important role in moving glucose from the blood to the cells by enhancing glucose transporters on the cell membrane (GLUT-4 transporters) and possibly by increasing blood flow. The reversibility principle states that when training is discontinued, adaptations are lost. The reversibility of metabolic adaptations can occur quickly; in fact, 7–10 days of detraining reduces glucose tolerance. However, it was not known whether this decrease is attributable to changes in GLUT-4 transporters only or whether blood flow is also altered in 7–10 days of detraining. Arciero et al. (1998) designed a study to determine whether 7–10 days of detraining (from a highly trained state) resulted in changes in blood flow that were associated with a decline in glucose tolerance and insulin sensitivity.

Arciero and coworkers tested highly trained male endurance athletes on two occasions: when the participants were in a highly trained state and after they refrained from exercise training for a period of 7–10 days (detrained). During the testing period, the athletes ingested a known amount of glucose (75 g) and had blood samples taken for the next 3 hours—this is known as an oral glucose tolerance test (OGTT). Blood flow was measured in the forearm and calf before and during the OGTT. The accompanying graphs present blood glucose and calf blood flow data obtained in the trained and detrained state. These data reveal the following:

1. There was a greater blood glucose response following the ingesting of 75 g of glucose in the detrained state compared to the trained state, despite higher insulin levels. This is consistent with earlier studies that showed that endurance training increases glucose tolerance.

2. Calf blood flow was lower at several time points during the OGTT after ingesting the glucose in the detrained state than in the trained state. Pre-OGTT calf blood flow was not different between the two conditions.

These data suggest that blood flow may be an important element in enhancing the ability of muscles to extract glucose from the blood in the trained state. As with most research, this study invites future inquiry, specifically to explore the relationship between blood flow and glucose tolerance in different populations and at different points in a training or detraining program.

Source: Arciero, P. J., D. L. Smith, & J. Calles-Escandon: Effects of short-term inactivity on glucose tolerance, energy expenditure, and blood flow in trained subjects. *Journal of Applied Physiology.* 74(4):1365–1373 (1998).

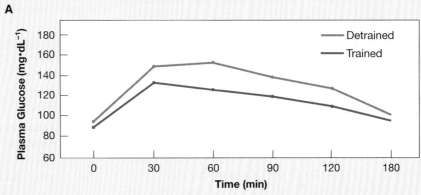

A

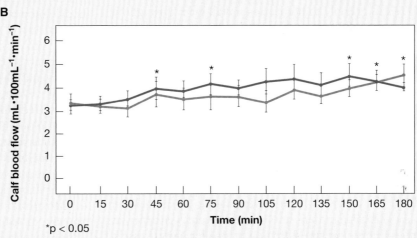

B

*p < 0.05

2–3 d·wk⁻¹ (American College of Sports Medicine/American Heart Association, 2010).

Exercise training for individuals with diabetes requires close monitoring and should be done in conjunction with medical personnel. Individuals with diabetes, especially Type 1 individuals, often have abnormal blood pressure and other cardiovascular responses to exercise. Insulin injections (the amount used and choice of injection site to avoid working muscles) and carbohydrate ingestion must be carefully adjusted to prevent an exercising diabetic from developing hypoglycemia (American College of Sports Medicine/American Heart Association, 2010; Colberg, 2001; Hanson, 1993).

TABLE 15.3 Classification of Blood Pressure for Adults and Adolescents

Category	Systolic (mmHg)	Diastolic (mmHg)
Adults (>19 yr)		
Normal	<120	<80
Prehypertension	120–139	80–89
Hypertension		
Stage I	140–159	90–99
Stage II	≥160	≥100
Adolescents*		
Mild-moderate	≥144	≥90
Severe	≥160	≥104

*Values at or above the 95th percentile for age and sex indicate hypertension.

Source: National High Blood Pressure Education Program: National Institutes of Health; National Heart, Lung, and Blood Institute. The Seventh Report of the Joint Committee on Detection, Evaluation, and Treatment of High Blood Pressure, Washington, DC (2003).

Hypertension

Nearly one in every three American adults has **hypertension**, or high blood pressure. The prevalence of hypertension increases with advancing age, reaching approximately 75% in those over 75 years. Furthermore, prevalence varies widely by race and sex. Black females have the highest prevalence (45.7%), followed closely by black males (43.0%). White males have a slightly higher prevalence (33.9%) than white females (31.3%) (American Heart Association, 2011). **Figure 15.4** presents the portion of the adult population with high blood pressure; currently, approximately 33% of the population suffers from hypertension, placing them at much higher risk for death from cardiovascular disease.

The stages of hypertension are presented in **Table 15.3**. These values apply to both sexes and all races throughout the entire adult life span. Note that although the cutoff for diagnosed hypertension is 140/90 mmHg, values between 120/80 and 140/90 mmHg, defined as **prehypertension**, should signal the beginning of lifestyle modifications. All stages of hypertension are associated with an increased risk of cardiovascular disease. The higher the stage of hypertension, the higher the risk of CHD and the more aggressive monitoring and treatment should be (American College of Sports Medicine, 2004). Hypertension imposes an afterload on the heart, thus increasing ventricular muscle hypertrophy (thickness) and reducing early diastolic filling. Hypertension is a leading factor in endothelial injury and calcium deposition in the coronary arteries, as well as thickening and stiffening of smaller blood vessels. Atherosclerosis occurs in hypertensive individuals two to three times more quickly than in normotensive individuals (Kannel and Wilson, 1999; Stewart, 1998). Hypertension is associated with increased mortality from CVD; 69% of those suffering their first heart attack and 77% of those suffering their first stroke had hypertension (American Heart Association, 2011). Hypertension can also cause left ventricular hypertrophy and increases the risk of sudden cardiac death (Levy et al., 1990). Ninety to ninety-five percent of the cases of hypertension lack a known cause.

Such hypertension is called *primary or essential hypertension*. However, for blood pressure to reach the levels of hypertension, either cardiac output (Q̇) or total peripheral resistance (TPR), or both, must be elevated. The resulting high blood pressure may injure the endothelium and begin the process of atherosclerosis. Further evidence indicates that increased pulse pressure (SBP-DBP) may be an independent predictor of CVD disease morbidity and mortality (American College of Sports Medicine, 2004).

THE INFLUENCE OF EXERCISE AND EXERCISE TRAINING ON HYPERTENSION Research strongly demonstrates the role of exercise training in the primary prevention, treatment, and control of moderate hypertension. Individuals at high risk for developing hypertension—because of genetics, body composition, primary disease status, or an exaggerated blood pressure response to acute exercise—can reduce their risk through an endurance training program. Longitudinal studies show that high levels of both physical activity and physical fitness are associated with decreased risk of developing hypertension (American College of Sports Medicine, 2004). Dynamic aerobic training reduces resting blood pressure in both individuals with normal or hypertensive values. The decrease is higher in hypertensive individuals (6–7 mmHg systolic/5–6 mmHg diastolic) than in normotensive individuals (2–3 mmHg systolic/1–2 mmHg diastolic).

Most studies have found that blood pressure responds quickly to exercise training. Blood pressure decreases within 3 weeks to 3 months after training starts, often does not become fully normalized, and does not decrease further with continued training. Decreased total peripheral resistance (TPR) appears to be the primary mechanism for the reduction in blood pressure with exercise training (American College of Sports Medicine, 2004). If the training is stopped, the resting blood pressure returns to the elevated level. At least part of the reduction in blood pressure may be a function of each individual exercise session rather than a permanent training adaptation, for even a single session of submaximal exercise reduces blood pressure for 1–22 hours postexercise (American College of Sports Medicine, 2004; Hagberg, 1990). That is, blood pressure exhibits a last-bout and a chronic adaptation to training (American College of Sports Medicine, 2004; Hagberg, 1990). The decrease in blood pressure following an acute bout of exercise is termed *postexercise hypotension (PEH)*. It occurs in both normotensive and hypertensive males and females of all ages and races, with the greatest reductions again occurring in those with hypertension (American College of Sports Medicine, 2004).

Dynamic aerobic endurance exercise training can also benefit individuals with severe or very severe hypertension. In this case, however, pharmacological therapy should be initiated first and the exercise program then added. Such sequencing leads to a further reduction in blood pressure and ultimately a decreased reliance on antihypertensive medication (Hagberg, 1990; Simons-Morton, 1999).

The pressor response accompanying dynamic resistance training has always been of great concern, and individuals with hypertension have historically been discouraged from doing weight lifting. Studies on resistance exercise, however, have failed to substantiate an adverse effect on blood pressure. Dynamic resistance training reduces blood pressure in normotensive and hypertensive individuals chronically by approximately 3 mmHg for both systolic and diastolic pressure. However, the limited evidence suggests that it has no postexercise hypotensive affect. Limited evidence also suggests that static exercise reduces blood pressure in adults with elevated blood pressures (American College of Sports Medicine, 2004). Therefore, although the cardiovascular changes elicited by endurance training are more desirable than those from resistance training, dynamic resistance training can be done by hypertensive individuals as part of a comprehensive training program. Strength training should not be the only exercise program, however, and it is most effective added after 2 or 3 months of typical aerobic endurance training.

The following exercise prescription is recommended for individuals with hypertension:

Type: primarily aerobic endurance exercise supplemented with dynamic resistance exercise.
Frequency: most, if not all, days of the week.
Intensity: moderate: for adults, this should equal 40–59% HRR or $\dot{V}O_2R$.
Duration: 30–60 minutes, either performed continuously or accumulated in 10-minute bouts (American College of Sports Medicine, 2004).

Hypertension High blood pressure, defined as adult values equal to or greater than 140/90 mmHg.

Metabolic Syndrome A cluster of interrelated risk factors of metabolic origin that directly promote the development of atherosclerotic CVD and increase the individual's risk of diabetes.

Obesity

Obesity is now a common feature of American society. **Figure 15.4** reveals that in 2008, approximately 67% of adults were overweight or obese, and the rate of increase in overweight and obesity has yet to level off. Based on data from 2005 to 2008, just over 32% of adult men and 35% of adult women are obese (American Heart Association, 2011). A body mass index of >30 kg·m⁻², and a waist girth >102 cm (40 in.) for males and >88 cm (35 in.) for females, are field measures to determine obesity as a risk factor for disease (American College of Sports Medicine, 2010). Body composition measures are fully discussed in this text in Chapter 7.

The relationship between obesity and CVD is both independent of and interrelated to the other cardiovascular risk factors in a disease process known as the metabolic syndrome (Gordon, 1998; Kannel and Wilson, 1999; Welk and Blair, 2000). The **metabolic syndrome** is a cluster of interrelated risk factors of metabolic origin that directly promote the development of atherosclerotic CVD and increase the individual's risk of diabetes. The predominant underlying risk factors for the metabolic syndrome appear to be abdominal obesity (high amounts of upper body visceral fat) and insulin resistance (Grundy, 2007). Under the stimulation of the enzyme lipoprotein lipase, visceral abdominal adipocytes readily release free fatty acids (FFA) into the circulation. FFA have two possible fates: (1) they may be transported to the liver, where they are converted to VLDL and ultimately LDL cholesterol; or (2) they may be taken up by other cells, including skeletal muscle cells, and oxidized to provide ATP energy by cellular respiration. This enhancement of lipid oxidation may lead to a reduced use of glucose as fuel. At the same time, the increased FFA levels act directly in the liver to inhibit insulin clearance, resulting in hyperinsulinemia. Hyperinsulinemia combined with high levels of blood glucose (hyperglycemia) leads to a reduction in insulin sensitivity. The combination of high glucose and hyperinsulinemia can hasten the development of cardiovascular disease (see **Figure 15.6**). Hyperinsulinemia also increases sodium retention and in susceptible salt-sensitive individuals may precipitate hypertension. Thus, high visceral abdominal obesity is directly related to dyslipidemia (low HDL-C and high triglycerides), reduced glucose tolerance, insulin resistance, hypertension, and inflammation, which together form the cluster of risk factors for cardiovascular disease known as the metabolic syndrome (Balagolpal et al., 2011; Buemann and Tremblay, 1996; Gordon, 1998; Kannel and Wilson, 1999; Welk and Blair, 2000). Treatment of the "syndrome" is no different from treatment for each of its individual components. However, at the very least, the concept of a syndrome may help the individual realize that all risk factors need to be identified and treated simultaneously (Marks, 2006; Venkat Narayan, 2006).

THE INFLUENCE OF EXERCISE TRAINING ON OBESITY AND THE METABOLIC SYNDROME Exercise training, or fitness level, has a large influence on obesity, metabolic syndrome, and cardiovascular disease. **Figure 15.7** presents

FOCUS ON APPLICATION

The Impact of a Change in Physical Fitness on Cardiovascular Disease Mortality

This chapter describes the inverse relationship between physical activity and mortality from coronary heart disease and the positive impacts of exercise training on each cardiovascular disease risk factor. The cited studies relating physical activity or physical fitness to mortality, however, generally used only a single baseline evaluation of activity or fitness with subsequent follow-up to determine the incidence of death from cardiovascular causes. Although extremely important, these results could have been influenced both by genetics and by changes in risk factor status between the baseline testing and time of death. Conversely, the studies of exercise training had both pretraining and posttraining evaluations but did not examine the overall impact on cardiovascular mortality. From a public health, exercise professional, and personal perspective, the overall goal of exercise training is to enhance both the quality and quantity of life. It is important to determine whether improving and maintaining physical fitness can attain these goals. Therefore, a linkage between the two types of studies is important.

Blair et al. (1995) studied the mortality and relative risk of death ratios from cardiovascular disease of 9777 males who had at least two complete examinations at the Cooper Institute for Aerobics Research between 1970 and 1989. The average interval between the two testing sessions was 4.0 ± 4.1 years, and the average follow-up for mortality was 5.1 ± 4.2 years, but the range was 1–18 years for both. Treadmill time to volitional fatigue, converted to maximal oxygen uptake, was the measure of cardiovascular physical fitness. Individuals whose results fell into the bottom quintile (lowest 20%) based on age-adjusted results were labeled unfit. The unfit group had the following $\dot{V}O_2$max values for each age group:

<35.0 mL·kg^{-1}·min^{-1}, 20–39 years
<32.2 mL·kg^{-1}·min^{-1}, 40–49 years
<29.4 mL·kg^{-1}·min^{-1}, 50–59 years
<24.5 mL·kg^{-1}·min^{-1}, 60+ years

All individuals in quintiles (Q) 2, 3, 4, and 5 were labeled fit. Men who were unfit at both testing times had the highest death rate from CVD; men who were fit at both testing times had the lowest death rate; and men who changed fitness status between testing sessions had intermediate death rates, as shown in panel A of the accompanying graph. Although the values for the men who changed fitness status appear to be similar, these must be interpreted relative to the direction of the change. The unfit men who moved out of the lowest quintile died at a rate less than half that of those who remained unfit, whereas those who moved from fit to unfit had an increased death rate of approximately 25%. When changes in status occurred among the four upper quartiles, a dose-response relationship was seen. A low mortality rate was evident in men who remained in quintiles 2 and 3; a lower mortality rate was seen in men who moved from quintiles 2 and 3 to 4 and 5; and the lowest mortality rate was seen in men in the upper two quintiles (4 and 5) who remained there.

The comparable results in terms of relative risk are shown in panel B of the graph. The unfit men who moved into the fit category reduced their risk of death from cardiovascular disease

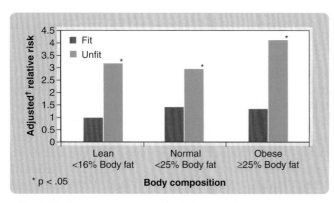

FIGURE 15.7 Cardiovascular Disease Mortality by Cardiorespiratory Fitness and Percent Body Fat.
†adjusted for age, exam year, smoking, alcohol, and heredity.
Source: Based on data from Lee, C. D., S. N. Blair, & A. S. Jackson: Cardiorespiratory fitness, body composition, and all-cause and cardiovascular disease mortality in men. *American Journal of Clinical Nutrition*. 69:373–380 (1999).

a study showing the relative risk of cardiovascular disease mortality (adjusted for age, exam year, smoking, alcohol intake, and heredity) by percent body fat (lean, normal, obese) and cardiorespiratory fitness (fit, unfit) (Lee et al., 1999). Relative risk (RR) indicates how much more likely a group of individuals with the risk factor are to develop the outcome. A value of 1.0 is the baseline for the group without the risk factor; in this case 1.0 represents lean fit males. Statistically significant numbers higher than 1.0 mean than individuals with that risk factor have a higher "relative risk" of dying from CVD. For example, a RR = 3.16 (as for the unfit, lean group) means that these individuals are 316% more likely to die of CVD than individuals in the fit, lean group! Importantly, unfit, lean males had a higher risk of CVD mortality than fit males in all body fat categories. Unfit obese males had the highest relative risk (4.11). Fit obese males had a lower risk of CVD mortality than did unfit, lean men.

The effect of exercise training on visceral and total body obesity is detailed in the metabolic unit of this text. The effect of exercise training on each of the other risk by 52% (relative risk = .48). After adjustment for potential confounders, each minute of increase in treadmill time (equivalent to $\dot{V}O_2$max increase of only 1.75 mL·kg⁻¹·min⁻¹ in the protocol used) was associated with a reduced risk of 8.6% for CVD mortality. Those who changed from fit to unfit had a risk less than half that of the consistently unfit, but almost twice that of those who remained fit.

A follow-up analysis of these data (Kampert, 2004) confirmed that mortality risk was inversely related to change in fitness after correction for measurement error and adjustment for initial CVD, fitness level, age, health status, and exam year.

The message is clear. Individuals who are unfit must be encouraged and helped to attain at least a minimal level of fitness. This minimal level can be achieved by engaging in at least 30 minutes of moderate physical activity 5 days of the week or vigorous activity 3 days per week in bouts of at least 10 minutes (Haskell et al., 2007). Individuals who are already fit must be equally encouraged and helped to maintain or improve their level of fitness. Although Blair and his colleagues' results were compiled only on males (because of an insufficient number of female subjects), Manson et al. (1999) have reported similar findings from the Nurses' Health Study, which followed 72,488 women 40–65 years of age.

It is never too late to try to become fit; it is never too soon to make a lifetime commitment to activity and fitness.

Sources: Blair et al. (1995), Kampert (2004), Manson et al. (1999).

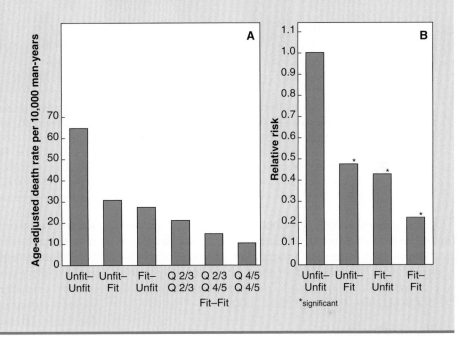

factors in the cluster of metabolic syndrome is described in the appropriate sections of this chapter. A sedentary lifestyle, poor cardiovascular fitness (Lakka et al., 2003), and poor muscular strength (Jurca et al., 2005) have all been shown to be associated with the metabolic syndrome. Regular physical activity can improve the metabolic risk profile and reduce the risk of cardiovascular disease.

Figure 15.8 presents the results of 20 weeks of aerobic training on men and women with the metabolic syndrome. As the figure shows, significant improvements occurred in all risk factors but HDL-C (which often requires more vigorous exercise to change). The overall result was that 30.5% of the participants classified as having metabolic syndrome at the beginning of the exercise training were no longer classified this way at the end of the training (Katzmarzyk et al., 2003). Research continues to identify the optimal training program to improve cardiovascular risk associated with the metabolic syndrome (Ciolac et al., 2010; Stensvold et al., 2010; Strasser et al., 2010). Cardiorespiratory training reduces several metabolic syndrome risk factors. The magnitude of the effect of exercise on risk factors varies based on the training program employed and may not be consistent among risk factors (American College of Sports Medicine, 2011).

A significant dose-response relationship has been observed between cardiorespiratory fitness and mortality in males with metabolic syndrome. In one study of 3757 men with metabolic syndrome, men in the middle and lower tertiles of cardiorespiratory fitness had 2.08 and 3.48 times the risk of cardiovascular disease mortality than the men in the upper tertile of CVD fitness (Katzmarzyk et al., 2004). Another study categorized men into low (lowest 20%), moderate (middle 40%), and high (highest 40%) cardiorespiratory fitness based on age and treadmill test results. For any given level of waist circumference, visceral fat, or subcutaneous fat, the high fitness group had lower TG levels and higher HDL-C than either the moderate- or low-fitness groups. The relative risks of having the metabolic syndrome were 1.8 and 1.6 times higher in the low- and moderate-fitness groups than in the high-fitness group after adjusting for age, visceral fat, and subcutaneous fat (Lee et al., 2005).

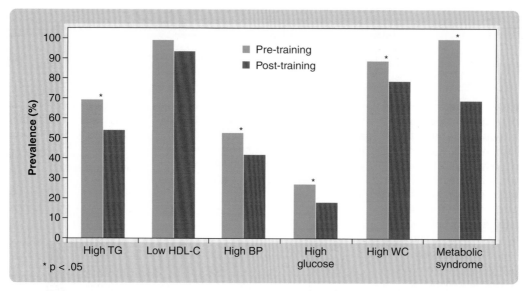

FIGURE 15.8 Effect of Aerobic Training on Individual Risk Factors and the Metabolic Syndrome.
TG, triglycerides; HDL-C, high-density lipoprotein cholesterol; BP, blood pressure; WC, waist circumference. *p < 0.05.
Source: Katzmarzyk, P. T., A. S. Leon, J. H. Wilmore, J. S. Skinner, D. C. Rao, T. Rankinen, & C. Bouchard: Targeting the Metabolic Syndrome with exercise: Evidence from the Heritage Family Study. *Medicine & Science in Sports & Exercise*. 35(10):1703–1709 (2003). Reprinted with permission.

In general, physical activity, exercise training, and cardiovascular-respiratory fitness bring about beneficial changes that limit the progression of metabolic syndrome, with or without changes in total body weight and composition (Buemann and Tremblay, 1996; Carroll and Dudfield, 2004; Welk and Blair, 2000).

Physical Inactivity

In the last decade emphasis has shifted from the product of physical fitness (typically defined as cardiorespiratory fitness as measured by $\dot{V}O_2max$) to the behavior of physical activity to achieve health benefits. There is, of course, evidence that both *physical fitness* and *physical activity* lead to health benefits and decreased negative health outcomes. The Physical Activity and Public Health recommendations (American College of Sports Medicine, 2011; U.S. Department of Health and Human Services, 2008) updated from the 1996 Surgeon General's report (SGR) (U.S. Department of Health and Human Services) suggest that adults from 18 to 65 years participate in at least 30 minutes of moderate aerobic activity 5 days of the week (for a total of 150 minutes) or vigorous aerobic activity for 20–60 minutes 3 d·wk⁻¹ (for a total of 75 minutes). These guidelines also point out that additional health benefits accrue as activity levels increase. Such activities must be in addition to routine activities of daily living that are of light intensity such as casual walking or grocery shopping. However, moderate or vigorous activities performed as part of daily life such as brisk walking or heavy manual labor can be counted toward the activity recommendations. In addition, muscle strengthening

activity consisting of 8–10 exercises involving the major muscle groups for 8–12 repetitions, 2–3 d·wk⁻¹ should be included. Individuals not participating in a regular exercise program or not meeting these minimal physical activity guidelines are considered to have the risk factor of a sedentary lifestyle (American College of Sports Medicine, 2011). It was thought that it would be easier to motivate the public to accumulate lifestyle moderate activity than to undergo the regimented vigorous exercise usually prescribed for physical fitness enhancement. Therefore the risk factor for cardiovascular disease is labeled *physical inactivity* rather than *lack of physical fitness*. **Figure 15.9** documents the prevalence of individuals who meet physical activity guidelines among men and women of different ethnic backgrounds. Unfortunately the data indicate that a relatively small percentage (~25–40%) of the population is meeting current guidelines for physical activity. Furthermore, within each ethnic group, women are less likely to meet current guidelines than men.

Figure 15.10 presents findings from a single study investigating cardiovascular risk reduction based on total physical activity. In this study, the third quintile (Q3) represents the level of activity recommended in the Surgeon General's Report (U.S. Department of Health and Human Services, 1996), the equivalent of walking briskly for 30 min·d⁻¹, 5 d·wk⁻¹. Note that the baseline relative risk of 1.0 represents the relative risk of those with no physical activity (Q1), and that relative risk values less than 1.0 represent a lower risk with more activity. Participants in this study were postmenopausal females. As the figure shows, women with the recommended level of activity had a 19% lower

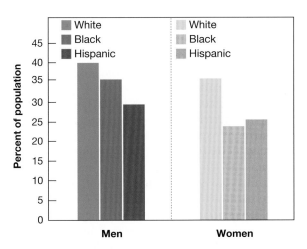

FIGURE 15.9 Prevalence of Regular Leisure-time Physical Activity Among Adults Aged 18 and Older by Race/Ethnicity and Sex.

("Regular leisure-time physical activity" was defined as engaged in moderate leisure-time physical activity for at least 150 minutes per week or vigorous activity at least 75 minutes per week or an equivalent combination.)

Source: Roger, V. L., A. S. Go, D. M. Lloyd-Jones, E. J. Benjamin, J. D. Berry, W. B. Borden, et al.: Heart Disease and Stroke Statistics—2012 Update: A Report from the American Heart Association. *Circulation*. 125:e02–e220 (2011). Reprinted with permission.

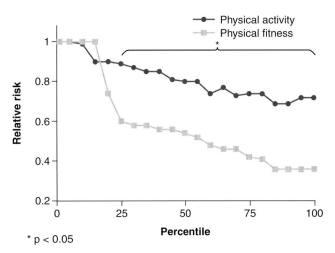

* p < 0.05

FIGURE 15.11 Effects of Physical Fitness and Physical Activity on Heart Disease Risk Factors.

Source: Williams, P. T. Physical fitness and activity as separate heart disease risk factors: A meta-analysis. *Medicine Science in Sports and Exercise*. 33(5):754–761 (2001). Reprinted with permission.

---

risk for cardiovascular disease than those who engaged in no physical activity. Those who engaged in higher amounts of activity had even more reduction in risk, 22% and 28% in Q4 and Q5, respectively. Those with less than the recommended level of total activity had no significant ben-

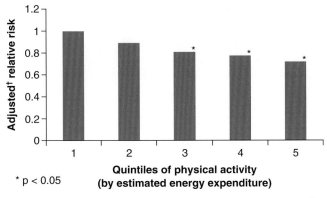

* p < 0.05

FIGURE 15.10 Relative Risk of Cardiovascular Disease by Quintile of Physical Activity.

†adjusted for age, personal habits, socioeconomic factors, heredity, and body composition.

Source: Based on data from Manson, J. E., P. Greenland, A. Z. LaCroix, M. L. Stefanick, C. P. Mouton, A. Oberman, M. G. Perri, D. S. Sheps, M. B. Pettinger, & D. S. Siscovick: Walking compared with vigorous exercise for the prevention of cardiovascular events in women. *The New England Journal of Medicine*. 347(10):716–725 (2002).

efit. Results were similar whether the women were normal weight, overweight, or obese, and whether their race was black or white (Manson et al., 2002).

Figure 15.11 is a composite graph of the effects of *physical activity* and *physical fitness* on relative risk of heart disease based on a meta-analysis of eight studies of physical fitness and 30 studies of physical activity. This graph reveals that (a) the RR of CHD/CVD decreases linearly with increasing amounts of physical activity; (b) the risks of CHD/CVD drop precipitously before the 25th percentile of physical fitness and then parallel the slope of the decline in physical activity; and (c) a significant difference in risk reduction is associated with being more physically fit than physically active (Williams, 2001). The author suggested that this might indicate that lack of physical fitness and physical inactivity are separate, distinct risk factors for CVD and that both physical fitness and physical activity should be measured and interventions followed if warranted. One of the issues is that physical fitness can be measured more accurately than physical activity and that this could at least partially explain the results. Whether the difference in risk reduction between physical fitness and physical activity is true or a measurement artifact needs more study. It is clear, however, that at least moderate physical activity should be undertaken by all, but that the attainment of physical fitness is certainly not to be discouraged once individuals have achieved the minimal level of physical activity (Plowman, 2005). Current recommendations explicitly encourage vigorous physical activity for those who are willing and able to do it (American College of Sports Medicine, 2011).

The degree of risk for those who are physically inactive, about twice that of those without this risk factor, is approximately the same as the risk associated with systolic hypertension, cigarette smoking, and hyperlipidemia. As has been discussed in the sections for each of these other risk factors, physical activity positively impacts the risk from these as well. Given the high prevalence of physical inactivity and the benefits derived from becoming more physically active, potentially more benefit overall could be achieved by increasing the activity level of US citizens than by changing any other single risk factor (American Heart Association, 2007; Caspersen and Heath, 1993; Froelicher, 1990). One of the most important facts about activity or exercise training is that the greatest health benefits occur when very sedentary individuals increase their endurance activity levels even minimally (Blair and Minocha, 1989).

The mechanisms by which physical activity achieves its protective effect are many and varied. Some are independent and a direct result of the adaptive changes that occur in the cardiovascular system and its neural control, as were documented earlier in this unit. For example, the increases in parasympathetic tone and decreases in sympathetic response reduce the resting and exercise heart rate in physically active individuals and possibly influence hypertension. These changes also enhance the electrical stability of the myocardial cells, reducing the risk of potentially fatal conduction system defects and coronary vessel spasms. Other indirect mechanisms are linked to the different risk factors (Caspersen and Heath, 1993). Obviously participating in physical activity directly eliminates physical inactivity as a risk factor. The impact of physical activity or exercise training on all of the major modifiable risk factors is summarized in **Table 15.4**.

Recently additional studies have raised the probability that extreme physical inactivity in the form of excessive sedentary behavior also has implications for health

and that too much sedentary behavior is distinct from too little exercise. In this context, *sedentary behavior* is used to characterize those behaviors for which energy expenditure is low, including prolonged sitting time in transit (driving/riding in a car), at work (computer/desk tasks), at home, and in leisure time (television watching/computer activities). Observational epidemiological studies strongly suggest that daily sitting time or low nonexercise activity levels (such as limited standing, getting up and down from a chair, and/or incidental walking) may have a significant direct relationship to mortality, cardiovascular disease, Type 2 diabetes, metabolic syndrome, obesity, depression, increased waist circumference, hypertension, depressed lipoprotein lipase activity, blood glucose, insulin, and lipoproteins. Even when adults meet physical activity guidelines, sitting for prolonged periods can compromise health. This is termed the *Active Couch Potato phenomenon*. When sedentary behavior is broken up even by short bouts of nonexercise physical activity, reduction of the adverse acute biological effect occur. Common sense suggests that it is prudent to try to minimize prolonged sitting with 5-minute breaks every hour to walk around, stretch, or do some activity of daily living (American College of Sports Medicine, 2011; Hamilton et al., 2007; Katzmarzyk et al., 2009; Owen et al., 2009, 2010). If you have been diligently sitting and studying for at least an hour, it's time for you to take such a short break.

Contributing and Selected Nontraditional Risk Factors

C-Reactive Protein

C-reactive protein (CRP) is a marker of systemic inflammation, tissue damage, and infection.

TABLE 15.4	Summary of Impact of Physical Activity or Exercise Training on Modifiable CHD Risk Factors
Risk Factor	**Impact of Exercise Training**
Cholesterol-Lipid factors	↑ HDL-C fraction ↓ TC (maybe)
Cigarette smoking	Indirect
Hypertension	↓ SBP; ↓ DBP (incomplete normalization)
Physical inactivity	Directly eliminates
Diabetes mellitus	↑ glucose tolerance ↑ insulin sensitivity
Obesity	↓ body fat ↓ visceral abdominal fat
Stress	Unknown on hostility component of type A behavior; TABP may ↓
Fibrinogen levels and fibrinolytic activity	↓ fibrinogen levels ↑ fibrinolytic activity

Note: The impact is the same for children, adolescents, and adults except for stress and fibrinogen level and fibrinolytic activity, where insufficient information is available.

↑, increased; ↓, decreased.

FOCUS ON APPLICATION: *Clinically Relevant*

Influence of Physical Activity on Mortality in Elderly with Coronary Artery Disease

This chapter describes the inverse relationship between physical activity and mortality from coronary heart disease and the positive impact of exercise training on each cardiovascular disease risk factor. The following study specifically investigated the dose-response relationship between physical activity and the relative risk of mortality in patients with coronary artery disease in an observational cohort study.

Jansenn and Jolliffe (2006) studied the dose-response relationship between baseline physical activity level and all-cause mortality risk over a 9-year period in 1045 men and women with coronary artery disease. Participants were stratified based on sex, age, smoking, adiposity, self-perceived health, number of risk factors, and coronary artery disease subtype so that the relationship between physical activity and mortality could be examined within each strata. Participants returned for a 3-year follow-up examination. A separate analysis was performed on a subset of participants ($n = 785$) who had changed their physical activity level (from baseline to the 3-year follow-up) to determine the relationship between changes in physical activity over the initial 3-year follow-up and mortality risk over the subsequent 6-year period.

The dose-response curve shown in panel A depicts the relationship between energy expenditure and relative risk of mortality for the entire group. The data are adjusted for age, sex, race, smoking, alcohol consumption, socioeconomic status, adiposity, prevalent disease, and type of coronary artery disease. As seen in other studies, the relative risk of mortality decreased with increasing levels of activity (expressed as energy expenditure). The data were then examined by strata. Independent of age, sex, smoking, adiposity, self-perceived health status, number of risk factors, or type of coronary artery disease, the relative risks of mortality were significantly lower in the active participants (>1500 kcal·wk⁻¹) compared to inactive participants (<1500 kcal·wk⁻¹). However, even those individuals who accumulated only approximately 1000 kcal·wk⁻¹ had a 19% reduction in mortality risk, again showing that some exercise is always better than no exercise.

The dose-response curve shown in panel B depicts the relationship between change in energy expenditure (from baseline to the 3-year follow-up) and relative risk of mortality at the study completion (9 years). Again, the data are adjusted for age, sex, race, smoking, alcohol consumption, socioeconomic

status, adiposity, prevalent disease, and type of coronary artery disease. Clearly, the risk of mortality was higher for individuals whose physical activity level decreased, and lower for those whose physical activity level increased.

The practical implications of this study are immense. This study reinforces the common finding of an inverse relationship between physical activity and mortality risk, and clearly demonstrates that in patients with coronary artery disease, regardless of age, sex, severity of disease, or other risk factors, there is a protective benefit to higher levels of physical activity. Finally, in a group of patients with coronary artery disease, an increase in physical activity level was associated with reduction in mortality risk. The bottom line is that physical inactivity increased mortality risk in study participants regardless of whether they were men or women, old or very old, smokers or nonsmokers, lean or overweight, or otherwise healthy or unhealthy. The take-home message is that physical activity should be encouraged for the vast majority of people, including coronary artery disease patients.

Source: Janssen and Jolliffe (2006).

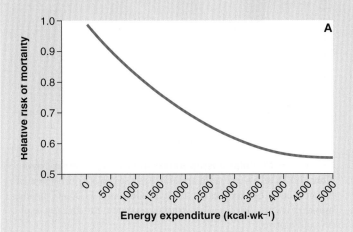

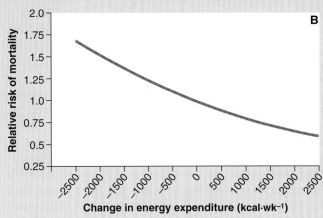

FIGURE 15.12 Relative Risk of Future Heart Attack Based on Selected Risk Factors Among Apparently Healthy Men and Women.
Source: Modified from Ridker, P. M.: Clinical application of C-Reactive Protein for cardiovascular disease detection and prevention. *Circulation.* 107(3):363–369 (2003).

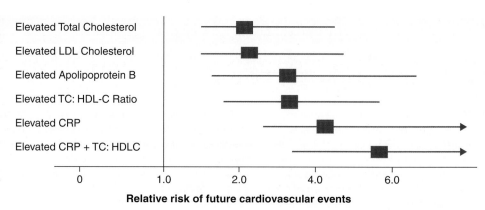

Prospective studies have repeatedly shown that CRP independently predicts heart attacks, stroke, and sudden cardiac death in apparently healthy men and women (Ridker and Libby, 2005). Importantly, CRP adds predictive value to traditional risk factors. **Figure 15.12** shows the relative risk of future heart attack associated with selected traditional and nontraditional risk factors in initially healthy middle-aged men and women. As discussed earlier, elevated total cholesterol (TC) is associated with an increased risk of heart disease. The mean relative risk in the highest quartile of individuals compared to the lowest quartile for TC was approximately 2.0, representing a 200% increase in the risk of heart attack in those with the highest TC. The predictive value was even greater when individuals in the highest quartile of TC:HDL-C ratio were compared to the lowest quartile. Elevated apolipoprotein B (discussed in the lipid section) is also associated with an increased relative risk for a heart attack. Of particular significance is the dramatic increase in risk associated with the highest quartile of CRP (RR = 4.0). Furthermore, when CRP and the TC:HDL-C ratio are both elevated, the combined risk is even greater (RR = 6.0). CRP has also been shown to predict recurrent coronary events, poor outcomes associated with angina, and vascular complications after bypass surgery (Ridker and Libby, 2005).

Inflammation plays a central role in atherosclerotic plaque development and in plaque rupture. As described previously, the early phase of atherosclerosis is characterized by an inflammatory response in the arterial wall. Research suggests that plaque rupture, leading to clot formation, is also associated with inflammation. A study using autopsy data found that individuals who suffered a plaque rupture had a higher CRP than those who died of nonvascular causes (Burke et al., 2002).

An acute bout of prolonged, strenuous aerobic exercise leads to an elevation in CRP that is evident 6 hours postexercise and appears to peak around 24 hours postexercise (Mooren et al., 2006; Sorichter et al., 2006).

However, regular endurance training is associated with reduced levels of CRP. **Figure 15.13** presents data in which CRP levels are reported based on fitness quartile. An inverse relationship between CRP levels and fitness quartile was present for both men and women. Furthermore, this inverse relationship was independent of other factors that influence CRP, including smoking, adiposity, and hormone replacement therapy (Aronson et al., 2004). A reduction in CRP levels is associated with chronic physical activity (Kasapis and Thompson, 2005). However, the mechanisms for this reduction are not clear. One study has found that exercise without weight loss does not reduce CRP (Church et al., 2010), thus suggesting that weight loss along with regular exercise may be an important factor in inflammatory levels.

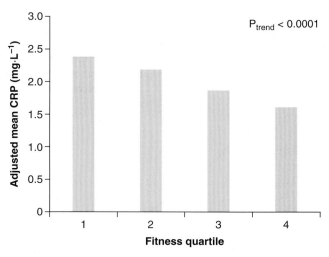

FIGURE 15.13 Relationship Between CRP and Fitness Level.
Note: CRP levels are adjusted for age, sex, BMI, presence of diabetes and hypertension, triglycerides and HDL-C levels, smoking status, and use of hormone replacement therapy, aspirin, and statins.
Source: Aronson, D., M. Sheikh-Ahmad, O. Avizohar, A. Kerner, R. Sella, P. Bartha, W. Markiewicz, Y. Levy, & G. J. Brook: C-Reactive protein is inversely related to physical fitness in middle-aged subjects. *Atherosclerosis.* 176(1):173–179 (2004). Reprinted with permission.

CHECK YOUR COMPREHENSION

Vivian is a 63-year-old female with the following characteristics:

WT = 76.4 kg

Waist circumference = 95 cm; hip circumference = 103 cm

RBP seated = 124/82 mmHg; RHR seated = 80 b·min⁻¹

Total cholesterol = 280 mg·dL⁻¹; HDL-C = 34 mg·dL⁻¹

Glucose (fasting) = 116 mg·dL⁻¹ and 118 mg·dL⁻¹

Her father died of a myocardial infarction at 52 years of age; her mother is alive. Vivian cares for her mother night and day. She has felt chest pain when moving her mother, doing housework, or walking briskly. She smoked two packs of cigarettes per day until one month ago. Vivian feels under pressure and claims to have no time to exercise. Recently she went to her physician and was diagnosed with "walking pneumonia." She is taking an antibiotic and a daily multivitamin. Complete the following CVD risk analysis for Vivian:

Name the six major modifiable risk factors.

Provide cutoff numerical values including units for each major modifiable risk factor.

Provide values for Vivian from her history and determine whether she has this risk factor.

How many total risk factors for CVD does Vivian have?

Check your answer in Appendix C.

Fibrinogen/Coagulation

As described at the beginning of this chapter, one of the major dangers of atherosclerotic plaque is that plaque rupture would lead to clot formation that could block an already narrowed blood vessel. Fibrinogen is a protein present in blood plasma that, under certain physiological circumstances, is converted into fibrin threads that form the basis of a blood clot. In addition, fibrinogen increases blood platelet aggregation and blood viscosity. Thus, fibrinogen is a thrombotic marker. High levels of fibrinogen increase the likelihood of internal clot formation. Fibrinogen levels are positively related to age, obesity, cigarette smoking, diabetes, and LDL-C and inversely related to HDL-C, alcohol use, physical activity, and exercise level (Margaglione et al., 1998; Wu, 1997). Much of the relationship between smoking and CHD and some of the association between psychological stress and CHD may be mediated through plasma fibrinogen levels. Prospective studies suggest that individuals with fibrinogen levels in the highest quartile have approximately twice the risk of coronary heart disease as those in the lowest quartile (Woo and Magliano, 2003).

It is unclear what effect a single bout of exercise has on fibrinogen levels, as various studies have reported increases, decreases, or no effect. Furthermore, evidence in the literature is conflicting about the effect of exercise training on fibrinogen levels. However, most well-designed studies suggest that aerobic training does not affect fibrinogen levels in healthy individuals or those with cardiovascular risk factors (El-Sayed et al., 2000; Womack et al., 2003).

While fibrinogen levels do not consistently change as a result of exercise or exercise training, other measures of blood coagulability do in fact change. A single acute bout of exercise is associated with increased coagulatory potential (potential for forming a clot). The magnitude of this change appears to be heavily influenced by exercise intensity (Hegde et al., 2001). Aerobic exercise training is associated with decreased platelet aggregation and a decrease in some clotting factors, suggesting that coagulatory potential may be decreased following an aerobic training program (Womack et al., 2003).

Fibrinolytic Activity

Fibrinolytic activity refers to the breakdown of fibrin clots. Enhanced fibrinolytic activity can reduce the risk of clots and thus the risk of CHD. Conversely, an inhibition of fibrinolysis increases the risk of arterial thrombosis. Prospective studies have reported that elevated levels of plasminogen activator inhibitor (PAI-1), a protein that inhibits fibrinolytic activity, are associated with increased risk of initial and recurrent myocardial infarction (Meade, 1995). Visceral abdominal obesity leads to increased PAI-1 production from adipocytes and thus is directly related to reduced fibrinolytic activity (Ridker and Libby, 2005).

A single bout of aerobic exercise (but not static exertion) has consistently been shown to increase fibrinolytic activity (Drygas, 1988; Womack et al., 2003). The change is greater in active than in sedentary individuals, and high-intensity exercise produces more change than moderate-intensity exercise.

Importantly, it appears that both coagulatory and fibrinolytic potential increase following exercise (Hegde et al., 2001; Menzel and Hilberg, 2009). However, they do not remain elevated for the same time period. There is evidence that coagulatory potential remains elevated for at least 60 minutes, whereas fibrinolytic activity quickly returns to normal values (Hegde et al., 2001). This may create an imbalance that favors clot formation in the postexercise period. Fibrinolytic potential is improved with aerobic exercise training in both healthy individuals and those with risk factors for cardiovascular disease (Buemann and Tremblay, 1996; Carroll et al., 2000; El-Sayed et al., 2000; Szymanski and Pate, 1994; Szymanski et al., 1994; Womack et al., 2003; Wood and Stefanik, 1990).

Stress

Stress (see Chapters 1 and 21) is probably the most controversial of the CHD risk factors. Many factors affect how stress impacts an individual, and these factors are difficult to identify and measure. How much stress any given stressor causes depends not just on the stressor but also on characteristics of the individual. For example, what vulnerabilities, or conversely, what coping strategies does the individual have?

The response to the stressor varies according to the individual's psychological and physiological level of reactivity. For example, among the acute physiological responses to fear or anger, mediated through the neural and hormonal systems, are increases in heart rate, blood pressure, respiratory rate, and blood viscosity, and decreases in clotting time and the breakdown of fats used as a fuel. In the short term, these responses (often called "fight or flight responses"), if appropriate to the level of need, are good. That is, from an evolutionary perspective, the individual might have to fight (and, if wounded, would need to clot blood quickly to prevent too great a loss of blood) or flee (and have sufficient energy and oxygen-carrying capacity to do so). However, if they are excessive or become chronic, these responses form a possible mechanism for the development of hypertension, atherosclerosis, thrombogenesis, and clinical heart disease.

The consequences of both the stressor and the response to the stressor can also vary, from extremely positive and health-enhancing effects to illness or injury or, ultimately, death. For example, adaptation to exercise training for an improved fitness level can enhance health. Conversely, as has been documented in several cases, bad news can precipitate sudden death from a heart attack in susceptible individuals (Caspersen and Heath, 1993; Landers, 1994; Plowman, 1994).

The type of stress primarily implicated in cardiovascular disease is psychosocial or emotional stress rather than physical stress (Holmes et al., 2006). Although life events, daily hassles, and occupational stresses, among other factors, have been considered in studies of stress, emphasis was originally placed on behavioral patterns known as Type A and Type B. The Type A behavior pattern (TABP) is characterized by hard-driving competitiveness; time urgency, haste, and impatience; a workaholic lifestyle; and hostility. The Type B behavior pattern (TBBP) is characterized by relaxation without guilt and less time urgency.

Research in the 1970s showed a positive relationship between Type A behavior and CHD. Research in the 1980s and 1990s, however, seemed to pinpoint only the hostility component. As a psychological concept, hostility includes cynicism, anger, mistrust, and aggression and is frequently associated with situations of "high demand and low control." Without hostility, the other Type A personality traits are now thought to be relatively benign (Landers, 1994; Plowman, 1994). Recently a new personality behavior pattern, Type D, has been investigated. Type D is characterized by the joint tendencies to experience negative emotions (negative affectivity) and

to inhibit these emotions while avoiding social contact with others (social inhibition). Type D individuals have been observed to have an increased risk for CVD morbidity and mortality (Sher, 2005). Stress may have a direct impact through neurohormonal changes (especially in catecholamine and serotonin levels) or an indirect effect through the use of unhealthy coping strategies, such as overeating, smoking, or excessive alcohol intake (Gordon, 1998; Habra et al., 2003).

Three studies have investigated the impact of exercise training on TABP, but none of them isolated the component of hostility. Two of the three did show, however, a decrease in TABP with dynamic endurance exercise training. These studies involved both higher-intensity and longer-duration exercise than the study that showed no significant response (Landers, 1994). In a randomized controlled trial that incorporated 16 weeks of aerobic exercise training and stress management in addition to routine medical care in patients with heart disease, those who received the additional treatment experienced reduced emotional distress and had improved markers of cardiovascular risk more than those who received only the usual medical care (Blumenthal et al., 2005). An acute bout of exercise is well-established as an effective stress management technique (Berger, 1994).

Children and the Cardiovascular Risk Factors

The concern about cardiovascular disease risk factors in children is not that children exhibit clinical cardiovascular disease but that atherosclerotic cardiovascular disease is a lifelong process that begins in childhood. Therefore, if risk factors can be prevented, modified, or counteracted in childhood, it may be possible to prevent or at least delay or reduce the severity of cardiovascular problems in adulthood.

In relation to physical activity, the intent is to establish patterns of participation in children that will continue throughout adulthood. To a large extent, the success of this strategy depends on a phenomenon called tracking. In this context **tracking** means that a characteristic is maintained, in terms of relative rank, over a long time span or even a lifetime. An example of tracking a nonrisk factor is height. Children in the upper percentiles of height at a very young age tend to maintain that relative position and be taller than average adults. Thus, in relation to children, it is important to determine the presence or absence of modifiable risk factors, the tracking strength of risk factors, and the impact of physical activity and exercise training on both short-term risk factor reductions and long-term lifestyle modifications (Rowland, 1991; Rowland and Freedson, 1994).

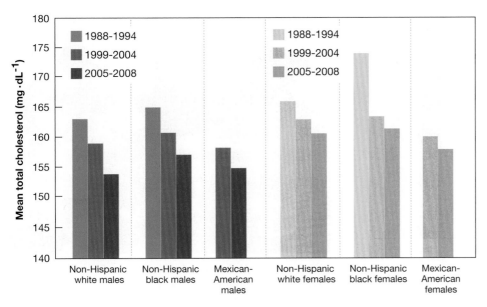

FIGURE 15.14 Trends in Mean Total Blood Cholesterol Among Adolescents Aged 12–17 years by Race and Sex.
Source: Roger, V. L., A. S. Go, D. M. Lloyd-Jones, E. J. Benjamin, J. D. Berry, W. B. Borden, et al.: Heart Disease and Stroke Statistics—2012 Update: A Report from the American Heart Association. *Circulation*. 125: e2–e220 (2011). Reprinted with permission.

Cholesterol-Lipid Fractions

At birth, total cholesterol levels are approximately 70 mg·dL⁻¹, with 35 mg·dL⁻¹ of that total being HDL. During the first few weeks, the level of TC rises rapidly to between 100 and 150 mg·dL⁻¹. By 2 years and until adulthood, the average value for males is about 160 mg·dL⁻¹ and for females about 165 mg·dL⁻¹, with HDL-C levels between 50 and 55 mg·dL⁻¹. At puberty males show a decline of HDL-C and females a decline in LDL-C values. In general, cholesterol levels do track from childhood to adulthood, although not all children with high juvenile levels of cholesterol will have elevated adult levels. In one study, 43% of children with cholesterol values above the 90th percentile also had adult values above the 90th percentile, and 81% had values above the 50th percentile (Armstrong and Simons-Morton, 1994; Mahoney et al., 1991). **Figure 15.14** depicts total cholesterol values for adolescent males and females of different ethnic backgrounds. Although not shown in the figure, approximately 8.5% of adolescents have total cholesterol values at or above 200 mg·dL⁻¹ (Roger et al., 2011).

Values that represent acceptable, borderline, and high-risk levels for children are included in **Table 15.2**. In adults, high TC, high LDL-C, and low HDL-C levels have been found to relate to the magnitude of early atherosclerotic lesions. Autopsy reports have confirmed that early signs of atherosclerosis are present in children as young as 3 years and are frequently evident by age 10. Poor lipid profiles often run in families because of both genetics and shared lifestyle factors. Insufficient evidence is available regarding the role of the apolipoproteins in children although it has been shown that as the number of metabolic syndrome component criteria increases so does the ratio of apolipoprotein B to apolipoprotein A1 (Retnakaran et al., 2006).

Cross-sectional studies of the relationship between physical activity and lipid levels have reported that active youngsters have higher HDL-C values and lower TG than inactive youngsters, but TC levels and LDL-C that do not differ with activity status. However, the relationship between physical fitness and lipid risk factors is stronger than that of physical activity and these factors. Studies indicate that high levels of cardiorespiratory fitness for both boys and girls and/or muscular fitness in girls are associated with a more favorable lipid-metabolic profile (Garcia-Artero et al., 2007; Janssen and LeBlanc, 2010; Ortega et al., 2008). Cardiorespiratory fitness in childhood and adolescence is a predictor of abnormal blood lipids later in life (Ruiz et al., 2009). Training studies, including clinical and school-based programs, have shown beneficial effects for HDL-C and TG if the intervention has been sufficient to also improve aerobic fitness, but not for TC or LDL-C. Youths who begin training studies with normal values for lipid levels are unlikely to show positive changes. A minimum of 40 min·d⁻¹, 5 d·wk⁻¹ of at least moderate to vigorous activity over 4 months is apparently needed to achieve beneficial effects in lipid levels in children and adolescents (Andersen et al., 2011; Mountjoy et al., 2011; Strong et al., 2005).

Cigarette Smoking

Figure 15.15 reports the prevalence of cigarette smoking among high school students (grades 9–12) by race/ethnicity and sex. Overall, 19.5% of students reported current cigarette use in 2009 (Roger et al., 2011). Approximately 80% of adult smokers started smoking before age 18 (American Heart Association, 2007); smoking definitely tracks from

> **Tracking** A phenomenon in which a characteristic is maintained, in terms of relative rank, over a long time span or even a lifetime.

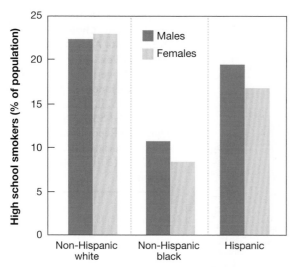

FIGURE 15.15 Prevalence of Smoking Among High School Students by Race/Ethnicity and Sex.
Source: Roger, V. L., A. S. Go, D. M. Lloyd-Jones, E. J. Benjamin, J. D. Berry, W. B. Borden, et al.: Heart Disease and Stroke Statistics—2012 Update: A Report from the American Heart Association. *Circulation*. 125:e2–e220 (2011). Reprinted with permission.

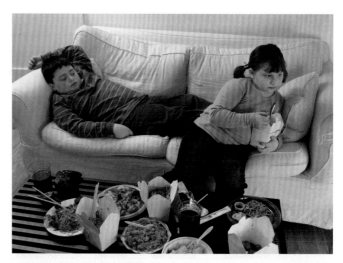

FIGURE 15.16 Unhealthy Food Choices Contribute to the High Level of Childhood Obesity.

adolescence to adulthood. The physiological effects of smoking and the indirect relationship between activity and smoking are the same regardless of the age of the smoker.

One study of Finnish youth showed that over a 6-year span, with individuals who were 12, 15, and 18 years old at the beginning of the study, higher activity levels were associated with less smoking in both boys and girls. Almost half of those who were sedentary smoked, but only about 10% of those who were active smoked (Raitakari et al., 1994). A 2011 study (Horn et al., 2011) investigated the effects of physical activity on teen smoking cessation. Individuals who had smoked in the previous 30 days were randomly assigned to brief intervention, Not on Tobacco (a proven teen cessation program) or Not on Tobacco plus a physical activity module. Smoking cessation rates were determined at 3 and 6 months after baseline. Results indicated that teens in the Not on Tobacco plus physical activity group had significantly higher cessation rates than either of the other two programs. While physical activity can assist in smoking cessation, it remains a primary goal of physical education and exercise science professionals to encourage an active lifestyle and discourage the onset of smoking in children and adolescents.

Diabetes Mellitus

Children with Type 1 and Type 2 diabetes are at risk of prematurely developing atherosclerosis. Furthermore, diabetes tracks into adulthood. The incidence of Type 2 diabetes mellitus has risen dramatically in children and adolescents in recent years—in large part paralleling

the incidence in obesity (**Figure 15.16**). There is only weak evidence of a positive relationship between physical activity and insulin sensitivity independent of adiposity in children and adolescents. However, the early establishment and maintenance of activity can benefit both glucose/insulin variables and body fatness (Bunt et al., 2003; Rowland, 2006). Additionally, regular physical activity has beneficial affects on the presence of glucose in the blood in Type 1 diabetes without increasing the risk of hypoglycemia (Herbst et al., 2006). The importance of and cautions related to physical activity and exercise training for individuals with diabetes were discussed earlier in the section on adults but also apply here for younger individuals.

Hypertension

Hypertension is evident in children as young as 6 years of age. In children, hypertension is defined as average SBP or DBP that is greater than or equal to the 95th percentile for age, sex, and height on three or more occasions (U.S. Department of Health and Human Services, 2005). **Table 15.5** provides mean blood pressure values for children based on age at the 50th and 75th percentile of height (National High Blood Pressure Education Program Working Group, 1996).

Although childhood blood pressures do not predict adult blood pressures per se, there is a definite tendency for both systolic and diastolic blood pressures to track from childhood to adulthood. In one study, children with blood pressures at the 90th percentile had three times the risk of having high adult systolic blood pressure and twice the risk of having high adult diastolic blood pressure as those whose childhood values were at the 50th percentile (Mahoney et al., 1991). There is strong evidence indicating that cardiorespiratory fitness in childhood and adolescence is a predictor of high blood pressure later in life (Ruiz et al., 2009). In addition, there is a dose-response

TABLE 15.5 Mean Blood Pressure Values for Girls and Boys Based on Height

Age (yr)	Girls' SBP/DBP		Boys' SBP/DBP	
	50th Percentile for Height	75th Percentile for Height	50th Percentile for Height	75th Percentile for Height
1	104/58	105/59	102/57	104/58
6	111/73	112/73	114/74	115/75
12	123/80	124/81	123/81	125/82
17	129/94	130/85	136/87	138/88

DBP, diastolic blood pressure; SBP, systolic blood pressure.

Source: Adapted from the National High Blood Pressure Education Program. Update on the 1987 Task Force Report on High Blood Pressure in Children and Adolescents: A working group report from the National High Blood Pressure Education Program. National High Blood Pressure Education Program Working Group on Hypertension Control in Children and Adolescents. *Pediatrics.* 98(Pt. 1):649–658 (1996).

relationship between aerobic fitness and blood pressure in youth. That is, the least fit boys and girls have been shown to be more likely to have hypertension than their high fit peers. This relationship is strongest in overweight children (Andersen et al., 2011). A similar inverse relationship has been found between physical activity and blood pressure (Gopinath et al., 2011).

Physical activity intervention of at least 30 minutes, three times per week with intensity sufficient to increase aerobic fitness, has been shown to reduce blood pressure in both boys and girls with essential hypertension (Andersen et al., 2011; Janssen and LeBlanc, 2010; Mountjoy et al., 2011). As with adults, the reductions that do occur rarely result in normal blood pressure levels, and regular physical activity or exercise is necessary to maintain the beneficial results. Dynamic resistance training used by itself, in one study, did not bring about a reduction in either systolic or diastolic pressure. However, when weight training was instituted after a period of aerobic endurance training that resulted in reduced blood pressures, the reduction in blood pressure was maintained with just the weight training (Andersen et al., 2011). Therefore, as with adults,

the best procedure is to begin young individuals with hypertension on a dynamic endurance activity regimen and add resistance training several months later, if desired (Alpert and Wilmore, 1994). There is neither a need for nor any evidence of a reduction in blood pressure in normotensive children and adolescents with exercise training (American College of Sports Medicine, 2004; Mountjoy et al., 2011; Rowland, 2006; Strong et al., 2005).

Overweight and Obesity

As seen in **Figure 15.17** the percentage of children 6–11 and adolescents 12–19 years old who are obese has increased dramatically in recent years. In addition, the prevalence of obesity in children 2 to 5 years now varies by sex and race from 7% to 19%. There is even a 7% prevalence of high weight in infants between 6 and 23 months old. Unfortunately, overweight and obesity shows evidence of tracking. An estimated 70% of overweight adolescents have a 70% chance of becoming overweight adults. This increases to an 80% chance if one or both parents are overweight or obese (Roger et al., 2011). Approximately 80% of obese adolescents become obese adults.

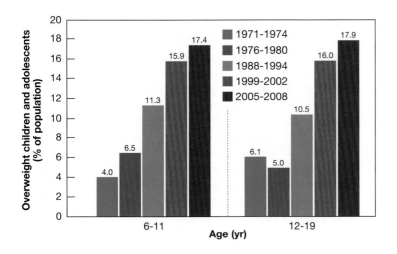

FIGURE 15.17 Trends in Prevalence of Obesity Over Time Among US Children and Adolescents by Age and Survey Year.
Source: Roger, V. L., A. S. Go, D. M. Lloyd-Jones, E. J. Benjamin, J. D. Berry, W. B. Borden, et al.: Heart Disease and Stroke Statistics—2012 Update: A Report from the American Heart Association. *Circulation.* 125:e2–e220 (2011). Reprinted with permission.

There is strong evidence that body composition in childhood and adolescence is a predictor of adult CVD risk factors. There is also strong evidence that high body mass index (BMI) in childhood and adolescence increase the risk of early adult death (Eisenmann et al., 2005; Ruiz et al., 2009). Furthermore, fatness has been determined to be a mediator of the relationship between physical activity and several other risk factors (Gutin and Owens, 2011). A significant relationship between adolescent cardiorespiratory fitness and adult body fatness has been demonstrated. The deleterious consequences of high fatness can to a meaningful extent be counteracted by having high levels of cardiorespiratory fitness (Ortega et al., 2008).

As for adults, the relationship between exercise training and reduced body weight and body fat is detailed in the metabolic unit of this text (see Chapter 8). A few brief comments are appropriate here, however. Recent research suggests that *prevention* of excess fatness in youths is primarily dependent on an adequate volume of vigorous intensity exercise. Youths of both sexes who participate in moderate to vigorous aerobic physical activity have less body fat than those who do not but vigorous physical activity is associated more with lower levels of fatness than is moderate physical activity. That is, there is a dose-response relationship between physical activity and obesity. Resistance exercise may also elicit favorable changes in body composition (Gutin and Owens, 2011; Janssen and LeBlanc, 2010; Ruiz et al., 2009). Exercise training of moderate intensity 30–60 min·d^{-1}, 3–7 d·wk^{-1} reduces total body and visceral fat in overweight children and adolescents. Limited evidence suggests that more intensive and longer duration (>80 min·d^{-1}) exercise training is needed to reduce the % body fat in normal-weight youths of both sexes (Strong et al., 2005). Although beneficial changes often occur in body composition in obese youngsters, decreases in body weight and body mass index are not consistently found (Watts et al., 2005).

Obese children have abnormalities in vascular function and structure, and exhibit biochemical markers of inflammation (Kapiotis et al., 2006). Research shows that 60% of overweight children between the ages of 5 and 10 years have at least one other major CV risk factor (Centers for Disease Control and Prevention, 1999). The clustering of risk factors known as the metabolic syndrome is evident in children and adolescents with a prevalence of 3–14% in the general population and 13–37% in obese children (Andersen et al., 2011; Weiss and Raz, 2006). The criterion for metabolic syndrome in children and adolescents requires the presence of on an increased central/abdominal obesity plus any two of the following: a raised triglyceride level, a reduced HDL-C level, hypertension, and elevated fasting plasma glucose (Zimmet et al., 2007). Both physical fitness and physical activity are inversely related to metabolic syndrome risk factors. Furthermore, an interaction between physical activity and physical fitness suggests a stronger relationship between activity and metabolic risk factors in those with low cardiorespiratory fitness. Thus, children and adolescents with the lowest levels of fitness should benefit most from increasing their physical activity (Andersen et al., 2011; Brage et al., 2004; Steele et al., 2008; Wedderkopp et al., 2003). Several exercise studies have shown improvements in specific elements of metabolic syndrome in both obese and nonobese youth (Strong et al., 2005).

Physical Inactivity

Neither lifestyle physical activity nor exercise training is likely to alter cardiovascular risk factor variables in children or adolescents whose values for these variables are normal. Maintenance of normal values, however, can be assisted by activity. Abnormal levels are consistently and positively impacted by physical activity or exercise interventions—thus deterring the continued development of that risk factor and establishing a lifestyle pattern for adulthood (Rowland, 2006). For example, significant tracking of physical activity was observed in a Finnish study of both boys and girls, with 44% remaining active from age 12 to 18 years, from 15 to 21 years, and from 18 to 24 years. Physical inactivity tracked even more closely, with 57% remaining inactive over the 6 years of the study. Those who remained active had better risk factor profiles than their inactive counterparts. They smoked less, were less fat, had higher HDL-C and lower TC values, and had favorable differences in insulin levels. They also had a healthier diet, which would, of course, have affected these results (Raitakari et al., 1994). Another study showed that physically active young male adults had had better physical fitness test results as children or adolescents (Dennison et al., 1988).

Twisk et al. (2002) summarized the results from five longitudinal observational studies investigating relationships between physical activity and cardiorespiratory physical fitness in youth and CVD risk factors later in life. Childhood physical fitness was found to be predictive of a healthy CVD risk profile later in life while physical activity was not. As with adults, the difficulty of accurately measuring physical activity may be partially responsible for these results. It may also be that physical fitness more directly indicates the quality of the cardiorespiratory system or that the predictive value of physical fitness may be caused by the relationship between physical fitness and % body fat. Or, as with adults, it may be that physical fitness and physical activity need to be considered separate risk factors in youth. This means that both physical fitness and physical activity need to be measured, evaluated, and acted on when an individual's results warrant improvement.

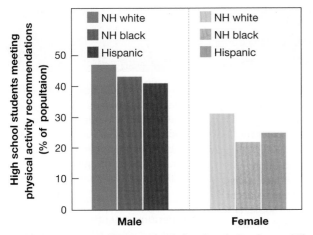

FIGURE 15.18 Prevalence of High-school Students Who Meet Recommended Levels of Physical Activity by Sex and Race/Ethnicity.

NH, non-Hispanic.

Note: "Recommended levels" is defined as activity that increased heart rate and made breathing harder some of the time for a total of at least 60 min·d⁻¹ on 5 or more of the 7 days preceding the survey. *Source*: Roger, V. L., A. S. Go, D. M. Lloyd-Jones, E. J. Benjamin, J. D. Berry, W. B. Borden, et al.: Heart Disease and Stroke Statistics—2012 Update: A Report from the American Heart Association. *Circulation*. 125:e2–e220 (2011). Reprinted with permission.

Figure 15.18 reveals that currently less than half of the males and approximately a fifth to a third of the females 12–17 years engage in the recommended level of physical activity. Additionally, the proportion of those meeting the activity recommendations declines from the 9th grade (~40%) to the 12th grade (~30%). Even more disconcerting, there is a marked discrepancy between those who self-reported being active (as shown in the figure) and those who actually were that active when measured objectively with portable motion sensors. Part of the problem is that only 33.3% of students in K-12 attend physical education classes daily (Roger et al., 2011).

Note that the recommended amount of activity for children and youths is 60 min·d⁻¹ (National Association for Sport and Physical Education, 2004; Strong et al., 2005; U.S. Department of Health and Human Services, 2008). Recent research not only has reinforced the 60-minute daily minimum but has indicated that physical activity levels might need to be at least 90 min·d⁻¹ to prevent insulin resistance, which appears to be a central component in the clustering of cardiovascular risk factors (Andersen et al., 2006). This does not mean that children and adolescents should be expected to participate in 90-minute exercise sessions. It does mean that a variety of options for accumulating physical activity should be available each day, including daily school physical education classes, free play, recess, before and after school programs, intramurals, recreational and educational athletic

programs, and lifestyle activities such as biking or walking for transportation (Pate et al., 2006; Weiss and Raz, 2006).

As with adults, there is now a large body of evidence showing that, independent of physical activity levels, sedentary behaviors exhibit a dose-response relationship with unfavorable health outcomes in children and adolescents. Similarly, there is evidence that decreasing any type of sedentary time (but especially limiting television time to under 2 hr · d⁻¹) is associated with lower health risks in youth aged 5–17 years. Thus, there is the need to advocate for both increases in physical activity and decreases in sedentary behavior in children and adolescents (Tremblay et al., 2011).

Nontraditional Risk Factors

CRP is a marker of inflammation and inflammation is central to all stages of atherosclerosis. Many pediatric studies have shown that elevated CRP is associated with CVD risk factors including excess body fat and blood pressure. High CRP levels are seen in children with metabolic syndrome, and high childhood CRP levels predict high adult CRP levels. A relationship between elevated CRP levels and reduced fitness in normal weight children has been reported. Despite these preliminary indications, it is not yet clear whether high CRP levels during childhood and adolescence lead to an increased risk of CVD in later life (Balagopal et al., 2011).

Fibrinogen is also a key player in the promotion of atherogenesis and may be an independent risk factor for CVD. Studies in children and adolescents have demonstrated a positive relationship between fibrinogen and obesity, and a negative relationship with physical fitness. Physical activity–based interventions in youths have shown consistent decreases in the level of fibrinogen. Fibrinolytic activity refers to the breakdown of fibrin clots. High levels of PAI-1 (a protein that inhibits fibrinolytic activity) have been reported in obese children. The effect of physical activity on levels of PAI-1 and the fibrinolytic system are mixed in children and adolescents. Thus, again, despite promising preliminary findings, the potential use of fibrinogen/fibrinolytic activity as markers of CVD risk in children and adolescents needs to be confirmed with longitudinal studies (Balagopal et al., 2011).

A 2009 study (Roemmich et al., 2009) is the first to study stress reactivity and exercise in children. It determined that DBP, SBP, and HR reactivity to a speech stressor was dampened after exercise compared to TV watching in a group of 8- to 12-year-old children. Surprisingly, physical fitness was positively associated with HR reactivity. Further research is needed to fully determine the impact of physical activity and physical fitness on the stress responses of children and adolescents.

FOCUS ON RESEARCH: *Clinically Relevant*

The Cardiovascular Risk Associated with Acute Exercise

As has been discussed throughout this chapter, regular physical activity is widely advocated because substantial research evidence suggests that physical activity and exercise training delay the development of CVD risk factors, atherosclerosis, and CHD events. Despite all of the positive benefits, however, vigorous physical exercise can also acutely and transiently increase the risk of heart attacks (acute myocardial infarctions) and sudden cardiac death in susceptible individuals. For example, studies have reported 1 death per 133,000 males and 1 death per 769,000 females for high school and college athletes, including all nontraumatic deaths. In older adults 1 death per 82,000 members for a mortality rate of 1 per 2.57 million workouts over 2 years has been reported by a large commercial fitness center chain. This is based on 71 deaths in that time with a mean age of 52 years. Nearly half of these deaths occurred in members who exercised infrequently or less than once a week.

Exercise-associated acute cardiac events generally occur in individuals with known or unknown cardiac disease. In young individuals this most commonly means hereditary or congenital cardiovascular abnormalities. In this population, the health risks of vigorous physical activity exceed the benefits, although moderate physical activity may be beneficial in terms of preventing other health risks or problems. In older individuals, coronary artery disease is the most common pathological finding. Habitual vigorous physical activity appears to reduce the risk of CHD death in patients with diagnosed

disease such that the benefits of physical activity appear to outweigh the risks.

Several strategies are suggested for reducing the likelihood of an exercise-induced cardiac event:

1. Maintain physical fitness through regular physical activity because a disproportionate number of events occur in the least physically active subjects performing unaccustomed vigorous physical activity.

2. Both young athletes and adults should undergo preparticipation screening before engaging in vigorous physical activity.

3. High-risk individuals may need to be excluded from or restricted in vigorous activity.

4. Physically inactive individuals and patients with known cardiovascular disease should avoid strenuous, unaccustomed exercise in both excessively cold and hot conditions and at altitude.

5. Individuals should be encouraged to monitor their bodies for early symptoms of cardiovascular events and seek medical attention. Such symptoms include but are not limited to chest pain, increasing fatigue, feelings of indigestion, and excessive breathlessness.

6. Health-fitness facilities should:

   a. Perform preentry screening by appropriately trained personnel
   b. Have written emergency policies
   c. Regularly conduct emergency drills and cardiopulmonary resuscitation practices
   d. Have an automatic external defibrillator available for use by trained personnel
   e. Establish a "hotline" to summon emergency medical care

Source: American College of Sports Medicine and American Heart Association: Joint Position Statement: Exercise and acute cardiovascular events: Placing the risks into perspective. *Medicine & Science in Sports & Exercise.* 39(5):886–897 (2007).

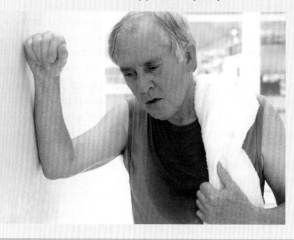

SUMMARY

1. Cardiovascular disease is a major cause of death in the United States, accounting for approximately 34% of all deaths. Coronary heart disease is the most prevalent type of cardiovascular disease. Coronary heart disease is characterized by the formation of atherosclerotic plaque in the coronary arteries.

2. Cardiovascular risk factors are classified as nonmodifiable (age, heredity, race, and sex); major modifiable (cholesterol-lipid fractions, cigarette smoking,

diabetes mellitus, hypertension, obesity, physical inactivity); and contributing and nontraditional (apolipoproteins, CRP, fibrinogen, fibrinolytic activity, and stress).

3. Triglycerides and a small amount of cholesterol are transported from the small intestines or liver to adipose tissue or muscles by chylomicrons and very low density lipoproteins (VLDL).

4. VLDLs are degraded into intermediate-density lipoproteins (IDL), which, in turn, are converted to low-density lipoproteins (LDL) in the liver. LDL

transports 60–70% of the total cholesterol (TC) in the body to all cells except liver cells.

5. High-density lipoproteins (HDL) may block cholesterol uptake at the cellular or tissue level. HDL definitely carries cholesterol away from the sites of deposit to the liver, where the cholesterol can be broken down and eliminated in the bile.

6. Arteriosclerosis is characterized by a thickening of the arterial wall, inflammation, loss of elastic connective tissue, and hardening of the vessel wall.

7. Atherosclerosis is a pathological process that results in the buildup of plaque (composed of connective tissue, smooth muscle cells, cellular debris, and cholesterol) inside the vessel. The buildup of plaque obstructs blood flow and increases the risk of thrombosis. Depending on the amount of obstruction, the result can be pain, a heart attack, or a stroke.

8. Active individuals generally have lipid profiles that indicate a reduced risk for coronary heart disease (CHD).

9. The atherosclerotic process is accelerated in individuals who smoke cigarettes. Smoking injures the arterial wall lining, increases the levels of circulating TC, and decreases the amount of HDL-C. Smoking also causes blood platelets to adhere to each other, speeds up the rate of internal blood clotting, and makes the clots tougher to dissolve.

10. Individuals who are at high risk for developing hypertension can reduce the risk by participating in an endurance training program. Most hypertensive individuals experience decreased blood pressure as a result of a consistent aerobic endurance exercise program.

11. Only about 30% of Americans report regular leisure-time activity. Therefore, potentially more benefit overall could be achieved by increasing the activity level of US citizens than by changing any other single CHD risk factor.

12. Metabolic syndrome is a progressive disease process in which high visceral abdominal obesity is directly related to dyslipidemia, inflammation, impaired glucose tolerance, insulin resistance, and hypertension, which together form a cluster of risk factors for CVD. Regular exercise results in favorable changes in each of these risk factors.

13. The beginnings of metabolic syndrome and cardiovascular disease occur during childhood and adolescence. In general, risk factors track into adulthood and can predict future CVD. Physical activity and physical fitness are important moderators of risk factor development and progression in childhood and adolescence.

REVIEW QUESTIONS

1. Describe the progression of atherosclerosis, indicating the role of lipids (specifically LDL-C) and inflammation.

2. Identify risk factors that cannot be changed, and discuss their relationship with cardiovascular disease.

3. Identify the major modifiable risk factors, and discuss their relationship with cardiovascular disease.

4. Identify contributing and nontraditional risk factors, and discuss their relationship with cardiovascular disease.

5. Discuss metabolic syndrome.

6. What is the impact of exercise training on each CHD risk factor?

7. What is the importance of identifying cardiovascular disease risk factors in children?

For further review and additional study tools, visit the website at http://thePoint.lww.com/Plowman4e ✳ ▶

REFERENCES

Alcazar, O., R. C. Ho, & L. J. Goodyear: Physical activity, fitness, and diabetes mellitus. In Bouchard, C., S. N. Blair, & W. L. Haskell (eds.): *Physical Activity and Health*. Champaign, IL: Human Kinetics, 191–204 (2006).

Alpert, B. S. & J. H. Wilmore: Physical activity and blood pressure in adolescents. *Pediatric Exercise Science*. 6(4):361–380 (1994).

American College of Sports Medicine: Position stand: Exercise and hypertension. *Medicine & Science in Sports & Exercise*. 36(3):533–553 (2004).

American College of Sports Medicine: Joint Position Statement: Exercise and Type 2 diabetes. *Medicine & Science in Sports & Exercise*. 32(7):2283–2303 (2010).

American College of Sports Medicine: Quantity and quality of exercise for developing and maintaining cardiorespiratory, musculoskeletal, and neuromotor fitness in apparently healthy adults: Guidance for prescribing exercise. *Medicine & Science in Sports & Exercise*. 43(7):1334–1359 (2011).

American College of Sports Medicine and American Heart Association: Joint Position Statements: Exercise and acute cardiovascular events; placing the risks into perspective. *Medicine & Science in Sports & Exercise*. 39(5):886–897 (2007).

American Heart Association: *Heart Disease and Stroke Statistics*. Dallas: Author (2007).

American Heart Association: Policy Statement: Forecasting the future of cardiovascular disease in the United States: A policy statement from the American Heart Association. *Circulation*. 123:933–944 (2011).

Andersen, L. B., M. Harro, L. B. Sardinha, K. Froberg, U. Ekelund, S. Brage, & S. A. Anderssen: Physical activity and clustered cardiovascular risk in children: a cross-sectional study (the European Youth Heart Study). *Lancet*. 368(9532):299–304 (2006).

Andersen, L. B., C. Riddoch, S. Kriemler, & A. Hills: Physical activity and cardiovascular risk factors in children. *British Journal of Sports Medicine*. 45:871–876 (2011).

Arciero, P. J., D. L. Smith, & J. Calles-Escandon: Effects of short-term inactivity on glucose tolerance, energy expenditure, and blood flow in trained subjects. *Journal of Applied Physiology*. 74(4):1365–1373 (1998).

Armstrong, N. & B. Simons-Morton: Physical activity and blood lipids in adolescents. *Pediatric Exercise Science*. 6(4):381–405 (1994).

Aronson, D. & E. J. Rayfield: Diabetes and obesity. In Fuster, V., R. Ross, E. J. Topol (eds.): *Atherosclerosis and Coronary Artery Disease* (2nd edition). Philadelphia, PA: Lippincott-Raven (2005).

Aronson, D., M. Sheikh-Ahmad, O. Avizohar, A. Kerner, R. Sella, P. Bartha, W. Markiewicz, Y. Levy, & G. J. Brook: C-Reactive protein is inversely related to physical fitness in middle-aged subjects. *Atherosclerosis*. 176(1):173–179 (2004).

Balagopal, P., S. D. deFerranti, S. Cook, S. R. Daniels, S. S. Gidding, L. L. Hayman, et al.: Nontraditional risk factors and biomarkers for cardiovascular disease: Mechanistic, research, and clinical considerations for youth. *Circulation*. 123:2749–2769 (2011).

Barter, P. J., C. M. Ballantyne, R. Carmena, M. C. Cabezas, M. J. Chapman, P. Couture, et al.: Apo B versus cholesterol in estimating cardiovascular risk and in guiding therapy: Report of the thirty-person/ten-country panel. *Journal of Internal Medicine*. 259:247–258 (2006).

Berger, B. G.: Coping with stress: The effectiveness of exercise and other techniques. *Quest*. 46:100–119 (1994).

Berkwits, M. & E. Guallar: Risk factors, risk prediction, and the apolipoprotein B-apolipoprotein A-I ratio. *Annals of Internal Medicine*. 146:677–679 (2007).

Blair, S. N., H. W. Kohl, C. E. Barlow, R. S. Paffenbarger, L. W. Gibbons, & C. A. Macera: Changes in physical fitness and all-cause mortality: A prospective study of healthy and unhealthy men. *Journal of the American Medical Association*. 273(14):1093–1098 (1995).

Blair, S. N. & H. C. Minocha: Physical fitness and all-cause mortality: A prospective study of healthy men and women. *Journal of the American Medical Association*. 262:2395–2401 (1989).

Blumenthal, J. A., A. Sherwood, M. A. Babyak, L. L. Watkins, R. Waugh, A. Georgiades, S. L. Bacon, J. Hayano, R. E. Coleman, & A. Hinderliter: Effects of exercise and stress management training on markers of cardiovascular risk in patients with ischemic heart disease. *JAMA*. 293(13):1626–1634 (2005).

Brage, S., N. Wedderkopp, U. Ekelund, P. W. Franks, N. J. Wareham, L. B. Andersen, & K. Froberg: Features of the metabolic syndrome are associated with objectively measured physical activity and fitness in Danish children. *Diabetes Care*. 27(9):2141–2148 (2004).

Briefel, R. R. & C. L. Johnson: Secular trends in dietary intake in the United States. *Annual Review of Nutrition*. 24:401–431 (2004).

Buemann, B. & A. Tremblay: Effects of exercise training on abdominal obesity and related metabolic complications. *Sports Medicine*. 21(3):191–212 (1996).

Bunt, J. C., A. D. Salbe, I. T. Harper, R. L. Hanson, & P. A. Tataranni: Weight, adiposity, and physical activity as determinants of an insulin sensitivity index in Pima Indian children. *Diabetic Care*. 26(9):2524–2530 (2003).

Burke, A. P., R. P. Tracy, F. Kolodgie, G. T. Malcom, A. Zieske, R. Kutys, J. Pestaner, J. Smialek, & R. Virmani: Elevated C-Reactive protein values and atherosclerosis in sudden coronary death: Association with different pathologies. *Circulation*. 105(17):2019–2023 (2002).

Carroll, S., C. B. Cooke, & R. J. Butterly: Leisure time physical activity, cardiorespiratory fitness, and plasma fibrinogen concentrations in nonsmoking middle-aged men. *Medicine & Science in Sports & Exercise*. 32(3):620–626 (2000).

Carroll, S. & M. Dudfield: What is the relationship between exercise and metabolic abnormalities? A review of the metabolic syndrome. *Sports Medicine*. 34(6):371–418 (2004).

Caspersen, C. J. & G. W. Heath. The risk factor concept of coronary heart disease. In J. L. Durstine, A. C. King, P. L. Painter, J. L. Roitman, L. D. Zwiren, & W. L. Kenney (eds.): *American College of Sports Medicine: Resource Manual for Guidelines for Exercise Testing and Prescription* (2nd edition). Philadelphia, PA: Lea & Febiger (1993).

Center for Disease Control and Prevention: National diabetes fact sheet: National estimates and general information on diabetes and prediabetes in the United States, 2011. Atlanta, GA: U.S. Department of Health and Human Services, Center for Disease Control and Prevention (2011).

Centers for Disease Control and Prevention: *Obesity epidemic increases dramatically in the United States*. www.cdc.gov/nccd-php/dnpa/obesity-epidemic.htm (1999).

Church, T. S., C. P. Earnest, A. M. Thompson, E. Priest, R. Q. Rodarte, T. Sanders, R. Ross, & S. N. Blair: Exercise without weight loss does not reduce C-Reactive protein: The INFLAME Study. *Medicine & Science in Sports & Exercise*. 42(4):708–716 (2010).

Ciolac, E. G., E. A. Bocchi, L. A. Bortolotto, V. O. Carvalho, J. Greve, & G. V. Guimaraes: Effects of high-intensity aerobic interval training vs. moderate exercise on hemodynamic, metabolic and neuro-humoral abnormalities of young normotensive women at high familial risk for hypertension. *Hypertension Research*. 33:836–843 (2010).

Colberg, S. R.: Exercise: A diabetes "cure" for many? *ACSM's Health and Fitness Journal*. 5(2):20–26 (2001).

Dannenberg, A. L., J. B. Keller, P. W. F. Wilson, & W. P. Castelli: Leisure time physical activity in the Framingham offspring study. *American Journal of Epidemiology*. 129:76–88 (1989).

Dennison, B. A., J. H. Straus, D. Mellits, & E. Charney: Childhood physical fitness tests: Predictor of adult physical activity levels? *Pediatrics*. 82(3):324–330 (1988).

Drygas, W. K.: Changes in blood platelet function, coagulation, and fibrinolytic activity in response to moderate, exhaustive, and prolonged exercise. *International Journal of Sports Medicine*. 9:67–72 (1988).

Eisenmann, J. C., E. E. Wickel, G. J. Welk, & S. N. Blair: Relationship between adolescent fitness and fatness and cardiovascular disease risk factors in adulthood: The Aerobics Center Longitudinal Study (ACLS). *American Heart Journal*. 149:46–53 (2005).

Elibero, A., K. J. VanRensburg, & D. J. Drobes: Acute effects of aerobic exercise and hatha yoga on craving to smoke. *Nicotine & Tobacco Research*. 13(1):1140–1148 (2011).

El-Sayed, M. S., C. Sale, P. G. W. Jones, & M. Chester: Blood hemostasis in exercise and training. *Medicine & Science in Sports & Exercise*. 32(5):918–925 (2000).

Froelicher, V. F.: Exercise, fitness, and coronary heart disease. In Bouchard, C., R. J. Shephard, T. Stephens, J. R. Sutton, & B. D. McPherson (eds.): *Exercise, Fitness, and Health: A Consensus of Current Knowledge*. Champaign, IL: Human Kinetics, 429–451 (1990).

Garcia-Artero, E., F. B. Ortega, J. R. Ruiz, J. L. Mesa, M. Delgado, M. González-Gross, et al.: Lipid and metabolic profiles in adolescents are affected more by physical fitness than physical activity. *Revista Española de Cardiologia.* 60(6):581–588 (2007).

Gaziano, M. J.: Global burden of cardiovascular disease. In Zipes, D. P., P. Libby, R. O. Bonow, & E. Braunwald (eds.): *Braunwald's Heart Disease: A textbook of cardiovascular medicine* (7th edition). Philadelphia, PA: Elsevier Saunders, 1–19 (2005).

Gielen, S., S. Erbs, G. Schuler, & R. Hambrecht: Exercise training and endothelial dysfunction in coronary artery disease and chronic heart failure. From molecular biology to clinical benefits. *Minerva Cardioangiologica.* 50(2):95–105 (2002).

Gielen, S. & R. Hambrecht: Effects of exercise training on vascular function and myocardial perfusion. *Cardiology Clinics.* 19(3):357–368 (2001).

Gopinath, B., L. L. Hardy, E. Teber, & P. Mitchell: Association between physical activity and blood pressure in prepubertal children. *Hypertension Research.* 34(7):851–855 (2011).

Gordon, N. F.: Conceptual basis for coronary artery disease risk factor assessment. In Roitman, J. L. (ed.): *ACSM's Resource Manual for Guidelines for Exercise Testing and Prescription* (3rd edition). Philadelphia, PA: Lippincott, Williams & Wilkins, 3–12 (1998).

Gordon, N. F., R. F. Leighton, & A. Mooss: Factors associated with increased risk of coronary heart disease. In Kaminsky, L. A. (ed.): *ACSM's Resource Manual for Guidelines for Exercise Testing and Prescription* (5th edition). Philadelphia, PA: Lippincott, Williams, & Wilkins, 95–114 (2006).

Grandjean, P. & S. F. Crouse: Lipid and lipoprotein disorders. In LeMura, L. M. & S. P. von Duvillard (eds.): *Clinical Exercise Physiology.* Philadelphia, PA: Lippincott, Williams & Wilkins, 55–85 (2004).

Grundy, S. M.: Metabolic syndrome: A multiplex cardiovascular risk factor. *Journal of Clinical Endocrinology and Metabolism.* 92(2):399–404 (2007).

Grundy, S. M., I. J. Benjamin, G. L. Burke, A. Chait, R. H. Eckel, B. V. Howard, W. Mitch, S. C. Smith, & J. R. Sowers: Diabetes and cardiovascular disease: A statement for healthcare professionals from the American Heart Association. *Circulation.* 100:1134–1146 (1999).

Gutin, B. & S. Owens: The influence of physical activity on cardiometabolic biomarkers in youths: A review. *Pediatric Exercise Science.* 23:169–185 (2011).

Habra, M. E., W. Linden, J. C. Anderson, & J. Weinberg: Type D personality is related to cardiovascular and neuroendocrine reactivity to acute stress. *Journal of Psychosomatic Research.* 55(3):235–245 (2003).

Hagberg, J. M.: Exercise, fitness and hypertension. In Bouchard, C., R. J. Shephard, T. Stephens, J. R. Sutton, & B. D. McPherson (eds.): *Exercise, Fitness, and Health: A Consensus of Current Knowledge.* Champaign, IL: Human Kinetics (1990).

Hahn, R. A., G. W. Heath, & M.-H. Chang: Cardiovascular disease risk factors and preventive practices among adults—United States, 1994: A behavioral risk factor atlas. *Morbidity and Mortality Weekly Report (MMWR).* 47(SS-5):35–69 (1998).

Hamilton, M. T., D. G. Hamilton, & T. W. Zderic: Role of low energy expenditure and sitting in obesity, metabolic syndrome, type 2 diabetes, and cardiovascular disease. *Diabetes.* 56:2655–2667 (2007).

Hanson, P.: Pathophysiology of chronic diseases and exercise. In Durstine, J. L., A. C. King, P. L. Painter, J. L. Rostman, L. K. Zwireu, & W. L. Kenney (eds.): *American College of Sports Medicine Resource Manual for Guidelines for Exercise Testing and Prescription* (2nd edition). Philadelphia, PA: Lea & Febiger, 187–196 (1993).

Haskell, W. L., I.-M. Lee, R. R. Pate, K. E. Powell, S. N. Blair, B. A. Franklin, C. A. Macera, G. W. Heath, P. D. Thompson, & A. Bauman: Physical activity and public health: Updated recommendation for adults from the American College of Sports Medicine and the American Heart Association. *Medicine & Science in Sports & Exercise.* 39(8):1423–1434 (2007).

Hegde, S. S., A. H. Goldfarb, & S. Hegde: Clotting and fibrinolytic activity change during the 1h after a submaximal run. *Medicine & Science in Sports & Exercise.* 33(6):887–892 (2001).

Heidenreich, P. A., J. G. Trogdon, O. A. Khavjou, J. Butler, K. Dracup, M. D. Ezekowitz, E. A. Finkelstein, Y. Hong, S. C. Johnston, A. Khera, D. M. Lloyd-Jones, S. A. Nelson, G. Nichol, D. Orenstein, P. W. Wilson, Y. J. Woo; American Heart Association Advocacy Coordinating Committee; Stroke Council; Council on Cardiovascular Radiology and Intervention; Council on Clinical Cardiology; Council on Epidemiology and Prevention; Council on Arteriosclerosis; Thrombosis and Vascular Biology; Council on Cardiopulmonary; Critical Care; Perioperative and Resuscitation; Council on Cardiovascular Nursing; Council on the Kidney in Cardiovascular Disease; Council on Cardiovascular Surgery and Anesthesia, and Interdisciplinary Council on Quality of Care and Outcomes Research: Forecasting the future of cardiovascular disease in the United States: a policy statement from the American Heart Association. *Circulation.* 123(8):933–944 (2011).

Herbst, A., R. Bachran, T. Kapellen, & R. W. Holl: Effects of regular physical activity on control of glycemia in pediatric patients with Type 1 diabetes mellitus. *Archives of Pediatric & Adolescent Medicine.* 160(6):573–577 (2006).

Holmes, S. D., D. S. Krantz, H. Rogers, J. Gottdiener, & R. J. Contrada: Mental stress and coronary artery disease: A multidisciplinary guide. *Progress in Cardiovascular Disease.* 49(2):106–122 (2006).

Horn, K., G. Dino, S. A. Branstetter, J. J. Zhang, N. Noerachmanto, T. Jarrett, & M. Taylor: Effects of physical activity on teen smoking cessation. *Pediatrics.* 128(4):E801–E811 (2011).

Janssen, I. & C. J. Jolliffe: Influence of physical activity on mortality in elderly with coronary artery disease. *Medicine & Science in Sports & Exercise.* 38(3):418–423 (2006).

Janssen, I. & A. G. LeBlanc: Systematic review of the health benefits of physical activity and fitness in school-aged children and youth. *Journal of Behavioral Nutrition and Physical Activity.* 7:40–56 (2010).

Jurca, R., M. J. Lamonte, C. E. Barlow, J. B. Kampert, T. S. Church, & S. N. Blair: Association of muscular strength with incidence of metabolic syndrome in men. *Medicine & Science in Sports & Exercise.* 37(11):1849–1855 (2005).

Kampert, J. B.: Sustained changes in cardiorespiratory fitness and mortality in the Aerobics Center Longitudinal Study [abstract]. *Medicine & Science in Sports & Exercise.* 36(Suppl.):S135 (2004).

Kannel, W. B. & P. W. F. Wilson: Cardiovascular risk factors and hypertension. In J. L. Izzo & H. R. Black (eds.): *Council on High Blood Pressure Research, American Heart Association, Hypertension Primer* (2nd edition). Baltimore, MD: Lippincott, Williams & Wilkins, 199–202 (1999).

Kapiotis, S., G. Holzer, G. Schaller, M. Haumer, H. Widhalm, D. Weghuber, B. Jilma, G. Roggla, M. Wolzt, K. Widhalm, & O. F. Wagner: A proinflammatory state is detectable in obese children and is accompanied by functional and morphological vascular changes. *Arteriosclerosis, Thrombosis, and Vascular Biology*. 26:2541–2546 (2006).

Kasapis, C. & P. D. Thompson: The effects of physical activity on serum C-Reactive protein and inflammatory markers: A systematic review. *Journal of the American College of Cardiology*. 45(10):1563–1569 (2005).

Katsanos, C.: Prescribing aerobic exercise for the regulation of postprandial lipid metabolism: Current research and recommendations. *Sports Medicine*. 36(7):547–560 (2006).

Katzmarzyk, P. T., T. S. Church, & S. N. Blair: Cardiorespiratory fitness attenuates the effects of the Metabolic Syndrome on all-cause and cardiovascular disease mortality in men. *Archives of Internal Medicine*. 164:1092–1097 (2004).

Katzmarzyk, P. T., T. S. Church, C. L. Craig, & C. Bouchard: Sitting time and mortality from all causes, cardiovascular disease, and cancer. *Medicine & Science in Sports & Exercise*. 41(5):998–1005 (2009).

Katzmarzyk, P. T., A. S. Leon, J. H. Wilmore, J. S. Skinner, D. C. Rao, T. Rankinen, & C. Bouchard: Targeting the metabolic syndrome with exercise: Evidence from the Heritage Family Study. *Medicine & Science in Sports & Exercise*. 35(10):1703–1709 (2003).

Kelley, G. & K. S. Kelley: Aerobic exercise and HDL2-C: A meta-analysis of randomized controlled trials. *Atherosclerosis*. 184(1):207–215 (2006).

Koplan, J. P., K. E. Powell, R. K. Sikes, R. W. Shirley, & C. C. Campbell: An epidemiological study of the benefits and risks of running. *Journal of the American Medical Association*. 248:3118–3121 (1982).

LaFontaine, T.: Preventing the progression of or reversing coronary atherosclerosis. *American College of Sports Medicine Certified News*. 4(3):1–6 (1994).

Lakka, T. A., D. E. Laaksonen, H.-M. Lakka, N. Mannikko, L. K. Niskanen, R. Rauramaa, & J. T. Salonen: Sedentary lifestyle, poor cardiorespiratory fitness, and the Metabolic Syndrome. *Medicine & Science in Sports & Exercise*. 35(8):1279–1286 (2003).

Landers, D. M.: Performance, stress, and health: Overall reaction. *Quest*. 46:123–135 (1994).

Lee, C. D., S. N. Blair, & A. S. Jackson: Cardiorespiratory fitness, body composition, and all-cause and cardiovascular disease mortality in men. *American Journal of Clinical Nutrition*. 69:373–380 (1999).

Lee, S., J. L. Kuk, P. T. Katzmarzyk, S. N. Blair, T. S. Church, & R. Ross: Cardiorespiratory fitness attenuates metabolic risk independent of abdominal subcutaneous and visceral fat in men. *Diabetes Care*. 28:895–901 (2005).

Levy, D., G. J. Garrison, D. D. Savage, W. B. Kannel, & W. P. Castelli: Prognostic implications of echocardiographically determined left ventricular mass in the Framingham Heart Study. *New England Journal of Medicine*. 323(24):1706–1707 (1990).

Libby, P.: Inflammation and cardiovascular disease mechanisms. *American Journal of Clinical Nutrition*. 83(Suppl.):456S–460S (2006).

Libby, P. & P. Theroux: Pathophysiology of coronary artery disease. *Circulation*. 111:3481–3488 (2005).

Linke, A., S. Erbs, & R. Hambrecht: Exercise and the coronary circulation—alterations and adaptations in coronary artery disease. *Progress in Cardiovascular Diseases*. 48(4):270–284 (2006).

Lippi, G., F. Schena, G. L. Salvagno, M. Montagnana, F. Ballestrieri, & G. C. Guidi: Comparison of the lipid profile and lipoprotein(a) between sedentary and highly trained subjects. *Clinical Chemistry and Laboratory Medicine*. 44(3):322–326 (2006).

Mahoney, L. T., R. M. Lauer, J. Lee, & W. R. Clarke: Factors affecting tracking of coronary heart disease risk factors in children: The Muscatine study. In Hyperlipidemia in Childhood and the Development of Atherosclerosis. *Annals of the New York Academy of Sciences*. 623:120–132 (1991).

Manson, J. E., P. Greenland, A. Z. LaCroix, M. L. Stefanick, C. P. Mouton, A. Oberman, M. G. Perri, D. S. Sheps, M. B. Pettinger, & D. S. Siscovick: Walking compared with vigorous exercise for the prevention of cardiovascular events in women. *The New England Journal of Medicine*. 347(10):716–725 (2002).

Manson, J. E., F. B. Hu, J. W. Rich-Edwards, G. A. Colditz, M. J. Stamfer, W. C. Willett, F. E. Speizer, & C. H. Hennekens: A prospective study of walking as compared with vigorous exercise in the prevention of coronary heart disease in women. *New England Journal of Medicine*. 341:650–658 (1999).

Margaglione, M., G. Cappucci, D. Colaizzo, L. Pirro, G. Vecchione, E. Grandone, & G. Di Minno: Fibrinogen plasma levels in an apparently healthy general population—relation to environmental and genetic determinants. *Thrombosis and Haemostasis*. 80(5):805–810 (1998).

Marks, J. B.: Metabolic syndrome: To be or not to be? *Clinical Diabetes*. 24(1):3–4 (2006).

Meade, T. W.: Fibrinogen in ischaemic heart disease. *European Heart Journal*. 16(Suppl. A):31–35 (1995).

Menzel, K. & T. Hilberg: Coagulation and fibrinolysis are in balance after moderate exercise in middle-aged participants. *Clinical and Applied Thrombosis/Hemostasis*. 15(3):348–355 (2009).

Mooren, F. C., A. Lechtermann, M. Fobker, B. Brandt, C. Sorg, K. Volker, & W. Nacken: The response of the novel proinflammatory molecules S100A8/A9 to exercise. *International Journal of Sports Medicine*. 27(9):751–758 (2006).

Mountjoy, M., L. B. Andersen, N. Armstrong, S. Biddle, C. Boreham, H.-P. B. Bedenbeck, et al.: International Olympic Committee consensus statement on the health and fitness of young people through physical activity and sport. *Sports Medicine*. 45:839–848 (2011).

National Association for Sport and Physical Education: Physical activity for children: A statement of guidelines for children ages 5–12 (2nd edition). Reston, VA: NASPE (2004).

National High Blood Pressure Education Program: National Institutes of Health; National Heart, Lung, and Blood Institute. The Fifth Report of the Joint Committee on Detection, Evaluation, and Treatment of High Blood Pressure: Washington, DC (1993).

National High Blood Pressure Education Program Working Group on Hypertension Control in Children and Adolescents: Update on the 1987 Task Force Report on High Blood Pressure in Children and Adolescents: A Working

Group Report from the National High Blood Pressure Education Program. *Pediatrics*. 98(4):649–658 (1996).

Nordstrom, C. K., K. M. Dwyer, C. N. Merz, A. Shorcore, & J. H. Dwyer: Leisure time physical activity and early atherosclerosis: The Los Angeles Atherosclerosis study. *American Journal of Medicine*. 115(1):19–25 (2003).

Ortega, F. B., J. R. Ruiz, M. J. Castillo, & M. Sjöström: Physical fitness in childhood and adolescence: A powerful marker of health. *International Journal of Obesity*. 32:1–11 (2008).

Owen, N., A. Bauman, & W. Brown: Too much sitting: A novel and important predictor of chronic disease risk? *British Journal of Sports Medicine*. 43(2):81–83 (2009).

Owen, N., G. N. Healy, C. E. Matthews, & D. W. Dunstan: Too much sitting: The population health science of sedentary behavior. *Exercise and Sport Sciences Reviews*. 38(3):105–113 (2010).

Pate, R. R., M. G. Davis, T. N. Robinson, E. J. Stone, T. L. McKenzie, & J. R. Young: Promoting physical activity in children and youth: A leadership role for schools. A Scientific statement from the American Health Association Council on Nutrition, Physical Activity, Metabolism (Physical Activity Committee) in collaborations with the Councils on Cardiovascular Disease in the Young and Cardiovascular Nursing. *Circulation*. 114:1214–1224 (2006).

Pfeiffer, M., C. Wenk, & P. C. Colombani: The influence of 30 minutes of light to moderate intensity cycling on postprandial lipemia. *European Journal of Cardiovascular Prevention and Rehabilitation*. 13(3):363–368 (2006).

Plowman, S. A.: Stress, hyperactivity, and health. *Quest*. 46:78–99 (1994).

Plowman, S. A.: Physical activity and physical fitness: Weighing the relative importance of each. *Journal of Physical Activity and Health*. 2:143–158 (2005).

Raitakari, O. T., K. V. K. Porkka, S. Taimela, R. Telama, L. Rasaneu, & J. S. A. Viikari: Effects of persistent physical activity and inactivity on coronary risk factors in children and young adults: The cardiovascular risk in young Finns study. *American Journal of Epidemiology*. 140(3):195–208 (1994).

Retnakaran, R., B. Zinman, P. W. Connelly, S. B. Harris, & A. J. G. Hanley: Nontraditonal cardiovascular risk factors in pediatric metabolic syndrome. *Journal of Pediatrics*. 148:176–182 (2006).

Ridker, P. M.: Clinical application of C-Reactive Protein for cardiovascular disease detection and prevention. *Circulation*. 107(3):363–369 (2003).

Ridker, P. M. & P. Libby: Risk factors for Atherothrombotic disease.. In Zipes, D. P., P. Libby, R. O. Bonow, & E. Braunwald (eds.): *Braunwald's Heart Disease: A Textbook of Cardiovascular Medicine* (7th edition). Philadelphia, PA: Elsevier Saunders, 939–958 (2005).

Roemmich, J. N., M. Lambiase, S. J. Salvy, & P. J. Horvath: Protective effect of interval exercise on psychophysiological stress reactivity in children. *Psychophysiology*. 46:852–861 (2009).

Roger, V. L., A. S. Go, D. M. Lloyd-Jones, E. J. Benjamin, J. D. Berry, W. B. Borden, et al.: Heart disease and stroke statistics—2012 update: A report from the American Heart Association. *Circulation*. 125(1): e2–e220 (2011).

Rowland, T. W.: Influence of physical activity and fitness on coronary risk factors in children: How strong an argument? *Pediatric Exercise Science*. 3(3):189–191 (1991).

Rowland, T. W.: Physical activity, fitness, and children. In: Bouchard, C., S. N. Blair, & W. L. Haskell (eds.): *Physical Activity and Health*. Champaign, IL: Human Kinetics, 260–270 (2006).

Rowland, T. W. & P. S. Freedson: Physical activity, fitness, and health in children: A close look. *Pediatrics*. 93(4):669–672 (1994).

Ruiz, J. R., J. Castro-Piñero, E. G. Artero, F. B. Ortega, M. Sjöström, J. Suni, & M. J. Castillo: Predictive validity of health-related fitness in youth: A systematic review. *British Journal of Sports Medicine*. 43:909–923 (2009).

Sacks, F. M.: The apolipoprotein story. *Atherosclerosis Supplements*. 7:23–27 (2006).

Schuler, G., R. Hainbrecht, G. Schlierf, J. Niebauer, K. Haver, J. Neumann, E. Hoberg, A. Drinkmann, F. Bacher, M. Grunze, & W. Kubler: Regular physical exercise and low-fat diet: Effects on progression of coronary artery disease. *Circulation*. 86:1–11 (1992).

Sher, L.: Type D personality: The heart, stress, and cortisol. *QJM*. 98(5):323–329 (2005).

Sigal, R. J., G. P. Kenny, D. H. Wasserman, C. Castaneda-Sceppa, & R. D. White: Physical Activity/Exercise and Type 2 Diabetes: A consensus statement from the American Diabetes Association. *Diabetes Care*. 29(6):1433–1438 (2006).

Simons-Morton, D. G.: Physical activity, fitness and blood pressure. In Izzo, J. L. & H. R. Black (eds.): *Council on High Blood Pressure Research, American Heart Association, Hypertension Primer* (2nd edition). Baltimore, MD: Lippincott, Williams & Wilkins, 259–262 (1999).

Sorichter, S., M. Martin, P. Julius, A. Schwirtz, M. Huonker, W. Luttman, S. Walterspacher, & A. Berg: Effects of unaccustomed and accustomed exercise on the immune response in runners. *Medicine & Science in Sports & Exercise*. 38(10):1739–1745 (2006).

Squires, R. W.: Coronary atherosclerosis. In Roitman, J. L. (ed.): *ACSM's Resource Manual for Guidelines for Exercise Testing and Prescription* (3rd edition). Philadelphia, PA: Lippincott, Williams & Wilkins, 225–230 (1998).

Squires, R. W. & W. L. Williams: Coronary atherosclerosis and acute myocardial infarction. In Durstine, J. L., A. C. King, P. L. Painter, J. L. Roctman, L. D. Zwiren, & W. L. Kenney (eds.): *American College of Sport Medicine Resource Manual for Guidelines for Exercise Testing and Prescription* (2nd edition). Philadelphia, PA: Lea & Febiger, 129–150 (1993).

Steele, R. M., S. Brage, K. Corder, N. J. Wareham, & U. Ekelund: Physical activity, cardiorespiratory fitness, and the metabolic syndrome in youth. *Journal of Applied Physiology*. 105:342–351 (2008).

Stensvold, D., A. E. Tjonna, E. Skaug, S. Aspenes, T. Stolen, U. Wisloff, & S. A. Slordahl: Strength training versus aerobic interval training to modify risk factors of metabolic syndrome. *Journal of Applied Physiology*. 108:804–810 (2010).

Stewart, K. J.: Exercise and hypertension. In Roitman, J. L. (ed.): *ACSM's Resource Manual for Guidelines for Exercise Testing and Prescription* (3rd edition). Philadelphia, PA: Lippincott, Williams & Wilkins, 275–280 (1998).

Strasser, B., U. Siebert, & W. Schobersberger: Resistance training in the treatment of the metabolic syndrome: A systematic review and meta-analysis of the effect of resistance training on metabolic clustering in patients with abnormal glucose metabolism. *Sports Medicine*. 40(5):397–415 (2010).

Strong, W. B., R. M. Malina, J. R. B. Cameron, S. R. Daniels, R. K. Dishman, B. Gutin, A. C. Hergenroeder, A. Must, P. A. Nixon, J. M. Pavarnik, T. Rowland, S. Trost, & F. Trudeau: Evidence based physical activity for school-age youth. *Journal of Pediatrics*. 146:732–737 (2005).

Summary of the Third Report of the National Cholesterol Education Program (NCEP): Expert panel on detection, evaluation and treatment of high blood cholesterol in adults (adult treatment panel II). *Journal of the American Medical Association*. 285:2486–2497 (2001).

Szymanski, L. M. & R. R. Pate: Effects of exercise intensity, duration, and time of day on fibrinolytic activity in physically active men. *Medicine and Science in Sports and Exercise*. 26(9):1102–1108 (1994).

Szymanski, L. M., R. R. Pate, & J. L. Durstine: Effect of maximal exercise and venous occlusion on fibrinolytic activity in physically active and inactive men. *Journal of Applied Physiology*. 77(5):2305–2310 (1994).

Tambalis, K., D. B. Panagiotakos, S. A. Kavouras, & L. S. Sidossis: Responses of blood lipids to aerobic, resistance, and aerobic with resistance exercise training: A systematic review of current evidence. *Angiology* 60(5):614–632 (2009).

Thomas, T. R. & T. LaFontaine: Exercise and lipoproteins. In Roitman, J. L. (ed.): *ACSM's Resource Manual for Guidelines for Exercise Testing and Prescription* (3rd edition). Philadelphia, PA: Lippincott, Williams & Wilkins, 294–301 (1998).

Tremblay, M. S., A. G. LeBlanc, M. E. Kho, T. J. Saunders, R. Larouche, R. C. Colley, G. Goldfield, & S. C. Gorber: Systematic review of sedentary behavior and health indicators in school-aged children and youth. *International Journal of Behavioral Nutrition and Physical Activity*. 8(1):98–120 (2011).

Twisk, J. W. R., H. C. G. Kemper, & W. van Mechelen: Prediction of cardiovascular disease risk factors later in life by physical activity and physical fitness in youth: General comments and conclusions. *International Journal of Sports Medicine*. 23:S44–49 (2002).

U.S. Department of Health and Human Services: *Physical Activity and Health: A Report of the Surgeon General*. Atlanta, GA: U.S. Department of Health and Human Services, Centers for Disease Control and Prevention, National Center for Chronic Disease Prevention and Health Promotion (1996).

U.S. Department of Health and Human Services: *The Fourth Report on the Diagnosis, Evaluation, and Treatment of High Blood Pressure in Children and Adolescents*. Atlanta, GA: U.S. Department of Health and Human Services (2005).

U.S. Department of Health and Human Services: *2008 Physical Activity Guidelines for Americans*. Atlanta, GA: U.S. Department of Health and Human Services, Centers for Disease Control and Prevention, National Center for Chronic Disease Prevention and Health Promotion (2008).

Ussher, M., R. West, R. Doshi, & A. K. Sampuran: Acute effect of isometric exercise on desire to smoke and tobacco withdrawal symptoms. *Human Psychopharmacology*. 21(1):39–46 (2006).

Van der Steeg, W. A., S. M. Boekholdt, E. A. Stein, K. El-Harchaoui, E. S. G. Stroes, M. S. Sandu, N. J. Wareham, J. W. Jukema, R. Luben, A. H. Zwinderman, J. J. P. Kastelein, & K. T. Khaw: Role of the apolipoprotein B-apolipoprotein A_I ratio in cardiovascular risk assessment: A case-control analysis in EPIC-Norfolk. *Annals of Internal Medicine*. 146:640–648 (2007).

Venkat Narayan, K. M.: The Metabolic Syndrome: Some second thoughts? *Clinical Diabetes*. 24(1):38–39 (2006).

Watts, K., T. W. Jones, E. A. Davis, & D. Green: Exercise training in obese children and adolescents: Current concepts. *Sports Medicine*. 35(5):375–392 (2005).

Wedderkopp, N., K. Froberg, H. S. Hansen, C. Riddoch, & L. B. Andersen: Cardiovascular risk factors cluster in children and adolescents with low physical fitness: The European Youth Heart Study (EYHS). *Pediatric Exercise Science*. 15(4):419–427 (2003).

Weiss, R. & I. Raz: Focus on childhood fitness, not just fatness. *Lancet*. 368:261–262 (2006).

Welk, G. J. & S. N. Blair: Physical activity protects against the health risks of obesity. *President's Council on Physical Fitness and Sports Research Digest*. 3(12):1–8 (2000).

Williams, P. T.: Relationship of distance run per week to coronary heart disease risk factors in 8283 male runners. *Archives of Internal Medicine*. 157:191–198 (1997).

Williams, P. T.: Physical fitness and activity as separate heart disease risk factors: A meta-analysis. *Medicine & Science in Sports & Exercise*. 33(5):754–761 (2001).

Womack, C. J., P. R. Nagelkirk, & A. M. Coughlin: Exercise-induced changes in coagulation and fibrinolysis in healthy populations and patients with cardiovascular disease. *Medicine & Science in Sports & Exercise*. 33(11):795–807 (2003).

Woo, K. M. & D. Magliano: Novel atherosclerotic risk factors and management. In Tonkin, A. (ed.): *Atherosclerosis and Heart Disease*. London: Martin Dunitz, 41–58 (2003).

Wood, P. D. & M. L. Stefanick: Exercise, fitness, and atherosclerosis. In Bouchard, C., R. J. Shephard, T. Stephens, J. R. Sutton, & B. D. McPherson (eds.): *Exercise, Fitness, and Health: A Consensus of Current Knowledge*. Champaign, IL: Human Kinetics, 409–423 (1990).

Wu, K. K.: Hemostatic tests in the prediction of atherothrombotic disease. *International Journal of Clinical and Laboratory Research*. 27:145–152 (1997).

Zimmet, P., K. Alberti, M. M. George, F. Kaufman, N. Silink, S. Arslanian, et al.: The metabolic syndrome in children and adolescents—an IDF consensus report. *Pediatric Diabetes*. 8:299–306 (2007).

Neuromuscular-Skeletal System Unit

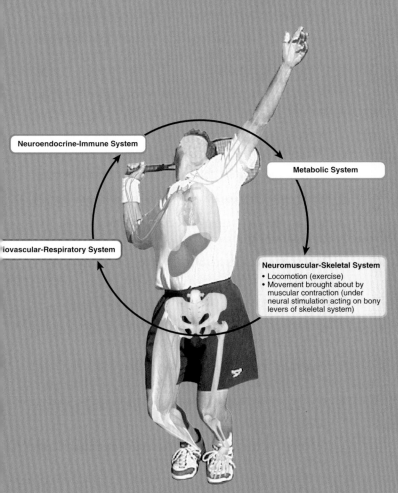

Neuroendocrine-Immune System

Metabolic System

Cardiovascular-Respiratory System

Neuromuscular-Skeletal System
- Locomotion (exercise)
- Movement brought about by muscular contraction (under neural stimulation acting on bony levers of skeletal system)

The contraction of skeletal muscles, pulling on the bony levers of the body, causes movement. The nervous system provides the electrical signal that causes the contraction of skeletal muscle. Hence, exercise is, by definition, the direct result of neuromuscular activity. This unit will address how the skeletal, muscular, and neural systems function together to bring about movement of any type, including exercise. These systems are not the only body systems that play a role in exercise and other movement, however. In order for muscles to contract, they must continually produce energy (ATP), which means that the metabolic system is also responsible for muscle contraction and, therefore, exercise. Furthermore, the cardiorespiratory system is responsible for supplying the muscle cells with oxygen, which supports the production of ATP necessary for continued contractions.

16

Skeletal System

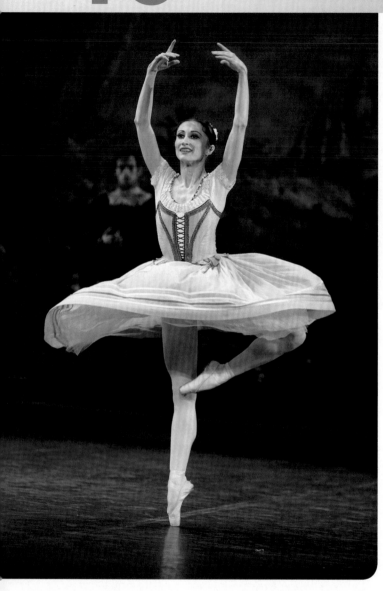

OBJECTIVES

After studying the chapter, you should be able to:

› Differentiate between cortical and trabecular bone.

› Define bone remodeling, and explain how bone mineral density is affected by the balance of bone resorption and deposition.

› Describe the hormonal control of bone remodeling and growth.

› Explain the criterion method of measuring bone mineral density.

› Identify age-related changes in bone mineral density.

› Identify male-female differences in bone mineral density.

› Discuss the factors involved in attaining peak bone mineral density.

› Discuss the factors involved in the rate of bone loss in adults.

› Describe the exercise response in skeletal tissue.

› Apply the training principles to the development of an exercise program to enhance bone health.

› Describe the skeletal adaptations that occur as a result of an exercise training program and with detraining.

› Describe the female athlete triad, particularly in relation to bone health.

› Describe micro- and macrotrauma skeletal injuries, and suggest ways of preventing them.

Introduction

The skeletal system includes the bones and cartilage that provide the framework for the muscles and organs of the body. Like other systems of the body, the skeletal system adapts to exercise training. A healthy skeleton is important for preventing sports-related injuries and major health problems, including osteoporosis.

Exercise physiologists are concerned with issues such as the maximization of peak bone mass, the prevention and treatment of osteoporosis, and the impact of heavy exercise training on the skeleton of growing prepubescent athletes. This chapter addresses these important issues after reviewing basic concepts of skeletal physiology and the influence of physical activity on bone tissue.

Skeletal Tissue

Bone tissue, also called osseous tissue, is a dynamic, living tissue that is constantly undergoing change. In fact, adults recycle 5–7% of their bone mass every week (Marieb, 2010). **Bone remodeling** (bone turnover) refers to the continual process of bone breakdown (resorption) and formation (deposition of new bone). Bone remodeling has important roles in regulating blood calcium levels and replacing old bone with new bone to ensure the integrity of the skeletal system. The mass and shape of bones depend largely on the stress placed on them. The more bones are stressed (by mechanical loading during physical activity), the more they increase in volume and mass, specifically at the site of mechanical loading. The concept that bone adapts to changes in mechanical loading is described by **Wolff's law** (Beck and Marcus, 1999).

Functions

The skeletal system provides a number of important structural and physiological functions. Structurally, the skeletal system provides rigid support and protection for vital organs and allows for locomotion. Physiologically, skeletal tissue provides a site for blood cell formation (hematopoiesis in bone marrow), plays a role in the immune function (providing the site for white blood cell formation), and serves as a dynamic storehouse for calcium and phosphate, which are essential for nerve conduction, heart and muscle contraction, blood clotting, and energy formation (Bailey and McColloch, 1990; Marieb, 2010).

Bone Remodeling The continual process of bone breakdown (resorption) and formation (deposition of new bone).

Wolff's Law Bone forms in areas of stress and is resorbed in areas of nonstress.

The ability of bone to perform its structural functions relates directly to its role in storing calcium. Because calcium is essential for many processes in the body, bone is broken down (resorbed) as needed to maintain blood calcium levels. The body sacrifices bone mineral (calcium) when it is needed to maintain blood calcium levels.

Regulation of Blood Calcium

As shown in **Figure 16.1**, the skeletal system (bone), the digestive system (stomach and intestines), and the urinary system (kidneys) operate together to regulate and maintain blood calcium levels. Adequate ingestion and absorption of calcium are required through the digestive system to provide the necessary calcium to be deposited in bone. In turn, because of the importance of calcium in so many vital processes of the body, bone mass is broken down to maintain blood calcium within normal limits (9–11 mg·dL^{-1}). The kidneys regulate blood calcium by filtering and reabsorbing it. The primary hormones involved in regulating blood calcium levels and bone remodeling are parathyroid hormone (PTH), calcitonin, and vitamin D (calcitriol).

Levels of Organization

Understanding the structure and physiology of the skeletal system helps one understand how the skeletal system responds to exercise and training.

Bones as Organs

The human body contains over 200 different bones joined together at articulations known as joints. Joints enable movement when muscles exert force on the bones. The skeleton is typically divided into two categories: the axial (or central) skeleton that includes the bones of the skull, vertebral column, and rib cage, and the appendicular (or peripheral) skeleton that includes the bones of the hips, shoulders, and extremities. Bones have several different shapes—long, short, flat, and irregular—and each shape is specific to its function. Furthermore, according to Wolff's law, a bone's shape reflects its response to the stress placed on it.

Bone Tissue

The two types of bone tissue are cortical and trabecular bone. Cortical bone, also called compact, dense, or lamellar bone, is densely packed. It makes up around 80% of the skeleton. Trabecular bone, also called spongy or cancellous bone, is more porous and is surrounded by cortical bone. Individual bones are composed of both types of bone tissue in varying relative proportions. **Table 16.1** presents relative percentages of trabecular and cortical bone tissue in various bones of the body. In general, bones of the axial skeleton have a much greater percentage of trabecular bone, whereas bones of the appendicular skeleton have a greater percentage of cortical bone. **Figure 16.2**

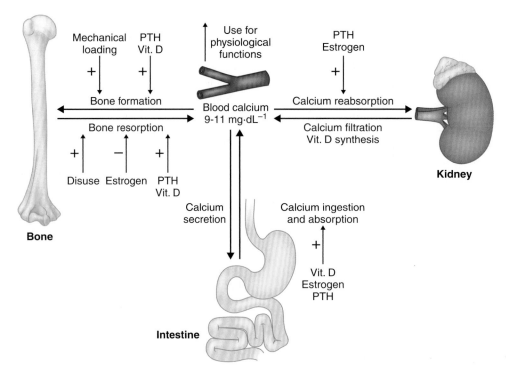

FIGURE 16.1 Regulation of Blood Calcium.
Blood calcium is a carefully controlled variable. Calcium is essential for the structure of bone (and teeth) and for numerous physiological functions (muscle contraction, nerve conduction, blood clotting). Blood calcium levels are maintained by the coordination of several systems, notably the digestive, urinary, skeletal, and hormonal systems. Bone loading affects bone formation and resorption. PTH = parathyroid hormone
Source: Modified from Borer, K. T.: Physical activity in the prevention and amelioration of osteoporosis in women; Interaction of mechanical, hormonal, and dietary factors. *Sports Medicine*. 35:779–830 (2005).

shows the humerus, a typical long bone. The shaft is composed primarily of cortical bone, and the epiphyses have a greater percentage of trabecular bone.

Cortical bone is composed of osteons, which are the functional units of bone (Haversian system). Osteons are organized into concentric layers of matrix called lamellae, which are surrounded by widely dispersed cells. The matrix, the intercellular space, is made up of organic and inorganic substances.

TABLE 16.1	Composition of Various Bones	
Measurement Site	**Cortical Percentage**	**Trabecular Percentage**
Calcaneus	5	95
Lumbar spine		
Anterior-posterior view	50	50
Lateral view	10	90
Proximal femur	60	40
Total body	80	20
Source: Highet, R. Athletic Amenorrhea: An update on etiology, complications and management. *Sports Medicine*. 7:82–108 (1989).		

Trabecular bone is composed of branching projections or struts, called trabeculae, which form a lattice-like network of interconnecting struts. Its appearance gives rise to another of its names, spongy bone. Trabecular bone has the same cells and matrix elements as cortical bone, but with more porosity. About 80–90% of the volume of cortical bone is calcified, while only 15–25% of trabecular bone is calcified (Baron, 1993). The remaining volume is occupied by bone marrow, blood vessels, and connective tissue. Cortical bone is best suited for structural support and protection, and trabecular bone is best suited for shock absorption and physiological functions.

Because of its large surface area, trabecular bone can remodel more rapidly than cortical bone. The greatest age-related loss of bone mineral density also occurs in trabecular bone. Therefore, most osteoporotic fractures occur in areas composed predominantly of trabecular bone (wrist, hip, and spine).

Bone Development

Bone development involves three processes: bone growth, bone modeling, and bone remodeling. Each process predominates at different times throughout an individual's life.

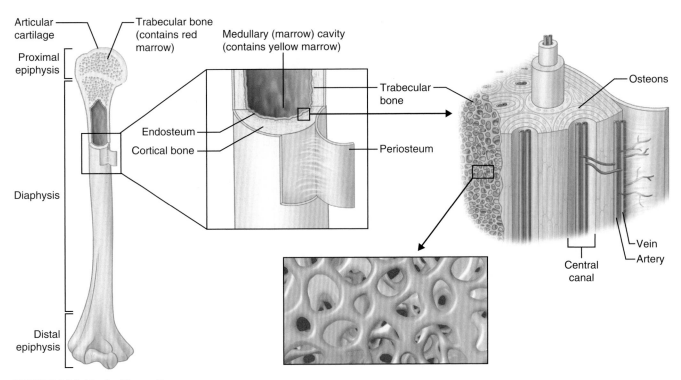

Articular cartilage
Proximal epiphysis
Diaphysis
Distal epiphysis

Trabecular bone (contains red marrow)
Medullary (marrow) cavity (contains yellow marrow)
Endosteum
Cortical bone

Trabecular bone
Periosteum

Osteons
Vein
Artery
Central canal

FIGURE 16.2 Typical Long Bone.
Structure and cross-sectional view of bone.

Growth

Bone growth refers to size increase caused by an increasing number of bone cells (Frost, 1991a). There are two types of bone growth. Appositional growth is an increase in thickness or mass. Longitudinal growth occurs at the epiphyseal plate until a person reaches adult stature. This is an area of interest because of concerns that excessive exercise might stunt a child's growth.

The longitudinal growth of bones results from the growth of cartilage, which is later replaced by bone. While growing, bone is also remodeling itself—that is, changing its shape and thickness. Bone growth and remodeling are distinct but closely related processes. In general, growth refers to the longitudinal growth of bone, and remodeling involves the balance between bone resorption and bone formation. If bone formation exceeds resorption, this process would also represent growth.

Modeling

Bone modeling is the process of altering the shape of bone and adjusting bone strength through bone resorption and bone formation (Frost, 1991a; Khan et al., 2001c). Micromodeling involves the microscopic

level of cell organization that occurs during formation; it determines what kind of tissue will be formed (Frost, 1991a). Macromodeling controls if, when, and where new tissue will form or old tissue will be removed. This process ensures that the bone's shape matches its role (Frost, 1988, 1991a,b; Khan et al., 2001c; Lanyon, 1989; Marcus, 1987). Modeling is largely responsible for bone growth during the years in which the skeleton is growing.

Remodeling

Bone remodeling involves a continual process of bone turnover, maintenance, replacement, and repair (Frost, 1991a). It reflects the balance between the coupled processes of bone resorption and bone formation. This ongoing process occurs because of the coupled actions of bone cells, with osteoclasts responsible for bone resorption and osteoblasts responsible for bone formation. Remodeling occurs in response to stress on the skeleton throughout the adult years. Physical activity influences bone strength and mass through remodeling, which is accomplished largely because of the activity of bone cells.

BONE CELLS The three types of bone cells are osteoclasts, osteoblasts, and osteocytes. These cells are the living part of bone. Although the cells represent a small fraction—less than 2% (Teitelbaum, 1993)—of the total composition of bone, they are responsible for its remodeling.

Bone Modeling The process of altering the shape of bone by bone resorption and bone deposition.

Osteoclasts are large, multinucleated bone cells that cause the resorption of bone tissue. Osteoclasts secrete enzymes that disintegrate bone matrix. As the bone is degraded, the mineral salts (primarily calcium and phosphate) dissolve and move into the bloodstream. **Osteoblasts** are bone cells that cause the deposition of bone tissue. Also called bone-forming cells, osteoblasts produce an organic bone matrix that becomes calcified and hardens as minerals are deposited in it. Hardening of the bone matrix is known as ossification. **Osteocytes,** which are mature osteoblasts surrounded by calcified bone, help regulate the process of bone remodeling. Osteocytes appear to initiate the process of calcification.

The actions of osteoclasts and osteoblasts are coupled; they work together to remodel bone. Osteoclasts must first cause bone resorption before the osteoblasts can form new bone. **Figure 16.3** outlines the major events of a bone-remodeling cycle (Marcus, 1987; Parfitt, 1987; Teitelbaum, 1993). From the resting phase (**Figure 16.3A**), the osteoclasts are stimulated and cause the resorption of bone, forming a cavity (**Figure 16.3B** and **C**). Osteoblasts then appear and deposit bone matrix where the cavity exists (**Figure 16.3D**). The matrix is called osteoid until it is calcified (**Figure 16.3E**). Calcification of the new bone occurs as calcium and phosphate minerals are deposited in the osteoid (**Figure 16.3F**). The bone then returns to the resting or quiescent phase.

Bone remodeling may result in greater bone mass, the same bone mass, or a reduction in bone mass. Through young adulthood, typically, more bone is formed than is resorbed, increasing bone mass. This increased mass strengthens the bone and accounts for the increase in bone mineral density (BMD) that commonly occurs during this period of life. When bone remodeling is in equilibrium, the amount of bone resorbed equals the amount of bone formed; thus, bone mineral density remains relatively constant. In older adults and those with certain diseases, the amount of bone resorbed is greater than the amount of bone formed, decreasing bone mineral density.

The remodeling of bone provides for skeletal growth and involves a constant turnover of bone throughout life. Bone remodeling is a complex process regulated by hormonal and local factors (Canalis, 1990).

HORMONAL CONTROL Bone remodeling reflects the interrelationship between the structural and physiological functions of bone. Calcium is necessary not only to provide structural integrity of bone but is also essential for the proper functioning of the heart, skeletal muscles, and nervous tissue. Only about 1 g of calcium is present in the extracellular fluid of the body, compared to approximately 1150 g of calcium present in bone tissue (Bailey and McColloch, 1990; Khan et al., 2001c).

Excess calcium in the blood leads to the release of calcitonin (from the thyroid gland), which causes deposition

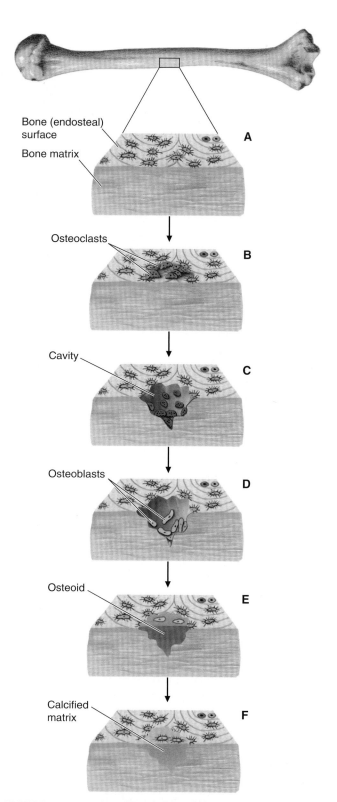

FIGURE 16.3 Stages of Bone Remodeling.
A. Resting cell surface. **B.** Osteoclasts (multinucleated) are activated and begin dissolving bone (minerals released to the blood). **C.** Osteoclasts produce a cavity in the blood matrix. **D.** Osteoblasts appear. **E.** Osteoblasts secrete the osteoid (uncalcified matrix). **F.** The matrix is calcified.

TABLE 16.2 Effect of Calcitonin and PTH on Bone and Blood Calcium Levels

Hormone	Stimulus for Release	Effect on Bone	Effect on Blood Calcium Levels
Calcitonin	Increased blood calcium levels	Bone deposition (increased calcium)	Decreased blood calcium levels
Parathyroid hormone (PTH)	Decreased blood calcium levels	Bone resorption (decreased calcium)	Increased blood calcium levels

of calcium in the bone. This deposition decreases the blood calcium level and increases bone mineral density. Conversely, when the blood calcium level drops below normal, parathyroid hormone stimulates osteoclast activity, causing calcium to be released from its storage site, bone. This release of calcium from the bone causes the blood calcium level to increase and bone mineral density to decrease. **Table 16.2** summarizes the effect of calcitonin and PTH on bone and blood calcium levels. Vitamin D (calcitriol) is important for the absorption of calcium from the intestines. Thus, it leads to an increased blood level of calcium.

Other hormones that play an important role in skeletal health are the sex steroids (estrogen and testosterone) and growth hormone. These hormones stimulate the protein formation necessary for bone growth and are responsible for the eventual closure of the epiphyseal plate, which determines bone length and thus a person's height (Bailey and McColloch, 1990). Estrogen promotes calcium retention and acts as an inhibiting agent of parathyroid hormone. The loss of the protective role of estrogen on the skeletal system after menopause or during secondary amenorrhea has important consequences for females. Decreased estrogen causes increased bone resorption. Growth hormone and insulin-like growth factor (IGF-1) also play an important role in bone formation and remodeling in children. Hormones are themselves stimulated by other factors, including physical activity and nutritional status.

Measurement of Bone Health

Bone strength is determined by bone mass, external geometry, and internal microstructure (Beck and Marcus, 1999; Frost, 1997; Heaney et al., 2000). Because it is difficult to quantify external geometry and microstructure, measures of bone mass and bone mineral density are most often used to describe bone strength. Bone strength refers to

Osteoclasts Bone cells that cause the resorption of bone tissue (bone-destroying cells).

Osteoblasts Bone cells that cause the deposition of bone tissue (bone-forming cells).

Osteocytes Mature osteoblasts surrounded by calcified bone that help regulate the process of bone remodeling.

bone's ability to withstand forces that may cause fracture. Bone strength is largely influenced by bone mass. A less dense bone will break with less force (Heaney et al., 2000). *Bone mineral content (BMC)* refers to the absolute amount of calcium and phosphate salts and is measured in grams. The calcium and phosphate salts are responsible for the hardness of the bone matrix. *Bone mineral density (BMD)* is defined as the relative value of bone mineral per measured bone area, expressed as grams per centimeter squared ($g \cdot cm^{-2}$) or milligrams per centimeter cubed ($mg \cdot cm^{-3}$), depending on the technology used to measure area.

Accurate measures of bone mineral content and bone mineral density can be obtained only in laboratory or clinical settings, primarily because of the cost of equipment and safety considerations. Nonetheless, these measurements have dramatically increased the information available to researchers, clinicians, and those in fitness professions. At present, no field tests validly predict bone mineral density.

Dual-Energy X-ray Absorptiometry

Dual-energy X-ray absorptiometry (DXA) is the standard method of measuring BMD for research and clinical purposes (American College of Sports Medicine, 2004). DXA uses an X-ray beam to measure regional and whole-body mineral content (**Figure 16.4**) and provides an areal bone mineral density (aBMD) value. Areal

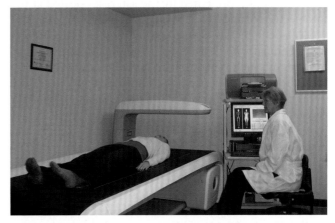

FIGURE 16.4 Dual-Energy X-ray Absorptiometer.
Subject is positioned for a total body scan.

FIGURE 16.5 Computer-Generated Printout of Whole-Body BMD for Healthy Young Female.
A. Whole body BMD scan. **B.** Graphical presentation of total body BMD compared to reference values and age. **C.** Print out of regional BMD values and compared to reference values.
Source: Data from the University of Connecticut Health Center, Osteoporosis Research Center.

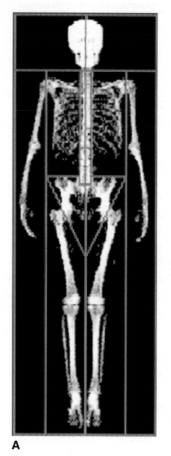

A

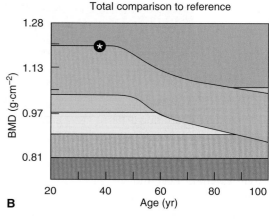

Total comparison to reference

B

Bone results			
Standard analysis – DEXA calibration			
Region	BMD g.cm^{-2}	% young adult	% age matched
Head	2.323	—	—
Arms	0.977	116	117
Legs	1.229	106	108
Trunk	0.971	106	108
Ribs	0.711	—	—
Pelvis	1.217	110	112
Spine	1.289	113	116
Thoracic	1.185	—	—
Lumbar	1.507	—	—
Total	1.197	106	108

C

BMD provides a two-dimensional measure of density. **Figure 16.5** shows a computer-generated printout of whole-body BMD and various regions of the body for a 37-year-old active female. **Figure 16.5A** represents regions of the body individually analyzed for BMD. The total body BMD is compared with standard references in **Figure 16.5B**. The blue area represents an average range across the age span of 20–100 years. Notice that the individual in the example is above average for total body BMD as represented by the asterisk (located at the intersection of age 37 years and BMD of 1.197 g·cm^{-2}).

Regional BMDs are shown in **Figure 16.5C** along with comparisons with young adult normative data. Notice that each region of the body has a unique BMD value because of the varying composition of bones. For example, the legs have a BMD of 1.229 g·cm^{-2}, whereas the pelvis has a BMD of 1.217 g·cm^{-2}. These values correspond to 106% and 110% of young adult values, respectively. In addition to these total body scans, clinicians and researchers often measure BMD at specific, clinically relevant sites, such as the hip or spine, where osteoporotic fractures are more likely. When scanning just a small area (e.g., a hip or spine), a better quality scan results. **Figure 16.6A** and **B** present a hip and spine scan of an active, older woman. These site-specific scans enable researchers to investigate differences in bone mineral

density at various sites, among various individuals, and as a result of adaptation to long-term exercise training.

Bone mineral density derived from DXA is the basis of the operational definitions of osteopenia and osteoporosis. BMD is normally distributed and is often expressed in standard deviation (SD) units related to its T or Z distribution. The T distribution has a mean score of zero (0). **Osteopenia** is a condition of decreased bone mineral density defined as a T-score of –1 to –2.5. This means a BMD value greater than one standard deviation below (but not more than 2.5 SD below) values for young, normal adults (25–35 years, sex-matched). **Osteoporosis** is a condition of porosity and decreased BMD defined as a T-score >–2.5, indicating a BMD more than 2.5 SD below values for young, normal adults (WHO, 1994). *Established osteoporosis* is the term for the condition of osteoporosis, as defined above, plus one or more fractures (Kanis et al., 1993). **Figure 16.7** indicates the relative risk of fracture at the spine, hip, and forearm based on T-scores.

The International Society for Clinical Densitometry (ISCD) recommends using T-scores for evaluating postmenopausal women and Z-scores for adolescents and premenopausal women. Both T- and Z-scores represent SDs from the average score, but the comparison group for Z-scores is age- and sex-matched while the T-score

Use of DXA to Measure BMD and Estimate Bone Strength

It is well established that the BMD of gymnasts' legs is greater than age-matched controls, yet bone health depends on both BMD and bone strength. A team of researchers from Canada, the United States, and Australia conducted a study to investigate structural variables of bone and estimate bone strength based on values derived from DXA measurements. They measured BMD and indices of bone strength of the femur in premenarcheal gymnasts and age-matched, physically active controls.

The researchers measured cross-sectional area (CSA) (believed to reflect the strength of bone), calculated an index of bending strength (how much bending force can be applied to a bone before it breaks), and derived a strength index (SI). Their goal was to find measures derived from current technology that provides information about bone strength beyond what can be determined by bone mass alone.

As shown in the figure below, when adjusted for body size, the gymnasts had greater BMD, axial strength, and bending strength. The gymnasts also had a greater CSA and strength index (SI) at the femoral shaft than age-matched controls.

These results suggest that the femur of gymnasts adapts to the loading imposed by competitive gymnastic activity. The data also suggest that DXA measures may be able to provide measures of bone strength in addition to measures of bone mineral density.

Source: Faulkner, R. A., M. R. Forwood, T. J. Beck, J. C. Mafukidze, K. Russell, & W. Wallace: Strength indices of the proximal femur and shaft in prepubertal female gymnasts. *Medicine & Science in Sports & Exercise.* 35(3):513–518 (2003).

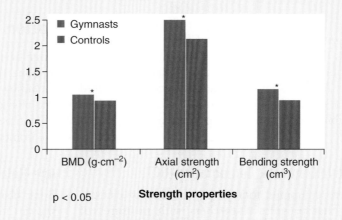

$p < 0.05$

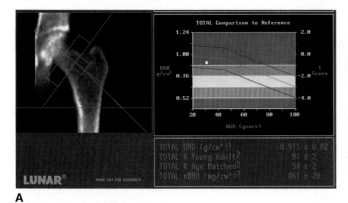

FIGURE 16.6 DXA Scan.
A. Hip (head of femur). **B.** Spine.

Osteopenia A condition of decreased bone mineral density (BMD) defined as a T-score of −1 to −2.5, which means a BMD value greater than one standard deviation (SD) below (but not more than 2.5 SD below) values for normal young adults.

Osteoporosis A condition of porosity and decreased bone mineral density defined as a T-score below −2.5, which indicates a BMD greater than 2.5 SD below values for young, normal adults.

compares with a single sex-matched young adult value. The ISCD defines a Z-score above −2 (<2 SDs below average) as a BMD "within the expected range for age." Z-scores of −2 or lower (more than 2 SDs below average) are defined as "below the expected range for age." Z-score comparisons with age-matched peers are especially important for individuals under the age of 20 years because they are still accumulating bone (Leib et al., 2004).

In addition to measures of bone mineral density, DXA measures have been used to estimate bone strength

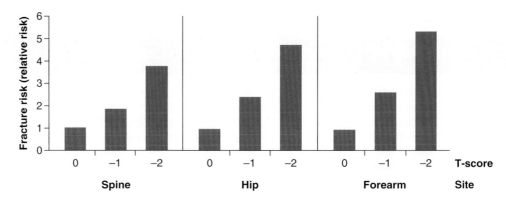

(see Focus on Research Box). As discussed earlier, *bone strength* refers to the ability of bone to resist fracture and is determined by bone mass, physical properties of bone, and bone geometry. Variables thought to reflect bone strength include directly measured variables, such as the cross-sectional area, and calculated variables, such as a bending index and a strength index.

Quantitative Computed Tomography (QCT)

Quantitative computed tomography (QCT) is a newer technique that provides researchers with measures of bone health in addition to BMD (**Figure 16.8**). QCT can determine the volumetric bone mineral density (vBMD) of trabecular and cortical bone. Volumetric BMD is a measure of three-dimensional volume. Since QCT appears more sensitive to bone changes than DXA, QCT measures will likely be used increasingly to assess bone adaptations to exercise (Khan et al., 2001c; Polidoulis et al., 2012).

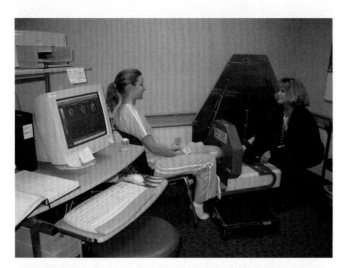

FIGURE 16.8 A peripheral QCT (pQCT) is Used to Determine the Volumetric Bone Mineral Density (vBMD) of Trabecular and Cortical Bone.

Factors Influencing Bone Health

Bone health is related to the mass, strength, and stiffness of bone (Burr, 2011) and is influenced by many factors, including nutrition, hormonal status, body composition, and physical activity. Bone health is largely related to peak bone mass attainment and bone loss rate. Both processes are influenced by age and sex.

Age-Related Changes in Bone

Bone changes in density throughout life. **Figure 16.9** shows the characteristic pattern between bone mass and age for males and females (Ott, 1990). The first 20 years of life are characterized by active growth in bone mass. About 25% of the final adult bone is accumulated from approximately 11.5 to 13.5 years (around the age of menarche) for girls and 13.0–15.0 (peri- to postpuberty) for boys. This approximates the amount of bone lost in females in postmenopausal years (MacKelvie et al., 2002). The skeletal consolidation phase occurs in early adulthood, and peak bone mass is generally attained by 30 years. Shortly after attainment of peak bone mass, bone mass loss begins. After a rapid-loss phase, the rate of bone loss decreases (Teitelbaum, 1993). The theoretical curves shown in **Figure 16.9** assume the attainment of full genetic potential. If environmental factors such as exercise, nutrition, and hormonal status are inadequate, full genetic potential for bone mass may not be realized, increasing fracture risk (Heaney et al., 2000). The specific affect of aging is difficult to know precisely because bone health is affected by many factors, especially physical activity level and nutritional patterns (Tucker et al., 2002; Wohl et al., 2000).

Male-Female Differences in Bone Mineral Density

BMD varies between males and females. As shown in **Figure 16.9**, total BMD changes throughout the life span for both sexes. Bone mineral density increases throughout childhood and early adult life for both sexes, but the peak bone mineral density attained is less in females than males (Ott, 1990).

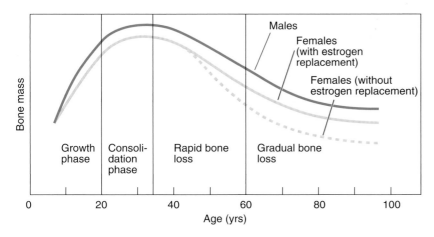

FIGURE 16.9 Comparison of BMD for Females and Males.
Bone mineral density values change throughout the life span. Female values are influenced by hormonal status.

In addition to differences in total BMD, BMD also varies between males and females according to measurement site. **Table 16.3** compares adult BMD at various sites for men and women (Beck and Marcus, 1999).

At menopause, females lose the protective influence of estrogen, and bone loss accelerates if estrogen is not pharmacologically replaced. The loss of the protective influence of estrogen explains the prevalence of osteoporotic fractures in older postmenopausal women.

Development of Peak Bone Mass

Peak bone mass is attained during the mid-30s in both sexes, although 95% of peak bone mass is achieved by age 20 (Beck and Marcus, 1999). The individual's peak bone mass developed in young adulthood is influenced by mechanical factors, nutrition, hormonal levels, and genetics (Heaney et al., 2000; Ott, 1990). Mechanical factors include physical activity and gravity. These forces are generally considered necessary stimuli for bone formation and growth (Frost, 1997). Studies done with astronauts and with individuals confined to bed rest clearly show a loss of bone mineral density when bone is not subjected to the force of gravity.

Although additional research is needed to specify exercise prescriptions for optimal skeletal development, children and adolescents should be encouraged to engage in physical activity to promote bone health along with other positive changes and development within the body. Specifically for bone development, children and adolescents should be encouraged to participate in high-impact activities (Greene and Naughton, 2006; Grimston et al., 1993; Khan et al., 2001b; Macdonald et al., 2007; Vicente-Rodriguez, 2006). Some have suggested that the time period of puberty is particularly important for the development of bone mass (Ackerman and Misra, 2011; MacKelvie et al., 2002). For girls, peak BMC velocity occurs on the average at about age 12.7 years (the average age of menarche); for boys it occurs about 1.5 years later. Of course, maturational age varies widely among individuals. Specific exercises for bone development are generally important from approximately 9 to 16 years.

Adequate nutrition is necessary for developing a strong skeletal system. Dietary calcium is essential for bone health but is often deficient in young athletes. **Table 16.4** shows the recommended Dietary Reference Intake (DRI) of calcium. Note that these are adequate intake (AI) values, that is, recommended amounts based on observed or experimentally determined approximations from healthy individuals when a more specific recommended dietary allowance (RDA) has not been determined. Unfortunately, many individuals fall well below the recommendations, particularly young women concerned about weight control. For instance, young women may eliminate dairy products from their diet because they are high in fat. But dairy products also are an excellent source of calcium. Thus, while trying to maintain weight, these athletes may be negatively affecting the attainment of peak bone mass. Exercise professionals must consider the need for dietary calcium when counseling young athletes (particularly females) about weight management (American College of Sports Medicine, 2004; Loucks, 1988). The availability of the many low-fat dairy products makes including calcium in the diet easier.

TABLE 16.3	Comparison of Adult Male and Female Bone Mineral Density at Various Sites	
	Males	**Females**
Hip (gm·cm⁻²)	1.033	0.942
Spine (L2–L4) (gm·cm⁻²)	1.115	1.079
Radius (gm·cm⁻²)	0.687	0.579

Source: Beck, B. & R. Marcus: Skeletal effects of exercise in men. In Orwoll, E. S. (ed.): *Osteoporosis in Men: The Effect of Gender on Skeletal Health.* San Diego, CA: Academic Press, 129–155 (1999).

TABLE 16.4 Recommendations for Dietary Intake

Age Group	Dietary Reference Intakes (AIs) (mg)
Infant	
Birth–6 mo	210
6 mo–1 yr	270
Children	
1–3 yr	500
4–8 yr	800
Adolescents and Young Adults	
9–18 yr	1300
Men	
19–50 yr	1000
>50 yr	1200
Women	
19–50 yr	1000
>50 yr	1200
Pregnant or nursing	1000–1300

Source: National Academy of Sciences. "Dietary Reference Intakes (DRIs): Recommended Intakes for Individuals, Elements." Food and Nutrition Board, Institute of Medicine, National Academies. 2004.

As mentioned previously, adequate estrogen levels are also needed to attain peak bone mass. This is discussed further in relation to older adults and female athletes later in this chapter.

Finally, there are genetically determined limits to the amount of BMD that an individual can attain. The only way to achieve genetic potential, however, is to pay careful attention to modifiable factors: nutritional status, hormonal status, and activity level.

Exercise Response

Physical activity increases mechanical forces on bones. This leads to physiological changes in bone cells that allow bone to be modeled and remodeled. **Mechanotransduction** is the process by which a bone responds to a mechanical force on it. Mechanical forces are converted into biological signals (primarily by osteocytes) that signal bone remodeling by osteoblast activity and osteoclast resorption (Bonnet and Ferrari, 2010). As illustrated in **Figure 16.10**, physical activity applies a mechanical force (e.g., bending or deformation) to bone. Bending causes both *compressive* and *tensile* stress that alters the hydrostatic pressure in different

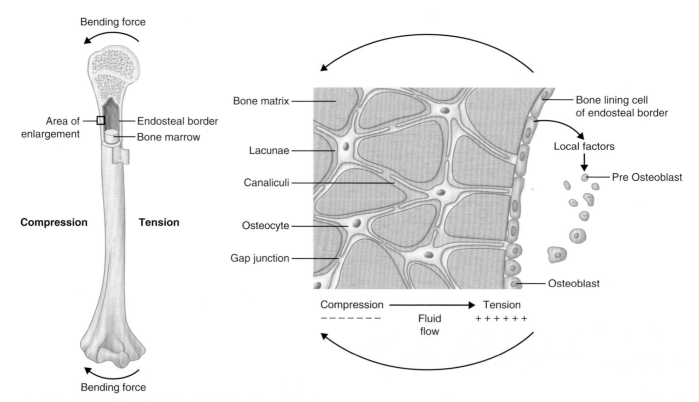

FIGURE 16.10 Effect of Bending Force on Bone Physiology.
Bending creates both compressive and tensile forces. Compression creates high hydrostatic pressure that facilitates movement of bone fluid to the area of tension, which has low hydrostatic pressure. The movement of fluid through the lacunocanalicular system aids in nutrient delivery and waste removal and plays an important role in the osteogenic response to loading.
Source: Modified from Zernicke, R. F., G. R. Wohl, & J. M. LaMothe: The Skeletal-Articular System. In Tipton, C. M., M. N. Sawka, C. A. Tate, & R. L. Terjung (eds.): *ACSM's Advanced Exercise Physiology*. Baltimore, MD: Lippincott Williams & Wilkins, 106 (2006).

regions of the bone tissue, causing movement of fluid in this tissue. Fluid flows through the small canals and spaces within the bone matrix (lacunocanalicular system) and around osteocytes; this flow aids in the transport of nutrients and waste. This fluid movement also exerts a shear stress that may stimulate an osteogenic response, resulting in the formation of new bone.

Physical activity causes specific changes in bone physiology within minutes. Soon after a mechanical load is placed on bone cells, they release prostacyclin; this is followed within minutes by an increase in enzymes related to metabolism. Six to twenty-four hours after activity, RNA synthesis increases. There is evidence of increased collagen and mineral deposition on the bone surface within 3–5 days after a bout of loading (Khan et al., 2001c). However, the relationship between levels of blood biomarkers of bone turnover and structural and mineral adaptations of bone is still not fully understood (Lester et al., 2009; Maïmoun and Sultan, 2011).

Application of the Training Principles

Bone's adaptation to physical activity depends on the type of loading. In other words, the response is specific to the type of activity performed. Stress (or load) refers to the external force applied to a bone, whereas strain (deformation) refers to changes in the bone tissue. Adaptations in any given physiological system are dependent on the extent to which exercise stresses that system. For instances, adaptations in the cardiovascular system depend on the intensity, duration, and frequency of predominantly aerobic exercise training. Similarly adaptations in skeletal muscle depend on the load, number of reps, rest period, number of sets, and frequency that load-bearing exercise is performed. The adaptation to a mechanical load (physical activity) in bone depends on the strain magnitude, strain rate, distribution of load on the bone, and number of cycles (Khan et al., 2001a). *Strain magnitude* is the amount of relative change in bone length under mechanical loading. *Strain rate* is the speed at which strain develops and releases. *Distribution of load* refers to how strain occurs across a section of bone. *Strain cycles* are the number of load repetitions.

Mechanotransduction The process by which a bone responds to a mechanical force on it.

Weight-Bearing Exercise A movement performed in which the body weight is supported by muscles and bones.

Non–Weight-Bearing Exercise A movement performed in which the body weight is supported or suspended and thereby not working against the pull of gravity.

The *mechanostat theory*, shown in **Figure 16.11**, suggests that bone adapts to set points of *minimal effective strain (MES)*. This theory suggests that a control system operates in which a MES is necessary to maintain bone and that a higher MES must be surpassed to overload bone appropriately for positive adaptations (increased bone mineral density and strength). Above the repair MES, bone enters a state of overuse. In the pathological overuse zone, bone suffers from microdamage, and woven (unorganized) bone is added as part of the repair process, leading to increased bone mass but not bone strength (Khan et al., 2001a).

The precise type and amount of activity for enhancing and maintaining bone health is not fully known at present. However, several recommendations can be made based on the mechanostat theory and research. The overall goals of physical activity relative to skeletal health are to (a) increase peak bone mass in adolescents, (b) minimize age-related bone loss, and (c) prevent falls and fractures (American College of Sports Medicine, 2004).

Specificity

The specificity principle applies to the particular bones being stressed, the composition of the bone being stressed (cortical versus trabecular), and the type of activity being performed. Research data suggest that the type of exercise or activity performed greatly influences skeletal adaptations. **Weight-bearing exercise** refers to movement in which the body weight is supported by muscles and bones, thereby working against gravity. **Non–weight-bearing exercise,** in contrast, refers to movement in which the body is supported or suspended and thereby not working against the pull of gravity. Weight-bearing or impact-loading activities, such as running, gymnastics, stair climbing, volleyball, and resistance training, are more likely to stimulate increased bone mass than non–weight-bearing activities, such as swimming and cycling (American College of Sports Medicine, 2004; Dalsky, 1993; Duncan et al., 2002; Grimston et al., 1993; Proctor et al., 2002). The best activity is chosen based on the individual's health and preference. When considering exercise for individuals with low bone mineral content, the risk of falling and causing a fracture is a major concern. Activities with a high risk of falls or collisions should not be recommended for certain populations, such as older adults. **Table 16.5** provides general guidelines for types of activities appropriate for various groups (American College of Sports Medicine, 2004; Dalsky, 1993).

Because dynamic resistance training is associated with positive adaptations in skeletal tissue as well as muscular fitness, exercise physiologists generally recommend this type of exercise for maintaining both muscular and skeletal health (American College of Sports Medicine, 2004; Layne and Nelson, 1999). Loading seems to have a localized effect (*Wolff's law*); thus, specific sites can be isolated for impact. Conversely, a

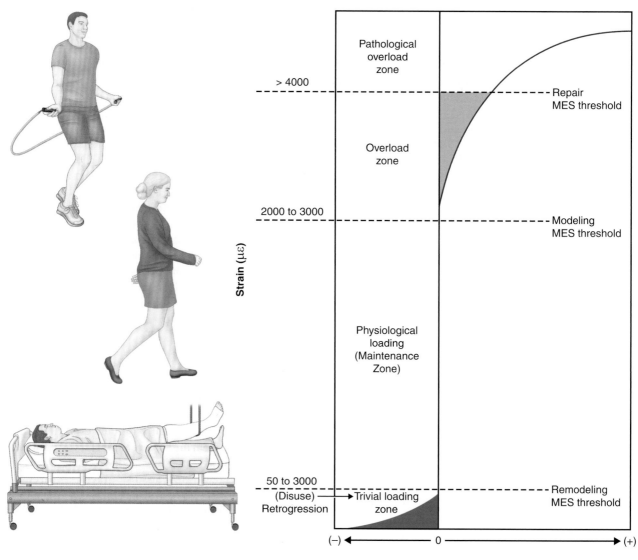

FIGURE 16.11 The Mechanostat Theory Relating Strain to Bone Mass.
MES = minimal effective strain
Source: Modified from Forwood, M. R. & C. H. Turner: Skeletal adaptations to mechanical usage: results from tibial loading studies in rats. *Bone*. 17:1975–2055 (1995).

TABLE 16.5	Recommended Activities for Skeletal Health			
	Children and Young Adults	**Adults, Premenopausal**	**Adults, Below-Normal BMD**	**Adults, Very Low BMD**
Goal	To attain peak bone mass	To slow the rate of bone loss and prevent musculoskeletal injury	To decrease risk of injury and/or slow rate of bone loss	To avoid injury
Type of activity	High-impact-loading movements Dynamic resistance exercise	Moderate-impact-loading movements Dynamic resistance exercise	Low- to moderate-impact-loading movements	Low-impact-loading movements
Examples	Sprinting, jumping, track and field, volleyball, basketball, gymnastics, soccer, weight training, rope skipping	Walking, jogging, running, hiking, stair climbing, stepping (machines), dancing, weight training, rope skipping, skiing	Stair climbing (machine), hiking, cross-country skiing, weight training	Walking, water aerobics, swimming, stationary cycling

Proposed "Osteogenic Index" to Measure the Effectiveness of Exercise on Bone Formation

Some researchers think that bone cells exhibit a desensitization when mechanical loading sessions are extended. Turner and Robling (2003) developed an "osteogenic index" (OI) to determine the effectiveness of the stimulation for bone formation based on the number of repetitions of high-impact exercise (such as jumping) per session and per week. This is presented in the figure below.

In this figure the cycles·wk^{-1} refers to the number of jumps completed. Such mild-impact loading represents three times the body weight. The dashed horizontal line represents the OI generated by 20 minutes of walking 5 d·wk^{-1} (800 load cycles per leg at 1.1 times body weight). According to this instrument, the OI increases threefold if the exercise is administered 5 d·wk^{-1} as opposed to 1 d·wk^{-1}. Clearly, based on this tool, adding more sessions per week improved the OI more than lengthening the exercise session by the number of jump cycles. Furthermore, the OI is increased as much as an additional 50% if the

daily exercise is divided into two shorter sessions separated by 8 hours. However, dividing the exercises into three sessions separated by 4 hours does not achieve a better OI. If the theory proposed by these researchers proves correct and the OI is a valuable tool for measuring bone stimulation, then load-induced bone formation would be

enhanced by regimens that incorporate rest periods between short vigorous bouts. For example, running short sprints should build more bone than an endurance run.

Source: Turner, C. H., & A. G. Robling: Designing exercise regimens to increase bone strength. *Exercise and Sport Sciences Reviews.* 31(1):45–50 (2003).

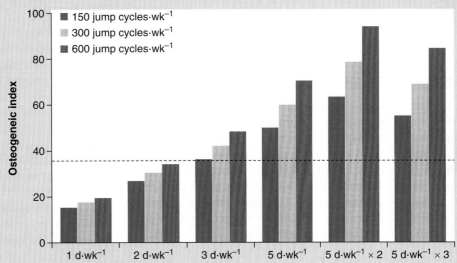

general dynamic resistance program that works all the major muscles of the body should benefit the total skeleton. Note that bone tissue does not appear to respond to static resistance exercise (Turner and Robling, 2003).

The Check Your Comprehension box provides you the opportunity to apply the information presented in this section. Check your answer in Appendix C.

CHECK YOUR COMPREHENSION

Use Table 16.5 to answer the following questions.

1. What type of activities would you recommend for your 45-year-old aunt who has just learned that she has low BMD? How is this program consistent with the goals for this population?

2. Because of your aunt's diagnosis of low BMD, what physical activities and dietary recommendations would you give to your 15-year-old cousin (your aunt's daughter)? Why?

Overload

As mentioned earlier, weight-bearing exercises result in positive skeletal adaptations. As shown in **Figure 16.11**, the threshold for a stimulus that initiates new bone formation is termed the minimal effective strain (MES) for remodeling (Frost, 1997). A load or force that exceeds this threshold and is repeated a sufficient number of times is thought to cause osteoblasts to secrete osteoid and lead to the formation of new bone. The MES for bone modeling, and thus the impact load necessary to induce positive skeletal adaptations in humans, is not precisely known, but the stimulus must include forces considerably greater than those of habitual activity. There is strong evidence that weight-bearing, impact-loading exercises can lead to an increase in bone mineral density in children and adolescents and also decrease the age-related loss of bone mineral density in adulthood (American College of Sports Medicine, 2004; Borer, 2005; Ernst, 1998).

Impact loads, and thus the strain applied to bones, can be manipulated by increasing repetitions or by increasing the strain magnitude as measured by ground reaction force or joint force. For example, running loads bones by high repetition, whereas rope jumping overloads the bones primarily by intensity (strain magnitude). For adaptations in skeletal tissue, intensity is apparently more important than repetition (Beck and Marcus, 1999).

Until the amount of exercise needed to impose an overload is known, the rate of adaptation or the ideal progression necessary to induce additional gains in bone density cannot be determined. However, any type of exercise overload (intensity, duration, or frequency) must begin at a level the individual can safely tolerate and progress gradually. Skeletal adaptations are unique in terms of the slow turnover rate of bone. Because it takes about 3–4 months for one remodeling cycle to complete the sequence of bone resorption, formation, and mineralization, a minimum of 6–8 months of exercise training are typically required to detect a measurable change in bone mass in humans, using current technology (American College of Sports Medicine, 2004).

Rest/Recovery/Adaptation

To date little research has been done with humans to determine the optimal amount of rest and recovery for positive bone adaptations. Some researchers have used information from animal studies to develop an osteogenic index (see Focus on Application Box) to guide exercise prescription for bone adaptations, but the utility of such a tool has not yet been proven. It is known that inadequate rest and recovery along with excessive repetitive loads can lead to stress fractures (discussed later in this chapter).

Individualization

The individual response principle applies to the skeletal system as well as other body systems; that is, different people respond to the same exercise stress differently depending on their genetic makeup, hormonal and nutritional status, and so on. Individuals with low BMD have the greatest potential for benefit.

Additionally, exercise interventions goals vary for individuals across the life span. During childhood, the primary goal is to improve bone acquisition and attain the highest peak bone mass genetically possible. High-impact activities, such as jumping and hopping, should be incorporated into activity starting in the prepubertal years. The goal through early adulthood is to build bone and through middle age to maintain bone. This requires weight-bearing activity with a force of impact greater than 2.5 times body weight. For older adults, the goal is to reduce bone loss and prevent falls. This means emphasizing activities that challenge the postural system and use resistance for loading muscles and bone. Dynamic resistance programs should promote balance and upper and lower body muscle strength to reduce the risk of falling and possible resulting bone fractures. Osteoporotic individuals should not engage in jumping activities. Although

walking in itself is not a strong bone stimulus (see Focus on Application Box), a lifetime of walking may beneficially reduce bone loss (Beck and Snow, 2003).

Retrogression/Plateau/Reversibility

The reversibility principle suggests that if you cease exercising for a time, you lose the benefits of exercising. Studies of immobilized patients (Donaldson et al., 1970; Vogel and Whittle, 1976) and discontinued training (Dalsky et al., 1988; Iwanton et al., 2001; Nordström et al., 2005; Winters and Snow, 2000) indicate that this principle also applies to bone. The effects of detraining on bone are discussed later in this chapter.

Maintenance

The increased BMD resulting from exercise training appears to be reduced with the cessation of training. The rate of bone loss is not known, however, nor is the level of activity needed to maintain bone mineral density or the threshold at which bone loss occurs. Intense exercise training during the pubertal years and early adulthood may lead to greater attainment of peak bone mass, which may protect against fractures later in life because more bone mass can be lost then before the bone is weakened to the point of fracture (Heaney et al., 2000; Karlsson, 2004). There is evidence that increases in BMC in the femoral neck gained during 7 months of high-impact training in prepubertal children were maintained during a 7-month detraining period (Fuchs and Snow, 2002). Clearly, activity is needed to maintain BMD, but additional research is necessary to determine the level of activity in various age groups for maintaining improvements in bone mineral density that resulted from exercise training.

Warm-Up and Cooldown

The effect of warming up and cooling down on bone density is not known. However, warming up and stretching are important for ligaments and tendons, which are part of the skeletal system.

In summary, the optimal exercise prescription for skeletal health is not currently known. However, this should not be used as an excuse not to exercise. Some weight-bearing or impact-loading exercise is clearly better than none. Most individuals should undertake an exercise program using weight-bearing activity and dynamic resistance exercise.

Skeletal Adaptations to Exercise Training

The adaptation of the skeletal system to exercise training is depicted in **Table 16.6**. As the table indicates, the adaptation of bone to exercise depends largely on the

FOCUS ON APPLICATION
Plyometrics

Again, high-impact activities are thought to be the key for bone development. *Plyometrics* is an exercise training method originally designed to develop explosive power. It consists of exercises involving powerful contractions following dynamic loading or pre-stretching of the contracting muscles. Plyometrics depth jumps can produce ground reaction forces of up to seven times body weight. In terms of skeletal loading, ground reaction forces less than two times body weight are considered to be low intensity, ground reaction forces two to four times body weight are moderate intensity, and ground reaction forces greater than four times body weight constitute a high-intensity load (Witzke and Snow, 2000). Thus, plyometrics provides a potentially excellent training modality for building bone mineral density.

Basic plyometric exercises include all the following:

- Bounds for horizontal distance

- Jumps for vertical height

- Hops for vertical height as rapidly as possible

- Leaps for maximal vertical plus horizontal distance

- Skips for vertical height plus horizontal distance

- Ricochets for rapid leg and foot movement while minimizing vertical and horizontal distance

- Swings for trunk movements with involvement of shoulders and arms

- Twists for lateral movement without shoulder or arm involvement

A program of plyometrics can be used with individuals as young as 12 years of age if designed carefully and applied progressively (Radcliffe and Farentinos, 1985). Witzke and Snow (2000) implemented a plyometrics training program in a freshman physical education class (3 d·wk^{-1}, 30–45 min·d^{-1}, for 9 months). All participants volunteered for this class. Despite the fact that the control subjects in a "traditional" physical education class were active more hours per week outside class than the plyometrics exercisers (5.6 versus 2.6 hr·wk^{-1}), the plyometrics exercisers had greater increases in bone mass measured at all sites. However, the difference between groups was statistically significant at only one site, the greater trochanter. The researchers reported that although some students worked harder in class than others, most enjoyed the plyometrics class and participated in it safely. Only one injury occurred during the entire program. Thus, plyometrics training may be a viable alternative activity for junior and senior high school physical education classes or after-school programs in fitness facilities. The implementation of such programs requires a knowledgeable instructor and a conscientiously constructed training program.

Sources: Radcliffe and Farentinos (1985), Witzke and Snow (2000).

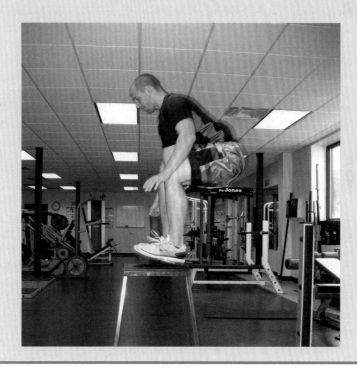

amount of activity and may be represented as a continuum. Measurable skeletal adaptation also depends on the type of bone being measured (trabecular or cortical) as well as the type of activity employed.

One approach to studying the effects of increased physical activity on bone density is to compare the dominant limb to the nondominant limb in sports such as tennis and baseball. These studies report that the dominant arm has greater bone mineral density or mass than the nondominant arm (Huddleston et al., 1980; Jones et al., 1977; Kontulainen et al., 2002). This seems true for both females and males and across a wide age range. Furthermore, the difference in BMD between the dominant and nondominant arm appears related to the age at which participants started playing the sport. Kontulainen et al. (2002) have reported that BMD measures of the humerus of the dominant arm are approximately 17% greater than those in the

TABLE 16.6 Effects of Physical Activity and Exercise Training on Bone Health

No or Too Little Activity	Acceptable Amounts of Activity	Too Much, High-Intensity, Long-Duration, Rapid Increment Activity
Low mineralization and density	Adequate mineralization or enhanced mineralization and density	Osteopenia or osteoporosis in amenorrheic athletes
Aging-associated osteoporosis	Normal rate of growth, stature, and proportion	Fragile bones, increased risk of fracture
Fragile bones, increased fracture potential	Delayed aging-associated osteoporosis	Overuse injuries include those to the elbow (bony spurs or bone disruption at joint surface), the vertebrae (microfractures leading to slippage), the knees (Osgood-Schlatter diseases: inflammation of the bones or cartilage), and the legs and feet (stress reactions and/or fractures)

nondominant arm in racquet sport players who began playing before menarche, compared to a 9% difference between dominant and nondominant limbs in players who began playing after menarche. The control group of nonathletic individuals evidenced a 3% difference in BMD between the dominant and nondominant arm (Kontulainen et al., 2002).

Another approach to studying skeletal adaptations to exercise training has been to compare different athletic groups with one another and with control groups (see accompanying Focus on Research). These studies collectively suggest that individuals involved in athletics or participating in vigorous fitness training have greater bone mineral density than sedentary controls. Furthermore, individuals involved in weight-bearing or impact-loading sports have higher BMD than those involved in non–weight-bearing activities (American College of Sports Medicine, 2004; Duncan et al., 2002; Proctor et al., 2002; Riser et al., 1990).

Training studies have also been conducted of sedentary individuals beginning an exercise program. BMD measurements were compared before and after the exercise training. A review of 21 longitudinal studies in which participants were randomly assigned to exercise treatment or control groups strongly suggests that regular physical exercise can delay the physiological decrease in bone mineral density that occurs with aging and reduce the risk of osteoporosis. Weight-bearing exercises, including weightlifting, jumping, and running, were associated with the greatest improvements in bone mass (Ernst, 1998).

Skeletal adaptation to exercise depends on the age of the participant. Vigorous exercise helps increase bone mass and strength in children and is thus important for the attainment of peak bone mass. Furthermore, bone mass tracks from childhood to adulthood, as shown by the following studies. One study (Barnekow-Bergkvist et al., 2006) tested female students at age 16.1 and 20 years

later. Active girls had higher BMD than inactive girls as adolescents. Those who continued to be active in weight-bearing activity had significantly higher BMD (5–19%) in adulthood than those who ceased participation or who had never been active. Membership in a sports club and site-specific physical performance in adolescence were significantly associated with higher adult BMD. Another study (Delvaux et al., 2001) tested males at ages 13 and 40 years. Static arm strength, running speed, and upper body muscular endurance as an adolescent contributed significantly to the prediction of adult bone mass. Additionally, no consistent evidence suggests that exercise training negatively affects either skeletal maturation (measured by ossification) or bone length in growing children. Although isolated studies have shown both retarded and accelerated growth in stature in young athletes, the consensus is that youngsters involved in exercise training grow at the same rate and to the same extent as their sedentary counterparts (Baxter-Jones and Maffulli, 2002; Caine, 1990; Malina, 1988; Plowman et al., 1991; Sprynarova, 1987).

A study by Welsh and Rutherford (1996) suggests that elderly men and women respond to exercise in a similar manner. High-impact aerobics, performed 2–3 $d \cdot wk^{-1}$, resulted in an increase in total body BMD and in hip and spine BMD. The increase in BMD was similar for the males and females who participated in the 12-month study.

Overall, studies suggest that weight-bearing and resistance exercise training play an important role in maximizing bone mass during childhood and adolescence, increasing or maintaining bone mass through adulthood, attenuating bone loss with aging, and reducing falls and fractures in the elderly (American College of Sports Medicine, 2004; Polidoulis et al., 2012). However, if some is good, more is not necessarily better when it comes to exercise training and bone health. Excessive physical activity, noted as the pathological overload zone in **Figure 16.11**, can exceed the adaptive ability of bone, resulting in overuse injuries.

FOCUS ON RESEARCH

Gymnastics Are Associated with Higher Upper Limb BMD

To examine the effect of high-impact-loading forces on BMD, Proctor and colleagues examined female college gymnasts (NCAA Division I) and age- and weight-matched controls. Gymnastics is a unique sport because the limbs of the upper body are weight-bearing and subject to high-impact loading.

Following are the BMD figures of the gymnasts and controls.

As found in earlier studies focusing on the lower body of weight-bearing athletes, this study found that gymnasts had higher BMD values at the lumbar spine and femur than controls. The major new finding was that female collegiate gymnasts had 17% higher arm BMD than controls. Furthermore, while the control group had the typical pattern of slightly greater BMD in the dominant arm, this difference was not evident in the gymnasts.

These results are consistent with the mechanostat theory and suggest that gymnastic training provides a sufficient training stimulus (overload) to elicit positive bone adaptations.

Source: Proctor, K. L., W. C. Adams, J. D. Shaffrath, & M. D. Van Loan: Upper-limb bone mineral density of female college gymnasts versus controls. *Medicine & Science in Sports & Exercise.* 34(11):1830–1835 (2002).

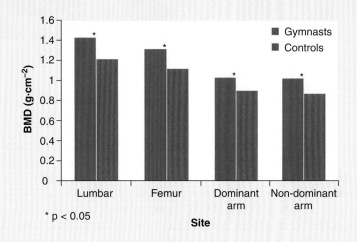

Skeletal Adaptations to Detraining

Research clearly shows that a cessation of weight-bearing exercise is detrimental to the skeleton because it results in a loss of bone mineral density. This effect has been clearly shown in astronauts and in patients confined to bed rest or immobilized in a cast. Studies have consistently indicated that weight-bearing bones are affected more and that trabecular bone (measured in the spine) is lost at a greater rate than cortical bone (Donaldson et al., 1970; Frost, 1988; Vogel and Whittle, 1976).

Research also suggests that discontinuing weight-bearing exercise results in a loss of the positive adaptation that occurs with training. Detraining is associated with a reversal of the positive effects of exercise on bone in young adult males 3 years after discontinuing intense hockey training (Nordström et al., 2005), in premenopausal women after 6 months of detraining following a year of impact and resistance training (Winters and Snow, 2000), and in postmenopausal women with osteoporosis after 1 year of detraining following a year of walking and gymnastic exercises (Iwamoto et al., 2001).

In a classic study that investigated changes in bone mineral content with training and subsequent detraining, Dalsky et al. (1988) reported that 22 months of weight-bearing exercise caused a significant increase (6.2%) in lumbar bone mineral content. When subjects discontinued exercise training (or trained <3 d·wk⁻¹), bone mineral content returned to baseline values. After 1 year of detraining, bone mineral content was only 1.1% above baseline values. Collective data strongly suggest that the increased bone mineral resulting from exercise is lost if exercise is not continued; bone responds to activity and inactivity.

Special Applications to Health and Fitness

The following sections discuss three practical implications of skeletal health of special interest to those involved in health and fitness: osteoporosis, the female athlete triad, and skeletal injuries.

Osteoporosis

Osteoporosis is a serious health problem affecting millions of Americans. An estimated 10 million individuals already have the disease, and an estimated additional 34 million have low bone mass placing them at increased risk for osteoporosis (National Osteoporosis Foundation, 2012). Osteoporosis, meaning "porous bones," is a condition characterized by compromised bone strength that increases the risk of fracture. Bone strength is determined by both bone density and bone quality (including external geometry and internal microstructure) (Seeman and Delmas, 2003). Osteoporosis results from an imbalance

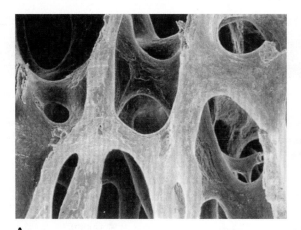

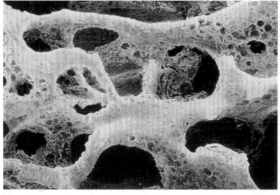

A

B

FIGURE 16.12 Trabecular Bone.
A. Normal. **B**. Osteoporotic.

between bone resorption and bone formation. Resorption occurs faster than formation, leading to a loss in BMD. Clinically, osteoporosis is defined by a BMD more than 2.5 SD (T-score ≥ –2.5) below the young normal adult average (Kanis et al., 1993). **Figure 16.12** shows normal and osteoporotic trabecular bone. Note the more porous trabeculae in the osteoporotic bone, a condition that weakens the bone.

The most common fracture sites related to osteoporosis are the hip, spine, and wrist. Approximately 300,000 hip, 550,000 vertebral, and 400,000 wrist osteoporosis-related fractures occur each year in the United States (Burge et al., 2007). Most hip fractures require surgery, with a 15–20% mortality rate following this surgery. The national direct cost for osteoporotic fractures was an estimated $13.8 billion in 1995 and is expected to exceed $25 billion by 2025 (Burge et al., 2007; National Osteoporosis Foundation, 2012). Spinal vertebral fractures occur when an osteoporotic bone is literally crushed by the weight of the body, resulting in a loss of height, curvature of the spine, and considerable pain.

The cause of osteoporosis is not known, although several risk factors have been identified (**Table 16.7**) (Carmona, 2004; Kleerekoper and Avioli, 1993; Lindsay, 1993; Loucks, 1988; National Institute of Health (NIH), 2001). Genetic risk factors include race, sex, heredity, and body build. Low body mass index (BMI) is associated with increased risk of osteoporotic fracture in the elderly. Low BMI may result in several factors, including low BMD, less soft tissue to protect bone from impact forces, and an increased risk of falling due to muscle weakness (Nielson et al., 2012). Nutritional risk factors include low calcium intake, excessive alcohol consumption, and consistently high protein intake. Lifestyle factors associated with osteoporosis include a lack of physical activity and smoking. Physiological factors include inadequate levels of estrogen (related to a delayed menarche, amenorrhea, or

an early menopause). Several research studies have indicated that the rapid loss of BMD following menopause is related to the decrease in estrogen levels. The low activity levels of females in the United States, particularly older women, also contribute to the risk of developing osteoporosis. Bone mineral content is positively related to long-term physical activity.

The American College of Sports Medicine recommends that older adults acquire 150 min·wk⁻¹ of physical activity per week. If older adults are not able to achieve 150 min·wk⁻¹ of moderate-intensity activity because of chronic health conditions, they should be as physically active as their abilities and conditions allow (American College of Sports Medicine, 2009). These recommendations are made based on the understanding of multiple benefits of exercise, including enhancing bone health. In addition to its positive effect on BMD, exercise also appears to help reduce the risk of fractures by increasing muscular strength and coordination, thereby decreasing the risk of falling (Kemmler et al., 2010). The risk of falling is affected by the individual's coordination, sight, and muscular strength. Environmental risk factors that increase the risk of falling include poor lighting, uneven or slippery floor surfaces, and inappropriate footwear. Exercise leaders must provide an exercise area that reduces the risk of falling for older adults.

While it is clear that physical activity is important for maintaining bone health in older adults, nutritional factors also play a role. Calcium and vitamin D have a permissive effect on bone that acts synergistically with exercise to influence bone remodeling. There is no evidence that excessive amounts of calcium or vitamin D will result in greater skeletal gains and in the absence of exercise, nutritional factors cannot adequately maintain bone mass or strength. However, adequate amounts of calcium and vitamin D are independently important for bone health (Daly and Kukulijan, 2010).

TABLE 16.7 Risk Factors Associated with Osteoporosis

Risk Factors	Relationship to Disease	Possible Explanations
Genetic		
Race	Whites are more likely to develop disease than African Americans	Unknown
Sex	Women are four times more likely to develop osteoporosis than men	Lighter bones of females; rapid bone loss following menopause; longer life span
Heredity	There appears to be a genetic predisposition to the disease	Unknown
Body build	Petite individuals are at greater risk	Less peak bone mass to lose
Lifestyle		
Lack of physical activity	Lack of weight-bearing activity increases risk of disease	No weight-bearing activities to stimulate bone formation
Smoking	Smoking increases risk of disease	May lower serum estrogen or cause early menopause
Sex hormones (late menarche, amenorrhea, or menopause)	Decrease in sex hormones is associated with increased risk	Loss of protective effect of estrogen on bone
Nutritional		
Calcium intake	Low calcium level interferes with bone formation	Insufficient calcium to adequately ossify bone
Alcohol use	Alcohol use may be damaging to bone	Resulting in poor diet from excessive alcohol consumption
Protein intake	High protein intake is associated with low BMD	Protein increases calcium loss in urine

The Female Athlete Triad

Postmenopausal females are not the only people at risk for developing osteoporosis and subsequent bone fractures. So too are young female athletes who exhibit components of a medical syndrome called the female athlete triad (Ackerman and Misra, 2011; American College of Sports Medicine, 2007; Beals and Meyer, 2007; DeSouza and Williams, 2004; International Olympic Committee, 2006).

The **female athlete triad** is a syndrome of interrelated conditions including disordered eating, menstrual dysfunction, and skeletal demineralization. The syndrome was once narrowly defined in terms of the extremes of each of these conditions, but it is now recognized that each ranges along a continuum from health to disease (Beals and Meyer, 2007; Loucks, 2003b; Zanker and Cooke, 2004). **Figure 16.13** shows the conditions that make up the triad, the continuum comprising each and arrows that indicate the interaction between the factors. Thus, disordered eating is directly related to both menstrual dysfunction and skeletal demineralization, while

> **Female Athlete Triad** A syndrome of interrelated conditions including disordered eating, menstrual dysfunction, and skeletal demineralization.
>
> **Energy availability** Dietary intake minus exercise energy expenditure.

menstrual dysfunction in turn can impact skeletal demineralization. There is increasing evidence for a potential fourth component, that is, endothelial dysfunction. Endothelial dysfunction is a well-established warning sign in the development of cardiovascular disease (Zach et al., 2011). Although eating and reproductive disorders can occur in male athletes (Loucks, 2006), no comparable syndrome has been identified in males.

Disordered Eating

Disordered eating is considered the key to the development of the female athlete triad. A female athlete who thinks that a lower body weight will improve her athletic performance begins to diet. Initially, this strategy may prove successful (although in the long run, it often is not), and so her dieting becomes more extreme. Alternatively, possibly unknowingly, she does not increase her caloric intake to meet her exercise energy requirements because she lacks time to prepare meals, lacks money for high-quality food, or has insufficient nutritional knowledge (Beals and Meyer, 2007). Regardless of the initial cause, she has reduced energy availability.

Energy availability is defined as dietary intake minus exercise energy expenditure. This is the amount of dietary energy remaining for all other physiological functions. Humans need dietary energy for five functions: cellular maintenance, thermoregulation, movement, growth, and

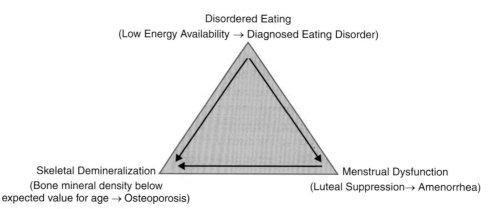

FIGURE 16.13 The Female Athlete Triad.
The female athlete triad is a syndrome consisting of a combination of some degree of disordered eating, menstrual dysfunction, and skeletal demineralization. In the extreme, these conditions can result in a diagnosed eating disorder, amenorrhea, and osteoporosis. The arrows indicate that disordered eating can directly impact both menstrual dysfunction and skeletal demineralization whereas menstrual dysfunction directly impacts only skeletal demineralization.

Sources: Based on information from Beals, K. A., & N. L. Meyer: Female Athlete Triad Update. *Clinics in Sports Medicine*. 26:69–89 (2007). Loucks, A.: Introduction of menstrual disturbances in athletes. *Medicine & Science in Sports & Exercise*. 35(9):1551–1552 (2003b)

reproduction. If a large proportion of the available energy is used for movement (exercise training), there may be insufficient energy available for the other functions. Reproductive functions seem particularly vulnerable to the effects of insufficient energy.

In exercising females, reproductive function and bone turnover are impaired when energy availability (that amount of dietary intake available for all other physiological functions after accounting for the amount used in exercise) is decreased more than 33%. Many amenorrheic athletes decrease their energy availability by 67%, well over the threshold 33%. The threshold for sufficient energy availability appears to be approximately 30 kcal·kg LBM^{-1}·d^{-1}. Thus, female runners may be able to sustain normal reproductive hormonal function while running up to 8 mi·d^{-1} as long as they maintain a dietary energy intake of at least 45 kcal·kg LBM^{-1}·d^{-1} (Ihle and Loucks, 2004; Loucks, 2006; Loucks and Thuma, 2003). For example, if the runner were 125 lb (56.8 kg) with a body fat of 20%, she would have 25 lb (11.4 kg) of fat and 100 lb (45.4kg) of lean body mass (LBM). Multiplying 45.4 kg by 45 kcal·kg LBM^{-1}·d^{-1} would require a caloric intake of 2043 kcal·d^{-1}.

Disordered eating involves a continuum of abnormal eating behaviors from low energy availability to clinically diagnosed eating disorders. Clinically diagnosed eating disorders include anorexia nervosa, bulimia nervosa, and eating disorders not otherwise specified (Beals and Meyer, 2007; International Olympic Committee, 2006). These are discussed more fully in Chapter 6.

Menstrual Dysfunction

Menstrual dysfunction is one mechanism through which low energy availability is thought to impact bone health. It is thought that insufficient fuel (especially carbohydrate) to meet energy requirements causes a change in brain function. The female reproductive system is controlled by the hypothalamus-pituitary-ovarian axis. A key role is the secretion of gonadotropin-releasing hormone (GnRH) from the hypothalamus. Low energy availability somehow decreases GnRH release. Inadequate GnRH results in the suppression of luteinizing hormone (LH) and follicle-stimulating hormone (FSH), which causes, in turn, inadequate secretion of estrogen (estradiol) and progesterone. The resultant disruptions in menstrual function can include (a) luteal suppression (phase defects in which ovulation occurs but implantation cannot), (b) anovulation, (c) oligomenorrhea (irregular and inconsistent menstrual cycles), and (d) amenorrhea. Amenorrhea may be either primary (the failure to achieve menarche by age 15) or secondary (no menses for a minimum of 3 consecutive months in a female who has attained menarche) (DeSouza and Williams, 2004; Loucks, 2006).

While the athlete often feels the absence of a regular menstrual cycle is a good thing, physiologically it is not. A major concern with amenorrhea is that the low levels of circulating estrogen (hypoestrogenia) can negatively impact bone (Giannopoulou and Kanaly, 2004). This is true for both primary amenorrhea (almost half of bone mass accrual occurs during adolescence and young adulthood) and secondary amenorrhea. An athlete who

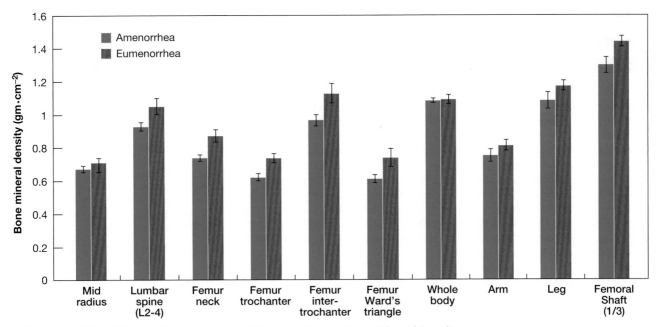

FIGURE 16.14 The Effects of Exercise-Induced Amenorrhea on Bone Mineral Density.
Source: Data from Myburgh, K.H., L.A. Bachrach, B. Lewis, K. Kent and R. Marcus: Low bone mineral density at axial and appendicular sites in amenorrheic athletes. *Medicine and Science in Sports and Exercise*. 25(11):1197–1202 (1993).

misses more than six consecutive menstrual periods has increased risk of failure to reach potential peak bone mass or premature bone loss. Indeed, athletes should have a BMD similar to or higher than (depending on the site and sport) sedentary individuals and nonmenstruating athletes, not lower, and regularly do (Ackerman and Misra, 2011; Beals and Meyer, 2007; DeSouza and Williams, 2004; Giannopoulou and Kanaly, 2004; International Olympic Committee, 2006). **Figure 16.14** presents data on bone mineral density at several sites in amenorrheic and eumenorrheic (regular menstrual cycling) athletes.

Skeletal Demineralization

The International Olympic Committee (IOC) (2006) suggests that any athlete identified with a current or past history of oligomenorrhea, amenorrhea, or fractures be further evaluated. Their osteoporosis decision tree is presented in **Figure 16.15**. Note that the IOC recommends that individuals with a Z-score of –1 or lower be referred for counseling or treatment. A Z-score of –2.0 or lower in an amenorrheic athlete 20 years of age or older is considered to be osteoporotic, placing the athlete at risk for fractures (Beals and Meyer, 2007; International Olympic Committee, 2006).

Skeletal demineralization is also linked directly to low energy availability—possibly in a dose-response relationship. A study by Ilhe and Loucks (2004) showed that markers of *bone formation* were suppressed at moderate levels of energy restriction, whereas markers of *bone resorption* increased only when the energy restriction was severe enough to suppress estrogen. The primary role of estrogen

in bone metabolism is to reduce the rate of bone resorption (Loucks, 2003b). Low energy availability likely initially affects metabolic substrates and hormones other than estrogen (insulin, growth hormone, insulin-like growth factor, cortisol, leptin, and thyroid) that are important in bone metabolism and, then, with more severe energy restriction, impacts estrogen as well (DeSouza and Williams, 2004).

Note that although exercise is a stressor and thus elicits neurohormonal responses in the body, exercise itself does not appear to cause the female athlete triad beyond the impact of its energy cost on energy availability. No particular body weight or body composition appears to be a critical threshold level beyond which a disruption of the hypothalamus-pituitary-ovarian axis occurs. Eumenorrheic and amenorrheic athletes both span a common range of body weight and composition (Beals and Meyer, 2007; Loucks, 2003a,b). Finally, while estrogen is important for both menstrual and bone health, estrogen supplementation alone has not been shown to restore BMD to normal in amenorrheic athletes. The Clinically Relevant Focus on Research box presents a case study demonstrating the roles of calcium, estrogen, and energy availability in treatment and recovery of low bone mineral density resulting from amenorrhea.

Skeletal Injuries

Skeletal injuries can be categorized as resulting from macrotrauma or microtrauma (Micheli, 1989). Macrotrauma injuries are sudden acute incidents, such as a broken leg or clavicle from impact or a fracture at the epiphyseal growth plate. Growth plate fractures have the greatest

FOCUS ON RESEARCH: *Clinically Relevant*
Reversing the Female Athlete Triad

The athlete in this case study was an elite Caucasian female distance runner. She started running competitively at age 12 (before menarche) and competed until age 25. Her personal best at the 26.2 mi marathon distance was 2:41. She began restrictive eating at age 13 years. At times her training volume was 90 mi·wk^{-1}. She exhibited primary amenorrhea until age 23, when she began calcium supplementation and estrogen replacement in the form of oral contraceptives. At that time her BMD (shown in the graph below) was only 74% (T-score = −2.5) and 80% (T-score = −1.54) of normal peak for her spine and hip, respectively. Her body weight was 107 lb (48.6 kg), and her body mass index (BMI) (shown in the graph accompanying) was 15.8 kg·m^{-2}. Over the next 2 years, her body weight increased 4 lb (1.8 kg), and menarche occurred. However, not until she increased her energy availability by adopting better nutritional habits and decreasing her training mileage did she gain weight and increased her BMD (see graph). By age 31, she weighed a healthy 144 lb (BMI = 21.3 kg·m^{-2}), and her BMD values were almost in the normal range (spine = 94%; T-score = −0.63 and hip = 96%; T-score = −0.33). As the authors state, convincing competitive athletes to gain weight is sometimes a "formidable challenge." Indeed, in this case, the individual was 25 years old before finally acting on the seriousness of her situation. It would, of course, have been better to avoid the female athlete triad in the first place.

The extent to which bone deficits can be reversed is unknown, especially in athletes with secondary amenorrhea. In the case presented here, the positive changes started to occur within 2 years of menarche. Hormone replacement (in conjunction with calcium intake) was insufficient to regain bone density. Improved nutrition, weight gain, and resumption of normal menstrual cycles were necessary for successful treatment.

Source: Fredericson, M. & K. Kent: Normalization of bone density in a previously amenorrheic runner with osteoporosis. *Medicine & Science in Sports & Exercise.* 37(9):1481–1486 (2005).

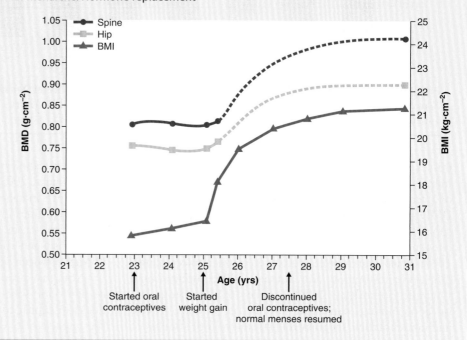

potential for harm. The probability of a growth plate injury is greatest in automobile accidents, falls, contact sports, and dynamic resistance training. Fractures of the growth plate can result in progressive bone shortening, deformity, or joint incongruity. Fortunately, acute traumatic growth plate injuries are less frequent than other injury types, and most such injuries appear not to result in growth disturbances (Caine, 1990).

Microtrauma injuries are overuse injuries from chronic repetitive overtraining (Micheli, 1989). The anatomical site of microtrauma depends on the sport. Microtrauma injuries to bone generally involve an uncoupling or imbalance between bone resorption and bone deposition, called a stress reaction. **Stress reactions** refer to maladaptive areas of bone hyperactivity where resorption progressively exceeds deposition.

Early minor stress reactions may have no clinical manifestations. The individual feels no pain and has no swelling or tenderness. As the overuse continues and the imbalance becomes more extreme, several clinical symptoms may occur, including degeneration and loosening of portions of bone from the joint capsules, the formation of bone spurs, inflammation of bone and cartilage, and/or stress fractures. A **stress fracture** is a hairline break in bone that occurs without acute trauma, is clinically symptomatic, and is detectable by X-rays or bone scans. It is often difficult to determine exactly when a bone's stress reaction becomes a stress fracture. The typical fine hairline fracture may be undetectable by X-rays or bone scans for 3–4 weeks after pain occurs.

Although exercise training can and does have a beneficial impact on bone growth and health, too much exercise training, usually in the form of repetitive overuse or rapid increments of intensity or duration, can be detrimental. Harm is more likely if the bone already has a low bone mineral density. The concern about overuse injuries therefore focuses on female athletes exhibiting the female athlete triad and young growing athletes of both sexes (Sterling et al., 1992).

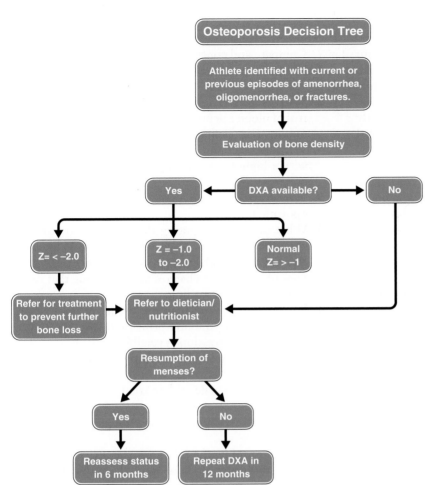

FIGURE 16.15 Osteoporosis Decision Tree. Algorithm to decide whether an athlete needs evaluation and possibly treatment for low bone density.

The concern for amenorrheic athletes is well founded. A higher prevalence of stress fractures has been documented in this population than in female athletes with normal menstrual cycles in a variety of sports (Lloyd et al., 1986; Maffulli, 1990; Micheli, 1989; Myburgh et al., 1990).

The exact incidence of microtrauma, including stress fractures, in youth athletes is difficult to document, although reports from orthopedists indicate that the number is growing as more children and adolescents participate in competitive sports (Faulkner et al., 1993). The highest incidence of stress fractures occurs between the ages of 10 and 15, at the time of peak growth (Lloyd et al., 1986; Sterling et al., 1992). Some researchers have suggested that a normal imbalance between bone matrix formation and mineralization occurs during the growth spurt. Furthermore, during this growth spurt, muscle imbalances can occur around joints as the muscles, tendons, and ligaments are stretched and become progressively tighter when the bones elongate. A muscle that is fatigued from overuse, is weak or out of balance with its antagonist, and/or is inflexible is less able to absorb shock, allowing abnormally high stress to be transmitted to the bone. This situation increases the risk of stress fractures, other repetitive stress reactions, and impact injuries (Jones et al., 1989; Kibler et al., 1992; Mafulli, 1990).

The primary risk factor for overuse injuries is training error, particularly abrupt increases in intensity, duration, and frequency (Micheli, 1989). Workload should not increase more than 10% per week in young training athletes. Other risk factors include the aforementioned musculoskeletal imbalances of strength, flexibility, or size; errors in technique or skills; anatomical malalignments; footwear that fits improperly; and running on hard surfaces such as concrete and asphalt. Parents and others involved in youth sports must give careful attention to these factors. For example, during periods of rapid growth, the intensity of training should be reduced and static stretching programs emphasized.

Although the skeletal system is often taken for granted, it should not be. When it is injured or malfunctioning, we quickly become aware of its importance. Adequate nutrition, reasonable training regimens, and maintenance of normal hormonal levels are keys to good bone health.

Stress Reactions Maladaptive areas of bone hyperactivity where the balance between resorption and deposition is progressively lost such that resorption exceeds deposition.

Stress Fracture A fine hairline break in bone that occurs without acute trauma, is clinically symptomatic, and is detectable by X-rays or bone scans.

SUMMARY

1. The skeletal system serves a number of important functions, including support, protection, movement, mineral storage, and hematopoiesis (blood cell formation).

2. Bone tissue is dynamic, living tissue that is constantly undergoing change. Bone remodeling is a continual process of bone resorption and formation of new bone.

3. Osteoclasts are bone cells that cause the resorption (breakdown) of bone tissue. Osteoblasts are bone-forming cells. Osteocytes are mature osteoblasts surrounded by calcified bone.

4. The two major types of bone tissue are cortical and trabecular bone; they differ in their microscopic appearance.

5. Studies generally show that physical activity has a positive effect on bone health. Exercise training can enhance the attainment of peak bone mass during late adolescence and early adulthood, can slow the rate of age-related bone loss in later adulthood, and may offset menopausal-related bone loss.

6. Weight-bearing and impact-loading activities lead to an acute osteogenic effect in bone.

7. The mechanostat theory of bone response posits that a minimal effect strain is necessary to elicit normal remodeling of bone tissue and that a higher threshold exists for the enhancement of bone strength. This is consistent with the overload principle of training.

8. Weight-bearing or impact-loading activities produce greater changes in bone mineral density than do non–weight-bearing or weight-supported activities.

9. An appropriate exercise prescription for skeletal health should take into account the individual's current skeletal health. On the basis of current status and individual desires, activities should be chosen from a continuum of impact-loading activities.

10. Osteoporosis means "porous bones," a condition characterized by a loss of bone mineral density, resulting in bones that are weak and susceptible to fracture. It is clinically defined as a bone mineral density greater than 2.5 standard deviations below young, normal adult averages.

11. The female athlete triad is a syndrome of interrelated conditions including disordered eating, menstrual dysfunction, and skeletal demineralization. Low energy availability is directly linked to menstrual dysfunction through low estrogen levels and to skeletal demineralization by affecting metabolic substrates and hormones including estrogen and other hormones. Any female athlete without a regular menstrual cycle for 6 consecutive months should be evaluated for possible treatment.

REVIEW QUESTIONS

1. Compare and contrast cortical and trabecular bone.
2. Diagram the stages of bone remodeling, citing the specific role of the different types of bone cells.
3. What is the relationship between the hormonal control of blood calcium levels and the hormonal control of bone remodeling?
4. Why are osteoporotic fractures more likely in bones with a higher percentage of trabecular than cortical bone?
5. Why are women more likely than men to suffer osteoporotic fractures?
6. What can be done during the growth years to optimize the attainment of peak bone mass? Why is the attainment of peak bone mass important?
7. Describe the acute changes in bone tissue that result from mechanical loading.
8. Explain how the mechanostat theory of bone relates to the following training principles: specificity, overload, and retrogression/reversibility.
9. What factors influence skeletal adaptations to exercise?
10. Describe the female athlete triad and recommended treatment.
11. Describe how physical activity helps prevent osteoporosis.
12. Defend or refute the following statements:
    a. Disturbances in bone growth frequently result from overtraining in young athletes.
    b. Young athletes are more susceptible to stress fractures during the time of peak growth than at other times.

For further review and additional study tools, go to http://thePoint.lww.com/Plowman4e ☀ ▶

REFERENCES

Ackerman, K. E. & M. Misra: Bone health and the female athlete triad in adolescent athletes. *The Physician and Sports Medicine*. 31(1):131–141 (2011).

American College of Sports Medicine: Position stand: Exercise and physical activity for older adults. *Medicine & Science in Sports & Exercise*. 41(7):1510–1530 (2009).

American College of Sports Medicine: Position stand: Female athlete triad. *Medicine & Science in Sports & Exercise*. 39(19):1867–1882 (2007).

American College of Sports Medicine: Position stand: Physical activity and bone health. *Medicine & Science in Sports & Exercise*. 36(11):1985–1996 (2004).

Bailey, D. A. & R. G. McColloch: Bone tissue and physical activity. *Canadian Journal of Sports Studies*. 15(4):229–239 (1990).

Barnekow-Bergkvist, M., G. Hedberg, U. Pettersson, & R. Lorentzon: Relationships between physical activity and physical capacity in adolescent females and bone mass in adulthood. *Scandinavian Journal of Medicine and Science in Sports*. 16(6):447–455 (2006).

Baron, R.: Anatomy and ultrastructure of bone. In Favus, M. J. (ed.): *Primer on the Metabolic Bone Diseases and Disorders of Mineral Metabolism* (2nd edition). New York, NY: Raven Press, 3–10 (1993).

Baxter-Jones, A. D. G. & N. Maffulli: Intensive training in elite young female athletes. *British Journal of Sports Medicine*. 36(1):13–15 (2002).

Beals, K. A. & N. L. Meyer: Female athlete triad update. *Clinics in Sports Medicine*. 26:69–89 (2007).

Beck, B. & R. Marcus: Skeletal effects of exercise in men. In Orwoll, E. S. (ed.): *Osteoporosis in Men: The Effect of Gender on Skeletal Health*. San Diego, CA: Academic Press, 129–155 (1999).

Beck, B. R. & C. M. Snow: Bone health across the lifespan—exercising our options. *Exercise and Sport Sciences Reviews*. 31(3):117–122 (2003).

Bonnet, N. & S. L. Ferrari: Exercise and the skeleton: How it works and what is really does. *International Bone and Mineral Society BoneKEy*. 7(7):235–248 (2010).

Borer, K. T.: Physical activity in the prevention and amelioration of osteoporosis in women; Interaction of mechanical, hormonal, and dietary factors. *Sports Medicine*. 35:779–830 (2005).

Burge, R., B. Dawson-Hughes, D. H. Solomon, J. B. Wong, A. King, & A. Tosteson: Incidence and economic burden of osteoporosis-related fractures in the United States, 2005–2025. *Journal of Bone and Mineral Research*. 22:465–475 (2007).

Burr, D. B.: Why bones bend but don't break. *Journal of Musculoskeletal and Neuronal Interactions*. 11(4):270–287 (2011).

Caine, D. J.: Growth plate injury and bone growth: An update. *Pediatric Exercise Science*. 2(3):209–229 (1990).

Canalis, E.: Regulation of bone remodeling. In Favus, M. J. (ed.): *Primer of Metabolic Bone Disorders*. Kelseyville, CA: American Society of Bone and Mineral Research Society Office, 23–26 (1990).

Carmona, R. H.: *Bone health and osteoporosis: A report of the surgeon general*. Rockville, MD: US Department of Health and Human Services, Office of the Surgeon General; 2004. Available at: www.hhs.gov/surgeongeneral/library/bone-health/content.html. Accessed December 13, 2006.

Dalsky, G. P.: The role of exercise in the prevention and treatment of osteoporosis. *Osteoporosis Report*. 8(4):2–3 (1993).

Dalsky, G. P., K. Stocke, A. Ehsani, E. Slatopolsky, W. Lee, & S. Birge: Weight-bearing exercise training and lumbar bone mineral content in post-menopausal women. *Annals of Internal Medicine*. 108:824–828 (1988).

Daly, R. M. & S. Kukuljan: Independent and combined effects of exercise and calcium on bone structural and material properties in older adults. In Burckhardt, P., B. Dawson-Hughes, C. Weaver (eds.): *Nutritional Influences on Bone Health*. Dordrecht, The Netherlands: Springer. 7:51–58 (2010).

Delvaux, K., J. Lefevre, R. Philippaerts, J. Dequeker, M. Thomis, B. Vanreusel, A. Claessens, B. V. Eynde, G. Beunen, & R. Lysens: Bone mass and lifetime physical activity in Flemish males: A 27-year follow-up study. *Medicine & Science in Sports & Exercise*. 33(11):1868–1875 (2001).

DeSouza, M. J. & N. I. Williams: Physiological aspects and clinical sequelae of energy deficiency and hypoestrogenism in exercising women. *Human Reproduction Update*. 10(5):433–448 (2004).

Donaldson, G. L., S. B. Hulley, J. M. Vogel, R. S. Huttner, J. H. Boyers, & D. E. MacMillan: Effect of prolonged bed rest on bone mineral. *Metabolism*. 19:1071–1084 (1970).

Duncan, C. S., C. J. R. Blimkie, C. T. Cowell, S. T. Burke, J. N. Briody, & R. Howman-Giles: Bone mineral density in adolescent female athletes: relationship to exercise type and muscle strength. *Medicine & Science in Sports & Exercise*. 34:286–294 (2002).

Ernst, E.: Exercise for female osteoporosis: A systematic review of randomised clinical trials. *Sports Medicine*. 25(6):359–368 (1998).

Faulkner, R. A., D. A. Bailey, D. T. Drinkwater, A. A. Wilkinson, C. S. Houston, & H. A. McKay: Regional and total body bone mineral content and bone mineral density, and total body tissue composition in children 8–16 years of age. *Calcified Tissue International*. 53(2):7–12 (1993).

Faulkner, R. A., M. R. Forwood, T. J. Beck, J. C. Mafukidze, K. Russell, & W. Wallace: Strength indices of the proximal femur and shaft in prepubertal female gymnasts. *Medicine & Science in Sports & Exercise*. 35:513–518 (2003).

Forwood, M. R. & C. H. Turner: Skeletal adaptations to mechanical usage: Results from tibial loading studies in rats. *Bone*. 17:197S–205S (1995).

Fredericson, M. & K. Kent: Normalization of bone density in a previously amenorrheic runner with osteoporosis. *Medicine & Science in Sports & Exercise*. 37(9):1481–1486 (2005).

Frost, H. M.: Vital biomechanics: Proposed general concepts for skeletal adaptations to mechanical usage. *Calcified Tissue International*. 42:145–156 (1988).

Frost, H. M.: Some ABC's of skeletal pathophysiology. The growth/modeling/remodeling distinction. *Calcified Tissue International*. 49:301–302 (1991a).

Frost, H. M.: Some ABC's of skeletal pathophysiology. 7. Tissue mechanisms controlling bone mass. *Calcified Tissue International*. 49:303–304 (1991b).

Frost, H. M.: Why do marathon runners have less bone than weight lifters? A vital-biomechanical view and explanation. *Bone*. 20(3):183–189 (1997).

Fuchs, R. K. & C. M. Snow: Gains in hip bone mass from high-impact training are maintained: A randomized controlled trial in children. *Journal of Pediatrics*. 141(3):357–362 (2002).

Giannopoulou, I. & J. Kanaly: Menstrual dysfunction. In Le Mura, L. M. & S. P. von Duvillard (eds.): *Clinical Exercise Physiology: Application and Physiological Principles*. Philadelphia, PA: Lippincott Williams & Wilkins, 347–367 (2004).

Greene, D. A. & G. A. Naughton: Adaptive skeletal responses to mechanical loading during adolescence. *Sports Medicine*. 36(9):723–732 (2006).

Grimston, S. K., N. D. Willows, & D. A. Hanley: Mechanical loading regime and its relationship to bone mineral density in children. *Medicine and Science in Sports and Exercise*. 25(11):1203–1210 (1993).

Heaney, R. P., S. Abrams, B. Dawson-Hughes, A. Looker, R. Marcus, V. Matkovic, & C. Weaver: Peak bone mass. *Osteoporosis International*. 11:985–1009 (2000).

Huddleston, A. L., D. Rockwell, D. N. Kulund, & R. B. Harrison: Bone mass in lifetime tennis athletes. *Journal of the American Medical Association*. 244:1107–1109 (1980).

Ihle, R. & A. B. Loucks: Dose-response relationship between energy availability and bone turnover in young exercising women. *Journal of Bone and Mineral Research*. 19(8):1231–1240 (2004).

International Olympic Committee Medical Commission Working Group Women in Sport. Position stand on the female athlete triad. 9/12/2006. Available: http://multimedia.olympic.org/pdf/en-report-917.pdf. Accessed 8/05/07

Iwamoto, J., T. Takeda, & S. Ichimura: Effect of exercise training and detraining on bone mineral density in postmenopausal women with osteoporosis. *Journal of Orthopedic Science.* 6(2):128–132 (2001).

Jones, B. H., J. M. Harris, T. N. Vinh, & C. Rubin: Exercise-induced stress fractures and stress reactions of bone: Epidemiology, etiology and classification. In Pandolf, K. B. (ed.): *Exercise and Sport Sciences Reviews.* Baltimore, MD: Williams & Wilkins. 17:379–422 (1989).

Jones, H. H., J. D. Priest, W. C. Hayes, C. C. Tichenor, & D. A. Nagel: Humeral hypertrophy in response to exercise. *Journal of Bone and Joint Surgery.* 59(2):204–208 (1977).

Kanis, J. A., P. Meunier, L. Alexeera, P. Burkhardt, C. Christiansen, C. Cooper, P. Delmas, O. Johnell, C. Johnston, P. Lips, L. J. Melton, E. Seeman, J. Stephan, & A. Tosteson: 1993 *Assessment of Osteoporotic Risk Fracture and Its Role in Screening for Postmenopausal Osteoporosis.* Geneva, Switzerland: World Health Organization (1993).

Karlsson, M. K.: Physical activity, skeletal health and fractures in a long term perspective. *Journal of Musculoskeletal and Neuronal Interactions.* 4(1):12–21 (2004).

Kemmler, W., S. von Stengel, K. Engelke, L. Häberle, & W. A. Kalender: Exercise effects on bone mineral density, falls, coronary risk factors, and health care costs in older women: The randomized controlled senior fitness and prevention study. *Archives of Internal Medicine.* 170(2):179–185 (2010).

Khan, K., H. McKay, P. Kannus, D. Bailey, J. Wark, K. Bennell, & A. Heinonen: *Physical Activity and Bone Health.* Champaign, IL: Human Kinetics (2001a).

Khan, K., H. McKay, P. Kannus, D. Bailey, J. Wark, K. Bennell, & K. MacKelvie: *Physical Activity and Bone Health.* Champaign, IL: Human Kinetics (2001b).

Khan, K., H. McKay, P. Kannus, D. Bailey, J. Wark, K. Bennell, & M. Forwood: *Physical Activity and Bone Health.* Champaign, IL: Human Kinetics (2001c).

Kibler, W. B., T. J. Chandler, & E. S. Stracener: Musculoskeletal adaptations and injuries due to overtraining. In Holloszy, J. O. (ed.): *Exercise and Sport Science Reviews.* Baltimore, MD: Williams & Wilkins. 20:99–126 (1992).

Kleerekoper, M., & L. V. Avioli: Evaluation and treatment of postmenopausal osteoporosis. In *Primer on the Metabolic Bone Diseases and Disorders of Mineral Metabolism* (2nd edition). New York, NY: Raven Press, 223–228 (1993).

Kontulainen, S., H. Sievänen, P. Kannus, M. Pasanen, & I. Vuori: Effect of long-term impact-loading on mass, size, and estimated strength of humerus and radius of female racquet-sports players: A peripheral quantitative computed tomography study between young and old starters and controls. *Journal of Bone and Mineral Research.* 17:1–9 (2002).

Layne, J. E. & M. E. Nelson: The effects of progressive resistance training on bone mineral density: A review. *Medicine & Science in Sports & Exercise.* 31(1):25–30 (1999).

Lanyon, L. E.: Strain-related bone modeling and remodeling. *Topics in Geriatric Rehabilitation.* 4(2):13–24 (1989).

Leib, E. S., Lewiecki, E. M., Binkley, N., & R. C. Hamdy: Official position of the international society for clinical densitometry. *Journal of Clinical Densitometry.* 7(1):1254–1259 (2004).

Lester, M. E., M. L. Urso, R. K. Evans, J. R. Pierce, B. A. Spiering, C. M. Maresh, D. L. Hatfield, W. J. Kraemer, & B. C. Nindl: Influence of exercise mode and osteogenic index on bone biomarker responses during short-term physical training. *Bone.* 45:768–776 (2009).

Lindsay, R.: Prevention of osteoporosis. In *Primer on the Metabolic Bone Diseases and Disorders of Mineral Metabolism* (2nd edition). New York, NY: Raven Press, 240–245 (1993).

Lloyd, T., S. J. Triantafyllou, E. R. Baker, P. S. Houts, J. A. Whiteside, A. Kalenak, & P. G. Stumpf: Women athletes with menstrual irregularities have increased musculoskeletal injuries. *Medicine and Science in Sports and Exercise.* 18(4):373–379 (1986).

Loucks, A. B.: Energy availability, not body fatness, regulates reproductive function in women. *Exercise and Sport Sciences Reviews.* 31(3):144–148 (2003a).

Loucks, A.: Introduction of menstrual disturbances in athletes. *Medicine & Science in Sports & Exercise.* 35(9):1551–1552 (2003b).

Loucks, A.: Osteoporosis prevention begins in childhood. In Brown, E. & C. Branta (eds.): *Competitive Sports for Children and Youth.* Champaign, IL: Human Kinetics (1988).

Loucks, A. B., N. S. Stachenfeld, & L. DiPietro: The female athlete triad: do female athletes need to take special care to avoid low energy availability? *Medicine & Science in Sports & Exercise.* 38:1694–1700 (2006).

Loucks, A. B. & J. R. Thuma: LH Pulsatility is disrupted at a threshold of energy availability in regularly menstruating women. *Journal of Clinical Endocrinology and Metabolism.* 88:297–301 (2003).

Macdonald, H. M., S. A. Kontulainen, K. M. Khan, & H. A. McKay: Is a school-based physical activity intervention effective for increasing tibial bone strength in boys and girls? *Journal of Bone and Mineral Research.* 22:434–446 (2007).

MacKelvie, K. J., K. M. Khan, & H. A. McKay: Is there a critical period for bone response to weight-bearing exercise in children and adolescents? A systematic review. *British Journal of Sports Medicine.* 36:250–257 (2002).

Maffulli, N.: Intensive training in young athletes: The orthopedic surgeon's viewpoint. *Sports Medicine.* 9(4):229–243 (1990).

Maïmoun, L. & C. Sultan: Effects of physical activity on bone remodeling. *Metabolism:—Clinical and Experimental.* 60: 373–388 (2011).

Malina, R. M.: Biological maturity status of young athletes. In Malina, R. M. (ed.): *Young Athletes: Biological, Psychological and Educational Perspectives.* Champaign, IL: Human Kinetics (1988).

Marcus, R.: Normal and abnormal bone remodeling in man. *Annual Review of Medicine.* 38:129–141 (1987).

Marieb, E.: *Human Anatomy and Physiology* (8th edition). Redwood City, CA: Benjamin Cummings (2010).

Micheli, L. T.: Sports injuries in children and adolescence. In Nudel, D. (ed): *Pediatric Sports Medicine.* New York, NY: PMA Publishing, 177–192 (1989).

Myburgh, K. H., L. K. Bachrach, B. Lewis, K. Kent, & R. Marcus: Low bone mineral density at axial and appendicular sites in amenorrheic athletes. *Medicine and Science in Sports and Exercise.* 25(11):1197–1202 (1993).

Myburgh, K. H., J. Hutchins, A. B. Fataar, S. F. Hough, & T. D. Noakes: Low bone density is an etiologic factor for stress fractures in athletes. *Annals of Internal Medicine.* 113:754–759 (1990).

Nielson, C. M., P. Srikanth, & E. S. Orwoll: Obesity and fractures in men and women: An epidemiological perspective. *Journal of Bone and Mineral Research*. 27(1):1–10 (2012).

NIH consensus development panel on osteoporosis prevention, diagnosis, and therapy. osteoporosis prevention, diagnosis, and therapy. *Journal of American Medical Association*. 285:785–795 (2001).

National Osteoporosis Foundation. http://www.nof.org/osteoporosis/stats.htm. Accessed March 27, 2012.

Nordström, A., T. Olsson, & P. Nordström: Bone gained from physical activity and lost through detraining: A longitudinal study in young males. *Osteoporosis International*. 16(7):835–841 (2005).

Ott, S.: Editorial: Attainment of peak bone mass. *Journal of Clinical Endocrinology and Metabolism*. 71(5):1082A–1082C (1990).

Parfitt, A. M.: Bone remodeling and bone loss: Understanding the pathophysiology of osteoporosis. *Clinical Obstetrics and Gynecology*. 30(4):789–811 (1987).

Plowman, S. A., N. Y. S. Lui, & C. L. Wells: Body composition and sexual maturation in premenarcheal athletes and nonathletes. *Medicine and Science in Sports and Exercise*. 23(1):23–29 (1991).

Polidoulis, I., J. Beyene, & A. M. Cheung: The effect of exercise on pQCT parameters of bone structure and strength in postmenopausal women—A systematic review and meta-analysis of randomized controlled trials. *Osteoporosis International*. 23:29–51 (2012).

Proctor, K. L., W. C. Adams, J. D. Shaffrath, & M. D. Van Loan: Upper-limb bone mineral density of female college gymnasts versus controls. *Medicine & Science in Sports & Exercise*. 34(11):1830–1835 (2002).

Radcliffe, J. C., & R. C. Farentinos. *Plyometrics: Explosive Power Training*. Champaign, IL: Human Kinetics (1985).

Riser, W. L., E. J. Lee, A. Leblanc, H. B. Poindexter, J. M. Risser, & V. Schneider: Bone density in eumenorrheic female college athletes. *Medicine and Science in Sports and Exercise*. 22:570–574 (1990).

Seeman, E., & P. D. Delmas: Bone quality: The material and structural basis of bone strength and fragility. *New England Journal of Medicine*. 354:2250–2261 (2006).

Sprynarova, S.: The influence of training on physical and functional growth before, during and after puberty. *European Journal of Applied Physiology*. 56:719–724 (1987).

Sterling, J. C., D. W. Edelstein, R. D. Calvo, & R. Webb II: Stress fractures in the athlete: Diagnosis and management. *Sports Medicine*. 14(5):336–346 (1992).

Teitelbaum, S. L.: Skeletal growth and development. In Favus, M. J. (ed.): *Primer on Metabolic Bone Diseases and Disorders of Mineral Metabolism*. Kelseyville, CA: American Society of Bone and Mineral Research Society (1993).

Tucker, K. L., C. Honglei Chen, M. T. Hannan, L. A. Cupples, P. W. F. Wilson, D. Felson & D. P. Kiel: Bone mineral density and dietary patterns in older adults: The Framingham osteoporosis study. *The American Journal of Clinical Nutrition*. 76(1):245–252 (2002).

Turner, C. H. & A. G. Robling: Designing exercise regimens to increase bone strength. *Exercise and Sport Sciences Reviews*. 31(1):45–50 (2003).

Vicente-Rodriguez, G.: How does exercise affect bone development during growth? *Sports Medicine*. 36:561–569 (2006).

Vogel, J. M. & M. W. Whittle: Bone mineral changes: The second manned skylab mission. *Aviation, Space, and Environmental Medicine*. 13:282–289 (1976).

Welsh, L. & O. M. Rutherford: Hip bone mineral density is improved by high-impact aerobic exercise in postmenopausal women and men over 50 years. *European Journal of Applied Physiology and Occupational Physiology*. 74:511–517 (1996).

Winters, K. M. & C. M. Snow: Detraining reverses positive effects of exercise on the musculoskeletal system in premenopausal women. *Journal of Bone and Mineral Research*. 15(12):2495–2503 (2000).

Wohl, G. R., S. K. Boyd, S. Judex, R. F. Zernicke: Functional Adaptations of bone to exercise and injury. *Journal of Science and Medicine in Sport*. 3(3):313–324 (2000).

World Health Organization. Assessment of fracture risk and its application to screening for postmenopausal osteoporosis. Geneva, Switzerland: WHO (1994).

Witzke, K. A. & C. M. Snow: Effects of plyometric jump training on bone mass in adolescent girls. *Medicine & Science in Sports & Exercise*. 32(6):1051–1057 (2000).

Zach, K. N., A. L. Smith, A. Z. Hoch: Advances in management of the female athlete triad and eating disorders. *Clinical Sports Medicine*. 30:551–573 (2011).

Zanker, C. L. & C. B. Cooke: Energy balance, bone turnover, and skeletal health in physically active individuals. *Medicine & Science in Sports & Exercise*. 36:1372–1381, 2004.

Zernicke, R. F., G. R. Wohl, & J. M. LaMothe: The Skeletal-Articular System. In Tipton, C. M., M. N. Sawka, C. A. Tate, & R. L. Terjung (eds.): *ACSM's Advanced Exercise Physiology*. Baltimore, MD: Lippincott Williams & Wilkins, p. 106 (2006).

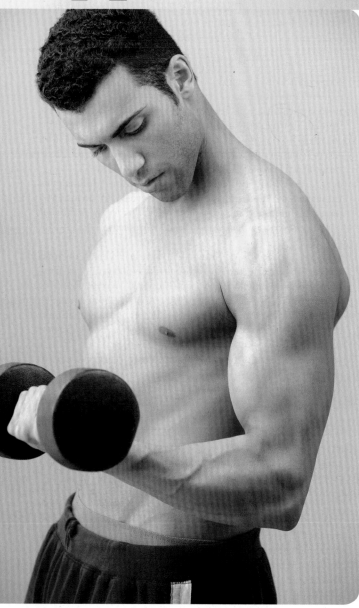

17

Skeletal Muscle System

OBJECTIVES

After studying the chapter, you should be able to:

> Describe the functions of skeletal muscle tissue.

> Identify the characteristics of muscle tissue that make movement possible.

> Describe the macroscopic and microscopic organization of skeletal muscle tissue.

> Relate the molecular structure of myofilaments to the sliding filament theory of muscle contraction.

> Identify the regions of a sarcomere, and explain the changes that occur in these regions during contraction.

> Discuss the importance of specialized organelles, specifically, the sarcoplasmic reticulum, the T tubules, and the myofibrils.

> Explain the events involved in excitation-contraction coupling.

> Describe the sequence of events in the generation of force within the contractile elements.

> Differentiate muscle fiber types based on their contractile and metabolic properties.

> Discuss the ramifications of fiber type distribution on the likelihood of success in a given athletic event.

Introduction

Muscle contractions provide the basis for all human movement. Movement also involves interactions among different body systems. For instance, the muscle cells (fibers) produce and utilize ATP to provide the energy for contraction and force production. The digestive, respiratory, endocrine, and cardiovascular systems must be operating effectively to provide muscle cells with the oxygen and nutrients needed to produce the energy. For the purposes of this chapter, it is assumed that these other body systems are functioning properly.

Overview of Muscle Tissue

Muscle tissue produces force through the interaction of its basic contractile elements—the myofilaments—which are composed primarily of protein. The three types of muscle tissue (skeletal, smooth, and cardiac) have different general functions. The force of contraction may be used for movement such as locomotion (skeletal muscle), the movement of materials through hollow tubes such as the digestive tract or blood vessels (smooth muscle), or the pumping action of the heart (cardiac muscle). Regardless of type, all muscle tissue can produce force because of certain basic characteristics. This chapter focuses on skeletal muscle (**Figure 17.1**).

Because skeletal muscles have various characteristics, they are often referred to by different names. Skeletal muscles are under conscious control and are often called *voluntary muscles*. Skeletal muscles are also sometimes referred to as *striated muscle* because of the repeating pattern of light and dark bands seen in their microscopic structure. Additionally, to differentiate skeletal muscle fibers from intrafusal fibers found in sensory organs of the muscle (proprioceptors; see Chapter 20), physiologists sometimes refer to skeletal muscle fibers as *extrafusal muscle fibers*.

Physiologist terms

Functions of Skeletal Muscle

Although movement is the primary function of muscle tissue, the muscular system also has other important roles. In addition to locomotion and manipulation, skeletal muscles maintain body posture, assist in the venous return of blood to the heart, and produce heat

Wide array of muscular uses

> **Irritability** The ability of a muscle to receive and respond to stimuli.
>
> **Contractility** The ability of a muscle to respond to a stimulus by shortening.
>
> **Extensibility** The ability of a muscle to be stretched or lengthened.
>
> **Elasticity** The ability of a muscle to return to resting length after being stretched.

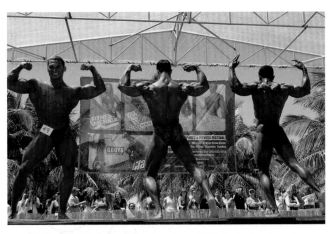

FIGURE 17.1 Bodybuilders.
Bodybuilding poses demonstrate muscle hypertrophy and definition.

(thermogenesis). Heat is a by-product of cellular respiration; because muscles use a great deal of energy for movement, they also generate a great deal of heat. Additionally, muscles act as energy transducers by converting biochemical energy from ingested food into mechanical and thermal energy. Skeletal muscles also help protect internal organs. Because muscles make up most of the protein in the body, they constitute a potential but rarely used form of stored energy. The use of protein as an energy substrate is discussed in the metabolism unit.

Rarely use protein

Striated because of light and dark bands

Characteristics of Muscle Tissue

The unique characteristics of muscle tissue are specifically suited to its primary function: converting an electrical signal into a mechanical event (contraction of muscle fibers). These characteristics include irritability, contractility, extensibility, and elasticity.

Chemical/Irrit.

Irritability refers to the ability of a muscle to receive and respond to stimuli. The stimulus is usually a chemical message (from a neurotransmitter), and the response is the generation of an electrical current (action potential) along the cell membrane. **Contractility** refers to the ability of a muscle to shorten in response to a stimulus. This shortening produces force. Muscle tissue is the only body tissue that can generate force. **Extensibility** refers to the ability of a muscle to be stretched or lengthened. Stretching occurs when a muscle is manipulated by another force. **Elasticity** refers to the ability of a muscle to return to its resting length after being stretched. Together, these characteristics of muscles allow for human movement.

Macroscopic Structure of Skeletal Muscles

The human body has over 400 skeletal muscles, which account for 40–45% of the adult male body weight and 23–25% of the adult female body weight (Hunter, 2000).

40–45% Male weight
23–25 % female weight

These muscles function together in remarkable ways to provide smooth, integrated movement for a wide variety of activities, many of which require little conscious thought. Muscle action is also the basis of sport and fitness activities. To understand how muscles function in various sports and exercise activity, or in any other activity, it is necessary to look beneath the skin.

Organization and Connective Tissue

Skeletal muscles are organized systematically, as shown in **Figure 17.2**. Some of this organization is apparent to the naked eye, but other aspects are apparent only when muscle fibers are viewed through a microscope.

Skeletal muscles are attached to bones by tendons, which allow the contraction of a muscle to move a bone. Each muscle is bound together by a thick layer (sheath) of connective tissue called *fascia*. Just beneath the fascia is a more delicate layer of connective tissue called *epimysium* that directly covers the muscle.

The interior of the muscle is subdivided into bundles of muscle fibers called *fasciculi* (singular: *fasciculus* or *fascicle*), which are also surrounded by connective tissue. The sheath of connective tissue that separates fasciculi within a skeletal muscle is called *perimysium*. The fasciculi are comprised of many individual muscle fibers (cells), each of which is surrounded by its own sheath of connective tissue called *endomysium*.

The three layers of connective tissue (the epimysium, the perimysium, and the endomysium) provide the framework that holds the muscle together. These layers of connective tissue come together at each end of the muscle to form the tendons that attach the muscle to bone. As a muscle contracts, it pulls on the connective tissue in which it is wrapped, causing the tendon to pull on the bone to which it is attached.

Architectural Organization

Different arrangements of fasciculi within a muscle account for the different shapes of muscles. Muscles can be described as longitudinal, fusiform, radiate, unipennate, bipennate, or circular, as shown in **Figure 17.3**. The shape of a muscle in part determines its range of motion

FIGURE 17.2 Organization of Skeletal Tissue.
A. Intact skeletal muscle. Biceps brachii are attached to bones through tendons. **B.** Connective tissue. The entire muscle is surrounded by connective tissue called epimysium. The muscle is organized into bundles called fasciculi, which are surrounded by connective tissue called perimysium. Each fasciculus contains many individual fibers surrounded by connective tissue called endomysium.

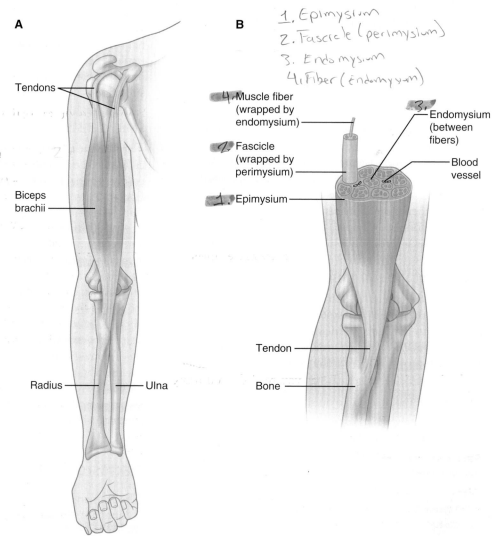

A

Tendons

Biceps brachii

Radius — Ulna

B

1. Epimysium
2. Fascicle (perimysium)
3. Endomysium
4. Fiber (Endomysium)

4. Muscle fiber (wrapped by endomysium)

1. Fascicle (wrapped by perimysium)

1. Epimysium

3.
Endomysium (between fibers)

Blood vessel

Tendon

Bone

Classification	Example	Diagram
Longitudinal	Sartorius	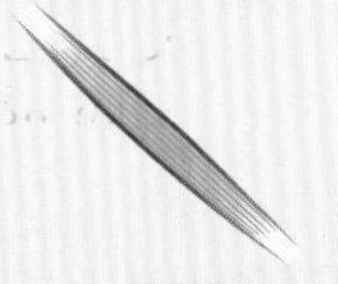
Fusiform	Biceps brachii	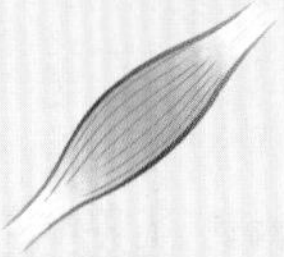
Radiate	Gluteus medius	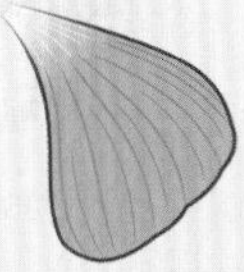
Unipennate	Tibialis posterior	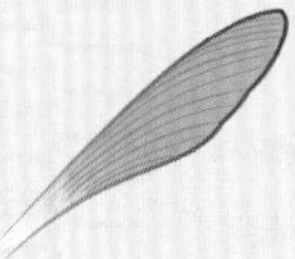
Bipennate	Gastrocnemius (calves)	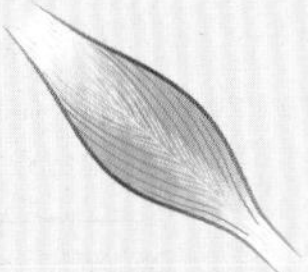
Circular	Orbicular oculi (and sphincters)	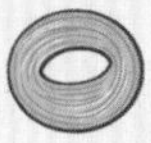

FIGURE 17.3 Arrangement of Fasciculi.

and influences its power production. Longer and more parallel muscle fibers, as are present in longitudinal muscles, allow for greater muscle shortening. Bipennate muscles, in contrast, shorten very little but are more powerful.

Microscopic Structure of a Muscle Fiber

Individual muscle fibers are composed primarily of smaller units called myofibrils, which are in turn made up of myofilaments. Refer to the organization of skeletal muscle shown in **Figure 17.4** as you read the following sections.

SR = calcium storage/release
TT = electrical

Sarcoplasmic Reticulum (SR) The specialized muscle cell organelle that stores and releases calcium.

Transverse Tubules (T Tubules) Organelles that carry the electrical signal from the sarcolemma into the interior of the cell.

Muscle Fibers

Muscle fibers, also called muscle cells, are long, cylinder-shaped cells ranging from 10 to 100 μm in diameter and 1–400 mm in length (Hunter, 2000; Marieb and Hoehn, 2010). The major structures of a muscle fiber and their functions are summarized in **Table 17.1**.

A skeletal muscle fiber contains many nuclei, which are located just below the cell membrane. The *sarcolemma is the polarized plasma membrane* of a muscle cell, whose properties account for the irritability of muscle. The *sarcoplasm* of a muscle cell is similar to the cytoplasm of other cells, but it has specific adaptations to serve the functional needs of muscle cells, namely, increased amounts of glycogen and the oxygen-binding protein myoglobin.

A muscle fiber contains the same organelles found in other cells (including a large number of mitochondria) along with some specialized organelles. Organelles of specific interest are the transverse tubules (T tubules), the sarcoplasmic reticulum (SR), and the myofibrils. Myofibrils are composed primarily of the protein myofilaments and are responsible for the contractile properties of muscles. Skeletal muscle cells also have a highly organized complex cytoskeleton that provides the framework for the organelles and plays an important role in transmitting force from muscle tissue to bone.

Sarcoplasmic Reticulum and Transverse Tubules

Figure 17.4 illustrates the relationship among the myofibrils, the sarcoplasmic reticulum, and the transverse tubules. The sarcoplasmic reticulum (SR) is a specialized organelle that stores and releases calcium. It is an interconnecting network of tubules running parallel with and wrapped around the myofibrils. (In **Figure 17.4** the sarcolemma has been partially removed to illustrate the SR and myofibrils.) The major significance of the sarcoplasmic reticulum is its ability to store, release, and take up calcium and thereby control muscle contraction. Calcium is stored in the portion of the sarcoplasmic reticulum called the *lateral sacs* or *cisterns*.

The transverse tubules (T tubules) are organelles that carry the electrical signal from the sarcolemma to the interior of the cell. T tubules are continuous with the sarcolemma and protrude into the sarcoplasm of the cell. As their name implies, T tubules run perpendicular (transverse) to the myofibril. Each T tubule runs between two lateral sacs of the sarcoplasmic reticulum, creating what is known as a triad; this ensures that that the spread of an electrical signal (action potential) through the T tubules causes the release of calcium from the lateral sacs of the sarcoplasmic reticulum. *(Triad)*

Myofibrils and Myofilaments

Each muscle fiber contains hundreds to thousands of smaller cylindrical units, or rod-like strands, called

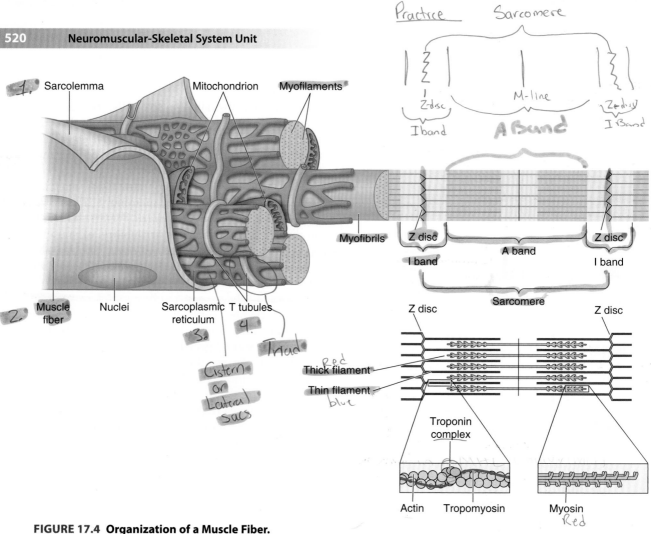

Handwritten annotations:
1. Sarcolemma
2. Muscle fiber
3. Cistern or Lateral Sacs
4. Triad

Practice Sarcomere
Z-disc   M-line   Z-disc
I band   A Band   I Band

Labels in figure: Sarcolemma, Mitochondrion, Myofilaments, Myofibrils, Z disc, A band, Z disc, I band, I band, Sarcomere, Muscle fiber, Nuclei, Sarcoplasmic reticulum, T tubules, Z disc, Z disc, Thick filament (Red), Thin filament (blue), Troponin complex, Actin, Tropomyosin, Myosin (Red)

FIGURE 17.4 Organization of a Muscle Fiber.
There is a close anatomical relationship among the organelles, specifically the myofibrils, T tubules, and sarcoplasmic reticulum (SR). The repeating pattern of the myofibrils is due to the arrangement of the myofilaments.

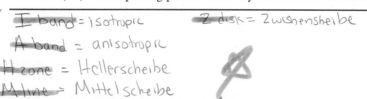

Handwritten notes:
Might be on test
I band = isotropic   Z disk = Zwischenscheibe
A band = anisotropic
H zone = Hellerscheibe
M line = Mittelscheibe

Cell Part	Description	Function
TABLE 17.1 Summary of Major Components of a Skeletal Muscle Cell		
Nucleus	Multinucleated	Is the control center for the cell
Sarcolemma	Polarized cell membrane	Is capable of receiving stimuli from the nervous system
Sarcoplasm	Intracellular material	Holds organelles and nutrients; provides the medium for glycolytic enzymatic reactions
Organelles		
Myofibrils	Rod-like structures composed of smaller units called myofilaments; account for 80% of muscle volume	Contain contractile proteins (myofilaments), which are responsible for muscle contraction
T tubules	Series of tubules that run perpendicular (transverse) to the cell and are open to the external part of cell	Spread polarization from the cell membrane into the interior of cell, which triggers the sarcoplasmic reticulum to release calcium
Sarcoplasmic reticulum	Interconnecting network of tubules running parallel with and wrapped around the myofibrils	Stores and releases calcium
Mitochondria	Sausage- or spherical-shaped organelles; numerous in a muscle cell	Are the major site of energy production

myofibrils (**Figure 17.4**). Myofibrils are specialized contractile organelles composed of myofilaments. These myofibrils, sometimes simply called fibrils, typically lie parallel to the long axis of the muscle cell and extend the entire length of the cell. Myofibrils account for approximately 80% of the volume of a muscle fiber.

As shown in **Figure 17.4**, each myofibril is composed of still smaller **myofilaments (or filaments)** arranged in a repeating pattern along the length of the myofibril. **Myofilaments** are contractile proteins (thick and thin) that are responsible for muscle contraction. Myofilaments account for most of the muscle protein. The repeating pattern of these myofilaments along the length of the myofibril gives skeletal muscle its striated appearance. Each repeating unit is referred to as a sarcomere.

Sarcomeres

A **sarcomere** is the functional unit (contractile unit) of a muscle fiber. As shown in **Figure 17.5**, each sarcomere contains two types of myofilaments. The *thick* filaments are composed primarily of the contractile protein **myosin**, and the *thin* filaments are composed primarily of the contractile protein actin. Thin filaments also contain the *regulatory proteins*, troponin and tropomyosin. Viewed with an electron microscope, the arrangement of myofilaments has the appearance of alternating bands of light and dark striations. The light bands are called *I bands* and contain only thin filaments. The dark bands are called *A bands* and contain thick and thin filaments, with the thick filaments running the entire length of the A band. The length of the thick filament thus determines the length of the A band.

The letter names of the various regions of the sarcomere derive from the first letter of the German word that describes the appearance of each. The names of the bands relate to the refraction of light through them. The I band is named for the word *isotropic*, which means that this area appears lighter because more light passes through it. The A band is named for its *anisotropic* properties, meaning that it appears darker because not as much light passes through. These properties relate to the types of filament present in the bands.

Each A band is interrupted in the midsection by an *H zone* (from the German *Hellerscheibe*, for "clear disk"), where there is no overlap of thick and thin filaments. Running through the center of the H zone is a dense line called the *M line* (from the German *Mittelscheibe*, for "middle disk"). The I bands are also interrupted

Myofibril Contractile organelles composed of myofilaments.

Myofilaments Contractile (thick and thin) proteins responsible for muscle contraction.

Sarcomere The functional unit (contractile unit) of muscle fibers.

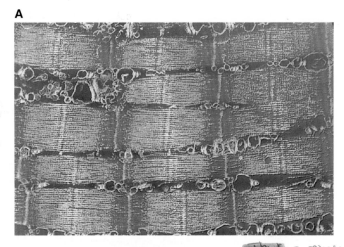

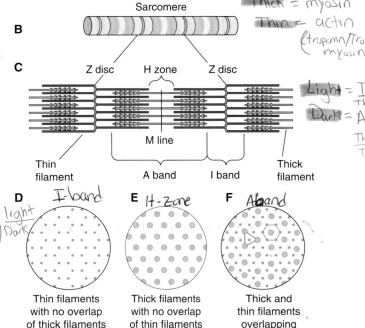

FIGURE 17.5 Arrangement of Myofilaments in a Sarcomere. A. Micrograph of sarcomeres. **B.** Model of sarcomeres. **C.** Relationship between thick and thin filaments. **D.** Cross-sectional view of thin filaments. **E.** Cross-sectional view of thick filaments. **F.** Cross-sectional view of thick and thin filaments.

at the midline by a darker area called the **Z disk** (from the German *Zwischenscheibe*, for "between disc"). A sarcomere extends from one Z disk to the successive Z disk. The Z disk serves to anchor the thin filaments to adjacent sarcomeres.

Myofilaments occupy three-dimensional space. The arrangement of the myofilaments at different points in the sarcomere is shown in **Figure 17.5D–F. Figure 17.5D** presents a cross section of thin filaments in regions where there is no overlap with thick filaments (i.e., the I band), whereas **Figure 17.5E** presents a cross section of thick filaments in a region where there is no overlap with thin filaments (H zone). Notice that

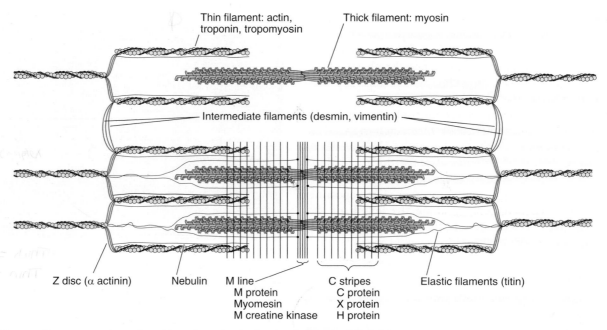

FIGURE 17.6 Representation of Auxiliary Proteins in the Sarcomere.
Source: From Billeter, R. & H. Hoppeler: Muscular basis of strength. In Komi, P. V. (ed.): *Strength and Power in Sport*. Champaign, IL: Human Kinetics. 45 (1992). Copyright 1992 by International Olympic Committee. Reprinted by permission.

myosin = MHC (Heavy chain)
MLC (Light chain)

in regions where the thick and thin filaments overlap (**Figure 17.5F**), each thick filament is surrounded by six thin filaments, and each thin filament is surrounded by three thick filaments.

A sarcomere consists of contractile, regulatory, and structural proteins. Structural proteins make up much of the cytoskeleton. In recent years, researchers have identified dozens of proteins that contribute to a highly organized and complex sarcomere (Caiozzo and Rourke, 2006). **Figure 17.6** diagrams some of the major auxiliary structural proteins in the cytoskeleton of the sarcomere and indicates the relationship between the structural and contractile proteins (Billeter and Hoppler, 1992). Proteins of the M line and the Z disk hold the thick and the thin filaments in place, respectively. Titan, an elastic filament, helps keep the thick filament in the middle of the sarcomere during contraction. Structural proteins also serve as mechanical links between sarcomeres and the extracellular matrix. Collectively, these connection sites are called costameres (Caiozzo and Rourke, 2006).

Molecular Structure of the Myofilaments

The contractile proteins of the myofilaments slide over one another during muscular contraction. Hence, the sliding filament theory of muscle contraction explains how muscles contract. Knowing the structure of the myofilaments is essential to understanding how muscles contract.

Thick Filaments

Thick filaments are composed of myosin molecules, primarily the contractile form, myosin heavy chain (MHC). Myosin light chain (MLC) molecules are also present and assist in regulating the rate of contractions (Caiozzo and Rourke, 2006). The term myosin as used in this text refers to the contractile form (MHC) unless otherwise specified. Each molecule of myosin has a rod-like tail and two globular heads (**Figure 17.7A**). A typical thick filament contains approximately 200–300 myosin molecules (Caiozzo and Rourke, 2006). These molecules are oriented so that the tails form the central rod-like structure of the filament (**Figure 17.7B**). The globular myosin heads extend outward and form *cross-bridges* when they interact with thin filaments. The myosin heads have two reactive sites: One allows it to bind with the actin filament, and one binds to ATP. Only when the myosin heads bind strongly to the active sites on actin, forming a cross-bridge, can contraction occur.

The myosin subunits are oriented in opposite directions along the filament, forming a central section that lacks projecting heads (**Figure 17.7C**). The result is a bare zone in the middle of the filament, which is the H zone seen in the middle of the A band (**Figure 17.5C** and **D**).

Thin Filaments

Thin filaments are composed primarily of the contractile protein actin. As illustrated in **Figure 17.8A** and **B**, actin is composed of small globular subunits (G actin) that form long strands called fibrous actin (F actin). A filament of

FOCUS ON APPLICATION: *CLINICALLY RELEVANT*

Increasing Protein Synthesis—Interaction of Training and Nutrition

Many athletes, especially those engaged in resistance training, are interested in increasing protein synthesis. Increased protein synthesis increases the amount of contractile proteins and thus makes the muscles larger and stronger. Protein synthesis is enhanced in several circumstances: (a) following resistance exercise, (b) when amino acid availability is increased, and (c) when blood insulin levels are high. Recent research by Rasmussen et al. (2000) suggests that when these three conditions occur together, their effect on protein synthesis is additive. Participants in this study ingested a drink containing six essential amino acids and 35 g of sucrose following a bout of resistance training. The participants consumed the drink at either 1 or 3 hours after training, and the results were compared to a control group that consumed a flavored placebo drink. The ingestion of sucrose caused an elevation in blood insulin levels.

The combination of essential amino acids, elevated insulin levels, and resistance training stimulated protein synthesis approximately 400% above predrink levels when the drink was consumed 1 or 3 hours after resistance exercise. This increase in protein synthesis is greater than that reported following resistance training alone (~100% increase in protein synthesis), increased amino acid availability alone (~150% increase in protein synthesis), and the combination of resistance training and increased amino acid availability (~200% increase in protein synthesis). Based on these results, fitness professionals may recommend that exercise participants interested in increasing muscle size consider consuming a drink containing essential amino acids and carbohydrate following resistance training workouts. The supplement is equally effective when consumed 1 or 3 hours after a workout.

Source: Rasmussen et al. (2000).

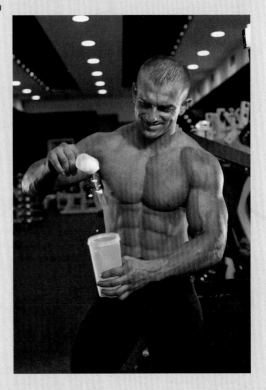

---

actin is formed by two strands of F actin coiled about each other to form a double-helical structure; this structure, which resembles two strands of pearls wound around each other, may be referred to as a *coiled coil* (**Figure 17.8C**). The actin molecules contain active sites to which myosin heads bind during contraction.

The thin filaments also contain the regulatory proteins called tropomyosin and troponin, which regulate the interaction of actin and myosin. *Tropomyosin* is a long, double-stranded, helical protein wrapped about the long axis of the actin backbone (**Figure 17.8D**). Tropomyosin blocks the active site on actin, thereby inhibiting actin and myosin from binding under resting conditions.

Troponin is a small, globular protein complex composed of three subunits that control the position of the tropomyosin (**Figures 17.8E** and **17.9**). The three units are troponin C (TnC), troponin I (TnI), and troponin T (TnT). TnC contains the calcium-binding sites,

Sliding Filament Theory of Muscle Contraction The theory that explains muscle contraction as the result of myofilaments sliding over each other.

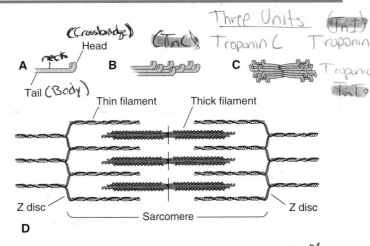

FIGURE 17.7 Molecular Organization of Thick Filaments. **A.** Individual myosin molecules have a rod-like tail and two globular heads. **B.** Individual molecules are arranged so that the tails form a rod-like structure and the globular heads project outward to form cross-bridges. **C.** Myosin subunits are oriented in opposite directions along the filament forming a central bare zone in the middle of the filament (H zone). **D.** Thick filament (myosin) within a single sarcomere showing the myosin heads extending toward the thin filament.

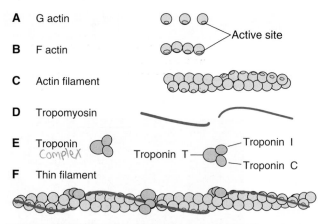

A G actin

B F actin

C Actin filament

D Tropomyosin

E Troponin
Complex

Troponin T — Troponin I / Troponin C

F Thin filament

FIGURE 17.8 Molecular Organization of Thin Filaments.
A. Individual actin subunits (globular, G actin) shown with active site for binding to myosin heads. **B.** Fibrous actin (F actin). **C.** Actin filament with two strands of fibrous actin wound around itself to form a coiled coil. Active sites are exposed. **D.** Tropomyosin is a regulatory protein that covers the binding sites on actin. **E.** Troponin is a regulatory protein that when bound to Ca^{2+} removes tropomyosin from its blocking position on actin. **F.** The thin filament is composed of actin, tropomyosin, and troponin.

TnT binds troponin to tropomyosin, and TnI inhibits the binding of actin and myosin in the resting state (**Figure 17.9B**). When calcium binds to the TnC subunit, the troponin complex undergoes a configurational change. Because troponin is attached to tropomyosin, the change in the shape of troponin causes tropomyosin to be removed from its blocking position, thus exposing the active sites on actin (Marieb and Hoehn, 2010). Once the active sites are exposed, the myosin heads can bind to the actin, forming the cross-bridges (**Figure 17.9C**). Thus, calcium is key to controlling the interaction of the filaments and, thus, muscle contraction.

Contraction of a Muscle Fiber

For a muscle to contract, three major events must happen:

1. An *action potential* must be generated in the motor neuron that innervates the muscle fibers.
2. The motor neuron must release a neurotransmitter that travels across the neuromuscular junction and binds to receptors on the muscle cell membrane (sarcolemma).
3. An action potential in the muscle fiber must lead to the sliding of the myofilaments—thus shortening the muscle cell.

The first two of these necessary events are discussed in detail in Chapter 20. The following section addresses the third event in the sequence: how a muscle fiber produces force when stimulated. The process whereby electrical events in the sarcolemma of the muscle fiber are linked to the movement of the myofilaments is called *excitation-contraction coupling.*

Before detailing the physiological changes within the muscle fiber (and their myofilaments) as a result of electrical stimulation, however, it is useful to consider the major tenets of the sliding filament theory as revealed through microscopic studies.

The Sliding Filament Theory of Muscle Contraction

The sliding filament theory of muscle contraction is commonly used to describe how muscle contraction generates force. A great deal of data have been amassed from X-ray, light microscopic, and electron microscopic studies to support the sliding filament theory of muscle contraction. This theory accounts for force production during concentric (shortening) contractions very well. However, there is some concern about the extent to which the sliding filament theory adequately explains force generation during eccentric (lengthening) contractions. The basic principles of this theory are as follows:

1. The force of contraction is generated by the process that slides the actin filament over the myosin filament.
2. The lengths of the thick and the thin filaments do not change during muscle contraction.
3. The length of the sarcomere decreases as the actin filaments slide over the myosin filaments and pull the Z disks toward the center of the sarcomere.

See animation [Sliding Filament Theory] at http://thePoint.lww.com/Plowman4e.

Changes in the Sarcomere during Contraction

Much of the evidence for the sliding filament theory comes from observed changes in the length of a sarcomere during muscular contraction. **Figure 17.10** diagrams the sarcomere during rest (**Figure 17.10A**) and during shortening with contraction (**Figure 17.10B**). Notice the following changes in the sarcomere:

1. The A band does not change length, but the Z disks do move closer together. The length of the A band is preserved because the thick filament length does not change.
2. The I band shortens and may disappear. The I band shortens because the thin filaments are pulled over the thick filaments toward the center of the sarcomere. Thus, there is little or no area where the thin filaments do not overlap the thick filaments.
3. The H zone shortens and may disappear because the thin filaments are pulled over the thick filaments toward the center of the sarcomere. If the thin filament overlaps the thick filament for the entire length of the thick filament, there is no H zone.

As detailed in the next section, the sarcomere shortens as the result of the attachment of the myosin heads with the active site on actin and the subsequent release of stored energy that swivels the myosin cross-bridges. This step causes the actin to pull the Z disk toward the center of the sarcomere, which in turn causes the sarcomere, and thus the muscle fiber, to shorten.

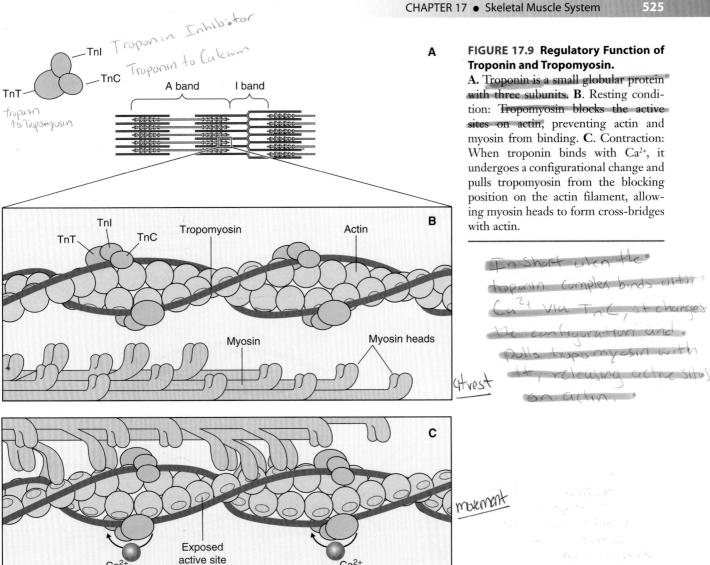

A

FIGURE 17.9 Regulatory Function of Troponin and Tropomyosin.

A. Troponin is a small globular protein with three subunits. **B**. Resting condition: Tropomyosin blocks the active sites on actin, preventing actin and myosin from binding. **C**. Contraction: When troponin binds with Ca^{2+}, it undergoes a configurational change and pulls tropomyosin from the blocking position on the actin filament, allowing myosin heads to form cross-bridges with actin.

In short when the troponin complex binds with Ca^{2+} via TnC, it changes the configuration and pulls tropomyosin with it, releasing active sites on actin.

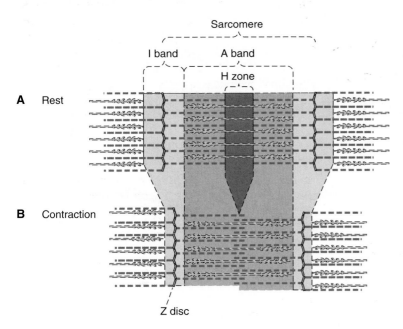

FIGURE 17.10 Changes in a Sarcomere during Contraction.

A. Sarcomere at rest. **B.** During contraction of the sarcomere, the lengths of actin and myosin filaments are unchanged. Sarcomere shortens because actin slides over myosin, pulling Z disks toward the center of the sarcomere. The H zone disappears, the I band shortens, and the A band remains unchanged.

Excitation-Contraction Coupling

Excitation-contraction coupling is the sequence of events by which an action potential (AP; an electrical event) in the sarcolemma of the muscle cell initiates the sliding of the myofilaments, resulting in contraction (a mechanical event). Excitation-contraction coupling occurs in three phases:

Phases of Excitation Contraction

1. The spread of depolarization
2. The binding of calcium to troponin
3. The generation of force (cross-bridge cycling)

Figure 17.11 summarizes what occurs in each phase of excitation-contraction coupling. In the resting state, the regulatory protein tropomyosin is covering the active sites on actin. Excitation-contraction coupling begins with depolarization and the spread of an action potential (AP) along the sarcolemma (labeled 1 in **Figure 17.11**) and continues with the propagation of the action potential into the T tubules. The action potential in the T tubules causes the release of calcium from the adjacent lateral sacs of the sarcoplasmic reticulum (labeled 1a **Figure 17.11**).

The calcium that is released from the SR binds to the troponin molecules (TnC subunit) on the thin filament during the second phase. This causes troponin to undergo a configurational change, thereby removing tropomyosin from its blocking position on the actin filament (labeled 2 in **Figure 17.11**).

The third phase of excitation-contraction coupling is the cross-bridging cycle (labeled 3 in **Figure 17.11** and

FIGURE 17.11 Phases of Excitation-Contraction Coupling.

Triad
Transverse Tubule Reticulum
R - Sarcoplasmic Reticulum
L - Sarcoplasmic Reticulum

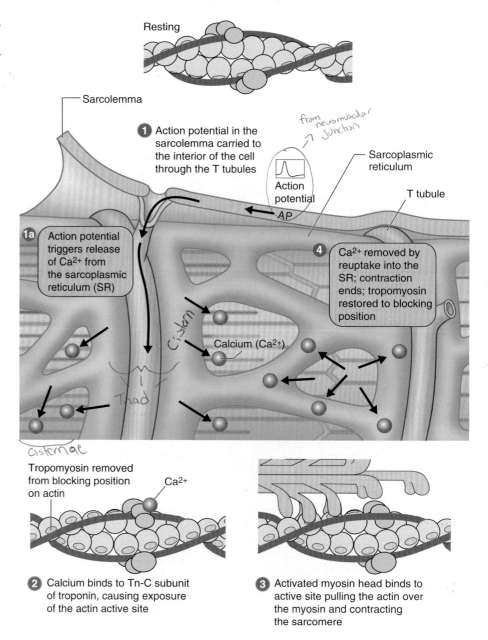

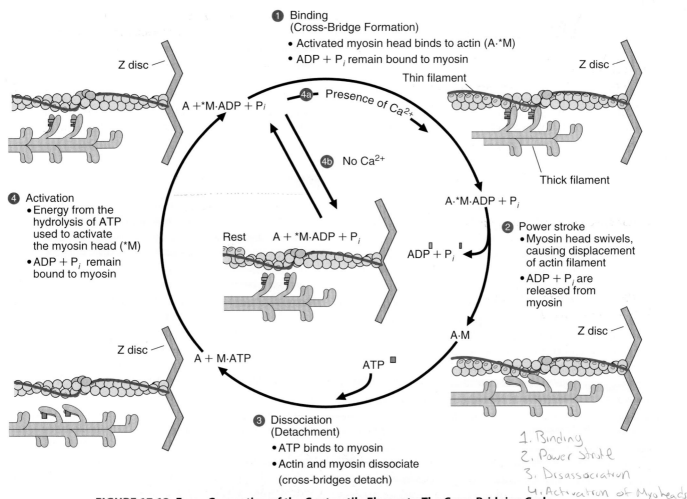

FIGURE 17.12 Force Generation of the Contractile Elements: The Cross-Bridging Cycle.

detailed fully in **Figure 17.12**). The **cross-bridging cycle** involves myosin heads binding to the active sites on actin and a series of cyclic events necessary for the generation of tension within the myosin heads during muscle contraction. The tension within the contractile elements results from the binding of the myosin heads to actin and the subsequent release of stored energy in the myosin heads.

As detailed in **Figure 17.12**, the cross-bridging cycle occurs in four steps (Marieb and Hoehn, 2010; Vander et al., 2001):

1. Binding of myosin heads to actin (cross-bridge formation)
2. Power stroke

Excitation-Contraction Coupling The sequence of events by which an action potential in the sarcolemma initiates the sliding of the myofilaments, resulting in contraction.

Cross-Bridging Cycle The cyclic events necessary for the generation of force or tension within the myosin heads during muscle contraction.

3. Dissociation of myosin and actin
4. Activation of myosin heads

The first step in the *cross-bridge cycle* is the binding of activated myosin heads (*M) with the active sites on actin, forming cross-bridges. In **Figure 17.12**, a centered dot (·) indicates binding, and an asterisk (*) indicates activated myosin heads. Thus, A·*M means that the activated myosin heads are bound to actin (A), whereas A + M indicates that actin and myosin are unbound.

The second step in the cross-bridging cycle is the power stroke. During this step, activated myosin heads swivel from their high-energy, activated position to a low-energy configuration (M with no*). This movement of the myosin cross-bridges results in a slight displacement (sliding) of the thin filament over the thick filament toward the center of the sarcomere. As shown in **Figure 17.12**, during the second step, ADP and Pi are released from the myosin heads, resulting in myosin bound only to actin (A·M).

The third step involves the binding of ATP to the myosin heads and the subsequent dissociation (detachment) of the myosin cross-bridges from actin, thus producing A + M·ATP.

Note the role of ATP in steps 3 and 4. The *binding of ATP* molecules to the myosin head in step 3 allows the myosin heads to detach from actin. In the fourth step, the *breakdown of ATP* provides the energy to activate the myosin heads (*M). The activation of the myosin head is extremely important because it provides the cross-bridges with the stored energy to move the actin during the power stroke. The breakdown of ATP at this step depends on the presence of myosin ATPase (also known as myofibrillar ATPase), as depicted in the following reaction:

$$M \cdot ATP \xrightarrow{\text{myosin ATPase}} {}^*M \cdot ADP + P_i$$

Notice that the products of ATP hydrolysis, ADP + P_i, remain bound to the myosin heads and that the myosin is now in its high-energy or activated state.

The cross-bridging cycle continues as long as ATP is available and calcium is bound to troponin (TnC), causing the active sites on actin to be exposed. On the other hand, activated myosin will remain in the resting state awaiting the next stimulus if calcium is not available in sufficient concentration to remove tropomyosin from its blocking position on actin (labeled 4b in **Figure 17.12**). Because each cycle of the myosin cross-bridges barely displaces the actin, the myosin heads must bind to the actin and be displaced many times for a single contraction to occur. Thus, myosin makes and breaks its bond with actin hundreds or even thousands of times during a single muscle twitch. For this make-and-break cycle to occur, the myosin heads must detach from actin and then be reactivated. This detaching and reactivating process requires the cycle to be repeated and requires the presence of ATP (step 3).

An analogy helps explain the role of ATP in providing energy to activate the myosin head. Visualize a spring-loaded mousetrap. It takes energy to set the trap, just as it takes the splitting of ATP to set or activate the myosin head. Once set, however, the trap will release energy when it is sprung. In a similar manner, the myosin head possesses stored energy that is released when the myosin heads bind to actin and swivel.

It may be useful to review the cycle of events in **Figure 17.12** several times, paying attention to a different aspect (the symbols, the wording, the diagrams, the role of ATP) in each review. Also, keep in mind that ATP plays several important roles in muscle contraction:

1. ATP breakdown provides the energy to activate and reactivate the myosin cross-bridge prior to binding with actin.
2. ATP binding to the myosin head is necessary to break the cross-bridge linkage between the myosin heads and the actin so that the cycle can repeat.
3. ATP is used for the return of calcium into the sarcoplasmic reticulum and restoration of the resting membrane potential once contraction has ended.

The final phase of muscular contraction is a return to muscular relaxation. Relaxation occurs when the nerve impulse ceases and calcium is pumped back into the sarcoplasmic reticulum by active transport (labeled 4, **Figure 17.12**). In the absence of calcium, tropomyosin returns to its blocking position on actin, and myosin heads are not able to bind to actin. While emphasis is usually placed on muscle contraction, relaxation of a muscle following contraction is just as important.

All-or-None Principle

According to the all-or-none principle, when a motor neuron is stimulated, all the muscle fibers in that motor unit contract to their fullest extent or do not contract at all. A motor unit is defined as a motor neuron (α_1 or α_2) and the muscle fibers it innervates. The minimal stimulus necessary to initiate that contraction is referred to as the *threshold stimulus*. When the threshold is reached, a muscle fiber contracts to its fullest extent. This principle involves the electrical properties of the stimulated cell membrane and thus applies to a motor unit or a single muscle fiber only, not to the entire muscle. Consider the analogy of a light switch. When enough pressure (threshold) is applied to the switch to flip it on, the light will turn on to its fullest extent. When the switch controls a group of lights (like a motor neuron innervating multiple muscle fibers), all the lights will turn on to their fullest extent. You cannot make the lights brighter by pushing the switch harder, because it is an all-or-none response. The same is true for an individual muscle fiber or a motor unit: Either a threshold stimulus is reached and contraction occurs or a threshold stimulus is not reached and contraction does not occur.

Muscle Fiber Types

Muscle fibers are typically described by two characteristics: their contractile (twitch) properties and their metabolic properties (**Figure 17.13**).

Contractile (Twitch) Properties

Based on differences in *contractile (twitch) properties*, human muscle fibers can be categorized as *slow-twitch (ST)* or *fast-twitch (FT) fibers*. Slow-twitch fibers are sometimes called Type I fibers, and fast-twitch fibers Type II fibers. The difference between ST and FT fibers appears to be absolute—like the difference between black and white. Some FT fibers contract and relax slightly faster than other fast-twitch fibers, but both of them are clearly much faster than ST fibers. Understanding the difference between twitch speeds begins with understanding the integration of muscles and nerves.

Skeletal muscle fibers are innervated by alpha (α) motor neurons, which exist in two categories, α_1 and α_2

Muscle Fibers			
Twitch properties	Slow	Fast	
Metabolic properties	Oxidative	Oxidative/ glycolytic	Glycolytic
Name based on twitch and metabolic properties	SO	FOG	FG
Other nomenclature	ST, Type I	FTa, FTA, Type IIA	FTx, FTX, Type IIX
Motor Neurons			
Neuron type	α_2	α_1	α_1
Neuron size	Small	Large	Large
Conduction velocity	Slow	Fast	Fast
Recruitment threshold	Low	High	High

FIGURE 17.13 Properties of Motor Units.

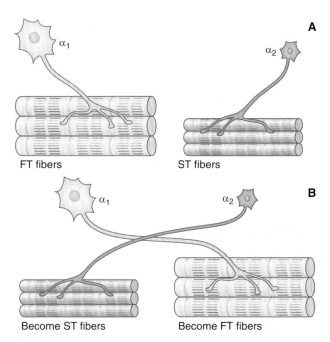

FIGURE 17.14 Results of Cross Innervation.
A. Under normal conditions, α_1 motor neurons innervate FT fibers and α_2 motor neurons innervate ST fibers. **B.** If the neurons supplying the muscles are switched (cross-innervated), the muscle fibers acquire the properties of the new motor neuron.

The α_1 motor neurons innervate FT fibers, and the α_2 motor neurons innervate ST fibers. **Figure 17.14** depicts the results of an experiment that manipulated the innervation of muscle fibers. The α_1 motor neuron was severed from the FT fibers and connected to the ST fibers, and the α_2 motor neuron was cut from the ST fibers and connected to the FT fibers. Importantly, the ST fibers became FT fibers when the α_1 motor neuron replaced the α_2 motor neuron, and vice versa. Therefore, it is logical to conclude that the contractile property of muscle depends on the type of motor neuron that innervates the muscle fibers (Buller et al., 1960; Noth, 1992).

Other elements in the muscle, especially the contractile enzyme myosin ATPase, also contribute to the variation in twitch speed. Indeed, when biopsied muscle fibers are typed, the amount of stain for myosin ATPase is often used to distinguish twitch speed, since the motor neurons are not typically biopsied.

Note that α_2 motor neurons are the smaller of the two nerves and innervate the ST muscle fibers; the α_1 motor neurons are the larger nerves and innervate the FT muscle fibers. The size difference is important because small motor neurons have low excitation thresholds and slow conduction velocities and are thus recruited at low workloads. In contrast, larger motor neurons have a higher excitation threshold and are not recruited until

All-or-None Principle When a motor neuron is stimulated, all of the muscle fibers in that motor unit contract to their fullest extent or do not contract at all.

Motor Unit A motor neuron and the muscle fibers it innervates.

high force output is needed. Thus, motor neurons are recruited according to the *size principle*. Smaller motor units (α_2 motor neurons innervating ST fibers) are recruited during activities that require low force output, such as maintaining posture. As the need for force production increases, such as lifting heavy weights, larger motor units (α_1 motor neurons innervating FT fibers) are recruited.

Metabolic Properties

On the basis of differences in *metabolic properties*, human muscle fibers can be described as *glycolytic, oxidative*, or a combination of both, *oxidative/glycolytic*. All muscle fibers can produce energy both anaerobically (without oxygen, labeled as glycolytic) and aerobically (with oxygen, labeled as oxidative). These processes and terms are fully explained in the unit on metabolism.

Despite the ability of all muscle fibers to produce energy by both glycolytic and oxidative processes, one or the other type of energy metabolism may predominate or the production may be balanced. Thus, the metabolic properties of muscle fibers are not absolute characteristics as much as a continuum (oxidative to glycolytic). This continuum involves shades of gray, unlike the black-or-white typing of slow or fast twitch fibers. The metabolic properties of a muscle specimen are determined by staining for key enzymes (often phosphofructokinase [PFK] for glycolytic processes and succinate dehydrogenase [SDH] for oxidative processes) (Saltin et al., 1977).

Integrated Nomenclature

Slow-twitch fibers rely primarily on oxidative metabolism to produce energy and are therefore referred to as **slow oxidative (SO) fibers** (Type I fibers). Fast-twitch fibers that can work under both oxidative and glycolytic conditions are called **fast oxidative glycolytic (FOG) fibers;** these fibers are also referred to as Type IIA or Type IIa fibers. Other fast-twitch fibers that perform predominantly under glycolytic conditions are called **fast glycolytic (FG) fibers** and are also known as Type IIX or Type IIx fibers.

Skeletal muscle has been classified in numerous ways based on the composition of the myosin molecules, particularly the isoforms of the myosin heavy chain (MHC) and to a lesser extent on the myosin light chain (MLC) isoform (Caiozzo and Rourke, 2006). This chapter primarily relies on the integrated nomenclature of SO, FOG, and FG for clarity but occasionally the designations Type I, IIA (or IIa), and IIX (or IIx) will be used. **Figure 17.13** and **Table 17.2** summarize the properties of motor units and muscle fibers (Caiozzo and Rourke, 2006; Harris and Dudley, 2000).

A motor unit consists of a motor neuron (α_1 or α_2) and the muscle fibers it innervates. As previously described, the twitch speed of a muscle fiber depends largely on the motor neuron that innervates it. Thus, all muscle fibers within a motor unit will be either FT or ST. In addition, because all muscle fibers in a motor unit are recruited to contract together, they have the same metabolic capabilities. Therefore, a motor unit is composed exclusively of SO, FOG, or FG muscle fibers. That means that references to muscle fiber types also refer to motor unit types.

Table 17.2 further compares the different muscle fiber types in reference to important structural, neural, functional, and metabolic characteristics (Harris and Dudley, 2000; Zierath and Hawley, 2004). The diameters of the individual ST and FT fibers differ. The size of the muscle fiber is related to the size of the motor neuron innervating it, but primarily its size reflects the amount of contractile proteins within the muscle cell. ST fibers are smaller than FT fibers and have smaller motor neurons. The larger size of FT fibers is the result of their having more contractile proteins, which, in turn, enables them to produce greater force. **Figure 17.15** shows functional differences in the three types of muscle fibers, including different force production curves (**A**), different fatigue curves (**B**), and different contractile force and power at various speeds (**C**).

Other structural differences among fiber types are related directly to their predominant metabolic pathway for energy production. The SO fibers, which rely mainly on oxidative pathways for energy production, have a high number of mitochondria, high capillary density, high myoglobin content, and high oxidative enzyme activity. The FG fibers, which rely primarily on glycolytic pathways for energy production, have few mitochondria, low capillary density, low myoglobin content,

TABLE 17.2 Characteristics of Muscle Fibers	Type I	Type II	
Contractile (Twitch):	ST	FTa	FTx
Metabolic:	SO	FOG	FG
Structural Aspects			
Muscle fiber diameter	Small	Intermediate	Large
Mitochondrial density	High	Intermediate	Low
Capillary density	High	Intermediate	Low
Myoglobin content	High	Intermediate	Low
Functional Aspects			
Twitch (contraction) time	Slow	Fast	Fast
Relaxation time	Slow	Fast	Fast
Force production	Low	Intermediate	High
Fatigability	Low	Intermediate	High
Metabolic Aspects			
Phosphocreatine stores	Low	High	High
Glycogen stores	Low	Intermediate	High
Triglyceride stores	High	Intermediate	Low
Myosin-ATPase activity	Low	Intermediate	High
Glycolytic enzyme activity	Low	Intermediate	High
Oxidative enzyme activity	High	Intermediate	Low

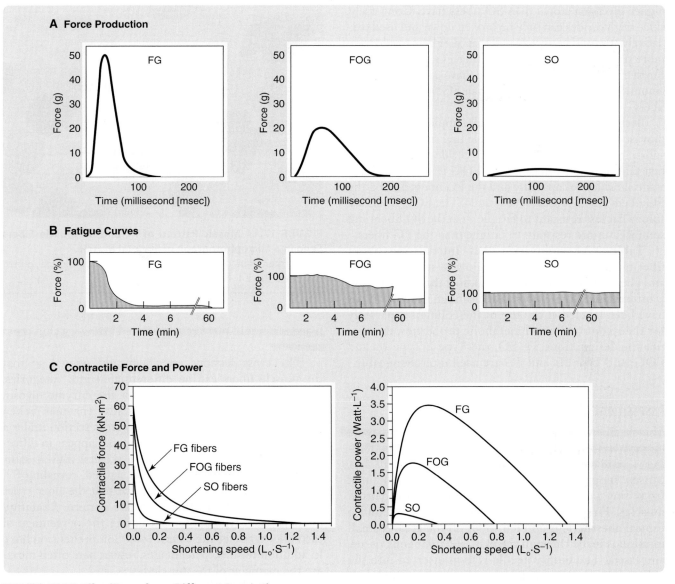

FIGURE 17.15 Fiber Types have Different Properties.
A. Force Production **B.** Fatigue Curves **C.** Contractile Force and Power at Different Contraction Speeds.
Sources: Adapted from Edington, D. W. & V. R. Edgarton: The Biology of Physical Activity. Boston: Houghton Mifflin (1986) and Caiozzo, V. J. & B. Rourke: The muscular system: Structural and functional plasticity. In: *ACSM's Advanced Exercise Physiology.* Philadelphia, PA: Lippincott, Williams & Wilkins (2006).

and high glycolytic enzyme activity. The FOG fibers share characteristics of both SO and FG but also have unique characteristics. Specifically, the FOG fibers have intermediate mitochondrial density, capillary density, myoglobin content, and oxidative enzyme activity and high PC stores, glycogen stores, and glycolytic enzyme activity.

The metabolic differences among muscle fibers both require and reflect differences in energy substrate availability. All muscles store and utilize glycogen; but since glycogen is the only substrate (along with its constituent parts—glucose) that can be used to fuel glycolysis, it makes sense that the FOG and FG fibers would have

Slow Oxidative (SO, Type I) Fibers Slow-twitch muscle fibers that rely primarily on oxidative metabolism to produce energy.

Fast Oxidative Glycolytic (FOG, Type IIA or IIa) Fibers Fast-twitch muscle fibers that can work under oxidative and glycolytic conditions.

Fast Glycolytic (FG, Type IIX or IIx) Fibers Fast-twitch muscle fibers that perform primarily under glycolytic conditions.

higher glycogen stores than SO fibers have. Conversely, since triglycerides can only be broken down and used oxidatively, it would be anticipated that SO fibers would have more triglyceride storage than either FG or FOG fibers. Furthermore, FOG fibers would have an intermediate amount of triglycerides—more than FG but less than SO fibers.

Because SO fibers are so well supplied by the cardiovascular system and have ample fuel supplies (energy substrate), particularly from triglycerides, they are very resistant to fatigue. Because the FOG fibers have a substantial oxidative capability and the FG fibers do not, the FG fibers are the quickest to fatigue. The FOG fibers are somewhat less resistant to fatigue than the SO fibers and somewhat more resistant to fatigue than the FG fibers.

Table 17.2 summarizes key information about fiber types. Take a few minutes now to study this table and check your understanding of how this information is interrelated. Remember that although the fiber types have been labeled at the top of the columns separately for their contractile and metabolic properties, in practice the designations ST, SO, and Type I; Type IIa and FOG; and Type IIx and FG are used interchangeably.

Assessment of Muscle Fiber Type

Muscle fiber type is typically determined by a needle biopsy, an invasive procedure that involves collecting a small sample of skeletal muscle (Figure 17.16). Muscle biopsy samples are most commonly obtained from the gastrocnemius, vastus lateralis, or deltoid muscles. First, the skin is thoroughly cleaned and a topical anesthetic is applied to numb the area. A small incision is made through the skin, subcutaneous tissue, and fascia. The biopsy needle is then inserted into the belly of the muscle to extract a small amount of skeletal muscle tissue (~20–40 mg). This sample is then

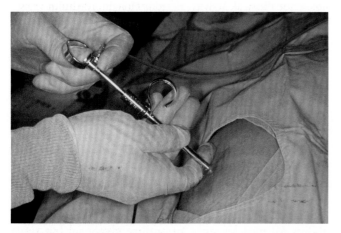

FIGURE 17.16 Muscle Biopsy
A biopsy needle is inserted into a small incision to obtain a sample of skeletal tissue.

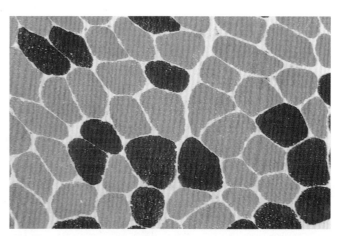

FIGURE 17.17 Mosaic Pattern of FT and ST Muscle Fibers Seen in a Microphotograph of Skeletal Muscle.
The darker stained fibers are the ST fibers, the lighter stained fibers are the FT Fibers.

frozen in liquid nitrogen and sliced into very thin cross sections.

The cross sections are chemically stained so that the muscle fibers can be differentiated into categories. Muscle samples may be stained for the enzyme myosin ATPase and for glycolytic and oxidative enzymes. When stained muscle fibers are viewed in cross section under a microscope, different muscle fiber types appear in different colors. Figure 17.17 shows a skeletal muscle sample that has been histochemically stained, revealing ST (dark) and FT (light) fibers. Notice that the fiber types are intermingled, creating a mosaic pattern. Counting fibers of each type allows calculating the percentage of each fiber type (see the Check your Comprehension box). In addition to these percentages, researchers often measure the diameter of the muscle fibers.

Muscle fibers also can be typed noninvasively by nuclear magnetic resonance spectroscopy (NMR), but this laboratory technique has not yet gained widespread acceptance (Baguet et al., 2011; Boicelli et al., 1989). Attempts to use the vertical jump as a field measure of fiber type have met with varying success (see the Focus on Application) (Costill, 1978; Fry et al., 2003).

Knowledge about fiber types is important for at least three reasons:

1. Fiber type differences help explain individual differences in performance and response to training.
2. Fiber type differences help explain what training can and cannot do.
3. The relationship between fiber types and training and performance in elite athletes helps in the design of training programs for others who wish to be successful in specific events even if they do not know their exact fiber type percentages or distribution.

FOCUS ON APPLICATION

The Relationship between Muscle Fiber Characteristics and Physical Performance

Athletes in strength or power sports have higher percentages of fast-twitch (FT) fibers than athletes in endurance events. Additionally, the cross-sectional area of FT fibers is larger in weightlifters and strength athletes than in sedentary individuals or endurance-trained athletes. Based on the structure-function relationship that underlies physiology, a strong relationship would be expected between fiber type percentage and performance variables. Indeed, when a group of researchers investigated the relationship (correlations) between fast oxidative glycolytic (FOG)

fibers (both percentage of fibers and area) and performance, they found several statistically significant correlations (see table below).

Correlations between Muscle Fiber Characteristics and Performance Variables		
	% FOG Fibers	% Area of FOG Fibers
1 RM snatch	0.94	0.83
Vertical jump	0.83	0.75

The high percentage and large cross-sectional area of fast oxidative fibers in weightlifters is strongly related to performance in both weightlifting and in vertical jump performance. These results support the theoretical relationship between muscle fiber characteristics and actual physical performance. The results also suggest that a simple test for lower-body power, the vertical jump, may be a useful field test to provide a noninvasive indicator of muscle fiber characteristics.

Source: Fry et al. (2003).

CHECK YOUR COMPREHENSION

Fiber typing involves determining the percentage of a sample's fast-twitch or slow-twitch fibers. Count how many total fibers are visible in **Figure 17.17**. Now count how many of those fibers are darkly stained (indicating, in this example, that they are ST fibers). Based on these two numbers, what is the percentage of ST fibers in this muscle sample? What is the percentage of FT fibers in this sample?
Check your answer in Appendix C.

Distribution of Fiber Types

All muscles in humans are composed of a combination of slow-twitch and fast-twitch muscle fibers arranged in a mosaic pattern. This arrangement is thought to reflect the variety of tasks that human muscles must perform. The relative distribution, or percentage, of these fibers, however, may vary greatly from one muscle to another. For example, the soleus muscle may have as much as 85% ST fibers, and the triceps and ocular muscles may have as few as 30% ST fibers. The distribution may also vary considerably among individuals for the same muscle group (Saltin et al., 1977). The following are general characteristics of the distribution of fiber types:

1. Although distribution of fiber type varies within and between individuals, most individuals possess between 45% and 55% ST fibers.
2. The distribution of fiber types is not different for males and females, although males tend to show greater variation than females.

3. After early childhood, the fiber distribution does not change significantly as a function of age.
4. Fiber type distribution is primarily genetically determined.
5. Muscles involved in sustained postural activity have the highest number of slow-twitch muscle fibers.

Fiber Type in Athletes

Few topics in exercise physiology evoke more interest and debate than issues of fiber type in athletes. **Figure 17.18** shows the distribution of fiber types in male and female athletes. Athletes in endurance activities typically have a higher percentage of slow-twitch fibers, while athletes in power activities have a higher percentage of fast-twitch muscle fibers. The distribution of fiber type ranges widely in each group, however, indicating that athletic success is not determined solely by fiber type.

Not only do endurance athletes differ in general fiber type from power or resistance athletes but often these differences relate to specific muscles within these athletic groups. The results of one study of fiber type distribution are reported in **Figure 17.19** (Tesch and Karlsson, 1985). According to this study, the vastus lateralis muscles of the legs possess a greater percentage of ST fibers in endurance athletes primarily using the legs for their activity (such as runners). In contrast, athletes whose sport requires endurance of the upper body possess a greater percentage of ST fibers in the deltoid muscle.

An interesting question arises from such comparisons of fiber type distribution in various athletes: Did training and participation in a given sport influence the fiber type, or did fiber type influence the type of athletic participation? Although some researchers have

FOCUS ON RESEARCH

Does Fiber Type Distribution Affect Maximal Oxygen Uptake?

Researchers have long been interested in the distribution of fiber type in athletes. At the time that Bergh et al. undertook this classic study, researchers knew that aerobically trained individuals were characterized by a high percentage of ST fibers (and hence a lower percentage of FT fibers) and that anaerobically trained individuals (e.g., sprinters) were more likely to have a high percentage of FT fibers. Researchers also knew that aerobic training was associated with a high $\dot{V}O_2$max. $\dot{V}O_2$max is the greatest amount of oxygen an individual can take in, transport, and use during strenuous work; it is considered the best measure of an individual's aerobic (or cardiovascular) fitness. Thus, Bergh et al. proposed that there would be a relationship between the percentage of slow-twitch fibers and a person's $\dot{V}O_2$max.

Their results, shown here in the graph, support their hypothesis.

These data lead to two important conclusions:

1. There is a strong linear relationship between $\dot{V}O_2$max and %ST fibers. This makes sense because the ST fibers have the greatest oxidative ability, that is, the ability to use oxygen to produce large amounts of ATP to support long-duration activities.

2. At any given %ST (above ~40%), an athlete has a greater $\dot{V}O_2$max than a non-athlete. This is consistent with what we know about the trainability of muscle fibers. Endurance training increases the oxidative capacity of muscle, thereby allowing the muscle to use more oxygen and thus achieve a higher $\dot{V}O_2$max.

Source: Bergh, U., A. Thorstensson, B. Sjodin, B. Hulten, K. Piehl, & J. Karlsson: Maximal oxygen uptake and muscle fiber types in trained and untrained humans. *Medicine and Science in Sports and Exercise.* 10(3):151–154 (1978).

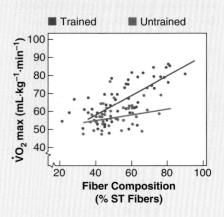

theorized that changes are possible in the contractile properties of muscle, most available evidence indicates that the distribution of ST and FT fibers (the types involving contractile properties) is genetically determined and cannot be altered in humans by exercise training (Kraemer, 2000; Saltin et al., 1977; Williams, 1994). Evidence does show, however, that training can alter the metabolic properties of the cell (enzyme concentration, substrate storage, and so on). These changes may lead

to a conversion of FT fiber subdivisions. Indeed, with endurance training, the oxidative potential of FOG and FG fibers can exceed that of SO fibers of sedentary individuals (Saltin et al., 1977).

In summary, the distribution of fiber types varies considerably within the muscle groups of an individual and among individuals. The basic distribution of fiber type appears to be genetically determined. It is generally thought that exercise training does not alter the

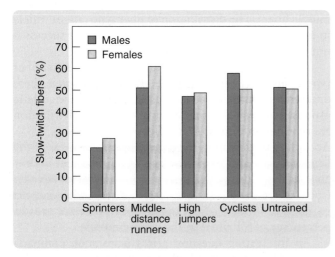

FIGURE 17.18 Fiber Type Distribution among Athletes.
Source: Data from Fox, E. L., R. W. Bowers, & M. L. Foss: *The Physiological Basis for Exercise and Sport.* Dubuque, IA: Brown & Benchmark, 94–135 (1993).

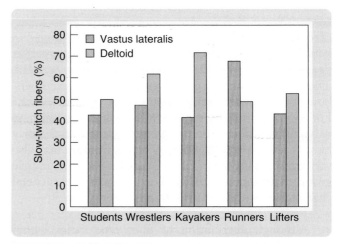

FIGURE 17.19 Fiber Type Distribution of Different Muscle Groups Among Athletes.
Source: Data from Tesch, P. A. & J. Karlsson: Muscle fiber types and size in trained and untrained muscles of elite athletes. *Journal of Applied Physiology.* 59:1716–1720 (1985).

FOCUS ON RESEARCH

Are There Sex Differences in Muscle Fiber Power Production in Older Adults?

It is well known that males are generally stronger than females. The purpose of this study was to determine if differences in power at the single muscle fiber level contribute to the sex difference in whole muscle power production in elderly individuals. Sixteen older adults (mean age = 72 years) participated in the study. A muscle biopsy procedure was performed to obtain muscle fibers.

As expected, the males were stronger in a double-knee press and had greater right knee extension power than females (although some measures of strength and power did not differ between these males and females). However, the slow oxidative (SO) and fast oxidative glycolytic (FOG) fibers of these males and females did not differ significantly in power production.

Thus, it appears that power-generating capacity differs by muscle fiber type (SO<FOG), but not by sex. Rather, it appears that the primary reason that males are stronger than females is that they possess greater muscle mass.

Source: Krivickas, L. S., R. A. Fielding, A. Murray, D. Callahan, A. Johansson, D. J. Dorer, & W. R. Frontera: Sex differences in single muscle fiber power in older adults. *Medicine & Science in Sports & Exercise.* 38(1):57–64 (2006).

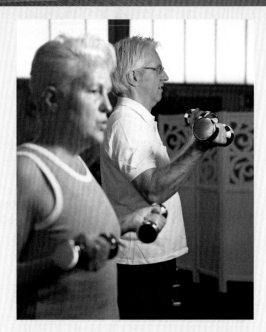

contractile properties of muscle fibers. The possibility remains, however, that training adaptations can alter the metabolic capabilities of muscle fibers sufficiently to change the classification of fiber types within the FT fibers (i.e., from FG to FOG or vice versa).

SUMMARY

1. Skeletal muscles provide for locomotion and manipulation, maintain body posture, and play an important role in heat generation.

2. The muscle characteristics that allow production of movement include irritability, contractility, extensibility, and elasticity.

3. A motor neuron along with the muscle fibers it innervates is called a motor unit. Because each muscle fiber in a motor unit is connected to the same neuron, the electrical activity in the motor neuron controls the contractile activity of all the muscle fibers in a given motor unit.

4. Skeletal muscle fibers are bundled together into groups of fibers called fasciculi. A muscle fiber is itself comprised of smaller units called myofibrils, which are made up of myofilaments.

5. The two types of myofilaments are the thick and thin filaments. The repeating pattern of these myofilaments along the length of the myofibril gives skeletal muscle its striated appearance.

6. The repeating unit, or sarcomere, is the functional unit of the muscle.

7. Tropomyosin is a regulatory protein that blocks the active site on actin, thereby inhibiting actin and myosin from binding under resting conditions. The position of tropomyosin is controlled by troponin.

8. Excitation-contraction coupling is the sequence of events by which an action potential in the sarcolemma initiates the contractile process of the myofilaments.

9. Excitation-contraction coupling has three phases: the spread of depolarization, the binding of calcium to troponin, and the generation of force (cross-bridge cycling).

10. Force is generated in the cross-bridging cycle. This cycle consists of the binding of myosin to actin, the power stroke, the dissociation of myosin and actin, and the activation of myosin heads.

11. The spread of depolarization (action potential) is carried into the interior of the muscle fiber by the T tubules. As the electrical signal moves into the cell, it causes the release of calcium, which is stored in the lateral sacs of the sarcoplasmic reticulum.

12. Calcium released from the sarcoplasmic reticulum binds to the troponin molecules, which undergo a configuration change, thereby removing tropomyosin from its blocking position on the actin filament. This allows the myosin cross-bridges (heads) to bind with the actin filaments.

13. The generation of tension within the contractile elements results from the binding of actin and myosin, which causes the release of stored energy in the myosin heads.

14. ATP plays several important roles in muscle contraction. The hydrolysis of ATP provides the energy to activate or reactivate the myosin head before binding with actin. ATP binding is also necessary to break the linkage between the myosin cross-bridge and actin so that the cycle can repeat. ATP is also used to return calcium to the sarcoplasmic reticulum and to restore the resting membrane potential.

15. During relaxation, calcium is pumped back into the sarcoplasmic reticulum (by active transport), and troponin no longer keeps tropomyosin from its blocking position.

16. When a muscle fiber or motor unit is stimulated to contract, it contracts to its fullest extent or does not contract at all. This is known as the all-or-none principle.

17. Human muscle fibers are categorized as two different types, ST and FT, based on their contractile properties. The FT fibers can be further classified as FOG or FG fibers based on their metabolic properties. ST fibers are metabolically oxidative or SO.

18. Athletes involved in endurance activities typically have a high percentage of slow-twitch fibers. Athletes involved in power activities typically have a high percentage of fast-twitch muscle fibers.

19. Training alters the metabolic capabilities of muscle fibers, but not their contractile properties. It is possible that metabolic alterations could be significant enough to change the classification of fibers with the FT fibers (FOG to FG, and vice versa).

REVIEW QUESTIONS

1. List, in order of largest to smallest, the major components of the whole muscle.
2. What causes the striated appearance of skeletal muscle fibers?
3. What are the T tubules and the sarcoplasmic reticulum? What is the function of each?
4. Relate each region of the sarcomere to the presence of thick and thin myofilaments.
5. Diagram a sarcomere at rest and at the end of a contraction, and identify each of the areas.
6. Describe the role of the regulatory proteins in controlling muscle contraction.
7. Describe the sequence of events in excitation-contraction coupling.
8. Identify the role of ATP in the production of force within the contractile unit of muscle.
9. What is the role of calcium in muscle contraction?
10. Describe the all-or-none principle as it relates to the contraction of a single muscle fiber.
11. Diagram the force production, twitch speed, and fatigue curve for the different fiber types.
12. Discuss the possibility of influencing fiber type distribution by exercise training.

For further review and additional study tools, visit the website at http://thePoint.lww.com/Plowman4e.

REFERENCES

Bergh, U., A. Thorstensson, B. Sjodin, B. Hulten, K. Piehl, & J. Karlsson: Maximal oxygen uptake and muscle fiber types in trained and untrained humans. *Medicine and Science in Sports and Exercise*. 10(3):151–154 (1978).

Baguet, A., I. Everaert, P. Hespel, M. Petrovic, E. Achten, & W. Derave: A new method for non-invasive estimation of human muscle fiber type composition. *Public Library of Science ONE*. 6(7):1–6 (2011).

Billeter, R. & H. Hoppler: Muscular basis of strength. In Komi, P. V. (ed.): *Strength and Power in Sport*. Oxford: Blackwell Scientific, 39–63 (1992).

Boicelli, C. A., A. M. Baldassarri, C. Borsetto, & F. Conconi: An approach to noninvasive fiber type distribution by nuclear magnetic resonance. *International Journal of Sports Medicine*. 10:53–54 (1989).

Buller, A. J., J. C. Eccles, & R. M. Eccles: Interactions between motoneurones and muscles in respect of the characteristic speeds of their responses. *Journal of Physiology*. 150:417–439 (1960).

Caiozzo, V. J. & B. Rourke: The muscular system: Structural and functional plasticity. In: Farrell, P., M. J. Joyner, and VJ Caiozzo (ed). *ACSM's Advanced Exercise Physiology*. Philadelphia, PA: Lippincott, Williams & Wilkins (2006).

Costill, D. L.: *Muscle Biopsy Research: Application of Fiber Composition to Swimming*. Proceedings from Annual Clinic of American Swimming Coaches Association, Chicago. Ft. Lauderdale, FL: American Swimming Coaches Association (1978).

Fox, E. L., R. W. Bowers, & M. L. Foss: *The Physiological Basis for Exercise and Sport*. Dubuque, IA: Brown & Benchmark, 94–135 (1993).

Fry, A. C., B. K. Schilling, R. S. Staron, F. C. Hagerman, R. S. Hikida, & J. T. Thrush: Muscle fiber characteristics and performance correlates of male Olympic-style weightlifters. *Journal of Strength and Conditioning Research*. 17:746–754 (2003).

Harris, R. T. & G. Dudley: Neuromuscular anatomy and physiology. In Baechle, T. R. & R. W. Earle (eds.): *Essentials of Strength and Conditioning*. Champaign, IL: Human Kinetics, 15–23 (2000).

Hunter, G. R.: Muscle physiology. In Baechle, T. R. & R. W. Earle (eds.): *Essentials of Strength Training and Conditioning*. Champaign, IL: Human Kinetics, 3–13 (2000).

Kraemer, W. J.: Physiological adaptations to anaerobic and aerobic training programs. In Baechle, T. R. & R. W. Earle (eds.): *Essentials of Strength Training and Conditioning*. Champaign, IL: Human Kinetics, 137–168 (2000).

Krivickas, L. S., R. A. Fielding, A. Murray, D. Callahan, A. Johansson, D. J. Dorer, & W. R. Frontera. Sex differences in single muscle fiber power in older adults. *Medicine & Science in Sports & Exercise*. 38(1):57–64 (2006).

Marieb, E. N. & K. Hoehn: *Human Anatomy and Physiology* (8th edition). San Francisco, CA: Benjamin Cummings (2010).

Noth, J.: Motor units. In Komi, P. V. (ed.): *Strength and Power in Sport*. Oxford: Blackwell Scientific, 21–28 (1992).

Rasmussen, B. B., K. D. Tipton, S. L. Miller, S. E. Wolf, & R. R. Wolfe: An oral essential amino acid-carbohydrate supplement enhances muscle protein anabolism after resistance exercise. *Journal of Applied Physiology*. 88:386–392 (2000).

Saltin, B., J. Henriksson, E. Nygaard, P. Anderson, & E. Jansson: Fiber types and metabolic potentials of skeletal muscles in sedentary man and endurance runners. *Annals of the New York Academy of Sciences*. 301:3–29 (1977).

Tesch, P. A. & J. Karlsson: Muscle fiber types and size in trained and untrained muscles of elite athletes. *Journal of Applied Physiology*. 59:1716–1720 (1985).

Williams, J.: Normal musculoskeletal and neuromuscular anatomy, physiology, and responses to training. In Hasson, S. M. (ed.): *Clinical Exercise Physiology*. St. Louis, MO: Mosby-Year Book Publishers (1994).

Zierath, J. R. & J. A. Hawley: Skeletal muscle fiber type: Influence on contractile and metabolic properties. *Public Library of Science Biology*. 2(10):1523–1527 (2004).

18 Muscular Contraction and Movement

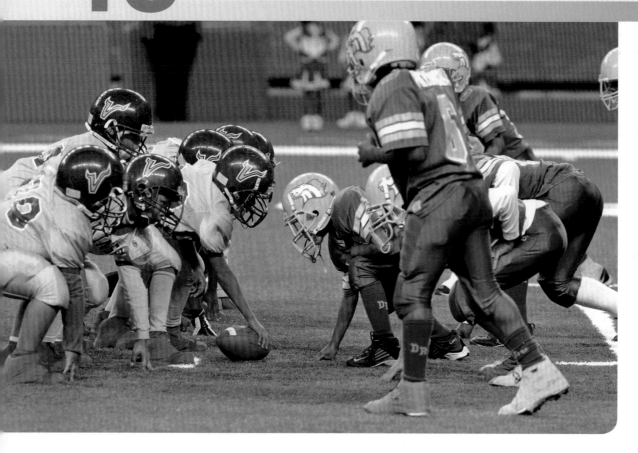

OBJECTIVES

After studying the chapter, you should be able to:

> Differentiate between force and load.

> Identify the different types of muscle contraction and the terms to describe muscle fiber contraction or whole-muscle contraction.

> Compare and contrast concentric and eccentric dynamic contractions.

> Describe neural and mechanical factors that affect force development.

> Differentiate between the length-tension relationship as it applies to a muscle fiber and as it applies to a whole muscle.

> Identify possible causes of muscle fatigue, and indicate the most probable cause of muscle fatigue for various types of activities.

> Outline the integrated model of delayed-onset muscle soreness and explain why DOMS can be a concern.

> Refute the popular belief that delayed-onset muscle soreness is caused by an accumulation of lactic acid in the muscle.

> Identify the different laboratory and field methods for measuring muscular function.

> Describe the basic pattern of strength development.

> Compare and contrast the expression of strength in males and females.

> Describe the impact of age on strength expression in children/adolescents and older adults, and explain the factors affecting older adult.

Introduction: Exercise—The Result of Muscle Contraction

Dictionaries generally define exercise as an activity performed using muscles. In other words, the contraction of muscles is exercise. Therefore, it is impossible to discuss the exercise response of the neuromuscular system in the same way that it is discussed for the cardiovascular-respiratory or metabolic systems.

Although not all muscle action results in exercise, all exercise is done by muscle action. An almost endless number of exercises result from the many ways different body muscles can contract. For example, imagine a basketball player taking off from the foul line for a slam dunk, a bodybuilder flexing in a pose, a swimmer doing a front crawl stroke, and the movement of your eyes across the pages of this book. All of these activities require different muscle actions—explosive dynamic power; controlled static activity; force against a resistance through a large range of motion; and highly coordinated, rapid, but minimal force movement. Although the individual actions involving muscle contractions vary widely, they can be classified in general ways. These classifications help us understand differences in how muscle contractions produce force.

Muscular Force Production

Tension Versus Load

The force developed when a contracting muscle acts on an object is called **muscle tension**. The force exerted on the muscle by the object is called the **load**. The load and muscle tension are opposing forces.

Muscle Tension Force developed when a contracting muscle acts on an object. *[handwritten: Tension = contracting on an object]*

Load Force exerted on the muscle. *[handwritten: Load = force on muscle]*

Contraction Tension-producing process of the contractile elements within muscle. *[handwritten: Contraction = tension produced within muscle]*

Torque The capability of a force to produce rotation of a limb around a joint. *[handwritten: Torque = rotation force]*

Isotonic Contraction A muscle fiber contraction in which the tension generated by the muscle fiber is constant through the range of motion. *[handwritten: Isotonic = tension constant]*

Dynamic Contraction A muscle contraction in which the force exerted varies as the muscle shortens to accommodate change in muscle length and/or joint angle throughout the range of motion while moving a constant external load. *[handwritten: Dynamic = accommodates change in muscle length]*

Concentric Contraction A dynamic muscle contraction that produces tension during shortening. *[handwritten: Concentric contraction = shortening]*

The term **contraction** refers to the tension-producing process of the contractile elements within muscle. However, not all contractions produce movement; movement depends on the magnitude of the load exerted and the tension produced by the muscle. In order for a muscle to move a load, the force of muscle tension must exceed the force of the load. Furthermore, muscle tension developed experimentally in an isolated muscle fiber, a motor unit, or even a whole muscle is not necessarily the same as the force developed by an intact muscle in the human body.

All human motion involves rotation of body segments about their joint axes. The capability of a force to produce rotation is referred to as **torque**. Thus, torque is force applied at some distance away from the center of the joint, causing the limb to rotate around the joint. Torque changes as a muscle moves bone through the range of motion.

Classification of Muscle Contractions

A classification of muscle contractions is presented in **Table 18.1**. This classification is based on three component characteristics: time (as duration and/or velocity), displacement (length change), and force production. Throughout this discussion, it is important to distinguish whether a contraction is being described in an isolated muscle fiber/motor unit or in intact, whole muscles.

As shown in **Table 18.1**, at the muscle fiber or motor unit level, the three basic types of contraction are isotonic, isokinetic, and isometric. At the whole-muscle level, contractions may be defined as dynamic, isokinematic, or static. The following paragraphs describe these different contractions in a muscle fiber and the corresponding types of contraction in an intact muscle.

An **isotonic contraction** is a muscle fiber contraction in which the tension generated by the muscle fiber is constant throughout the range of motion. The term isotonic indicates that the force production (tonus) is unchanged (iso means "same") when the muscle fiber contracts, causing movement of an external load. In the intact human system, such a contraction is practically impossible. What happens in intact whole muscle is that the muscle force varies as the muscle contracts. This variation is necessary to accommodate changes in muscle length and/or joint angles as limbs move through their ranges of motion. Thus, the load is constant, but the force produced to move it through the range of motion is not. Therefore, the term dynamic is more accurate to describe contraction within the intact human.

A **dynamic contraction** is a whole-muscle contraction that produces movement of the skeleton. If the movement results from a dynamic muscle contraction that produces tension during shortening, it is a **concentric contraction**. Concentric contractions result in positive external work and are primarily responsible for acceleration in movement. The lifting action of the biceps in curling a barbell is an example of a concentric dynamic contraction.

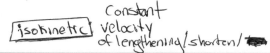

TABLE 18.1 Classification of Contractions

Type of Contraction			
Muscle Fiber or Motor Unit	**Intact Muscle in Humans**	**External Work in Intact Muscle in Humans**	**Function of Contraction**
Isotonic: constant-force production: shortening, or lengthening	**Dynamic concentric**: muscle force varies as muscle shortens to accommodate change in muscle length and/or joint angles as limb moves through ROM while moving a constant external load.	Positive: (work = force × distance); external load can be overcome.	Acceleration
	Dynamic eccentric: see above, except muscle lengthens	Negative: (work = force × distance); external load assists lengthening.	Deceleration
Isokinetic: constant velocity of lengthening or shortening	**Isokinematic (dynamic)**: rate of limb displacement or joint rotation is constant. Velocity varies with joint angle.	Positive or negative: see above	Acceleration or deceleration
Isometric: constant muscle length	**Static**: limb displacement or joint rotation does not occur; little muscle fiber shortening occurs.	Zero: (work = force × distance, where distance = 0); external load cannot be overcome.	Fixation

Note: ROM, range of motion.

Sources: Komi, P. V.: Physiological and biomechanical correlates of muscle function: Effects of muscle structure and stretch-shortening cycle of force and speed. In Terjung, R. (ed.): *Exercise and Sport Sciences Reviews* (Vol. 12). Lexington, MA: Collamore Press, 81–122 (1984); Williams, J. H.: Normal musculoskeletal and neuromuscular anatomy, physiology and responses to training. In Hasson, S. M. (ed.): *Clinical Exercise Physiology.* St. Louis, MO: Mosby (1994).

The sliding-filament theory describes this type of contraction (Chapter 17).

If movement occurs as a result of a dynamic muscle contraction that produces tension while lengthening, the contraction is referred to as an **eccentric contraction**. Eccentric contractions result in negative work and are primarily responsible for deceleration in movement. The lowering action of the biceps in curling a barbell is an example of an eccentric dynamic contraction. During an eccentric contraction, the cross-bridges are cycling as the filaments are being pulled apart. Because of this action of being pulled apart, strenuous eccentric activities can cause mechanical disruption of the sarcomeres, muscle damage, and soreness (Peake et al., 2005). Strenuous eccentric contractions also allow for a greater force of contraction at a lower energy cost than concentric contractions (Stauber, 1989). Skeletal muscle fibers produce 1.5–1.9 times more force during maximal eccentric contraction than during maximal isometric contraction, whereas an eccentric contraction in whole muscle is slightly greater than a concentric contraction (Aagaard and Bangsbo, 2006; Byrne et al., 2004).

Why can an eccentric contraction produce more force than a concentric one? During a concentric contraction, only about half of the available cross-bridges cycle. During an eccentric contraction, some of the cross-bridges do not cycle but are continually pulled backward. Because of this, the myosin heads do not rotate forward, and the actin and myosin remain bound (Stauber, 1989). As the contraction continues, a number of additional cross-bridges are formed that may exceed the number of

cross-bridges in a concentric contraction. Hence, more tension can be produced.

Why does eccentric (negative) work have a lower energy cost than concentric (positive) work? The answer to this question is not completely known, but two possibilities have been suggested (Stauber, 1989). First, fewer muscle fibers are recruited during eccentric contractions than during concentric contractions; fewer fibers use less oxygen, which translates to a smaller energy cost. Second, because some of the cross-bridges do not cycle, less ATP is broken down and used as energy. Researchers estimate that positive work uses three to nine times more energy than negative work. To appreciate the applicability of this information, mentally compare climbing up stairs in a high-rise building with walking down them.

An **isokinetic contraction** is a muscle fiber contraction in which the velocity of contraction is kept constant. Isokinetic contractions are also dynamic contractions in that movement occurs; the force generated is sufficient to overcome the external load. In the intact human, the velocity of the movement actually varies with the joint angle; however, the rate of limb displacement can be held constant with special exercise equipment. Hence, the term **isokinematic contraction** is more technically correct, although seldom used. What differentiates isokinetic contractions from other forms of dynamic contractions is that the rate of shortening or lengthening (kinesis means "motion") is constant (iso means "same").

An **isometric contraction** is a muscle fiber contraction without a length change in the muscle fiber. In an isometric contraction, the cross-bridges are cycling—hence producing tension—but sliding of the filaments does not occur. The actual length (metric derives from meter and refers to length) is constant. This kind of action is possible in an isolated fiber because the fiber can be stabilized at both ends in an experimental apparatus before being stimulated. However, an intact fiber has an elastic element (connective tissue and joints) to contend with, and so some fiber shortening actually does occur even though no limb displacement or joint rotation occurs. A **static contraction** is a muscle contraction that produces an increase in muscle tension but does not cause meaningful limb displacement or joint rotation and therefore does not result in movement of the skeleton. Thus, the term static, meaning "not in motion," is better than isometric for describing such a contraction that occurs in an intact muscle in humans. No external work is done by static contractions, but they often perform the important task of fixation or stabilization. Gripping a tennis racket or barbell is an example of a static contraction.

Force Development

All types of contractions exert tension; however, the amount of tension that can be generated is not the same for all contractions. In whole muscles, eccentric dynamic contractions produce the greatest force, followed by static contractions and then by dynamic concentric contractions.

The amount of force produced by each type of contraction depends on neural and mechanical factors (Komi, 1984). This is true on the level of the muscle fiber and also in the intact, whole muscle. The following sections discuss how neural and mechanical factors influence force development. Each section first discusses the muscle fiber and then the more complex environment of whole muscles.

Eccentric Contraction A dynamic muscle contraction that produces tension (force) while lengthening.

Isokinetic Contraction A muscle fiber contraction in which the velocity of the contraction is kept constant.

Isokinematic Contraction A muscle contraction in which the rate of limb displacement or joint rotation is held constant with the use of specialized equipment.

Isometric Contraction A muscle fiber contraction that does not result in a length change in muscle fiber. *Static*

Static Contraction A muscle contraction that produces an increase in muscle tension but does not cause meaningful limb displacement or joint displacement and therefore does not result in movement of the skeleton.

Neural Activation

* the all-or-nothing principle (threshold)

A single muscle fiber or motor unit that is stimulated to contract will contract maximally or not at all according to the all-or-none principle of muscle contraction described in Chapter 17). When stimulated, a muscle fiber produces a *twitch* and then relaxes (**Figure 18.1A**). If a second stimulus is applied before the fiber has completely relaxed, *temporal summation* results, producing slightly greater tension. If the frequency of stimulation is increased enough to prohibit relaxation, the individual contractions blend together to form first an *irregular* (or *unfused*) *tetanus* and then a *smooth* (*fused*) *tetanus* (**Figure 18.1B**). Unfused tetanic contractions produce greater tension than either single twitches or summations, and fused tetanic contractions produce the highest tension. *temporal summation = second stimulus hits before first relaxes.*

In intact muscle, contractions occur with tetanic contractions of motor units. Unlike single muscle fiber or motor unit contractions, whole-muscle contractions do not occur in an all-or-none fashion. Whole-muscle contractions can be graded, meaning a muscle contraction can produce little force (for instance, to move your hand while turning a page) or a lot of force (for instance, to lift a heavy barbell). Two neural factors determine force production in whole muscle. The first factor is the frequency of stimulation, or *rate coding* (Enoka, 1988). As shown in **Figure 18.1C**, as the frequency of stimulation increases, so does the force that the muscle produces. Notice that at frequencies less than 50 Hz, a small increase in frequency of firing can produce a large increase in muscle tension (Sale, 1992).

The second neural way of controlling force output is by varying the number of motor units activated, which is called recruitment, or *number coding*. In the intact human, some motor units are always contracting in an alternating manner. These contractions maintain what is called *muscle tone,* or *tonus*. When greater tension is needed, the processes of rate coding and number coding occur in tandem. As the firing of a given motor unit reaches its maximum, new motor units are recruited. Such activation or recruitment, and the subsequent deactivation or derecruitment, occurs according to the size principle. Remember that smaller motor neurons are easier to stimulate than larger ones. Therefore, in accordance with the size principle, the small α_2 motor neurons innervating slow oxidative (SO) motor units are recruited first (**Figure 18.1D**) (Sale, 1992). As the stimulus increases, the larger α_1 motor neurons that innervate the fast oxidative glycolytic (FOG) muscle fibers are activated, followed by the recruitment of fast glycolytic (FG) fibers as the stimulus increases. For example, the speed continuum of walk, jog, and run involves a continuum of SO, FOG, and FG muscle fiber recruitment. Once the neural stimulation ends, deactivation proceeds in reverse sequence. The larger, faster fibers (FG, then FOG) are inactivated first; finally, the slower, smaller fibers are deactivated until only muscle tonus remains.

muscle tone is muscles constantly contracting

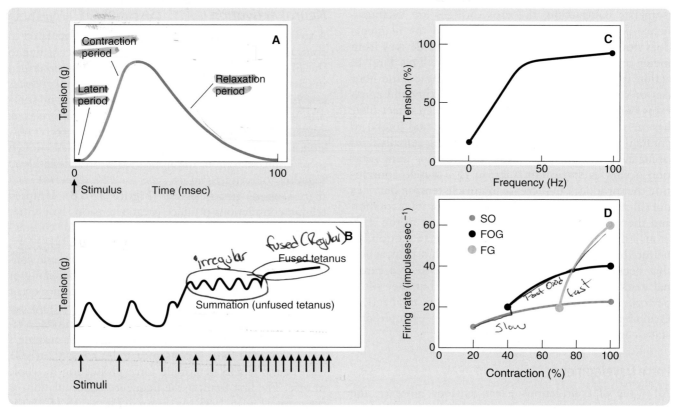

FIGURE 18.1 Muscle Response to Stimulation.
A. Myogram of a single muscle fiber twitch. **B.** Myogram of a series of muscle fiber twitches. **C.** Effect of frequency of stimulation on muscle tension in whole muscle. **D.** Firing rate and muscle tension in different fiber types in whole muscle. SO = slow oxidative; FOG = fast oxidative glycolytic; FG = fast glycolytic.

Mechanical Factors Influencing Muscle Contractions

Several mechanical factors influence the force produced during muscle contractions. This section discusses four mechanical factors: length-tension-angle relationships, force-velocity relationships, the elasticity-force relationship, and cross-sectional area/architectural design. Force production in a muscle fiber is discussed first, followed by the more complex situation in whole muscles.

LENGTH-TENSION-ANGLE RELATIONSHIPS Within a muscle fiber, the amount of tension that can be exerted is related to the initial length of the sarcomeres. As shown in **Figure 18.2A**, this relationship forms an inverted U (Edman, 1992). The amount of tension produced is directly related to the degree of overlap of the thick and thin filaments. In elongated fibers, there is little overlap of the actin and myosin filaments, making it hard for cross-bridges to form. In shortened fibers, where the thick and thin filaments already overlap almost completely, there is little room for further shortening. Thus, less force is produced in both the elongated and shortened positions. In contrast, the maximum number of cross-bridges coincides with the highest force production, which occurs at

approximately 100–120% of the resting sarcomere length (Edman, 1992).

In whole muscle, this length-tension relationship also holds, but its expression is complicated by many factors. These factors include the cross-sectional area of the muscle, the arrangement of the sarcomere in relation to the line of pull, the level of neural muscle activation, the degree of fatigue, the involvement of the elastic components of muscle, and the biomechanical aspects of how a muscle exerts force at a joint. The biomechanical aspects are most notable, as described below.

When whole-muscle tension (measured as muscle force or torque) is plotted against the joint angle at which it occurs, strength curves are generated (**Figure 18.2B**). Imagine the muscle action involved in performing a bicep curl. As the barbell is lifted through the joint's range of motion, different amounts of force are generated to compensate for biomechanical differences related to joint angle. Of course, the force produced depends on the length of the sarcomere, but force production is also greatly influenced by biomechanical aspects of the joint. **Figure 18.2B** shows the strength curve for this bicep curl (elbow flexion) example. The joint angle is plotted along the horizontal axis, and the force of the contracting

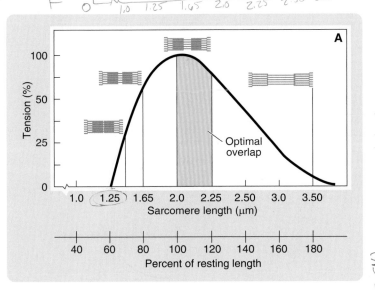

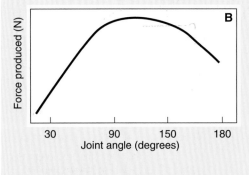
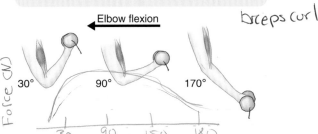

FIGURE 18.2 Length-Tension Relationship in Muscle.
A. Length-tension relationship in skeletal muscle fibers. **B.** Example of a strength curve illustrating the length-tension relationship in whole muscle.
Source: From Paul Edman, K. A: Contractile Performance of Skeletal Muscle Fibres. In Komi, P. V. (ed.): *Strength and Power in Sport*. Champaign, IL: Human Kinetics, 103. Copyright 1992 by International Olympic Committee. Reprinted by permission.

muscle is plotted along the vertical axis. In this graph the action of raising the barbell proceeds from right to left because the joint angle is greatest in the lowered position (~170°) and smallest with the barbell in the raised position (~30°). In this example, peak force occurs at approximately 100–120°.

As indicated in **Figure 18.3**, strength curves occur in three forms: ascending, descending, or ascending and descending. An *ascending strength curve* is characterized by an increase in torque as the joint angle increases. A *descending strength curve* is characterized by a decrease in torque as the joint angle increases. In an *ascending and descending strength curve*, the force initially increases and then decreases as a function of joint angle.

Figure 18.4A presents a generalized strength curve for knee flexion. Most studies describe this as an ascending curve, although some findings disagree (Kulig et al., 1984).

As shown in the figure, when the joint angle is greatest, the greatest force is exerted. This point also corresponds to the point at which the muscles of the hamstrings are longest.

Figure 18.4B presents a generalized strength curve for hip abduction (Kulig et al., 1984). This curve is generally described as descending. In this case, larger joint angles correspond to lower forces. In this example, the tensor fasciae latae (the muscle responsible for hip abduction) is longest at the lowest joint angle.

Both of these situations—**Figure 18.4A** and **B**—are in reality consistent: The longer the muscle length, the greater the force exerted. However, remember that it is not just, or even primarily, the length of the muscle itself that causes this variation.

There is general agreement that both elbow flexion (**Figure 18.4C**) and knee extension (**Figure 18.4D**)

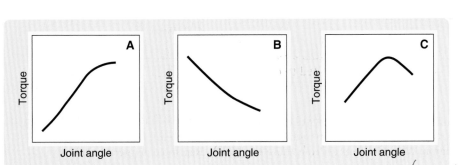

FIGURE 18.3 Classification of Strength Curves.
A. Ascending. **B.** Descending. **C.** Ascending and descending.
Source: K. Kulig, J. G. Andrews, & J. G. Hay: Human strength curves. In Terjung, R. (ed.): *Exercise and Sport Sciences Reviews* (Vol. 12). Lexington, MA: Collamore Press, 417–466 (1984). Reprinted by permission of Williams & Wilkins.

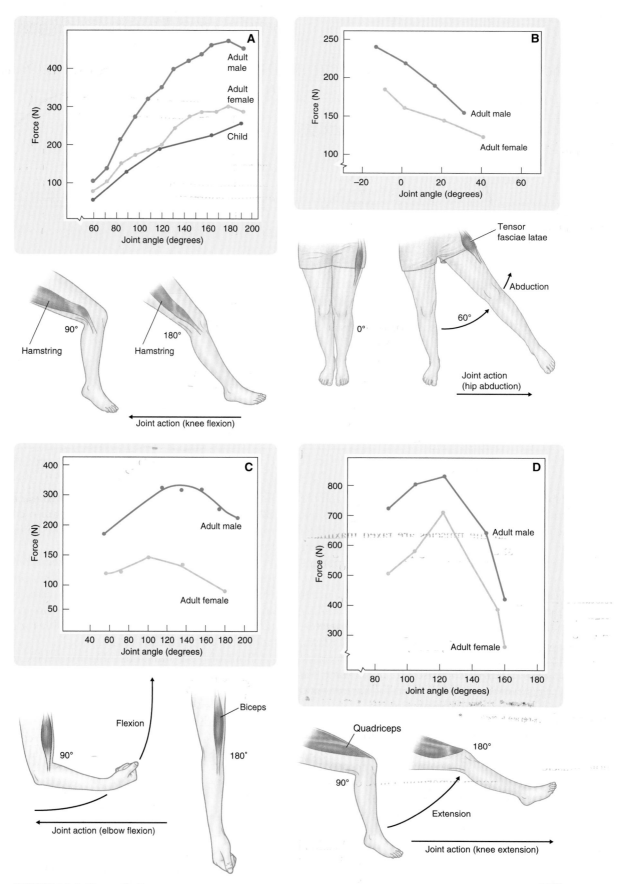

FIGURE 18.4 Strength Curves.
A. Knee flexion. **B**. Hip abduction. **C**. Elbow flexion. **D**. Knee extension.
Source: Kulig, K., J. G. Andrews, & J. G. Hay: Human strength curves. In Terjung, R. (ed.): *Exercise and Sport Sciences Reviews* (Vol. 12). Lexington, MA: Collamore Press, 417–466 (1984). Reprinted by permission of Williams & Wilkins.

exhibit ascending and descending strength curves (Kulig et al., 1984). The strongest angles for elbow flexion seem to be between 90° and 130°; for knee extension, the strongest angles are between 100° and 130°. As with the other configurations, the joint angle that coincides with the greatest force production is partially, but not entirely, a result of the muscle length and degree of overlap of the thick and thin filaments.

Although there are some differences, the strength curves are similar for males and females, and the young and the old. Injuries typically result in low strength curve values; thus, preinjury strength curves or strength curves from a comparable healthy individual are sometimes used as goals in rehabilitation. Standard norms for strength curves are not generally available.

Knowledge of strength curves has another practical application. When lifting an external load—for example, a barbell through the range of elbow flexion (bicep curl exercise)—the individual is limited by the weight that can be handled at the weakest point. The stronger angles are not overloaded as much as the weaker angles, and the muscle is taxed maximally only at its "sticking point."

Finally, strength curves have been used to design strength training equipment—specifically, variable-resistance equipment (Kulig et al., 1984). Nautilus developed the variable-radius cam to mimic the strength curve of selected single-joint exercises. The aim is to compensate for changes in mechanical leverage throughout the range of motion of a joint, thereby matching the load to the strength curve so that the muscles are taxed maximally at all angles, not just at the sticking point. Although this reasoning seems logical, training studies have not demonstrated that greater benefits are derived from variable-resistance training programs than from traditional free weight programs. On the contrary, it appears that training programs that employee free-weights produce superior strength gains (Stone et al., 2000).

FORCE-VELOCITY AND POWER-VELOCITY RELATIONSHIPS

The second major mechanical factor that influences the expression of muscle force or torque is the velocity at which the shortening occurs.

The relationship between force and velocity is similar for a single muscle fiber (**Figure 18.5A**) and an intact whole muscle (**Figure 18.5B**). The single muscle fiber does not exhibit the smooth hyperbolic curve of an intact muscle, but both show the basic relationship: The shortening velocity of a muscle increases as the force developed by the muscle decreases, which means that a muscle can shorten fastest when the load is the lightest. Maximal velocity occurs in an unloaded (zero force) situation, and a maximal load results in no movement (zero velocity). Between these two extremes, the velocity gradually decreases in a curvilinear fashion as the load increases. To apply this information, think about swinging a baseball bat. As the weight of the bat increases, the speed with which it can be swung decreases.

If the external force overcomes the ability of the muscle to resist it, the muscle lengthens (eccentric contraction) but only after producing additional tension (Stauber, 1989). The eccentric contraction is seen in **Figure 18.5A** where the force curve dips below the horizontal axis. Notice that the force produced continues to increase during this eccentric phase. This result is consistent with earlier statements made about eccentric dynamic contractions.

It is interesting to note that on the cellular level, the maximal velocity of shortening varies among individual

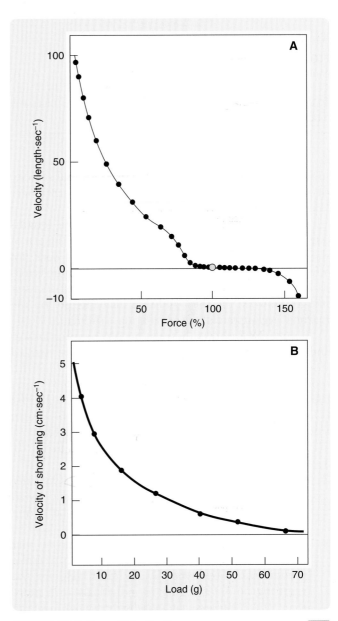

FIGURE 18.5 Force-Velocity Curves.
A. In a single muscle fiber. **B.** In a whole muscle.
Source: From Paul Edman, K. A: Contractile Performance of Skeletal Muscle Fibers. In Komi, P. V. (ed.): *Strength and Power in Sport.* Champaign, IL: Human Kinetics, 105. Copyright 1992 by International Olympic Committee. Reprinted by permission.

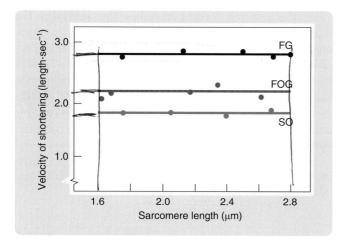

FIGURE 18.6 Velocity-Length Curves.
Source: Reprinted with permission from Edman, K. A. P.: Contractile performance of skeletal muscle fibers. In Komi, P. V. (ed.): *Strength and Power in Sport*. Boston, MA: Blackwell Scientific, 96–114 (1992).

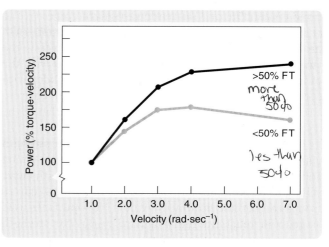

FIGURE 18.7 Influence of Fiber Type on Velocity-Power Relationship.
Source: Coyle, E. F., D. L. Costill, & G. R. Lesmes: Leg extension power and muscle fiber composition. *Medicine and Science in Sports*. 11(1):12–15 (1976).

muscle fibers, but within the same fibers, maximal velocity of shortening is constant regardless of the sarcomere length (**Figure 18.6**) (Edman, 1992).

Compare **Figure 18.6** with **Figure 18.2** (the length-tension curve). This comparison shows that the length of the sarcomere influences force production but does not affect the velocity of force production. The maximum velocity of shortening does not depend on the number of cross-bridges between the thick and thin filaments but on the maximal cycling rate of the cross-bridges (Edman, 1992).

Figure 18.7 shows the relationship between power and velocity in whole muscles. These data were derived from a study of two different groups of subjects: one with more than 50% FT muscle fibers (average = 58.5%) and the other with less than 50% FT fibers (average = 38.3%) (Coyle et al., 1976). Several conclusions can be drawn from this graph.

1. Power is positively related to velocity.
2. The shape of the relationship is curvilinear. Consider what this power-velocity relationship would mean if a heavier (rather than lighter) bat can be swung quickly enough to contact a fast pitch.
3. The graph in **Figure 18.7** shows that the power that can be generated at any given velocity varies with the predominant fiber type. At any given velocity, the resulting power is higher in individuals with more than 50% FT fibers than in individuals with less than 50% FT fibers. Thus, individuals with high percentages of FT fibers would seem to be genetically predisposed, given sufficient training and practice, to be more successful in power events such as sprinting, power lifting, and jumping and in field events such as shot, javelin, and discus.

4. The power curve of the predominantly ST fiber individuals (those with <50% FT) not only levels off but also makes a downturn at the higher velocities. Although such a downturn is not evident at the tested speeds for the FT group, it is likely that there is a fiber-type–specific optimal speed of movement for the generation of power.

ELASTICITY-FORCE RELATIONSHIP Elasticity is the third mechanical factor involved in the force development capabilities of muscles. Both the muscle fibers and their tendinous attachments contain elastic components. When a muscle fiber is stretched and then contracted, the resultant contraction is stronger than it would have been without prestretching. In the intact human, the relationship between prestretch and force of contraction is expressed as a stretch-shortening cycle (SSC), where the preactivated muscle is first stretched (eccentric action) and then followed by the shortening (concentric) action (Komi, 1992; Nicol et al., 2006). Stretch-shortening cycles do not occur in all human movements, however. They are most evident in activities such as running, jumping, and (to a lesser extent) bicycling. **Figure 18.8** shows that the calf muscles and Achilles tendon are stretched while contracting eccentrically as a runner's foot impacts the ground (Komi, 1992). The push-off, or concentric-shortening phase, is aided by the release of the potential energy stored during the stretch phase. To feel the impact of the SSC, stand up and see how high you can jump with a little flexion as possible and then with moderate flexion at your hip, knee, and ankle joints. Finally, try a rebound jump from a small stool. This latter task is an example of a *plyometric exercise*. A plyometric exercise is one in which a concentric contraction is immediately preceded by an

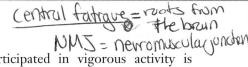

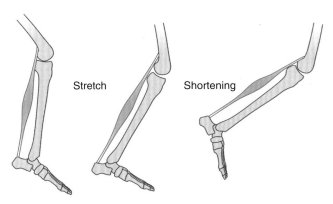

FIGURE 18.8 Stretch-Shortening Cycle.
Source: Komi, P. V.: Physiological and biomechanical correlates of muscle function: Effects of muscle structure and stretch-shortening cycle of force and speed. In Terjung,R. (ed.): *Exercise and Sport Sciences Reviews* (Vol. 12). Lexington, MA: Collamore Press, 81–122 (1984). Reprinted by permission of Williams & Wilkins.

eccentric contraction (such as the eccentric contraction upon landing and absorbing the force from jumping off a stool before the concentric contraction of jumping up). Plyometrics will be discussed more thoroughly in the section on flexibility in Chapter 20, because more than just elasticity is involved in the physiological basis for their execution. As a result of additional power generation with increasing stretch-proceeding contraction, you should be able to jump successively higher in the three examples.

The stretch-shortening cycle not only leads to more powerful muscle contractions but also affects mechanical efficiency. Efficiency is discussed at length in Chapter 4. The point here is that more work can be done with less energy expenditure following a prestretch.

CROSS-SECTIONAL AREA/ARCHITECTURAL DESIGN The maximal force that can be developed within a muscle fiber is related to its cross-sectional area. The force that can be developed by a whole muscle is also related to its cross-sectional area. However, this relationship is not as strong as the one within a single muscle fiber, largely owing to different arrangements of the muscle fibers within a muscle. Muscles that are designed for a high force generation (pennate, bipennate, and multipennate muscles) are arranged anatomically to maximize their cross-sectional area. Muscles designed for high-velocity shortening have parallel fibers and are arranged in a fusiform manner (Goldspink, 1992).

Muscular Fatigue and Soreness

Despite all the benefits and enjoyment of exercise, unaccustomed muscular activity can also lead to some unpleasant outcomes. The following section discusses two such consequences: muscular fatigue and muscular soreness.

Muscular Fatigue

Anyone who has participated in vigorous activity is familiar with muscular fatigue. Although exercise physiologists have studied fatigue for a long time, many questions remain about the basic cellular causes of fatigue. The National Heart Lung and Blood Institute (NHLBI) defines fatigue as "a condition in which there is a loss in the capacity for developing force and/or velocity of a muscle, resulting from muscle activity under load which is reversible by rest" (NHLBI, 1990). This means that fatigue results in a transient loss in the ability of the muscle to develop force and or velocity, often leading to a cessation of muscular work or an inability to maintain a given intensity of work. The muscle is not damaged, and restoration and recovery are possible (Fitts, 2008).

But what causes muscle fatigue? Muscle fatigue is a complex and still controversial phenomenon that appears to include failure at one or more of the sites along the chain of events that leads to muscular contraction. As diagramed in **Figure 18.9**, fatigue can be classified as central or peripheral based on the site of fatigue. Central sites refer to the nervous system (brain and spinal cord), whereas peripheral sites include specific sites in the skeletal muscle. **Table 18.2** lists the possible sites of fatigue and summarizes the proposed mechanisms for the muscle fatigue at each site. In reality, fatigue is a complex phenomenon that likely results from an interaction of these mechanisms at one or more sites. Fatigue depends on the type of exercise performed, the fiber type of the muscle involved, and the exerciser's fitness and nutritional status.

Central fatigue may be related to neurons in the brain or spinal cord, inhibitory input from muscle afferents innervating neurons in the brain, or alterations in motor neurons. Central fatigue may also be influenced by psychological factors and motivation involving how much effort the individual makes, particularly when continuing the activity causes pain.

Peripheral fatigue refers to fatigue at a site beyond the central nervous system (CNS), anywhere from the neuromuscular junction (NMJ) to the skeletal muscle. Peripheral fatigue can occur at several specific sites: the neuromuscular junction, the sarcolemma-T tubules-sarcoplasmic reticulum system, and the myofilaments. Failure of neuromuscular transmission is a possible cause of fatigue. This failure could include depletion of the neurotransmitter and/or problems with the binding of the neurotransmitter to the receptors on the motor end plate. Fatigue could also result from a failure of the electrical excitation along the sarcolemma and T tubules and an inability of the sarcoplasmic reticulum (SR) to release sufficient calcium. Likewise, fatigue could result from any alteration in the ability of calcium to bind to troponin and thereby remove tropomyosin from its blocking position on actin. Fatigue might also result from biochemical and metabolic changes within the contractile elements (myofilaments of the muscle cell).

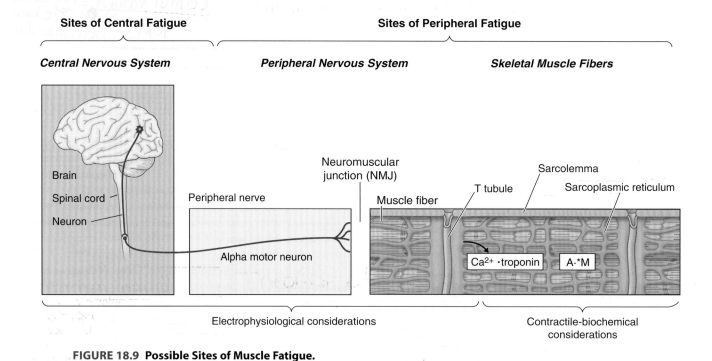

FIGURE 18.9 Possible Sites of Muscle Fatigue.

Notice in **Figure 18.9** that fatigue can also be categorized in relation to electrophysiological or contractile biochemical considerations. Electrophysiological considerations involve steps within the central nervous system, the peripheral nervous system, or the muscle fiber leading up to the binding of the actin and myosin filaments (A·*M). These include the initial neural impulse from the motor cortex, transmission of the impulse across the synapse, propagation of the neural impulse along

the motor neuron, transmission of the impulse across the neuromuscular junction, and subsequent spread of an action potential along the sarcolemma and into the T tubules. Contractile considerations involve the ability of actin and myosin to continue their cross-bridge attachment-detachment cycles, thus producing force. The reduced peak force with fatigue can be explained by both a decline in the force per cross-bridge and the number of cross-bridges that are formed (Fitts, 2008; Nocella et al., 2011).

Two primary hypotheses attempt to explain the causes of fatigue within the contractile elements of the muscle: the depletion (or exhaustion) hypothesis and the accumulation hypothesis (MacLaren et al., 1989). The depletion hypothesis suggests that fatigue results from decrease in certain metabolites, specifically, ATP, phosphocreatine (PC), and glycogen. Thus, the muscle fibers are no longer able to produce force. The accumulation hypothesis suggests that fatigue is caused by the accumulation of certain metabolites that are known to impair force generation within muscles, specifically, lactate, hydrogen ions, ammonia, and phosphate.

Current research suggests that the primary site of fatigue usually is within the muscle itself. The factors that contribute to fatigue are complex and interrelated and depend on the muscle fibers involved and the type of activity being performed. The depletion of PC leads to fatigue in FG fibers that rely on this substrate to regenerate ATP for explosive-type events. The depletion of glycogen leads to fatigue in SO fibers that rely on this substrate to produce ATP aerobically during prolonged activity. The accumulation of lactate and the H+

TABLE 18.2 Site of Muscle Fatigue and Proposed Mechanism

Site of Fatigue	Proposed Mechanism
Central	
CNS	① Malfunction of neurons
	② Inhibition of voluntary effort (motor cortex)
	③ Psychological factors
Peripheral	
NMJ	① Inhibition of axon terminal
	② Depletion of neurotransmitter
	③ Altered neurotransmitter binding to receptors
T tubule/SR	① Inability to release Ca^{2+}
	② Inability of Ca^{2+} to bind to troponin
Contractile elements	① Depletion of ATP
	② Depletion of PC
	③ Depletion of glycogen
	④ Accumulation of lactate, H^+, PO_4^-, etc.

FOCUS ON APPLICATION

The Effects of Caffeine on Exercise and Sports Performance

Caffeine has been used for many centuries and is well known for increasing wakefulness. Caffeine is also used as an ergogenic aid to enhance sport performance. Caffeine is readily absorbed through the gastrointestinal tract and appears in the blood stream 15–45 minutes after ingestion, with peak blood concentrations occurring approximately 1 hour after ingestion. The effectiveness of caffeine as an ergogenic aid varies with the type of activity performed.

Caffeine has a well-documented beneficial effect on endurance performance. It is acknowledged that caffeine's effect on endurance exercise is multifactorial, and there is evidence that caffeine has an effect on both the central nervous system and the excitation contraction coupling of skeletal muscle (Tarnopolsky, 2008). Improvements in sustained endurance events are apparent after low-to-moderate doses of caffeine (3–6 mg·kg^{-1}).

More recently, the impact caffeine has on short-term, high-intensity performance, such as sprinting, team sports, and resistance training, has been studied with varying results. The discrepancies in published studies may be due to differences in testing protocols, the caffeine dose, training status, and habitual caffeine use. Astorino and Roberson reviewed the impact of acute caffeine use on short-term, high-intensity exercise and found that a majority of the studies reported an increase in performance for team sport exercise and power-related sports. However, the results were more pronounced in elite athletes who did not regularly use caffeine. Similarly, the benefit of caffeine ingestion was noted in the studies that employed resistance training. A study conducted by Beck et al. (2006) tested 37 resistance trained men (mean age 21 years) on the Wingate Anaerobic Test, a one-repetition max test, and a muscle endurance test after ingesting 2.5 mg·kg^{-1} of caffeine or placebo. There was a 2.1% increase in the one-repetition max test for the caffeine group while there was no change for the placebo group. There were no changes in the Wingate Anaerobic Test or the muscle endurance test for either group. In general, research suggests that moderate caffeine ingestion (4–6 mg·kg^{-1}) is advantageous for short-term, high-intensity performance in trained athletes.

While research indicates a benefit of acute caffeine ingestion for various types of activity, the exact mechanism of action remains unknown. As with other ergogenic aids, it should be noted that it is rare that a single mechanism fully explains physiological effects of a supplement (Goldstein et al., 2010). It has been proposed that caffeine exerts its beneficial effects on sports performance through several potential mechanisms. Possible mechanisms include stimulation of the central nervous system and alteration of substrate utilization, β-endorphin release, and neuromuscular function. Astorino and Roberson (2010) have proposed a model to explain the impact caffeine has on the central nervous system and skeletal muscles to improve short-term, high-intensity performance. This model, presented in the accompanying figure, reinforces the fact that there are multiple ways that caffeine may affect both the central nervous system and the muscular system to improve performance and prevent fatigue. The model also notes areas where research evidence is more robust.

Given that caffeine supplementation can significantly enhance athletic performance, the International Olympic Committee (IOC) has mandated an upper limit on caffeine (12 μg·mL^{-1} in the urine). Caffeine ingestion of 9–13 mg·kg^{-1} (6–8 cups of brewed coffee) approximately 1 hour before testing would correspond to maximal urinary concentrations. The National Collegiate Athletic Association (NCAA) has set a value of greater than 15 μg·mL^{-1} as illegal.

The International Society of Sports Nutrition (ISSN) has concluded that caffeine has an ergogenic affect that is specific to the condition of the athlete and the type of exercise being performed (Goldstein et al., 2010). Based on the available scientific literature, they have drawn the following conclusions:

1. Caffeine should be ingested 60 minutes prior to the onset of activity to ensure optimal absorption.

2. Caffeine should be ingested in low-to-moderate doses (~3–6 mg·kg^{-1}). There is no further benefit when consumed in higher amounts (≥9 mg·kg^{-1}).

3. Caffeine has been shown to be an effective ergogenic aid in maximal endurance and time trial events.

4. Caffeine has been shown to be an effective ergogenic aid in prolonged, high-intensity team sports, such as soccer, rowing, or field hockey.

5. Research is inconsistent regarding the effectiveness of caffeine as an ergogenic aid in strength and power performance. These inconsistencies may be due to differences in training protocols, fitness of the participants, or caffeine dosage. More research is still needed in this area.

6. Limited research has shown a positive benefit of caffeine on strength/power of trained women and a moderate increase in performance for the recreationally trained women.

7. Caffeine is more effective when consumed in a capsule/tablet form as compared to drinking coffee.

Sources: Astorino et al. (2010), Beck et al. (2006), Ganio et al. (2009), Goldstein et al. (2010), Tarnopolsky (2008).

Proposed mechanisms for caffeine's ergogenic effects during short-term, high-intensity exercise

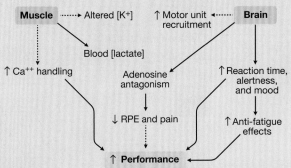

RPE = rate of perceived exertion

associated with lactic acid may lead to fatigue by interfering with the contractile process in several places, decreasing the amount of calcium released, interfering with calcium-troponin binding, disrupting the Na^+–K^+ pump, inhibiting anaerobic glycolysis (by inhibiting the rate-limiting enzyme PFK), or interfering with cross-bridging. The detrimental effects of H^+ accumulation appear most evident in FOG fibers that produce large amounts of lactic acid. But the role lactic acid in muscular fatigue is far from clear. Several recent studies suggest that lactate and acidosis during exercise are beneficial. While the controversy about the role or roles of lactate remain to be resolved, what is certain is that lactate/H^+ may contribute to fatigue but is not the sole cause of muscular fatigue (Bangsbo, 2006; Cairns, 2006; Lamb, 2006).

Because many types of activity involve more than one fiber type, several of the mechanisms described in this section may be involved in muscle fatigue for any given activity (Conley, 2000; Fitts, 2006).

Type of Activity and Muscle Fatigue

Fatigue is now thought to result from different mechanisms in different types of activity. Furthermore, the fiber type involved in a given activity greatly influences the most probable mechanism of fatigue for that activity. Table 18.3 summarizes the most probable causes of fatigue for different types of activity. Note that any given activity may have several possible causes and that the proposed mechanisms often interact. Investigation in this area is ongoing.

[handwritten: – all of them have depletion of glycogen]
[handwritten: – inhibits glycolysis]
[handwritten: Theories of Fatigue]

TABLE 18.3 Most Probable Causes of Muscle Fatigue	
Type of Activity	**Probable Causes of Fatigue**
Long-term, moderate to heavy, submaximal aerobic	Depletion of glycogen Accumulation of H^+ Inhibits glycolysis Decreases Ca^{2+} release from SR Interferes with Ca^{2+}-troponin binding La^- interferes with cross-bridging
Incremental aerobic exercise to maximum	Depletion of glycogen Accumulation of H^+ Inhibits glycolysis Decreases Ca^{2+} release from SR Interferes with Ca^{2+}-troponin binding Depletion of PC La^- interferes with cross-bridging
Static	Depletion of PC Accumulation of H^+ Inhibits glycolysis Decreases Ca^{2+} release from SR Interferes with Ca^{2+}-troponin binding Occlusion of blood flow Inhibition of motor cortex via sensory fibers in muscle La^- interferes with cross-bridging
Dynamic resistance	Depletion of PC stores
Low repetitions	Depletion of glycogen
High repetitions	Accumulation of H^+ Inhibits glycolysis Decreases Ca^{2+} release from SR Interferes with Ca^{2+}-troponin binding La^- interferes with cross-bridging
Anaerobic (sprint)	Depletion of PC stores Accumulation of H^+ Inhibits glycolysis Decreases Ca^{2+} release from SR Interferes with Ca^{2+}-troponin binding La^- interferes with cross-bridging

Long-Term, Moderate to Heavy, Submaximal Aerobic Exercise

Steady-state activities that are performed at moderate workloads rely almost exclusively on SO fibers to produce ATP. As a result, lactic acid levels do not increase substantially during these activities. The most probable cause of fatigue during steady-state activities is the depletion of glycogen stores, resulting in peripheral fatigue. During prolonged activities performed at an intensity high enough to recruit FOG fibers, a significant amount of lactic acid is formed. In this case, the high levels of H^+ likely produce fatigue (Conley, 2000).

Central fatigue is also thought to play a significant role in fatigue during prolonged activities. The "central fatigue" hypothesis suggests that an alteration in brain neurotransmitters (specifically the ratio of serotonin to dopamine) is associated with reduced motor unit recruitment and feelings of tiredness and lethargy during prolonged activity (Meeusen et al., 2006; Newsholme et al., 1987). Central fatigue may be especially important in prolonged activities in warm environments (Nybo and Nielson, 2001).

Incremental Aerobic Exercise to Maximum

Incremental aerobic exercise to maximum involves recruiting all muscle fiber types in the order of SO, FOG, and FG corresponding to the increasing intensity of effort. All of the mechanisms described above likely play a role in fatigue during this type of exercise. Furthermore, the cardiovascular system may be unable to provide blood supply to the working muscle adequate to support aerobic energy production (Conley, 2000).

Static Exercise

When a person maintains a static contraction at a given intensity (expressed as a percentage of maximal voluntary contraction, %MVC), force decreases over time because of fatigue. **Figure 18.10** depicts the force a muscle can produce statically as a function of time. This figure suggests that if the individual sustains a static contraction (in this case, a handgrip exercise) at less than 20% MVC, the load can be maintained indefinitely. However, as the %MVC increases, the time that the contraction can be maintained decreases rapidly. A force equal to 50% MVC can be maintained only for approximately 1 minute in a handgrip exercise. The precise shape of the fatigue curve varies among muscle groups, reflecting differences in fiber type distribution and architectural design.

Fatigue likely results from several factors: depletion of PC in FG fibers (if the intensity of effort is great enough to recruit them), the accumulation of H^+, and inhibition of the CNS by afferent fibers that are sensitive to the buildup of H^+ and other metabolites (Conley, 2000).

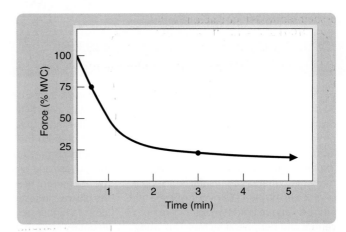

FIGURE 18.10 Hypothetical Fatigue Curve for Handgrip.

Dynamic Resistance Exercise

Dynamic resistance exercises that involve very few repetitions employ FG fibers. Fatigue is therefore likely due to a depletion of PC. In resistance exercise involving a high number of repetitions or a high total volume of work, fatigue is more likely caused by an accumulation of H^+ (and perhaps P_i and ADP) acting at the cross-bridges to reduce force, velocity, and power (Conley, 2000; Fitts, 2006).

Very Short-Term, High-Intensity Anaerobic Exercise

When an individual performs a high-intensity exercise, the amount of force that can be developed decreases rapidly due to fatigue. **Figure 18.11** depicts the change in force production on a Wingate Anaerobic Test (described fully in Chapter 3). During this test, the participant pedaled as

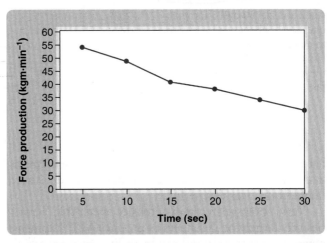

FIGURE 18.11 Force Decrement During Short-Term, High-Intensity Exercise (30 seconds. WAT).

fatigue affects both central/peripheral (handwritten)

Effect of Glucose Supplementation on Fatigue

Glucose is an important substrate during muscular work, and decreased levels of blood glucose during prolonged activity have been linked to fatigue. Ingestion of carbohydrates during prolonged exercise may improve performance, whereas an insufficient supply of glucose may lead to hypoglycemia and fatigue. Fatigue is known to involve both central and peripheral factors. This study investigated the effects of glucose supplementation during 3 hours of cycling and subsequent force production during a 2-minute sustained maximal static contraction of the knee extensors. During the trial, subjects cycled at 60% of their $\dot{V}O_2$max. In the glucose trial, they ingested a 6% glucose drink and in the placebo trial, they ingested an equal volume of a noncaloric placebo drink. A total of 200 g of carbohydrate was ingested in the glucose trial, and a total of 3.3 L of fluid was ingested in both trials.

During the maximal knee extension task, subjects were instructed to attempt to maintain maximal contraction throughout the 2-minute period. An electrical stimulation was superimposed every 30 seconds to assess the subjects' ability to voluntarily produce activation of the motor neurons.

This study demonstrated that prolonged exercise was associated with decreased blood glucose levels and elevated RPE and that glucose supplementation was able to maintain blood glucose and lessen perceived exertion during the exercise bout. As expected, maximal force generation decreased

during the 2 minutes of sustained maximal voluntary contraction in all conditions (baseline, after glucose ingestion, and after a placebo trial). At the onset of the maximal contraction, force was similar in the glucose and placebo trials. However, in the last minute of sustained contraction, the glucose ingestion trial subjects maintained a higher percentage of maximal voluntary force than the placebo subjects. Furthermore, the glucose subjects achieved a higher voluntary activation percentage at 60, 90, and 120 seconds of contraction.

This study found that the development of hypoglycemia during prolonged

exercise is associated with impaired neuromuscular performance, and the lower force generated during a subsequent sustained maximal contraction seems to be related to "central fatigue." This suggests that hypoglycemia impairs the ability to maintain high neural drive to the muscles. The observed "central fatigue" seems to be alleviated by carbohydrate supplementation.

Source: Nybo, L.: CNS fatigue and prolonged exercise: Effect of glucose supplementation. *Medicine & Science in Sports & Exercise.* 35(4):589–594 (2003).

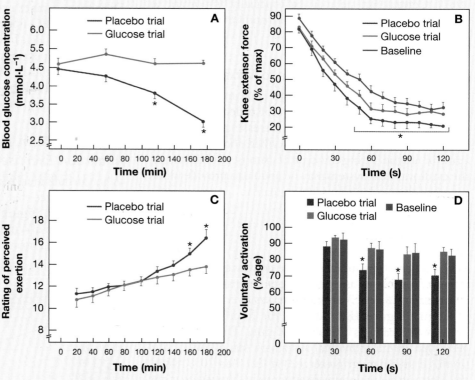

hard as possible for 30 seconds. Despite continued maximal effort, the force that could be developed decreased dramatically over this period.

Very short-term, high-intensity anaerobic activities rely largely on FT fibers to produce ATP. Explosive power events rely more heavily on FG, whereas activities that continue 1–3 minutes rely more heavily on FOG fibers. During explosive-type activities involving a predominance of FG fibers, fatigue most likely results

from the depletion of PC stores and the subsequent inability to regenerate ATP. During anaerobic activities that rely on anaerobic metabolism and use FOG fibers, the primary factor limiting performance appears to be the accumulation of H^+ associated with increased lactic acid. The accumulation of H^+ interferes with the contractile process (see explanation above) and inhibits the production of ATP by anaerobic glycolysis (Conley, 2000; Fitts, 2006).

lactic acid not a reason for muscle soreness

Muscle Soreness

Muscle soreness is a familiar consequence of overexertion. The two generally recognized types of muscle soreness are immediate and delayed onset. *Immediate-onset soreness* is characterized by pain during and immediately after exercise, which may persist for several hours. This type of soreness is thought to be caused by stimulation of the pain receptors by metabolic by-products of cellular respiration, especially the H^+ associated with increased lactic acid levels. It is generally relieved by discontinuing exercise or subsides shortly thereafter.

Delayed-onset muscle soreness (DOMS) is characterized by muscle tenderness, pain on palpitation, and mechanical stiffness that appears approximately 8 hours after exercise, increases and peaks over the next 24–48 hours, and usually subsides within 96 hours (Byrne et al., 2004). Delayed-onset muscle soreness is generally considered an adult phenomenon. Children experience less muscle damage from excessive exercise than adults and may recover more quickly (Rowland, 2005). The age in adolescence when this changes has not been determined.

DOMS is of concern to exercise professionals because it affects athletic performance and exercise participation. Despite its importance and considerable research attention, the precise causative factors and cellular mechanisms of DOMS remain elusive. However, there is widespread agreement that muscle damage and inflammation play important roles in DOMS. Eccentric muscle action has been documented as the principle factor responsible for muscle damage (Byrne et al., 2004).

Etiology and Mechanisms

The model most likely to explain DOMS combines at least three theories: the mechanical trauma, muscle damage, and inflammation theories. The sequence of events in this integrated model is still hypothetical but is backed by considerable research (Armstrong, 1984; Byrne et al., 2004; Cheung et al., 2003; Smith, 1991):

1. Unaccustomed high-force activity, particularly during eccentric muscle contraction, causes disruption of structural proteins in muscle fibers, especially along the Z lines of the sarcomeres. At the same time, damage occurs to the connective tissue at the muscle-tendon junction.
2. Damage to the sarcolemma of the cell leads to an accumulation of calcium, which in turn inhibits ATP production and causes a disruption in calcium homeostasis. (Remember that ATP is needed to return calcium to its storage locations.) High calcium concentrations lead to further degradation of the Z lines, troponin, and tropomyosin and ultimately tissue necrosis (death).
3. Structural damage initiates inflammation and activation of the immune system. Fluid moves into the muscle and causes swelling (edema).
4. The accumulation of by-products and debris from the cellular deaths and the immune system response in addition to increased pressure from the edema ultimately stimulate pain nerve endings, resulting in the sensations associated with DOMS.

Figure 18.12 summarizes the integrated model of DOMS. The sequence of events whereby muscle trauma leads to inflammation and activation of the immune system is described fully in Chapter 22. In fact, the cytokine hypothesis of overtraining proposes that muscle damage, inflammation, and the immune response are central to explaining the symptoms of overtraining (Smith, 2000). In addition to the well-established theories that contribute to the integrated model of DOMS, researchers have also provided evidence that oxidative stress (Ascensão et al., 2008), the release of bradykinin (Murase et al., 2010), and restricted blood flow (Umbel et al., 2009) may play a role in DOMS.

One of the popular misconceptions about DOMS is that it is caused by the accumulation of lactic acid. Although this theory was originally proposed by researchers (Asmussen, 1956; Edington and Edgerton, 1976), it remains popular only with the lay public. Considerable research evidence now argues against this theory, including the fact that individuals with McArdle's syndrome, who do not produce lactic acid, also suffer from DOMS. Additional evidence against lactic acid as the cause of muscle soreness is that the type of activity that produces the greatest degree of soreness, eccentric contractions, produces lower lactic acid levels than concentric contractions of the same power output (Armstrong et al., 1983; Bonde-Petersen et al., 1972; Davies and Barnes, 1972). Perhaps the most compelling evidence is that lactic acid has a half-life of 15–25 minutes and is fully cleared from muscle within an hour (see Chapter 3). Since lactic acid is not present at elevated levels 24–48 hours later, it cannot cause soreness then.

Effect on Muscle Function

While the sensation of soreness (DOMS) is important, many athletes are equally concerned with the functional impairments related to muscle damage. Exercise-induced muscle damage, especially with eccentric exercise, has a detrimental effect on muscle function. Muscle damage reduces strength, power, and performance. Unusual patterns of muscle recruitment during any given movement

---

Delayed-Onset Muscle Soreness (DOMS) is a condition characterized by muscle tenderness, pain on palpitation, and mechanical stiffness that appears approximately 8 hours after exercise, increases and peaks over the next 24–48 hours, and usually subsides within 96 hours.

FIGURE 18.12 An Integrated Model to Explain Delayed-Onset Muscle Soreness (DOMS).
This integrated model of DOMS recognizes that mechanical trauma leads to muscle damage, resulting in an inflammatory response that causes swelling and pain.

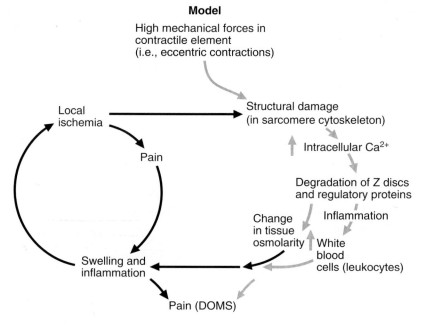

may include alteration in temporal sequencing of muscles. Altered joint mechanics and reduced joint range of motion have also been reported. These impairments are immediate but may persist for a prolonged period even though the athlete or exerciser may perceive no change. Reduced strength and power may lead to an individual working at a higher intensity than normal. Altered coordination or segment motion as well as reduced force output may lead to compensatory recruitment of muscles unused to such work. An inaccurate perception of impairment may lead to a premature return to high-intensity exercise (Cheung et al., 2003).

Evidence suggests that the time course of functional impairment is not the same as the time course of the sensation of DOMS (Byrne et al., 2004). The severity of muscle function impairment and time course of recovery greatly depend on the muscle group studied and the exercise protocol. An eccentric exercise protocol resulted in a 57% loss in strength immediately after exercise with strength measures remaining 33% below baseline after 5.5 days of recovery (Sayers and Clarkson, 2001). Performing the eccentric phase of a barbell squat exercise resulted in a 30–40% reduction in knee extensor strength immediately after exercise, which recovered to 95% of baseline strength by day 7 of recovery (Byrne and Eston, 2002). Marathon running has been shown to result in a 30% reduction in ankle extensor strength, which recovered fully 2 days after the race (Avela et al., 1999). A soccer match has also resulted in evidence of muscle damage and impaired function (Ascensão et al., 2008). Importantly, the time course of recovery varies substantially among individuals.

An athlete, coach, or clinician must be sensitive to individual differences when planning workouts after a stressful bout of exercise, particularly when it includes a large eccentric component, because recovery varies considerably. DOMS may otherwise lead to more substantial injury.

Treatment for Relief and Prevention

Several different treatment strategies have been researched to prevent DOMS or decrease the severity of the symptoms and restore function to the affected muscles as quickly as possible. Anti-inflammatory drug use has been suggested to prevent or treat muscle soreness, since inflammation is clearly part of the DOMS cycle. Although nonsteroidal anti-inflammatory drugs (NSAIDS) (such as aspirin, naproxen, and ibuprofen) do help relieve DOMS symptoms, their effect on muscle damage is less clear because muscle damage generates a local proinflammatory response, but the systemic response is tightly regulated by anti-inflammatory mediators (Peake et al., 2005). Current evidence suggests that NSAIDS may be beneficial for short-term recovery from muscle damage and soreness in healthy individuals (Cheung et al., 2003; Lanier, 2003). Research has also found that branched-chain amino acid supplementation administered before heavy resistance exercise can lessen the functional impairment associated with DOMS (Shimomura et al., 2010).

Acute exercise also diminishes DOMS (Armstrong et al., 1983). Indeed, exercise is the most effective technique for decreasing the pain of DOMS. Unfortunately, this analgesic effect ends quickly when the activity is stopped. Compression of the sore area may be of some value. Massage has shown varying results that warrant further research. Research is needed to determine whether manual manipulation of injured tissue enhances healing or delays it. Static stretching is thought to initiate the inverse myotatic reflex (by stimulation of the Golgi

Muscle Damage and DOMS

While it seems clear that exercise-induced muscle damage is related to the sensation of DOMS, the timelines of recovery from muscle damage and DOMS may be very different. Exercise-induced muscle damage (within the contractile elements, the sarcolemma, and the cytoskeleton) leads to inflammation that is believed responsible for the sensation of pain, tenderness, and stiffness that characterize DOMS and result in impairment of muscle function. In many studies, the sensation of DOMS is used as the primary marker of muscle damage. However, several studies have shown that measures of muscle function do not correspond with the sensation of DOMS. The accompanying figures report changes in maximal isometric force production, plasma levels of CK (representing muscle damage), and sensation of DOMS for 96 hours following 12 maximal eccentric contractions of the elbow flexors.

It can be seen clearly in these graphs that muscle function (strength) was impaired immediately after exercise without an immediate change in plasma CK level or an immediate sensation of pain (measured as a visual analog scale from 0 to 50 mm). On the other hand, by 96 hours after exercise, the sensation of pain was beginning to subside while the measure of muscle damage remained at its highest level. The lack of a temporal association among DOMS, muscle damage, and muscle function has important implications for athletes and fitness participants alike. Eccentric exercise can cause muscle damage and impairment of muscle function that last far longer than the sensation of pain or discomfort associated with DOMS. The fact that muscular pain recedes does not guarantee that muscle repair is complete or that function is restored. Thus, it seems prudent to avoid another bout of strenuous eccentric work as soon as pain is no longer a limiting factor. In fact, a hasty return to strenuous work—without adequate recovery time—may be an important factor in overtraining.

Sources: Nosaka et al. (2002), Byrne et al. (2004), Warren et al. (1999).

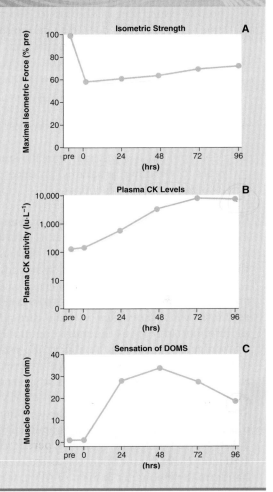

tendon organs, GTO), which results in relaxation of the stretched muscle (DeVries and Housh, 1994). (Reflexes are discussed in detail in Chapter 20.) Although some research (DeVries and Housh, 1994) has demonstrated a reduced soreness resulting from stretching, other research has not (McGlynn et al., 1979). Icing, ultrasound, and electrical current modalities have not been shown to consistently eliminate DOMS symptoms (Cheung et al., 2003) although there is evidence that cold water immersion or contrast water therapy may be of benefit (Vaile et al., 2008).

Repeated Bout Effect

As discussed previously, a single bout of unaccustomed, predominately eccentric exercise causes DOMS, symptoms of muscle damage, and a loss of muscle function. However, it is well established that a repeated bout of similar eccentric exercise results in markedly reduced symptoms of damage compared to the initial bout of exercise. This protective adaptation to a single bout of exercise is referred to as the *repeated bout effect* (McHugh, 2003; McHugh et al., 1999; Nosaka and Clarkson, 1995). The protective adaptation has been shown to last for several weeks and possibly up to 6 months when the initial bout of eccentric exercise was performed at near maximal intensity. While the existence of the repeated bout effect is well known, and the conditions necessary to induce it are fairly well characterized, the mechanisms of its protective effect are not well understood (McHugh, 2003).

Measurement of Muscular Function

Accurate measurement of the strength, endurance, and power a muscle can generate is important for five reasons:

1. Measurement aids screening to determine the extent of muscle weaknesses and/or imbalances. Both weakness

and imbalance can make an individual more prone to injury. Measurement also establishes baseline values for an individual.

2. Measurement can be used as a guide to rehabilitation. Measurement of the loss of function after an injury or accident is needed to determine rehabilitation workloads and to monitor progress.

3. Measurement is necessary for exercise prescription. Both athletes and fitness participants need realistic programs based on their own performance capabilities.

4. Measurement aids selection of the best exercises for working on specific problems.

5. Measurement is a research tool for studying which types of training programs produce the greatest changes in muscle function.

Strength is the ability of a muscle or muscle group to exert force against a resistance. It is usually measured as one maximal effort. For dynamic resistance exercise, this is often called a one-repetition maximum (1-RM), whereas for static exercise it is referred to as a maximal voluntary contraction (MVC). Torque is the more correct term when movement is made through a range of motion, but strength is the more commonly used term. **Muscular endurance** is the ability of a muscle or muscle group to repeatedly exert force against a resistance; the activity is typically performed at a given percentage of the 1-RM (for resistance exercise) or MVC (for static exercise). For example, an exerciser wishing to improve muscle endurance might lift a weight equal to 60% of her 1-RM for 12 repetitions. Similarly, a researcher studying static muscle endurance may ask an individual to hold a handgrip dynamometer at 50% of MVC for 90 seconds. **Power** is the amount of work done per unit of time and is the product of force and velocity ($P = F \times V$). Thus, power is the expression of strength exerted quickly.

Strength and muscular endurance can be expressed as either absolute or relative values. Absolute values refer to the actual external load commonly measured in pounds (lb), kilograms (kg), newtons (N), or newton-meters (N·m). Relative values are expressed in relation to body weight. Both values are useful. For example, if two individuals are doing a two-arm curl and individual A can lift 70 kg and individual B can lift only 60 kg, it might seem that individual A is stronger. However, if individual A weighs 55 kg and individual B weighs 47 kg, then both are lifting 1.27 kg per kg of body weight—and on a relative basis, neither is considered stronger. When a comparison is made between individuals, a relative expression of strength is generally preferred. In contrast, absolute values are preferred for comparisons made of the same person under different conditions or at different times, for example, before and after a training program.

In terms of muscular endurance, if individual A has a handgrip strength of 70 kg and individual B has a handgrip strength of 60 kg, and both are asked to hold a handgrip dynamometer at 40 kg, you would assume that individual A could do so for a longer period of time, because that load represents 57% MVC (40/70) for individual A and 67% MVC (40/60) for individual B. An absolute load thus puts the weaker individual at a disadvantage. However, if both are asked to hold a load representing a 50% MVC (35 kg for individual A, 30 kg for individual B), you would expect that both individuals could hold that load for the same length of time, assuming equal motivation. To confirm your understanding of the influence of body weight on the expression of strength, complete the Check Your Comprehension 1 box.

CHECK YOUR COMPREHENSION 1

Listed below are the body weight (BW) and MVC for a handgrip task.

Name	Gender	BW (kg)	Absolute Strength MVC (kg)	Relative Strength kg·kg⁻¹	50% MVC
Jody	F	60.0	40.0		
Jill	F	68.0	60.0		
Pat	F	70.0	36.0		
Scott	M	63.0	50.0		
Tom	M	82.0	72.0		
Mike	M	70.0	71.0		

1. Calculate the relative strength for each individual (strength ÷ BW).

2. Calculate the load that would need to be held for each of the subjects to be working at 50% MVC (absolute strength × 0.5).

3. Who is the strongest person on an absolute basis? On a relative basis?

4. For whom would 50% MVC represent the most absolute force?

Check your answers in Appendix C.

Laboratory Methods

To quantify the several aspects of muscular function, exercise physiologists use various laboratory and field methods. Laboratory methods are generally more accurate and precise for measuring different aspects of muscular function but are more expensive and inaccessible to many people.

Electromyography

Electromyography (EMG) is the measurement of the electrical activity, known as muscle action potentials, that brings about muscle contraction. Motor unit activity can be recorded using needle electrodes, or whole-muscle activity can be recorded using surface electrodes. The EMG voltage is proportional to the force of a static contraction, to the tension developed in constant-velocity contractions (Lippold, 1952), and to velocity in dynamic contractions (Bigland and Lippold, 1954). Therefore, one can obtain a reasonably valid estimation of tension development in a muscle by EMG.

EMG provides not an absolute value of force or torque but a direct functional indication of muscle activity. If it is plotted against incremental loads or values resulting from a submaximal hold, it can be used to predict strength or endurance, respectively. Such submaximal testing using EMG is particularly important in situations where an individual either cannot or is not motivated to perform maximally. In addition, because weak individuals produce a greater EMG signal than strong individuals for any absolute load (Fischer and Merhautova, 1961), EMG activity can be used to monitor rehabilitation or training progress.

Perhaps the most valuable role of EMG in muscle function assessment is showing which muscles are primarily responsible for specific actions. For example, when training or testing individuals for abdominal strength, an exercise should be selected that maximizes the involvement of the abdominal muscles (the rectus abdominis and the external obliques) and that minimizes the involvement of the hip flexors and thigh muscles (rectus femoris). EMG helps in this selection.

The Check Your Comprehension 2 box provides an example of the EMG activity of these muscles during a sit-up with the feet supported and unsupported and the knees at various angles (Hall et al., 1990; Halpern and Bleck, 1979). Work through the questions in the box to confirm your understanding.

Strength The ability of a muscle or muscle group to exert maximal force against a resistance in a single repetition.

Muscular Endurance The ability of a muscle or muscle group to repeatedly exert force against a resistance.

Power The amount of work done per unit of time; the product of force and velocity; the ability to exert force quickly.

Electromyography (EMG) The measurement of the neural or electrical activity that brings about muscle contraction.

CHECK YOUR COMPREHENSION 2

Study the EMG data for each of the muscle groups with the feet supported (●) and with the feet unsupported (●), and answer the following questions:

● Feet supported   ● Feet unsupported

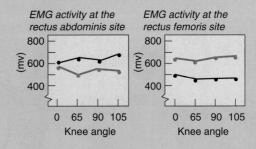

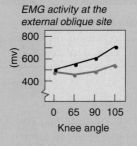

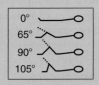

Knee angle designation for sit-up variations

1. Does bending the knees eliminate the involvement of thigh muscles (rectus femoris) if the feet are held down? Which muscles are more active if the feet are held—the abdominal or thigh muscles?

2. Which muscle group does the angle of knee bend affect most?

3. Should the feet be held or not held to maximize the involvement of the abdominal muscles?

4. On the basis of your answers in 1–3, which sit-up form (feet held or not held) and which knee angle would you recommend?

Check your answers in Appendix C.

Isokinetic Machines

Isokinetic machines, such as a Cybex or MERAC (**Figure 18.13**), allow the velocity of limb movement to be kept nearly constant throughout a contraction. These devices provide accurate and reliable measurements of muscular strength, muscular endurance, and power while the speed of the limb is kept constant at a predetermined velocity. Any increase in muscular force results in increased resistance rather than increased acceleration of the limb (Heyward, 1991). Measurements obtained on isokinetic machines serve as a reference against which other methods of measurement can be compared. These devices can be configured to test the limbs of the upper or the lower body.

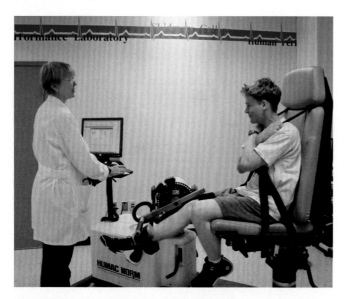

FIGURE 18.13 Isokinetic Exercise Equipment.
The measurement of isokinetic strength of the quadriceps is recorded throughout the normal range of motion.

Force Transducers

Force transducers measure static strength and endurance. The deformation of the transducer sends an electrical signal to a computer, which displays the force output. When the subject exerts as much force as possible in a single trial, this device measures maximal strength. It can also measure static muscular endurance when the subject holds a given percentage of the predetermined maximal value (%MVC). Static muscular endurance is then calculated by determining either how long the individual can maintain the predetermined value or how long it takes the individual to drop to a specified percentage of the maximal contraction.

Laboratory and Field Methods

Several other methods of measuring muscle function require only relatively simple testing devices. They may be used in a laboratory or field test.

Dynamometers

Dynamometers measure static strength and static muscular endurance. Two commercially available dynamometers are the handgrip dynamometer and the back and leg dynamometer. As force is applied to the dynamometer, its spring is compressed and moves the needle to indicate force produced. Like the force transducer, these devices can be used to measure maximal strength when the subject exerts as much force as possible in a single maximal voluntary contraction (MVC). Because of its availability and ease of administration, the handgrip dynamometer has been extensively used to measure grip strength.

Dynamometers can also be used to measure static muscular endurance when the subject performs at a given percentage of the predetermined maximal value. Muscular endurance is then calculated by determining how long the individual can maintain the predetermined (submaximal) value.

Constant-Resistance Equipment

The most common method of measuring dynamic strength is to determine the maximal amount an individual can lift in a single repetition against constant resistance using free weight or weight machines. Known as a one-repetition max (1-RM), this is a trial-and-error method of determining how much an individual can lift. If the selected weight is too heavy to be lifted, a lower weight is used. If the weight is successfully lifted, then additional weight is added. Care must be taken because too many trials will cause fatigue, thereby decreasing the true maximal strength value.

Constant-resistance equipment can also be used to measure dynamic muscular endurance by determining how many times an individual can lift a submaximal load. The submaximal load is usually a predetermined load (such as the 80-lb bench press test for males or the 35-lb test for females used in the YMCA assessment battery), or it may be expressed as a percentage of body weight or as a percentage of 1-RM.

Field Tests

Several easily administered tests are commonly used in the field to measure muscle function. Common field tests include calisthenic and jumping activities.

Calisthenic Activities

Calisthenic activities are often used in field settings to measure muscular endurance and, to a lesser extent, muscular strength. The most common tests include some version of sit-ups or curl-ups, push-ups, and pull-ups or flexed-arm hang. Although these tests are often reported to measure strength, they are in fact usually endurance tests; that is, they measure the maximum number of times an individual can perform a given test (often within a specified time period, such as the number of curl-ups per minute). If the participant can complete more than one repetition, the result represents muscular endurance. If the subject can complete only one repetition (or sometimes no repetitions), the result represents strength (or lack thereof). Note that these tests indicate relative strength or endurance, because the amount of resistance depends on the individual's body size and mass.

Vertical Jump/Standing Broad Jump

Jump tests are used to measure the explosive muscular power of the legs. Although they are easy to administer, they are influenced by the individual's weight. Furthermore, these tests may have a strong neural component and have a definite alactic anaerobic metabolic component (see Chapter 3).

Although all of these calisthenic (performance) tests are commonly used, they have not been definitively validated as tests of strength, muscular endurance, and/or power. Therefore, it may be better to consider them what they are—a push-up test, for example—rather than asserting they are a substitute for a laboratory assessment.

The Influence of Age and Sex on Muscle Function

Male-Female Differences

Adult females on average have about 56% of the static strength values of adult males in upper-body locations, about 64% in trunk strength, and about 72% in lower-body locations (Lauback, 1976). As shown in **Figure 18.14**, the variation between upper- and lower-body strength occurs also in the bench press and the leg press (Wells and Plowman, 1983). Note the considerable overlap in the distribution of leg strength even in untrained males and females (**Figure 18.14A**), whereas virtually no overlap exists in arm strength (bench press) distributions (**Figure 18.14B**).

Although field tests are not pure tests of muscle function, differences in these tests parallel those seen in strength with growth and maturation and between boys and girls. **Figure 18.15** illustrates these relationships for the flexed-arm hang and the standing long jump. Adult performances also appear to parallel adolescent male-female strength differences. **Figure 18.16** shows that throughout the adult age span, males can perform more push-ups than females, even inactive males. With a leg-lift exercise, however, the performance gap is smaller, with considerable overlap between inactive males and active females.

Why do these differences occur? Strength and other muscle functions increase as children grow because muscle mass increases in parallel with increases in body mass.

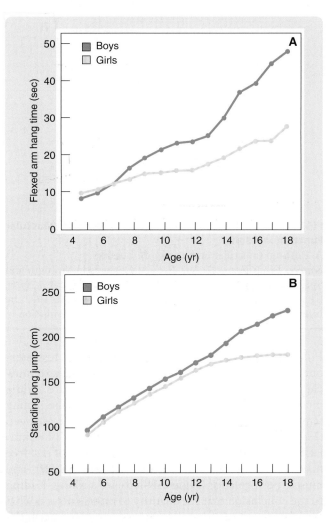

FIGURE 18.15 Performance on Field Tests of Muscular Function in Children.
A. Flexed-arm hang (muscular endurance). **B**. Standing long jump (muscular power).
Source: From Malina, R. M. & C. Bouchard: *Growth, Maturation, and Physical Activity* (2nd edition). Champaign, IL: Human Kinetics, 220, 221. Copyright 2004 Robert M. Malina and Claude Bouchard. Reprinted by permission.

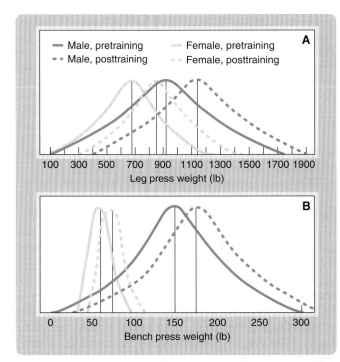

FIGURE 18.14 Frequency Distribution for Leg Press (A) and Bench Press (B) Values for Males and Females before and after a Training Program.
Source: Reprinted with permission from Wells, C. L. & S. A. Plowman: Sexual differences in athletic performance: Biological or behavioral? *The Physician and Sports Medicine.* 11(8):52–63 (1983).

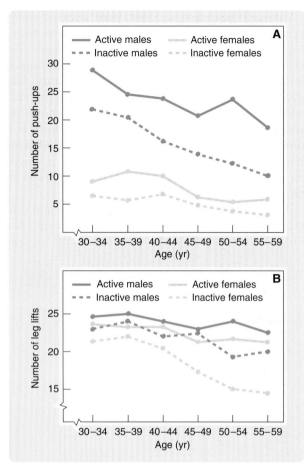

FIGURE 18.16 Performance on Field Tests of Muscular Function in Adults.
A. Push-up (muscular endurance). **B**. Leg lifts.
Source: From Israel, S.: Age-Related Changes in Strength and Special Groups. In Komi, P. V. (ed.): *Strength and Power in Sport*. Champaign, IL: Human Kinetics, 323. Copyright 1992 by International Olympic Committee. Reprinted by permission.

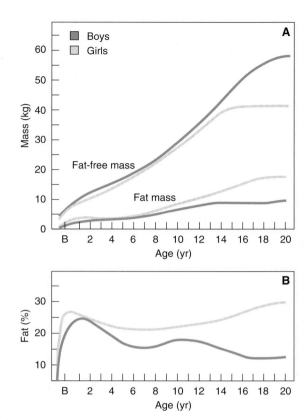

FIGURE 18.17 Growth Curves for Mass and Percent Fat in Children.
A. Mass. **B**. Fat.
Source: From Malina, R. M., C. Bouchard, & O. Bar-Or: *Growth, Maturation, and Physical Activity* (2nd edition). Champaign, IL: Human Kinetics, 114 (2004); Growth curves for Fat, B: Data from Malina, R. M.: *Growth and maturation*: Normal variation and effects of training. In Gisolfi, C. V. & D. R. Lamb (eds.): *Perspectives in Exercise Science and Sports Medicine: Youth, Exercise, and Sport* (Vol. 2). Indianapolis, IN: Benchmark Press, 223–265 (1989) and Malina, R. M., C. Bouchard, & G. Beunen: Human growth: Selected aspects of current research on well-nourished children. *Annual Review of Anthropology*. 17:187–219 (1988). Reprinted with permission.

Pubertal hormonal changes—particularly in testosterone, which is involved with the anabolic process of muscle growth—favor males. While young males are adding muscle mass under the influence of testosterone, young females are adding fat under the influence of estrogen (**Figure 18.17**) (Malina and Bouchard, 1991). The similarities among the graphic representations of fat-free mass (**Figure 18.17A**), strength (**Figure 18.18**), and muscle performance (**Figure 18.15**) are striking, leading to the conclusion that the quantity of muscle mass is what accounts for the difference in the expression of strength.

That it is muscle quantity rather than quality that is responsible for these male-female inequities is emphasized by calculating relative strength values (Wells and Plowman, 1983; Wilmore, 1974). In one study the percentage of handgrip strength exhibited by the females in relation to the males increased from 57% in absolute strength terms to relative values of 73% (absolute strength divided by total body weight) and 83% (absolute strength divided by lean body mass) (Wilmore, 1974). For the bench press, the corresponding figures were 37%, 46%, and 53%, and for the leg press, they were 73%, 92%, and 106%. Thus, in leg strength relative to lean body mass, female performance actually exceeded that of males.

In addition, studies relating strength to cross-sectional area of muscle show no inequities between the sexes. Overall then, all these studies show that the larger size of males in general, their greater muscle mass, and their larger fiber size are physiologically responsible for their greater strength, rather than any inherent difference in the potential or function of the muscle fibers per se.

Another important factor is cultural expectations. Many adolescent girls become less active as they grow up, detraining to some extent. Some detraining may be anatomically selective. Although males and females of all ages experience gravity equally when walking, climbing stairs, sitting down, and standing up, individuals can selectively avoid upper-body activities, such as lifting heavy loads, opening jars, hammering, and weight lifting. Thus, differences in upper-body versus lower-body activities in males and females may in part be cultural. Future studies may note a change in these relationships as more girls have the opportunity to enter sports at an early age and continue to be active into middle age and old age.

Children and Adolescents

Strength generally develops in humans from infancy through maturity. **Figure 18.18** shows a common pattern of development. Strength increases rectilinearly from early childhood (3–7 years) through early adolescence (13–14 years) for both sexes. A marked increase in strength then occurs during the rest of adolescence and into early adulthood (15–20 years) for boys. Girls, however, do not have an accelerated increase in strength in late adolescence. They either maintain a slow rectilinear rise, as shown for grip strength (**Figure 18.18B**), or decline

after age 16, as shown for both elbow flexion and knee extension (**Figure 18.18C** and **D**) (Malina and Bouchard, 1991). The increase in strength during childhood and adolescence, even without training, is more than can be accounted for just from growth in size, although other causative factors have not been determined. In males, the average muscle mass increases from 42% at age 5 to 53% at age 17 years of total body mass. In females, comparable values are 41% at age 5 and 42% at age 17 (Rowland, 2005). This growth occurs by increasing protein content in the existing muscle fibers, not by increasing the number of muscle fibers.

In early childhood, there is virtually no difference in strength measurements between boys and girls. As puberty begins and progresses though, a gap appears and progressively widens. On the average, at 11–12 years of age, girls have approximately 90% of boys' strength; at 13–14 years, this percentage has decreased to 80%, and at 15–16 years, to 75%. These percentages vary not only with age but also with the muscle group being measured.

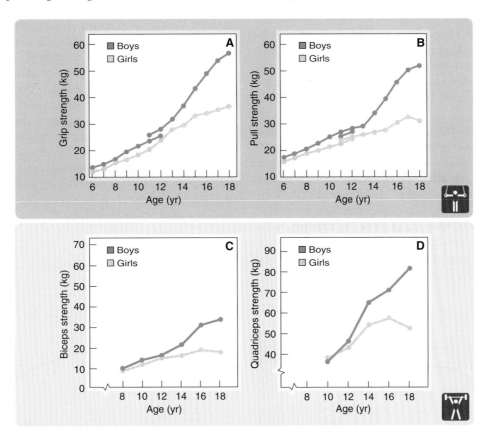

FIGURE 18.18 Strength Development in Boys and Girls.
A. Grip strength in young children. **B**. Pull strength in children 6–18 years old. **C**. Biceps strength. **D**. Quadriceps strength.
Source: From Malina, R. M., C. Bouchard, & O. Bar-Or: *Growth, Maturation, and Physical Activity.* (2nd edition). Champaign, IL: Human Kinetics, pp. 191, 219 (2004); Data for Gripping and Pulling from Malina, R. M., & A. F. Roche: *Manual of Physical Status and Performance in Childhood: Physical performance* (Vol. 2). New York: Plenum (1983).; Data for biceps from Rodahl, K., P.-O. Åstrand, N. C. Birkhead, T. Hettinger, B. Issekutz, D. M. Jones, & R. Weaver: Physical work capacity: A study of some children and young adults in the United States. *Archives of Environmental Health*. 2:499–510 (1961). Data for quadriceps from Bouchard et al. (unpublished). Reprinted with permission.

Because most research documents static strength measures in children and adolescents, there is still a clear need to measure and interpret isokinetic muscle strength and muscle power during growth and maturation (De Ste Croix et al., 2003; Van Praagh and Doré, 2002).

Older Adults

Significant declines in muscular strength in both males and females are well documented from middle age to old age, but the rate of loss varies substantially among muscle groups (Rogers and Evans, 1993). **Figure 18.19** shows a generalized change in strength (grip strength) over the normal life span for males and females (Komi, 1992). From the peak values in late adolescence or early adulthood, strength is maintained until approximately 45–50 years, followed by a fairly gradual decline into and beyond the 70s. The decline in muscle strength generally amounts to about 15% per decade in the sixth and seventh decades of life and 30% per decade after that (Rogers and Evans, 1993). Relative static endurance (at ~40–50% MVC) is similar between older and younger individuals. **Figures 18.16** and **18.19** show parallel declines in performance and show that different muscle groups decline at different rates, even between the sexes.

What causes the age-related decline in strength? Three possibilities are (1) a loss of muscle mass, (2) a loss of mechanical or contractile properties (fiber type changes, fiber size changes, fiber number changes), and/or (3) reduced activation of motor units or denervation.

Muscle mass is clearly lost with age. Between the ages of 30 and 70 years, almost 25% of muscle mass is lost in both males and females (Rogers and Evans, 1993). This reduces force production. Some evidence, however, supports the contention that the decline in strength with aging is greater than can be accounted for just by the loss of muscle mass. The capacity to exert force per unit of cross-sectional area also declines (Rogers and Evans, 1993).

Early studies using traditional biopsy techniques seemed to show a preferential loss of FT and, especially, FG fibers. Since these are the high-force fibers, this result was intuitively logical. More definitive studies using whole-muscle cross-sectional techniques have shown, however, that both ST and FT fibers are lost equally with aging (Lexell et al., 1988).

As shown in **Figure 18.20**, the loss of muscle fibers begins at about age 30, and by age 80, a reduction of between 25% and 40% has occurred in females and males (Rogers and Evans, 1993). The genetically predetermined percentages of ST and FT fibers remain constant. The SO fibers appear to maintain their size longer than do FT fibers. Thus, although FT fibers are not lost at a faster rate than SO fibers, they do atrophy faster, and FG fibers atrophy faster than FOG fibers. Since FT fibers are generally the larger fibers, the preferential loss in size of these fibers largely accounts for the overall decrease in muscle size and strength with aging.

Of great concern is the practical meaning of these changes. Weakened respiratory muscles restrict aerobic activity. Weakened muscles around joints lead to instability, difficulty in restoring balance, and a greater potential for falls (Aoyagi and Shephard, 1992). Insufficient strength to get in and out of chairs, carry groceries, or take caps off medicine or food jars can lead to a loss of independent living. The most effective way to prevent these difficulties is systematic exercise training. Muscle aging cannot be prevented but can be delayed. Thus, maintaining and/or increasing muscular strength, endurance, and power is important for different reasons throughout the life span. Nonetheless, muscles respond to exercise training in basically the same fashion at all ages; that is, trained muscles produce greater force.

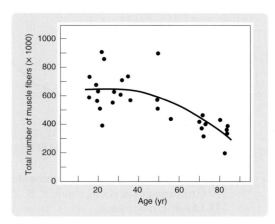

FIGURE 18.20 Loss of Muscle Fibers with Age.
Source: Rogers, M. A. & W. J. Evans: Changes in skeletal muscle with aging: Effects of exercise training. In Holloszy, J. O. (ed.): *Exercise and Sport Sciences Reviews* (Vol. 21). Baltimore, MD: Williams & Wilkins, 65–107 (1993). Reprinted by permission.

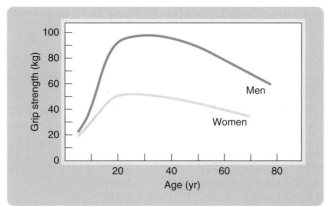

FIGURE 18.19 Theoretical Maximal Handgrip Strength.

FOCUS ON APPLICATION

Effect of Different Training Programs on Muscle Size and Strength

The cross-sectional area of muscle is related to the force it can generate. This implies that if a training program causes muscle hypertrophy (increase in size), it will also result in increased strength. However, there is considerable uncertainty about the optimal training program for improving muscle strength, and it has been speculated that not all populations may experience muscle hypertrophy. Postmenopausal women who are estrogen deficient, for example, may benefit tremendously from increased strength because independent living is related to strength. Yet it has not been established how this group would respond to different resistance training programs. Bemben et al. (2000) investigated the effects of high-load (80% of 1-RM; 8 reps) and high-repetition (40% of 1-RM; 16 reps) resistance training protocols on the musculoskeletal system of early postmenopausal, estrogen-deficient females. The accompanying graphs display changes in only two of the many variables investigated: rectus femoris muscle cross-sectional area (CSA) (measured by ultrasound) and leg press strength.

These graphs show that both training protocols effectively increased muscle strength (measured by the leg press) and increased muscle cross-sectional area (CSA). Based on these and other data, these authors concluded that both high-load and high-repetition resistance training programs are effective for improving muscular strength and size in postmenopausal women. This finding is important for exercise professionals because it indicates that postmenopausal women do adapt positively to exercise training and that a low-intensity, high-repetition training program can be beneficial for developing muscular fitness in women for whom a high-intensity program may not be appropriate.

Source: Bemben et al. (2000).

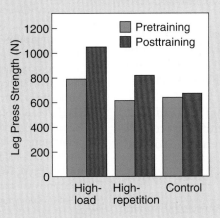

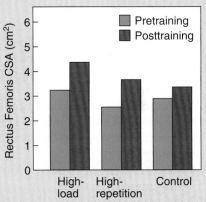

SUMMARY

1. Muscle tension is the force developed when a contracting muscle acts on an object. Load is the force exerted on the muscle by the object. For a muscle to move a load, muscle tension must exceed the force of the load.

2. In isotonic contractions of muscle fibers, force production is constant as the muscle fiber contracts. In the intact human system, such a contraction is practically impossible. Instead, the load is constant but the force needed to move it through the range of motion is not. Thus, the term dynamic more accurately describes contraction within the intact human.

3. If movement results from a contraction in which muscle shortening occurs, it is a concentric dynamic contraction. If movement results from a contraction in which muscle lengthening occurs, the contraction is referred to as an eccentric dynamic contraction.

4. In isokinetic contractions of muscle fibers, the velocity of contraction is constant. In the intact human, the velocity of movement varies with joint angle. Specialized equipment can hold the rate of limb displacement constant, resulting in isokinematic contraction.

5. A muscle fiber contraction that does not result in a meaningful length change in the muscle fiber is termed isometric. An intact fiber has an elastic element, such that some fiber shortening actually occurs with contraction even though no limb displacement occurs. Thus, the term static is preferable to isometric to describe this type of contraction in humans.

6. The amount of force produced by muscles depends on neural and mechanical factors. Important mechanical factors include length-tension-angle relationships, force-velocity relationships, elasticity-force relationships, and architectural design.

7. Muscular fatigue may be caused by a variety of factors, which can be described as central or peripheral, or as electrophysiological or biochemical in nature. The cause is determined largely by the muscle fiber type and therefore varies with different types of activity. Muscular fatigue results in a loss of muscle function.

8. Muscular soreness probably results from a combination of mechanical trauma, muscle damage, and inflammation.

9. Differences in strength between the sexes are largely due to the greater muscle mass of males. The magnitude of the difference in strength between males and females depends on the absolute or relative expressions

of strength, the region of the body where strength is measured, and the training status of the individuals.

10. Strength development occurs from infancy through maturity. The increase in strength during childhood and adolescence is more than can be accounted for just from growth in size.

11. Muscular strength declines in both males and females from middle age to old age, due in part to loss in both ST and FT fibers. Aging of muscles cannot be prevented, but loss of strength can be delayed with appropriate exercise training.

REVIEW QUESTIONS

1. Define isotonic, isokinetic, and isometric contractions. Discuss how they relate to dynamic and static contractions.

2. Diagram the force-length relationship in a muscle fiber. Diagram a strength curve for biceps flexion, knee flexion, and knee extension. Discuss the relationship between force and length in the muscle fiber and in the whole muscle.

3. Graph the force-velocity relationship in (a) a muscle fiber and in (b) a whole muscle. Identify the eccentric contraction on graph (a) and identify a static contraction on graph (b).

4. Create a schematic representation of the possible sites of muscular fatigue.

5. Indicate the most probable cause of muscle fatigue for the following categories of exercise: long-term, moderate to heavy, submaximal aerobic, incremental aerobic exercise to maximum, static, dynamic resistance, and very short-term, high-intensity anaerobic exercise.

6. Discuss the integrated model of delayed-onset muscle soreness (DOMS). How can DOMS be prevented or treated?

7. What are the primary laboratory methods for measuring muscular function? What are the primary field tests to measure muscular function? What are the limitations of these methods? What determines the appropriate test to administer?

8. Compare male and female strength development during childhood and adolescence.

9. Discuss differences in strength between adult males and females. How is the difference in strength affected by absolute or relative units used to express strength? How do differences vary among different regions of the body? What are the most likely causes of sex-related differences in muscular function?

10. What factors account for the age-related decline in muscular strength? Can this loss be minimized or slowed? If so, how?

For further review and additional study tools, visit the website at http://thePoint.lww.com/Plowman4e ✳ ▶

REFERENCES

Aagaard, P. & J. Bangsbo: The muscular system: Design, function, and performance relationships. In *ACSM's Advanced Exercise Physiology*. Philadelphia, PA: Lippincott, Williams & Wilkins, 144–160 (2006).

Aoyagi, Y. & R. J. Shephard: Aging and muscle function. *Sports Medicine*. 14(6):376–396 (1992).

Armstrong, R. B.: Mechanisms of exercise-induced delayed onset muscular soreness: A brief review. *Medicine and Science in Sports and Exercise*. 16(6):529–538 (1984).

Armstrong, R. B., M. H. Laughlin, L. Rome, & C. R. Taylor: Metabolism of rats running up and down an incline. *Journal of Applied Physiology*. 55:518–521 (1983).

Ascensão, A., A. Rebelo, E. Oliveira, F. Marques, L. Pereira, & J. Magalhães: Biochemical impact of a soccer match—analysis of oxidative stress and muscle damage markers throughout recovery. *Clinical Biochemistry*. 41:841–851 (2008).

Astorino, T. A., & D. W. Roberson: Efficacy of acute caffeine ingestion for short-term high-intensity exercise performance: A systematic review. *Journal of Strength and Conditioning Research*. 24(1):257–265 (2010).

Asmussen, E.: Observations on experimental muscular soreness. *Acta Rheumatologica Scandinavica*. 2:109–116 (1956).

Avela, J., H. Kyröläinen, P. V. Komi, & D. Rama: Reduced flex sensitivity persists several days after long-lasting stretch-shortening cycle exercise. *Journal of Applied Physiology*. 86(4):1292–1300 (1999).

Bangsbo, J., M. Mohr, & P. Krustrup: Physical and metabolic demands of training and match-play in the elite football player. *Journal of Sports Sciences*. 24(7):665–674 (2006).

Beck, T. W., T. J. Housh, R. J. Schmidt, G. O. Johnson, D. J. Housh, J. W. Coburn, & M. H. Malek: The acute effects of a caffeine-containing supplement on strength, muscular endurance, and anaerobic capabilities. *Journal of Strength and Conditioning Research*. 18(1):506–510 (2006).

Bemben, D. A., N. L. Fetters, M. G. Bemben, N. Nabavi, & E. T. Koh: Musculoskeletal responses to high- and low-intensity resistance in early menopausal women. *Medicine & Science in Sports & Exercise*. 32(11):1949–1957 (2000).

Bigland, B., & O. C. J. Lippold: The relation between force, velocity, and integrated electrical activity in human muscles. *The Journal of Physiology*. 123:214–224 (1954).

Bonde-Petersen, F., H. G. Knuttgen, & J. Henriksson: Muscle metabolism during exercise with concentric and eccentric contractions. *Journal of Applied Physiology*. 33:792–795 (1972).

Byrne, C., C. Twist, & R. Eston: Neuromuscular function after exercise-induced muscle damage. *Sports Medicine*. 34(1): 49–69 (2004).

Byrne, C. & R. Eston: Maximal intensity isometric and dynamic exercise performance following eccentric muscle actions. *Journal of Sports Sciences*. 20(12):951–959 (2002).

Cairns, S. P.: Lactic acid and exercise performance: Culprit or friend? *Sports Medicine*. 36(4):279-291 (2006).

Cheung, K., P. A. Hume, & L. Maxwell: Delayed onset muscle soreness: Treatment strategies and performance factors. *Sports Medicine*. 33(2):145–164 (2003).

Conley, M.: Bioenergetics of exercise training. In Baechle T. R, & R. W. Earle (eds.): *Essentials of Strength Training and Conditioning*. Champaign, IL: Human Kinetics, 73–90 (2000).

Coyle, E. F., D. L. Costill, & G. R. Lesmes: Leg extension power and muscle fiber composition. *Medicine and Science in Sports.* 11(1):12–15 (1976).

Davies, C. T. M, & C. Barnes: Negative (eccentric) work. II. Physiological responses to walking uphill and downhill on motor-driven treadmill. *Ergonomics.* 15:121–131 (1972).

De Ste Croix, M. B. A., M. A. Deighan, & N. Armstrong: Assessment and interpretation of isokinetic muscle strength during growth and maturation. *Sports Medicine.* 33(10):727–743 (2003).

DeVries, H. A. & T. J. Housh: *Physiology of Exercise: For Physical Education, Athletics and Exercise Science.* Madison, WI: Brown & Benchmark (1994).

Edington, D. W. & V. R. Edgerton: *The Biology of Physical Activity.* Boston, MA: Houghton Mifflin, 282 (1976).

Edman, K. A. P.: Contractile performance of skeletal muscle fibers. In Komi, P. V. (ed.): *Strength and Power in Sport.* Boston, MA: Blackwell Scientific, 96–114 (1992).

Enoka, R. M.: *Neuromechanical Basis of Kinesiology.* Champaign, IL: Human Kinetics, 31–64 (1988).

Fischer, A. & J. Merhautova: Electromyographic manifestations of individual stages of adapted sports technique. In *Health and Fitness in the Modern World.* Chicago, IL: Athletic Institute, 134–147 (1961).

Fitts, R. H.: The cross-bridge cycle and skeletal muscle fatigue. *Journal of Applied Physiology.* 104:551–558 (2008).

Fitts, R. H.: The muscular system: Fatigue process. In *ACSM's Advanced Exercise Physiology.* Philadelphia, PA: Lippincott, Williams & Wilkins, 178–196 (2006).

Ganio, M. S., J. F. Klau, D. J. Casa, L. E. Armstrong, & C. M. Maresh: Effect of caffeine on sport-specific endurance performance: A systemic review. *Journal of Strength and Conditioning Research.* 23(1):315–324 (2009).

Goldspink, G.: Cellular and molecular aspects of adaptation in skeletal muscles. In Komi, P. V. (ed.): *Strength and Power in Sport.* Boston, MA: Blackwell Scientific, 211–229 (1992).

Goldstein, E. R., T. Ziegenfuss, D. Kalman, R. Kreider, B. Campbell, C. Wilborn, L. Taylor, D. Willoughby, J. Stout, B. S. Graves, R. Wildman, J. Ivy, M. Spano, A. Smith, & J. Antonio: International society of sports nutrition position stand: Caffeine and performance. *Journal of International Society of Sports Nutrition.* 7:5 (2010).

Hall, S. J., J. Lee, & T. M. Wood: Evaluation of selected sit-up variations for the individual with low back pain. *Journal of Applied Sport Science Research.* 4(2):42–46 (1990).

Halpern, A. A. & E. E. Bleck: Sit-up exercises: An electromyographic study. *Clinical Orthopaedics and Related Research.* 145:172–178 (1979).

Heyward, V. H.: *Advanced Fitness Assessment and Exercise Prescription.* Champaign, IL: Human Kinetics (1991).

Komi, P. V.: Physiological and biomechanical correlates of muscle function: Effects of muscle structure and stretch-shortening cycle of force and speed. In Terjung, R. (ed.): *Exercise and Sport Sciences Reviews* (Vol. 12). Lexington, MA: Collamore Press, 81–122 (1984).

Komi, P. V.: Stretch-shortening cycle. In Komi, P. (ed.): *Strength and Power in Sport.* London: Blackwell Scientific, 169–180 (1992).

Kulig, K., J. G. Andrews, & J. G. Hay: Human strength curves. In Terjung, R. (ed.): *Exercise and Sport Sciences Reviews* (Vol. 12). Lexington, MA: Collamore Press, 417–466 (1984).

Lamb, G. D., D. G. Stephenson, J. Bangsbo, & C. Juel: Point: Counterpoint: Lactic acid accumulation is an advantage/ disadvantage of muscle activity. *Journal of Applied Physiology.* 100(4):1410–1412 (2006).

Lexell, J., C. C. Taylor, & M. Sjöström: What is the cause of the ageing atrophy? Total number, size and proportion of different fiber types studied in whole vastus lateralis muscle from 15- to 83-year-old men. *Journal of Neurological Sciences.* 84(2–3):275–294 (1988).

Lauback, L. L.: Comparative muscle strength of men and women: A review of the literature. *Aviation, Space and Environmental Medicine.* 47:534–542 (1976).

Lippold, D. C. J.: The relation between integrated action potentials in a human muscle and its isometric tension. *Journal of Physiology.* 117:492–499 (1952).

MacLaren, D. P., H. Gibson, M. Parry-Billings, & R. H. T. Edwards: A review of metabolic and physiological factors in fatigue. *Exercise and Sport Sciences Reviews.* 17:29–66 (1989).

Malina, R. M.: *Growth and maturation*: Normal variation and effects of training. In Gisolfi, C. V. & D. R. Lamb (eds.): *Perspectives in Exercise Science and Sports Medicine: Youth, Exercise, and Sport* (Vol. 2). Indianapolis, IN: Benchmark Press, 223–265 (1989).

Malina, R. M., & A. F. Roche: *Manual of Physical Status and Performance in Childhood: Physical performance* (Vol. 2). New York: Plenum (1983).

Malina, R. M. & C. Bouchard: *Growth, Maturation, and Physical Activity.* Champaign, IL: Human Kinetics (1991).

Malina, R. M., C. Bouchard, & G. Beunen: Human growth: Selected aspects of current research on well-nourished children. *Annual Review of Anthropology.* 17:187–219 (1988).

McGlynn, G. H., N. T. Laughlin, & V. Rowe: Effect of electromyographic feedback and static stretching on artificially induced muscle soreness. *American Journal of Physical Medicine.* 58:139–148 (1979).

McHugh, M. P., D. A. J. Connonlly, R. G. Eston, & G. W. Gleim: Exercise-induced muscle damage and potential mechanisms for the repeated bout effect. *Sports Medicine* 27(3):157–170 (1999).

McHugh, M. P.: Recent advances in the understanding of the repeated bout effect: The protective effect against muscle damage from a single bout of eccentric exercise. *Scandinavian Journal of Medicine and Science in Sports.* 13:88–97 (2003).

Meeusen, R., P. Watson, H. Hasegawa, B. Roelands, & M. F. Piacentini: Central fatigue: The serotonin hypothesis and beyond. *Sports Medicine.* 36(10):881–909 (2006).

Murase, S., E. Terazawa, F. Queme, H. Ota, T. Matsuda, K. Hirate, Y. Kozaki, K. Katanosaka, T. Taguchi, H. Urai, & K Mizumura: Bradykinin and nerve growth factor play pivotal roles in muscular mechanical hyperalgesia after exercise (delayed-onset muscle soreness). *The Journal of Neuroscience.* 30(10):3752–3761 (2010).

National Heart, Lung and Blood Institute (NHLBI) Workshop Summary. *American Review of Respiratory Diseases* 142:474–480 (1990).

Newsholme, E. A., I. Acworth, & E. Blomstrand. Amino-acids, brain neurotransmitters and a functional link between muscle and brain that is important in sustained exercise. In Benzi, G. (Ed.): *Advances in Biochemistry.* London: John Libbey Eurotext Ltd., 127–133 (1987).

Nicol, C., J. Avela, & A. V. Komi: The strength-shortening cycle: A model to study naturally occurring neuromuscular fatigue. *Sports Medicine.* 36(11):977–99 (2006).

Nosaka, K., M. Newton, & P. Sacco: Muscle damage and soreness after endurance exercise of the elbow flexors. *Medicine & Science in Sports & Exercise.* 34(6):920–927 (2002).

Nocella, M., B. Colombini, G. Benelli, G. Cecchi, M. A. Bagni, & J. Bruton: Force decline during fatigue is due to both a decrease in the force per individual cross-bridge and the number of cross-bridges. *Journal of Physiology.* 589(13):3371–381 (2011).

Nosaka, K. & P. M. Clarkson: Muscle damage following repeated bouts of high force eccentric exercise. *Medicine and Science in Sports and Exercise.* 27:1263–1269 (1995).

Nybo, L.: CNS fatigue and prolonged exercise: Effect of glucose supplementation. *Medicine & Science in Sports & Exercise.* 35(4):589–594 (2003).

Nybo, L. & B. Nielsen. Hyperthermia and central fatigue during prolonged exercise in humans. *Journal of Applied Physiology.* 91:1055–1060 (2001).

Peake, J., K. Nosaka, & K. Suzuki: Characterization of inflammatory responses to eccentric exercise in humans. *Exercise Immunology Review.* 11:64–85 (2005).

Rodahl, K., P.-O. Åstrand, N. C. Birkhead, T. Hettinger, B. Issekutz, D. M. Jones, & R. Weaver: Physical work capacity: A study of some children and young adults in the United States. *Archives of Environmental Health.* 2:499–510 (1961).

Rogers, M. A. & W. J. Evans: Changes in skeletal muscle with aging: Effects of exercise training. In Holloszy, J. O. (ed.): *Exercise and Sport Sciences Reviews* (Vol. 21). Baltimore, MD: Williams & Wilkins, 65–102 (1993).

Rowland, T. W.: *Children's Exercise Physiology.* (2nd edition). Champaign, IL: Human Kinetics (2005).

Sale, D. S.: Neural adaptations to strength training. In Komi, P. V. (ed.): *Strength and Power in Sport.* Boston, MA: Blackwell Scientific, 249–265 (1992).

Sayers, S. P. & P. M. Clarkson: Force recovery after eccentric exercise in males and females. *European Journal of Applied Physiology.* 84(1–2):122–126 (2001).

Shimomura, Y., A. Inaguma, S. Watanabe, Y. Yamamoto, Y. Muramatsu, G. Bajotto, J. Sato, N. Shimomura, H. Kobayashi, & K. Mawatari: Branched-chain amino acid supplementation before squat exercise and delayed-onset muscle soreness. *International Journal of Sport Nutrition and Exercise Metabolism.* 20:236–244 (2010).

Smith, L. L.: Acute inflammation: the underlying mechanism in delayed onset muscle soreness? *Medicine and Science in Sports and Exercise.* 23(5):542–551 (1991).

Smith, L. L.: Cytokine hypothesis of overtraining. *Medicine & Science in Sport & Exercise.* 32(2):317–331 (2000).

Stauber, W. T.: Eccentric action of muscles: Physiology, injury, and adaptation. *Exercise and Sport Sciences Reviews.* 17:157–186 (1989).

Stone, M. H., D. Collins, S. Plisk, G. Haff, & M. E. Stone: Training principles: Evaluation of modes and methods of resistance training. *National Strength and Conditioning Journal.* 22(3):65–76 (2000).

Tarnopolsky, M. A.: Effect of caffeine on the neuromuscular system-potential as an ergogenic aid. *Applied Physiology Nutrition and Metabolism.* 33:1284–1289 (2008).

Umbel, J. D., R. L. Hoffman, D. J. Dearth, G. S. Chleboun, T. M. Manini, & B. C. Clark: Delayed-onset muscle soreness induced by low-load blood flow-restricted exercise. *European Journal of Applied Physiology.* 107(6):687–695 (2009).

Vaile, J., S. Halson, N. Gill, & B. Dawson: Effect of hydrotherapy on the signs and symptoms of delayed onset muscle soreness. *European Journal of Physiology.* 102:447–455 (2008).

Van Praagh, E. & E. Doré: Short-term muscle power during growth and maturation. *Sports Medicine.* 32(11):701–728 (2002).

Warren, G. L., D. A. Lowe, & R. B. Armstrong: Measurement tools used in the study of eccentric contraction-induced injury. *Sports Medicine.* 27(1):43–59 (1999).

Wells, C. L. & S. A. Plowman: Sexual differences in athletic performance: Biological or behavioral? *The Physician and Sports Medicine.* 11(8):52–63 (1983).

Wilmore, J. H.: Alterations in strength, body composition, and anthropometric measurements consequent to a 10-week weight training program. *Medicine and Science in Sports.* 6:133–138 (1974).

Muscular Training Principles and Adaptations

19

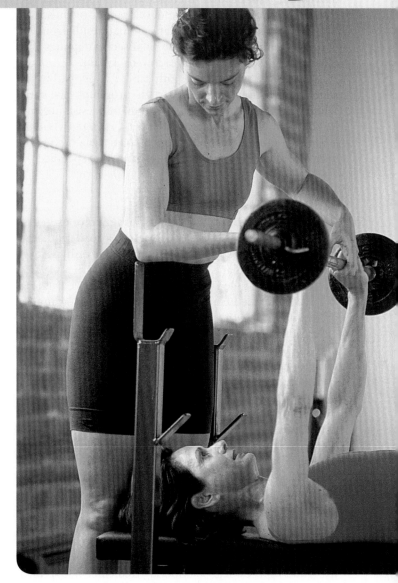

OBJECTIVES

After studying the chapter, you should be able to:

> Apply each of the training principles to the development of a resistance training program.

> Describe muscular adaptations to resistance training.

> Identify similarities and differences in training adaptations between males and females, children and adults, and young and older fitness participants.

> Discuss the relationship between muscle function and low-back pain.

Introduction

The previous chapters have discussed how isolated muscle fibers and intact muscles contract to produce coordinated movement. This chapter discusses specific applications of the training principles for the development of muscular fitness and the training adaptations that result from an exercise training program. The final section applies this information to the problems of low-back pain.

Although a training program can be developed using static contractions, in reality such programs are rare. Therefore, this chapter focuses on dynamic resistance and isokinetic training programs. The term *resistance training program* is used inclusively to encompass dynamic resistance and isokinetic training unless otherwise specified.

Overview of Resistance Training

Resistance training is a systematic program of exercises involving the exertion of force against a load, with the goal of developing strength, endurance, and/or hypertrophy of the muscular system (Davies and Barnes, 1972). It is commonly called *weight training*. Resistance training is a recommended component of a well-rounded fitness program for healthy children, adolescents, adults, and older adults. A resistance training program should be individualized, be progressive, and involve all the major muscle groups (American College of Sports Medicine, 2009; Haskell et al., 2007; Nelson et al., 2007).

The scientific and medical community accepts that muscular strength is a necessary trait for health, functional ability, athletic performance, and an enhanced quality of life. Resistance training is acknowledged as an effective way to develop musculoskeletal health and is now routinely recommended by health and fitness professionals. Especially when incorporated as part of a comprehensive fitness program, resistance training helps reduce the risk factors associated with coronary artery disease, type 2 diabetes, and colon cancer; maintains muscle mass in weight loss; and improves dynamic stability and preserves functional capacity (American College of Sports Medicine, 2009; Bird et al., 2005). The American College of Sports Medicine (ASCM) position stand titled "Progression Models in Resistance Training for Healthy Adults" provides guidelines for progression models of resistance training that can be applied to novice, intermediate, and advanced training levels (American College of Sports Medicine, 2009).

When done under skilled supervision with proper instruction in form, breathing, body mechanics, and prescription of loads, resistance training can be enjoyed by all individuals. It carries a relatively low risk of harm for prepubescent children (Behm et al., 2008; Faigenbaum and Myer, 2010a; Faigenbaum et al., 2009). Resistance training is also appropriate and effective in older adults as long as training principles are properly applied (Nelson et al., 2007; Steib et al., 2010).

Application of the Training Principles

The training principles for a safe and effective resistance training program are the same as for other types of exercise programs.

Specificity

As in any training program, a plan for muscular fitness must be specific to the individual's goals. Individuals may pursue resistance training as part of a comprehensive fitness program, to improve overall health, to enhance functional capacity, to change personal appearance, or to improve athletic performance. For muscular fitness, the goals of a resistance training program may include the development of muscular strength, hypertrophy, power, muscular endurance, or any combination of the above. Of course, these goals overlap. A person who gains muscle mass (hypertrophy), for example, is certainly stronger. However, the resistance training program should emphasize the goal that is most important to the individual. Many individuals focus on different components of muscular fitness at different times as part of a well-designed periodization plan.

Muscles respond specifically to different types of contraction and loads imposed. Athletes in many sports, including basketball, football, hockey, volleyball, etc., use dynamic resistance programs to increase muscle strength, mass, and power. Athletes in other sports, including swimming, are more likely to use isokinetic training programs to develop strength through a specified range of motion.

The specificity training principle applies to the muscle groups being trained, the type of contraction performed, the selection of single- or multiple-joint exercises, and the velocity of contraction. Because resistance training is specific to the muscle groups being trained, a resistance training program should include at least one exercise for all the major muscle groups of the body. It is recommended that all resistance training programs include a concentric and eccentric component. Although most resistance training programs should include single-joint and multiple-joint exercises, programs designed to develop muscular power should emphasize multiple-joint exercises (American College of Sports Medicine, 2009).

Specificity also applies to the velocity of contraction in isokinetic exercises (American College of Sports Medicine, 2009; Kawamori and Haff, 2004; Perrin, 1993). Exercise performed at slow velocities generally increases torque specific to the training velocity. Training at high velocities generally increases strength at and below the exercise velocity and is thus not as specific as slow-velocity training. Furthermore, it is a misconception that the velocity of isokinetic exercise should be specific to athletic events (Perrin, 1993). In reality, the angular velocities of joint movements in many athletic events (such as throwing) far exceed what can be performed during isokinetic exercise.

TABLE 19.1 Application of Overload Principle to Resistance Training Program

Goal/Level	Order	Loading	Volume	Rest Intervals
Strength				
Novice		60–70% of 1-RM	1–3 sets, 8–12 reps	2–3 min for core, 1–2 min for others
Intermediate	Large → small	70–80% of 1-RM	Multiple sets, 6–12 reps	2–3 min for core, 1–2 min for others
	Multiple joint → single joint			
	High intensity → low intensity			
Advanced		70–100% of 1-RM periodized	Multiple sets, 1–12 reps—periodized	2–3 min for core, 1–2 min for others
Hypertrophy				
Novice		60–70% of 1-RM	1–3 sets, 8–12 reps	1–2 min
Intermediate	Large → small	70–80% of 1-RM	Multiple sets, 6–12 reps	1–2 min
	Multiple joint → single joint			
	High intensity → low intensity			
Advanced		70–80% of 1-RM with emphasis on 70–85%—periodized	Multiple sets, 1–12 reps with emphasis on 6–12 reps—periodized	2–3 min—very heavy, 1–2 min—light to medium heavy
Power				
Novice		Heavy loads (>80% of 1-RM)—strength	Train for strength	2–3 min for core, 1–2 min for others
Intermediate	Large → small	Light (30–60% of 1-RM) velocity—periodized	1–3 sets, 3–6 reps	2–3 min for core, 1–2 min for others
Advanced	High intensity → low intensity		3–6 sets, 1–6 reps—periodized	2–3 min for core, 1–2 min for others
Endurance				
Novice		50–70% of 1-RM	1–3 sets, 10–15 reps	1–2 min for high-rep sets
Intermediate	Variety recommended	50–70% of 1-RM	Multiple sets, 10–15 reps or more	1–2 min for high-rep sets
Advanced		30–80% of 1-RM—periodized	Multiple sets, 10–25 reps or more—periodized	>1 min for 10–15 reps

Source: American College of Sports Medicine: Position stand on progression models in resistance training for healthy adults. *Medicine & Science in Sports & Exercise.* 41(3): 687–708 (2009).

Overload

Successfully applying the overload principle in resistance training requires the manipulation of intensity (load), volume, frequency, and rest intervals. The *intensity* of the workout can be expressed as a relative load (a percentage of an individual's 1-RM) or an absolute load (a specific amount of weight). *Volume* is a measure of total amount of work done in an exercise session and can be expressed several ways, for example, total number of repetitions, number of repetitions × number of sets, or number of repetitions × number of sets × intensity (Wernbom et al., 2007). **Table 19.1** provides recommendations for the manipulation of these variables depending on the individual's goal and fitness level. The amount of stress, or load, applied to the muscle largely determines the response of the muscle. A muscle exposed to near-maximal load will develop greater strength than a muscle experiencing many repetitions of a lighter load. In contrast, a muscle that performs many repetitions of a lighter load will develop relatively more muscular endurance than one exposed to a small number of near-maximal repetitions. There is an

Resistance Training A systematic program of exercises involving the exertion of force against a load, used to develop strength, endurance, and/or hypertrophy of the muscular system.

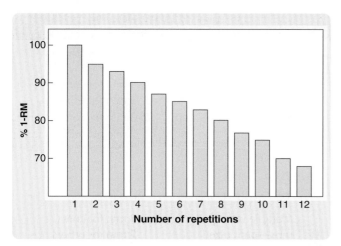

FIGURE 19.1 Estimated Repetitions that Can Be Performed at a Particular % of 1-RM.

inverse relationship between the load (weight) that can be lifted and the number of repetitions that can be performed. By definition, the most weight that can be lifted one time is the **one-repetition maximum (1 rep max; 1-RM)**. **Figure 19.1** provides guidelines for estimating the number of repetitions that are possible at various loads, expressed as a percentage of 1-RM (Baechle et al., 2000). When using **Figure 19.1**, keep in mind that the number of repetitions that can be performed at any given load is only an estimate. The actual number of repetitions that can be performed at any given load varies among individuals (resistance-trained athletes often can exceed the predicted repetitions) and among muscle groups.

CHECK YOUR COMPREHENSION 1

A college basketball player is in the specific preparation phase of her periodization plan, preparing for her fourth season as a forward. What volume should she emphasize to increase her strength? What rest interval is appropriate?

Check your answer in Appendix C.

Historically, programs based on the overload principle began in 1948 when DeLorme and Watkins introduced *progressive resistance exercise*. The DeLorme and Watkins program uses 30 repetitions per training session for each muscle group exercised. The 30 repetitions are broken down into 3 sets of 10 repetitions (reps) each, as follows:

Progressive resistance

set 1 = 10 repetitions at 50% of 10-RM
set 2 = 10 repetitions at 75% of 10-RM
set 3 = 10 repetitions at 100% of 10-RM

Since the 1950s, considerable research has been done to determine the optimal number of repetitions and sets, the workload, and the frequency for developing muscular strength, endurance, and power. This research has led to the development of many training systems. No single combination of repetitions and sets produces the best results, however; the ideal number of sets depends on the individual's goals and differences. To elicit improvements in both muscular strength and endurance, the ACSM recommends that a minimum of one set of 8–12 repetitions be performed with each of the major muscle groups 2–3 d·wk^{-1} (American College of Sports Medicine, 2009). It may be more appropriate for older or more frail individuals to perform 10–15 repetitions per muscle group (Nelson et al., 2007). Although greater gains in strength may result from performing more than one set of exercise, for the general public, the incremental strength gains from additional sets are offset by the longer period needed to complete the exercise and the increased risk of orthopedic injury. A meta-analysis compiled evidence that increasing training volume leads to improved muscle hypertrophy. This dose-response curve was characterized by an increase in the rate of hypertrophy in the initial part of the curve, followed by peak rate of hypertrophy, and in turn, followed by a plateau (Wernbom et al., 2007). Thus, athletes and individuals wishing to optimize muscular fitness (and hypertrophy in particular) may benefit from performing more than one set; this is reflected in current recommendations (see **Table 19.1**).

Core exercises develop the strength and endurance of the muscles of the trunk and pelvis, which are responsible for body stability and essential for most human movement. Core strengthening has received greater emphasis in recent years, and it is currently recommended that all resistance training programs include core strengthening exercises.

To avoid fatigue, it is recommended that exercises be arranged in a specific order, alternating lower-body with upper-body exercises. This tactic allows the muscles to recover between exercises or exercise sessions. Generally, large muscle groups should be exercised first, followed by smaller muscle groups. For example, if an exerciser wants to work the latissimus dorsi (lats) and the biceps, the lats should be worked first (pull-downs), because they involve a larger muscle group. This approach helps ensure that the fatigue of the smaller muscle group (the biceps) does not limit the work that can be performed by the larger muscle group (the lats).

CHECK YOUR COMPREHENSION 2

A 22-year-old collegiate football player is writing out his next resistance training workout. If he wants to avoid fatiguing his muscles too early and allow himself to recover as much as he can between exercises, in what order should he put the following exercises?

Bench press, calf raises, shrugs, sit-ups, shoulder press, power cleans, leg extensions, calf raises, forearm curls, back squats, and lat pull-downs.

Check your answer in Appendix C.

The length of rest periods between exercise sets is also related to the overload placed on the muscles. If the goal is maximal strength gains, relatively long (several minutes) rest periods should be used between sets. If endurance is the primary goal, shorter rest periods should be used (American College of Sports Medicine, 2009; Baechle et al., 2000).

The optimal frequency of resistance training also depends on the individual's goals and training status. Additionally, frequency varies depending on training stage (periodization). Obviously, a competitive bodybuilder trains more frequently than an adult fitness participant hoping to derive the health-related benefits of resistance training. The ACSM recommends strengthening exercises at least 2 days a week to achieve the health-related benefits of such exercises (American College of Sports Medicine, 2009; Haskell et al., 2007). Additional training leads to additional benefits. Training from 2 to 4 days a week appears to be most popular with weight lifters. Twice a week is considered the minimum necessary to improve muscular strength; training less than twice a week may predispose the individual to muscle soreness and injury. Athletes who train 4 days a week often follow a program that alternates an upper-body workout day with a lower-body workout day, so that 2 days a week are devoted to each anatomical area.

Competitive resistance-trained athletes often follow a training program in which they train 3 or 4 days consecutively and then take a day off. With such a program, they follow a split routine: each muscle group is exercised only twice a week. A split routine emphasizes a single muscle group in a workout. This muscle group is then rested for 48–72 hours. A variation of this program is the double-split routine in which two exercise sessions are performed on each workout day.

The frequency of training also depends on the individual's periodization plan. An athlete may engage in resistance training 4–6 d·wk⁻¹ in the general preparatory stage (off-season), 3 or 4 d·wk⁻¹ in the specific preparatory stage (preseason), 1 or 2 d·wk⁻¹ in the competitive season (in-season), and 1–3 d·wk⁻¹ in the transition (active rest) stage of periodization.

The duration—the amount of time spent in the weight room—depends largely on the number of repetitions, the number of sets, and the number of exercises performed. In itself, time spent on resistance training is not a critical component of the exercise prescription.

Overloading for prepubescent children should involve the same factors as outlined for adults, with some modification. A beginning program should stress learning proper form, techniques, and safety considerations, such as spotting (Behm et al., 2008; Faigenbaum and Myer, 2010b). The equipment should fit the child, which may

mean that some exercise machines (designed primarily for adult males) should not be used. Exercises should include major muscle groups and work both agonist and antagonist muscles at each joint. Children should begin with a program consisting of a single set for the first several (2–6) weeks while skill development is emphasized. Rest periods should be between 2 and 3 minutes. Low-intensity work of 8- to 15-RM is the best starting point. Initially children should perform 1–2 sets, progressing to 4 sets of 8–15 repetitions (Behm et al., 2008). A frequency of 2 or 3 d·wk⁻¹ is recommended. Historically there has been concern about having children perform maximal lifts. However, studies (see Focus on Application: Clinically Relevant box) have shown that children can safely perform a 1-RM test to guide a lifting program.

Older adults also benefit from resistance exercise in many ways (including improved overall health, strength, and functional ability). Many professional organizations, including the American College of Sports Medicine and the American Heart Association, recommend resistance training for older individuals. Current recommendations for older individuals include 1 set of 10–15 repetitions of exercises involving all the major muscle groups at least 2 days a week (Nelson et al., 2007). However, research evidence suggests that older individuals seeking more strength gain have superior adaptations to 3-set resistance training than with 1-set training in leg exercises (Paulsen et al., 2003; Steib et al., 2010).

CHECK YOUR COMPREHENSION 3

A 48-year-old woman has recently read an article in a health magazine that extols the benefits of resistance training. Hoping to improve her strength, she joins the local YMCA and now is seeking advice on how to design and implement her program. Based on the overload principle and her individual goals, what would you recommend?

Check your answer in Appendix C.

Rest/Recovery/Adaptation

Muscles adapt to the stress placed on them. The most obvious changes that result from a resistance training program are increased muscle strength and size. However, the extent to which muscles adapt to training by becoming stronger and bigger depends on the training program that is followed. For example, at some point during a resistance training program, individuals will realize that their initial 10-repetition maximum can now be lifted more than 10 times. This indicates that adaptation has occurred. The rate of adaptation depends on several factors, including rest periods and adequate diet, and the rate may not be the same for all muscle groups trained. The importance of rest (recovery) between exercise sessions to allow for the positive adaptations of exercise training

One-Repetition Maximum (1 rep max; 1-RM) The most weight that can be lifted one time.

FOCUS ON APPLICATION: *Clinically Relevant*

Is It Safe to Determine 1-RM in Children?

Establishing a 1-RM load is necessary to develop a resistance training program based on a percentage of maximal capacity. The safety of maximal testing has been explored for many populations, including older adults, and patients with cardiac and pulmonary disease. However, many clinicians and researchers have been cautious about maximal testing in children for fear of injury.

Faigenbaum and colleagues addressed the safety and efficacy of 1-RM testing in healthy children. The participants were healthy boys ($n = 64$) and girls ($n = 32$) between the ages of 6.2 and 12.3 years (mean age = 9.3 years). The children had no previous history of resistance training. The children participated in an introductory training session and were taught proper lifting technique for each exercise. Each participant's 1-RM was then determined for an upper-body exercise (either standing chest press or seated chest press) and a lower-body exercise (either leg extension or leg press). All testing was performed on a weight machine. Before attempting a 1-RM, participants performed 6 reps with a relatively light load, then 3 reps with a heavier load, and finally a series of single reps with increasing loads. If the weight was lifted with proper form, the load was increased by 0.5–2.3 kg. On average, the upper-body 1-RM was determined within 7 trials and the lower-body 1-RM was determined within 11 trials. An NCSA-certified Strength and Conditioning Specialist supervised all testing.

No injuries occurred during the study period, and the participants tolerated all testing well. No complaints of severe muscle soreness were reported. This study supports other smaller studies that found that children can perform 1-RM with no apparent adverse consequences when properly supervised. Since resistance training is becoming more popular and helps increase health and overall fitness in this population, a 1-RM strength test would be beneficial for practitioners to evaluate the effectiveness of a resistance program, assess the participant's strengths and weaknesses, base the training program on, and motivate progress. Of course, the authors rightly note that any testing with children must be properly supervised and that great care must be taken to teach proper form and ensure that it is used—both during testing and during lifting exercises.

Source: Faigenbaum et al. (2003).

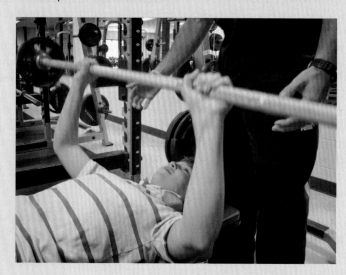

cannot be overemphasized. At least 1 day of rest should follow a day of training for a particular muscle group. Adequate rest periods and alternating heavy and light days are important to allow training adaptations to occur and to prevent injury and soreness. As mentioned earlier, many competitive athletes who lift high volumes allow 72-hour rest periods before training the same muscle group again.

McLester et al. (2003) have investigated the time course of muscle endurance recovery in a group of young (18–30 years) and older (50–65 years) men using the number of repetitions that can be performed after a given time as a measure of recovery. The authors report that after 24 hours of recovery neither of the groups could perform as many repetitions as they did on the initial day of testing. By 48 hours, both groups could perform the same number of repetitions, and by 72 hours the younger subjects could perform more repetitions. This study reported large individual variability and suggests that individual recovery testing is practical.

Adaptation occurs in children as it does in adults. Careful monitoring of recovery between sessions is probably even more important for children to ensure they rest adequately (at least 48 hours).

Progression

Once the body has adapted to the current training level, exercise stress should be increased following the overload principle if further adaptations are desired. This principle is the basis of progressive resistance exercise.

Progression should be done gradually. Progression can be accomplished by increasing the load, the repetitions, the number of sets, or the frequency of the workout, or by decreasing the rest period between sets. Load and the number of repetitions are the variables most

Does Supervision of a Strength Training Program Make a Difference?

Many individuals seek the assistance of an exercise professional when implementing their training programs. A personal trainer may provide important information and advice and serve as a motivator. But does the supervision of a training program lead to improved performance? Mazzetti et al. (2000) investigated the influence of direct supervision of resistance training on strength performance. Their results suggest that supervision does make a difference. These researchers randomly assigned volunteers with 1–2 years of lifting experience to a supervised group or an unsupervised group for a 12-week training period. The supervised group was trained one-on-one by a personal trainer. The unsupervised group attended one private fitness consultation at the beginning of the training and performed subsequent training without direct supervision, although the personal trainer was present at all training sessions to answer questions concerning the program and to confirm the participants' adherence to the program. Both groups followed identical periodized resistance training programs consisting of pre-paratory (10- to 12-RM), hypertrophy (8- to 10-RM), strength (5- to 8-RM), and peaking (3- to 6-RM) phases using free weights and variable resistance equipment. At the end of 12 weeks, there was no difference between the number of training sessions, sets, or repetitions performed per week for the squat and bench exercises. However, the supervised group had lifted more weight per set than the unsupervised group. Both training groups experienced increases in strength, but the supervised group had greater increases than the unsupervised group. These results clearly show that personal training (one-on-one supervision) can affect the strength gains achieved by participants, even if they have been lifting on their own for 1–2 years.

Source: Mazetti et al. (2000).

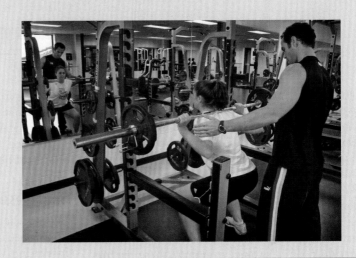

often manipulated. Again, the choice depends largely on the individual's goals. If strength is the primary goal, then a heavier weight should be used. If endurance is the goal, then the same weight should be lifted more times. Often a combination of these two variables is used. For instance, many people begin with a weight they can lift for 6 repetitions. As they adapt to this stress, they progress to 7 repetitions, then 8 repetitions, and so on. Once they can perform 8–10 repetitions, they increase the weight to something they can again only lift for 6 repetitions. As recommended earlier, a novice lifter should begin by doing more repetitions with a lighter load. Once the body has adapted, the individual can lift heavier weights. Although it has been recommended that acute increases in training volume should be small (2.5–5%), advanced athletes often exceed this recommendation (American College of Sports Medicine, 2009; Kraemer and Ratamess, 2004).

As in adults, progression in prepubescent children should be done slowly, especially in terms of intensity. Moderate loads of 8- to 15-RM are recommended for the first 2–6 months; after that, heavier loads of 6- to 10-RM can be introduced.

Individualization

The first step in individualizing a resistance training program is to determine the participant's personal goals, followed by evaluating the individual's current strength level. This assessment is usually done by determining the individual's one-repetition maximum (1-RM). A 1-RM should be established for each muscle group exercised; it is then used to determine the work intensity. For example, a program may call for an individual to do 6 repetitions per set at 80% of the 1-RM.

The final step is determining the training cycle to be used. This technique is often referred to as periodization (see Chapter 1), and it is a common step among athletes who use resistance training as an integral part of their training programs for athletic competition. For instance, a player who is conditioning for basketball would follow a different weight training program during the transition phase, general preparatory phase, and specific preparatory phase than during the competitive season. Periodization is also important to individuals who use weight training to maintain health-related muscular fitness; it prevents

TABLE 19.2 Developing a Resistance Training Program

Step	Special Considerations	Applicable Training Principles
1. Goal identification	Desired outcome Component of muscular fitness to be stressed Mode of contraction most appropriate Muscle groups to be stressed	Specificity Individualization
2. Evaluation of initial strength or muscular endurance levels	Each muscle group to be used Proper lifting techniques	Specificity
3. Determination of the training cycle (periodization)	Prevention of boredom Peaking	Adaptation Progression Retrogression/Plateau Individualization
4. Determination of the training system (design of a single session)	Exercises to be included Load Number of sets Rest periods Order in which exercises are to be done Warm-up and cooldown	Specificity Overload Individualization Warm-up and cooldown

boredom by regularly changing the training program. Competitive resistance-trained athletes also use periodization techniques to vary their training and to prepare for a peak season. **Table 19.2** provides an outline for developing a training program based on the individualization of the training principles.

Even if different individuals follow the same program, training adaptations should be expected at different rates. The principle of individualization states that responses to exercise vary among individuals because of factors unique to the individual. In resistance training, these factors include age, body size and type, initial strength, and, perhaps most importantly, genetic makeup (including fiber type distribution).

A coach or exercise leader must be sensitive to differences in the rate of individual adaptation because it directly affects the progression of training. Unfortunately, it is a common mistake for a coach to design a program for the entire team and expect everyone's adaptations to occur at the same rate. The result is often frustration for both the coach and athletes and sometimes even overtraining and/or injuries.

Individually prescribing a resistance training program is probably even more important for prepubescent children than for adults. Children are growing both physiologically and psychologically, and their rate of growth varies greatly. Periodization should be used with children as well as adults. Competition between children should be discouraged.

Maintenance

Once the desired level of muscular strength and endurance is achieved, it can be maintained by reduced amounts of work as long as the intensity (workload) is maintained;

that is, as long as the same weight is lifted, the individual can maintain strength with only one session per week. A reasonable program to maintain muscular strength and endurance would allow individuals to train at a similar workload but with fewer days per week.

Retrogression/Plateau/Reversibility

Despite the best plans of coaches, training improvements do not occur in a linear fashion. Even with progressively increasing workloads, at times performance will stay at the same level (plateau) or show a decrease (retrogression). The causes may be overtraining or individual differences. If overtraining is suspected, it is wise to include more rest days or include light days in the training regimen. It may also be beneficial to alter the training program using the periodization technique discussed earlier.

Warm-Up and Cooldown

A proper warm-up raises body temperature and is often recommended to prevent injury and muscle soreness. Although a warm-up has not been conclusively proven to decrease the incidence of injury, some evidence is consistent with this theory. A higher temperature decreases the viscosity of the joint capsule and increases the speed of muscle contraction and relaxation and enzymatic reactions (Enoka, 1988).

General and specific warm-ups for resistance training are recommended for weight lifting and isokinetic exercises (American College of Sports Medicine, 2009; Perrin, 1993). A general warm-up involves the major muscles of the body; it is similar to the warm-up used for aerobic exercise and includes activities such as jumping rope or jogging. Specific warm-up activities for weight training involve performing the same lifts that are part of the normal program but at a weight well below the training level. The duration and the intensity of the warm-up should be suited to the individual and the task to be performed. A proper warm-up should cause a rise in core body temperature of 0.5–1.0°C but should not be so strenuous that it causes fatigue. Generally, a warm-up is considered adequate when the individual begins to sweat.

A cooldown period, followed by stretching, is recommended after a training session. Cooling down may prevent muscle soreness and lead to an increase in flexibility, an aspect of muscular fitness often overlooked in resistance training programs. Importantly, cooling down helps prevent venous pooling of blood in the lower extremities.

A warm-up and cooldown are just as important for children as for adults. The same pattern of activities should be followed to increase body temperature and to stretch the muscles.

The Application of Training Principles to Bodybuilding

The sport of competitive bodybuilding has gained great popularity in the past several decades. Furthermore, many individuals engage in resistance training programs to enhance their physique. For these athletes, weight lifting is not only about gaining strength, but also about "sculpting" the body. The goals of bodybuilding are to develop superior muscularity and mass, to develop symmetry and harmony between different body parts, and to enhance muscle density and visual separation of muscles. The effect of such programs is shown in **Figure 19.2**. To achieve their goals, bodybuilders follow specific training strategies and a strict diet.

The training strategies for bodybuilding are designed to increase muscle hypertrophy. As discussed earlier, this means that bodybuilders use a very high volume (load times repetitions) of training. The frequency of training varies, but split routines or double-splits are most common among competitive bodybuilders. These programs often allow for training on 3 or 4 consecutive days, followed by a day of rest. This schedule allows for more than 48 hours of recovery for each muscle group. The overall cycle of training (periodization) is important to bodybuilders. Bodybuilders commonly do more strength training in the general preparatory phase of their periodization plan to build muscle mass. As the season approaches, the load is reduced and more repetitions are performed in an attempt to gain muscle symmetry.

Diet is perhaps as important in bodybuilding as an appropriate resistance training program. To enhance muscle definition and promote visual separation of the

Cutting Decreasing body fat and body water content to very low levels in order to increase muscle definition.

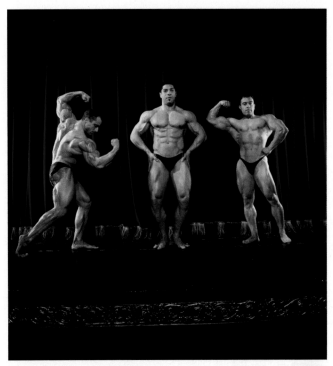

FIGURE 19.2 Bodybuilders.
A goal of bodybuilding is to "sculpt" the body.

various muscle groups, bodybuilders maintain a low percentage of body fat through a combination of training and diet. Bodybuilders follow a strict low-fat diet, despite the large number of calories. The practice of **cutting** or *ripping* refers to the bodybuilder's attempt to decrease body fat and body water to very low levels before a competition in order to increase muscle definition.

Neuromuscular Adaptations to Resistance Training

Resistance training programs are important for health, fitness, and performance and are widely recommended by leading health organizations. This section addresses neuromuscular training adaptations from resistance training, with an emphasis on changes that occur within muscle tissue. Human skeletal muscle readily adapts to changes in the loading state. The hallmark adaptations to resistance training are increases in muscle strength and size (hypertrophy). **Table 19.3** summarizes neuromuscular adaptations to resistance training.

Muscle Function

Resistance exercise leads to increased muscular strength, endurance, and power. Increased strength is the most obvious result of a resistance training program and the reason many individuals participate in resistance training.

TABLE 19.3   Neuromuscular Adaptations to Resistance Training

1. Muscle Function
   a. ↑ Strength
   b. ↑ Endurance
   c. ↑ Power
2. Muscle Size and Structure
   a. Muscle Fibers
      i. ↑ Whole muscle CSA
      ii. ↑ Muscle fiber CSA
      iii. ↑ Myofibril protein content
      iv. Conversion of FOG to FG fibers
   b. Connective Tissue
      i. ↑ Collagen synthesis
      ii. = Portion of connective tissue to skeletal muscle
      iii. ↑ Collagen stiffness
3. Neural Adaptations
   a. ↑ Motor unit recruitment
   b. ↑ Synchronization
   c. ↓ Golgi tendon organ reflex
4. Metabolic Adaptations
   a. ↑ Glycogen
   b. ↑ PC
   c. ↑ Creatine phosphokinase (CPK)
5. Hormonal Adaptations
   a. Inconsistent findings for testosterone
   b. No change in GH
   c. Inconsistent findings for cortisol
   d. ↑ Insulin-like growth factor (IGF-1)

Strength gains following a resistance training program vary widely, owing largely to differences in initial strength and the training program. Resistance training at least twice a week improves muscle strength and endurance by approximately 25–100% (Haskell et al., 2007).

The increase in muscle strength from a resistance training program depends on the particular resistance training program and the muscle group(s) trained. **Figure 19.3** shows the percent change in 1-RM during 11 weeks of training using two different training programs—one using 1 set of lower-body exercises and 3 sets of upper-body exercise (1L-3UB) and one using 3 sets of lower-body exercises and 1 set of upper-body exercise (3L-1UB). Notice that the percent changes were greater for the leg exercises (shown in panel A) when a greater number of sets using the lower body was used. However, for the upper-body exercises (panel B) there was no difference between groups, with both training groups increasing arm strength approximately 25% (Rønnestad et al., 2007).

The intensity of training also affects the magnitude of adaptation. A 12-week training program that compared low-intensity (15% of 1-RM) and high-intensity (70% 1-RM) contractions while carefully equalizing the total volume of training found that 1-RM quadriceps strength increased by 36% following high-intensity contractions and by 19% with low-intensity contractions (Holm et al., 2008).

Muscle Size and Structure

Resistance training increases muscle size and strength. The hypertrophic response to resistance training is affected by the individual factors, such as genetic background, age, and gender, and by the training protocol (Schoenfeld, 2010). Increases in muscle cross-sectional area (CSA) of 7–15% have been reported with 10–14 weeks of resistance training when intensity greater than 60% of 1-RM was used (Holm et al., 2008; Rønnestad et al., 2007). The increase in cross-sectional area of the whole muscle reflects an increase in individual muscle fiber cross-sectional area. The increased cross-sectional area of muscle results from hypertrophy of all three muscle fiber types, although the fast-glycolytic (FG) fibers exhibit the greatest increase (Bird et al., 2005). The hypertrophy that occurs is due to an increase in the total contractile protein (actin and myosin), in the size and number of the myofibrils per fiber, and in the amount of connective tissue surrounding the muscle fibers (Folland and Williams, 2007; Schoenfeld, 2010). Resistance training results in increased collagen synthesis and a strengthening of the connective tissue around the muscle. However, the ratio of connective tissue to skeletal muscle appears relatively consistent between trained and untrained individuals. There is also evidence of increased tendon stiffness with resistance training, which could enhance the rapid application of force (Folland and Williams, 2007).

Figure 19.4 presents data from a study in which muscle biopsies were taken from a group of resistance trained (RT) and untrained (UT) men. Each major subdivision of muscle fiber type clearly had a greater cross-sectional area in the RT group than the untrained group. Furthermore, each of the muscle fiber types could produce greater force in the trained group (Shoepe et al., 2003).

Resistance training causes a conversion of muscle fiber subtypes in humans. High-intensity resistance training induces a change from fast oxidative glycolytic (FOG) to fast glycolytic (FG) in the early phases of training, with transitions being complete by approximately 12 weeks of training (Kraemer et al., 1995). It appears that intensity of training is an important stimulus for this adaptation (Holm et al., 2008).

Resistance training can theoretically lead to *hyperplasia*—an increase in number of muscle fibers. Hyperplasia could occur as a result of muscle fiber splitting or branching with subsequent hypertrophy or myogenesis, or a combination of the two. However, the contribution of hyperplasia to increased muscle cross-sectional area (and strength) remains relatively unknown because of measurement difficulties. The exact role of hyperplasia in increased muscle size is highly controversial. However, given the magnitude of changes in muscle size attributable to hypertrophy, it seems that the contribution of hyperplasia to increased muscle cross-sectional area is minimal (Folland and Williams, 2007).

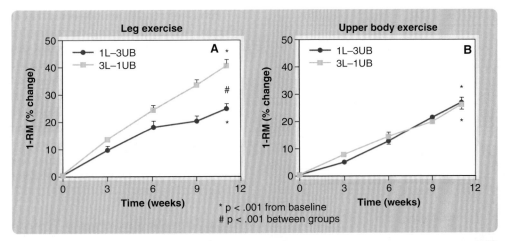

FIGURE 19.3 Relative Changes in 1-RM in Leg Exercise (A) and Upper-Body Exercise (B) During 11-Week Training Program.

Note: 1L-3UB, 1 set of leg exercises and 3 sets of upper-body exercises; 3L-1UB, 3 sets of leg exercises and 1 set of upper-body exercises. *Significant difference from baseline (p < 0.001). #Significant difference between groups (p < 0.001). Reprinted with permission of Williams & Wilkins.

Source: Ronnestad, B. R., W. Egeland, N. H. Kvamme, P. E. Refsnes, F. Kadi, & T. Raastad: Dissimilar effects of one-and three-set strength training on strength and muscle mass gains in upper and lower body in untrained subjects. *Journal of Strength and Conditioning Research*. 21(1):157–163 (2007).

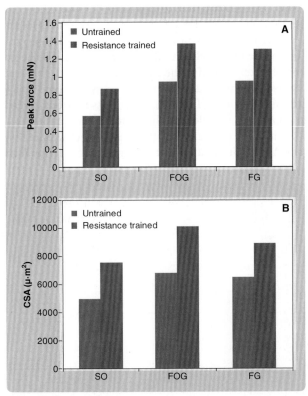

FIGURE 19.4 Peak Force (A) and Cross Sectional Area (CSA) (B) of Muscle Fibers in Untrained (UT) and Resistance-Trained (RT) Individuals.

Source: Shoepe, T. C., J. E. Stelzer, D. P. Garner, & J. J. Widrick: Functional adaptability of muscle fibers to long-term resistance exercise. *Medicine & Science in Sports & Exercise*. 35(6):944–951 (2003).

Neural Adaptations

While it is generally accepted that neural adaptations have a critical role in the increased force production resulting from resistance training, the precise changes that occur are not completely understood. This is, in large part, because of methodological difficulties associated with measuring neurological adaptations (Folland and Williams, 2007). Resistance training programs typically result in strength gains within the first few weeks despite modest changes in muscle mass, suggesting that neural factors are largely responsible for early strength gains (Gabriel et al., 2006; Sale, 1988). **Figure 19.5** illustrates the relative contributions of neural and muscular adaptations to strength gains.

Neural adaptations to resistance training include increased neural drive to the muscle, increased synchronization of the motor units, and an inhibition of the protective mechanism of the Golgi tendon organs (Fleck and Kraemer, 1987; Gabriel et al., 2006). Increased neural drive indicates that greater muscle activation can occur because more motor units can be recruited. Evidence suggests that resistance-trained individuals exhibit greater synchronization—a higher correlation between timing of action potentials of concurrently active motor units that allows for greater force production. Indirect evidence also suggests that resistance training leads to changes in intermuscular coordination of agonists, antagonists, and synergists, which dampens inhibitory reflexes and allows for greater force production. Activation of Golgi tendon organs results in inhibition of the agonist via inhibitory motor neurons,

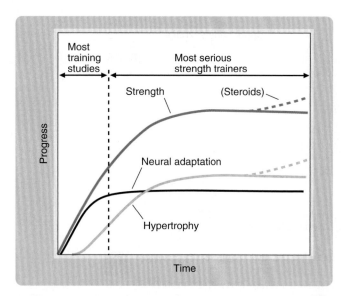

FIGURE 19.5 Contribution of Neural and Muscular 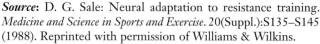 **Adaptations to Strength Gains.**
Source: D. G. Sale: Neural adaptation to resistance training. *Medicine and Science in Sports and Exercise*. 20(Suppl.):S135–S145 (1988). Reprinted with permission of Williams & Wilkins.

thus providing an important protective reflex that limits excessive force generation within muscle (see Chapter 20). Resistance training dampens the reflex action of the Golgi tendon organ, although it is not clear whether this occurs by changing the receptor or the neural pathways (Gabriel et al., 2006).

Metabolic Adaptations

In addition to greater strength and hypertrophy, metabolic adaptations occur within muscle fibers that increase the ability of the muscle to generate ATP. These changes are characterized by an increased ability to generate ATP from anaerobic metabolism; thus, there is an increase in phosphocreatine (PC) and glycogen stores and an increase in the enzyme creatine phosphokinase that breaks down PC (MacDougall et al., 1977). Refer to Chapters 2 and 3 for a review of anaerobic metabolism.

Hormonal Adaptations

An acute bout of resistance exercise results in a catabolic state in which muscle proteins are broken down. During recovery, anabolism predominates, leading to muscle repair and growth. This coupled process of catabolism and anabolism is responsible for the remodeling of muscle tissue in response to resistance training. Many anabolic and catabolic processes are controlled by the neuroendocrine system, with numerous acute hormonal responses to resistance exercise. In contrast, resistance training causes relatively few hormonal adaptations.

Published reports are not consistent about the chronic effect of resistance training on resting testosterone levels. Several studies have reported elevated resting testosterone levels, whereas many others have reported no change in resting levels of testosterone following resistance training. Similarly, findings are inconsistent regarding the effect of resistance training on resting cortisol levels. It appears that resistance training does not change resting growth hormone concentration. Evidence suggests, however, that resistance training leads to an increased resting level of insulin-like growth factor (IGF-1) (Kraemer and Ratamess, 2005).

Male-Female Resistance Training Adaptation Comparisons

Although men are typically stronger than women, both sexes respond to resistance training in a similar manner (Bird et al., 2005; Cureton et al., 1988; Tesch, 1992; Wilmore, 1974;). Typically, sedentary males and females can attain strength gains of 25–100% in a training program, although the actual increase in strength varies among muscle groups and is affected by the individual's initial strength (Haskell et al., 2007). **Figure 19.6** shows the percentage change in muscle strength for men and women for the elbow flexors, elbow extensors, knee flexors, and knee extensors after 16 weeks of participation in a weight training program (Cureton et al., 1988). In addition to having similar patterns of strength gains, the men and women in this study both had similar changes in muscle cross-sectional area (as determined from CT scans). The cross-sectional area of the upper-arm muscles for the men and women increased 15% and 23%, respectively, after the 16-week training program. Although the men had a greater cross-sectional area

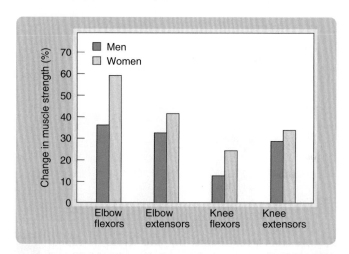

FIGURE 19.6 Improvement in Muscular Strength After **16 Weeks of Weight Training.**
Source: Cureton, K. J., M. A. Collins, D. W. Hill, & F. M. McElhannon: Muscle hypertrophy in men and women. *Medicine and Science in Sports and Exercise*. 20(4):338–344 (1988).

FOCUS ON RESEARCH

Got Milk? Protein Ingestion Enhances Protein Synthesis Following Resistance Exercise

A primary goal of many resistance training programs is to build muscle mass. As discussed in this chapter, manipulating program variables, particularly the load and volume, is an important factor influencing the extent of muscle hypertrophy. However, nutrients are also essential for the building of muscle mass, which is composed primarily of protein. For this reason, the scientific community and practitioners have long been interested in the role of various nutrients in increasing muscle mass. Much attention has recently focused on determining the ideal mix of nutrients to stimulate protein synthesis during recovery from resistance training.

In this study, the authors sought to determine the effect of drinking milk on net protein synthesis after a resistance exercise. Furthermore, the researchers investigated different types and quantities of milk (fat-free versus whole milk) to determine if these factors affected protein synthesis. Participants were young, healthy men and women who were not resistance trained in the past 5 years. Participants were placed into one of three groups: a group that ingested 237 g (8 oz) of fat-free milk (FFM), a group that ingested 237 g of whole milk (WM), and a group that ingested 393 g (13 oz) of fat-free milk with the same number of kcals as the whole milk (iso-FFM). The two quantities of fat-free milk allowed investigators to compare FFM and WM when the total calories consumed was the same (since 237 g of WM and 393 g of FFM provide the same number of kcals). Participants completed 10 sets of 8 repetitions of leg extensions at 80% of 1-RM. Each set was completed in approximately 30 seconds, with a 2-minute rest period between sets. Blood samples and blood flow were measured for 5 hours after exercise (muscle biopsies were also obtained but are not discussed here).

The study revealed that the uptake of the amino acids threonine and

phenylalanine was significantly greater than 0 following the ingestion of WM and iso-FFM (panels A and B). Furthermore, threonine uptake was significantly greater (2.8 fold higher) following WM ingestion versus FFM (panel B).

The primary finding of the study was that milk ingestion stimulated net uptake of the amino acids threonine and phenylalanine. Since threonine and phenylalanine are not oxidized in muscle, the uptake of these amino acids represented net protein

synthesis following resistance exercise. This clearly suggests that milk is an appropriate recovery drink to stimulate protein synthesis following resistance training.

Next time you're looking to replace fluids after a workout, grab a container (8 oz) of whole milk!

Source: Elliot, T. A., M. G. Cree, A. P. Sanford, R. R. Wolfe, & K. D. Tipton: Milk ingestion stimulates muscle protein synthesis following resistance exercise. *Medicine & Science in Sports & Exercise.* 38(4):667–674 (2006).

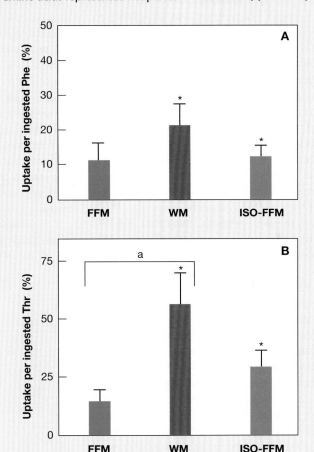

Ratio of amino acid uptake relative to amount ingested for phenylalanine **(A)** and threonine **(B)** following ingestion of milk during recovery. *p < 0.05; versus 0; a p < 0.05; versus FFM.

than the women, both before and after training, in both sexes the muscle strength and muscle cross-sectional area of the upper arm increased with training.

A review article analyzing the results of studies in which groups of men and women followed the same training program also found that men and women respond to resistance training with similar increases in muscle cross-sectional area. This review found that on average, muscle cross-sectional area increases an average 0.13% per day in males and 0.14% per day in females (Wernbom et al., 2007).

Resistance Training Adaptations in Children and Adolescents

Resistance training produces strength gains in prepubescents and adolescents and is recognized as an important component of youth fitness programs (Faigenbaum et al., 2009). Research suggests that strength gains of approximately 30% (range 13–40%) are typical following short-term resistance training programs (up to 20 weeks) in children. Increases in strength seem fairly consistent between prepubescents and adolescents. There is no apparent difference in the relative strength (percentage) increases between boys and girls (Faigenbaum et al., 2009) nor between children/adolescents and adults (Rowland, 2005).

In one study, fourteen 8- to 12-year-old boys and girls trained twice a week for 8 weeks using 3 sets of 10–15 repetitions on 5 exercises, with intensities varying between 50% and 100% of their 1-RM (Faigenbaum et al., 1993). After the training period, strength increased 74.3%, whereas strength in a control group increased only 13%. The increase in strength reported in the control group was probably related to growth and maturation of the subjects.

Although the strength improvement in this study is consistent with improvements documented in adults, the underlying physiological adaptations that account for increased strength appear somewhat different. Resistance training does not appear to induce muscle fiber hypertrophy in preadolescents, possibly because of the lack of testosterone. Changes do occur in the ability of the nervous system to activate motor units, as shown by increased EMG activity with training. Improved motor coordination is also thought to be a contributing neural factor. Thus, neurological factors rather than muscular factors are believed to be responsible for the strength changes in this age group (Faigenbaum et al., 2009; Rowland, 2005).

Resistance Training Adaptations in Older Adults

Resistance exercise is widely acknowledged as beneficial for older adults, and many agencies actively promote resistance exercise for this age group (American College of Sports Medicine, 2009; Nelson et al., 2007). Resistance training is also safe and effective for increasing muscular strength and cross-sectional area in older individuals (Aagaard et al., 2007; Charette et al., 1991; Frontera et al., 1991; Larsson, 1982; Nelson et al., 2007). In fact, older men and women have similar or even greater strength gains than young individuals from resistance training. Resistance training is a recommended component of fitness programs for older adults and is considered important for minimizing or reversing physical frailty, which is prevalent among the elderly (American College of Sports Medicine, 2009; Kraemer and Ratamess, 2004). Chronic resistance training over a long period results in greater strength, rate of force development, and muscle fiber cross-sectional area than is evidenced in untrained individuals (Aagaard et al., 2007). Short-term resistance training programs are also successful in leading to muscular adapations in the elderly. **Figure 19.7** shows the improvements in dynamic strength of the knee extensors (quadriceps) and the knee flexors (hamstrings) following 12 weeks of training in older men (Rogers and Evans, 1993). By the end of the training period, strength in both muscle groups had increased over 100%. Additionally, these men demonstrated an 11% increase in muscle cross-sectional area, accompanied by a 34% increase in ST fiber area and a 28% increase in FT fiber area. A similar response to resistance training has been shown in older women (Wilmore, 1974). For example, following a resistance training program of 12 weeks, elderly women had improved their strength 28–115%, depending on the muscle group tested (Charette et al., 1991).

Resistance training is also beneficial for frail, institutionalized men and women (Fiatarone et al., 1990). A group of 90- to 100-year-old men and women who engaged in

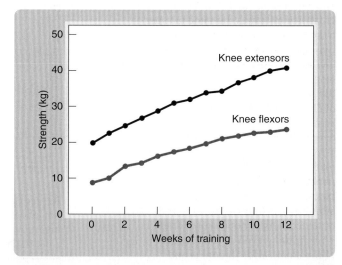

FIGURE 19.7 Effects of Dynamic Resistance Exercise on Muscular Strength in Older Men.
Source: M. A. Rogers. & W. J. Evans. Changes in skeletal muscle with aging: Effects of exercise training. In Holloszy, J. O. (ed.): *Exercise and Sport Sciences Reviews* (Vol. 21). Baltimore, MD: Williams & Wilkins, 65–102 (1993). Reprinted by permission.

a resistance training program for 8 weeks increased their strength 174% (from an average initial value of 8 to 21 kg). Their muscle cross-sectional area increased 15%. These improvements demonstrate rather remarkably the capacity of the muscular system to adapt to progressive resistance exercise as long as a person is willing to participate in a program at an appropriate intensity.

Figure 19.8 summarizes the results of several studies that investigated changes in muscle strength and cross-sectional area that occur in the quadriceps of males and females of various ages after a resistance training program. These values indicate a percentage change from the initial values; they do not imply that females are stronger than males as adults nor that the elderly are stronger than the younger subjects. In fact, those who are weakest initially may be in the best position to show a high percentage improvement.

Muscular Adaptations to Aerobic Endurance Training Programs

Muscle fibers respond differently to aerobic training than to resistance training. Aerobic training is characterized by increased aerobic power ($\dot{V}O_2$max) with little or no change in muscle strength or power. Similarly, the structural and metabolic changes in muscle fibers facilitate the production of large quantities of ATP, primarily by aerobic means, following an aerobic training program, thus enhancing muscular endurance.

Aerobic endurance training results in an increase in ST fiber size in adult males and no change in FT fiber size (Gollnick et al., 1972). There is also evidence that aerobic endurance training can result in the transformation of FG muscle fibers to FOG muscle fibers (Fleck and Kraemer, 1987). Aerobic endurance training in older men and women also results in an increase in the cross-sectional area of the ST fibers (averaging 12%) and an increase in the percentage of FOG fibers (Coggan et al., 1990).

Muscular Adaptations to Concurrent Training

Many sports require a combination of muscular strength and aerobic endurance, and thus a combination of resistance and aerobic endurance training is required to improve performance. The integration of endurance- and resistance-based training into a training program is called **concurrent training**. The most consistent finding from studies of concurrent training is that increases in strength and power are lower than with strength training alone but changes in aerobic fitness are only slightly lower

> **Concurrent Training** The integration of endurance- and resistance-based training into a training program.

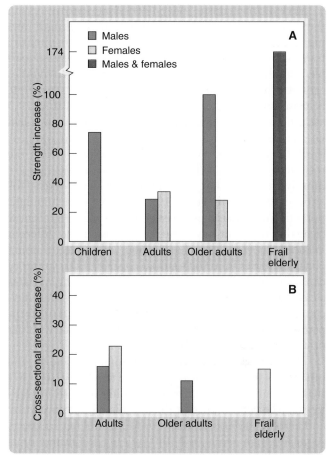

FIGURE 19.8 Strength and Cross Sectional Area Increases in Quadriceps Following Resistance Training.
A. Strength increase. **B.** Cross sectional area increase.
Sources: Charette, S. L., L. McEvoy, G. Pyka, C. Snow-Harter, D. Guido, R. A. Wiswell, & R. Marcus: Muscle hypertrophy response to resistance training in older women. *Journal of Applied Physiology.* 70:1912–1916 (1991); Cureton, K. J., M. A. Collins, D. W. Hill, & F. M. McElhannon: Muscle hypertrophy in men and women. *Medicine and Science in Sports and Exercise.* 20(4):338–344 (1988); Faigenbaum, A. D., L. D. Zaichkowsky, W. L. Westcott, L. J. Micheli, & A. F. Fehlandt: The effects of a twice-a-week strength training program on children. *Pediatric Exercise Science.* 5:339–346 (1993); Fiatarone, M. A., E. C. Marks, N. D. Ryan, C. N. Meredith, L. A. Lipsitz, & W. J. Evans: High intensity strength training in nonagenarians. Effects on skeletal muscle. *Journal of the American Medical Association.* 263:3029–3034 (1990); Frontera, W. R., V. A. Hughes, K. J. Lutz, & W. J. Evans: A cross-sectional study of muscle strength and mass in 45- to 78-yr-old men and women. *Journal of Applied Physiology.* 71:644–650 (1991).

than those found with aerobic training alone. However, research findings are not consistent. Other studies have shown that concurrent training has no inhibitory effect on the development of strength or aerobic endurance. Finally, at least one study has shown that the development of aerobic fitness but not strength is compromised by concurrent training (Leveritt et al., 1999; Nader, 2006).

Several mechanisms have been suggested to explain the more prevalent finding of inhibition of strength during concurrent training. If individuals do high-intensity training in both modalities, overtraining may be responsible. The chronic hypothesis contends that skeletal muscles cannot adapt to both types of training at the same time because many of the adaptations shown in **Table 19.3** are different. The acute hypothesis contends that residual fatigue from the aerobic endurance component compromises the ability to work as hard as necessary during the resistance training. While both of these hypotheses are intuitively reasonable, only limited evidence exists for either one (Leveritt et al., 1999). Newer data highlight potential molecular mechanisms (Hawley, 2009). It is now clear that different modalities of exercise cause different intracellular signaling mechanisms; endurance training elicits increases in mitochondrial content and respiratory capacity of muscle fibers and resistance training initiates a cascade of events leading to increased synthesis of muscle contractile protein. The stimulation of the different pathways may result in inhibition or interference with the other pathway (Hawley, 2009; Nader, 2006).

Periodization programs that emphasize one or the other type of training throughout the training year rather than concurrent high-intensity training in both modalities may be very important for optimizing both muscular and aerobic endurance adaptations for athletes in sports requiring high levels of both. Training for fitness typically involves exercise sessions on different days for the different modalities, as opposed to true concurrent training. Also peak levels of performance are not generally the goal. Therefore, inhibition of one type of training by the other is not typically a major concern.

Neuromuscular Adaptations to Detraining

Detraining can be defined as a partial or complete loss of training-induced adaptations as a result of training reduction or cessation. Detraining may occur due to lack of compliance with a training program, injury or illness, or a planned periodization cycle especially in the transition (active rest) phase.

Detraining leads to loss of neuromuscular adaptations. As with the other systems, the time course for the loss of adaptation depends on the individual's training status and the extent to which training load is decreased. Strength-trained athletes retain strength gains during short periods of inactivity (2 weeks) and retain significant portions of strength gains (88–93%) during inactivity lasting up to 12 weeks (Mujika and Padilla, 2000a). Thus, it appears that strength gains are preserved longer than many other training adaptations.

The effect of detraining on muscle strength is not consistent in all muscle groups or for all exercises. In one study, squat exercise strength decreased by only 13% following

30–32 weeks of detraining, whereas leg press strength decreased by 32% (Staron et al., 1991). There appears to be no differences in strength loss between the sexes during detraining, but there is evidence that older individuals lose strength gains more rapidly than younger people (Lemmer et al., 2000). There is some evidence in trained swimmers that muscular power (defined as a swim test) may decrease substantially during 4 weeks of inactivity even when muscular strength is maintained (Neufer et al., 1987). On the other hand, vertical jump (a field measure of muscle power) has been shown to be unchanged with 8 or 12 weeks of detraining (Häkkinen et al., 1981, 1985).

Short-term detraining (2 weeks) in resistance-trained athletes has resulted in a significant decrease in fast twitch (FT) muscle fiber cross-sectional area, whereas longer periods of detraining (12 weeks) have been associated with a significant decrease in cross-sectional area of both FT and slow twitch (ST) muscle fibers (Häkkinen et al., 1985; Hortobágyi et al., 1993). Diminished neural activation (as measured by integrated electromyography [IEMG]) has been shown to occur with detraining (Häkkinen et al., 1981, 1985; Häkkinen and Komi, 1983).

The impact of detraining in children is confounded by the concomitant effects of growth-related strength increases. The actual gains above this growth level do appear to be lost once training ceases (Blimkie, 1988).

Special Application: Muscular Strength/ Endurance and Health

Athletes have long used resistance training programs to increase muscular function and to improve performance. There is now increasing evidence for both children/adolescents and adults that enhanced neuromuscular fitness, especially muscular strength/endurance, is also associated with an improvement in overall health status and, conversely, a reduction of risk for chronic disease, disability and, in adults, mortality (Warburton et al., 2006).

Mortality rates have been found to be lower in adult males and females when individuals with moderate/high muscular fitness (primarily measured by grip strength, sit-ups, leg and bench press) were compared with individuals with low muscular fitness, even after adjusting for cardiorespiratory fitness, body composition, and other potentially confounding variables (FitzGerald et al., 2004; Katzmarzyk and Craig, 2002). In one large-scale study, researchers assessed muscular fitness in over 9100 men and women between the ages of 20 and 82 years over an 8-year period (FitzGerald et al., 2004). Muscular fitness was based on a composite score from a maximal bench press, maximal leg press, and the number of sit-ups completed in 1 minute. For each individual test, participants were divided into tertiles, and a combined score from the three tests was used as an indicator of muscular fitness—defined as low, medium, high. A mortality follow-up was conducted 7 years after the completion of the muscular fitness evaluation, revealing that 194 participants had died since their evaluation. A statistical analysis was performed comparing the relative risk of all-cause mortality across all three groups in which the relative risk was set at 1.0 for the low muscular fitness group. Participants in the moderate and high muscular fitness groups had a relative risk of 0.64 (95% CI = 0.44–0.93) and 0.80 (95% CI = 0.49–1.31) compared with the low muscular fitness group after statistically adjusting for differences in age, health status, body mass index, cigarette smoking, and cardiorespiratory fitness.

Muscular fitness has also been shown to have a positive influence on several measures of health including cardiovascular risk factors (Ortega et al., 2008; Warburton et al., 2001a) and metabolic health. Specifically, resistance training has been shown to lower LDL-C, raise HDL-C, and reduce both SBP and DBP (Phillips and Winett, 2010; Strasser et al., 2010).

Several lines of research indicate the positive effects of resistance training on metabolic health. Substantial improvements in blood glucose, glycosylated hemoglobin (an index of glucose control), insulin sensitivity, and insulin stabilization have been reported in individuals with diabetes who have weight trained (Phillips and Winett, 2010; Strasser et al., 2010). Evidence is also emerging that indicates a positive impact of neuromuscular fitness on metabolic syndrome/metabolic health risk factors in both adults (Strasser et al, 2010) and youths (Artero et al., 2011; Benson et al., 2008; Steene-Johannessen et al., 2009). This relationship appears to operate independently of, or in addition to, cardiorespiratory fitness and/or body mass/body composition. A large, multicenter European study examined the independent associations of muscular and cardiorespiratory fitness with clustered metabolic risk in over 700 adolescents (aged 12.7–17.5) (Artero et al., 2011). In this study, adolescents in the lowest muscular fitness quartile (based on handgrip score) had a significantly elevated metabolic risk compared to all other fitness quartiles. Additional analysis revealed that the participants who were in the lowest quartile for muscular fitness and the lowest quartile for cardiorespiratory fitness had a significantly higher metabolic risk score than all other groups.

High levels of muscular strength and muscular endurance and/or resistance training improvements have also been shown to positively impact or predict long-term changes in body composition (Strasser et al., 2010; Warburton et al, 2001b, 2006). In general, resistance training programs are associated with a decrease in fat mass and visceral adipose tissue (a component of the metabolic syndrome). Because resistance training decreases fat mass and increases lean mass, it results in positive health benefits even in the absence of overall changes in body weight.

In addition to the evidence of a role of resistance training in improving cardiometabolic health and body composition, there is also extensive literature indicating that muscular fitness is an important determinant of quality of life, including measures of functional status and psychological well-being.

Because of the numerous benefits of muscular fitness, many organizations are promoting resistance training as a part of every complete fitness program. In fact, as described in the preceding paragraphs, there are many well-documented health benefits of resistance training programs, some of which are summarized in **Table 19.4**.

Special Application: Muscular Strength and Endurance and Low-Back Pain

At some point in their lives, 60–80% of all people experience low-back pain (LBP). The condition is disabling in 1–5% of the population. Most cases of LBP occur between the ages of 25 and 60 years, but 12–26% of children and adolescents are LBP sufferers. Males and females are affected equally.

The exact causes and risk factors for LBP have not been identified. However, there has been great interest in the link between muscular fitness and the absence or occurrence of LBP. Some tests of health-related physical fitness have included sit-and-reach, sit-ups or curl-ups, and trunk extension tests as means of testing low-back function. The theoretical link between physical fitness and LBP is largely based on functional anatomy (**Table 19.5**), and at this time the anatomical logic is stronger than the research evidence.

To have a healthy, well-functioning back, an individual must have flexible low-back (lumbar) muscles, hamstrings, and hip flexors and strong, fatigue-resistant abdominal and back extensor muscles. The goal is to keep the vertebrae aligned properly without excessive disk pressure, allowing a full range of motion in all directions. In addition, the pelvis must freely rotate both posteriorly and anteriorly without straining the muscle or fascia.

Research evidence shows that individuals suffering from LBP have less strength in both abdominal and back extensors. EMG activity is also increased in the back muscles of individuals with LBP. These differences, however, are more likely to be the result of LBP rather than the cause. Studies that have attempted to predict who might get LBP, either for a first time or in recurrent episodes, based on strength and muscular endurance measures have identified back extension endurance as the critical variable. That is, individuals with low levels of back extension endurance are more likely to develop LBP than individuals with high levels of back extensor endurance. Although high levels of back extensor strength and abdominal flexion strength or endurance have not been shown to have this same predictive value, they have never

TABLE 19.4 Comparison of Adaptations to Aerobic and Resistance Training

Variable	Aerobic Training	Resistance Training
Functional and Structural		
Physical endurance	↑↑↑	↑↑
Strength	↔	↑↑↑
Bone mineral density	↑	↑↑↑
Metabolic		
Body composition		
Fat mass	↓↓	↓
Muscle mass	↔	↑↑
Basal metabolism	↑	↑↑
Glucose metabolism		
Insulin response to glucose challenge	↓↓	↓↓
Basal insulin levels	↓	↓
Insulin sensitivity	↑↑	↑↑
Serum lipids		
High-density lipoprotein	↑↔	↑↔
Low-density lipoprotein	↓↔	↓↔
Cardiovascular		
Resting heart rate	↓↓	↔
Blood pressure at rest		
Systolic	↓↓	↓
Diastolic	↓↓	↓

Based on Braith, R. W. & K. J. Stewart: Resistance exercise training: Its role in the prevention of cardiovascular disease. *Circulation*. 113: 2642–2650 (2006).

TABLE 19.5 Theoretical Relationship between Physical Fitness Components and Healthy or Unhealthy Low-Back or Spinal Function

Physical Fitness Component (Neuromuscular)	Normal Anatomical Function in Low-Back: Healthy	Dysfunction	Results of Dysfunction: Unhealthy
Lumbar flexibility	Allows the lumbar curve to almost be reversed in forward flexion	Inflexible	Disrupts forward and lateral movement; places excessive stretch on hamstrings, leading to low-back and hamstring pain
Hamstring flexibility	Allows anterior rotation (tilt) of the pelvis in forward flexion and posterior rotation in the sitting position	Inflexible	Restricts anterior pelvic rotation and exaggerates posterior tilt; both cause increased disk compression; excessive stretching causes strain and pain
Hip flexor flexibility	Allows achievement of neutral pelvic position	Inflexible	Exaggerates anterior pelvic tilt if not counteracted by strong abdominal muscles, thereby increasing disk compression
Abdominal strength or endurance	Maintains pelvic position; reinforces back extensor fascia and pulls it laterally on forward flexion, providing support	Weak, easily fatigued	Allows abnormal pelvic tilt; increases strain on back extensor muscles
Back extensor strength or endurance	Provides stability for the spine; maintains erect posture; controls forward flexion	Weak, easily fatigued	Increases loading on the spine; causes increased disk compression

FOCUS ON RESEARCH: *Clinically Relevant*
Low-Back Strengthening

This review article examines the effect of specific resistance training for back extension (lumbar extension) in the treatment of chronic low-back pain (CLBP). As Carpenter and Nelson point out, there is a great need for exercise leaders to understand the appropriate use of exercise to prevent and treat low-back pain, because low-back pain is the fifth most frequent reason for hospitalization and third most frequent reason for surgical procedures. Acute low-back pain (pain lasting <3 weeks) usually resolves itself without any intervention; by 3 weeks, 75% of individuals have recovered from acute low-back pain, and by 2 months, 90% of individuals have recovered from low-back pain. However, patients with CLBP (symptoms lasting more than 7 weeks) do not enjoy the same prognosis. In fact, CLBP is the number-one cause of disability in the United States. Furthermore, the longer an individual suffers from CLBP, the worse the prognosis. Patients with CLBP are characterized by the deconditioning syndrome: a cyclical pattern of pain, followed by avoidance of activity, followed by deconditioning, which leads to more pain. Therefore, the general consensus is that patients with CLBP need active reconditioning exercises that progressively apply overload to strengthen the back (lumbar) extensors. Research data

reviewed by Carpenter and Nelson support the following exercise prescription for individuals who suffer from CLBP.

- Specific exercise—Resistance exercise of lumbar extensors with the pelvis stabilized

- Overload—1 set of 6–15 repetitions to fatigue

- Frequency—1 d·wk^{-1}

A rehabilitation program using an exercise program similar to this for patients who had suffered CLBP for an average of 26 months resulted in improved lumbar strength and range of motion and substantial improvements in low-back pain and leg pain. Furthermore, the patients who demonstrated the greatest gains in muscle strength also experienced the greatest decrease in pain. Exercise programs that apply progressive overload to strengthen the lumbar extensors have also been shown to prevent low-back pain. The graph summarizes the results of a study that examined the incidence of back injuries in a group of strip mine workers who participated in a program of isolated low-back muscle strengthening. Data are also presented for the industry average and the average incidence of low-back injury in this coal mine for the past 9 years.

This review article clearly shows that a progressive resistance training program aimed at strengthening the lumbar extensors can significantly help prevent and treat low-back pain. Given the extremely high incidence of low-back pain, all exercise professionals should understand the potential beneficial effect of exercise. This information applies not only to individuals working in occupational settings but also to anyone who routinely recommends exercise to individuals—that is, to all exercise professionals.

Source: Carpenter, D. M. & B. W. Nelson: Low back strengthening for the prevention and treatment of low back pain. *Medicine & Science in Sports & Exercise.* 31(1):18–24 (1999).

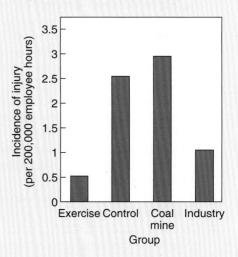

---

been shown to be detrimental. Thus, a total body workout for strength and muscular endurance should include exercises for the back and abdominals, even though such a program does not absolutely protect individuals from LBP (Plowman, 1992).

SUMMARY

1. Resistance training is used to improve overall health, improve athletic performance, rehabilitate injuries, and change physical appearance. Resistance training is also the primary activity in the sports of power lifting and bodybuilding.

2. A plan for muscular fitness should be specific to the individual's goals, which may include the development of muscular strength, hypertrophy, power or endurance, or any combination of these properties.

3. Overload of the muscular system is achieved by manipulating the load, volume, rest intervals, and frequency of training. Volume is determined by load (intensity) and repetitions (volume = load × reps × sets).

4. If different individuals use the same training program, adaptation will occur at different rates because of individual differences in age, body size and type, initial strength, and genetic makeup.

5. A coach or exercise leader must be sensitive to the differences in rates of individual adaptation, which directly affect the progression of training. A common mistake is for coaches to design a program for the entire team and expect adaptations to occur at the same rate.

6. Adaptation to resistance training in children and older adults is very similar to adaptations that occur in young and middle-aged adults.

7. Periodization within a training program can help prevent the inhibitions of strength gains during concurrent training.

8. Strength gains are preserved for longer periods of time compared to other training adaptations. The impact of detraining on muscle strength varies by muscle group and exercise type.

9. Resistance training provides multiple health benefits, including decreased mortality, improved cardiometabolic health, and improved functional measures.

10. Functional back health requires flexibility in the lumbar muscles, hamstrings, and hip flexors and strength of the abdominals and back extensor muscles.

REVIEW QUESTIONS

1. Give several reasons why an individual may engage in a resistance training program and specify different goals of such programs.

2. Discuss how each of the training principles can be applied in the development of a resistance training program. How do these applications vary if the exerciser is a child?

3. Is there an ideal number of repetitions and sets that should be performed by everyone? Defend your answer.

4. Discuss the importance of adequate recovery time for training adaptations to a resistance training program.

5. Do all individuals respond to a training program with the same adaptation (or magnitude of adaptation)? Why or why not?

6. What is the importance of a warm-up period before resistance training?

7. Compare and contrast the training adaptations that occur in skeletal muscle as a result of resistance training and endurance training.

8. Describe the health benefits of muscular strength and endurance training.

9. What is the relationship between muscle function and low-back pain?

10. Identify three research questions about resistance training for which scientists have yet to provide answers.

For further review and additional study tools, visit the website at http://thePoint.lww.com/Plowman4e ✳ ▶

REFERENCES

Aagaard, P., P. S. Magnusson, B. Larsson, M. Kjaer, & P. Krustrup: Mechanical muscle function, morphology, and fiber type in lifelong trained elderly. *Medicine & Science in Sports & Exercise.* 39(11):1989–1996 (2007).

American College of Sports Medicine: Position stand on progression models in resistance training for healthy adults. *Medicine & Science in Sports & Exercise.* 41(3):687–708 (2009).

Artero, E. G., J. R. Ruiz, F. B. Ortega, V. España-Romero, G. Vicente-Rodríguez, D. Molnar, F. Gottrand, M. González-Gross, C. Breidenassel, L. A. Moreno, & A. Gutiérrez: Muscular and cardiorespiratory fitness are independently associated with metabolic risk in adolescents: The HELENA study. *Pediatric Diabetes.* 12:704–712 (2011).

Baechle, T. R., R. W. Earle, & D. Wathen: Resistance training. In Baechle T. R., & R. W. Earle (eds.): *Essentials of Strength Training and Conditioning.* Champaign, IL: Human Kinetics, 393–426 (2000).

Behm, D. G., A. D. Faigenbaum, B. Falk, & P. Klentrou: Canadian society for exercise physiology position paper: resistance training in children and adolescents. *Applied Physiology, Nutrition, and Metabolism.* 33:547–561 (2008).

Benson, A. C., M. E. Torode, & M. A. Fiatarone: Effects of resistance training on metabolic fitness in children and adolescents: A systematic review. *Obesity Reviews.* 9:43–66 (2008).

Bird, S. P., K. M. Tarpenning, & F. E. Marino: Designing Resistance Training Programmes to Enhance Muscular Fitness: A Review of the Acute Program Variable. *Sports Medicine.* 35(10):841–851 (2005).

Blimkie, C. J. R.: Resistance training during preadolescence: Issues and controversies. *Sports Medicine.* 15(6):389–407 (1988).

Braith, R. W. & K. J. Stewart: Resistance exercise training: Its role in the prevention of cardiovascular disease. *Circulation.* 113:2642–2650 (2006).

Carpenter, D. M. & B. W. Nelson: Low back strengthening for the prevention and treatment of low back pain. *Medicine and Science in Sports and Exercise.* 31(1):18–24 (1999).

Charette, S. L., L. McEvoy, G. Pyka, C. Snow-Harter, D. Guido, R. A. Wiswell, & R. Marcus: Muscle hypertrophy response to resistance training in older women. *Journal of Applied Physiology.* 70:1912–1916 (1991).

Coggan, A. R., R. J. Pina, D. S. King, M. A. Rogers, M. Brown, P. M. Nemeth, & J. O. Holloszy: Skeletal muscle adaptations to endurance training in 60- to 70-year-old men and women. *Journal of Applied Physiology.* 68:1896–1901 (1990).

Cureton, K. J., M. A. Collins, D. W. Hill, & F. M. McElhannon: Muscle hypertrophy in men and women. *Medicine and Science in Sports and Exercise.* 20(4):338–344 (1988).

Davies, C. T. M. & C. Barnes: Negative (eccentric) work. II. Physiological responses to walking uphill and downhill on motor-driven treadmill. *Ergonomics.* 15:121–131 (1972).

DeLorme, T. L. & A. L. Watkins: Techniques of progressive resistance exercise. *Archives of Physical Medicine.* 29:263–273 (1948).

Elliot, T. A., M. G. Cree, A. P. Sanford, R. R. Wolfe, & K. D. Tipton: Milk ingestion stimulates muscle protein synthesis following resistance exercise. *Medicine & Science in Sports & Exercise.* 38(4):667–674 (2005).

Enoka, R. M.: *Neuromechanical Basis of Kinesiology.* Champaign, IL: Human Kinetics, 31–64 (1988).

Faigenbaum, A. D., L. D. Zaichkowsky, W. L. Westcott, L. J. Micheli, & A. F. Fehlandt: The effects of a twice-a-week strength training program on children. *Pediatric Exercise Science.* 5:339–346 (1993).

Faigenbaum, A. D., L. A. Milliken, & W. L. Westcott: Maximal strength testing in healthy children. *Journal of Strength and Conditioning Research*. 17:162–166 (2003).

Faigenbaum, A. D. & G. D. Myer: Pediatric resistance training: Benefits, concerns, and program design considerations. *Current Sports Medicine Reports*. 9(3):161–168 (2010)

Faigenbaum, A. D. & G. D. Myer: Resistance training among young athletes: Safety, efficacy and injury prevention effects. *British Journal of Sports Medicine*. 44:56–63 (2010)

Faigenbaum, A. D., W. J. Kramer, C. J. R. Blimkie, I. Jeffreys, L. J. Micheli, M. Nitka, & T. W. Rowland: Youth resistance training: Updated position statement paper from the national strength and conditioning association. *National Strength and Conditioning Association*. 0(0):1–20 (2009)

Fiatarone, M. A., E. C. Marks, N. D. Ryan, C. N. Meredith, L. A. Lipsitz, & W. J. Evans: High intensity strength training in nonagenarians. Effects on skeletal muscle. *Journal of the American Medical Association*. 263:3029–3034 (1990).

FitzGerald, S. J., C. E. Barlow, J. B. Kampert, J. R. Morrow, A. W. Jackson, & S. N. Blair: Muscular fitness and all-cause mortality: Prospective observations. *Journal of Physical Activity and Health*. 1:7–18 (2004).

Fleck, S. J. & W. J. Kraemer: *Designing Resistance Training Programs*. Champaign, IL: Human Kinetics (1987).

Folland, J. P. & A. G. Williams: The adaptations to strength training. *Sports Medicine*. 37(2):145–168 (2007).

Frontera, W. R., V. A. Hughes, K. J. Lutz, & W. J. Evans: A cross-sectional study of muscle strength and mass in 45- to 78-yr-old men and women. *Journal of Applied Physiology*. 71:644–650 (1991).

Gabriel, D. A., G. Kamen, & G. Frost: Neural adaptations to restive exercise: Mechanisms and recommendations for training practices. *Sports Medicine*. 36:133–149 (2006).

Gollnick, P. D., R. B. Armstrong, C. W. Saubert IV, K. Piehl, & B. Saltin: Enzyme activity and fiber composition in skeletal muscle of untrained and trained men. *Journal of Applied Physiology*. 33(3):312–319 (1972).

Häkkinen, K., M. Alén, & P. V. Komi: Changes in isometric force- and relaxation-time, electromyographic and muscle fibre characteristics of human skeletal muscle during strength training and detraining. *Acta Physiologica Scandinavica*. 125:573–585 (1985).

Häkkinen, K., P. V. Komi, & P. A. Tesch: Effect of combined concentric and eccentric strength training and detraining on force-time, muscle fiber and metabolic characteristics of leg extensor muscles. *Scandinavian Journal of Sports Science*. 3:50–58 (1981).

Häkkinen, K. & P. V. Komi: Electromyographic changes during strength training and detraining. *Medicine and Science in Sports and Exercise*. 15:455–460 (1983).

Haskell, W. L., I. M. Lee, R. R. Pate, K. E. Powell, S. N. Blair, B. A. Franklin, C. A. Macera, G. W. Heath, P. D. Thompson, & A. Bauman: Physical activity and public health: Updated recommendation for adults from the American College of Sports Medicine and the American Heart Association. *Medicine & Science in Sports & Exercise*. 39(8):1423–1434 (2007).

Hawley, J. A.: Molecular responses to strength and endurance training: Are they incompatible? *Applied Physiology, Nutrition, and Metabolism*. 34:355–361 (2009).

Holm, L., S. Reitelseder, T. G. Pedersen, S. Doessing, S. G. Petersen, A. Flyvbjerg, J. L. Andersen, P. Aagaard, & M. Kjaer: Changes in muscle size and MHC composition in response to resistance exercise with heavy and light loading intensity. *Journal of Applied Physiology* 105:1454–1461 (2008).

Hortobágyi, T., J. A. Houmard, J. R. Stevenson, D. D. Fraser, R. A. Johns, & R. G. Israel: The effects of detraining on power athletes. *Medicine and Science in Sports and Exercise*. 25:929–935 (1993).

Katzmarzyk, P. T. & C. L. Craig: Musculoskeletal fitness and risk of mortality. *Medicine & Science in Sports & Exercise*. 34:740–744 (2002).

Kawamori, N. & G. Haff: The optimal load for the development of muscular power. *Journal of Strength and Conditioning Research*. 18(3):675–684 (2004).

Kraemer, W. J., J. F. Patton, S. E. Gordon, E. A. Harman, M. R. Deschenes, K. Reynolds, R. U. Newton, N. T. Triplett, & J. E. Dziados: Compatibility of high-intensity strength and endurance training on hormonal and skeletal muscle adaptations. *Journal of Applied Physiology*. 78(3):976–989 (1995).

Kraemer, W. J. & N. A. Ratamess: Fundamentals of resistance training: Progression and exercise prescription. *Medicine & Science in Sports & Exercise*. 36(4):674–688 (2004).

Kraemer, W. J. & N. A. Ratamess: Hormonal responses and adaptations to resistance exercise and training. *Sports Medicine*. 35(4):339–336 (2005).

Larsson, L.: Physical training effects on muscle morphology in sedentary males at different ages. *Medicine and Science in Sports and Exercise*. 14:203–206 (1982).

Lemmer, J. T., D. E. Hurlbut, G. F. Martel, B. L. Tracy, F. M. Ivey, E. J. Metter, J. L. Fozard, J. L. Fleg, & B. F. Hurley: Age and gender responses to strength training and detraining. *Medicine & Science in Sports & Exercise*. 32:1505–1512 (2000).

Leveritt, M., P. J. Abernethy, B. K. Barry, & P. A. Logan: Concurrent strength and endurance training: A review. *Sports Medicine*. 28(6):413–427 (1999).

Mazzetti, S. A., W. J. Kraemer, J. S. Volek, N. D. Duncan, N. A. Ratamess, A. L. Gomez, R. U. Newton, K. Hakkinen, & S. J. Fleck: The influence of direct supervision of resistance training on strength performance. *Medicine & Science in Sports & Exercise*. 32(6):1175–1184 (2000).

MacDougal, J. D., G. R. Ward, D. G. Sale & J. R. Sutton: Biochemical adaptation of human skeletal muscle to heavy resistance training and immobilization. *Journal Applied Physiology*. 43(4):700–703 (1977).

McLester, J. R., P. A. Bishop, J. Smith, L. Wyers, B. Dale, J. Kozusko, M. Richardson, M. E. Nevett & R. Lomax: A series of studies-a practical protocol for testing muscular endurance recovery. *Journal of Strength and Conditioning Research*. 17(2):259–273 (2003).

Mujika, I. & S. Padilla: Detraining: Loss of training-induced physiological and performance adaptations. Part I. *Sports Medicine*. 30(2):79–87 (2000a).

Nader, G. A.: Concurrent strength and endurance training: From molecules to man. *Medicine & Science in Sports & Exercise*. 38(11):1965–1970 (2006).

Nelson, M. E., W. J. Rejeski, S. N. Blair, P. W. Duncan, J. O. Judge, A. C. King, C. A. Macera, & C. Castaneda-Sceppa: Physical activity and public health in older adults: Recommendation from the American College of Sports Medicine and the American Heart Association. *Medicine & Science in Sports & Exercise*. 39(8):1434–1445 (2007).

Neufer, P. D., D. L. Costill, R. A. Fielding, M. G. Flynn, & J. P. Kirwan: Effect of reduced training on muscular strength and endurance in competitive swimmers. *Medicine and Science in Sports and Exercise*. 19:486–490 (1987).

Ortega, F. B., R. R. Ruiz, M. J. Castillo, & M. Sjöström: Physical fitness in childhood and adolescence: a powerful marker of health. *International Journal of Obesity*. 32:1–11 (2008).

Paulsen, G., D. Myklestad, & T. Raastad: The influence of volume of exercise on early adaptations to strength training. *Journal of Strength and Conditioning Research*. 17(1):115–120 (2003).

Perrin, D. H.: *Isokinetic Exercise and Assessment*. Champaign, IL: Human Kinetics (1993).

Phillips, S. M., & R. A. Winett: Uncomplicated resistance training and health-related outcomes: Evidence for a health mandate. *Current Sports Medicine Reports*. 9(4)208–213 (2010).

Plowman, S. A.: Physical activity, physical fitness, and low back pain. In Holloszy, J. O. (ed.): *Exercise and Sport Sciences Reviews*. 20:221–242 (1992).

Rogers, M. A. & W. J. Evans: Changes in skeletal muscle with aging: Effects of exercise training. In Holloszy, J. O. (ed.): *Exercise and Sport Sciences Reviews* (Vol. 21). Baltimore, MD: Williams & Wilkins, 65–102 (1993).

Rønnestad, B. R., W. Egeland, N. H. Kvamme, P. E. Refsnes, F. Kadi, & T. Raastad: Dissimilar effects of one- and three-set strength training on strength and muscle mass gains in upper and lower body in untrained subjects. *Journal of Strength and Conditioning Research*. 21(1):157–163 (2007).

Rowland, T. W.: *Children's Exercise Physiology*. Champaign, IL: Human Kinetics, (2005).

Sale, D. G.: Neural adaptation to resistance training. *Medicine and Science in Sports and Exercise*. 20(suppl):S135–S145 (1988).

Schoenfeld, B. J.: The mechanisms of muscle hypertrophy and their application to resistance training. *Journal of Strength and Conditioning Research*. 24(10):2857–2872 (2010).

Shoepe, T. C., J. E. Stelzer, D. P. Garner, & J. J. Widrick: Functional adaptability of muscle fibers to long-term resistance exercise. *Medicine & Science in Sports & Exercise*. 35(6):944–951 (2003).

Staron, R. S., M. J. Leonardi, D. L. Karapondo, E. S. Malicky, J. E. Falkel, F. C. Hagerman, & R. S. Hikida: Strength and skeletal muscle adaptations in heavy-resistance-trained women after detraining and retraining. *Journal of Applied Physiology*. 70:631–640 (1991).

Steene-Johannessen, J., S. A. Anderssen, E. Kolle, & L. B. Andersen: Low muscle fitness is associated with metabolic risk in youth. *Medicine & Science in Sports & Exercise*. 41:1361–1367 (2009).

Steib, S., D. Schoene, & K. Pfeifer: Dose-response relationship of resistance training in older adults: a metaanalysis. *Medicine & Science in Sports & Exercise*. 42(5):902–914 (2010).

Strasser, B., W. Siebert, & W. Schobersberger: Resistance training in the treatment of the metabolic syndrome: A systematic review and meta-analysis of the effect of resistance training on metabolic clustering in patients with abnormal glucose metabolism. *Sports Medicine*. 40(5):397–415 (2010).

Tesch, P. A.: Training for body building. In Komi, P. V. (ed.): *Strength and Power in Sport*. London: Blackwell Scientific, 357–369 (1992).

Warburton, D. E. R., N. Gledhill, & A. Quinney: Musculoskeletal fitness and health. *Canadian Journal of Applied Physiology*. 26(2):217–237 (2001a).

Warburton, D. E. R., N. Gledhill, & A. Quinney: The effects of changes in musculoskeletal fitness on health. *Canadian Journal of Applied Physiology*. 26(2):217–237 (2001b).

Warburton, D. E. R., C. W. Nicol, & S. D. Bredin: Health benefits of physical activity: The evidence. *Canadian Medical Association Journal*. 174:801–809 (2006).

Wernbom, M., J. Augustsson, & R. Thomee: The influence of frequency, intensity, volume and mode of strength training on whole muscle cross-sectional area in humans. *Sports Medicine*. 37(3):225–264 (2007).

Wilmore, J. H.: Alterations in strength, body composition, and anthropometric measurements consequent to a 10 week weight training program. *Medicine and Science in Sports*. 6:133–138 (1974).

Neuromuscular Aspects of Movement

20

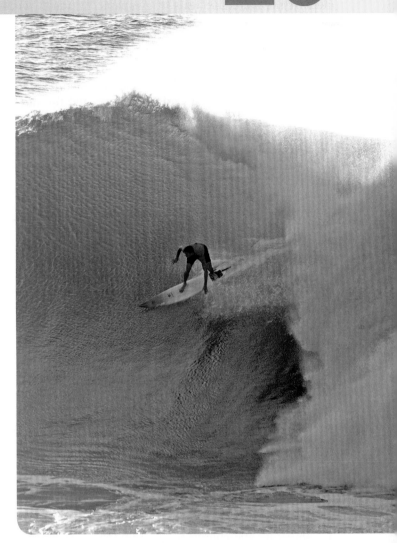

OBJECTIVES

After studying the chapter, you should be able to:

> Describe the nerve supply to muscle.

> Describe the sequence of events at the neuromuscular junction.

> Identify the components of a reflex arc.

> Describe the structure and innervation of the muscle spindle, and explain how the muscle spindle functions in the myotatic reflex.

> Describe the structure and innervation of the Golgi tendon organ, and explain how it functions in the inverse myotatic reflex.

> Provide research and clinical evidence that individual motor units can be volitionally controlled.

> Diagram the sequence of events involved in volitional control of movement.

> Differentiate between dynamic and static flexibility.

> Identify the anatomical factors that influence flexibility.

> Describe the basic methods of measuring flexibility.

> Discuss the relationship between flexibility and low-back pain.

> Differentiate among the different types of flexibility training.

> Describe the acute responses to static stretching.

> Identify the benefits of a balance training program.

> Apply the training principles to the development of a flexibility program and a balance program.

Introduction

As spectators watching the Olympic Games, we marvel at the grace and skill of figure skaters and stare in amazement at the incredible feats of gymnasts. As adults, we look on with wonder as a child learns a new task—rolling over, walking, tying a shoe—or an injured individual relearns basic skills. As coaches or fitness leaders, we experience the satisfaction of seeing individuals incorporate our suggestions to improve their skill. Understanding the awe-inspiring accomplishments of athletes and the simple movements that are often taken for granted requires knowledge of the nervous system.

The nervous system is made up of the brain, spinal cord, and nerves. It is the primary control and communication center for the entire body. The nervous system functions with the endocrine system to control and regulate the body's internal environment; that is, it helps maintain homeostasis. All human movement depends on the nervous system; skeletal muscles will not contract unless they receive a signal from the nervous system.

This chapter introduces some basic neuroanatomy and examines the role of the somatic nervous system in controlling human movement. It also discusses the influence of the nervous system on flexibility and flexibility training and on balance and balance training.

The Nervous System

The nervous system is a fast-acting control system that regulates a virtually endless list of bodily functions. The nervous system has three primary functions:

1. Monitoring the internal and external environment through sensory receptors
2. Integrating the information it has received
3. Initiating and coordinating a response by activating muscles (skeletal, smooth, and cardiac) and glands (including endocrine glands)

These functions are accomplished by the cells of the nervous system (neurons) that communicate with each other and with effector organs (muscle and glands). Communication within a neuron occurs by electrical signals (action potentials). Communication between neurons or between neurons and an effector organ (e.g., skeletal muscle) occurs by chemical signals (neurotransmitters).

The Basic Structure of the Nervous System

As shown in **Figure 20.1**, the nervous system can be structurally divided into the central nervous system (CNS), which consists of the brain and spinal cord, and the peripheral nervous system (PNS), which consists of all neural tissue outside the CNS. The PNS contains *afferent*

and *efferent neurons. Afferent neurons* relay information about the internal and external environment (from sensory receptors in the periphery) to the CNS. The CNS integrates information it receives from afferent neurons and responds by activating the efferent division. *Efferent neurons* relay signals from the CNS to effector organs in the periphery.

The somatic (or motor) system, shown on the left side of **Figure 20.1**, sends signals from the CNS to skeletal muscle to initiate muscle contraction and thus movement. This is the focus of this chapter. Although we may not always achieve the desired result from such movement (think about your last golf outing), the somatic system is under voluntary control. The autonomic nervous system (ANS) is involuntary, meaning we do not consciously control its activity. The autonomic nervous system, depicted on the right side of **Figure 20.1**, carries information from the CNS to cardiac muscle, smooth muscle, and endocrine glands, thereby providing subconscious neural regulation of the internal environment of the body. The autonomic nervous system is discussed more fully in the following chapter.

Activation of the Nervous System

The somatic nervous system may be activated by conscious thought or by afferent input from the periphery. Afferent signals involved in regulating nervous control of muscle contraction rely on different types of sensory receptors: mechanoreceptors (pressure, stretch, or contraction) and proprioceptors (spatial orientation), located primarily in skeletal muscle, tendons, and joints. Activation of these receptors often results in a reflex movement. A *reflex* is a rapid, involuntary movement in response to a stimulus (discussed in more detail later in this chapter).

The Nerve Cell

The neuron, or nerve cell, is the functional unit of the nervous system. In addition to the afferent and efferent neurons described above, the central nervous system also has connection or association neurons. Neurons vary considerably in size and shape, depending on their function and location in the body. However, the neurons described in this text generally contain three distinct regions (**Figure 20.2**). The dendrites, highly branched extensions of the neuron, are receptor sites that receive information and convey it to the cell body. The cell body is the control center. It integrates information that it receives from the dendrites and, if the signal is strong enough (at or above threshold level), passes it along to the axon. A cluster of cell bodies in the CNS is called a nucleus; a cluster of cell bodies in the PNS is called a ganglion.

The axon of a motor neuron is a single extension of the neuron. The axon has two important functions: conducting the action potential and secreting the

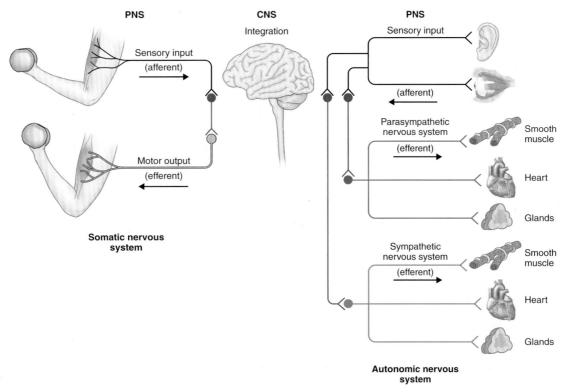

FIGURE 20.1 Major Divisions of the Nervous System.
The nervous system can be divided anatomically into the central (brain and spinal cord) nervous system (CNS) and the peripheral (sensory organs and nerves) nervous system (PNS). The nervous system can be functionally divided into the somatic nervous system and the autonomic nervous system (ANS). The somatic nervous system leads to contraction of muscle fibers through efferent (motor) neurons. The autonomic nervous system controls the heart, glands, and hollow organs and is essential in maintaining homeostasis.

neurotransmitter. An action potential causes the axon to release a neurotransmitter (a chemical signal) from its axon terminal. The release of neurotransmitters allows neurons to communicate with one another. The length of axons varies according to the body location that is being innervated, but they may be very long. Axons that extend from the spinal cord to the feet may be over a meter long. A long axon is called a nerve fiber, and a bundle of axons is called a nerve. The axon may be myelinated (wrapped with Schwann cells) or unmyelinated.

Nerve cells have the functional characteristic of irritability (the ability to respond to a stimulus). That characteristic is evident in the dendrites and cell body. Nerve cells also have the characteristic of conductivity (the transmission of an electrical impulse from one location to another). The axon conducts an electrical impulse. In general, large-diameter nerves conduct an impulse faster than small-diameter nerves. A myelin sheath protects and electrically insulates axons and increases the rate

Impulse An electrical charge transmitted through certain tissue that results in the stimulation or inhibition of physiological activity.

at which electrical impulses can be conducted. For example, the nerve conduction velocity in an unmyelinated neuron is 13.5–22.5 mi·hr^{-1}; in a myelinated skeletal muscle neuron of the same diameter, the speed is 135–225 mi·hr^{-1} (Robergs and Roberts, 1997)!

The Neural Impulse

An **impulse** is a charge transmitted through certain tissue that results in the stimulation or inhibition of physiological activity. A neuron carries an electrical impulse, called the action potential. Neurons, and all cells, possess an electrical resting membrane potential. The resting membrane potential is the difference between the electrical charge on the inside of the cell and the charge on the outside of the cell (**Figure 20.2A**). This resting potential results from the unequal distribution of positively and negatively charged ions. Negatively charged ions (anions [An$^-$]) predominate along the inside of the cell membrane and attract positively charged ions (cations) along the outside of the cell membrane. In a typical neuron at rest, sodium (Na$^+$) and chloride (Cl$^-$) ions predominate extracellularly. Potassium ions (K$^+$) and negatively charged protein anions predominate intracellularly.

Resting (Polarized) State   **A**

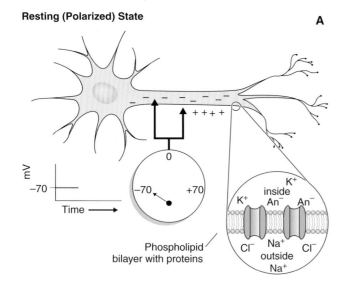

Phospholipid bilayer with proteins

Action Potential   **B**

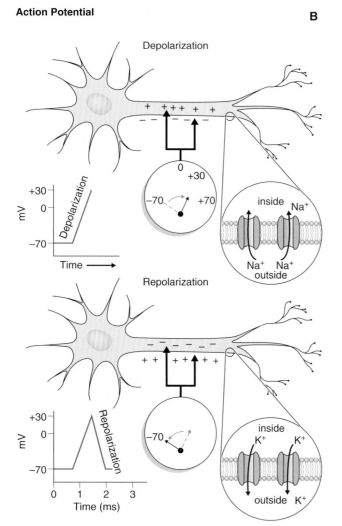

FIGURE 20.2 Generation of Action Potential.
A. Resting (polarized) state. **B.** Action potential. In the resting state, the neuron cell membrane is polarized (the inside is negative relative to the outside). During an action potential, the membrane polarity is reversed and the inside of the cell becomes positive.

The cell membrane itself is composed of proteins floating in a bilayer of lipids. The membrane is permeable, or capable of allowing ions to pass through it, some by diffusion and some through specific protein channels. Channels may be passive (always open so that they allow a leakage) or active (requiring a chemical or electrical change to open their gates).

At rest, potassium (K^+) "leaks" out through passive channels, and a sodium-potassium pump, which actively transports sodium out across the membrane and potassium back into the cell, removes three sodium ions from the cell for each two potassium ions it brings into the cell. Thus, at rest there is a net loss of positive ions from the interior of the cell, making the interior negatively charged (–65 to –85 μV) relative to the exterior (**Figure 20.2A**). Thus the resting neuron is said to be polarized.

When a sufficient stimulus (usually a chemical stimulus from other neurons) is applied to the cell, sodium (Na^+) channels open, and positive ions flow into the neuron. Polarity in this region of the neuron is reversed; that is, the cell membrane is depolarized, meaning that the inside of the cell is now positive relative to the outside (**Figure 20.2B**). This process takes about 1 millisecond, at which time the sodium gates close and potassium gates open. Potassium exits the cell, bringing about repolarization, or a return to a net negative charge inside. Sodium is returned to the outside of the cell and potassium to the inside by the sodium-potassium pump, which restores the ionic balance and resting membrane potential. This sequence of events is repeated down the length of the axon. The reversal of polarity or change in electrical potential across a nerve membrane that generates an electrical current is an **action potential**. The propagation of an action potential along the axon of a neuron is the mechanism by which electrical signals are sent within a neuron. Once generated in the axon, the action potential moves along the entire length of the axon and causes a neurotransmitter to be released from the terminal end of the axon. The terminal end of the axon communicates with other neurons, muscle cells, or glands across junctions known as **synapses**. If the synapse is between a neuron and a muscle cell, it is known as a neuromuscular junction.

Neural Control of Muscle Contraction

Both the somatic nervous system and the autonomic nervous system play important roles in controlling and regulating the body's response to exercise. However, this chapter focuses on the role of the somatic nervous system in initiating and controlling skeletal muscle contraction. The role of the somatic nervous system in exercise is straightforward. Skeletal muscle will not contract unless it receives a signal from a motor neuron. The action potential in the neuron causes the neuron to release its neurotransmitter, which acts as the signal to initiate contraction. Thus the somatic nervous system directly regulates exercise. (Chapter 19 explains the events involved in muscle contraction in detail.)

Nerve Supply

All skeletal muscles require nervous stimulation to produce the electrical excitation in the muscle cells that leads to contraction. *Efferent neurons* carry information from the central nervous system to the muscle. *Motor neurons* are efferent neurons that innervate skeletal muscle and are classified as alpha motor neurons or gamma motor neurons. Alpha (α) motor neurons are relatively large motor neurons that innervate skeletal muscle fibers and result in contraction of muscles. Recall from Chapter 17 that α_1 motor neurons innervate fast twitch (FT) muscle fibers, whereas α_2 motor neurons innervate slow twitch (ST) muscle fibers. *Gamma (γ) motor neurons* innervate proprioceptors.

As a nerve enters the connective tissue of the muscle, it divides into branches that all end near the surface of a muscle fiber. Because the axon of the motor neuron branches, each neuron is connected to several muscle fibers. As defined in Chapter 17, a motor neuron and the muscle fibers it innervates is called a *motor unit* (**Figure 20.3**). The motor unit is the basic unit of contraction. Because each muscle fiber in a motor unit is innervated by the same neuron, the electrical activity in that neuron controls the contractile activity of all the muscle fibers in that motor unit. The number of muscle fibers controlled by a single neuron (i.e., the number of muscle cells in a motor unit) varies tremendously, depending on the size and function of the muscle. Although a single neuron may innervate many muscle fibers, each muscle fiber is only innervated by a single motor neuron.

Figure 20.4 illustrates the relationship between the motor neuron (originating in the central nervous system-labeled 1 in **Figure 20.4**) and muscle fibers. The cell body of the motor neuron is located within the gray matter of the spinal cord (labeled 2 in **Figure 20.4**), and the axon extends out through the ventral root of the spinal nerve (labeled 3 in **Figure 20.4**) to carry the electrical signal to the muscle fiber (labeled 4 in **Figure 20.4**). Each branch of the motor neuron terminates in a slight bulge called the axon terminal, which lies very close to but does not touch the underlying muscle fiber.

The space between the membrane of the neuron and the muscle cell membrane at the *motor end plate* is called the neuromuscular (or synaptic) cleft. The entire region

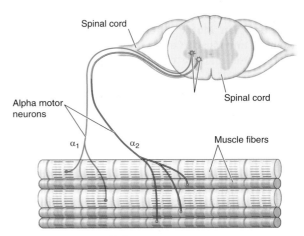

FIGURE 20.3 Motor Units.
Two motor units are depicted. Notice that the muscle fibers of the two motor units are intermingled.

is referred to as the neuromuscular junction. The *neuromuscular junction* is important because the electrical signal from the motor neuron is transmitted here, via a neurotransmitter, to the surface of the muscle cell that is to contract.

Muscle cells also have afferent (sensory) nerve endings, which are sensitive to mechanical and chemical changes in the muscle tissue and which relay this information back to the central nervous system. The information carried by afferent neurons is used by the central nervous system to make adjustments in muscular contractions.

The Neuromuscular Junction

The neuromuscular junction is a specialized synapse formed between a terminal end of a motor neuron and a muscle fiber. **Figure 20.5** summarizes the events that occur at the neuromuscular junction. When a neuronal action potential reaches the axon terminal, the membrane of the neuron increases its permeability to calcium, and calcium is taken up into the cell (**Figure 20.5A**). The increased level of calcium causes the synaptic vesicles to migrate to the cell membrane and release the neurotransmitter (acetylcholine, ACh) into the synaptic cleft by the process of exocytosis (**Figure 20.5B**). The ACh then diffuses across the synaptic cleft and binds to receptors on the sarcolemma, causing changes in the ionic permeability (especially to the inward flow of Na^+) and leading to the depolarization of the sarcolemma (**Figure 20.5C**). This change in permeability and subsequent depolarization leads to the generation of an action potential in the sarcolemma of the muscle fiber. The action potential spreads in all directions from the neuromuscular junction, depolarizing the entire sarcolemma. The action potential then spreads into the interior of the cell through the T tubules (**Figure 20.5D**) as described in Chapter 17.

Action Potential Reversal of polarity or change in electrical potential.

Synapses The gap, or junction, between terminal ends of the axon and other neurons, muscle cells, or glands.

FIGURE 20.4 Functional Relationship between Motor (Efferent) Neurons and Muscle Cells.
A motor neuron and the muscle cells it innervates is called a motor unit. (1) Schematic of central nervous system, (2) cross-sectional view of the spinal cord, (3) cross-sectional view of peripheral nerve emphasizing axon of motor neuron, and (4) the motor neuron branching near its terminal end where it forms the neuromuscular junction with the muscle fibers it innervates.

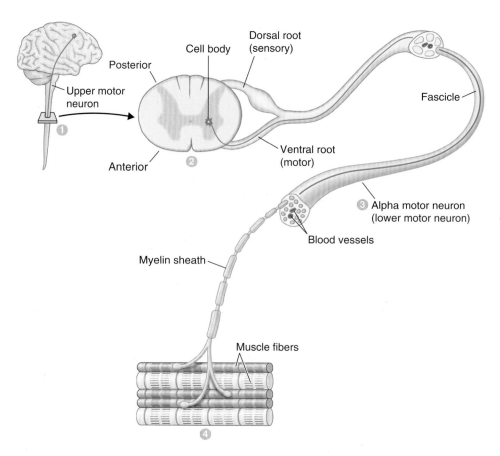

Although the neuromuscular junction functions much like other synapses, there are three important differences.

1. At a neuromuscular junction, a single presynaptic action potential leads to a postsynaptic action potential.
2. The synapse can only be excitatory.
3. A muscle fiber receives synaptic input from only one motor neuron.

Note the two distinct roles that calcium plays in controlling muscular contraction. The first is to facilitate the release of ACh from the synaptic vesicles in the motor neuron terminal. The second (and most often discussed) role of calcium is to control the position of the regulatory proteins troponin and tropomyosin on actin.

Reflex Control of Movement

Reflexes play important roles in maintaining an upright posture, responding to movement in a coordinated fashion, and mediating responses to stretching. A **reflex** is a rapid, involuntary response to stimuli in which a specific stimulus results in a specific motor response. Reflexes can be classified as *autonomic reflexes*, which activate cardiac

and smooth muscle and glands, or *somatic reflexes*, which result in skeletal muscle contraction. This section focuses on somatic reflexes, which play an important role in movement.

Many spinal reflexes do not require the participation of higher brain centers to initiate a response. Higher brain centers, however, are often notified of the resultant movement by neurons that synapse with the afferent neuron.

Spinal Cord

The spinal cord is involved in both involuntary and voluntary movements. The spinal cord connects the peripheral nervous system with the brain and serves as the site of reflex integration.

Figure 20.6 shows a cross-sectional view of the spinal cord. Note the spinal nerves extending from each side of the cord. Each spinal nerve contains afferent (sensory) fibers and efferent (motor) fibers. The cell bodies of the afferent neurons are located in the dorsal root ganglion of the spinal nerve, which is part of the peripheral nervous system. The cell bodies of the efferent neurons, however, are located within the central nervous system, and the axon exits through the ventral root of the spinal nerve. The most familiar efferent neurons are the alpha motor

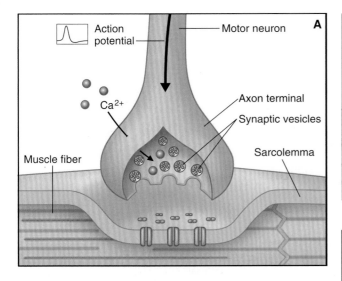

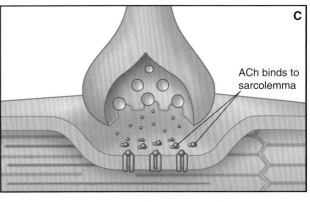

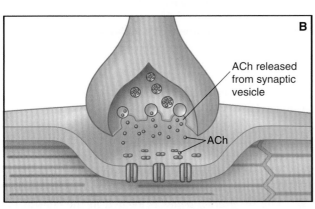

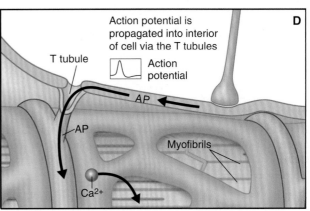

FIGURE 20.5 Events at the Neuromuscular Junction.
A. An action potential (AP) in the axon terminal causes the uptake of Ca^{2+} into the axon terminal and the subsequent release of the neurotransmitter. **B.** The neurotransmitter (ACh) is released from the synaptic vesicles and diffuses across the synaptic cleft. **C.** Generation of action potential: The binding of ACh to receptors on the sarcolemma causes a change in membrane permeability, causing an AP to be initiated in the sarcolemma. **D.** The AP is propagated into the interior of the cells via the T tubules.

neurons that innervate skeletal muscles leading to muscle contraction. The dorsal root and ventral root of the spinal nerve carry only afferent and efferent fibers, respectively. The two roots join to form a spinal nerve. Therefore, even though individual neurons have only sensory or motor functions, a nerve typically contains both afferent and efferent neurons and so has both sensory and motor functions.

Information is carried up and down the spinal cord through a series of tracts. A tract is a bundle of fibers in the central nervous system. The tracts that carry sensory (afferent) information are called ascending tracts. The tracts that carry motor (efferent) information are called descending tracts. Specific tracts are responsible for

Reflex Rapid, involuntary response to stimuli in which a specific stimulus results in a specific motor response.

carrying different types of sensory information (such as pressure and temperature) and motor information (such as fine distal movement).

The descending pathways of the spinal cord can be divided into the pyramidal and extrapyramidal pathways. Both include several descending tracts that carry specific information. Voluntary motor impulses are transmitted from the motor area of the brain to somatic efferent neurons leading to skeletal muscles via the *pyramidal pathways*.

Pyramidal System

The pyramidal (corticospinal) system is composed of neurons with cell bodies that originate in the cerebral cortex and axons that travel through the spinal cord. The neurons that extend from the brain down through the descending tract are called the upper motor neurons (see **Figure 20.4**). These neurons synapse with

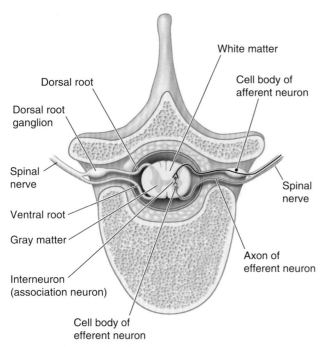

FIGURE 20.6 Cross-sectional View of the Spinal Cord Showing the Relationships between the Spinal Cord and Vertebra.

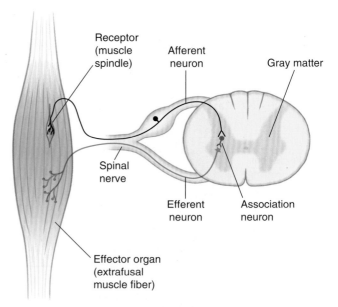

FIGURE 20.7 Components of a Reflex Arc.

the lower motor neurons, also known as the alpha (α) motor neurons, in the anterior gray matter of the spinal cord. The lower motor neurons then carry the message to specific skeletal muscles that control precise, discrete movement.

Both the lateral and anterior corticospinal (pyramidal) tracts decussate, or cross over, as they descend from the brain. Therefore, the motor cortex of the right side of the brain controls the muscles on the left side of the body, and vice versa. Thus, a patient who has had a cerebral vascular accident (stroke) on the right side of the brain may lose the motor function of the left side of the body.

Extrapyramidal System

The extrapyramidal system consists of all descending tracts not included in the pyramidal system. Typically, the neurons found in these tracts have cell bodies located in the basal nuclei or reticular formation of the brain. The extrapyramidal system carries information that controls muscle tone and posture as well as head movements in response to visual stimuli and changes in equilibrium.

Components of a Reflex Arc

Many of our movements depend on spinal reflexes. Spinal reflexes also play an important role in stretching activities. The neural pathway over which a reflex occurs is called

a reflex arc. The basic components of a reflex arc are as follows (**Figure 20.7**).

1. The *receptor* organ responds to the stimulus by converting it into a neural (electrical) signal.
2. The *afferent* (sensory) neuron carries the signal to the central nervous system.
3. The *integration center* is located in the central nervous system. Here the incoming neural signal is processed through the connection of the afferent neuron with *association neurons* (also called interneurons) and efferent neurons. The incoming afferent neuron may synapse directly with the efferent neuron or with association neurons, depending on the complexity of the reflex.
4. The *efferent* (motor) neuron carries the impulse from the central nervous system to the body organ that is to respond to the original stimulus.
5. The *effector organ* responds to the original stimulus. The effector organ may be a muscle or a gland.

Proprioceptors and Related Reflexes

Proprioceptive sensations provide an awareness of the activities of the muscles, tendons, and joints and provide a sense of equilibrium. Although all of the senses are important, this section emphasizes the role of the proprioceptive senses in order to explain the somatosensory system. Although the emphasis here is on proprioceptive receptors, the other senses and receptors also play a major role in human movement. For example, we use the visual sense to gain important information regarding the speed and direction of a tennis ball during a tennis match. We also listen to the sound of the impact of the ball on the opponent's racket to help judge the return. Remember that human movement is not only extremely complex but also affected by a host of factors, including sensory receptors of all types.

Stimulation of the proprioceptors gives rise to kinesthetic perceptions. Historically, *kinesthesis* was defined as a person's perception of his or her own motion, specifically the motion of the limbs relative to each other and the body as a whole. *Proprioception* was defined as the perception of movement of the body plus its orientation in space. Over the years, these terms have become practically synonymous (Schmidt, 1988).

Vestibular Apparatus

Specialized equilibrium receptors in the inner ear, called the vestibular apparatus, provide important proprioceptive sensations. The primary function of the vestibular apparatus is to maintain equilibrium and to preserve a constant plane of head position by modifying muscle tone (Sage, 1971). Receptors of the vestibular apparatus are located in the vestibule and in the semicircular canals.

The vestibule is comprised of two fluid-filled, saclike structures called the utricle and saccule. The receptors in these structures, the maculae, sense information about the position of the head when the body is not moving or is accelerating linearly. The semicircular canals are oriented in three planes of space; that is, each of the semicircular canals is positioned at right angles to the other. This arrangement allows the equilibrium receptors in the semicircular canals, the crista ampullaris, to detect angular movement of the head in any plane. The receptors in the semicircular canals are sensitive to changes in the velocity of head movements—that is, to angular acceleration.

Information from the vestibular apparatus is transmitted to the brain via the vestibulocochlear nerve. The information is carried to the vestibular nuclear complex and the cerebellum. Here it is processed along with information from visual receptors and the somatic receptors of the muscles, tendons, and joints. Although the vestibular receptors are very important, they can be overruled by information from other receptors. For example, the spotting technique (keeping the eyes focused on one spot) used by figure skaters allows them to perform spins without becoming dizzy.

Muscle Spindles and the Myotatic Reflex

Muscle spindles (sometimes called neuromuscular spindles, NMS) are located in skeletal muscle. They lie parallel to and are embedded in the skeletal muscle fibers. These receptors are stimulated by stretch and provide information to the central nervous system regarding the length and rate of length change in skeletal muscles. Stimulation of the muscle spindles results in reflex contraction of the

stretched muscle via a myotatic reflex, also known as a stretch reflex (Guyton and Hall, 2011). Thus the muscle spindle performs both a sensory and a motor function.

Figure 20.8 represents a muscle spindle and its nerve supply. The muscle spindle consists of a fluid-filled capsule composed of connective tissue; it is long and cylindrical with tapered ends. The typical spindle is 4–7 mm long and approximately 1/5 the diameter of a muscle fiber (extrafusal fiber) (Sage, 1971). The capsule contains specialized muscle fibers called *intrafusal muscle fibers*. In contrast to intrafusal fibers, skeletal muscle fibers that produce muscular movement are sometimes called *extrafusal fibers*. Each end of the spindle is attached to extrafusal muscle fibers.

Two types of intrafusal fibers are located within the muscle spindle: nuclear bag fibers and nuclear chain fibers. *Nuclear bag fibers* are thicker and contain many centrally located nuclei. These fibers extend beyond the spindle capsule and attach to the connective tissue of the extrafusal fibers. *Nuclear chain fibers* are shorter and thinner and have fewer nuclei in the central area of the fiber. Both types of intrafusal fibers contain contractile elements at their distal poles. The central region of the fibers does not contain contractile elements; this is the sensory receptor area of the spindle.

A typical muscle spindle contains 1–3 nuclear bag fibers and 3–9 nuclear chain fibers (Guyton and Hall, 2011). The intrafusal fibers of the spindle are innervated by sensory nerves called annulospiral and flower-spray neurons. The branches of the *annulospiral neurons* wrap around the nucleated parts of both types of intrafusal fibers. These annulospiral fibers are large, myelinated fibers (Standring, 2005).

The branches of the *flower-spray neurons* wrap around only the nuclear chain fibers (Standring, 2005). The flower-spray fibers are smaller than and conduct impulses slower than the annulospiral fibers. Both types of afferent fibers are stimulated when the central portion of the spindle is stretched. Since the intrafusal fibers are arranged in parallel with the extrafusal fibers, they are stretched or shortened with the whole muscle. The flower-spray nerve endings have a higher threshold of excitation than the annulospiral nerve endings. The flower-spray nerve endings provide information about relative muscle length; the annulospiral nerve endings respond primarily to the rate of length change.

The contractile intrafusal fibers also receive motor innervation from the central nervous system. The efferent fibers that terminate on the intrafusal fibers are called gamma efferents (γ motor neurons), or fusimotor neurons. The axons of the gamma motor neurons travel in the spinal nerve and terminate on the distal ends of the intrafusal fibers. Stimulation of the gamma motor neurons produces contraction of the intrafusal fiber, which causes the central region of the spindle to be stretched. Gamma motor neurons are important

FIGURE 20.8 Muscle Spindle and Its Nerve Supply.
Muscle spindles transmit sensory information through flower-spray neurons and annulospiral neurons. The muscle spindle also receives motor (efferent) information from gamma efferent fibers.

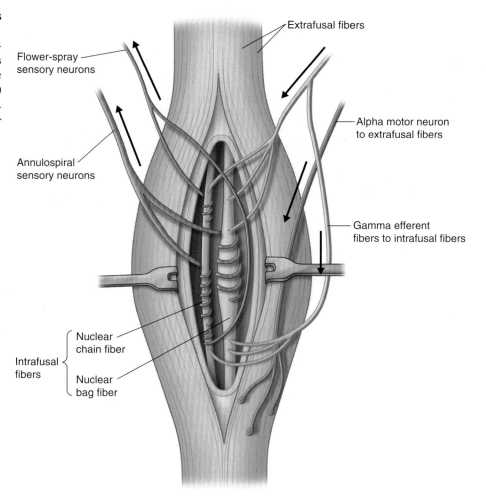

Flower-spray sensory neurons

Annulospiral sensory neurons

Extrafusal fibers

Alpha motor neuron to extrafusal fibers

Gamma efferent fibers to intrafusal fibers

Intrafusal fibers
{ Nuclear chain fiber
Nuclear bag fiber

enough to comprise almost a third of all motor neurons in the body.

MYOTATIC REFLEX The myotatic or stretch reflex has two separate components: a dynamic reaction and a static reaction. The dynamic reaction occurs in response to a sudden change in length of the muscle. When a muscle is quickly stretched, the annulospiral nerve endings (but not the flower-spray endings) transmit an impulse to the spinal cord, which results in an immediate strong reflex contraction of the same muscle from which the signal originated (Guyton and Hall, 2011). This is what happens in the knee-jerk response, diagramed in **Figure 20.9**, or in the head-jerk response when you fall asleep sitting up reading a book not nearly as interesting as this one. Because this reflex does not require that information be processed by the brain, it occurs very quickly.

Stretching of the skeletal muscle results in the stimulation of the muscle spindle fibers, which monitor changes in muscle length. In the knee-jerk response, the stretch is initiated by a tapping on the patellar tendon, causing a deformation that stretches the quadriceps muscle group

([1] in **Figure 20.9**). Sudden stretching of the muscle spindle causes an impulse to be sent to the spinal cord by way of the annulospiral nerve fibers ([2] in **Figure 20.9**). In the gray matter of the spinal cord this sensory fiber bifurcates, with one branch synapsing with an alpha motor neuron ([3a] in **Figure 20.9**). The other branch synapses with an association neuron ([3b] in **Figure 20.9**). The alpha motor neuron exits the spinal cord and synapses with the skeletal muscle, which was originally stretched ([4a] in **Figure 20.9**), resulting in a contraction that is roughly equal in force and distance to the original stretch ([5] in **Figure 20.9**). The inhibitory association neuron synapses with another efferent neuron, which innervates the antagonist muscle (hamstring group in this example), where it causes inhibition; this reflex relaxation of the antagonist muscle in response to the contraction of the agonist is called **reciprocal inhibition**. This response facilitates contraction of the agonist muscle that was stimulated; the inhibited antagonist cannot resist the contraction of the agonist ([4b] in **Figure 20.9**). The muscle spindle is also supplied with a gamma efferent neuron; for clarity, this neuron is shown on the opposite side of the spinal cord ([6] in **Figure 20.9**).

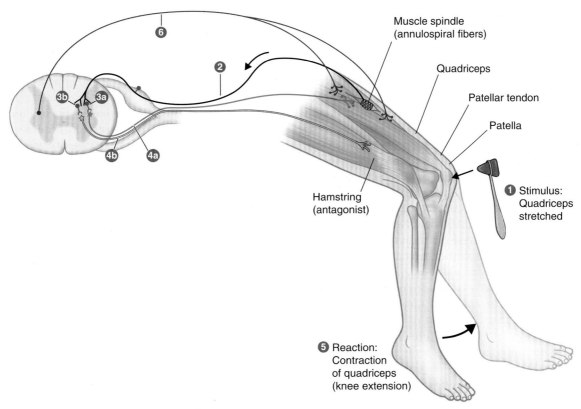

FIGURE 20.9 Myotatic (Stretch) Reflex.
A stimulus (1) is transmitted to the CNS via the afferent neuron (2). In the CNS, association neurons (3a and 3b) activate efferent neurons (4a and 4b) that result in contraction of the agonist and relaxation of antagonist (5). Gamma efferent neurons (6) innervate the muscle spindles and help provide smooth, coordinated movements.

As soon as the lengthening of the muscle stops increasing, the rate of impulse discharge returns to its original level, except for a small static response that is maintained as long as the muscle is longer than its normal length. The static response is elicited by both the annulospiral and flower-spray nerve endings. The resultant low-level muscle contractions oppose the force that is causing the excess length, with the ultimate goal of returning to the resting length. A static response is also invoked if the sensory receptor portion of the neuromuscular spindle is stretched slowly.

Normally, muscle spindles emit low-level sensory nerve signals that help maintain muscle tonus and postural adjustments. **Muscle tonus** is a state of low-level muscle contraction at rest. Muscle spindles also respond to stretch by an antagonistic muscle, to gravity, or to a load being applied to the muscle. The head jerk is an example of the response to gravity, but other muscles such as the back extensors and quadriceps function the same way for unconscious postural adjustments. As an example of the load stimulus, think about what happens if you stand with your elbows at 90°, palms up, and someone places a 10-lb weight in your hands. Before you can consciously adjust to this weight, and because the weight stretches your biceps, the muscle spindles cause a reflex contraction that stops your hands from dropping too far.

In addition to providing maintenance of muscle tone and adjustments for posture and load, the neuromuscular spindle also serves as a damping mechanism that facilitates smooth muscle contractions. This is accomplished by a *gamma loop*.

In a gamma loop, the stretch reflex is activated by the gamma motor neurons ([6] in **Figure 20.9**). Recall that the gamma motor neurons originate in the spinal cord and innervate the distal contractile portions of the intrafusal fibers. Pick up a rubber band and hold it at its maximal, unstretched length with your fingers. Now pull on both ends. What happens to the rubber band in the middle? Obviously, it is stretched. This is precisely what happens when the gamma motor neurons stimulate contractions at both ends of the intrafusal fibers. The central, noncontractile portion of the fibers is stretched, deforming the sensory nerve endings and eliciting the myotatic stretch response.

Reciprocal Inhibition The reflex relaxation of the antagonist muscle in response to the contraction of the agonist.

Muscle Tonus A state of low-level muscle contraction at rest.

What stimulates gamma motor neurons, and why? When signals are transmitted to the alpha motor neurons from the motor cortex or other areas of the brain, gamma motor neurons are almost always simultaneously stimulated. This action is called *coactivation*, and it serves several purposes. First, it provides damping, as mentioned earlier. Alpha and gamma neural signals to contract sometimes arrive asynchronously. But because the response to the gamma motor neuron stimulation is contraction anyway, the gaps can be filled in by reflex contractions, thereby smoothing out the force of contraction. Second, coactivation maintains proper load responsiveness regardless of the muscle length. If, for example, the extrafusal fibers contract less than the intrafusal fibers owing to a heavy external load, the mismatch would elicit the stretch reflex and the additional extrafusal fiber excitation would cause more shortening (Guyton and Hall, 2011). Similarly, because the intrafusal and extrafusal lengths are adjusted to each other, the neuromuscular spindle may be able to help compensate for fatigue by recruiting additional extrafusal fibers by reflex action. Finally, sensory information from neuromuscular spindles is always carried to higher brain centers, where it is unconsciously integrated with other sensory information. If the muscle spindles were not adjusted to the length of the extrafusal fibers during contraction, information on muscle length and the rate of length change could not be transmitted (Guyton and Hall, 2011). Since gamma fibers do adjust the muscle spindle fibers, the gamma loop can assist voluntary motor activity, but it does not actually control voluntary motor activity.

PLYOMETRICS *Plyometrics*, also known as depth jumping or rebound training, is a training exercise in which a concentric contraction is immediately preceded by an eccentric contraction. Plyometrics is an explosive form of physical training used to enhance power output, force production, and velocity. It involves such activities as jumping off a box with both feet together and then immediately performing a maximal jump back onto the box. Plyometric training, alone or in combination with other training modalities, has been shown to be effective in improving power output, force production, jumping height, athletic performance, and bone mineral density (Bobbert, 1990; Markovic and Mikulic, 2010; Robinson et al., 2004; Wilson et al., 1993). While plyometric training has proven effective in improving lower-extremity strength, power, and stretch-shortening muscle function, the mechanisms responsible for the improved performance have not been fully elucidated. However, it appears that the adaptive neuromuscular changes are the result of several factors, including increased neural drive, changes in muscle activation, changes in the mechanical properties of the muscle-tendon complex, and changes in muscle size and/or architecture (Markovic and Mikulic, 2010).

The stretch reflex is caused by activation of the muscle spindles in the agonist muscle. As the agonist is stretched during the eccentric phase of the movement, the muscle spindles activate a reflex arc culminating in stimulation of the alpha-motor neuron and enhanced concentric contraction of the agonist. That is, stretching a muscle before concentrically contracting results in a more forceful contraction than if no prestretch occurred. In addition, as described in Chapter 18 (see Stretch Shortening Cycle, **Figure 18.8**), elastic proteins in the muscle act in a similar manner as a rubber band to enhance the force of contraction. During the eccentric phase, these series elastic components are stretched and stored as potential energy. The stored energy is released on initiation of the concentric phase, allowing a more forceful contraction (Potach and Chu, 2000).

During planned landing activity, such as during plyometric training, there is the potential for the CNS to predict the time of ground contact and to contribute to the control of muscular activity at the time of ground contact. Such CNS-mediated programmed muscular activity may interact with components of reflex responses. Thus, the CNS may initiate jumping movement and participate with reflexes in modifying muscular response to landing (Taube et al., 2012).

Golgi Tendon Organs and Inverse Myotatic Reflex

Golgi tendon organs (GTOs) are receptors activated by stretch or active contraction of a muscle. They transmit information about muscle tension. Activation of these receptors results in a reflex inhibition of the muscle via the inverse myotatic reflex (Marieb and Hoehn, 2010). GTOs are located in the tendons, close to the point of muscular attachment. As shown in **Figure 20.10**, each Golgi tendon organ consists of a thin capsule of connective tissue enclosing collagenous fibers. The collagenous fibers within the capsule are penetrated by fibers of sensory neuron whose terminal branches intertwine with the collagenous fibers. This afferent neuron relays information about muscle tension to the spinal cord. The information is then transmitted to muscle efferents and/or to higher brain centers, particularly the cerebellum.

The Golgi tendon organ is in series with the muscle. The Golgi tendon organ therefore can be stimulated by either stretch or contraction of the muscle. Because of elongation properties of the muscle during stretch, however, active contraction of a muscle is more effective in initiating action potentials within the Golgi tendon organ.

INVERSE MYOTATIC REFLEX As with the myotatic reflex, the inverse myotatic reflex has both a static and dynamic component. When tension increases abruptly and intensely, the dynamic response is invoked. Within milliseconds this dynamic response becomes a lower-level static response within the GTO that is proportional to

The Role of Plyometrics in the Prevention of Lower-Extremity Injuries

Plyometric training is often used to increase muscle strength and improve athletic performance. However, there is compelling evidence that plyometric training can decrease the risk lower-extremity injuries, specifically, anterior-cruciate ligament (ACL) tears in female athletes that participate in sports that involve jumping and pivoting. The results from training studies indicate a reduction in the *rate of injuries* or a *decrease in the risk factors* associated with ACL injuries (such as knee instability, imbalance between quadriceps and hamstring ratio). Hewett et al. (1999) prospectively monitored high school female athletes (soccer, volleyball, and basketball) to access the effectiveness of plyometric training on the rate of injuries. Fifteen sports team participated in a 6-week plyometric training program during their preseason training. Fifteen sports teams did not participate in the structured preseason plyometric training program and served as the control group. The plyometric training consisted of jump and landing techniques designed to increase vertical jump height and increase lower-extremity strength. Training sessions lasted 6 weeks and were led by trained coaches and physical therapists. The training sessions lasted 60–90 minutes a day, 3 d·wk⁻¹. Following the training program the researchers monitored the athletes during their competitive season by compiling weekly injury data. Injury data included reporting of all injuries and in-depth information regarding lower-extremity injuries. Serious injuries were defined as a loss of at least 5 consecutive days of practice or competition. All ACL ruptures were confirmed by arthroscopy. The study found a significantly lower rate of lower-extremity injuries in female athletes who engaged in plyometric training compared to those who did not engage in plyometric training. In fact untrained female athletes had a 3.6 times higher incidence of knee injury than the trained females. This study clearly suggests the preventative role plyometric training can play in reducing the number of knee injuries. Encouragingly, many other studies have replicated this finding.

Sources: Hewett et al. (1999), Markovic and Mikulic (2010), Myer et al. (2006).

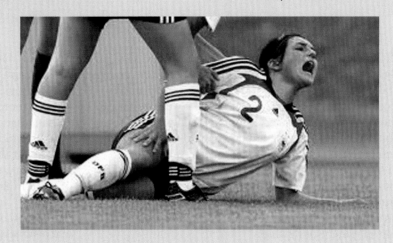

---

the muscle tension. The sequence of events in the inverse myotatic reflex is diagrammed in **Figure 20.11**.

Contraction of a skeletal muscle (or stretching) results in tension that stimulates the Golgi tendon organs in the tendon attached to the skeletal muscle ([1] in **Figure 20.11**). Stimulation of the Golgi tendon organ results in the transmission of impulses to the spinal cord by afferent neurons ([2] in **Figure 20.11**). In the spinal cord, the afferent neuron synapses with an inhibitory association neuron and an excitatory motor neuron ([3] in **Figure 20.11**). In turn, the inhibitory association neuron synapses with a motor neuron that innervates the muscle attached to the tendon; the inhibitory impulses lead to the relaxation of the contracted muscle ([4a] in **Figure 20.11**). The excitatory association neuron synapses with a motor neuron that innervates the antagonist muscle ([4b] in **Figure 20.11**).

Note that as the muscle group originally exhibiting the tension (the agonist) is relaxed, the opposing muscle group (or antagonist) is reciprocally activated. The relaxing action of the Golgi tendon organ serves several important functions. First, the Golgi tendon organ protects against muscle and tendon damage. Excessive tension that might cause muscles and tendons to be torn or pulled away from their attachments is prevented by action of the Golgi tendon organ. For example, a weight lifter who manages to

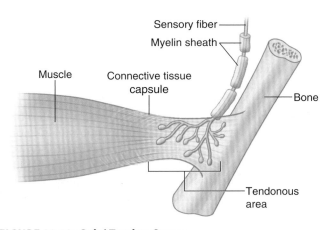

FIGURE 20.10 Golgi Tendon Organ.

Sensory fiber
Myelin sheath
Muscle
Connective tissue capsule
Bone
Tendonous area

FIGURE 20.11 Inverse Myotatic Reflex.
A stimulus (1) is transmitted to the CNS via the afferent neuron (2). In the CNS, association neurons (3) activate efferent neurons (4a and b) that result in relaxation of the agonist (5).

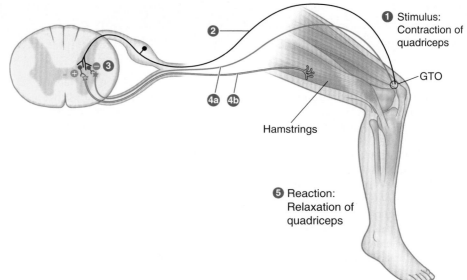

get a heavier barbell off the ground than he or she can really handle may suddenly find his or her muscle giving out because of the action of the Golgi tendon organs. It is speculated that increases in the amount of weight that can be lifted following resistance training are in part due to an inhibition of the Golgi tendon organs, allowing for a more forceful muscle contraction (Gabriel et al., 2006).

The second important advantage of Golgi tendon organ–mediated relaxation is that muscle fibers that are relaxed can be stretched further by opposing muscles or external force without damage. This response is useful in the development of flexibility.

Third, the sensory information regarding tension, which is provided to the cerebellum, allows for muscle adjustment so that only the amount of tension needed to complete the movement is produced. This feature ensures both a smooth beginning and a smooth ending to a movement and is particularly important in movements such as running that involve a rapid cycling between flexion and extension (Biering-Sorensen, 1984).

Volitional Control of Movement

Although reflexes are important for controlling human movement, the volitional control of movement is more important for skilled movement. This section discusses the volitional control of motor units and of whole muscles.

Volitional Control of Individual Motor Units

Healthy people often take the ability to move for granted; they assume that if their brain sends the proper signal, the desired action will simply occur. One discovers that it is not quite that simple when attempting to learn a new sport or when illness or injury intervenes. We normally do not think about conscious control of single motor units. Most people consider reflex action the most basic, albeit unconscious, form of muscle action. But even reflexes involve more than one motor unit and result in muscle activity that can be felt by the individual. In reality, motor unit control is the most basic level of volitional control of movement that can be achieved.

Basmajian (1967) and colleagues performed a series of experiments using intramuscular electrodes attached to a tape recorder and audio-amplifier for sound and an oscilloscope and camera for visual feedback. Initially, when subjects were asked to activate a motor unit, say, in the little finger, they moved the finger and got a typical EMG tracing such as the one shown in **Figure 20.12D**. Gradually, as movement was decreased to virtually nothing but neural signals were still being sent, a single motor unit (identifiable by a characteristic sound and spike pattern) (**Figure 20.12A**) was isolated. Once one motor unit had been isolated, the frequency of its recruitment could be varied. Other motor units could also be isolated (**Figure 20.12B** and **C**), and firings could be varied between the motor units. Thus it has been shown that one truly can control motor units. Precisely *how* this control is achieved is unclear both to the subjects doing it and to the scientists observing it, although some type of proprioceptive feedback is suspected.

Such delicate, discrete control has obvious implications for the refinement of motor skills. Perhaps its greatest benefit, however, is in the area of therapeutic rehabilitation. For example, bioengineers can use trained motor units to control myoelectric prostheses and orthoses. Individuals disabled with conditions such as cerebral palsy can learn better motor control. And some individuals whose spinal cords have been injured but not totally destroyed can learn through such biofeedback to control first one motor unit and then another to regain muscle movement.

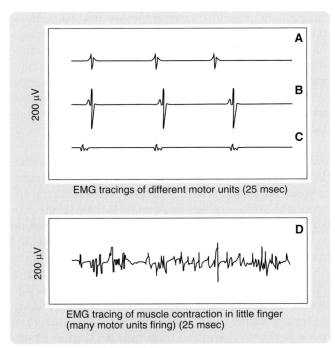

FIGURE 20.12 **Volitional Control of a Single Motor Unit.**
Source: Basmajian, J. V.: Control of individual motor units. *American Journal of Physical Medicine*. 48(1):480–486 (1967). Reprinted by permission of Williams & Wilkins.

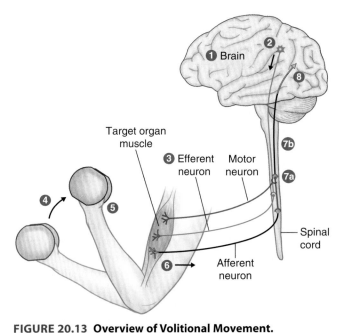

FIGURE 20.13 **Overview of Volitional Movement.**
Voluntary movement is initiated by the brain. Coordinated movement also requires integration of information from several reflexes that monitor muscle length, tension, and joint position.

Volitional Control of Muscle Movement

Figure 20.13 provides an overview of volitional movement. The brain initiates movement ([1] in **Figure 20.13**); that is, the plan for a desired movement, whether to lift a book or perform the high jump, originates in the brain. This information is transmitted down the appropriate descending tract ([2] in **Figure 20.13**). The neurons of the descending tract synapse with the motor neurons in the gray matter of the spinal cord. The efferent motor neuron then carries the impulse to the muscle, the effector organ ([3] in **Figure 20.13**).

On receiving the signal from the nervous system, the muscle contracts and produces movement ([4] in **Figure 20.13**). Changes in muscle length, tension, and position stimulate receptors in the muscles and joints of surrounding muscles ([5] in **Figure 20.13**). This information is transmitted to the central nervous system through afferent sensory neurons ([6] in **Figure 20.13**). The afferent neurons synapse with various association neurons in the gray matter of the spinal cord. In some instances, the neurons synapse with association neurons, which synapse with efferent motor neurons to reflexively control movement ([7a] in

Figure 20.13). In other cases, the association neurons synapse with neurons of the ascending tract, which will carry the information to the brain ([7b] in **Figure 20.13**).

The signals from the ascending pathway are transmitted to the brain, where the information is perceived, compared, evaluated, and integrated in light of past experience, desired outcome, and additional sensory information ([8] in **Figure 20.13**). The brain then adjusts its original message, which is again sent to the muscles via the descending pathway and the motor neuron.

This cycle continues throughout the duration of a given activity. The speed at which the information is transmitted is as remarkable as the degree of integration that occurs. What seems an instantaneous response, on, say, a racquetball court (such as reaction to a powerful serve), actually requires a vast amount of communication within the neuromuscular system.

As already stated, many movements rely on both involuntary reflex action and volitional control of movement. An example is flexibility exercise. Although we decide to initiate stretches, the responses to them depend largely on reflexes.

Flexibility

Flexibility The range of motion in a joint or series of joints that reflects the ability of the musculotendon structures to elongate within the physical limits of the joint.

Flexibility is the range of motion (ROM) in a joint or series of joints that reflects the ability of the musculotendon structures to elongate within the physical limitations of the joint (Hubley-Kozey, 1991). The two basic types of flexibility are static and dynamic. *Static flexibility* is the range of motion about a joint without considering how easily or quickly the range of motion is achieved. *Dynamic flexibility* is the resistance to motion in a joint that affects how easily and quickly a joint can move through its range of motion. Dynamic flexibility is also defined as the rate of increase in tension in a contracted or relaxed muscle as it is stretched. Thus, dynamic flexibility accounts for the resistance to stretch (Knudson et al., 2000). Dynamic flexibility is undoubtedly more important than static flexibility in relation to athletic performances (especially speed events) and the health or diseased condition of the joints (such as arthritis). Resistance to stretch is measured as *stiffness*. The opposite of stiffness is compliance (alteration in response to force). Stiffness is determined by the slope of a curve that plots the load (torque) against elongation (range of motion) for the individual. The steeper the line, the stiffer the muscle is. This testing requires specialized laboratory equipment (Gleim and McHugh, 1997). No standardized measurement technique exists for evaluating dynamic flexibility in practical settings (Plowman, 1992), and very little information is available about dynamic flexibility (Shellock and Prentice, 1985). Therefore, unless specifically stated otherwise, the discussion that follows is limited to static flexibility.

Several anatomical factors affect the range of motion in any given joint. The first is the actual structural arrangement of the joint—that is, the way the bones articulate. Each joint has a specific bony configuration that generally cannot and should not be altered. The soft tissue surrounding the joint, including the skin, ligaments, fascia, muscles, and tendons, also affects joint range of motion. The skin normally has very little influence on the range of motion. The ligaments provide joint stability, and their restriction of range of motion is generally considered necessary and beneficial. Thus, the muscles and their connective tissues are the critical factors that determine flexibility and that can be altered by flexibility training.

Muscles actively resist elongation through contraction and passively resist elongation because of the noncontractile elements of elasticity and plasticity. The difference between elastic and plastic properties is similar to the difference between a rubber band and a balloon. If the rubber band is stretched and then let go, it should rebound to its original length—at least when it is new and has not been frequently stretched. That is elasticity. Blowing up a balloon also stretches it, but when the air is let out of a previously fully inflated balloon, it does not return to its original size. That is plasticity. With flexibility training, one attempts to influence the plastic deformation so that a degree of elongation remains when the force causing the stretch is removed (Plowman, 1992). Flexibility is affected by neuromuscular disorders characterized by spasticity and rigidity, any injuries resulting in scar tissue, and adaptive muscle shortening caused by casting.

Flexibility and stretching are important for everyday living (putting on shoes, reaching the top shelf) and for muscle relaxation and proper posture. Flexibility is obviously important also for sport performance. How important flexibility is depends on the sport. **Table 20.1** lists some popular sports and fitness activities according to

---

TABLE 20.1   Flexibility in Sport and Fitness Activities

Skills Requiring Extreme Range of Motion in Specific Joints	Skills Requiring Greater-Than-Normal Range of Motion in One or More Joints	Skills Requiring Only Normal Range of Motion in Involved Joints
Figure skating	Jumping	Boxing
Gymnastics	Swimming	Long-distance jogging or running
Diving	Wrestling	Archery
Hurdles	Sprinting	Shooting
Pitching	Racquet sports	Curling
Dancing (ballet, modern)	Most team sports	Basketball
Karate		Cross-country skiing
Yoga		Bicycling
		Stair stepping
		Skating (in-line, roller)
		Horseback riding
		Resistance training

Note: If the skills involved with a particular sport do not require greater-than-normal flexibility it does not mean that stretching exercises should not be included in the exercise program.

Source: Modified from Hubley-Kozey, C. L.: Testing flexibility. In MacDougall, J. D., H. A. Weuger, & H. J. Green (eds.): *Physiological Testing of the High-Performance Athlete*. Champaign, IL: Human Kinetics (1991).

the degree of flexibility required. The three degrees of flexibility listed are a normal range of motion, a slightly above-average range of motion in one or more joints, and an extreme range of motion in specific joints.

Gymnasts obviously need to be more flexible than long-distance runners and cyclists. However, no definitive scientific studies directly link selected flexibility values with performance in athletes who can move through the required range of motion (Gleim and McHugh, 1997; Plowman, 1992). For example, a bicyclist with normal range of motion in the ankle, knee, hip, and trunk will not become a better cyclist just by increasing flexibility in those joints.

Measuring Flexibility

The measurement of flexibility is not an exact, standardized procedure with a well-established criterion test. Direct measurement in the laboratory usually measures angular displacement (in degrees) between adjacent segments or from a reference point. Such measurements are usually performed with a goniometer or flexometer. A goniometer resembles a protractor with two arms, one of which is movable. As seen in **Figure 20.14**, the center of the goniometer is placed over the joint about which movement occurs, and the arms are aligned with the body segments on both sides of the joint. For a measurement of the range of motion at the knee joint, the center of the goniometer would coincide with the knee, the stationary arm would be aligned with the upper leg, and the movable arm would be aligned with the lower leg. The angle would be measured at the extreme range of motion for extension and flexion—that is, with the leg completely extended and completely flexed. The range of motion for this joint is the difference between the angles measured.

Flexibility can also be measured with a flexometer. This instrument has a weighted 360° dial and pointer. Range of motion is measured relative to gravity. The instrument is

attached to the body segment to be moved, and the dial is locked at 0° at one extreme of the range of motion. The individual then performs the movement and the pointer is locked at the other extreme range of motion. The range of motion can then be read from the dial.

Flexibility measurements can be made passively, when an external force causes the movement through the range of motion, or actively, when the individual uses muscle action to produce the movement. Testers should note which technique is used because passive measurements are generally higher than active ones (Plowman, 1992).

Field methods for measuring flexibility typically involve linear distances between segments or from an external object. Variations of the stand or sit-and-reach test are the most popular field test of flexibility. To perform the sit-and-reach test, the individual sits with one (now recommended) or both (previously used) stocking feet flat against a testing box. The hands are positioned fully extended from the shoulders onto a scale on top of the testing box. The individual flexes as far forward as possible in a controlled fashion, sliding the fingertips along the scale. The point of maximum reach is recorded.

From the mid-1940s until the mid-1980s, the stand or sit-and-reach test was described as a test of low-back (lumbar) and hip (hamstring) flexibility, mobility, or extensibility. In the mid- to late 1980s, several studies were published showing clearly that although the stand or sit-and-reach test is a valid test of hamstring flexibility, it is *not* a valid test of low-back flexibility (Biering-Sorensen, 1984; Jackson and Baker, 1986; Jackson and Langford, 1989; Kippers and Parker, 1987; Nicolaisen and Jorgensen, 1985).

Because of its widespread use as the only flexibility test in physical fitness test batteries, the sit-and-reach test has often been misinterpreted as a measure of total body flexibility. That is, if an individual has good flexibility in this test, equally good flexibility is assumed in other joint-muscle units. Although this idea is appealing in terms of simplicity and ease of testing, it is not accurate (Clarke, 1975; Shephard et al., 1990). Joint flexibility is highly specific to individual locations; it is not a general trait common to all joints. If the goal of testing is to determine whether an individual is flexible, therefore, a profile of major joints must be compiled because no one test indicates total body flexibility (Araújo, 2004). Joint specificity for flexibility is true throughout the age span of childhood to old age.

The Influence of Sex and Age on Flexibility

Male-Female Comparisons

The specificity of flexibility to each joint makes it difficult to generalize about sex differences. One study has shown that across the entire age spectrum from 10 to 75 years, males exhibited greater anterior trunk flexion (also called lumbar mobility or low-back flexibility) than

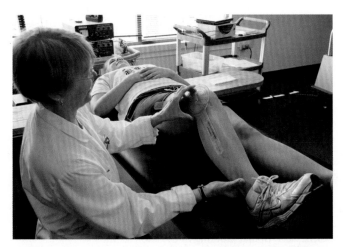

FIGURE 20.14 Use of a Goniometer to Measure Flexibility.

females (**Figure 20.15A**). Conversely, across most of the same age span, females exhibited greater right lateral trunk flexibility than males (**Figure 20.15B**). Although not shown in this figure, females also had greater left lateral flexibility than males, at least in adults.

The differences graphed in **Figure 20.15A** and **B** did not reach statistical significance at all ages and/or were not always tested for significance, so it may be that there really aren't any differences in flexibility between the sexes. Either way, these observations contradict the usual assumption that females are more flexible than males. Other data have shown that adult males are more flexible than adult females in trunk extension (Moll and Wright, 1971) and left and right trunk rotation (Gomez et al., 1991). However, adult males and females do not significantly differ in trunk flexion, trunk extension, left or right lateral trunk flexion (Gomez et al., 1991), left or right head rotation, external shoulder rotation, or plantar or dorsi ankle flexion. Adult males are less flexible than adult females in internal shoulder rotation and hip flexion (Sullivan et al., 1992).

The often-stated but apparently insupportable assumption that females are more flexible than males can probably be attributed to results from the sit-and-reach test. Because studies have shown that females have greater hip flexibility (Shephard et al., 1990), females would be expected to score better than males on the sit-and-reach test. **Figure 20.16** clearly shows that from 5 to 18 years, girls do have a higher sit-and-reach score than boys.

Despite the sit-and-reach results, the results of many other studies show there is no consistent generalized pattern of sex differences in flexibility. Depending on which joint is being measured, females may have a larger, equal, or smaller range of motion than males.

Influence of Age

The impact of age on flexibility is only slightly less confusing. **Figure 20.15A** and **B** illustrates specificity through the pubertal growth years. The general trend is for lumbar flexibility to decrease between 10 and 15 years of age, while lateral flexion generally increases during the same period. The sit-and-reach data (**Figure 20.16**) show an interaction of age and sex (Malina and Bouchard, 1991). Basically, girls show a consistent improvement from age 5 to 18 years, while boys show a U-shaped response—that

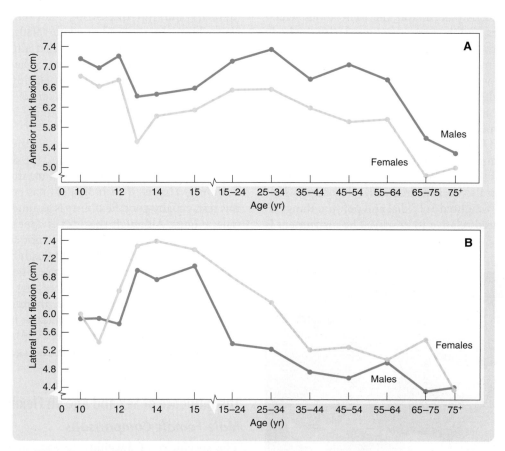

FIGURE 20.15 Flexibility in Males and Females.
A. Anterior trunk flexion (lumbar mobility). **B.** Lateral trunk flexibility.
Sources: Plotted from data of Moran H.M., M.A. Hall, A. Barr: Spinal mobility in the adolescent. *Rheumatology Rehabilitation*. 18:181–185 (1971). Moll, J. M. H. & V. Wright: Normal range of spinal mobility: An objective clinical study. *Annals of Rheumatic Diseases*. 30:381–386 (1971).

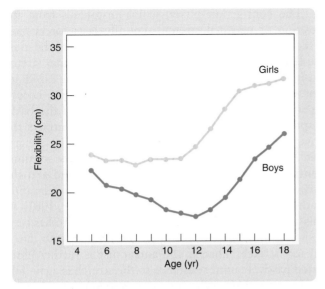

FIGURE 20.16 Flexibility as Measured by the Sit-and-Reach Test.
Source: From Malina, R. M. & C. Bouchard: *Growth, Maturation, and Physical Activity* (2nd edition). Champaign, IL: Human Kinetics, 223, (1991). Copyright 2004 by Robert M. Malina and Claude Bouchard. Reprinted by permission.

is, a gradual decline from age 5 to 13 years and then an improvement from 13 to 18 years, such that they are more flexible in the hip and posterior thigh by adulthood. Whether and how range of motion changes through the growing years is therefore joint specific.

Although **Figure 20.15** shows a pattern of declining flexibility as people progress from young adulthood through middle age and into old age, other studies investigating different joints suggest that flexibility does not change (Gomez et al., 1991; Shephard et al., 1990). An increase in range of motion with age through the adult years has not been shown to occur without training. Therefore, flexibility either declines or stays the same through the adult years. This is probably joint specific in terms of both direction and magnitude. Changes in flexibility with aging may also be confounded by the decreasing activity that often accompanies aging. Most flexibility studies are cross-sectional rather than longitudinal, and this information has not been analyzed taking activity level into account.

All ages appear to be trainable in terms of flexibility (Clarke, 1975; Rider and Daly, 1991). This adaptation may be especially important to the elderly, for whom healthy, independent living is at stake.

> **Ballistic Stretching** A form of stretching, characterized by an action-reaction bouncing motion, in which the involved joints are placed into an extreme range of motion by fast, active contractions of agonist muscle groups.

Flexibility and Low-Back Pain

The theoretical link between muscle function and low-back pain (LBP) was described in Chapter 19 (**Table 19.5**), with particular emphasis there on muscle strength and endurance. Here the emphasis is on the flexibility needs for a healthy, well-functioning back. Flexibility of the low-back and hip area and strong and balanced lumbar, hamstrings, and hip flexor muscles are crucial for controlled pelvic movement. Controlled pelvic movement means having neither an exaggerated anterior tilt (lordotic curve) nor a restricted anterior tilt (no low-back curvature). Either an exaggerated or a restricted pelvic tilt can increase vertebral disc compression and cause pain and strain in the low-back area.

Research shows that individuals suffering from LBP have less range of motion, particularly in the low-back and hamstring areas. As with the reduced strength and endurance, however, these differences are more likely the result of LBP than a cause of it.

One study found that first-time low-back pain could be predicted from lumbar flexibility (Jackson and Baker, 1986). However, in this study, high lumbar flexibility predicted LBP, not low flexibility, as might be expected; and it was predictive only in males. On the other hand, recurrent LBP has been found to be predictable from both low lumbar extension (not flexion) range of motion and low hamstring flexibility (Biering-Sorensen, 1984).

What exact values constitute too low or too high a range of motion are unknown. From the existing research, however, it can be recommended that flexibility of the hip, low back, and hamstrings be part of a general overall fitness program. Flexibility should be developed specifically for athletes as needed. However, flexibility should not be taken to extremes, nor should one expect that flexibility will mean absolute protection from LBP.

Stretching Techniques to Improve Flexibility

The biggest decision in setting up a *flexibility training program* is choosing a stretching technique. Three techniques have been used to increase flexibility: ballistic stretching, static stretching, and proprioceptive neuromuscular facilitation (PNF). **Ballistic stretching**, characterized by an action-reaction bouncing motion, is a form of stretching in which the joints involved are moved to the extremes of the joint range of motion by fast, active contractions of agonist muscle groups. As a result, the antagonistic muscles are stretched quickly and forced to elongate. This quick stretch distorts the intrafusal fibers of the neuromuscular spindle and activates the annulospiral nerve endings, which transmit an impulse to the spinal cord, resulting in an immediate strong reflex contraction (the myotatic reflex) of the muscles that had been stretched (Etnyre and Lee, 1987). This rebound bounce is proportional in force and distance to the original move. Although ballistic action occurs frequently in sports—for example, punting a football or a high kick in dance—and although ballistic stretching has been shown to be effective in increasing flexibility, this type of stretching is generally not recommended. Ballistic stretching may cause muscle soreness. In addition, although virtually no research or clinical evidence supports this, some fear that the forces generated by the series of pulls will exceed the extensibility limits of involved tissues and cause injury (Shellock and Prentice, 1985). Fortunately, alternative means of increasing flexibility do not invoke this (real or imagined) fear of injury.

Static stretching is a form of stretching in which the muscle to be stretched (the antagonist) is slowly put into a position of controlled maximal or near-maximal stretch. The position is held for 10–30 seconds. Because the rate of change in muscle length is slow as the individual gets into position and then stops as the position is held, the annulospiral nerve endings of the neuromuscular spindle (NMS) are not stimulated to fire, and a strong reflex contraction does not occur. That is, the dynamic phase of the NMS response is bypassed. Instead, if the stretch continues for at least 6 seconds, the Golgi tendon organs (GTOs) respond, leading to the inverse myotatic reflex and causing relaxation in the stretched muscle group. This response is called *autogenic inhibition* (Etnyre and Lee, 1987). This relaxation is easily felt by the exerciser, and it allows the muscle to be elongated even further. The impulses from the GTO can override the weaker static response impulses coming from the NMS to allow this reflex relaxation and a continuous sustained stretch. If a maximal stretch is held long enough, the muscle being stretched ultimately reaches a point of **myoclonus**—twitching or spasm in the muscle group—indicating the endpoint of an effective stretch.

Because no uncontrolled sudden forces are involved, injury is unlikely with this type of stretch (Shellock and Prentice, 1985). Indeed, static stretch has been touted as a means not only of avoiding injury but also of relieving muscle soreness. Static stretch before or after dynamic activity involving eccentric muscle contractions does not appear to prevent muscle soreness or delayed-onset muscle soreness (DOMS) (High et al., 1989; Knudson, 1998).

Proprioceptive neuromuscular facilitation (PNF) is a stretching technique in which the muscle to be stretched is first contracted maximally. The muscle is then relaxed and is either actively stretched by contraction of the opposing muscle or is passively stretched by an outside force. A number of different proprioceptive neuromuscular techniques are currently being used for stretching, but the two most popular are the contract-relax (CR) and contract-relax-agonist-contract (CRAC) techniques. In both the CR and CRAC techniques, the muscle to be stretched (the antagonist) is first placed in a position of maximal stretch by action of the agonist and then is contracted maximally, using either a dynamic concentric or static contraction. Both techniques also require the assistance of a partner or an implement to provide resistance and elongation.

The contraction phase, which originates from the position of maximal stretch, typically lasts for at least 6 seconds. Because of the slow rate of change of the muscle length as the individual gets to the maximal stretch position, the annulospiral nerve endings of the NMS are not stimulated to fire, and no reflex contraction occurs. As with a static stretch, the dynamic phase of the NMS response is bypassed. The exerciser then contracts the antagonists against the resistance provided by a partner. As tension is created in the muscle by the maximal contraction, the Golgi tendon organs respond and the inverse myotatic reflex is initiated, causing a relaxation in the stretched muscle group (Etnyre and Lee, 1987). At this point in the CR technique, the partner who has been resisting the contraction moves the relaxed limb into a greater stretch. That is, the antagonist is further elongated passively until resistance to the stretch is again felt.

In the CRAC technique, the exerciser actively contracts the agonist to assist the stretching of the antagonist. By reciprocal inhibition, the contraction of the agonist is thought to aid in the relaxation of the antagonist, allowing it to be stretched further. PNF stretching carries some risk of injury if the partner attempts to push the relaxed limb too far. However, if the partner stops at the point of myoclonus, which can be easily felt with proper hand placement, injury should be avoided.

The role of the Golgi tendon organ in bringing about an inhibitory relaxation of stretched muscle has generally been supported by research studies (Etnyre and Abraham, 1988; Etnyre and Lee, 1987; Hutton, 1992). When needle electrodes were implanted in the stretched muscles, very little EMG activity was recorded, indicating relaxation.

Table 20.2 summarizes the three stretching techniques. Although you have probably used all three techniques in the past, try them again now as described below. Be very conscious of what you are feeling and why.

1. Stand with your feet shoulder's width apart, legs straight, and quickly attempt to place your palms (or if that is easy, your elbows) on the floor. You should bounce back up, but might not have if you didn't go down forcefully because you didn't want to pull your hamstring. Review the action of the NMS in your mind.

2. Stand up with your feet shoulder's width apart, legs straight, and bend over at the waist with your head and arms dangling down. Hold that position until you feel your hamstring muscles relax and allow you to bend even further. Repeat until your hamstrings starts to quiver (myoclonus) or you can't go any further. If you can easily touch the floor initially, stand on a stable box that allows you to reach beyond your feet. Think about the interaction of the GTO and NMS.

3. Lie supine on the floor and place a towel around the heel of one foot so that you can pull on it. Elevate

TABLE 20.2 Summary of Stretching Techniques

	Ballistic	Static	PNF: CR	PNF: CRAC
Action	Antagonist stretched by dynamic contraction of agonist	Antagonist moved slowly to limit of ROM and held	Antagonist moved slowly to limit of ROM by action of agonist, where it contracts maximally for about 6–10 sec	Antagonist moved slowly to limit of ROM by action of agonist, where it contracts maximally for about 6–10 sec
Reaction	Bounce back proportional to force of original contraction	Relaxation and further elongation, usually gravity assisted	Relaxation and further passive elongation by partner or implement, such as towel or jump rope	Relaxation and further passive elongation by active dynamic concentric contraction of agonist
Mechanism	Neuromuscular spindle (myotatic reflex)	Golgi tendon organ, autogenetic inhibition (inverse myotatic reflex)	Golgi tendon organ, autogenetic inhibition (inverse myotatic reflex)	Golgi tendon organ, autogenetic inhibition (inverse myotatic reflex) plus reciprocal inhibition
Advantages	Improves flexibility; may mimic action in sport performance	Improves flexibility and is safest; may provide relief from delayed-onset muscle soreness	Improves flexibility and is safe	Improves flexibility and is safe
Disadvantages	Muscle soreness or injury may result		Requires partner or implement, such as towel, jump rope, or sweats	Requires partner or implement

Note: ROM, range of motion.

that leg straight until you feel resistance. Statically, contract the hamstrings for 6 seconds against the resistance being provided by your towel. Then pull on the towel with your arms to further stretch the hamstrings. This is the CR PNF technique. From the new position, repeat the static contraction for another 10 seconds. This time, stretch the hamstrings by actively contracting the quadriceps of that leg. This is the CRAC PNF technique. Think about the interaction of the NMS, GTO, and reciprocal inhibition needed to perform these actions.

Static Stretching A form of stretching in which the muscle to be stretched is slowly put into a position of controlled maximal or near-maximal stretch by contraction of the opposing muscle group and held for 30–60 seconds.

Myoclonus A twitching or spasm in a maximally stretched muscle group.

Proprioceptive Neuromuscular Facilitation (PNF) A stretching technique in which the muscle to be stretched is first contracted maximally. The muscle is then relaxed and either is actively stretched by contraction of the opposing muscle or is passively stretched.

Work through the exercises provided in the Check Your Comprehension box to ensure that you understand these concepts.

CHECK YOUR COMPREHENSION

Describe an exercise using each of the following techniques for the gastrocnemius (calf) muscle. Then perform the exercise.

1. Ballistic
2. Static
3. CR PNF
4. CRAC PNF

Check your answers in Appendix C.

Physiological Response to Stretching

Coaches and exercise professionals often recommend stretching before activity to prevent injury, improve performance, and prevent delayed-onset muscle soreness (DOMS). Unfortunately, these recommendations, though common, are not based on research evidence. This section describes the acute effects of stretching on flexibility, injury protection, performance, and the sensation of DOMS. The evidence may surprise exercise science students who are familiar with long-standing traditions in this area. As you read, it is important to distinguish between acute responses to pre-exercise stretching and a general program of flexibility training done at another time in terms of positive versus negative responses or adaptations.

Range of Motion

The obvious and well-known response to an acute bout of stretching exercises is increased range of motion of muscles around a joint—an increase in flexibility. To achieve this, muscle relaxation actually occurs within the sarcomeres. Evidence seems to suggest that this relaxation is the combined result of a decline in passive tension that results from the mechanical viscoelastic properties of the muscle and the neural actions for the inverse myotatic reflex (Gleim and McHugh, 1997; McHugh et al., 1999; Smith, 1994). All types of stretching appear to result in an increased range of motion, and no clear evidence suggests that one type of stretching is better than the others (Fields et al., 2007; Larouche and Connolly, 2006). Holding a stretch for 15–30 seconds appears to be more effective than shorter periods, but there is no apparent additional benefit for longer duration stretches. The increased range of motion resulting from an acute bout of stretching lasts for approximately 60–120 minutes (Fields et al., 2007; Fowles et al., 2000; Power et al., 2004).

Performance

Many coaches and exercise leaders suggest that pre-exercise stretching can enhance performance. However, the scientific literature appears to contradict this claim if the performance has a major strength or power component. Several research studies report a decrease in muscle strength following an acute bout of pre-activity stretching. In fact, this phenomenon has been termed the *stretching-induced force deficit* (Fowles et al., 2000). Strength decrements have been reported between 4.5% and 28%, regardless of the testing mode (i.e., isometric, isotonic, or isokinetic) (Rubini et al., 2007). Evidence suggests that the strength decrement may be greater with prolonged stretching than with moderate stretching. One study (Rubini et al., 2007) reported a 8.9% and 12.3% reduction in hip adductor strength following four 30-second sets of static or PNF:CR stretching exercises, respectively. Other studies have reported decreases in maximal voluntary contraction of 23.2% and 28% following static stretches of the plantar flexors for a total of 35–60 minutes, respectively (Avela et al., 1999; Fowles et al., 2000). There is some evidence, however, that ballistic stretching does not cause the same decrement in force that has been consistently reported with static stretching (Herda et al., 2008).

Prestretching may also negatively affect jumping. Several studies have shown that static and PNF stretching results in

a decrease in vertical jump by 3–7.3% (Church et al., 2001; Cornwell et al., 2001, 2002; Di Cagno et al., 2010; Young and Behm, 2003). However, other studies have failed to detect a significant change in vertical jump following acute stretching (Knudson et al., 2001; Power et al., 2004; Unick et al., 2005). Static stretching has been reported to result in significantly lower vertical jump values than a dynamic warm-up in adolescent boys and girls (Faigenbaum et al., 2006a,b). Other performance changes reported as a result of an acute bout of static stretching include a decrease in static balance and reaction time (Behm et al., 2004).

There are two primary hypotheses to explain stretching-induced force deficit. One suggests that mechanical factors within the musculotendinous unit, such as decreases in muscle stiffness or a deformation in the connective tissue, may limit the muscles maximal force production. The other hypothesis proposes that central nervous system factors, such as activation of motor units or reflex sensitivity, is altered by static stretching in a way that impairs maximal force production (Behm et al., 2001; Herda et al., 2008).

Delayed-Onset Muscle Soreness

Static stretching has also been advocated by coaches and exercise professionals as a way to prevent or minimize delayed-onset muscle soreness (DOMS). Unfortunately, the research literature does not support this contention. Meta-analyses investigating the effect of stretching immediately before or after exercise on subsequent delayed muscle soreness found that stretching had no significant effect on soreness (Herbert and Gariel, 2002; Herbert and de Noronha, 2007).

In summary, acute stretching increases range of motion around a joint. However, research suggests that stretching immediately before exercise may result in force decrements that impair other aspects of performance, and it does not appear to prevent or minimize muscle soreness. Therefore, at this point, the best advice may be to conduct flexibility training at times other than before exercise, to warm up before exercise (to increase muscle tendon compliance), and to use individual preference and judgment to decide if a pre-exercise stretch is warranted.

Application of the Training Principles to Flexibility Training

The application of the training principles to flexibility development has not received as much research attention as has the application of training principles to aerobic training programs and resistance training programs. Nonetheless, there is sufficient evidence of the health benefits of flexibility training that the American College of Sports Medicine (ACSM) recommends that flexibility training be included in a well-rounded fitness program

(American College of Sports Medicine, 2011). Guidelines for developing a flexibility training program are given in the following sections.

Specificity

Flexibility is joint specific (Marshall et al., 1980; Shephard et al., 1990) and therefore is also task or sport specific. The first step in developing a flexibility program is to analyze the task or sport to determine the degree of flexibility needed, the specific joint(s) involved, and the plane of action involved. For example, hurdling requires flexion and extension at both the hip and the knee joints and also hip adduction, abduction, and rotation. Swimming requires the same hip flexibility as hurdling; but instead of knee flexion and extension, swimming requires ankle flexion and extension plus inversion, eversion, and shoulder flexion and extension, adduction, abduction, and rotation (Hubley-Kozey, 1991). A general fitness participant should emphasize a total body workout of the major joints and muscle groups.

The response to stretching is not specific to the type of stretching performed or the type of movement that is to follow. How muscle and connective tissue are elongated does not matter as long as the elongation occurs. Because a movement will be done ballistically does not mean that ballistic flexibility work should be done (Etnyre and Lee, 1987; Hardy and Jones, 1986).

Overload

Overload in flexibility training is achieved by placing the muscle and connective tissue at or near the normal limits of extensibility and manipulating the NMS and GTO by holding the position or contracting the muscle to achieve an elongation. A static stretch should be held between 10 and 30 seconds (American College of Sports Medicine, 2011; Fields et al., 2007; Knudson, 1998). PNF stretches with 3–6 seconds of contraction at 20–75% of maximal voluntary contraction followed by 10–30 seconds of assisted stretch is recommended (American College of Sports Medicine, 2011).

A high number of repetitions is not necessary. Two to five are frequently recommended for both the static and PNF flexibility techniques. A reasonable target is to perform 60 seconds of total stretching time for each flexibility exercise (American College of Sports Medicine, 2011).

The intensity of the stretching exercises should be monitored by both myoclonus and pain. Stretched muscles that begin to twitch or spasm (myoclonus) are stretched too far and are fighting that stretch by reflexly trying to contract. Before proceeding, such a muscle should be shortened to the point where the myoclonus ceases. Pain also means the stretch is too intense; pain should not be tolerated. Both the rate of stretch and amount of force should be minimized.

The frequency of the workout should be at least 2–3 d·wk^{-1} in the development phase (American College

of Sports Medicine, 2011; Sharman, et al. 2006). However, stretching 3–5 days a week is an effective way to improve flexibility, and reasonable daily stretching should have no detrimental effects. Indeed, daily stretching is associated with the greatest gains in flexibility.

Rest/Recovery/Adaptation and Progression

Short-term improvements in flexibility have been shown to occur after as little as 1 week of daily sessions (Hardy and Jones, 1986). On the other hand, anecdotal evidence suggests that some people do not improve at all. At any rate, since the individual begins both static and PNF stretching exercises at the limit of extensibility, progression will naturally follow whatever adaptation does occur. Most importantly, except in the case of specific athletic requirements, progression should not continue to extreme flexibility.

Individualization

As stated previously, the most important consideration in flexibility training is that the individual's goals and technique preferences be considered. In a school program, the maturity of the individuals might also need to be considered. For example, if a PNF technique with a partner is going to be used, the partner has to be able to detect the onset of myoclonus and not try just to push as far as possible. Otherwise, individualization is inherent in the flexibility exercises themselves. Each individual stretches to his or her own limits at his or her own rate. Joint looseness is an individual characteristic (Marshall et al., 1980).

Maintenance

Once the appropriate or desired level of flexibility has been attained, it can apparently be maintained by just 1 d·wk^{-1} of training at the same intensity level. These data are based on a study that trained participants three times per week, using five reps of PNF stretching, over a 30-day period. Improvements in flexibility were maintained with only 1 day a week of training, although training three times per week resulted in continued improvements in range of motion (Wallin et al., 1985).

Retrogression/Plateau/Reversibility

Little is known about when or even if a plateau occurs in flexibility training, although there will be a point, probably set by genetics, when further improvement ceases (Etnyre and Lee, 1987). Improvements in flexibility have been shown to continue for at least 8 weeks after the cessation of exercise (Clarke, 1975).

Warm-Up and Cooldown

Considerable confusion exists about the relationship between warming up and stretching before an activity and flexibility training. A *flexibility training program* is a planned, deliberate, and regular program of exercises that can permanently and progressively increase the usable range of motion of a joint or set of joints over time (Alter, 1988). A *warm-up and cooldown stretching program* is a planned, deliberate, and regular program of exercises that are done immediately before and after an activity, with the intent to improve performance and reduce the risk of injury (Alter, 1988). Considerable evidence shows that a flexibility training program can and does improve flexibility, and some evidence suggests that it may decrease injuries in some activities. However, stretching immediately before an exercise may cause performance decrements even while improving joint range of motion.

Stretching does not cause an elevation in body temperature and therefore it is not a warm-up. A cardiovascular warm-up to elevate body temperature should precede stretching exercises regardless of the reason for stretching. The warm-up increases body temperature and therefore makes the muscles and joints more viscous and responsive to stretch. Stretching in conjunction with a warm-up is likely more important and beneficial to individuals whose sport or activity requires greater than normal or extreme range of motion (see **Table 20.1**) but not maximal force production.

Elevated body temperature is believed to decrease the viscous resistance of muscle fibers and tendons, thus leading to increased range of motion. Increased body temperature is also associated with increased nerve conduction rate, which may be important for complex motor tasks or those tasks that require a fast reaction time (Bishop, 2003). Despite the fact that increased body temperature should make stretching more effective, studies have not shown that flexibility gains after 3–4 minutes of warm-up are any different from flexibility gains after 3–4 minutes of warm-up plus 20–30 minutes of aerobic work (Cornelius et al., 1988).

Adaptation to Flexibility Training

Improved Range of Motion

Flexibility exercises and flexibility training improve range of motion, whether the technique used is ballistic, static, or one of the PNF techniques (Etnyre and Lee, 1987; Hutton, 1992; Shellock and Prentice, 1985). A recent randomized controlled clinical trial found that the current ACSM recommendations for flexibility training are effective for improving flexibility in young adults (Sainz de Baranda and Ayala, 2010). Many studies have explored the question of which technique brings about the greatest improvement. All types of flexibility are effective in bringing about changes in range of motion around a joint, but PNF stretching techniques appear to yield the greatest gains. Stretching programs using PNF techniques twice a week for up to 12 weeks have resulted in increases in range of motion of 21–32° in long-lever hip flexion (Sharman et al., 2006). The physiological

basis of training-induced changes in range of motion is not well understood. It has been speculated that relatively permanent anatomical changes occur in connective tissue, but these changes have not been documented. Changes in neural sensitivity or simply an increase in "stretch perception or tolerance modulation" may be involved (Gleim and McHugh, 1997; McHugh et al., 1999; Sharman et al., 2006; Smith, 1994).

Despite expressed concern about the effect of resistance training on flexibility, little scientific or empirical evidence suggests that resistance training decreases flexibility. In fact, studies have shown that heavy resistance training results in either an improvement or no change in flexibility in some joints (Massey and Chaudet, 1956; Monteiro et al., 2008). Furthermore, competitive weight lifters have average or above-average flexibility in most joints (Leighton, 1957). So that flexibility is not lost, those engaged in resistance training should stress the full range of motion of both the agonists and the antagonists.

Delayed-Onset Muscle Soreness

Muscle damage and resulting soreness and performance impairments are common in exercise and sport situations. As discussed in Chapter 18, delayed-onset muscle soreness (DOMS) is characterized by muscle soreness and stiffness that appears approximately 8 hours after exercise and increases and peaks over the next 24–48 hours. Because of the unpleasant sensations of muscle soreness and its interference with subsequent training and performance there is considerable interest in finding modalities to lessen muscle soreness. As discussed earlier in this chapter, several authors have suggested that an acute bout of stretching may lessen the soreness associated with exercise—especially eccentric exercise. However, research studies have not supported the notion that acute stretching can attenuate muscle soreness. In contrast, a program of flexibility training has been shown to decrease muscle soreness and muscle damage (measured by plasma CK levels) following a bout of eccentric exercise (Chen et al., 2011). Participants were assigned to a static stretching, proprioceptive neuromuscular facilitation (PNF), or control group. Participants in the stretching group performed stretching activity three times a week for 8 weeks. Both stretching groups improved their range of motion compared to the control group. Furthermore, both groups had smaller decrements in force production following the eccentric exercise than the control group and both stretching groups suffered less soreness. These results demonstrate that a flexibility training program, consisting of either static stretching or PNF, is protective against muscle damage and soreness.

Injury Prevention

Exercise professionals routinely recommend pre-exercise stretching as a way to prevent injury. The rationale for this is that stretching increases the compliance (decreases the stiffness) of the tendon unit and thus theoretically makes it less prone to injury (Witvrouw et al., 2004). In fact, there is evidence that 8 weeks of stretching can alter the viscoelastic properties of tendons, making them more compliant (Kabo et al., 2002).

However, despite this theoretical rationale and current widespread recommendations, the precise effects of pre-activity stretching on injury are not fully documented, largely because of major difficulties in conducting definitive studies. To determine the actual effect of pre-exercise stretching on risk of injury, a researcher would have to (1) randomly assign large numbers of athletes, exercisers, or workers of similar physical and fitness characteristics into groups that do and do not stretch before activity; (2) devise stretching routines that were completely standardized, carefully monitored, and did not include other confounding variables such as a warm-up period; and (3) continue the study long enough to ensure that an adequate number of injuries occurred for statistical analysis to be meaningful (including an analysis of the frequency of injuries and the types of injuries). Furthermore, when trying to determine the effect of stretching on risk of injury, a distinction must be made between long-term stretch programs that lead to adaptations (including increased flexibility) and an acute bout of stretching performed before the exercise. In fact, studies that investigate the effect of an acute bout of prestretching almost always do so as part of an ongoing training program.

Muscles, tendons, and ligaments are the tissues injured most frequently in work and in fitness and sports participation. Presently, there are no data available on an acute bout of stretching and injury incidence. There are data on flexibility training and injury rates. However, there is no conclusive evidence that high levels of flexibility or improvements in flexibility either protect against injury or reduce the severity of injury, including low-back pain (Hart, 2005; Park and Chou, 2006; Plowman, 1992; Shrier, 2004; Small et al., 2008; Thacker et al., 2004; Witvrouw et al., 2004). Indeed, there is some indication that hypermobility, or loose ligamentous structure, may predispose some individuals to injury or low-back pain (Gleim and McHugh, 1997; Plowman, 1992). However, as described in the accompanying Focus on Research Box, some studies have found no decreased risk of injury following a stretch program, whereas other studies have documented decreased injury risk. Many practitioners continue to believe that stretching is an important part of preparing for activity (Fields et al., 2007), but the available evidence does not uniformly back the suggestion that stretching prevents injury.

Nevertheless, individuals with poor flexibility for the task they will perform probably have a greater risk of exceeding the extensibility limits of the musculotendon unit. Such individuals should work on improving their flexibility. Likewise, individuals whose sports may cause maladaptive shortening in certain muscles should perform stretching exercises to counteract this tendency. Individuals who are shown to be hypermobile need to concentrate on strengthening the musculature around those joints.

Balance

All human movement requires continual muscular adjustments in posture to accommodate changes in the center of gravity as we move. Even the apparently simple act of standing motionless requires a continual process of minute adjustments of body position to keep the center of gravity over the base of support. As with flexibility, balance may be classified as static or dynamic. **Static balance** is the ability to make adjustments to maintain posture while standing still, whereas **dynamic balance** is the ability to make necessary adjustments while the center of gravity and the base of support are in motion. Clearly dynamic balance is more important during activities, from relatively simple activities like walking to more complex movements like a balance bar routine. Balance has traditionally been viewed as an important component of sport-specific fitness, and in fact many sports do require a great deal of balance. However, balance is also an essential skill of daily living. Good balance is critical for preventing falls, a leading cause of injury and mortality among older adults. Some authors have therefore argued that balance should be included as a component of health-related fitness (Claxton et al., 2006).

Balance is highly dependent on the nervous system and involves continuous feedback from visual, vestibular, and somatosensory inputs as well as rapid and coordinated activation of the muscular system. Postural control is a complex motor skill involving multiple sensorimotor processes. The two main functional goals of postural control are postural orientation and postural equilibrium. Postural orientation involves the control of body alignment and tone with respect to gravity, the support surface, the environment, and internal senses. This orientation relies heavily on sensory information received from the visual, somatosensory, and vestibular sensory organs. Postural equilibrium involves the integration and coordination of sensorimotor strategies to stabilize the body's center of mass during both voluntary and externally triggered disturbances in postural stability (Horak, 2006). When considering factors that affect an individual's risk of falling, it is important to realize that balance is a complex skill influenced by multiple factors. Not surprisingly, no single test adequately assesses balance, and probably no single type of exercise training can improve all components of balance.

Static Balance The ability to make adjustments to maintain posture while standing still.

Dynamic Balance The ability to make necessary postural adjustments while the center of gravity and the base of support are in motion.

Conflicting Views on Flexibility Training and Injury Risk

Prestretching Has No Apparent Effect on Risk of Injury

Military recruits undergo rigorous physical training shortly after enlisting in the service. The large number of new recruits in training makes this a good environment for a study investigating different strategies to prevent injury. In the study presented here, researchers investigated the effect of a stretching program on lower-limb injury in a large group of male recruits who enlisted in the Australian Army. The authors randomly assigned 1538 male recruits to a stretching or control group. During the following 12 weeks of training, both groups performed active warm-up exercises before physical training. In addition, the stretch group performed one 20-second stretch for each of six leg muscle groups. During the 12 weeks of training, 333 lower-limb injuries were reported: 158 injuries in the stretching group and 175 injuries in the control group, with no statistically significant difference between the groups. The authors concluded that typical muscle stretching performed before physical training does not produce clinically meaningful reductions in risk of exercise-related injuries in army recruits.

Importantly, however, the authors did find that a low level of fitness was a consistent and strong predictor of injury. In this study, the least fit participants (based on a 20-m shuttle run/PACER) were 14 times more likely to sustain a lower-limb injury than the fittest participants. Thus, while pre-exercise stretching does not appear to provide much protection against injury, high levels of fitness do help prevent injuries.

Source: Pope, R. P., R. D. Herber, J. D. Kirwan, & B. J. Graham: A randomized trial of preexercise stretching for prevention of lower-limb injury. *Medicine & Science in Sports & Exercise.* 32(2):271–277 (2000).

Flexibility Decreases Overuse Injuries

Although it has long been proposed that increased flexibility is associated with a lower injury rate, only limited scientific data have supported this hypothesis. Decreasing the incidence of injury is important for obvious reasons, including the fact that injuries that occur with the initiation of a fitness program often cause participants to discontinue exercise. In the military, basic training is often interrupted because of injuries sustained during training. To test the hypothesis that increased hamstring flexibility would decrease lower-extremity overuse injury in military basic trainees, Hartig and Henderson (1999) incorporated flexibility training in the scheduled fitness training of a company going through basic training. This group's change in flexibility and subsequent rate of lower-extremity injury were compared to another group (control group) that went through basic training at the same time. Both the intervention and control groups participated in 13 weeks of basic training program with the normal routine of stretching before physical training, including hamstring stretching. The intervention group added three hamstring stretching sessions (before lunch, dinner, and bedtime) each day. The stretching routine involved a partner holding the leg to be stretched at approximately 90°, while the participant moved his trunk forward with an anterior tilt at the pelvis until he perceived a hamstring muscle stretching sensation without pain. Each stretch was performed five times for each extremity and held for 30 seconds. At the completion of basic training, the control group had increased their hamstring flexibility by 3°, whereas the intervention group had increased their hamstring flexibility by 7°. Forty-three lower-extremity overuse injuries occurred in the control group, an incidence of 29.1%, compared with 25 injuries in the intervention group, an incidence of 16.7%. These researchers concluded that a simple stretching program that requires little time is effective in improving flexibility and decreasing the incidence of injury.

Source: Hartig, D. E. & J. M. Henderson: Increasing hamstring flexibility decreases lower extremity overuse injuries in military basic trainees. *The American Journal of Sports Medicine.* 27(2):173–176 (1999).

Given the conflicting evidence presented in these two studies, and reflected more generally in the literature, what advice should an exercise professional give about stretching before an event to decrease risk of injury? At this point, it seems prudent to recognize that stretching has not consistently been shown to prevent injury, but that there is some evidence that it may. However, the evidence clearly suggests that the application of the training principles, discussed throughout this text, is appropriate. In this case, it is particularly important to progress gradually, that is, to build fitness level progressively as a way to lessen risk of injury, and to accept that individuals may respond to stretching differently.

Measurements of Balance

The most sophisticated laboratory measurements of balance include the use of a force platform that can measure movement of the center of pressure and provide an indication of postural sway. Software used with these instruments can calculate various parameters during a stationary balance test, such as area outlined by the center of pressure path, the total distance traversed, and the maximum excursion in a particular plane, which are assumed to provide an indication of balance (Hrysomallis, 2007).

Field methods for assessing balance typically involve measuring static balance. The most common technique is the timed, single-limb balance test. The individual stands one foot on a flat, stable surface with eyes closed for as long as he or she can without moving. Another technique to assess static balance is the flamingo balance test in which balance is assessed in terms of the number of trials it takes for the participant to balance on one leg on a narrow balance beam for 1 minute with eyes open. Dynamic balance can be assessed using a modification of the timed, single-limb balance test described above, but in the dynamic balance test the individual stands on an unstable surface such as a foam balance mat (Hrysomallis, 2007). There is little consensus about which of the various tests is most appropriate for measuring balance, and not enough information is available to categorize balance based on the values derived from a balance test. In other words, although a person who could maintain the balance for 80 seconds on a timed, single-limb balance test would be considered to have better balance than a person who could maintain the balance for only 55 seconds, it is not clear what represents a "normal" or "good" level of balance. The lack of standard test techniques and appropriate normative category scales makes it difficult to interpret much of the literature about the relationship between balance and injury.

The Influence of Sex and Age on Balance

Balance improves as children mature. Both the sensory and motor processes involved with balance seem to undergo developmental maturation. The influence of proprioceptive function on stance stability has been reported to be completely developed by 4 years, whereas visual and vestibular influence reached adult levels by 16 years (Steindl et al., 2004). Research suggests possible differences between the sexes in balance parameters in children. A study that investigated several balance parameters in children who were approximately 10, 13, and 16 years found that boys exhibited greater and faster movements in the center of pressure than girls in the youngest age group. Furthermore, the boys showed age-related improvements in sway parameters (Nolan et al., 2005).

Older adults have an increased risk of falling, making balance a particular concern in this population. Falls are a common and devastating problem, causing tremendous amounts of morbidity, mortality, and use of health care services, including nursing home admissions (Rubenstein, 2006). Prospective studies indicate that 30–60% of independent living older adults fall each year and approximately 5–10% of falls result in serious injuries such as fractures or head trauma requiring hospitalization (Granacher et al., 2012). In 2007, there were nearly 1.5 million reported falls in the United States in patients over 75 years, with 400,000 requiring hospitalizations (Siracuse et al., 2012). In addition to medical complications associated with falling, the economic impact is enormous—the health care cost of older adults (>75 years) is about 5.5 times great than younger adults (25–34 years), in large part due to the incidence of fall-related injuries (Granacher et al., 2012). Given the dramatic effects of a serious fall and related injury on an individual, and the staggering health care

costs associated with serious injury, decreasing the risk of falling has become a major public health concern. Good balance depends on feedback from the visual, somatosensory, and vestibular senses and relies on muscle strength, reflex control, and reaction time. With increasing age, a progressive loss of functioning occurs in these systems, causing an increased risk of falling (Carter et al., 2001; Lord and Sturnieks, 2005).

Studies investigating balance in adults routinely report that balance decreases as an individual ages (Carter et al., 2006; Era et al., 2002; Holviala et al., 2006; Punakallio, 2003). A cross-sectional study found that older adults (over 50 years) had a lower functional balance and higher postural sway balance than younger adults (<39 years) (Punakallio, 2003). A longitudinal study that investigated balance in a group of older adults at age 75 years and again 5 years later (at age 80 years) found that balance deteriorated markedly in both sexes. However, women in this study scored better on the balance test than the men at both points in time (Era et al., 2002). Underscoring the importance of balance, the simple balance test of having individuals stand with their eyes open was a significant predictor of survival over the 5-year follow-up period.

Balance Techniques

Balance training programs may involve performing basic balance tasks such as alternating one-leg stands, standing on one leg with eyes closed, backward walking, and the use of a stability ball (**Figure 20.17**). Balance training

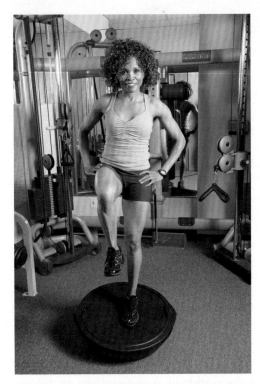

FIGURE 20.17 Stability Ball Training to Improve Balance.

FOCUS ON APPLICATION
A Safe Exercise Environment

The diagram outlines how intrinsic factors (related to the individual) and extrinsic factors (related to the environment) may influence the risk of falling and the risk of serious injury from a fall. This figure distinguishes between impairments (the loss or abnormality of psychological, physiological, or anatomical structure or function) and disability (a restriction or lack of ability to perform an activity in the manner or within the range that is considered normal) (Schuntermann, 1996).

Exercise professionals have a responsibility to do what they can to minimize the risk of falls and injury when working with any individuals, especially older adults or those at risk for falling.

This requires understanding intrinsic factors that increase the risk for falling and being mindful of environmental factors (such as a slippery floor, poor lighting) that may increase the risk of injury.

Source: Carter et al. (2001).

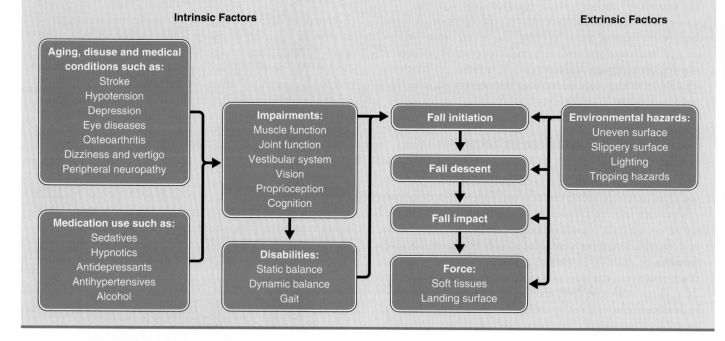

Intrinsic Factors

Extrinsic Factors

Aging, disuse and medical conditions such as:
Stroke
Hypotension
Depression
Eye diseases
Osteoarthritis
Dizziness and vertigo
Peripheral neuropathy

Impairments:
Muscle function
Joint function
Vestibular system
Vision
Proprioception
Cognition

Fall initiation

Fall descent

Fall impact

Force:
Soft tissues
Landing surface

Environmental hazards:
Uneven surface
Slippery surface
Lighting
Tripping hazards

Medication use such as:
Sedatives
Hypnotics
Antidepressants
Antihypertensives
Alcohol

Disabilities:
Static balance
Dynamic balance
Gait

---

may also use a specialized training aid such as the wobble board. The wobble board consists of a round section fixed to the top of a hemispherical section allowing for multiplanar movement. The wobble board is common in rehabilitative settings and has traditionally been used to help injured athletes work on strength, flexibility, and balance following a lower-limb injury.

Tai Chi is a form of training that employs self-initiated slow but continuous rhythmical movements and emphasizes multidirectional weight shifting, awareness of body alignment, and abdominal and lower-extremity muscle function. Both cross-sectional and controlled studies have shown that Tai Chi can lead to improved functional balance, with a reduction in falls in older persons (Li et al., 2004).

Physiological Responses to Balance Techniques

The vast majority of studies related to balance focus on long-term adaptations in the neuromuscular system related to injury reduction. The short-term physiological responses to a single bout of balance training exercises have received little attention.

Application of the Training Principles to Balance

Because balance involves the nervous and muscular systems and is influenced by flexibility and strength, balance training programs can be expected to follow the well-established training principles. However, relatively little scientific work has tested how best to apply the training principles to balance training. See the Focus on Research—Clinically Relevant study for when it might be best to do balance training. Remember, however, that much of the motivation for balance training comes from practitioners who work with older adults and seek to reduce the risk of

The Timing of Balance Training on Balance Ability

This study was designed to determine whether a single soccer practice/training session affected the player's balance ability and whether a balance training program was more effective when performed before or after the regular soccer practice/training. Thirty-nine high school–aged male soccer players (age = 16 ± 1 years; weight = 66 ± 6 kg; height = 174 ± 6 cm) were randomly divided into a control group (C = 13), a training group that followed a balance program before the regular soccer practice sessions (TxB = 13), and a training group that followed the same balance program after the soccer practice sessions (TxA = 13). Thirty-one of the subjects were right leg dominant for kicking the soccer ball. Training lasted 12 weeks and was performed three times per week for 20 minutes each session.

Balance was assessed before and after practice and before and after balance training by three different balance boards and the Biodex Stability System. Board 1a restricted movement to the anteroposterior direction only; board 1b restricted movement to the mediolateral direction only; board 1c allowed movement in both anteroposterior and mediolateral directions. On each board, the player maintained a single-limb stance for as long as possible. The best of three trials was recorded and used for analysis. In the Biodex test, the player maintained a single-limb stance for 20 seconds with the platform set to move freely by up to 20° from level in any direction. From the variance of the platform displacement, an instability index (Ii) was computed. Maximal effort isokinetic knee extension-flexion contractions were performed at angular velocities of 60° per second and 180° per second on a Cybex machine before and after a single soccer practice. These measurements were intended to determine the extent of muscular fatigue from a single soccer practice.

The balance training program consisted of five postural stability exercises in random order:

1. A 3-minute attempt to move a cursor depicting the position of the center of foot pressure (COP) to a specific target on a screen while standing on the Biodex platform.

2. A 45-second attempt to maintain a single-leg stance on board 1a.

3. A 45-second attempt to maintain a single-leg stance on board 1b.

4. A 45-second attempt to maintain a single-leg stance on board 1c.

5. A 45-second attempt to maintain a single-leg stance on a mini trampoline.

In all tasks, the players were asked to kick back a soccer ball thrown at them by the trainer with their nonsupporting leg. Both legs were worked, 15 seconds apart.

Results showed only an approximately 10%, statistically nonsignificant, decrease in maximal isokinetic joint measurements from before to after practice, meaning that there was no substantial muscle fatigue from the single soccer practice session. What minor changes did occur had no impact on any of the balance performances.

No differences in balance ability were found in the control (C) group before and after the 12 weeks. Conversely, the 12-week balance training program improved all the balance performance tests in both the before (TxB) and after (TxA) training groups. As seen in the accompanying figures, balance tested on the board 1a and board 1b tests improved in both groups that participated in balance training (both the group that did balance training before soccer practice [TxB] and the group that did balance training after soccer practice [TxA]). Additional analyses revealed that the improvement in balance measured using the board 1a test was greater in the TxA (after) group than the TxB (before) group for both legs. Furthermore, the improvement in balance measured on board 1b was greater in the after group than the before group but only for the left leg. These results indicate that balance exercises are most effective in improving balance when performed after rather than before the sport-specific practice. While this is only one study, it may mean that balance, much like flexibility, is best trained for after exercise.

Source: Gioftsidou, A., P. Malliou, G. Pafis, A. Beneka, G. Godolias, & C. N. Maganaris: The effects of soccer training and timing of balance training on balance ability. *European Journal of Applied Physiology.* 96:659–664 (2006).

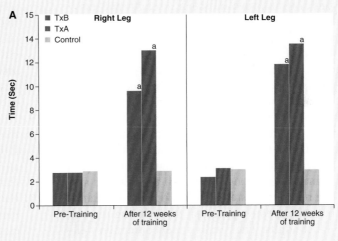

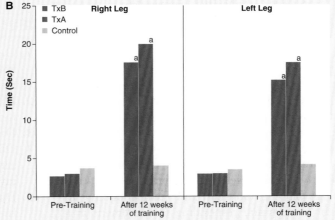

falls and injuries in this population. Thus, it is important that balance training, whether done by itself or as part of a multifaceted exercise program like Tai Chi that also seeks enhanced balance, be initiated at a level the participant can safely perform and be progressed slowly.

Adaptation to Balance Training

It is difficult to quantify the effect of balance training on balance because most studies using a balance training program have focused on the effect of training balance on injury prevention rather than on balance itself. A recent examination of six studies investigating the effect of balance training on injury prevention in active young adults (Hrysomallis, 2007) reported that balance training significantly reduced the incidence of recurrent ankle sprains in soccer players, recreational athletes, and volley ball players. However, not all studies have shown a decrease in ankle sprains. More importantly, two studies (Söderman et al., 2000; Verhagen et al., 2004) reported an increase in knee injuries in the groups that underwent balance training. Clearly additional research is warranted to better understand what constitutes an appropriate balance training program and the potential such a program has to reduce the risk of injury in young active adults.

Several studies have focused on multifaceted intervention studies to improve muscular strength and functional balance in older adults to reduce the risk of falling (Barnett et al., 2003). A program of heavy resistance exercise in a group of elderly women led to increased maximal strength, increased walking speed, and improved balance (Holviala et al., 2006). Both cross-sectional and controlled studies have provided evidence that Tai Chi results in improved functional balance and fewer falls in older persons (Li et al., 2004). While the studies cited above did not investigate balance training programs in isolation, they focused on neuromuscular training that is likely to influence components of both the nervous system and the muscular system that contribute to balance and that have the greatest potential for reducing the risk of falls in older adults. The results are encouraging: well-designed exercise programs that increase strength and improve balance can foster greater independence in older adults and lessen the risk of fall injury.

SUMMARY

1. The spinal cord performs the essential functions of connecting the peripheral nervous system with the brain and serving as a site of reflex integration.
2. Voluntary motor impulses are transmitted from the motor area of the brain to somatic efferent neurons, leading to skeletal muscles via the pyramidal pathways.
3. Reflexes play an important role in maintaining an upright posture and responding to movement in a coordinated fashion. Reflexes are rapid, automatic responses to stimuli in which a specific stimulus results in a specific motor response.
4. The myotatic reflex is initiated in response to a sudden change in length of the muscle. When a muscle is quickly stretched, the annulospiral nerve endings in the NMS transmit an impulse to the spinal cord, which results in an immediate strong reflex contraction of the same muscle from which the signal originated.
5. The inverse myotatic reflex is initiated when tension increases abruptly and intensely and stimulates Golgi tendon organs; it results in inhibition of the tensed muscle group, causing relaxation.
6. Volitional control of movement can function at the level of the motor unit as well as at the whole muscle level.
7. Flexibility is joint specific, and the degree of flexibility is specific to the individual. Stretching prior to exercise may decrease muscular power, strength, reaction time, and balance while increasing range of motion. Static stretching or proprioceptive neuromuscular facilitation techniques are recommended to enhance flexibility. Flexibility training improves range of motion. The decreases in performance components that occur after acute stretching do not occur as adaptations to flexibility training.
8. Researchers disagree considerably about the extent to which stretching before an activity decreases risk of injury: stretching has not been convincingly demonstrated to be associated with decreased risk of injury, although many athletes and coaches with considerable experience continue to believe in its effectiveness. Flexibility training has been shown to attenuate eccentric-induced muscle damage.
9. Despite popular belief, scientific evidence suggests that resistance training is not detrimental to flexibility. In fact, studies have shown that heavy resistance training results in either an improvement or no change in flexibility.
10. Balance is an important fitness component of particular interest because of its relationship to falls in the elderly.

REVIEW QUESTIONS

1. Describe the anatomical relationship between nerves and muscles. What is the functional significance of this relationship?
2. Diagram the sequence of events that occur at the neuromuscular junction.
3. Diagram the components of a generalized reflex arc.
4. Diagram the components of the myotatic reflex. Pay careful attention to the afferent and efferent neurons involved.
5. Diagram the components of the inverse myotatic reflex.

6. Outline the sequence of events involved in volitional control of movement.

7. Provide a rationale for incorporating a flexibility training program into an overall fitness program.

8. Critique the appropriateness of the sit-and-reach test to predict low-back pain.

9. What are the anatomical requirements of a healthy low back?

10. Describe static stretching, and explain the involvement of reflexes in muscle elongation during this type of stretching.

11. Describe the proprioceptive neuromuscular facilitation technique, and explain the involvement of reflexes in muscle elongation during this type of stretching.

12. Describe the responses to an acute bout of static stretching.

13. Discuss the application of the individual training principles to the development of a flexibility program and the training adaptations that occur.

14. Discuss the components of balance, how an alteration in these components can increase the risk of falling with aging, and how a training program may decrease the risk of falling.

For further review and additional study tools, visit the website at http://thePoint.lww.com/Plowman4e ✳ ◉

REFERENCES

Alter, M. J.: *The Science of Stretching*. Champaign, IL: Human Kinetics (1988).

American College of Sports Medicine: Position stand on the quantity and quality of exercise for developing and maintaining cardiorespiratory, musculoskeletal, and neuromotor fitness in apparently healthy adults: Guidance of prescribing exercise. *Medicine & Science in Sports & Exercise*. 43(7):1334–1359 (2011).

Avela, J., H. Kyröläinen, & P. V. Komi: Altered reflex sensitivity after repeated and prolonged passive muscle stretching. *Journal of Applied Physiology*. 86(4):1283–1291 (1999).

Barnett, A., B. Smith, S. R. Lord, M. Williams, & A. Baumand: Community-based group exercise improves balance and reduces falls in at-risk older people: a randomized controlled trial. *Age and Ageing*. 32:407–414 (2003).

Basmajian, J. V.: Control of individual motor units. *American Journal of Physical Medicine*. 48(1):480–486 (1967).

Behm, D. G., A. Bambury, F. Cahill, & K. Power: Effect of Acute Static Stretching on Force, Balance, Reaction Time, and Movement Time. *Medicine & Science in Sports & Exercise*. 36(8):1397–1402 (2004).

Behm, D. G. D. C., Button, & J. C. Butt. Factors affecting force loss with prolonged stretching. *Canadian Journal of Applied Physiology*. 26(3):261–272 (2001).

Biering-Sorensen, F.: Physical measurements as risk indicators for low-back trouble over a one year period. *Spine*. 9(2):106–119 (1984).

Bishop, D.: Warm up I: Potential mechanisms and the effects of passive warm up on exercise performance. *Sports Medicine*. 33(6):929–939 (2003).

Bobbert, M. F.: Drop jumping as a training method for jumping ability. *Sports Medicine*. 9(1):7–22 (1990).

Carter, N. D., P. Kannus, & K. M. Khan: Exercise in the prevention of falls in older people: A systematic literature review examining the rationale and the evidence. *Sports Medicine*. 31(6):427–438 (2001).

Chen, C. H., K. Nosaka, H. L. Chen, M. J. Lin, K. W. Tseng & T. C. Chen: Effects of flexibility training on eccentric exercise-induced muscle damage. *Medicine & Science in Sports & Exercise*. 43(3): 491–500 (2011).

Church, J. B., M. S. Wiggins, F. M. Moode, & R. Crist: Effect of warm-up and flexibility treatments on vertical jump performance. *Journal of Strength and Conditioning Research*. 15(3):332–336 (2001).

Clarke, H. H.: Joint and body range of motion. In *Physical Fitness Research Digest* (series 5, no 4). Washington, DC: President's Council on Physical Fitness and Sports (1975).

Claxton, D. B., M. Troy, & S. Dupree: A question of balance. *Journal of Physical Education, Recreation and Dance*. 77(3):32–37 (2006).

Cornelius, W. L., R. W. Hagemann, & A. W. Jackson: A study on placement of stretching within a workout. *Journal of Sports Medicine and Physical Fitness*. 28:234–236 (1988).

Cornwell, A., A. G. Nelson, G. D. Heise, & B. Sidaway: Acute effects of passive muscle stretching on vertical jump performance. *Journal of Human Movement Studies*. 40:307–324 (2001).

de Araújo, G. G. S.: *Flexitest: An Innovative Flexibility Assessment Method*. Champaign, IL: Human Kinetics (2004).

Cornwell, A., A. G. Nelson, & B. Sidaway: Acute effects of stretching on the neuromechanical properties of the triceps surae complex. *European Journal of Applied Physiology*. 86:428–434 (2002).

Di Cagno, A., C. Baldari, C. Battaglia, M. C. Gallotta, M. Videira, M. Piazza, & L. Guidetti: Preexercise static stretching effect on leaping performance in elite rhythmic gymnasts. *Journal of Strength and Conditioning Research*. 24(8):1995–2000 (2010).

Era, P., E. Heikkinen, I. Gause-Nillson, & M. Schroll: Postural balance in elderly people: Changes over a five-year follow-up and its predictive value for survival. *Aging Clinical and Experimental Research*. 14(3 Suppl):37–46 (2002).

Etnyre, B. R. & L. D. Abraham: Antagonist muscle activity during stretching: A paradox reassessed. *Medicine and Science in Sports and Exercise*. 20:285–289 (1988).

Etnyre, B. R. & E. J. Lee: Dialogue: Comments on proprioceptive neuromuscular facilitation stretching techniques. *Research Quarterly for Exercise and Sport*. 58:184–188 (1987).

Faigenbaum, A., J. Kang, J. McFarland, J. M. Bloom, J. Magnatta, N. A. Ratamess, & J. Hoffman: Acute effects of different warm-up protocols on anaerobic performance in teenage athletes. *Pediatric Exercise Science*. 18(1):64–75 (2006a).

Faigenbaum, A. D., J. E. McFarland, J. A. Schwerdtman, N. A. Ratamess, J. Kang, & J. R. Hoffman: Dynamic warm-up protocols, with and without a weighted vest, and fitness performance in high school female athletes. *Journal of Athletic Training*. 41(4):357–363 (2006b).

Fields, K. B., C. M. Burnworth, & M. Delaney: Sports Science Exchange # 104: Should athletes stretch before exercise? *Gatorade Sports Science Institute*. 14 June 2007.

Fowles, J. R., D. G. Sale, & J. D. MacDougall: Reduced strength after passive stretch of the human plantar flexors. *Journal of Applied Physiology*. 89:1179–1188 (2000).

Gabriel, D. A., G. Kamen, & G. Frost: Neural adaptations to restive exercise: Mechanisms and recommendations for training practices. *Sports Medicine*. 36:133–149 (2006).

Gleim, G. W. & M. P. McHugh: Flexibility and its effects on sports injury and performance. *Sports Medicine*. 24(5):289–299 (1997).

Gioftsidou, A., P. Malliou, G. Pafis, A. Beneka, G. Godolias, & C. N. Maganaris: The effects of soccer training and timing of balance training on balance ability. *European Journal of Applied Physiology*. 96:659–664 (2006).

Gomez, T. G., G. Beach, C. Cooke, W. Hrudey, & P. Goyert: Normative database for trunk range of motion, strength, velocity, and endurance with the Isostation B-200 Lumbar Dynamometer. *Spine*. 16:15–21 (1991).

Granacher, U., T. Muehlbauer, & M. Gruber: A qualitative review of balance and strength performance in healthy older adults: Impact for testing and training. *Journal of Aging Research*. Article ID 708905, 16 pages (2012).

Guyton, A. C. & J. E. Hall: *Textbook of Medical Physiology* (12th edition). Philadelphia, PA: Elsevier Saunders (2011).

Hardy, L. & D. Jones: Dynamic flexibility and proprioceptive neuromuscular facilitation. *Research Quarterly for Exercise and Sport*. 57:150–153 (1986).

Hart, L.: Effect of stretching on sport injury risk: A review. *Clinical Journal of Sports Medicine*. 15(2):113 (2005).

Hartig, D. E. & J. M. Henderson: Increasing hamstring flexibility decreases lower extremity overuse injuries in military basic trainees. *The American Journal of Sports Medicine*. 27(2):173–176 (1999).

Herbert, R. D. & M. de Noronha: Stretching to prevent or reduce muscle soreness after exercise. *Cochrane Database of Systematic Reviews*. Issue 4. Art. No.: CD004577 (2007). DOI: 10.1002/14651858.CD004577.pub2.

Herbert, R. D. & M. Gabriel: Effects of stretching before and after exercising on muscle soreness and risk of injury: A systematic review. *British Medical Journal*. 325:468–470 (2002).

Herda, T. J., J. T. Cramer, E. D. Ryan, M. P. McHugh, & J. R. Stout: Acute effects of static versus dynamic stretching on isometric peak torque, electromyopgraphy, and mechaniomyography of the bicep femoris muscle. *Journal of Strength and Conditioning Research*. 22(3):809–817 (2008).

Hewett, T. E., T. N. Lindenfeld, J. V. Riccobene, & F. R. Noyes: The effect of neuromuscular training on the incidence of knee injury in female athletes a prospective study. *The American Journal of Sports Medicine*. 27:699–706 (1999).

High, D. M., E. T. Howley, & B. D. Franks: The effects of static stretching and warm-up on prevention of delayed-onset muscle soreness. *Research Quarterly for Exercise and Sport*. 60:356–361 (1989).

Holviala, J. H. S., J. M. Sallinen, W. J. Kraemer, M. K. Alen, & K. K. T. Häkkinen: Effects of strength training on muscle strength characteristics, functional capabilities, and balance in middle-aged and older women. *Journal of Strength and Conditioning Research*. 20(2):336–344 (2006).

Horak, F. B.: Postural orientation and equilibrium: What do we need to know about neural control of balance to prevent falls? *Age and Ageing*. 35(S2):ii7–ii11 (2006).

Hrysomallis, C.: Relationship between balance ability, training and sports injury risk. *Sports Medicine*. 37(6):547–556 (2007).

Hubley-Kozey, C. L.: Testing flexibility. In MacDougall, J. D., H. A. Weuger, & H. J. Green (eds.): *Physiological Testing of the High-Performance Athlete*. Champaign, IL: Human Kinetics (1991).

Hutton, R. S.: Neuromuscular basis of stretching exercises. In Komi, P. V. (ed.): *Strength and Power in Sport*. London, UK: Blackwell Scientific, 39–65, (1992).

Jackson, A. W. & A. A. Baker: The relationship of the sit and reach test to criterion measures of hamstring and back flexibility in young females. *Research Quarterly for Exercise and Sport*. 57:183–186 (1986).

Jackson, A. W. & N. J. Langford: The criterion-related validity of the sit and reach test: Replication and extension of previous findings. *Research Quarterly for Exercise and Sport*. 60:384–387 (1989).

Kabo, K., H. Kanechisa, & T. Fukunaga: Effects of resistance and stretching training programmes on the viscoelastic properties of human tendon structures in vivo. *Journal of Physiology*. 538:219–226 (2002).

Kippers, V. & A. W. Parker: Toe-touch test: A measure of its validity. *Physical Therapy*. 67:1680–1684 (1987).

Knudson, D.: Stretching: From science to practice. *Journal of Physical Education Recreation and Dance*. 69(3):38–42 (1998).

Knudson, D., K. Bennett, R. Corn, D. Leick, & C. Smith: Acute effects of stretching are not evident in the kinematics of the vertical jump. *Journal of Strength and Conditioning Research*. 15(1):98–101 (2001).

Knudson, D. V., P. Magnusson, & M. McHugh: Current issues in flexibility fitness. *President's Council on Physical Fitness and Sports Research Digest Series*. 3(10):1–8 (2000).

LaRouche, D. P. & J. Connolly: Effects of stretching on passive muscle tension and response to eccentric exercise. *The American Journal of Sports Medicine*. 34:1000–1007 (2006).

Leighton, J.: Flexibility characteristics of three specialized skill groups of champion athletes. *Archives of Physical Medicine and Rehabilitation*. 36:580–583 (1957).

Li, F., P. Harmer, K. J. Fisher, & E. McAuley: Tai Chi: Improving functional balance and predicting subsequent falls in older persons. *Medicine & Science in Sports & Exercise*. 36(12):2046–2052 (2004).

Lord, S. R. & D. L. Sturnieks: The physiology of falling: Assessment and prevention strategies for older people. *Journal of Science and Medicine in Sport*. 8(1):35–42 (2005).

Malina, R. M. & C. Bouchard: *Growth, Maturation, and Physical Activity*. Champaign, IL: Human Kinetics (1991).

Marieb, E. N. & K. Hoehn: *Human Anatomy and Physiology* (8th edition). San Francisco, CA: Benjamin Cummings (2010).

Markovic, G. & P. Mikulic: Neuro-musculoskeletal and performance adaptations to lower-extremity plyometric training. *Sports Medicine*. 40(10):859–895 (2010).

Marshall, J. L., N. Johnson, T. L. Wickiewicz, H. M. Tischler, B. L. Koslin, S. Zeno, & A. Meyers: Joint looseness: A function of the person and joint. *Medicine and Science in Sports*. 12(3):189–194 (1980).

Massey, B. H. & N. L. Chaudet: Effects of heavy resistance exercise on range of joint movement in young male adults. *Research Quarterly*. 27:41–51 (1956).

McHugh, M. P., D. A. J. Connolly, R. G. Eston, I. J. Kreminic, S. J. Nichols, & G. W. Gleim: The role of passive muscle stiffness in symptoms of exercise-induced muscle damage. *The American Journal of Sports Medicine*. 27(5):594–599 (1999).

Moll, J. M. H. & V. Wright: Normal range of spinal mobility: An objective clinical study. *Annals of Rheumatic Diseases*. 30:381–386 (1971).

Monteiro, W. D., R. Simão, M.D. Polito, C.A. Santana, R.B. Chaves, E. Bezerra, S. J. Fleck: Influence of strength training on adult women's flexibility. *Journal of Strength & Conditioning Research*. 22 (3):672–677 (2008).

Myer, G. D., K. R. Ford, J. L. Brent, & T. E. Hewett: The effects of plyometric vs. dynamic stabilization and balance training on power, balance, and landing force in female athletes. *Journal of Strength and Conditioning Research*. 20(2):345–353 (2006).

Nicolaisen, T. & K. Jorgensen: Trunk strength, back muscle endurance and low-back trouble. *Scandinavian Journal of Rehabilitation Medicine*. 17:121–127 (1985).

Nolan, L., A. Grigorenko, & A. Thorstensson: Balance control: Sex and age differences 9- and 16-year-olds. *Developmental Medicine and Child Neurology*. 47:449–454 (2005).

Park, D. Y. & L. Chou: Stretching for prevention of Achilles tendon injuries: A review of the literature. *Foot and Ankle International*. 27(12):1086–1095 (2006).

Plowman, S. A.: Physical activity, physical fitness and low back pain. In Holloszy, J. O. (ed.): *Exercise and Sport Science Reviews*. 20:221–242 (1992).

Pope, R. P., R. D. Herber, J. D. Kirwan, & B. J. Graham: A randomized trial of preexercise stretching for prevention of lower-limb injury. *Medicine & Science in Sports & Exercise*. 32(2):271–277 (2000).

Potach D. H. & D. A. Chu: Plyometric training. In Baechle, T. R., Earle, R. W. (eds.): *Essentials of Strength Training and Conditioning*. Champaign, IL: Human Kinetics, 427–470 (2000).

Power, K., D. Behm, F. Cahill, M. Carroll, & W. Young: An acute bout of static stretching: Effects of force and jumping performance. *Medicine & Science in Sports & Exercise*. 38(8):1389–1396 (2004).

Punakallio, A.: Balancing abilities of different-aged workers in physically demanding jobs. *Journal of Occupational Rehabilitation*. 13(1):33–43 (2003).

Rider, R. A. & J. Daly: Effects of flexibility training on enhancing spinal mobility in older women. *Journal of Sports Medicine and Physical Fitness*. 31:213–217 (1991).

Robergs, R. A. & S. O. Roberts: *Exercise Physiology: Exercise, Performance and Clinical Applications*. St. Louis, MO: Mosby-Year Book (1997).

Robinson, L. E., S. T. Devor, M. A. Merrick, & J. Buckworth: The effects of lands vs. aquatic plyometrics on power, torque, velocity, and muscle soreness in women. *Journal of Strength and Conditioning Research*. 18(1):84–91 (2004).

Rubenstein, L. Z.: Falls in older people: Epidemiology, risk factors an strategies for prevention. *Age and Ageing*. 35(Suppl 2):ii37–ii41 (2006).

Rubini, E. C., L. L. Costa, & P. S. Gomes: The effects of stretching on strength performance. *Sports Medicine*. 37(3):213–224 (2007).

Sage, G: *Introduction to Motor Behavior: A Neurophysiological Approach*. Reading, MA: Addison-Wesley (1971).

Sainz de Baranda, P. & F. Ayala: Chronic flexibility improvement after 12 week of stretching program utilizing the ACSM recommendations: Hamstring flexibility. *International Journal of Sports Medicine*. 31:389–396 (2010).

Schmidt, R. A.: *Motor Control and Learning: A Behavioral Emphasis*. Champaign, IL: Human Kinetics (1988).

Schuntermann, M. F.: The international classification of impairments, disabilities and handicaps (ICIDH)—results and problems. *International Journal of Rehabilitation Research*. 19:1–11 (1996).

Sharman, M. J., A. G. Cresswell, & S. Riek: Proprioceptive neuromuscular facilitation stretching. *Sports Medicine*. 36(11):439–454 (2006).

Shellock, F. G. & W. E. Prentice: Warming-up and stretching for improved physical performance and prevention of sports-related injuries. *Sports Medicine*. 2(4):267–278 (1985).

Shephard, R. J., M. Berridge, & W. Montelpare: On the generality of the "sit and reach" test: An analysis of flexibility data for an aging population. *Research Quarterly for Exercise and Sport*. 61:326–330 (1990).

Shrier, I.: Does stretching improve performance? A systematic and critical review of the literature. *Clinical Journal of Sports Medicine*. 14(5):267–273 (2004).

Siracuse, J. J., D. D. Odell, S. P. Gondek, S. R. Odom, E. M. Kaspar, C. J. Hauser, & D. W. Moorman: Health care and socioeconomic impact of falls in the elderly. *The American Journal of Surgery*. 203:335–338 (2012).

Small, K., L. McNaughton, & M. Matthews: A systematic review into the efficacy of static stretching as part of a warm-up for the prevention of exercise-related injury. *Research in Sports Medicine*. 16:213–231 (2008).

Smith, C. A.: The warm-up procedure: To stretch or not to stretch. *Journal of Orthopedic Sports and Physical Therapy*. 19(1):12–17 (1994).

Söderman, K., S. Werner, T. Pietilä, B. Engström, & H. Alfredson: Balance board training: prevention of traumatic injuries of the lower extremities in female soccer players? *Knee Surgery, Sports Traumatology, Arthroscopy*. 8(6):356–363 (2000).

Standring, S.: *Gray's Anatomy—The Anatomical Basis of Clinical Practice* (39th edition). Oxford, UK: Elsevier Churchill Livingstone (2005).

Steindl, R., H. Ulmer, & A.W. Scholtz: Standing stability in children- and young adults. Influence of proprioceptive, visual and vestibular systems in age- and sex-dependent changes (abstract). *HNO*. 52(5):423–430. (2004).

Sullivan, M. K., J. J. DeJulia, & T. W. Worrell: Effect of pelvic position and stretching method on hamstring muscle flexibility. *Medicine and Science in Sports and Exercise*. 24:1383–1389 (1992).

Taube, W., C. Leukel, & A. Gollhofer: How neurons make us jump: The neutral control of stretch-shortening cycle movement. *Exercise and Sport Science Reviews*. 40(2):106–115 (2012).

Thacker, S. B., J. Gilchrist, D. F. Stroup, & D. Kimsey: The impact of stretching on sports injury risk: A systematic review of the literature. *Medicine & Science in Sports & Exercise*. 36(3):371–378 (2004).

Unick, J., H. S. Kieffer, W. Cheesman, & Feeney, A.: The acute effects of static and ballistic stretching on vertical jump performance in trained women. *Journal of Strength and Conditioning Research*. 19(1):206–212 (2005).

Verhagen, E., A. van der Beek, J. Twisk, L. Bouter, R. Bahr, & W. van Mechelen: The effect of a proprioceptive balance board training program for the prevention of ankle sprains: a prospective controlled trial. *American Journal of Sports Medicine*. 32(6):1386–1393 (2004).

Wallin, D., B. Ekblom, R. Grahn, & T. Nordenborg: Improvement of muscle flexibility: A comparison between two techniques. *American Journal of Sports Medicine*. 13:263–268 (1985).

Wilson, G. J., R. U. Newton, A. J. Murphy, & B. J. Humphries: The optimal training load for the development of dynamic athletic performance. *Medicine and Science in Sports and Exercise*. 25(11):1279–1286 (1993).

Witvrouw, E., N. Mahieu, L. Danneels, & P. McNair: Stretching and injury prevention. *Sports Medicine*. 34(7):443–449 (2004).

Young, W. B. & D. G. Behm: Effects of running, static stretching and practice jumps on explosive force production and jumping performance. *Journal of Sports Medicine and Physical Fitness*. 43:21–27 (2003).

Neuroendocrine-Immune System Unit

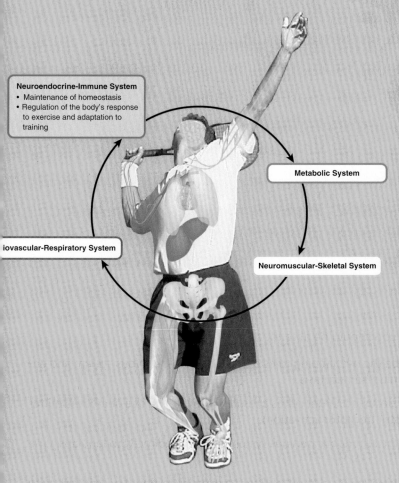

Neuroendocrine-Immune System
- Maintenance of homeostasis
- Regulation of the body's response to exercise and adaptation to training

Metabolic System

iovascular-Respiratory System

Neuromuscular-Skeletal System

The neural, endocrine and immune systems play a vital role in regulating and coordinating the body's response to exercise and the adaptations to exercise training. The autonomic nervous system and endocrine systems function to control cardiovascular and metabolic responses and adaptations. Recent evidence has made it increasingly clear that there is considerable communication between the chemical mediators of the endocrine system (hormones) and the cells and chemical mediators (cytokines) of the immune system. While these systems are essential for coordinating the positive adaptations to exercise training, there is also evidence that these same systems can reflect the pathological condition of overtraining.

Neuroendocrine Control of Exercise

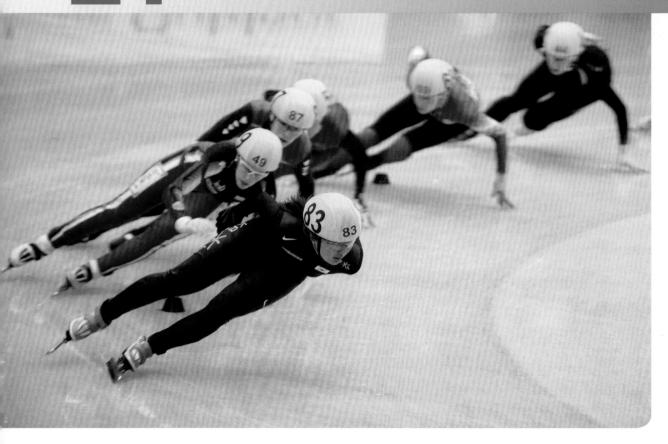

OBJECTIVES

After studying the chapter, you should be able to:

> Identify and briefly describe the overlapping roles of the autonomic nervous system and endocrine system in maintaining homeostasis.

> Identify changes that may occur in a target cell as a result of the binding of a neurotransmitter or hormone to a cell receptor (receptor activation).

> Describe the functions of the autonomic nervous system that relate directly to regulating the exercise response.

> Identify the primary hormones involved in regulating the exercise response and describe the exercise response of these hormones.

> Identify the adaptations that occur in the hormonal system as a result of exercise training.

Introduction

You know from your own experience that when you exercise, certain changes take place in your body. You consciously initiate the most obvious change—contraction of the muscles—by activating the nervous system, which in turn signals the muscles to contract. You may also be aware of other changes, such as an increased breathing rate, increased heart rate, and increased sweating; these responses you do not consciously initiate. Still other changes—fuel mobilization, enzyme actions, and energy utilization—also occur during exercise without conscious initiation, or even awareness of their occurrence. These changes are all part of an ongoing internal effort to maintain homeostatic balance. **Homeostasis** is the dynamic state of equilibrium in the internal functioning of the body. It is controlled and coordinated by the nervous and endocrine (hormonal) systems of the body. Furthermore, these two complementary and often overlapping systems regulate the body's response to any disruption in homeostasis, such as the disruption created by exercise. The nervous system is the faster-acting regulator of the body, whereas the endocrine system is the slower-acting regulator. The two systems interact and overlap in multiple ways to support exercise. Because these two systems function so closely together, they are often referred to as the *neuroendocrine* (or *neurohormonal*) system. While Chapter 20 examines the role of the nervous system in initiating exercise, this chapter addresses the role of the neuroendocrine system in regulating the body's responses to exercise. Because the neuroendocrine system controls body systems, including those described in this book (cardiorespiratory, metabolic, and neuromusculoskeletal), the basic principles of neuroendocrine control are critical for understanding the exercise response, training adaptations, and the integrated nature of all the systems studied in exercise physiology.

Both the nervous system and the hormonal system rely on chemical messengers to communicate with target cells. While neurons rely on electrical signals to conduct messages within a cell, they communicate with adjacent cells via chemical messengers called **neurotransmitters**. **Figure 21.1** depicts the cells of the nervous and hormonal systems and the chemical messengers they use. Neurons are secretory cells that release neurotransmitters at the site of the target cell. Endocrine glands, or hormone-producing tissues, release chemical messengers called **hormones** into the bloodstream or another body fluid. These hormones, in turn, have systemic or local effects. Thus, a hormone can be defined as a chemical substance that originates in glandular tissue (or cells) and is transported through body fluids to a target cell to influence physiological activity.

The effect of hormones on target cells can be further delineated as autocrine, paracrine, or endocrine. Autocrine function refers to the action of a hormone on the cell that secreted the hormone. Paracrine function refers to the action of a hormone released into the body fluids that has an effect on a nearby cell, and endocrine function refers to a hormone released into the bloodstream that has an effect on target cells at a distant site. If a neuron releases a chemical substance into the bloodstream, this substance is called a *neurohormone*.

The effect of chemical messengers (neurotransmitters, hormones, and neurohormones) on target cells is mediated by the substance's binding to a receptor on (or in) the target cells. The chemical messenger binds to the receptor because of the complementary shape of the messenger and the receptor. Thus, chemical messengers bind only to very specific receptors. The messenger-receptor binding is known as *receptor activation*. It results in one or more changes within the target cell:

1. Change in permeability, electrical state, or transport properties of the cell
2. Change in enzyme activity of the cell (altering metabolism)
3. Change in secretory activity of the cell
4. Muscle contraction
5. Protein synthesis

Table 21.1 summarizes the nervous and endocrine systems within a comparative framework.

Exercise as a Stressor that Activates the Neural and Hormonal Systems

As detailed in Chapter 1 and discussed throughout this text, exercise causes a disruption in homeostasis and simultaneously creates the need for the body to increase oxygen and nutrient delivery to the working muscles to support the metabolic demands of activity. These needs are met by the joint action of the neural and hormonal systems. Understanding the neurohormonal response to exercise is necessary for understanding how the bodily systems respond to exercise or any stressor (Hackney, 2006; Selye, 1956).

Homeostasis A dynamic state of equilibrium in the internal functioning of the body.

Neurotransmitters Chemical messengers with which neurons communicate with target cells of either other neurons or effector organs.

Hormones Chemical substances that originate in glandular tissue (or cells) and are transported through body fluids to a target cell to influence physiological activity.

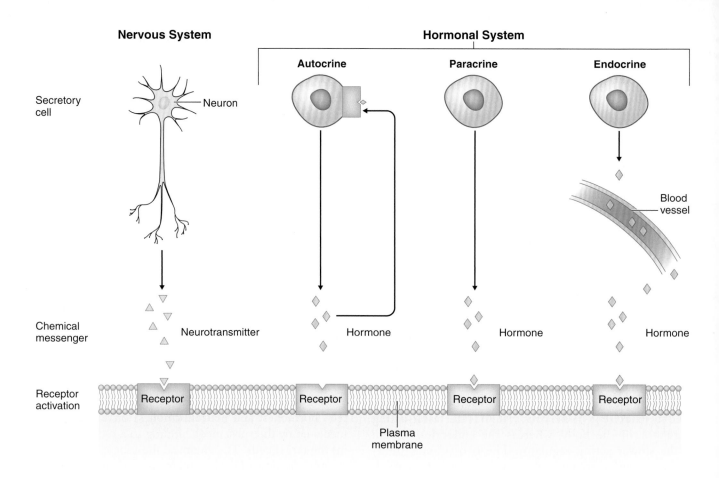

FIGURE 21.1 Chemical Messengers of the Nervous and Hormonal Systems.
Both the nervous system and the hormonal system rely on chemical messengers to communicate with target organs. Neurons release neurotransmitters in close proximity to the target organ. Endocrine glands release hormones into body fluids (often the blood) and may have an effect on target organs throughout the body.

TABLE 21.1	Outline of Nervous and Endocrine Systems	
	Nervous System	**Endocrine System**
Basic structure	Central and peripheral nervous system composed of neurons	Endocrine gland/tissue, which releases hormones
Chemical messenger	Neurotransmitter (NT)	Hormones
Mechanism of chemical release	Action potential in axon causes release of NT	Endocrine gland/tissue secretes hormone into blood/body fluid
Chemical/receptor binding	NT binds to receptor on target cell because of complementary shape and affinity	Hormone binds to receptor on target cell because of complementary shape and affinity
Mechanism of action	Change in membrane permeability Second messenger system Direct gene activation	Second messenger system Direct gene activation

Role in exercise	1. Contraction of skeletal muscle
	2. Regulation of cardiovascular-respiratory systems
	3. Coordination with endocrine system to
	  • Mobilize fuel for energy production
	  • Transport fuel, oxygen, and waste
	  • Maintain fluid and electrolyte balance
	  • Maintain thermal balance
		1. Regulate metabolic system
		  • Mobilize fuel for energy production
		  • Increase rate at which fuel is broken down to produce ATP
		  • Maintain blood glucose levels
		2. Regulate cardiovascular system
		  • Transport fuel, oxygen, and waste
		  • Maintain fluid and electrolyte balance
		  • Maintain thermal balance

Both the neural and the hormonal regulatory systems are involved in the stress response system, as shown in the schematic outline in **Figure 21.2**. The primarily neural component is called the brain stem (locus ceruleus)–sympathetic nervous system pathway, shown on the left. The primarily hormonal component is called the hypothalamus-pituitary-adrenal axis and is the pathway on the right. Notice, however, the overlap of the two systems. The *hypothalamus* is both a neural and endocrine organ, and activation of the sympathetic nervous system stimulates many target organs by direct innervation and causes the release of epinephrine and norepinephrine from the adrenal medulla. When the individual encounters a stressor, the hypothalamus coordinates the response. As both a neural structure and an endocrine gland, the hypothalamus orchestrates the body's response by stimulating both the sympathetic nervous system and the endocrine glands.

The sympathetic nerve fibers originate in the brain stem and travel throughout the body to a variety of target sites. The sympathetic nerve fibers also go to and control the adrenal medulla. Norepinephrine (NE) is released by

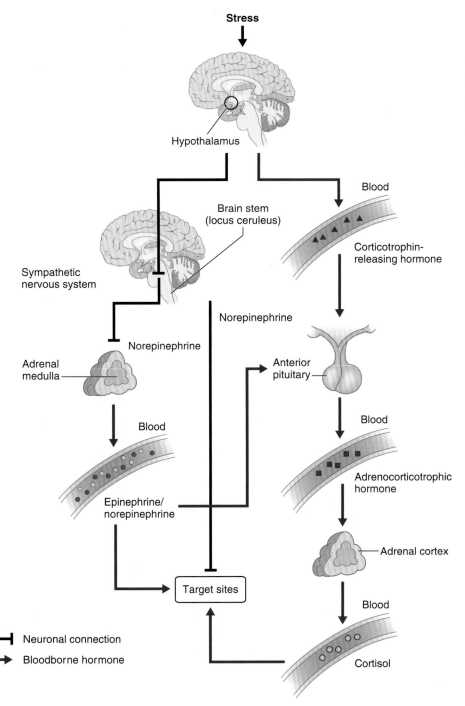

FIGURE 21.2 Neurohormonal Regulation of the Exercise Stress Response.
The nervous and hormonal systems have multiple, and often overlapping, roles in regulating the exercise response. The hypothalamus serves as both a neural tissue (activating the brain stem) and a hormone-secreting gland.

sympathetic nerve fibers, and both NE and epinephrine (E) are secreted by the adrenal medulla. The NE released from the sympathetic nerve endings and from the adrenal medulla is the same chemical. However, when NE is released by the nerves, it is considered to be a neurotransmitter, and when it is released by the adrenal medulla, it is considered to be a hormone. The NE and E secreted by the adrenal medulla circulate in the bloodstream to the target sites, where they mimic and reinforce the actions of the sympathetic nerve fibers that innervate these same target sites, for example, in elevating the heart rate. This response pattern is often referred to as sympathoadrenal activation. Both NE and E may also influence other endocrine glands, as indicated by the connecting line to the anterior pituitary gland in **Figure 21.2** (Chrousos and Gold, 1992).

The hypothalamus directly regulates endocrine glands both neurally and hormonally through a series of releasing factors, sometimes called releasing hormones. In the generic stress response, corticotrophin-releasing hormone (CRH) is released by the hypothalamus and stimulates the anterior pituitary to secrete adrenocorticotropic hormone (ACTH). ACTH in turn stimulates the adrenal cortex to release cortisol, which acts on specific target sites.

The following sections discuss the neural and hormonal responses to exercise separately in greater detail, but it is useful to remember the considerable overlap between these systems.

The Nervous System

The nervous system is a fast-acting control system that regulates an almost endless list of bodily functions. In general, the nervous system has three primary functions:

1. Monitoring the internal and external environment through sensory receptors
2. Integrating the information it receives
3. Initiating and coordinating a response by activating muscles (skeletal, smooth, and cardiac) and glands (including endocrine glands and sweat glands)

These functions are accomplished by the cells of the nervous system (neurons) communicating with each other and with *effector organs* (muscle and glands). Communication within a neuron occurs by electrical signals (action potentials). Communication between neurons or between neurons and an effector organ (e.g., skeletal muscle, cardiac muscle, glands) occurs by chemical signals (neurotransmitters).

The Autonomic Nervous System

As described in Chapter 20, the nervous system can be structurally divided into the *central nervous system*

(CNS) and the *peripheral nervous system* (PNS) (see **Figure 20.1**). Recall that functionally the *somatic nervous system* innervates skeletal muscles and is responsible for controlling their contraction. In contrast, *the autonomic nervous system* (ANS) provides subconscious neural regulation of the internal environment of the body by innervating cardiac muscle, smooth muscle, and endocrine glands.

The ANS has two branches, which work in opposition to each other through dual innervations. **Figure 21.3** is a schematic overview of major body organs influenced by the two divisions of the ANS; organs directly involved in regulating the response to exercise are highlighted by being shown in color. The sympathetic nerves exit the spinal cord in the thoracic and lumbar region, whereas parasympathetic nerves exit the spinal cord from the cranial nerves and the sacral area. The *sympathetic nervous system* (SNS) supports activities associated with the "fight or flight" stress response and is vital in regulating the body's integrated response to exercise (including increased oxygen delivery to the working muscles, fuel utilization in support of increased metabolic demands, and heat dissipation). The *parasympathetic nervous system* (PSNS) supports activities associated with "rest and digest" and is vital in the process of recovering from exercise. Changes in the balance of SNS and PSNS activity are responsible for many of the adjustments made during exercise and adaptations resulting from exercise training.

Neural Communication and Responses

Neurons are the functional unit of the nervous system. Excitation of a neuron leads to the generation of an electrical signal—termed an action potential (see Chapter 20 for full discussion). Once generated in the axon, the action potential moves along the entire length of the axon, causing a neurotransmitter to be released from the terminal end of the axon. The terminal end of the axon communicates with other neurons, muscle cells, or glands across junctions known as **synapses**. A synapse between a neuron and a muscle cell is known as a *neuromuscular junction*.

The dominant form of synapse is a chemical synapse, which involves the release of a neurotransmitter from the neuron. (The sequence of events involved in the release of a neurotransmitter at the neuromuscular junction is detailed in Chapter 20.) Acetylcholine (ACh) is the neurotransmitter released from somatic motor neurons, parasympathetic and sympathetic preganglionic fibers, and parasympathetic postganglionic fibers (**Figure 21.4**). Acetylcholine is always excitatory to skeletal muscle, but may be inhibitory or excitatory to target cells of the autonomic nervous system (smooth muscle, cardiac muscle, glands), depending on the target cell receptors to which it binds. Norepinephrine (NE) is the neurotransmitter released by most sympathetic postganglionic neurons;

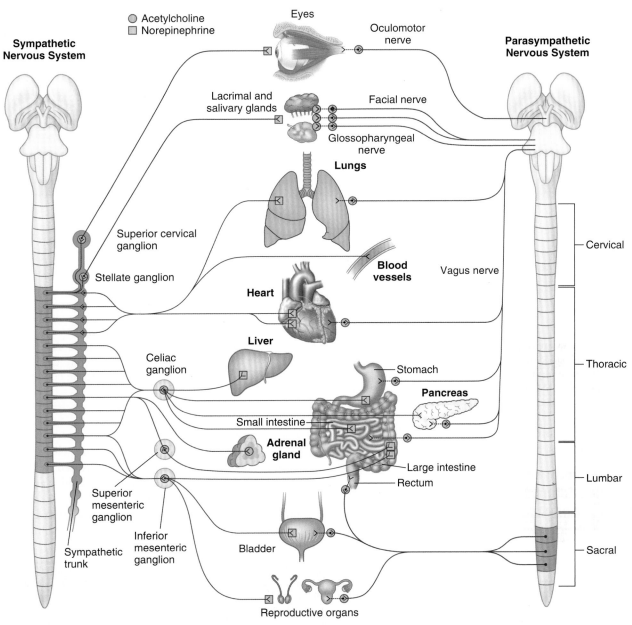

FIGURE 21.3 Components of the Autonomic Nervous System.
Sympathetic fibers exit the spinal cord at the thoracic and lumbar regions, whereas parasympathetic fibers exit from cranial nerves and the sacral region of the spinal cord. Parasympathetic preganglionic neurons are longer than sympathetic preganglionic neurons and synapse with postganglionic fibers near or within target organs.

neurons innervating sweat glands are an important exception. NE is also inhibitory or excitatory depending on the receptors to which it binds. Neurons that release ACh are called *cholinergic fibers*; neurons that release NE are called *adrenergic fibers*.

The response of the target organ depends not only on the neurotransmitter but also on the receptor to which it binds.

Synapse The gap, or junction, between terminal ends of the axon and other neurons, muscle cells, or glands.

Receptors that bind ACh are called cholinergic receptors, and receptors that bind NE are called adrenergic receptors. The two types of *cholinergic receptors* are nicotinic and muscarinic receptors, and the two types of *adrenergic receptors* are termed alpha (α) and beta (β). These latter are further subdivided into α_1, α_2, β_1, β_2, and β_3 receptors (Guyton and Hall, 2011). Because target organs may have more than one type of receptor, they may have different responses. **Table 21.2** outlines the effects of the SNS and PSNS on selected effector organs. This table shows the general principle that activation of the SNS supports activities associated with the

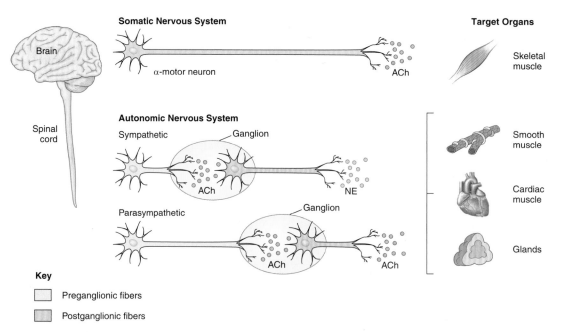

FIGURE 21.4   Neurotransmitters of the Somatic and Autonomic Divisions of the Nervous System.
Neurons of the somatic nervous system (α-motor neurons) release acetylcholine (ACh), which causes skeletal muscle to contract. Neurons of the parasympathetic division of the autonomic nervous system secrete (ACh). Preganglion fibers of the sympathetic nervous system also secrete (ACh), but postganglionic fibers secrete norepinephrine (NE). Autonomic fibers innervate smooth muscle, cardiac muscle, and glands.

"fight or flight" stress response, while the PSNS is associated with the "rest and digest" mode.

Measuring Autonomic Nervous System Activity

Changes in parasympathetic and sympathetic activity have profound effects. However, autonomic responses are not easily measured. The most direct measure, muscle sympathetic nerve activity (MSNA), measures electrical activity, typically in the peroneal nerve (located in the lower leg); this is an invasive method that provides an index of sympathetic excitement (Vallbo, 1979). More commonly, autonomic nervous system function is estimated by measuring heart rate variability (HRV) and heart rate recovery

TABLE 21.2 Effect of Autonomic Nervous Stimulation on Various Organs		Effect of Sympathetic Stimulation	Effect of Parasympathetic Stimulation
Cardiovascular	Heart	↑ Rate of contraction ↑ Force of contraction	↓ Rate of contraction Slight ↑ force of contraction
	Arterioles		
	Coronary	Dilation (β₂), constriction (α)	Dilation
	Skeletal	Constriction (α), dilation (β₂ and cholinergic)	None
	Skin and internal organs	Constriction (α)	None
Metabolic	GI motility	Decrease (β₂)	Increase
	Adipose tissue	Lipolysis	None
	Liver	Glycogenolysis Gluconeogenesis	Glycogen synthesis
Fluid balance and thermoregulation	Sweat glands	↑ Sweating (cholinergic)	None
	Kidney	↑ Renin secretion (α, β₁)	None
	Posterior pituitary	↑ ADH secretion	None
	Adrenal medulla secretion	Increase	None
	Coagulation	Increase	None
Sources: Seifter et al. (2005) and Guyton and Hall (2011).			

FOCUS ON RESEARCH: *Clinically Relevant*
Effect of Training Status on ANS Recovery

Exercise results in activation of the sympathetic nervous system and a shift in autonomic balance. The rate of recovery from this shift in autonomic balance depends on the intensity and duration of the activity and the training status of the individual. The quantification of heart rate variability (HRV) is a noninvasive tool to investigate changes in autonomic balance. HRV analysis can provide several useful variables, including mean HR, mean HR interval, and the root mean square of sequential deviations (RMSSD). RMSSD is often expressed as a percentage of pre-exercise values. A return to 100% indicates that pre-exercise autonomic balance has been restored.

As part of a larger study to investigate autonomic recovery from different exercise training regimens, Sieler et al. compared autonomic recovery from a high-intensity training session in highly trained athletes with recreationally trained athletes. The highly trained group (n = 9) had a mean age of 23 years, HRmax of 189 b·min^{-1}, and a $\dot{V}O_2$max of 72 mL·kg^{-1}·min^{-1}; they trained an average of 14 hr·wk^{-1}. The recreationally trained group (n = 8) had a mean age of 27 years, HRmax of 189 b·min^{-1}, and a $\dot{V}O_2$max of 60 mL·kg^{-1}·min^{-1}; they trained an average of 7 hr·wk^{-1}. Both groups performed

high-intensity interval exercise on a treadmill. Participants first performed a 20-minute warm-up, then completed a 30-minute interval session consisting of 6 × 3 minute intervals at a velocity eliciting 95–100% of $\dot{V}O_2$max with 2 minutes of active recovery periods, followed by a 10-minute warm-down. The RPE associated with the exercise session was 18 in both groups.

The figure below presents the RMSSD for the group of recreationally and highly trained athletes for the 4-hour postexercise period. The recovery of parasympathetic control after the intense interval exercise session was significantly

slower (60–90 minutes) in the recreationally trained versus the highly trained subjects.

Highly trained subjects had a more accelerated recovery from intense interval work than recreationally trained athletes. This adaptation may be an important factor in the ability of highly trained athletes to tolerate typical twice-daily training regimens common among elite endurance athletes.

Source: Seiler, S., O. Haugen, & E. Kuffel: Autonomic recovery after exercise in trained athletes: Intensity and duration effects. *Medicine & Science in Sports & Exercise.* 39(8):1366–1373 (2007).

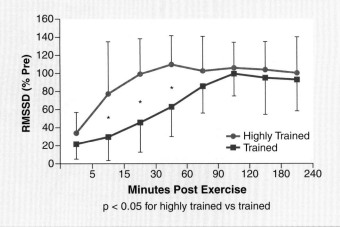

p < 0.05 for highly trained vs trained

(HRR) from exercise. **Heart rate variability** is the beat-to-beat variation in the time of the R to R intervals on a standard ECG. A healthy heart rate is not fixed but rather varies moment to moment in response to physiological stimuli. For instance, in a healthy individual with a resting heart rate of 60 b·min^{-1}, the interval between beats is not exactly 1 second but varies in a range of different times that average 1 second. Heart rate variability is typically determined using a standard ECG and a computer to assess interbeat variability over a specified time period. Lower variability reflects poor autonomic tone and is associated with a poor cardiovascular risk profile, elevated risk of coronary heart disease, and increased risk of all-cause mortality (Dekker et al., 2000; Thayer et al., 2010; Tsuji et al., 1994).

Heart rate recovery following a graded exercise test is also an easily obtained measure that is frequently used to estimate autonomic response to a challenge. Heart rate recovery is the difference between maximum heart rate and the heart rate after a specified time (usually 1 or 2 minutes) of recovery. The primary determinant of heart rate recovery is thought to be parasympathetic reactivation; thus, a faster heart rate recovery indicates a greater parasympathetic response (Carnethon and Craft, 2008). A delayed decrease in heart rate during the first minute after a graded exercise test is a powerful predictor of overall mortality, independent of workload, presence or absence of ischemia, and changes in heart rate during exercise (Cole et al., 1999; Nishime et al., 2000).

Autonomic Nervous System Control During Exercise

The role of the autonomic nervous system in regulating the exercise response is very diverse. As previously stated, the exercise response is mediated primarily through

> **Heart rate variability** The beat-to-beat variation in the time of the R to R intervals on a standard ECG.

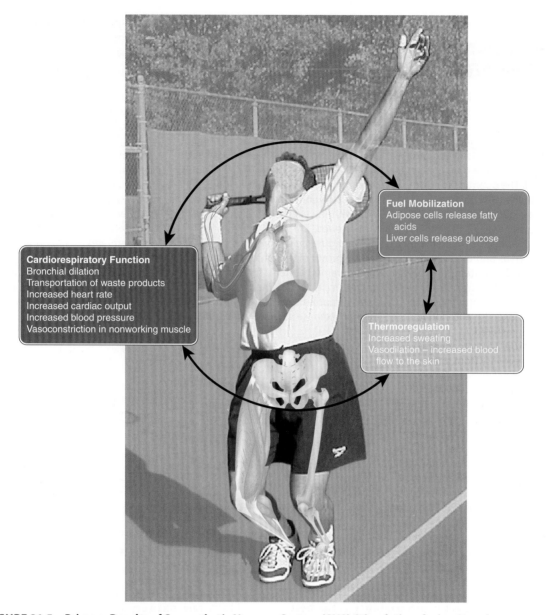

FIGURE 21.5   Primary Results of Sympathetic Nervous System (SNS) Stimulation during Exercise.
Activation of the sympathetic nervous system during exercise is responsible for many of the acute exercise responses.

the sympathetic branch of the autonomic nervous system. In addition to direct nerve stimulation via innervation of multiple organs (see **Figure 21.2**), sympathetic nerve stimulation leads to the release of epinephrine and norepinephrine from the adrenal medulla. These circulating hormones serve to augment the response of the sympathetic nervous fibers that directly innervate various organs. As summarized in **Figure 21.5**, the primary functions of the sympathetic branch of the ANS during exercise are to

1. Enhance cardiorespiratory function:
    a. Increase cardiac output
    b. Regulate blood flow and maintain blood pressure and blood volume
    c. Ensure that the body can stop any unnecessary bleeding

2. Maintain thermal balance
3. Increase fuel mobilization for the production of energy

Autonomic nerve fibers innervate the respiratory system and the heart. Stimulation of the SNS causes a decrease in airway resistance (bronchial dilation), facilitating movement of air into and out of the lungs. Stimulation of the SNS also increases heart rate and force of contraction, causing an increase in cardiac output and an increase in blood pressure. The increased cardiac output is important for transporting fuel and oxygen necessary to support muscular contraction and for transporting waste products that build up as a result of contraction and must be eliminated from the body.

Related to enhancing cardiovascular function, the SNS also plays an integral role in redirecting blood flow during exercise and maintaining blood pressure. These functions are achieved by controlling the diameter of blood vessels. Sympathetic nerve stimulation causes blood vessels (arterioles) in visceral organs, skin, and nonworking muscles to vasoconstrict (decrease in diameter). This allows more blood to be redirected to the contracting muscles to support their metabolic needs. Sympathetic nerve stimulation also plays an important role in maintaining fluid balance during exercise by causing the release of renin and antidiuretic hormone—two hormones directly involved in fluid balance (see Chapter 11).

Additionally, in response to SNS activation, the blood has an increased tendency to clot. This appears to be a protective mechanism associated with the increased risk of injury in situations in which the body is stressed. Furthermore, the increased clotting potential during SNS activation is balanced by an increased ability to breakdown clots (fibrinolysis) in healthy individuals. However, in individuals with cardiovascular disease, especially endothelial dysfunction, this increased coagulatory potential can be dangerous (see Chapter 17).

The ANS also helps maintain thermal balance by controlling blood flow to the skin and by regulating sweat glands. During exercise, particularly exercise performed in the heat, vasodilation of skin blood vessels facilitates heat loss by increasing blood flow in cutaneous vascular beds near the surface of the body where heat can be more easily dissipated. Sympathetic nerve stimulation also causes sweat gland secretion. Interestingly, the sympathetic nerve fibers that innervate sweat glands release ACh (unlike most sympathetic nerve fibers that release NE). The evaporation of sweat is the primary mechanism for heat loss during most exercise (see Chapter 14).

Finally, sympathetic nerve stimulation also helps to support the increased metabolic needs of exercise. The metabolic effects of the SNS are broad and include an increase in lipolysis in adipose tissue and an increase in glycogenolysis and gluconeogenesis in the liver. Thus, both fatty acids and glucose are mobilized to support the working muscles.

In addition to the activation of the sympathetic nervous system described above, the parasympathetic nervous system is simultaneously inhibited in the immediate pre-exercise anticipation stage and during exercise. The inhibition of the parasympathetic nervous system is often referred to as parasympathetic withdrawal. It is the withdrawal of parasympathetic nervous input that is responsible for the initial rise in heart rate seen with exercise and why immediate preexercise heart rates (such as might be taken before a treadmill test) are not accurate resting values.

The Endocrine System

The endocrine system, along with the nervous system, regulates the body's response to exercise. Although many hormones have changed blood concentrations during exercise, this textbook concentrates only on those hormones that play a primary role in regulating the exercise response or training adaptations. The primary role of the hormonal system during exercise is to help regulate the metabolic and cardiovascular systems (Bunt, 1986). Secondarily, hormones are involved in muscle, bone, and adipose tissue functions.

The Basic Structure of the Endocrine System

The endocrine system is composed of a series of ductless glands, other tissues, and the hormones they secrete. Hormones are chemical substances that originate in glandular tissue (or cells) and are transported through body fluids to a target cell to influence physiological activity. The major endocrine glands involved in exercise or training (**Figure 21.6**) include the hypothalamus, pituitary, thyroid, parathyroid, adrenal, pancreas, and gonads (ovaries and testes). Other tissues that secrete hormones include the heart, kidneys, liver, and gastrointestinal tract, as well as endothelial, immunological, and adipose cells. Hormones released from ductless glands are released directly into the bloodstream and travel throughout the body. Hormones released from tissue cells are excreted into the surrounding extracellular fluid, from which they may diffuse into nearby cells to exert an autocrine or a paracrine function (see **Figure 21.1**). Although a complete inventory and description of all hormones is beyond the scope of this book, **Table 21.3** lists those hormones directly involved in regulating exercise responses, training adaptations, or other functions discussed in this text.

Activation of the Hormonal System

SECRETION OF HORMONES Endocrine glands and tissues can be activated to secrete hormones in three ways: neural, hormonal, or humoral. Regardless of the type, the activation of an endocrine gland or hormone-secreting tissue always depends on a chemical signal. Furthermore, the synthesis

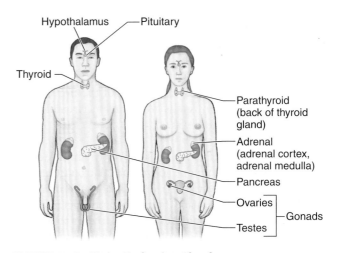

FIGURE 21.6 Major Endocrine Glands.

and release of most hormones are regulated by *negative feedback* mechanisms; that is, the output (the hormone or a variable controlled by the hormone) shuts off the original stimulus or reduces its intensity. Negative feedback mechanisms cause the variable to change in a direction opposite to the original change, returning the variable to its "set point" and thus helping to maintain homeostasis.

Neural activation occurs directly when a neuron releases a neurotransmitter that signals the endocrine tissue to release a hormone. For example, sympathetic neurons release the neurotransmitter NE, which stimulates the adrenal medulla to release the hormones E and NE.

Hormonal activation literally means that one hormone (sometimes called hormone-releasing factor) stimulates another gland to release a hormone in a *feedforward* control system. Hormones that stimulate the release of another hormone are called trophic hormones. The hypothalamus secretes numerous *trophic* hormones, including corticotrophin-releasing hormone (CRH). CRH in turn stimulates the anterior pituitary to release adrenocorticotrophic hormone (ACTH). ACTH then stimulates the adrenal cortex to release cortisol (the long-term stress hormone). When hormones from one gland cause the target gland to secrete a hormone, which affects yet another gland, this is called an axis. The example given above describes the hypothalamus-pituitary-adrenal axis diagrammed in **Figure 21.2**.

The term *humoral* refers to blood or other body fluids. *Humoral activation* thus refers to stimulation of an endocrine gland by blood levels of nutrients, electrolytes, water, ions, or other factors. For example, the pancreas responds to blood levels of glucose (a nutrient) by releasing the hormone insulin. Likewise, the thyroid gland and parathyroid glands are stimulated to release calcitonin and parathyroid hormone, respectively, in response to blood levels of calcium (an electrolyte).

BLOOD HORMONE LEVELS The plasma concentration of a hormone depends on several factors including:

1. The rate at which the hormone is secreted
2. The rate at which it is broken down and removed from the blood
3. For some hormones, the effective, or biologically active amount; that is, how much of the hormone is bound to a protein versus how much is circulating in the free or unbound state

Hormones can be secreted in pulsatile (or rhythmic), circadian (day/night or 24-hour periodization), entropic (random moment-to-moment variation), or cyclical (often monthly) patterns as well as on demand. Some hormones act instantaneously; others require minutes to hours to days to have an impact. Hormones can be broken down and cleared from the body by the kidney, liver, or target cells. In addition, many hormones (primarily the steroids) circulate in blood bound to protein. However, to interact with a receptor, the hormone must be unbound, or "free." In these cases, it is the amount of free hormone, not the total amount circulating that determines the biological effectiveness of the hormone.

In addition to the factors listed above, hormonal blood levels are affected by disease, temperature, altitude, nutritional status, age, sex, exercise, hydration level, and training status.

EXTENT OF CELLULAR RESPONSE As stated earlier, hormones affect a target cell by binding to a receptor on or in the target cell. This binding requires complementary shapes between the hormone and the receptor. The hormone-receptor binding is known as *receptor activation*. The extent of cellular response to receptor activation depends on three factors (Marieb and Hoehn, 2010):

1. The blood levels of the hormone
2. The relative number of receptors
3. The strength (affinity) of the bond between the hormone and receptor

Factors influencing the blood level of the hormone are described in the preceding section. The number of receptors on a cell for any given hormone can vary over time and in response to acute exercise and chronic exercise training. Hormone-receptor binding often destroys the receptor; as a result, replacement receptors are needed. High-affinity receptors produce a more pronounced hormonal effect than low-affinity receptors. High blood levels of a hormone may cause either an increase in the number of receptors (*up-regulation*) or a decrease in the number of receptors (*down-regulation*). Up-regulation increases the cell's ability to bring about the hormone-specific cellular response; down-regulation prevents the target cells from overreacting to persistently high hormonal levels. Low blood levels of a hormone may also result in up-regulation. The more receptors, the lower the hormone concentration required to cause any given physiological response.

Mechanism of Hormonal Action

Hormones are divided into three general classifications: (1) proteins and polypeptides, (2) steroid-based hormones, and (3) derivatives of the amino acid tyrosine. Protein and polypeptide hormones include those released from the anterior and posterior pituitary gland, the pancreas, the parathyroid gland, and dozens of others. Steroid-based hormones are derived from cholesterol and include only those hormones secreted from the adrenal cortex (aldosterone and cortisol) and gonads (estrogen and testosterone). Derivatives of tyrosine include the hormones released from the thyroid (T3 and T4) and the adrenal medulla (epinephrine and norepinephrine).

For a hormone to bring about an action within a cell, it must first bind to a cellular receptor. Receptors

TABLE 21.3 Hormones Involved in Regulating Exercise

Site produced (Endocrine Gland/Tissue)	Hormone(s)	Selected Functions Relative to Exercise Physiology
Adipose tissue	Leptin	Food intake, metabolic rate
Adrenal gland		
• Adrenal cortex	Cortisol, aldosterone	Metabolism, stress response, immune function, anti-inflammatory, catabolic to muscle tissue
• Adrenal medulla	Epinephrine, norepinephrine	Na$^+$, K$^+$, and acid secretion by kidneys, fluid balance
Gonads		
• Ovaries (female)	Estrogen	Fat deposition, bone remodeling
	Progesterone	Catabolic to muscular tissue, bone remodeling
• Testes (male)	Testosterone	Bone and muscle growth and development
Hypothalamus		
	Hypothalamic trophic hormones (general)	Controls secretions of hormones of anterior pituitary (in general): see anterior pituitary.
	• Corticotrophin-releasing hormone (CRH)	Stimulates anterior pituitary (Ant.Pit.) to secrete adrenocorticotrophic hormone (ACTH)
	• Thyrotrophin-releasing hormone (TRH)	Stimulates Ant.Pit. to secrete thyroid-stimulating hormone (TSH)
	• Growth hormone–releasing hormone (GHRH)	Stimulates Ant.Pit. to secrete growth hormone (GH)
	• Growth hormone–inhibiting hormone (GHIH)	Inhibits secretion of GH
	• Gonadotrophin-releasing hormone (GnRH)	Stimulates Ant.Pit. to secrete luteinizing hormone (LH) and follicle-stimulating hormone (FSH)
	Production of antidiuretic hormone (ADH), which is released by posterior pituitary gland	Water retention, fluid balance
Kidneys	Erythropoietin	Erythrocyte (RBC) production
Leukocytes (WBC) and endothelial cells	Cytokines	Immune functions
Liver	Somatomedins (insulin-like growth factors [IGFI])	Anabolic to muscle tissue
Pancreas	Insulin, glucagon	Metabolism, regulates blood glucose levels
Parathyroid	Parathyroid hormone (PTH)	Plasma Ca^{2+}, PO$_4^-$ levels
Pituitary		
• Anterior	Growth hormone	Bone and muscle growth, metabolism, stimulates IGF release
	Thyroid-stimulating hormone (THS)	Secretion of hormones from thyroid gland
	Adrenocorticotrophic hormone (ACTH)	Secretion of hormones from adrenal cortex
	Follicle-stimulating hormone (FSH) and Luteinizing hormone (LH)	Sex hormone secretion
• Posterior	Antidiuretic hormone (ADH, also called vasopressin)	Water excretion by kidneys, fluid balance, cardiovascular function
Thyroid	Thyroxine (T$_4$) triiodothyronine (T$_3$)	Metabolic rate
	Calcitonin	Plasma Ca^{2+} levels

may be on the cell membrane (often a transmembrane protein), in the cytoplasm, or in the nucleus of the cell. Once a hormone binds to a receptor on or in the target cell, a response is initiated. The sequence of steps from receptor activation to cellular response is known as the *signal transduction pathway* or *mechanism of action*. A hormone may exert its action through numerous transduction pathways; a full description of these pathways is beyond the scope of this text. However, as shown in **Figure 21.7**, signal transduction pathways may be

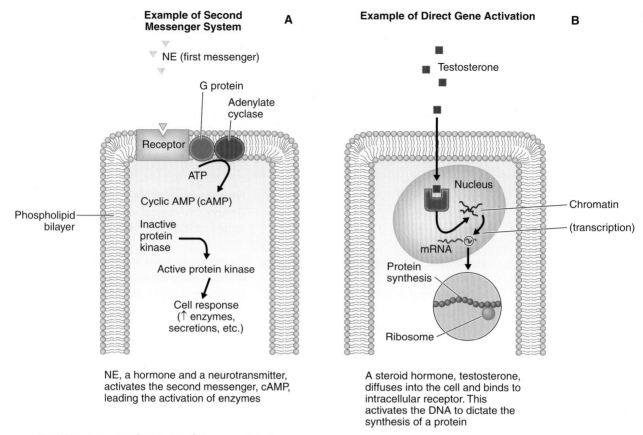

Example of Second Messenger System **A**

NE, a hormone and a neurotransmitter, activates the second messenger, cAMP, leading the activation of enzymes

Example of Direct Gene Activation **B**

A steroid hormone, testosterone, diffuses into the cell and binds to intracellular receptor. This activates the DNA to dictate the synthesis of a protein

FIGURE 21.7   Mechanisms of Hormonal Action.
Hormones may exert their effect on target organs (**A**) using a second messenger system (one example is shown) or (**B**) through direct gene activation.

broadly categorized into second messenger systems and gene activation pathways (Guyton and Hall, 2011; Marieb and Hoehn, 2010).

Because they are lipid insoluble and cannot diffuse into a cell, many hormones exert their influence primarily through a *second messenger system*. This mechanism begins when a hormone, known as the *first messenger* because it is delivering a chemical message from another tissue, binds to its specific receptor on the cell membrane. The binding of the first messenger to the receptor activates another membrane protein (e.g., G protein), which in turn activates a *second messenger* within the cell (e.g., adenylate cyclase). The second messenger initiates a cascade of chemical reactions (e.g., changing a protein kinase enzyme in the cell from an inactive to an active form) as shown in **Figure 21.7A**.

Steroid hormones and a few protein hormones are lipid soluble and diffuse easily into target cells. Once inside the cell, they operate by *direct gene activation*. Lipid-soluble hormones enter the cell and bind to receptors either in the nucleus or in the cell cytoplasm (forming a complex that must then migrate into the nucleus). The activated hormone-receptor complex signals the chromatin portion of the DNA, a gene, to be transcribed

to messenger RNA (mRNA). The mRNA carries the code from the nucleus to the cytoplasm, where a specific protein is synthesized (see **Figure 21.7B**). The protein produced may be a muscle filament or an enzyme that regulates cell metabolism.

Hormonal Communication and Responses

The hormonal system regulates and integrates a dizzying array of bodily functions. All hormones exert their influence by binding to a specific receptor on or in the cell. Several additional principles help explain how these hormone-receptor complexes translate into physiological responses that result from exercise. **Figure 21.8** summarizes these essential principles:

- A target cell may (and usually does) have many different receptor types on its surface (**Figure 21.8A**). Furthermore, as noted earlier, the number of any given type of receptor may change over time based on cell needs.
- A hormone may have several different functions within a cell (**Figure 21.8B**). For example, when insulin binds to receptors on skeletal muscle cells, it may cause several things to happen, depending on

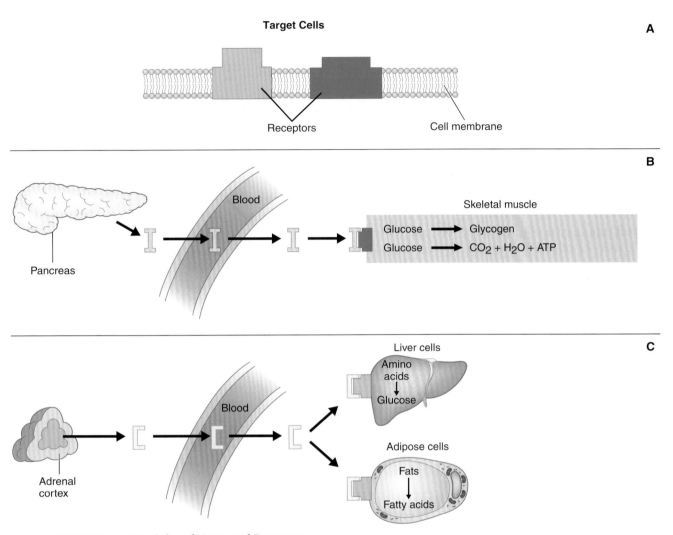

FIGURE 21.8   Principles of Hormonal Response.
A. Hormones bind to receptors because of complimentary structures. **B.** A hormone may have multiple effects within a single target organ. **C.** A hormone may affect multiple target organs.

metabolic conditions within the cell. These include an increase in the uptake of glucose into the cell, the formation of glycogen from glucose (by a process known as glycogenesis), or an increase in the rate at which glucose is broken down to produce ATP within the cell (glycolysis).

- A hormone may affect multiple target cells (**Figure 21.8C**). For example, when cortisol binds to receptors on the membrane of liver cells, it causes glycogen to be broken down into glucose through the process of glycogenolysis. Glucose levels in the blood thus increase, and glucose can be utilized as a fuel for active muscle cells and nervous tissue. However, when cortisol binds to receptors on adipose cells, it stimulates the breakdown of fats into free fatty acids and glycerol through the process of lipolysis. Thus, free fatty acid levels in the blood increase and can be utilized as a fuel for active muscle cells.

Interaction of Hormones

Many cellular responses require the joint action of many hormones. In a *synergistic response*, the combined effect of the hormones may be greater than the sum of their individual effects. In a *complementary response*, both or all hormones are needed to accomplish the task. *Permissive* hormones facilitate or potentiate the actions of another hormone, making their response more effective. In some situations, the actions of one hormone oppose another. These hormones are said to be antagonistic.

Role of the Endocrine System in Exercise

Exercise presents a physical stress that challenges homeostasis. In response, the neuroendocrine system, particularly the autonomic nervous system and the hypothalamic-pituitary-adrenal axis, react to help maintain homeostasis

(Mastorakos and Pavlatou, 2005). This section describes the hormonal response to exercise. The primary role of the endocrine system during an acute bout of exercise is to regulate the metabolic and cardiovascular systems (Bunt, 1986). The following sections therefore primarily describe how the endocrine system helps regulate the metabolic and cardiovascular systems, with secondary emphasis on muscle, bone, and adipose tissue.

Hormonal Regulation of Metabolism

Hormones play a critical role in regulating metabolism by controlling GI tract motility and the absorption of foodstuff, the storage and release of fuel, and the metabolic activity of cells. The overall goal of hormonal regulation of metabolism is to ensure that metabolic fuels (carbohydrate, fat, and protein) are available continuously to meet the metabolic needs of the organism and that excess fuels are stored. Additionally, the hormonal regulation of metabolism ensures that blood glucose levels are maintained at levels necessary to supply the nervous tissue with required amounts of glucose. The challenge of maintaining appropriate blood glucose and mobilizing lipids and amino acids when needed occurs because we ingest food only periodically (typically 2–6 times a day) but the cells constantly need fuel available to support metabolic activity—and the metabolic needs of the body may change drastically, as they do with exercise.

The goals of the endocrine system relative to metabolic activity are to:

1. Mobilize fuel for the production of ATP energy needed to support muscle contraction
2. Maintain blood glucose levels (because neural tissue can use only glucose to produce energy)

Glucagon, epinephrine, norepinephrine, growth hormone, and cortisol operate together under the permissive influence of triiodothyronine (T_3) to accomplish the first goal. Glucagon and insulin act antagonistically; glucagon levels increase and insulin levels are simultaneously suppressed during exercise. As shown in **Figure 21.9**, glucagon, NE, E, growth hormone (GH), and cortisol affect three primary target cells: adipose, liver, and skeletal muscle cells. When these hormones bind to receptors on adipose cells, fat storage is inhibited and fat mobilization and uptake enhanced. When these hormones bind to receptors on the liver, glycogen (chains of glucose molecules chemically linked together) is broken down to glucose, and additional glucose is synthesized from other sources, such as alanine (an amino acid), glycerol, or lactate. When these hormones bind to receptors on skeletal muscle, stored glycogen is broken down to glucose. These hormones also cause skeletal muscles to increase their uptake and utilization of fatty acids, which aids in providing substrate for ATP resynthesis.

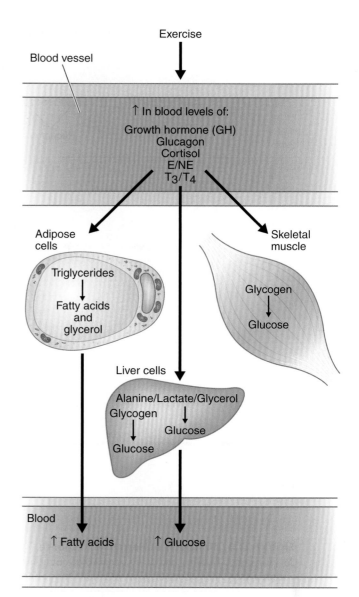

FIGURE 21.9   Effect of Metabolic Hormones.
Metabolic hormones affect adipose cells, liver cells, and skeletal muscle. The net effect of the metabolic hormones is to increase fuel availability.

Hormonal Regulation of Cardiovascular Function

The goals of the hormonal system relative to cardiovascular function are to:

1. Enhance cardiac function
2. Distribute blood to active tissues
3. Maintain blood pressure by stabilizing fluid and electrolyte balance

Enhanced cardiac function and distribution of blood to working muscles are primarily accomplished by E and NE released from the adrenal medulla. These adrenal hormones reinforce the actions of the sympathetic nervous system (see earlier section on ANS Control During

Exercise). In general, the two hormones have similar effects, but E is more important in increasing blood flow to skeletal muscle and the heart and NE is more influential in causing vasoconstriction and increasing blood pressure.

Two hormones predominate in the stabilization or maintenance of fluid and electrolyte balance: antidiuretic hormone (ADH), sometimes called vasopressin, and aldosterone. These hormones act on the kidneys to increase water resorption and retain or excrete specific electrolytes (Bunt, 1986). By maintaining fluid and electrolyte balance, these hormones positively affect blood volume and blood pressure as well (see Chapter 11).

Hormonal Involvement in Muscle, Bone, and Adipose Tissue

Hormones involved in the structure and function of muscle, bone, and adipose cells are beyond the immediate goals of supporting acute exercise, but they may be important during recovery and thus generally facilitate training adaptations (Bunt, 1986; Kraemer, 1992b); therefore they will be discussed briefly. Tissue repair mechanisms are activated during recovery after all exercise sessions. Hormones that impact muscle, bone, and adipose tissue include growth hormone, insulin-like growth factors (IGF), testosterone, estrogen, progesterone, calcitonin, parathyroid hormone (PTH), and leptin. The role of PTH, calcitonin, and estrogen in bone health is detailed in Chapter 16.

The impact of GH on protein synthesis in muscle is mediated through IGF. Growth hormone stimulates the release of IGF from the liver, and both muscle and connective tissue produce IGF. Specific effects of IGF include amino acid uptake, muscle synthesis, connective tissue (collagen) synthesis, bone and cartilage growth, and maintenance of fat-free muscle mass. Testosterone is responsible for the high ratio of muscle mass to fat mass that occurs in males at adolescence. Testosterone stimulates the release of GH and influences neural factors contributing to anabolic processes.

Adipose tissue has long been thought of as a mere storage depot for body fat, but we now know that adipose tissue is also an endocrine organ that plays an important role in regulating energy metabolism (Berggren et al., 2005; Galic et al., 2010; Greenberg and Obin, 2006; McMurray and Hackney, 2005; Ronti et al., 2006). As shown in **Figure 21.10**, adipose tissue secretes a number of cytokines, specifically termed adipokines because they are released from adipose tissue, although they are chemically identical to cytokines released from immune cells. Adipokines have diverse functions throughout the body. **Adipokines** are bioactive peptides released from adipose tissue that act locally and systemically through autocrine, paracrine, and endocrine effects with multiple of physiological roles, including mediating appetite and energy balance, influencing insulin sensitivity and lipid metabolism, and regulating immune function and hemostasis. The most prominent adipokine is the satiety hormone, leptin. Deficiencies in leptin or leptin receptors are associated with obesity (Tomas et al., 2004) (Chapter 8). Adiponectin is another adipokine and is associated with insulin resistance and the metabolic syndrome. Other adipokines are important mediators of inflammation and are discussed throughout this text in relation to vascular inflammation (Chapter 15), muscle damage (Chapter 19), and overtraining (Chapter 22). Adipose tissue thus functions as an endocrine organ and plays an important role in integrating the functions of the neuroendocrine system, the immune system, and metabolism. These physiological links help explain the role of increased adiposity in the development of atherosclerosis, hemostatic imbalance, insulin resistance, and the development of the metabolic syndrome.

Hormonal Responses to Exercise

It should be fairly obvious that the action of most of the aforementioned hormones increases during exercise (except for insulin). Without an increase in hormonal secretion, the enhanced functions just described would not occur. What is not so obvious is the pattern of response seen in blood concentrations of each of these hormones to exercises of different intensities, durations, and metabolic demands. Recall that changes in blood concentration of hormones may not simply indicate an increase in secretion, because hormonal levels are affected by changes in clearance rates, blood volume, receptor-binding turnover, and other factors (Bunt, 1986; Kraemer, 1992a). The following section presents what is known about hormonal response patterns in relation to the six categories of exercise used throughout this text:

1. Short-term light-to-moderate submaximal aerobic exercise
2. Long-term moderate-to-heavy submaximal aerobic exercise
3. Incremental aerobic exercise to maximum
4. Static exercise
5. Dynamic resistance exercise
6. Very short-term, high-intensity anaerobic exercise

In many instances, the hormonal responses in all six categories of exercise have not been identified. In general, much more is known about long-term moderate-to-heavy aerobic exercise and incremental exercise to maximum than other categories of exercise.

Although it might seem overwhelming to consider how different hormones respond to various categories of exercise, it is important to appreciate the differences in hormonal response based on the type of exercise performed. Indeed, many of the metabolic and cardiorespiratory responses described earlier in this text are determined in large part by these endocrine responses.

FIGURE 21.10 Adipose Tissue as an Endocrine Gland.
A. Adipose tissue secretes several peptides, collectively called adipokines, which have widespread and coordinated functions throughout the body **(B). C.** Adipokines also help modulate a multitude of neurohormonal factors that, in turn, regulate the secretion of adipokines from adipose tissue **(D).**

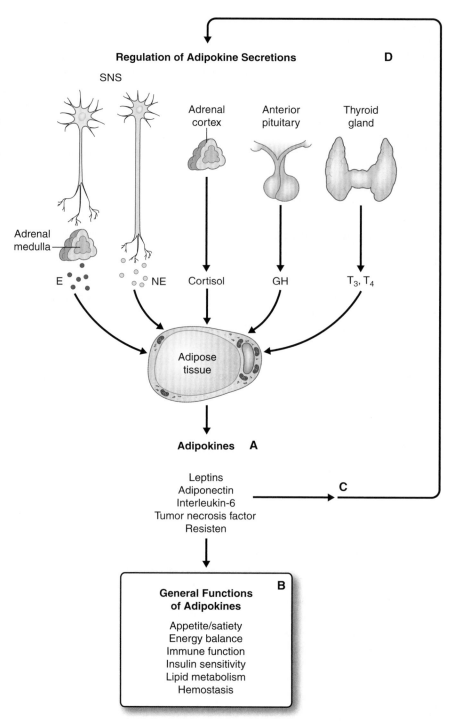

Metabolic and Cardiovascular Hormones

Epinephrine and Norepinephrine (Catecholamines)

Epinephrine (E) and norepinephrine (NE) are released from the adrenal medulla as a result of sympathetic nervous system stimulation. These hormones have widespread actions throughout the body and affect both the metabolic and cardiorespiratory responses to exercise. When interpreting the responses of E and NE to exercise, remember that NE is also released from sympathetic nerve endings. Because neural stimulation occurs more quickly than the endocrine response, the initial increase in NE in response to exercise is from the sympathetic nervous system (see **Figure 21.2**). Both E and NE are later released from the adrenal medulla. In this light, it should not be surprising that NE shows an elevation at lower workloads than E and that blood levels are generally higher for NE than E (Galbo, 1983).

The catecholamines are often called the "stress hormones," and they have widespread effects throughout the body and play an important role in coordinating adjustments to exercise, particularly intense exercise. Cardiovascular adjustments such as an increased heart rate and force of contraction and vasoconstriction in nonworking muscles are accomplished by the actions of the sympathetic nervous system and augmented and reinforced by circulating E and NE. Catecholamines are critical to the control of circulation, blood clotting, and immune defense and thus warrant considerable attention.

Minimal increases in both E and NE occur during short-term light-to-moderate submaximal aerobic exercise (**Figure 21.11A** and **B**). During long-term moderate-to-heavy submaximal aerobic exercise, the increase depends on time and is gradual if energy is supplied aerobically up to the point of fatigue (**Figure 21.11C** and **D**). Incremental aerobic exercise to maximum elicits positive exponential increases in both E and NE (**Figure 21.11E** and **F**), clearly indicating that a lower limit of submaximal intensity must be exceeded before a response is achieved and that above that point the increase in hormonal level depends on intensity (Acevedo et al., 2007). NE starts to spill out of organs by sympathetic nerve stimulation at intensities close to 70% of $\dot{V}O_2$max. E and NE from the adrenal medulla are secreted at intensities above 80–90% of $\dot{V}O_2$max (Borer, 2003). The E and NE response to static exercise (**Figure 21.11G** and **H**) is larger than during dynamic resistance exercise of equal heart rate or aerobic energy demand (oxygen consumption), and the rise in plasma E seems to be larger relative to NE than during aerobic exercise (Galbo, 1983). The response of E and NE to dynamic resistance exercise appears to be related to the force of muscle contraction, the amount of muscle tissue stimulated, and the amount of rest between repetitions (**Figure 21.11I** and **J**) (Kraemer, 1988; Kramer and Ratamess, 2005). Very short-term, high-intensity anaerobic work, such as in the Wingate anaerobic test (WAT), results in a large increase in both E and NE (Vincent et al., 2004).

Fluid Balance Hormones

Exercise causes rapid shifts in body fluid compartments, including a rapid decrease in plasma volume. Plasma volume may decrease by approximately 15% in the first few minutes of exercise, largely because the increase in blood pressure leads to an increase in capillary filtration pressure that pushes plasma into the interstitial space. Additionally, sweat loss during prolonged exercise can cause further reductions in plasma volume. Protecting against excessive fluid loss is important to maintain an aqueous environment for metabolic reactions, to maintain thermal balance, and to support cardiovascular function. Several hormones function together to help maintain fluid balance in response to exercise stress.

Antidiuretic hormone, released from the posterior pituitary, increases water retention, whereas aldosterone, released from the adrenal gland, increases salt and water retention. Thus, these two hormones act to maintain plasma volume. Aldosterone is linked with angiotensin II and renin. Renin converts angiotensinogen to angiotensin I, which is subsequently converted to angiotensin II, which initiates a signal for the adrenal glands to release aldosterone. Angiotensin II is also a potent vasoconstrictor helping to maintain blood pressure during vasodilation in working muscles. Thus, renin, antidiuretic hormone, and aldosterone work in concert to help maintain fluid balance, and thereby cardiovascular function, during exercise. (see Chapter 11 for a discussion of the hormonal control of blood volume.) Changes in renin, antidiuretic hormone, and aldosterone—known as fluid balance hormones—occur parallel to each other. They highly correlate with changes in NE and have similar time courses. **Figure 21.13E** depicts the positive exponential response of ADH to incremental exercise to maximum (Wade, 2000).

Metabolic Hormones

A number of overlapping hormonal responses help ensure that skeletal muscles can increase their metabolic activity during exercise. As discussed earlier, the catecholamines play an important role regulating metabolic responses to exercise (by increasing lipolysis, stimulating insulin, and suppressing glucagon). This section focuses on several other metabolic hormones directly involved in regulating the metabolic response to exercise.

The exercise responses of the metabolic hormones have been studied most extensively during long-term moderate-to-heavy submaximal aerobic exercise and incremental aerobic exercise to maximum. Therefore, what is known about the exercise response of these hormones applies primarily to these categories of exercise. Although plasma levels are presented for each hormone in the figures, keep in mind that changes in plasma levels may reflect not changes in secretion but rather changes in clearance rates. The responses might also reflect autonomic nervous system changes.

Insulin and Glucagon

Insulin operates to store fuel, whereas glucagon's role is to mobilize fuel. Therefore, in general, the responses of these two hormones are close to mirror images of each other. The ratio of glucagon to insulin primarily controls fuel mobilization, however. Insulin has multiple actions, including increasing glucose and free fatty acid uptake and decreasing glycogenolysis and gluconeogenesis. In contrast, glucagon stimulates glycogenolysis and gluconeogenesis and is important for maintaining blood glucose levels during prolonged exercise.

During short-term light-to-moderate submaximal aerobic exercise, insulin declines a small amount initially

FOCUS ON RESEARCH

Catecholamine Response to Resistance Exercise

The responses of the adrenal medullary hormones, epinephrine (E) and norepinephrine (NE), have been relatively well studied. However, little was known about the response of these hormones to the stress of heavy resistance exercise. Therefore, Bush and colleagues designed a study to examine the effect of dynamic resistance exercise on the response of the adrenal medullary hormones immediately after different protocols of resistance exercise and during recovery. Each participant was tested on 2 days: on one day, participants performed a high-force protocol (using a 10-repetition maximum), and on the other day, they performed a high-power protocol (using 15 repetitions). The total work performed on each day was equal. Blood was drawn at four different times: before each resistance training session, immediately postexercise (0-minute recovery), after 15 minutes of recovery, and after 4 hours of recovery. The concentration of norepinephrine and epinephrine in the plasma at each time with the two protocols is shown in the figures below.

Statistical analysis revealed the following:

1. Norepinephrine was significantly higher postexercise in both protocols.

2. Epinephrine increased significantly following exercise in both protocols and returned to near baseline levels by 15 minutes of recovery.

These results indicate that heavy resistance exercise activates the adrenal medulla. Because the activation of the sympathetic nervous system, the "fight or flight" response, is thought to be an important mediator of acute stress, the elevation of norepinephrine and epinephrine after a bout of heavy resistance exercise suggests that the neuroendocrine system helps regulate the body's response to the stress of resistance exercise. Furthermore, the similar response of NE and E in the two protocols suggests that, as long as the total work is equal, subtle differences in mean force and mean power characteristics of a workout do not affect this hormonal response.

Source: Bush, J. A., W J. Kraemer, A. M. Mastro, N. T. Triplett-M Bush, J. A., W. J. Kraemer, A. M. Mastro, N. T. Triplett-McBride, J. S. Volek, M. Putukian, W. J. Sebastianelli, & H. G. Knuttgen. Exercise and recovery responses of adrenal medullary neurohormones to heavy resistance exercise. *Medicine & Science in Sports & Exercise.* 31(4):554–559 (1999).

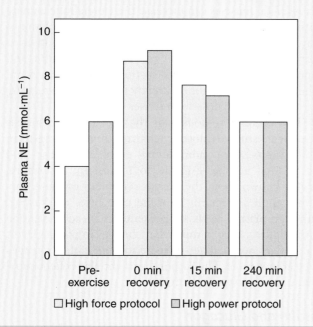

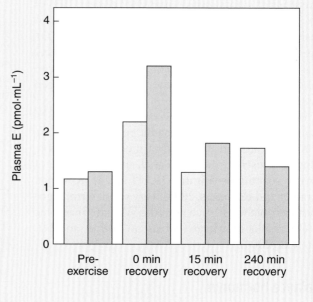

□ High force protocol   □ High power protocol

before leveling off, and glucagon rises a small amount initially before leveling off (Galbo, 1983). Long-term moderate-to-heavy submaximal aerobic exercise causes an initial rapid increase in glucagon followed by a gradual increase (**Figure 21.12A**) and a complementary initial rapid drop in insulin followed by gradual decline (**Figure 21.12B**) (Galbo, 1983). During incremental exercise to maximum, glucagon increases in a positively exponential manner. The increase in glucagon is proportionally greater as exercise intensity increases than is the decline in insulin (**Figure 21.13A and B**). Indeed, at high workloads (>60% $\dot{V}O_2$max), plasma insulin levels begin to rise again, resulting overall in a truncated U-shaped curve that remains below resting levels. Neither static activity nor short-term high-intensity exercise (such as sprinting or dynamic resistance exercise) appears to affect either insulin or glucagon much, because fuel demands for these activities do not require extensive mobilization. However,

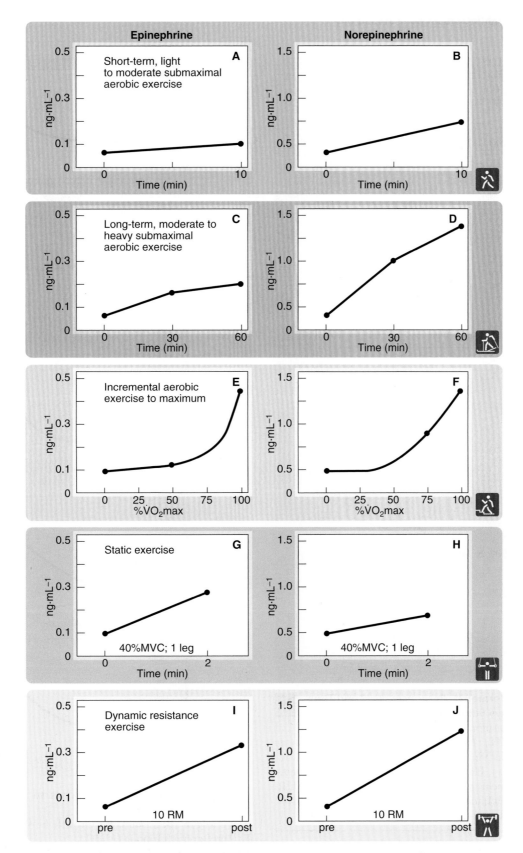

FIGURE 21.11 Epinephrine and Norepinephrine Responses to Various Categories of Exercise.
(**A, B**) Short-term, light to moderate submaximal aerobic exercise. (**C, D**) Long-term, moderate to heavy submaximal aerobic exercise. (**E, F**) Incremental aerobic exercise to maximum. (**G, H**) Static exercise. (**I, J**) Dynamic resistance exercise.

Sources: Galbo, H.: *Hormonal and Metabolic Adaptation to Exercise.* New York, NY: Thieme-Stratton (1983); Kraemer, W. J.: Endocrine responses to resistance exercise. *Medicine and Science in Sports and Exercise.* 20(5):S152–S157 (1988).

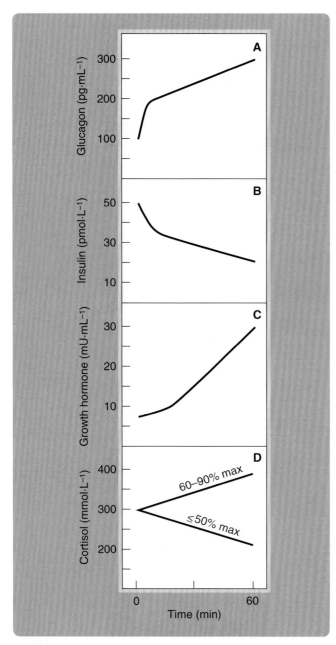

FIGURE 21.12 Hormonal Responses to Long-Term Moderate-to-Heavy Submaximal Aerobic Exercise.
A. Glucagon. **B.** Insulin. **C.** Growth hormone. **D.** Cortisol.
Sources: Galbo, H.: *Hormonal and Metabolic Adaptation to Exercise*. New York, NY: Thieme-Stratton (1983); Sutton, J. R., P. A. Farrell, & V. J. Harber: Hormonal adaptations to physical activity. In Bouchard, C., R. J. Shephard, T. Stephens, J. R. Sutton, & B. D. McPherson (eds.): *Exercise, Fitness, and Health*. Champaign, IL: Human Kinetics, 217–257 (1990).

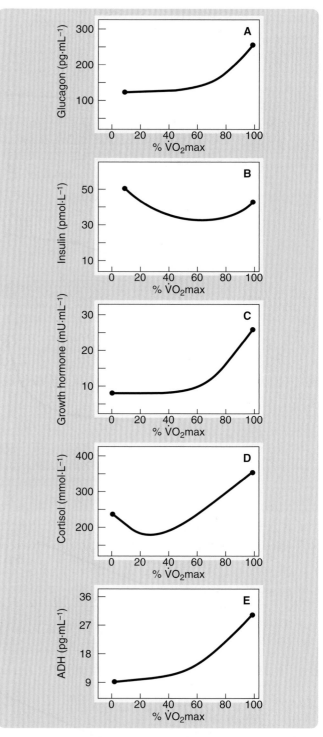

FIGURE 21.13 Hormonal Responses to Incremental Aerobic Exercise to Maximum.
A. Glucagon. **B.** Insulin. **C.** Growth hormone. **D.** Cortisol. **E.** Antidiuretic hormone (ADH).
Sources: Galbo, H.: *Hormonal and Metabolic Adaptation to Exercise*. New York, NY: Thieme-Stratton (1983); Sutton, J. R., P. A. Farrell, & V. J. Harber: Hormonal adaptations to physical activity. In Bouchard, C., R. J. Shephard, T. Stephens, J. R. Sutton, & B. D. McPherson (eds.): *Exercise, Fitness, and Health*. Champaign, IL: Human Kinetics, 217–257 (1990); Wade, C. E.: Hormonal regulation of fluid homeostasis during and following exercise. In Warren, M. P, & N. W. Constantini (eds.): *Sports Endocrinology*. Totowa, NJ: Humana Press, 207–226 (2000).

some authors have reported decreased insulin levels following a bout of resistance exercise (Raastad et al., 2000).

Growth Hormone

As a protein hormone, growth hormone (GH) has a slow rate of response, secretion, and clearance (Galbo, 1983).

FOCUS ON APPLICATION

Multiple Factors Affect Energy Balance and Adiposity

Exercise professionals routinely prescribe exercise to increase caloric expenditure (energy output) in an attempt to maintain caloric balance or to create an energy deficit (calorie expenditure > calorie intake) to decrease adiposity. Much of Chapters 8 in this text is devoted to such issues. This chapter focuses on hormonal responses to exercise, including the hormones that regulate hormonal adjustments to exercise.

Below is a schematic illustration of factors that influence energy intake and output and their relationship to adiposity.

Exercise professionals prescribing exercise for energy balance must consider many factors. The schematic above reminds us:

1. A large number of factors affect energy balance

2. The various factors interact extensively

3. Hormones have a central role in the body's responses to exercise and as regulators of hunger

4. Adipose tissue releases hormones and adipokines that in turn affect other hormones, the exercise response, and hunger

Source: McMurray and Hackney (2005).

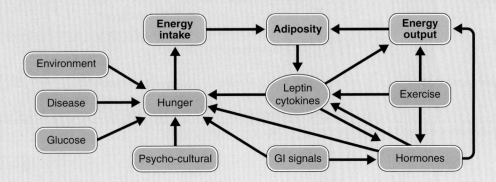

Thus there is a delay between the onset of exercise and changes in blood hormonal levels. The greater the intensity of the exercise, the shorter this delay. Short-term light-to-moderate submaximal aerobic exercise and static exercise are too brief for any changes to become apparent. A short but high-intensity exercise causes a peak value in GH that may occur from 15 to 30 minutes into recovery.

Long-term moderate-to-heavy submaximal aerobic exercise leads to a gradual increase in GH over 30–60 minutes (**Figure 21.12C**) (Galbo, 1983). If the activity continues much longer, however, as in a marathon, GH concentrations return to near baseline levels. With incremental aerobic exercise to maximum (**Figure 21.13C**), GH concentration increases with increasing workloads in a positive exponential fashion after the initial delay.

GH release increases during and following resistance exercise. High total work and short rest periods are associated with a much larger increase in GH than low total work volume and long rest periods (Kraemer, 1992a). Similarly, exercise using large muscle mass results in greater elevations of GH than those using a small muscle mass. Research suggests that the metabolic properties of the muscle affect the GH response. That is, protocols that cause high lactate levels (e.g., programs that use moderate- to high-intensity and high-volume exercise, that stress large muscle mass, and that use relatively short rest intervals, thus stressing the

fast glycolytic fibers) produce the most substantial increases in GH in both men and women (Kramer and Ratamess, 2005). Evidence also suggests that GH response is affected by menstrual state (normal cycling or disordered menstrual cycle) (Nakamura et al., 2011).

Cortisol

Like growth hormone, the steroid-based cortisol is a slow-acting hormone. In addition to multiple roles in metabolism, cortisol has numerous biological functions throughout the body, as outlined in **Table 21.4**. Cortisol is also considered a "stress hormone" because it mediates many responses to stress, particularly chronic or long-term stress. As such, cortisol is an important mediator of immune response to exercise (see Chapter 22).

It is difficult to generalize a pattern of cortisol's exercise response because of the initial delay in exercise-enhanced concentrations and because in short-duration and/or low- to moderate-intensity activity, clearance of the hormone exceeds secretion. This means that although secretion may increase, blood concentrations actually decrease (Sutton et al., 1990). This outcome can be seen in **Figure 21.12D**, which depicts the response of cortisol to long-term moderate-to-heavy exercise. Work intensity less than or equal to 50% of $\dot{V}O_2$max results in a steady decrease in blood cortisol level, whereas intensity loads

TABLE 21.4 Multiple Effects of Cortisol on Various Bodily Functions

Category of Function	Cortisol Activities
Metabolism	↑ Protein degradation in muscle and connective tissue
	↓ Protein synthesis in muscle and connective tissue
	↓ Amino acid transport into muscle
	↑ Amino acid transport into liver
	↑ Gluconeogenesis
	↑ Glycogen synthesis in liver
	↓ Glucose uptake and utilization
	↑ Lipolysis
Immunity	↓ Inflammatory cytokines (IL-1 and IL-6)
	↓ Capillary permeability
	↓ Phagocytosis
	↓ T lymphocytes
Circulation and blood	↑ Vasoconstriction
	↑ Blood volume (body fluid retention)
	↑ Erythrocyte and leukocyte synthesis
Kidney function	↑ Glomerular filtration rate
	↑ Sodium retention
Brain functions	↑ Mood (euphoria) ↓ Mood (depression)
	↓ Taste, hearing, and smell
	↓ Food intake

Source: Modified from Borer, K.T.: *Exercise Endocrinology.* Champaign, IL: Human Kinetics (2003).

from approximately 60 to 90% of V̇O₂max cause a gradual rise in blood cortisol level over time, despite a constant workload. The truncated U pattern for incremental exercise to maximum seen in **Figure 21.13D** reinforces the importance of intensity in the cortisol response. Indeed, cortisol may not increase until anaerobic metabolism makes a significant contribution to the total energy supply. Anaerobic exercise causes greater increases in cortisol than aerobic exercise, even at the same total work output, probably because of the greater intensity (Kraemer, 1988, 1992a). Dynamic resistance exercise causes large increases both during and after high-intensity sessions, probably because of its large anaerobic component. Cortisol levels in the blood remain elevated up to several hours after exercise. Exercise programs causing the greatest change in GH (and lactate) also result in the most substantial changes in cortisol (Kramer and Ratamess, 2005).

CHECK YOUR COMPREHENSION 1

Liz, a graduate student in kinesiology, takes a break from her research duties and goes out for a 60-minute bike ride. What hormones are involved in regulating the metabolic response to her exercise and what is the general goal of these hormones?

Check your answer in Appendix C

Thyroid and Parathyroid Hormone

The pattern of thyroid and parathyroid hormonal responses to the different categories of exercise is unclear (Galbo, 1983). Numerous studies have reported no change in blood concentrations of triiodothyronine (T₃) or thyroxine (T₄). However, it is possible that free T₃ and free T₄ change without resulting in changes in the total concentration of thyroid hormone; this lack of change does not mean an unchanged turnover (Berent and Wartofsky, 2000). With long-term heavy aerobic exercise, free T₄ increases slightly, while free T₃ declines gradually over time, but little more can be concluded. The data are insufficient to draw any conclusions regarding calcitonin or parathyroid hormone responses to exercise.

Hormones Related to Muscle, Bone, and Adipose Tissue

Muscle

There is no clear pattern of response of IGF to acute aerobic exercise, although there is some indication of an early (at about 10 minutes of exercise) increase in IGF that is unrelated to intensity and declines with increasing duration of exercise. A single bout of resistance exercise leads to acute changes in the hormonal environment (an increase in catecholamines and IGF) that is linked to the cellular processes involved in protein turnover and muscle

FOCUS ON APPLICATION: *Clinically Relevant*

The Influence of Menstrual Cycle Hormonal Fluctuations on Physiological Responses to Exercise

Although this chapter focuses on the effects of exercise and exercise training on the neurohormonal system, fluctuations in estrogen and progesterone during the menstrual cycle can potentially cause changes in exercise performance or the physiological responses and adaptations to exercise/exercise training. Current literature suggests that fluctuations in female reproductive hormones do not affect muscle contractile characteristics or $\dot{V}O_2$max (and its determinants). Similarly, neither maximal strength nor intense anaerobic activities appear affected by the menstrual cycle. During prolonged exercise in the heat, however, the exercise time to exhaustion decreases during the mid-luteal phase (when progesterone is increased and body temperature is elevated) (Janse de Jonge, 2003; Marsh and Jenkins, 2002).

There is some controversy concerning the lactate response to exercise during various phases of the menstrual cycle that may be the result of different analysis techniques.

Forsyth and Reilly (2005) studied 11 endurance-trained eumenorrheic (regularly cycling) female athletes not taking oral contraceptives at the mid-follicular (6–10 days after menses) and mid-luteal (6–10 days after the LH surge) phases of the menstrual cycle. Menstrual phase was confirmed by blood hormonal analyses. Subjects were tested at 06:00 and 18:00 hours on a Concept II rowing machine using an incremental test to maximum. Lactate threshold (LT1) was determined three ways: by a mathematical curve-fitting procedure, by the visual procedure shown in Chapter 3 (Figure 3.16), and at the fixed blood lactate concentration [La] of 4.0 mmol·L⁻¹ (LT2). Ventilatory threshold (VT1) was also determined. At rest and a fixed exercise intensity, La was significantly lower in the mid-luteal phase than in the mid-follicular phase. In the mid-luteal phase, LT at 4.0 mmol·L⁻¹ occurred at a significantly higher exercise intensity, heart rate, and oxygen consumption than in the mid-follicular phase. Blood lactate concentrations at VT1 and LT1 (but not power output, heart rate, $\dot{V}O_2$, or ratings of perceived exertion) using the mathematical curve-fitting procedure were significantly lower in the mid-luteal phase, but no changes were observed in any variable when LT1 was determined by the visual curve fitting technique. The curve fitting techniques provide information regarding the balance between lactate production and clearance. Below the LT1 threshold, production and clearance are equal. The glycogen-sparing effect of estrogen in the luteal phase likely causes a decrease in lactate production above LT1. This impact is masked when a set concentration is used for the lactate threshold.

These findings suggest that the menstrual cycle phase must be carefully considered when a fixed value of blood lactate is used to establish responses to training or even training load. Workouts linked to absolute lactate values may need adjustment throughout the menstrual cycle. When lactate thresholds are of interest, testing should be performed during the same menstrual cycle phase for each testing session. Alternately, use of the visual curve fitting techniques should eliminate the problem.

Sources: Janse de Jonge (2003), Marsh and Jenkins (2002), Forsyth and Reilly (2005).

---

growth (Kraemer and Ratamess, 2005). Muscle protein turnover is an important part of protein metabolism and is necessary for muscle breakdown (during exercise) and subsequent muscle repair (during recovery) (Crewther et al., 2006). Resistance training programs designed primarily to produce muscle hypertrophy cause large acute increases in growth hormone and the catabolic hormone, cortisol. On the other hand, programs designed primarily to increase dynamic power cause little or no change in GH and modest changes in cortisol. During and following high-intensity dynamic aerobic and resistance exercise, testosterone levels in men are elevated and remain so for a couple of hours during recovery. Prolonged exercise results in an initial increase, followed by a return to baseline or below during recovery (Cumming, 2000). Women have much lower basal levels of testosterone than men, and there are inconsistencies in the literature as to the extent that testosterone increases in women following resistance exercise (Enea et al., 2011). There is strong evidence that menstrual cycle state (normal cycling or disordered menstrual cycle) affects resting testosterone levels (Nakamura et al., 2011).

Bone

Acute submaximal aerobic and resistance exercise results in elevated blood levels of estrogen and progesterone (Chilibeck, 2000; McMurray and Hackney, 2005). Kemmier and colleagues (Kemmier et al., 2003) have shown that free testosterone, estradiol, and GH increase as a result of a single bout of high-impact exercise in postmenopausal females. IGF does not change, but the insulin-like growth factor–binding protein-3 increases biphasically during exercise and then 22 hours after exercise. This could be important for osteoporosis prevention.

Adipose Tissue

Testosterone may suppress leptin in an acute bout of exercise, but this is confounded by the duration and intensity of the exercise. In general, serum leptin concentrations are unchanged by short-duration (< ~40 minutes) light-to-moderate submaximal exercise. However, both very short-duration high-intensity anaerobic exercise (including resistance exercise) and long-duration moderate-to-heavy submaximal aerobic exercise appear to reduce serum leptin concentrations. These findings may also be related to changes in nutrient availability or flux at the adipocytes. The clinical relevance of the effects of exercise on circulating leptin concentration has not yet been established (Hulver and Houmard, 2003; Zafeiridis et al., 2003). Low and moderate aerobic exercise do not cause a change in adiponectin, but levels (corrected for plasma volume changes) increase 30 minutes after heavy or maximal aerobic exercise (Ferguson et al., 2004; Jürimäe et al., 2005, 2006a,b; Kraemer and Castracane, 2007)

Hormonal Adaptations to Training

Training programs are not usually deliberately designed to bring about adaptations in the hormonal system. No research-based training principles have been established, and few systematic attempts have been made to vary intensity, duration, frequency, length of training period, and modality in large numbers of subjects. Some information has been derived from cross-sectional studies that compared untrained (or sedentary) individuals to trained (or fit) individuals. Some information has also been derived from testing individuals before and after a training period. More information and consensus exists about hormonal responses to a long-term absolute submaximal aerobic exercise training program that is moderate to heavy in intensity. This section describes those changes and what training adaptations are known to result from resistance training programs. It is important to understand that adaptations in one hormone may impact plasma levels of another, and changes in receptor sensitivity may not be reflected in circulating hormone levels. Furthermore, adaptations in sympathetic nervous system responses may cause changes in hormonal levels. As with hormonal responses to exercise, training adaptations in the metabolic, cardiorespiratory, and neuromuscular systems often result from adaptations in the endocrine system.

Adaptations Related to Metabolic Function

Most of what is known about hormonal training adaptations comes from studies comparing the response of individuals to a prolonged bout of exercise before and after exercise training (**Figure 21.14**). The major hormones involved in fuel mobilization (glucagon, insulin, NE, E, cortisol) all show a dampening effect as a result of exercise training; that is, the change from resting levels that occurs during exercise represents a smaller disruption of homeostasis than in the untrained state (Bunt, 1986). Given that endurance training decreases the sympathetic nervous system response to an absolute workload, epinephrine and norepinephrine are expected to have muted responses (**Figure 21.14A**).

The decline in insulin is less in the trained than in the untrained state (**Figure 21.14B**). The rise in glucagon is also less: so much less that 60 minutes of submaximal exercise may not be long enough or intense enough to cause a glucagon response in a trained individual (**Figure 21.14C**) (Coggan and Williams, 1995; Sutton et al., 1990). Increased insulin sensitivity compensates for these changes. Growth hormone and cortisol have the same dampening effect, although both of these appear to have higher resting levels in aerobically trained than in untrained individuals (**Figure 21.14D** and **E**). Resistance-trained individuals appear to have unchanged resting GH concentrations (Kraemer, 1992a; Kraemer and Ratamess, 2005).

Adaptations Related to Cardiovascular Function

Neither of the hormones primarily responsible for fluid and electrolyte balance (ADH and aldosterone) show any clear training adaptation. However, plasma volume is higher in trained versus untrained individuals. The thyroid hormones adapt with an enhanced turnover rate, but too little is known about parathyroid hormone to draw any conclusion.

At the end of incremental exercise to maximum, E, NE, and cortisol are increased post training. Higher values reflect the trained individual's ability to do more high-intensity work (Borer, 2003; Bunt, 1986; Kjaer and Lange, 2000; Sutton et al., 1990).

Adaptations Related to Muscle, Bone, and Adipose Tissue

Muscle

It has been hypothesized that IGF initially decreases as a result of training but that after an unknown length of time (probably longer than 5 weeks), resting levels of both GH and IGF increase, indicating an anabolic (tissue growth) internal environment (Eliakim et al., 2000). Resistance training programs designed to increase muscle mass result in increases in GH and IGF (Crewthers, 2006).

The impact of chronic training on testosterone is controversial, possibly depending on the level of training. Moderate training results in an increase and extreme training a decrease (Urhausen and Kindermann, 2000). Together, a training increase in testosterone and growth

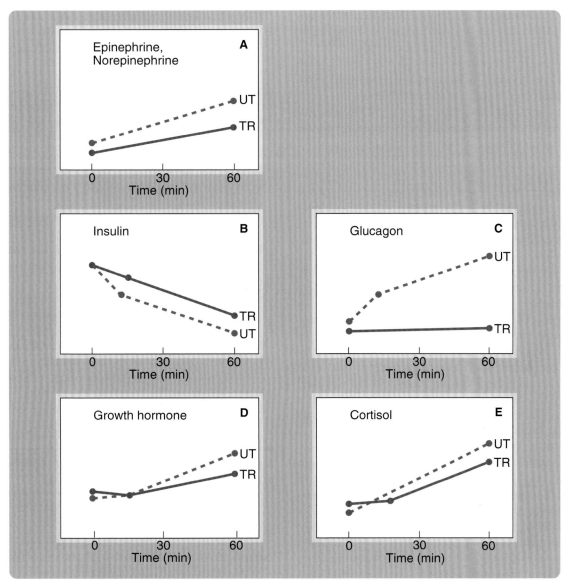

FIGURE 21.14 Training Adaptations Exhibited During Long-Term Submaximal Aerobic Exercise.
A. Epinephrine, norepinephrine. **B.** Insulin. **C.** Glucagon. **D.** Growth hormone. **E.** Cortisol.
Sources: Bunt, J. C.: Hormonal alterations due to exercise. *Sports Medicine*. 3:331–345 (1986); Coggan, A. R., & B. D. Williams: Metabolic adaptations to endurance training: Substrate metabolism during exercise. In Hargraves, M. (ed.): *Exercise Metabolism*. Champaign, IL: Human Kinetics, 177–210 (1995); Kjaer, M., & K. Lange: Adrenergic regulation of energy metabolism. In Warren, M. P. & N. W. Constantini (eds.): *Sports Endocrinology*. Totowa, NJ: Humana Press, 181–188 (2000); Sutton, J. R., P. A. Farrell, & V. J. Harber: Hormonal adaptations to physical activity. In Bouchard, C., R. J. Shephard, T. Stephens, J. R. Sutton, & B. D. McPherson (eds.): *Exercise, Fitness, and Health*. Champaign, IL: Human Kinetics, 217–257 (1990).

hormone could contribute to increases in muscle mass (Kraemer, 1992b).

Bone

Moderate exercise training appears to result in elevated resting levels of estrogen and progesterone, whereas severe training results in decreased resting levels. Male and female athletes reportedly have lower PTH levels and higher bone mineral density than nonathletes (Chilibeck, 2000).

Adipose Tissue

Training suppresses leptin levels (Gleim and Glace, 2000). Exercise training leads to a decrease in overall body fat. Levels of leptin are generally low in athletes of both sexes as well as in recreational runners, consistent with low levels of body fat. Also, in the general population, activity levels and leptin have been shown to be negatively related in both sexes (Popovic and Duntas, 2005). Finally, some studies have reported decreased resting concentrations of leptin with endurance or resistance training (McMurray and Hackney, 2005). Acute low-to-moderate physical activity causes hormonal changes that facilitate lipolytic activity, but trained individuals may be more sensitive to hormonal signals for the mobilization of fat as a fuel source (McMurray and Hackney, 2005). Training increases resting adiponectin levels in previously sedentary individuals (Blüher et al., 2006) but not elite rowers after a volume-extended training season (Jürimäe et al., 2006a,b).

SUMMARY

1. The nervous system and hormonal system both help maintain homeostasis and respond to the stress of exercise. These systems interact and overlap in multiple ways, so much so that they are often referred to collectively as the neurohormonal system. Both systems communicate with target cells by chemical messengers.

2. A target cell is activated when the chemical message from the nervous system (neurotransmitter) or endocrine system (hormone) binds to receptors on or in the target cell. Receptor activation can cause one or more of the following: change in the electrical state of the cell, change in enzyme activity, change in secretory activity of the cell, muscle contraction, or protein synthesis.

3. The autonomic nervous system (ANS) carries information from the CNS to cardiac muscle, smooth muscle, and endocrine glands. The two branches of the ANS, the sympathetic and parasympathetic nervous system, work in opposition to each other. The sympathetic nervous system plays a critical role in directing the body's response to exercise, whereas the parasympathetic nervous system is particularly important during recovery from exercise.

4. The exercise response is mediated primarily through the sympathetic nervous system. Its primary functions during exercise are to enhance cardiorespiratory function, regulate blood flow and maintain blood pressure, maintain thermal balance, and increase fuel mobilization for the production of energy.

5. During exercise, several metabolic hormones (glucagon, insulin, growth hormone, epinephrine [E], and norepinephrine [NE]) function together to mobilize fuel for the production of adenosine triphosphate (ATP) and to maintain blood glucose levels.

6. During exercise, several hormones help enhance cardiac function (E, NE), distribute blood to active tissue (E, NE), and maintain fluid and electrolyte balance (antidiuretic hormone [ADH], renin, and aldosterone).

7. Hormonal adaptations may result from exercise training, or individuals may become more sensitive to a lower level of hormone so that the same effect occurs following training even without a changed baseline hormonal level. The most common pattern is a blunted hormonal response to exercise following training (glucagon being an important exception).

REVIEW QUESTIONS

1. Define homeostasis, and identify the role of the nervous system and hormonal system in maintaining homeostasis.

2. Why are the nervous system and the endocrine system often referred to collectively as the neuroendocrine system?

3. What role does the autonomic nervous system play in regulating the exercise response?

4. Describe receptor activation and list five changes that may occur in a target cell as a result of receptor activation.

5. Discuss the primary role of exercise-induced hormonal changes relative to the cardiovascular system and the metabolic system.

6. Is adipose tissue an endocrine tissue? Explain.

7. Create a table that shows how the hormones involved in regulating metabolism and fluid balance respond to exercise.

8. How does the hormonal system adapt as a result of exercise training?

For further review and additional study tools, visit the website at http://thePoint.lww.com/Plowman4e ✳ ▶

REFERENCES

Acevedo, E. O., R. R. Kraemer, G. H. Kamimori, R. J. Durand, L. G. Johnson, & V. D. Castracane: Stress hormones, effort sense, and perceptions of stress during incremental exercise: An exploratory investigation. *Journal of Strength and Conditioning Research.* 21(1):283–288 (2007).

Berent, V. J. & L. Wartofsky: Thyroid function and exercise. In Warren, M. P. & N. W. Constantini (eds.): *Sports Endocrinology.* Totowa, NJ: Humana Press, 97–118 (2000).

Berggren, J. R., M. W. Hulver, & J. A. Houmard: Fat as an endocrine organ: Influence of exercise. *Journal of Applied Physiology.* 99:757–764 (2005).

Blüher, M., J. W. Bullen, J. H. Lee, S. Kralisch, M. Fasshauer, N. Klöting, J. Niebauer, M. R. Schön, C. J. Williams, & C. S. Mantzoros: Circulating adiponectin and expression of adiponectin receptors in human skeletal muscles: Associations with metabolic parameters and insulin resistance and regulation by physical training. *Journal of Clinical and Endocrinology and Metabolism.* 91(6):2310–2316 (2006).

Borer, K. T.: *Exercise Endocrinology.* Ann Arbor, MI: Human Kinetics, 2003.

Bunt, J. C.: Hormonal alterations due to exercise. *Sports Medicine.* 3:331–345 (1986).

Bush, J. A., W. J. Kraemer, A. M. Mastro, N. T. Triplett-M Bush, J. A., W. J. Kraemer, A. M. Mastro, N. T. Triplett-McBride,

J. S. Volek, M. Putukian, W. J. Sebastianelli, H. G. Knuttgen. Exercise and recovery responses of adrenal medullary neurohormones to heavy resistance exercise. *Medicine & Science in Sports & Exercise*. 31(4):554–559 (1999).

Carnethon, M. R. & L. L. Craft. Autonomic regulation of the association between exercise and diabetes. *Exercise and Sport Sciences Reviews*. 36(1):12–18 (2008).

Chilibeck, P. D.: Hormonal regulations of the effects of exercise on bone: Positive and negative effects. In Warren, M. P. & N. W. Constantini (eds.): *Sports Endocrinology*. Totowa, NJ: Humana Press, 239–252 (2000).

Chrousos, G. P., & P. W. Gold: The concepts of stress and stress system disorders. *Journal of the American Medical Association*. 267(4):1244–1252 (1992).

Coggan, A. R., & B. D. Williams: Metabolic adaptations to endurance training: Substrate metabolism during exercise. In Hargraves, M. (ed.): *Exercise Metabolism*. Champaign, IL: Human Kinetics, 177–210 (1995).

Cole, C. R., E. H. Blackstone, F. J. Pashkow, C. E. Snader, & M. S. Lauer: Heart-rate recovery immediately after exercise as a predictor of mortality. *New England Journal of Medicine*. 341:1351–1357 (1999).

Crewther, B., J. Keogh, J. Cronin, & C. Cook: Possible stimuli for strength and power adaptation. *Sports Medicine*. 36(3):215–228 (2006).

Cumming, D. C.: The male reproductive system, exercise, and training. In Warren, M. P. & N. W. Constantini (eds.): *Sports Endocrinology*. Totowa, NJ: Humana Press, 119–132 (2000).

Dekker, J. M., R. S. Crow, A. R. Folsom, P. J. Hannan, D. Liao, C. A. Swenne, & E. G. Schouten: Low heart rate variability in a 2-minute rhythm strip predicts risk of coronary heart disease and mortality from several causes. The ARIC study. *Circulation*. 102:1239–1244 (2000).

Eliakim, A., J. A. Brasel, & D. M. Cooper: Exercise and the growth hormone–insulin-like growth factor-I axis. In Warren, M. P. & N. W. Constantini (eds.): *Sports Endocrinology*. Totowa, NJ: Humana Press, 77–96 (2000).

Enea, C., N. Boisseau, M. A. Fargeas-Gluck, & V. Diaz: Circulating androgens in women: Exercise-induced changes. *Sports Medicine*. 41(1):1–15 (2011).

Ferguson, M. A., L. J. White, S. McCoy, H. W. Kim, T. Petty, & J. Wilsey: Plasma adiponectin response to acute exercise in healthy subjects. *European Journal of Applied Physiology*. 91(2–3):324–329 (2004).

Forsyth, J. J. & T. Reilly: The combined effect of time of day and menstrual cycle on lactate threshold. *Medicine & Science in Sports & Exercise*. 37(12):2046–2053 (2005).

Galbo, H.: *Hormonal and Metabolic Adaptation to Exercise*. New York, NY: Thieme-Stratton (1983).

Galic, S., J. S. Oakhill, & G. R. Steinberg: Adipose tissue as an endocrine organ. *Molecular and Cellular Endocrinology*. 316:129–139 (2010).

Gleim, G. W., & B. W. Glace: Energy balance and weight control: Endocrine considerations. In Warren, M. P. & N. W. Constantini (eds.): *Sports Endocrinology*. Totowa, NJ: Humana Press, 189–206 (2000).

Greenberg, A. S. & M. S. Obin: Obesity and the role of adipose tissue in inflammation and metabolism. *The American Journal of Clinical Nutrition*. 83:461S–465S (2006).

Guyton, A. C. & Hall, J. E.: *Textbook of Medical Physiology* (12th edition). Philadelphia, PA: W. B. Saunders (2011).

Hackney, A. C.: Exercise as a stressor to the human neuroendocrine system. *Medicina*. 42(10):788–797 (2006).

Hulver, M. W. & J. A. Houmard: Plasma leptin and exercise: recent findings. *Sports Medicine*. 33(7):473–482 (2003).

Janse de Jonge, X. A.: Effects of the menstrual cycle on exercise performance. *Sports Medicine*. 33(11):833–851 (2003).

Jürimäe, J., P. Hofmann, T. Jürimäe, J. Mäestu, P. Purge, M. Wonisch, R. Pokan, & S. P. von Duvillard: Plasma adiponectin response to sculling exercise at individual anaerobic threshold in college level male rowers. *International Journal of Sports Medicine*. 27(4):272–277 (2006a).

Jürimäe, J., P. Purge, T. Jürimäe: Adiponectin and stress hormone responses to maximal sculling after volume-extended training season in elite rowers. *Metabolism*. 55(1):13–19 (2006b).

Jürimäe, J., P. Purge, & T. Jürimäe: Adiponectin is altered after maximal exercise in highly trained male rowers. *European Journal of Applied Physiology*. 93(4):502–505 (2005).

Kemmier, W., L. Wildt, K. Engelke, R. Pintag, M. Pavel, B. Bracher, J. Weineck, & W. Kalender: Acute hormonal responses of a high impact physical exercise session in early postmenopausal women. *European Journal of Applied Physiology*. 90(1–2):199–209 (2003).

Kjaer, M., & K. Lange: Adrenergic regulation of energy metabolism. In Warren, M. P. & N. W. Constantini (eds.): *Sports Endocrinology*. Totowa, NJ: Humana Press, 181–188 (2000).

Kraemer, R. R., & V. D. Castracane: Exercise and humoral mediators of peripheral energy balance: ghrelin and adiponectin. *Experimental Biology and Medicine*. 232(2):184–194 (2007).

Kraemer, W. J.: Endocrine responses and adaptations to strength training. In Komi, P. V. (ed.): *Strength and Power in Sport*. London: Blackwell Scientific Publications, 291–304 (1992a).

Kraemer, W. J.: Endocrine responses to resistance exercise. *Medicine and Science in Sports and Exercise*. 20(5):S152–S157 (1988).

Kraemer, W. J.: Hormonal mechanisms related to the expression of muscular strength and power. In Komi, P. V. (ed.): *Strength and Power in Sport*. London: Blackwell Scientific Publications, 64–76 (1992b).

Kraemer, W. J. & Ratamess, N. A.: Hormonal responses and adaptations to resistance exercise and training. *Sports Medicine*. 35(4):339–361 (2005).

Marieb, E. N. & K. Hoehn: *Human Anatomy and Physiology* (8th edition). San Francisco, CA: Benjamin/Cummings (2010).

Marsh, S. A. & D. G. Jenkins: Physiological responses to the menstrual cycle: Implications for the development of heat illness in female athletes. *Sports Medicine*. 32(10):601–614 (2002).

Mastorakos, G. & M. Pavlatou: Exercise as a stress model and the interplay between the hypothalamus-pituitary-adrenal and the hypothalamus-pituitary-thyroid axes. *Hormone and Metabolic Research*. 37:577–584 (2005).

McMurray, R. G. & A. C. Hackney: Interactions of metabolic hormones, adipose tissue and exercise. *Sports Medicine*. 35(5):393–412 (2005).

Nakamura, Y., K. Aizawa, T. Imai, I. Kono, & N. Mesaki: Hormonal responses to resistance exercise during different menstrual cycle states. *Medicine & Science in Sports & Exercise*. 43(6):967–973 (2011).

Nishime, E. O., C. R. Cole, E. H. Blackstone, F. J. Pashkow, & M. S. Lauer: Heart rate recovery and treadmill exercise score as predictors of mortality in patients referred for exercise ECG. *Journal of American Medical Association*. 284(11):1392–1398 (2000).

Popovic, V., & L. H. Duntas: Leptin TRH and ghrelin: Influence on energy homeostasis at rest and during exercise. *Hormone and Metabolic Research*. 37(9):533–537 (2005).

Raastad, T., T. Bjøro, & J. Hallén. Hormonal responses to high- and moderate-intensity strength exercise. *European Journal of Applied Physiology*. 82(1):121–128 (2000).

Ronti, T., G. Lupattelli, & E. Mannarino: The endocrine function of adipose tissue: An update. *Clinical Endocrinology*. 64:355–365 (2006).

Seifter, J., A. Ratner, & D. Sloane: Concepts in Medical Physiology. Baltimore, MD: Lippincott Williams & Wilkins (2005).

Seiler, S., O. Haugen, & E. Kuffel: Autonomic recovery after exercise in trained athletes: Intensity and duration effects. *Medicine & Science in Sports & Exercise*. 39(8):1366–1373 (2007).

Selye, H.: *The Stress of Life*. New York, NY: McGraw-Hill (1956).

Sutton, J. R., P. A. Farrell, & V. J. Harber: Hormonal adaptations to physical activity. In Bouchard, C., R. J. Shephard, T. Stephens, J. R. Sutton, & B. D. McPherson (eds.): *Exercise, Fitness, and Health*. Champaign, IL: Human Kinetics, 217–257 (1990).

Thayer, J. F., S. S. Yamamoto, & J. F. Brosschot: The relationship of autonomic imbalance, heart rate variability and cardiovascular disease risk factors. *International Journal of Cardiology*. 141:122–131 (2010).

Tomas, E., M. *Kelly*, X. *Xiang*, T. S. *Tsao*, C. *Keller*, P. *Keller*, Z. *Luo*, H. *Lodish*, A. K. *Saha*, R. *Unger*, N. B. *Ruderman*: Metabolic and hormonal interactions between muscle and adipose tissue. *Proceedings of the Nutrition Society*. 63:381–385 (2004).

Tsuji, H., F. J. Venditti, E. S. Manders, J. C. Evans, M. G. Larson, C. L. Feldman, & D. Levy: Reduced heart rate variability and mortality risk in an elderly cohort: The Framingham heart study. *Circulation*. 90:878–883 (1994).

Urhausen, A. & W. Kindermann: The endocrine system in overtraining. In Warren, M. P, & N. W. Constantini (eds.): *Sports Endocrinology*. Totowa, NJ: Humana Press, 347–370 (2000).

Vallbo, A. B., T. E. Hagbarth, H. E. Torebjork, & B. G. Wallin: Somatosensory, proprioceptive, and sympathetic activity in human peripheral nerves. *Physiological Reviews*. 59:919–957 (1979).

Vincent, S., P. Berthon, H. Zouhal, E. Moussa, M. Cathliine, D. Bentue-Ferrer, & A. Gratas-Delamarche: Plasma glucose, insulin and catecholamine responses to a Wingate test in physically active women and men. *European Journal of Applied Physiology*. 61:15–21 (2004).

Wade, C. E.: Hormonal regulation of fluid homeostasis during and following exercise. In Warren, M. P, & N. W. Constantini (eds.): *Sports Endocrinology*. Totowa, NJ: Humana Press, 207–226 (2000).

Zafeiridis, A., I. Smilios, R. V. Considine, & S. P. Tokmakidis: Serum leptin responses after acute resistance exercise protocols. *Journal of Applied Physiology*. 94(2):591–597 (2003).

The Immune System, Exercise, Training, and Illness

22

OBJECTIVES

> After studying the chapter, you should be able to:

> Identify the primary cells of the innate and adaptive branches of the immune system, and indicate the mechanisms by which they lead to antigen destruction.

> Describe the sequence of events in inflammation.

> Differentiate between the immune responses to moderate aerobic exercise and exhaustive exercise.

> Describe the role of cytokines in regulating inflammation.

> Differentiate between overreaching and overtraining.

> Identify the causes of the overtraining syndrome, and describe actions designed to attempt to prevent it.

> Respond to this question: Does exercise increase or decrease the likelihood of upper respiratory tract infection?

> Describe the extent to which physical activity decreases the risk of certain cancers.

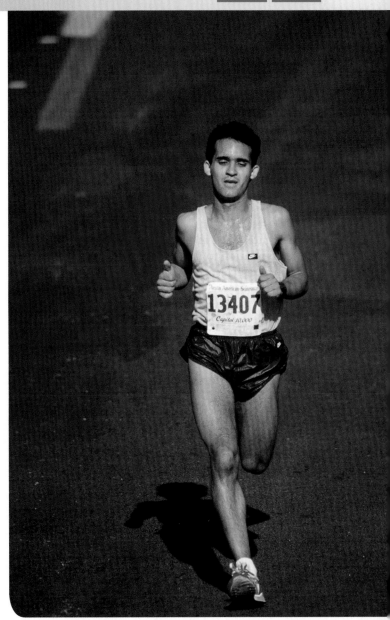

Introduction

Exercise training has many health benefits. Often active individuals, perhaps yourself included, claim they feel better and are healthier than their sedentary friends. They claim these benefits not just because they have altered their risk factors for major diseases, but also because they have colds, flu, sore throats, and other common illnesses less often. On the other hand, one hears about Olympic and professional athletes competing despite an illness, or conversely, being unable to compete at all because of illness—not injury. Indeed, a common cause of poor physical performance at athletic events is acute respiratory infection. Acute respiratory conditions such as the common cold or influenza annually affect 90 out of 100 persons, causing substantial morbidity and economic cost. The relationship between exercise and immune function thus has important implications for public health and for athletes (Brolinson and Elliott, 2007). In addition, many are interested in the role of exercise and exercise training in relation to diseases involving the immune system, such as cancer or HIV/AIDS. Does physical activity protect against certain cancers? Should individuals with disease be physically active?

Definitive answers to these questions are not yet possible. This chapter provides an overview of the functioning of the immune system, explores the acute immune response to exercise, considers adaptations in the immune system that occur as a result of exercise training, and, finally, addresses beneficial and detrimental influences of exercise on immune function and disease susceptibility.

The Immune System

Humans are constantly exposed to bacteria, viruses, and parasites capable of causing mild to serious disease. The fact that most of the time these foreign invaders do not overcome us is a testimony to the importance and efficiency of the body's defense mechanisms, comprised primarily of the immune system. The **immune system** is a complex and precisely ordered system of cells, hormones, and chemicals that regulate susceptibility to, severity of, and recovery from infection and illness (Nash, 1994). *Immunology* is the study of the body's physiological responses to destroy or neutralize foreign matter (Smith, 1995). The immune system operates with the nervous system and the endocrine system to maintain homeostasis. Although these systems operate independently, each with its own collection of highly specific cells and regulatory factors, they overlap considerably, and each system depends on the others for normal development and function (Pedersen et al., 2007). These three interrelated systems interact in complex, bidirectional, anatomical, and physiological ways (Miles, 2005), and are studied by the growing field known as psychoneuroimmunology or neuroimmunology.

In its organization and operation, the immune system parallels the nervous and endocrine systems. For example, all three systems consist of identifiable cells and chemical substances. All three systems react to stimuli; each has a network for communication within itself and with the other systems; and all three control and interact with other cells and organs. One major difference, however, is a gradient of mobility. The nervous system functions through fixed nerves and locally released neurotransmitters. The major endocrine glands are also fixed in place, but their hormones travel throughout the body, primarily via the bloodstream. The immune system consists primarily of free mobile cells that move within and outside the bloodstream, although some may be anatomically specific (Roitt et al., 1998).

As with the nervous and hormonal systems, one must understand the parts and processes of the immune system to understand how it functions. **Figure 22.1** outlines the basics of the immune system. All immune responses involve recognizing a threat to the body and reacting to eradicate that threat while minimizing damage. The most common threat or stimulus to the immune system is an infectious microbe or pathogen; such microorganisms include bacteria, fungi, parasites, protozoa, and viruses. Some pathogens (all viruses, some bacteria, and small protozoan parasites) invade the body's cells and replicate there, while others (most bacteria and larger parasites) reside primarily in body fluids and extracellular spaces. The site of the infection and the specific pathogen determine how the immune system responds. The immune system can also be stimulated by cellular damage, such as muscle damage. In this case, the goal of the immune response, mediated largely through the process of inflammation, is to bring immune cells to the site of local tissue damage to clear cellular debris and set the stage for tissue repair. Recent data also suggest that immune mediators play a role in regulating metabolism.

Structure and Function of the Immune System
Cells

The primary immune cells are *leukocytes*, or white blood cells. Leukocytes are subdivided into *lymphocytes* and *phagocytes*, each of which has three major subdivisions (**Figure 22.1**).

B lymphocytes and T lymphocytes (B cells and T cells) specifically recognize individual pathogens. Any pathogen that can be specifically recognized by B cells and/or T cells is called an *antigen*. Both B cells and T cells are derived from bone marrow cells, but B cells mature in the bone marrow, whereas T cells mature in the thymus. Each B and T cell is genetically programmed to recognize only one particular antigen. Once an antigen is recognized, B cells proliferate into plasma cells that produce an antibody to act immediately and memory cells that will ultimately provide lasting immunity. Vaccinations confer

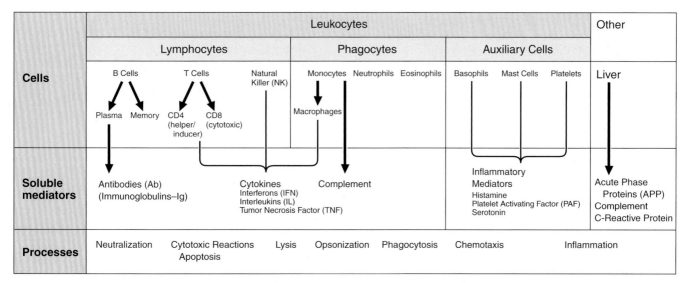

FIGURE 22.1 Components of the Immune System.
Source: Based on Roitt, I., J. Brostoff, & D. Male: *Immunology* (4th edition). Baltimore, MD: Mosby (1998).

immunity against diseases such as polio or measles by altering an antigen such that it becomes harmless but still brings about an antibody reaction.

Antigens recognized by T cells have been processed first in some way. Sensitized T cells enlarge and divide into two functionally separate classifications: CD8 cells, also called cytotoxic or killer cells, destroy infected cells directly. CD4 cells, which are helper or inducer cells, stimulate the action of cytotoxic cells and increase antibody production by B plasma cells. Through a variety of feedback mechanisms, both CD4 and CD8 cells can also act as suppressor T cells that inhibit cytotoxic T cells and antibody production, thus preventing excessive destruction (Roitt et al., 1998). Although they are classified as large granular lymphocytes, *natural killer (NK) cells* are different from other lymphocytes in that they act spontaneously against any target, apparently by recognizing surface changes on a variety of tumor cells and virally infected cells. As their name implies, these cells directly destroy infected host cells.

Phagocytes are leukocytes that bind to pathogenic microorganisms and antigens, internalize them, and then kill them. When they are in the bloodstream, mononuclear phagocytes are called *monocytes*; when they migrate into tissue, they evolve into *macrophages*. Macrophages often

"process" an antigen and then present it to T lymphocytes. *Neutrophils* are the most abundant blood leukocytes. Large numbers are necessary because when neutrophils engulf and destroy foreign material, they also die. *Eosinophils* are specialized to act against large extracellular parasites.

The role of the *auxiliary cells* is to release mediators to produce inflammation. *Mast cells* lie close to blood vessels; *basophils* and *platelets* circulate in the blood. The main purpose of inflammation is to attract leukocytes and their resultant soluble mediators to a site of infection or injury.

Soluble Mediators

Soluble mediators are intervening agents dissolved in a solution. These substances are produced primarily, but not exclusively, by immune cells that act either directly on the target pathogen or indirectly by signaling other immune cells to act or release additional mediators. Each immune cell produces and secretes only one particular set of mediators, although more than one cell type may produce the same classification of mediator. **Figure 22.1** shows representative soluble mediators but there are many others.

Antibodies produced by B plasma cells are also known as *immunoglobulins (Ig)*. Antibodies do not directly destroy antigens. Instead, they identify the invader by forming an antigen-antibody complex, and they then activate other soluble mediators and immune cells that perform the actual destruction. **Cytokines** are proteins or peptides that are released from immune cells and other tissues (notably skeletal muscle and adipose tissue). Cytokines are involved in communication between immune cells (especially lymphocytes and phagocytes) and other cells of the body. **Table 22.1** presents the major cytokines involved in the exercise immune response. Cytokines stimulate the

Immune System A precisely ordered system of cells, hormones, and chemicals that regulate susceptibility to, severity of, and recovery from infection and illness.

Cytokines Proteins or peptides that are released from immune cells and other tissues (notably skeletal muscle and adipose tissue) and are involved in communication between immune cells (especially lymphocytes and phagocytes) and other cells of the body.

TABLE 22.1 Major Cytokines Involved in the Exercise Immune Response		
Cytokine	**Released From**	**Primary Function**
Interleukin IL-1α, IL-1β	Macrophages	T-cell activation Macrophage function Proinflammatory function Fever
IL-2	T cells	T-cell activation T-cell proliferation
IL-4	T cells	Anti-inflammatory function
IL-6	Activated T cells Macrophages, Muscle	T- and B-cell growth Stimulates acute phase proteins Anti-inflammatory function Proinflammatory function
IL-10	T cells, B cells Macrophages, Mast cells	Anti-inflammatory and immunosuppressive functions
Interferon IFNα IFNγ	Leukocytes T cells, NK cells	Antiviral activity Stimulates cytotoxicity Stimulates cytotoxicity Macrophage activation Proinflammatory function
Tumor necrosis factor TNFα	Macrophages, NK cells	Stimulates cytotoxicity against tumor cells Proinflammatory function

proliferation of various immune cells and are important regulators of inflammation and the immune response. Among the principal types of cytokines are *interferons* (IFNs), which are important in limiting the spread of certain viral infections; *interleukins (ILs)*, each of which acts on a specific group of immune cells to divide and differentiate; and *tumor necrosis factors (TNFs)*, which are particularly important in inflammation and cytotoxic reactions. Cytokines are thought to be important in the exercise immune response because certain ones (IL-1, IL-6, IFNγ, and TNFα) are proinflammatory factors that probably play a role in coordinating the responses to muscle damage that may result from strenuous exercise. Other cytokines (IL-4, IL-10, and IL-6 in a dual role) are anti-inflammatory and suppress the activity of inflammatory cells, allowing normal structure and function to be restored. The release of these anti-inflammatory cytokines follows the proinflammatory response to vigorous physical activity (Moldoveanu et al., 2001; Petersen and Pedersen, 2005). Cytokines are also released following exercise that does not result in muscle damage, in which case they seem to play a role in regulating metabolism (Petersen and Pedersen, 2005).

Complement is a group of serum proteins whose overall function is to control inflammation. Complement activation results in a series of reactions, including increased blood flow to the site and increased permeability of capillaries to plasma molecules, which ultimately leads to destruction of the stimulating antigen (Mackinnon, 1999; Marieb and Hoehn, 2010).

Acute phase proteins (APP) are produced in and secreted from the liver, as are some complement proteins (Mackinnon, 1992; Marieb and Hoehn, 2010). APP are stimulated by proinflammatory cytokines and are so named because they increase rapidly during an infection. For example, chronically elevated levels of C-reactive protein reflect systemic infection and are associated with increased risk of type II diabetes and cardiovascular disease. APP stimulate an increase in the number of leukocytes and play an important role in tissue repair following muscle cell damage.

Inflammatory mediators are molecules that, as the name implies, control the development of inflammation. For example, *histamine*, *platelet activating factor (PAF)*, and *serotonin* (**Figure 22.1**) all bring about increased vascular permeability and smooth muscle contraction. Other inflammatory mediators not released from basophils, mast cells, or platelets include *fibrinopeptides* (the substance removed from fibrinogen during blood coagulation) and *fibrin breakdown products* plus *prostaglandins (PGE₂)*. These substances make the actions of other inflammatory mediators more effective.

Processes

The immune system can destroy or inactivate a pathogen in numerous ways. The defense mechanism(s) employed in response to an immune challenge vary according to the type of pathogen and its life cycle stage. In *cytotoxic reactions* complete cells are killed, primarily by punching holes in their outer membranes. A target cell may be signaled to self-destruct, a process that is termed *apoptosis*. *Lysis* is a form of cytotoxic reaction in which a cell is killed by destruction of its cell membrane. *Neutralization* occurs when antibodies block the binding site on antigens so that they cannot bind to tissues and cause damage. *Opsonization* is the coating of the membrane of an antigen, making it easier for phagocytes to adhere to and engulf the antigen. *Phagocytosis* is the engulfing and digesting of a pathogen. Additionally, intracellular granules (small grain-like bodies) may be released in a *respiratory oxidative burst*, which is a potent killer.

Functional Organization of the Immune System

As depicted in **Figure 22.2** functionally, the immune system can be divided into two separate but interrelated and overlapping branches: the innate (nonspecific) and the adaptive (specific) branches (Marieb and Hoehn, 2010; Smith, 1995). **Table 22.2** provides a glossary of the cells, soluble mediators, and processes that play an important role in the immune response.

The Innate Branch

The *innate branch* protects against foreign substances or cells without having to recognize them. It is nonselective and provides an initial line of defense against microbial invasion. The innate system consists of both a cellular component and physical barriers. Intact skin and mucous membranes are the major physical barriers. The primary cells of the innate system are the NK lymphocytes, neutrophils, and macrophages. Complement and acute phase proteins are the major soluble mediators. The innate system works through the processes of lysis, opsonization, and phagocytosis.

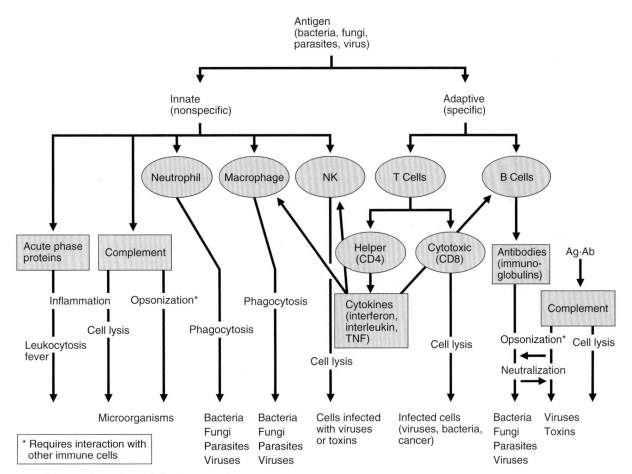

FIGURE 22.2 Overview of the Immune System.
The immune system is divided into the innate and adaptive branches, and is comprised of cells and chemical mediators that attack foreign antigens through several mechanisms. Immune cells are represented by circles, and soluble mediators (chemicals) are represented by boxes. The mechanisms of destruction are labeled within the arrows that point to the pathogen destroyed by the mechanism.
Sources: Modified from Marieb, E. N. & K. Hoehn: *Anatomy and Physiology* (4th edition). Redwood City, CA: Benjamin Cummings (2010); Smith, J. A.: Guidelines, standards, and perspectives in exercise immunology. *Medicine and Science in Sports and Exercise.* 27(4):497–506 (1995).

TABLE 22.2 Glossary of Cells, Molecules, and Processes Involved in the Immune Response

Branch of Immune System	Processes	Cells	Molecules/Chemical Factors
Innate and adaptive	*Lysis* is the killing of a cell via destruction of the cell membrane. *Phagocytosis* is the process of engulfing and digesting an antigen. *Inflammation* is the process that prevents the spread of damaging agents, disposes of pathogens and cellular debris, and sets the stage for tissue repair.	*Macrophages* are immune cells that (1) phagocytize pathogens, (2) present parts of the engulfed antigen on its plasma membrane to activate the T-cell response, and (3) secrete cytokines. They are important in both the innate and adaptive immune responses.	*Antigens* are substances capable of provoking an immune response. *Complement* is a group of ~20 plasma proteins. When activated, complement lyses microorganisms, enhances phagocytosis, and enhances the inflammatory response. Complement may be activated and function in either the innate or adaptive immune response. *Cytokines* are chemicals released from sensitized T cells, NK cells, and activated macrophages to help regulate the immune response.
Innate		*Natural killer (NK)* cells are innate immune cells that destroy virus-infected and cancerous body cells by cell lysis. *Neutrophils* are innate immune cells that phagocytize pathogens.	*Acute phase proteins (APPs)* are blood proteins produced in the liver that function in the innate immune response. APPs are important in the response to infection and inflammation.
Adaptive	*Neutralization* is a process that occurs when antibodies block the binding site on antigens so that they cannot bind to tissues and cause damage. *Opsonization* is the process of coating the membrane of an antigen, making it easier for phagocytes to adhere to and engulf the antigen.	*B cells* are lymphocytes that are part of the adaptive immune response and are responsible for the production of antibodies to a specific antigen. *T cells* are lymphocytes that are responsible for cell-mediated responses of the adaptive immune system. Functionally, there are two classes of T cells: cytotoxic T cells (CD8 cells), which destroy virus-infected and cancer cells directly via cell lysis; and helper T cells (CD4 cells), regulatory cells that influence the activity of cytotoxic T cells, B cells, NK, and macrophages. Cytotoxic and helper T cells can act as suppressor cells once the infection is controlled.	*Antibodies* are proteins produced by B cells to attack antigens.

Inflammation

Central to the functioning of the innate branch of the immune system is the *inflammatory response* (**Figure 22.3**). The cells of the immune system are widely dispersed in the body. When a thermal or physical injury or an infection occurs, immune cells must concentrate at the site of the emergency. Muscle or tissue damage following strenuous exercise can be a potent signal for inflammation. As shown in **Figure 22.3**, immune cells converge through four processes:

1. Vasodilation and an increased blood supply to the area
2. Increased capillary permeability
3. Chemotaxis
4. Leukocytosis (an increased number of leukocytes)

Increased blood flow and increased capillary permeability help bring leukocytes to the site of tissue damage or infection. *Chemotaxis* is the increased directional migration of immune cells. **Figure 22.4** depicts the sequence

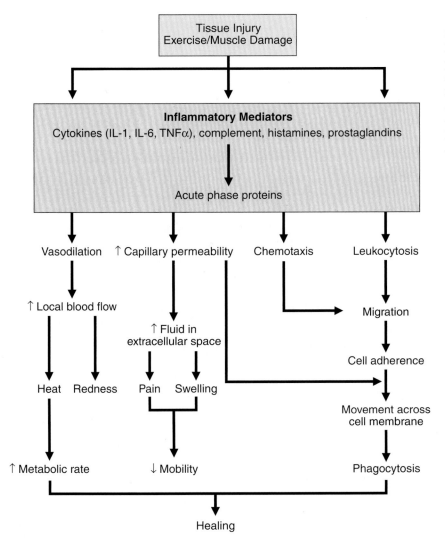

FIGURE 22.3 Sequence of Events in Inflammation.
Inflammation is characterized by heat, redness, pain, and swelling. These familiar responses occur because of the action of inflammatory mediators. Inflammation ensures immune cells are concentrated at the site of injury and that metabolic activity is increased to facilitate healing.

of events by which muscular damage can initiate chemotaxis and set the stage for repair of the damaged tissue. Chemotaxis occurs in response to the release of chemotactic factors, inflammatory mediators, and acute phase proteins. Neutrophils are the first cells to arrive at the injury site and do so within an hour. Neutrophils are followed by monocytes, which become macrophages once they enter the tissue. Macrophages dominate at the site of the injury 5–6 hours after the inflammatory response begins. On their arrival, these phagocytes adhere to the walls of the capillaries, a process facilitated by cell adhesion molecules (CAM). Eventually the phagocytes push between the endothelial cells in the capillary and cross the membrane. They then squeeze through the cell membrane by a process called diapedesis and move to the actual site of the inflammation. Once there, both neutrophils and macrophages phagocytize the foreign antigens and/or cellular debris.

Inflammation is characterized by redness, heat, swelling, and pain. The increased blood flow to the area resulting from vasodilation leads to the redness and heat. The increased capillary permeability allows fluid to seep into

extracellular spaces, creating swelling that activates pain receptors. The pain and swelling can result in lack of mobility. Although immobility may be inconvenient, it forces the injured part to rest, which aids in healing. Thus, inflammation can destroy foreign pathogens, prevent the spread of damaging agents, dispose of cellular debris due to tissue damage, and set the stage for tissue repair. Although part of the innate system, inflammation is also an important component of the adaptive immune response.

CHECK YOUR COMPREHENSION 1

During soccer practice, Nick collided with another player, and both fell to the turf. After practice, Nick realized that he had scraped his knee on the turf (turf burn). The next day Nick realized the area around his turf burn was red, swollen, and painful. What caused these responses? How do these responses help promote tissue repair?

Check your answer in Appendix C

Capillary   **Muscle Cell**

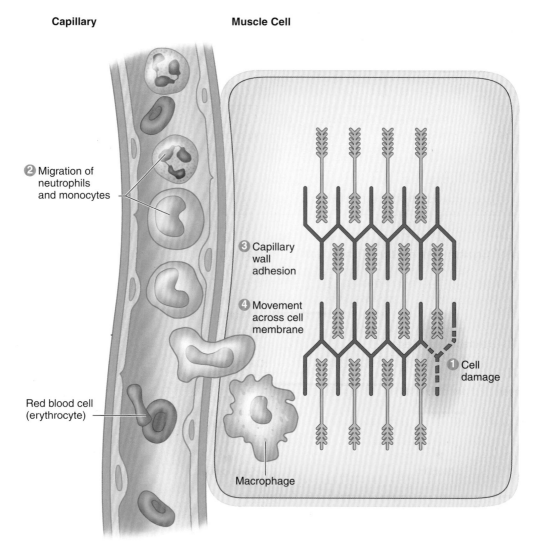

FIGURE 22.4 Events by Which Tissue Damage Leads to Increased Leukocytes in Tissues.
Muscle damage (1) produces a chemical signal that attacks neutrophils and monocytes to the area (2). The immune cells then adhere to the capillary wall (3) and move into the tissue area through the process of diapedesis (4).

The Adaptive Branch

In contrast to the innate branch, in the *adaptive branch* of the immune system, immune cells recognize a foreign material and react specifically and selectively to destroy it. The adaptive branch is antigen specific, is systemic, and has memory. The adaptive branch includes humoral (from the Latin word *humor*, meaning "fluids") and cell-mediated immunity. Antibodies produced from B cells provide *humoral immunity*. The antibodies circulate in the blood and lymph, where they bind to bacteria, toxins, and free viruses; inactivate them temporarily; and mark them for destruction by phagocytes or complements. *Cell-mediated immunity* is provided by T lymphocytes that directly attack and lyse cells infected by viruses, parasites, cancer cells, or grafts; release chemical mediators to enhance inflammation; and activate lymphocytes and macrophages.

The body's ability to mount a specialized immune response involves specific proteins called *major histocompatibility complex (MHC)* that exist on the membranes of the body's own cells and pathogens. MHCs are different in each individual except in identical twins. With an organ transplant, therefore, the recipient's immune system must be suppressed because otherwise it would not recognize the donor MHC and would "attack" the transplanted cells, resulting in the "rejection" of the organ. As can be seen in **Figure 22.2**, the major cells of the adaptive branch are the B and T cells. The major soluble mediators are antibodies, cytokines, and complement. The processes of action include lysis, neutralization, opsonization, and, indirectly, phagocytosis. **Figure 22.5** shows how the innate and adaptive branches work together for a generalized immune response, emphasizing the role of

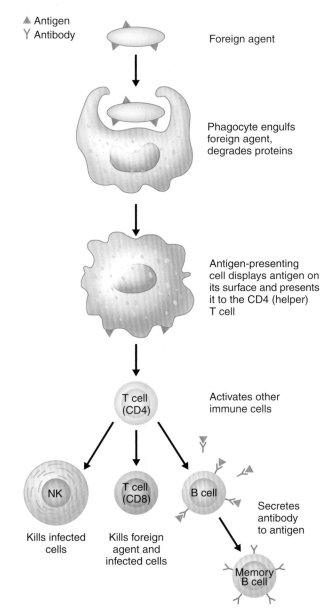

Antigen
Antibody

Foreign agent

Phagocyte engulfs
foreign agent,
degrades proteins

Antigen-presenting
cell displays antigen on
its surface and presents
it to the CD4 (helper)
T cell

T cell
(CD4)

Activates other
immune cells

NK

T cell
(CD8)

B cell

Secretes
antibody
to antigen

Kills infected
cells

Kills foreign
agent and
infected cells

Memory
B cell

FIGURE 22.5 Central Role of Macrophages in the Innate and Adaptive Immune Responses.
Macrophages are phagocytes that ingest foreign agents as part of the innate immune response. Once a macrophage has ingested a foreign invader it activates the adaptive branch of the immune system by "presenting" portions of the foreign invader to adaptive cells.

macrophages in phagocytizing the foreign invader and activating the adaptive immune response by serving as antigen-presenting cells.

The body's many defenses against tissue injury and infection are amazing and, admittedly, can seem overwhelming. Remember that the functions of different structures and substances in the immune system overlap and are in some ways redundant. This ensures an effective immune response to most pathogens and is essential for health.

The Immune Response to Exercise

An acute bout of exercise causes an immune response. Exercise physiologists, other exercise professionals, clinicians, and the general public are interested in the relationship between exercise and immune function. Indeed, much research has focused on this issue, although much about this relationship remains unanswered. **Figure 22.6** depicts the complexities involved in trying to address this important question (Woods et al., 1999). As with the effect of exercise on other body systems, the immune response to exercise depends largely on the intensity and duration of the exercise. Furthermore, because the physiological stress of exercise is additive with other stresses in one's life, including psychological, environmental, and nutritional stress, these factors must also be considered (Steinacker et al., 2004; Walsh and Whitham, 2006). Further complicating the relationship between exercise and immune function is a vast array of immune functions. Exercise appears to affect all of the cells of the immune system, but in different ways. Furthermore, each immune cell may perform several functions, and exercise may affect these functions differently. Researchers investigating the effects of exercise on immune function typically have subjects engage in an acute bout of exercise in a laboratory setting. They may then report resulting changes in blood levels of an immune cell, tissue levels of an immune cell, or functioning of an immune cell. Such studies may compare the acute response of the immune system in individuals with different characteristics (age, fitness status, etc.).

Although it is interesting to know how exercise affects individual cells of the immune system, most people are concerned about how exercise relates to health outcomes, such as the rate and severity of an infection or the risk of developing cancer. To answer these questions researchers typically use an epidemiological approach that relies on subjects reporting incidence of illness. Many of the original studies investigating the relationship between exercise and infection rates were epidemiological studies that quantified training level (as a measure of exercise stress) and collected self-reported data on incidence of symptoms of upper respiratory tract infections (URTI) (Nieman et al., 1990; Peters and Bateman, 1983). Generally, these studies found that individuals who ran marathons or competed in endurance events had a higher incidence of URTI (Nieman, 1997a,b). More recent studies have also reported that training volume influences upper respiratory tract infection incidence (Gleeson et al., 2011). However, these data must be interpreted cautiously because they are based on self-reports and because the symptoms of an URTI, such as a sore throat, may be caused by something other than an infection (e.g., airway inflammation due to drying of the mucosal membrane or inhalation of dry air or pollutants) (Gleeson, 2007; Pedersen and Hoffman-Goetz, 2000). Further complicating an understanding of

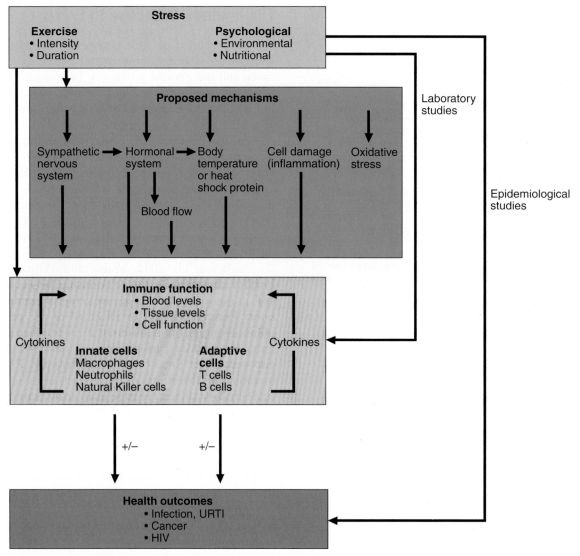

FIGURE 22.6   Relationships Among Exercise, Immune Function, and Health.
Exercise is one of many factors that activates the immune system and it does so through multiple mechanisms. There are multiple immune responses to exercise and they may have a positive or negative impact on health.

the effect of exercise on upper respiratory tract infections is the fact that these, because they rely on self-reports, do not provide actual evidence of an infection. This has prompted leading experts in the field to recommend that the phrase upper respiratory symptoms be used in studies that lack physician diagnosed infection or the lack of pathogen identification (Walsh et al., 2011). The precise relationship between exercise and the immune system will be better understood with controlled prospective studies that investigate immune function and health outcomes simultaneously.

A final challenge to understanding the relationship between exercise and immune function is the number of possible mechanisms that may mediate the effect of exercise on the immune system. Exercise may alter immune function directly or through any combination of the

mechanisms listed below (Fleshner, 2005; Pedersen and Ullum, 1994; Steinacker et al., 2004; Woods et al., 1999):

1. Directly stimulating immune function
2. Stimulating the sympathetic nervous system
3. Altering hormones (especially epinephrine, norepinephrine, cortisol, growth hormone, prolactin, and thyroxine)
4. Increasing body temperature
5. Exercise-induced cell damage (and the release of acute phase proteins or heat shock proteins)
6. Increasing oxidative stress

Another important factor that must be considered when describing the effect of exercise on the immune system is the recovery period from exercise. A strenuous bout

FOCUS ON RESEARCH

What Causes the Immune Response?

Aerobic exercise causes leukocytosis (an increase in circulating leukocytes). Leukocytes respond in different ways to exercise; some leukocytes increase in number and remain elevated during recovery, whereas other leukocytes increase during exercise but decrease during recovery. Furthermore, studies have clearly demonstrated that immune cell changes depend on exercise intensity and duration. Researchers have long been interested in determining the mechanisms responsible for the changes in leukocyte number and distribution in response to exercise. The most frequently proposed mechanism is the action of the sympathoadrenal-mediated stress hormones. Increased body temperature (exertional hyperthermia) has also been proposed as a possible mechanism. To better understand the relative influence of these mechanisms, Rhind et al. (1999) designed a study to examine changes in stress hormone levels and lymphocyte redistribution during exercise with and without a rise of rectal temperature. To control for temperature, participants exercised in water. One trial was performed in cold water (18°C, 64.4°F), and the other in hot water (39°C, 102.2°F), each involving the same amount of exercise. Rectal temperature increased only during the trial in hot water. The accompanying graphs present changes in the stress hormones (epinephrine, norepinephrine, and cortisol) and changes in immune cells (total leukocyte number and lymphocyte number).

These results demonstrate convincingly that hyperthermia affects hormone concentrations (increases in epinephrine, norepinephrine, and cortisol were all significantly higher in the hot trial) and thus leukocyte number and distribution (both total leukocyte number and lymphocyte number were higher in the hot trial). Furthermore, these data suggest that the influence of hyperthermia on leukocyte number and distribution is indirect; it is not the increase in temperature itself that influences leukocytes, but rather that the increase in temperature affects the hormonal system, which in turn affects the immune system. This research reinforces the interdependence of several systems of the body.

Source: Rhind, S. G., G. A. Gannon, P. N. Shek, I. K. M. Brenner, Y. Severs, J. Zamecnik, A. Buguet, V. M. Natale, R. J. Shephard, & M. W. Radomski: Contribution of exertional hyperthermia to sympathoadrenal-mediated lymphocyte subset redistribution. *Journal of Applied Physiology.* 87(3):1178–1185 (1999).

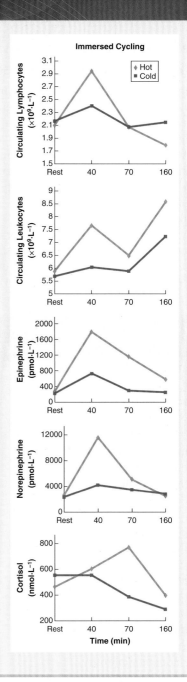

of exercise alters immune function for several hours or days. In fact, the suppression of several immune cells in the postexercise period is often proposed as the cause of more upper respiratory tract infections among high-volume, endurance-trained athletes (Mackinnon et al., 1987; Nieman, 1997b; Tomasi et al., 1982).

Clearly, the type of exercise is also a primary factor in determining the exercise response of the immune system. Most research on the effects of exercise on the immune system has studied prolonged aerobic exercise because of the epidemiological data linking high-volume endurance training with a greater incidence of upper respiratory tract infection. Thus, the following sections deviate somewhat from the exercise categories used throughout this textbook being limited to two variations of long-term, moderate to heavy submaximal aerobic exercise and very short-term, high-intensity anaerobic exercise. Specifically, the immune response is detailed in relation to "medium-duration" (45 minutes), moderate- and high-intensity aerobic exercise; "prolonged" (1–3 hours), moderate- and high-intensity exercise; and intense interval exercise.

Medium-Duration (<45 minutes), Moderate-to High-Intensity Aerobic Exercise

Table 22.3 reports the changes in immune cell numbers (reported as a percentage) during or immediately after exercise and during recovery from medium-duration, moderate- and high-intensity exercise (Mackinnon, 1999). Exercise results in **leukocytosis**, an increased number of white blood cells. Leukocytosis is evident during most forms of physical activity and depends on the intensity and duration of the exercise. In most cases, the leukocytosis persists for at least 1–4 hours after exercise.

Neutrophils increase in number as a result of endurance exercise. The increases are greater after high-intensity exercise than moderate exercise. The increase in neutrophils is evident for 2–4 hours after exercise

and is likely evident during moderate exercise, although research data are lacking. It appears that medium-duration aerobic exercise also enhances neutrophil function. Both the phagocytic activity and the oxidative burst activity of neutrophils are reportedly enhanced (Woods et al., 1999).

Circulating levels of monocytes are not altered by medium-duration moderate exercise but increase modestly during high-intensity exercise. This elevation persists for at least 2 hours after exercise. Recall that when monocytes leave the bloodstream, they are transformed to macrophages, which perform several roles in the immune response. Research suggests that macrophage functions are enhanced following medium-duration exercise. These functions include phagocytic activity, oxidative burst activity, and antitumor activity (Nieman, 1997a; Woods and Davis, 1994; Woods et al., 1993, 1997, 1999).

Circulating levels of natural killer (NK) cells increase during medium-duration bouts of both moderate- and high-intensity exercise, with the more intense exercise causing a larger increase in NK cell numbers. Of greater

TABLE 22.3 Exercise Response of Immune Cell Number to Medium-Duration (45 min), Moderate- and High-Intensity Aerobic Exercise

Variable/Exercise Intensity	During or Immediately After Exercise	Recovery
Total Leukocytes		
Moderate-intensity	↑ 0–40%	Unknown
High-intensity	↑ 50%	↑ 50–100% 2 hr postexercise
Innate Immune System		
Neutrophils		
Moderate-intensity	↑ 30–50%	Unknown
High-intensity	↑ 30–150%	Unknown up to 2 hr postexercise 25–100% 2–4 hr postexercise
Monocytes		
Moderate-intensity	No Change	Unknown
High-intensity	↑ 0–20%	↑ 0–50% 2 hr postexercise
Natural Killer cells		
Moderate-intensity	↑ 0–50%	Normal by 1 hr postexercise
High-intensity	↑ 100–200%	↓ 40% 2–4 hr postexercise
Adaptive Immune System		
T cells		
Moderate-intensity	No change	Unknown
High-intensity	↑ 100%	↓ 30% 1–2 hr postexercise
B cells		
Moderate-intensity	No change	Unknown
High-intensity	No change	↓ 0–25% 1–2 hr postexercise
Serum Ig		
Moderate-intensity	No change	No change
High-intensity	No change	No change
Salivary IgA		
Moderate-intensity	No change	No change
High-intensity	No change	No change

Source: Based on data from Mackinnon, L. T.: *Advances in Exercise Immunology.* Champaign, IL: Human Kinetics (1999).

importance, however, are the different responses during recovery. Following moderate-intensity exercise, blood levels of NK cells return to normal within 1 hour. Following high-intensity exercise, in contrast, NK cell levels drop approximately 40% below normal levels and remain depressed for 2–4 hours. Natural killer cell activity (NKCA) mimics the changes in NK cell numbers (Mackinnon, 1999; Woods et al., 1999). **Figure 22.7** depicts the changes in NKCA after 45 minutes of intense (80% $\dot{V}O_2$max), 2.5–3 hours of running (~76% $\dot{V}O_2$max), and during recovery. For now, concentrate on the 45-minute bout of exercise. Notice the large increase in NKCA immediately after exercise, followed by a reduction in NKCA below preexercise levels and a subsequent return to preexercise values by the fourth hour (Nieman et al., 1990, 1995a,b; Woods et al., 1999).

T-cell numbers do not change during moderate-intensity, medium-duration exercise but increase markedly as a result of high-intensity exercise. During recovery from intense exercise, a suppression in T-cell numbers is evident for 1–2 hours of recovery. As with NK cells, this suppression in T cells after exercise may make one more susceptible to infection.

B-cell numbers do not appear to change immediately after medium-duration bouts of moderate- or high-intensity dynamic exercise. However, B-cell numbers decrease 1–2 hours following intense exercise. Daughter cells of the B cells, plasma cells, produce antibodies (immunoglobulins) that lead to destruction of antigens. Serum or salivary levels of immunoglobulins apparently do not change following aerobic exercise lasting less than 45 minutes (Mackinnon, 1999).

Prolonged (1–3 hours) Moderate- to High-Intensity Aerobic Exercise

Table 22.4 reports the changes in immune cell numbers during or immediately after exercise and during recovery from prolonged moderate- and high-intensity aerobic exercise (Mackinnon, 1999). Prolonged high-intensity exercise results in the greatest leukocytosis immediately after exercise and in recovery.

Neutrophils increase in number as a result of aerobic exercise. The increases are greater following high-intensity exercise. Prolonged high-intensity exercise causes a significantly greater increase in neutrophils than shorter exercise bouts of the same intensity. Large increases in neutrophil numbers are evident for 2–6 hours after high-intensity exercise. Despite the increase in neutrophil numbers after prolonged moderate- and high-intensity exercise, there is evidence that neutrophil function may not respond uniformly (Mackinnon, 1999). Prolonged

Leukocytosis An increase in circulating leukocytes (WBC).

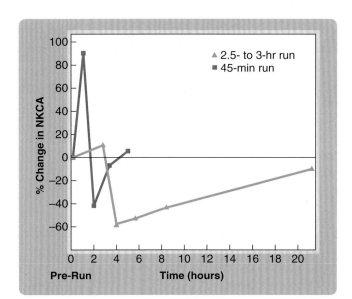

FIGURE 22.7 Natural Killer Cell Activity (NKCA) during and following Exercise of Different Durations.
NKCA is greater after 45 minutes of running (~80% $\dot{V}O_2$max) than after 2.5–3 hours of running (~76% $\dot{V}O_2$max). However, NKCA is suppressed longer after prolonged running (2.5–3 hours) than after 45 minutes of running.
Sources: Modified from Woods, J. A., J. M. Davis, J. A. Smith, & D. C. Nieman: Exercise and cellular innate immune function. *Medicine & Science in Sports & Exercise.* 31(1):57–66 (1999). Based on data from Nieman, D. C., L. M. Johanssen, J. W. Lee, & K. Arabatzis: Infectious episodes in runners before and after the Los Angeles Marathon. *Journal of Sports Medicine and Physical Fitness.* 30:316–328 (1990); Nieman, D. C., J. C. Ahle, D. A. Henson, B. J. Warren, J. Suttles, J. M. Davis, K. S. Buckley, S. Simandle, D. E. Butterworth, O. R. Fagoaga, & S. L. Nehlsen-Cannarella: Indomethacin does not alter natural killer cell response to 2.5 h of running. *Journal of Applied Physiology.* 79:748–755 (1995a); Nieman, D. C., K. S. Buckley, D. A. Henson, B. J. Warren, J. Suttles, J. C. Ahle, S. Simandle, O. R. Fagoaga, & S. L. Nehlsen-Cannarella: Immune function in marathon runners versus sedentary controls. *Medicine and Science in Sports and Exercise.* 27:5986–5992 (1995b).

moderate-exercise is associated with enhanced neutrophil function (phagocytic activity, oxidative burst activity, and antimicrobial activity). In contrast, prolonged high-intensity exercise is associated with a suppression of neutrophil function (Nieman, 1997a; Woods et al., 1999).

Circulating levels of monocytes are not altered by moderate-intensity aerobic exercise but increase substantially during intense aerobic exercise. The elevation persists for at least 2 hours after exercise. Furthermore, the increase in monocytes after prolonged high-intensity exercise is considerably greater than the increase in monocytes after medium-duration, high-intensity exercise, as is the postexercise elevation. Research suggests that macrophage function is enhanced following prolonged

TABLE 22.4 Exercise Response of Immune Cell Number to Prolonged (1–3 hr) Moderate- and High-Intensity Aerobic Exercise

Variable/Exercise Intensity	During or Immediately After Exercise	Recovery
Total Leukocytes		
Moderate-intensity	↑ 25–50%	↑ 25–65% 2 hr postexercise
High-intensity	↑ 200–300%	↑ 200–300% 2–6 hr postexercise
Innate Immune System		
Neutrophils		
Moderate-intensity	↑ 20–50%	↑ 50–150% 2 hr postexercise
High-intensity	↑ 300%	↑ 300–400% 2–6 hr postexercise
Monocytes		
Moderate-intensity	No Change	No Change
High-intensity	↑ 50–100%	↑ 50–100% 2–3 hr postexercise
Natural Killer cells		
Moderate-intensity	↑ 70–100%	↓ 0–50% 1–2 hr postexercise
High-intensity	↑ 100–200%	↓ 30–60% 1–2 hr postexercise
Adaptive Immune System		
T cells		
Moderate-intensity	↑ 20–30%	↓ 20% 2 hr postexercise
High-intensity	↑ 30–60%	↓ 30–40% 1–6 hr postexercise
B cells		
Moderate-intensity	No Change	No Change
High-intensity	No Change	No Change
Serum Ig		
Moderate-intensity	No Change	No Change
High-intensity	No Change	No Change
Salivary IgA		
Moderate-intensity	No Change	No Change
High-intensity	↓ 20–60%	↓ 20–60% 1 hr postexercise

Source: Based on data from Mackinnon, L. T.: *Advances in Exercise Immunology.* Champaign, IL: Human Kinetics (1999).

moderate-intensity aerobic exercise. However, the effect of high-intensity exercise on macrophage function is unclear. Some functions appear enhanced (phagocytosis, lysing, and antiviral activity), whereas other activities (oxidative burst) may be suppressed (Kohut et al., 1998; Nieman, 1997a; Woods et al., 1997, 1999).

Circulating levels of NK cells increase considerably following prolonged bouts of both moderate- and high-intensity aerobic exercise, with the intense exercise causing a larger increase in NK cell numbers. After prolonged moderate- or high-intensity exercise NK cell numbers are reduced, more so after high-intensity exercise. As with medium-duration exercise, NKCA mimics the changes in NK cell numbers. Look again at **Figure 22.7**, this time paying attention to the change in NKCA after 2.5–3 hours of intense (76% $\dot{V}O_2max$) running and during recovery (Nieman et al., 1990, 1995a,b; Woods et al., 1999). Notice the smaller increase in NKCA immediately postexercise for the prolonged run (2.5–3 hours) compared to the shorter run (45 minutes). However, during recovery from the prolonged run, NKCA is severe and

persistently reduced below preexercise levels. NKCA remained suppressed in excess of 20 hours following the prolonged, high-intensity run.

T-cell numbers increase after prolonged moderate-intensity and high-intensity exercise. During recovery from prolonged exercise (both moderate- and high-intensity) T-cell numbers are suppressed.

B-cell numbers do not appear to change immediately after prolonged bouts of moderate- or high-intensity exercise or during recovery from exercise. However, salivary levels of immunoglobulin A (IgA) are depressed after prolonged high-intensity exercise (Mackinnon, 1999; Novas et al., 2003; Tomasi et al., 1982) and there is a consensus that reduced salivary IgA levels are associated with increased risk of upper respiratory tract infections during heavy training (Walsh et al., 2011). The depression that is seen in cell number and function is transient with values typically returning to baseline values within 24 hours. However, inadequate recovery periods may not allow for fully immune recovery and may play a role in overtraining syndrome (see discussion later in this chapter).

TABLE 22.5 Exercise Response of Immune Cell Number to Intense Interval Exercise		
Variable	**During Exercise or Immediately After Exercise**	**Recovery**
Total Leukocyte Number	↑ 65–80%	↑ 75% 2–6 hr postexercise
Innate Immune System		
Neutrophils	↑ 25%	↑ 60–100% 2–6 hr postexercise
Monocytes	↑ 40–50%	↑15–60% 2–6 hr postexercise
Natural Killer cells	↑ 100–200%	Normal by 1–2 hr postexercise
Adaptive Immune System		
T cells	↑ 60–100%	↓ 30–40% 1–2 hr postexercise
B cells	↑ 0–7%	Normal by 1–6 hr postexercise

Source: Based on data from Mackinnon, L. T.: *Advances in Exercise Immunology.* Champaign, IL: Human Kinetics (1999).

Intense Interval Exercise

Table 22.5 reports the changes in immune cell numbers during or immediately after exercise and during recovery from intense interval exercise (Mackinnon, 1999). Again, exercise results in leukocytosis for at least 2–6 hours after exercise.

Neutrophils increase in number as a result of intense interval exercise and remain elevated for 2–6 hours afterward. Similarly, the circulating levels of monocytes increase following intense interval exercise and remain elevated for 2–6 hours. NK cell numbers increase markedly following intense interval exercise but return to pre-exercise levels within 2 hours.

T-cell numbers increase following intense interval exercise. During recovery, T-cell numbers are suppressed for 1–2 hours. B-cell numbers increase immediately after intense interval exercise but return to normal levels within 1–6 hours.

Cytokine Response to Exercise

Exercise is a potent activator of the immune system leading to changes in many cytokine concentrations. **Figure 22.8** is a schematic graph of the relative magnitude of changes in plasma cytokines during and after strenuous exercise. The most notable cytokine response to strenuous exercise is a large, rapid increase in IL-6. Plasma IL-6 concentrations increase exponentially, up to 100-fold, as exercise continues. This increase is related to exercise intensity, duration, muscle mass, and the individual's aerobic capacity (Gokhale et al., 2007; Miles in Kraemer and Rogol, 2005; Petersen and Pedersen, 2005). Importantly, the increase in IL-6 does not require muscle damage, suggesting that cytokines likely play important regulatory roles in addition to mediating inflammation. Plasma levels of IL-6 typically return to baseline levels within a few hours after exercise if muscle damage has not occurred (Miles, 2005). Following the increase in IL-6, the concentration in other cytokines

begins to increase. IL-1ra and IL-10 increase after IL-6, suggesting that IL-6 plays an important role in regulating the release of these anti-inflammatory cytokines. Importantly, the proinflammatory cytokines, TNFα and IL-1β, which increase during infection, do not increase after exercise in the absence of muscle damage (Petersen and Pedersen, 2005). Taken together, these data suggest that while exercise may evoke both inflammatory and anti-inflammatory cytokines, the anti-inflammatory cytokine response predominates, providing a possible mechanism for the observation that physically active individuals have less systemic inflammation than their sedentary counterparts.

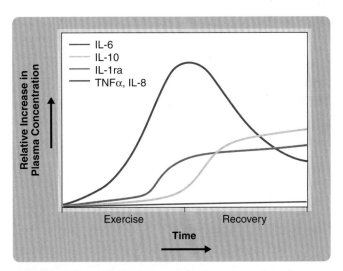

FIGURE 22.8 Cytokine Response to Strenuous Exercise.
Sources: Modified from Febraio, M. A. & B. K. Pedersen: Muscle-derived interleukin-6: Mechanisms for activation and possible biological roles. *The Federation of American Societies for Experimental Biology.* 16:1335–1347 (2002); Petersen, A. M. W. & B. K. Pedersen: The anti-inflammatory effect of exercise. *Journal of Applied Physiology.* 98:1154–1162 (2005).

Skeletal Muscle as an Endocrine Tissue that Releases Regulatory Cytokines (Myokines)

An acute bout of exercise is known to have a profound effect on the immune system. As discussed earlier, much recent research has focused on the effect of exercise on cytokines and their role in regulating the immune response. Recent studies have discovered that cytokines are released from contracting muscle as well as from immune cells (Pedersen et al., 2007; Steensberg et al., 2000). This discovery has important implications because it provides a mechanistic link between muscle contraction and the regulation of the immune response to exercise. Furthermore, evidence is growing that the cytokines released from exercising skeletal muscles also play an important role in metabolism.

To underscore the important role of skeletal muscle in producing and releasing cytokines that help provide an integrated response to exercise, some leading researchers have suggested that cytokines that are produced, expressed, and released from skeletal muscle and exert either paracrine or endocrine effects should be classified as myokines (Pedersen et al., 2007). This classification would parallel the use of the term "adipokines" for cytokines released specifically from adipose tissue.

Interleukin-6 (IL-6) is an important cytokine usually identified as a proinflammatory cytokine. However, IL-6 also plays an anti-inflammatory role (Petersen and Petersen, 2005). During contraction, skeletal muscle fibers produce and release IL-6. In fact, skeletal muscle production of IL-6 can account entirely for the exercise-induced increase in IL-6 (Steensberg et al., 2000). **Figure 22.9** is a schematic of how IL-6 may function as a myokine. IL-6 released from exercising skeletal muscle exerts its immunoregulatory role by its anti-inflammatory and proinflammatory actions. Anti-inflammatory effects include an increase in anti-inflammatory cytokines (IL-1ra, IL-10) and suppression of the proinflammatory cytokine TNFα. IL-6 also exerts a neuroendocrine influence by stimulating the hypothalamus and leading to the subsequent release of GH (from the anterior pituitary) and epinephrine and cortisol (from the adrenal glands). IL-6 also plays a metabolic role by increasing lipolysis and fat oxidation and increasing glucose uptake in skeletal muscle. Thus, IL-6 appears to play a central role in regulating a coordinated response to exercise that facilitates both the hormonal and immune responses necessary to balance inflammation and provide for the metabolic needs of working muscle (Pedersen et al., 2007).

CHECK YOUR COMPREHENSION 2

What tissue is primarily responsible for the increase in circulating IL-6 following exercise?
   What are some of the functions of IL-6?

Check your answer in Appendix C

While extensive research efforts have provided information about plasma levels of the proinflammatory and anti-inflammatory cytokines (see **Figure 22.8**) after strenuous exercise, these data must be interpreted cautiously. Cytokines have different rates of production and clearance, and their localization and use is important for assessing their contribution to overall immune function (Mastro and Bonneau, 2005). It is therefore fair to say that while cytokines play an important role in neurohormonal regulation and immune response to exercise, many questions still remain regarding the precise role of individual cytokines.

In summary, an acute bout of exercise has profound effects on many immune variables, including cell number

FIGURE 22.9 Regulatory Roles of Muscle-Derived Interleukin-6 (IL-6).
Interleukin 6 plays an important regulatory role in the immune, neuroendocrine, and metabolic responses to exercise.

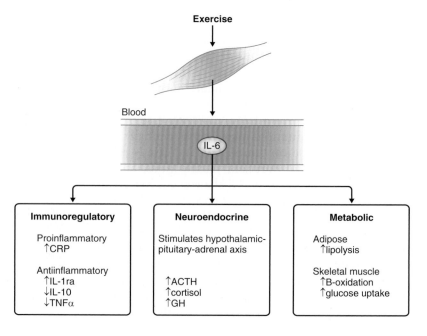

and function and circulating levels of cytokines. In general, moderate exercise appears to cause transient increases in immune function, with immune cell number and function returning to baseline within a couple of hours. Strenuous exercise, however, causes greater disruption of the immune system and a decrease in some cells and cellular function (especially NK cells and T cells) that may last for many hours into recovery. This reduction in cell number and function is the theoretical link to the greater incidence of upper respiratory tract infections reported in high-volume, endurance-trained individuals.

Neuroendocrine Control of Immune Response to Exercise

As discussed in the previous chapter, exercise is a stressor that stimulates both neuroendocrine and immune responses. **Figure 22.10** builds on **Figure 21.2** and extends the basic stress response to depict the neuroendocrine

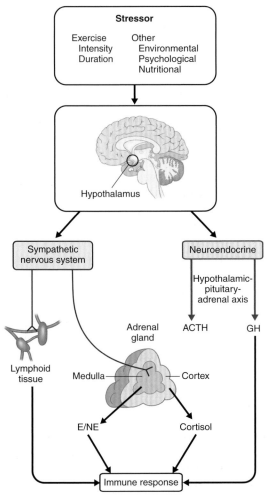

FIGURE 22.10 Neuroendocrine Regulation of Immune Function.
The immune response to exercise is mediated largely through the nervous and endocrine systems.

influence on immune function. This figure emphasizes that the body's response to exercise stress is a system-wide effort that is largely coordinated by the integration of the immune system with the neuroendocrine system (Fragala et al., 2011). Much of the influence on the immune system depends on the hypothalamic-pituitary-adrenal axis, which results in the release of cortisol from the adrenal cortex, and the sympathetic-adrenal medulla axis, which results in the release of the catecholamines from the adrenal medulla. Sympathetic nerve stimulation also directly innervates lymphoid organs. Exercise also causes the release of cytokines from skeletal muscle and immune cells, which help regulate the immune response.

As stated previously, moderate aerobic exercise appears to enhance immune function, and the cells of the immune system return to resting levels soon after exercise. Severe, exhaustive aerobic exercise, in contrast, causes an enhanced immune function followed by a suppression of cell activity. These different responses appear to depend largely on the hormones epinephrine and cortisol. During exercise at greater than 60% of $\dot{V}O_2$max, epinephrine and cortisol levels in the blood begin to increase rapidly, reaching their highest level after maximal exercise. Epinephrine is associated with a substantial increase in the number of lymphocytes in the blood. Cortisol causes an increased number of neutrophils but a decreased number of lymphocytes. Immediately after exercise, the blood concentrations of epinephrine fall rapidly to preexercise levels, whereas cortisol levels remain elevated for 2 hours or more (see Chapter 21). Researchers therefore hypothesize that after intense exercise, epinephrine is responsible for the increase in circulating lymphocytes, and the longer-acting cortisol is responsible for the prolonged increase in neutrophils and the decrease in lymphocytes (Nieman, 1994).

Training Adaptation and Maladaptation

The relationship of training to athletic performance involves a continuum best described as an inverted U (**Figure 1.10**) (Fry et al., 1991; Kuipers, 1998; Rowbottom et al., 1998). As described in Chapter 1, the goal of optimal periodized training is the attainment of peak fitness and/or performance. However, with too great or improperly applied training overload, maladaptation is possible.

Table 22.6 summarizes training adaptations in the immune system of moderately trained and highly trained or overtrained individuals. The resting immune system of moderately trained aerobic athletes is usually within normal parameters, although neutrophil function and serum immunoglobulins may be relatively low (Mackinnon, 2000; Nieman, 1994; Shephard et al., 1995). In general, moderate training appears to enhance some functions of the immune system, especially natural killer cell count and activity (Mackinnon, 2000; Matthews et al., 2002;

TABLE 22.6 Effects of Moderate and Intense Training/Overtraining on Immune Function and Resistance to Illness

	Moderate Training	Intense Training/Overtraining
Cells		
Leukocytes	No change in resting number	↓ Resting number in circulation of athletes after intense exercise
Neutrophils	No change in resting number	No change in resting number (or decrease) ↓ Activation at rest and after exercise
NK cells	No change in resting number ↑ NKCA at rest	↓ Resting number in circulation ↓ NKCA at rest
T cells	No change	No change, or decrease
B cells	No change in resting number	No change in resting number
Chemical Mediators		
Cytokines	No change in resting concentration ↑ Resting IL-1 in plasma of athletes compared with nonathletes	No change in resting concentrations ↑ Resting 1L-1 in plasma of athletes compared with nonathletes
APP	↓ Acute phase protein release after exercise	↓ Acute phase protein release after exercise
Antibodies (Ig)	No change in serum and secretory Ig levels ↑ Specific antibody response	↓ Serum Ig levels in athletes after intensified training ↓Salivary IgA levels in athletes after intensified training
Resistance to Illness	↑ Survival rate following viral infection ↑ Survival rate following bacterial infection ↓ Incidence of URTI ↓ Incidence of cancer	↑ Incidence of URTI ↑ Rate of paralysis following polio infection

Sources: Based on data from Mackinnon, L. T.: Chronic exercise training effects on immune function. *Medicine & Science in Sports & Exercise.* 32(7):S369–S376 (2000); Mackinnon, L. T.: *Advances in Exercise Immunology.* Champaign, IL: Human Kinetics (1999); Nieman, D. C.: Immune response to heavy exertion. *Journal of Applied Physiology.* 82(5):1385–1394 (1997a); Nieman, D. C.: Risk of upper respiratory tract infection in athletes: An epidemiologic and immunologic perspective. *Journal of Athletic Training.* 32(4):344–349 (1997b).

Shephard et al., 1995; Woods et al., 1999). In contrast, strenuous training or overtraining is associated with a suppression of several immune variables. Most notable among changed immune functions following severe training is a suppression of leukocyte numbers, a decrease in neutrophil function, a decrease in natural killer cell activity, and a reduction in lymphocytes (B cells, T cells, and NK cells) (Mackinnon, 1999, 2000; Nieman, 1997a; Woods et al., 1999). As seen in **Table 22.6**, training-induced adaptations also occur in several cytokines, acute phase proteins, and antibodies (immunoglobulins). Intense training or overtraining is associated with a reduction in acute phase proteins, serum Ig, salivary IgA, and complement (Mackinnon, 1999; Nieman, 1997a; Papacosta and Nassis, 2011; Woods et al., 1999).

One of the greatest research challenges in this area is to define more clearly what constitutes "moderate" training and "strenuous" training. Furthermore, there is a need to understand more fully whether strenuous training in itself results in immune suppression or whether immune suppression occurs only with more severe overtraining. While many chapters in this text focus on the beneficial adaptations that result from exercise training, the following sections address the serious condition of maladaptation.

The first step toward maladaptation may be **overreaching (OR)**, a short-term decrement in performance capacity that generally lasts only a few days to 2 weeks and from which the individual easily recovers. Overreaching can result from planned shock microcycles (see Chapter 1) or inadvertently from too much stress and too little planned recovery (Fry and Kraemer, 1997; Fry et al., 1991; Kuipers, 1998; Meeusen et al., 2006). If overreaching is planned and recovery is sufficient, positive adaptation and improved performance, sometimes called supercompensation, result (**Figure 22.11A**) This type of overreaching is called *functional overreaching (FOR)*. However, if recovery is insufficient and takes longer than desired, *nonfunctional overreaching (NFOR)* is said to occur. If NFOR is left unchecked or the individual or coach interprets the decrement in performance as an indication that more work must be done with less rest and recovery, NFOR may develop into overtraining (**Figure 22.11B**). Overtraining, more properly called the **overtraining syndrome (OTS)** (or staleness), is a state of chronic decrement in performance and ability to train, in which restoration may take several months, or even years. Indeed, the distinction between NFOR and OTS is based primarily on the amount of time needed for performance restoration (approximately several weeks to months for

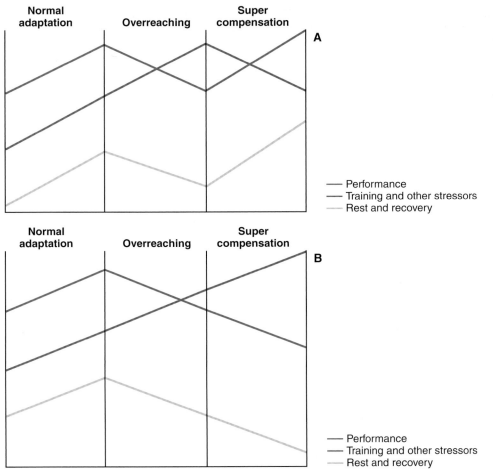

FIGURE 22.11 Exercise Training Adaptations (A) and Maladaptation (B).
Sources: Fry, R. W., A. R. Morton, & D. Keast: Periodization and the prevention of overtraining. *Canadian Journal of Sport Sciences.* 17:241–248 (1992); Kreider, R. B., A. C. Fry, & M. L. O'Toole: Overtraining in sport: Terms, definitions, and prevalence. In Kreider, R. B., A. C. Fry, & M. L. O'Toole (eds.): *Overtraining in Sport.* Champaign, IL: Human Kinetics, vii–ix (1998); Kuipers, H.: Training and overtraining: An introduction. *Medicine & Science in Sports & Exercise.* 30:1137–1139 (1998).

NFOR and several months to years with OTS). This is assuming that all other possible causes of prolonged underperformance have been eliminated (Armstrong and vanHeest, 2002; Bosque et al., 2008; Fry and Kraemer, 1997; Fry et al., 1991; Kreider et al., 1998; Meeusen et al., 2006, 2010; Nederhof et al., 2008; Schmikli et al., 2011).

The relationship between overreaching and the overtraining syndrome is often depicted as a continuum, as shown in **Figure 1.10** (Fry et al., 1991; Meeusen et al., 2006, 2010). As the imbalance between training and recovery increases, the complexity of the symptoms also increases and the athlete progresses from overreached to overtrained. It is thought that the symptoms of OTS are more severe than those of NFOR. No experimental data

exist, however, to either confirm or refute this assumption (Halson and Jeukendrup, 2004; Meeusen et al., 2006, 2010). Coaches and athletes often use shock microcycles to induce overreaching in the normal periodization of training, making it possible for scientists to follow and test athletes in such a situation. However, it is neither ethical nor reasonable to deliberately induce a state of OTS. Scientific data on OTS have therefore largely been derived retroactively from case studies of athletes with unexplained underperformance. Data on meaningful numbers of subjects in both resistance and endurance activities followed from adaptation and performance improvement through overreaching to the overtraining syndrome are not available.

Nonetheless, a very long list of signs and symptoms has been observed in athletes exhibiting unexplained performance decrements (Fry et al., 1991; Urhausen and Kindermann, 2002). **Table 22.7** lists some, but not all, signs and symptoms that may be observed by athletes, coaches, and athletic trainers. This list is complicated by the fact that apparently there are two forms of the OTS: a sympathetic form and a parasympathetic form (Flynn, 1998; Fry and Kraemer, 1997; Kenttä and Hassmén, 1998; Lehmann et al., 1993, 1998a,b; Meeusen et al., 2006; Urhausen and

Overreaching (OR) A short-term decrement in performance capacity that generally lasts only a few days to 2 weeks and from which the individual easily recovers.

Overtraining Syndrome (OTS) A state of chronic decrement in performance and ability to train in which restoration may take several weeks, months, or even years.

TABLE 22.7 Signs and Symptoms of the Overtraining Syndrome

Type	Signs and Symptoms
Performance related	• Consistent decrement in performance • Persistent fatigue and sluggishness that leads to several days of poor training • Prolonged recovery from training sessions or competitive events • Reappearance of already corrected errors • Increased occurrence of muscular accidents/injuries
Physiological	• Decreased maximal work capacities and markers • Increased disruption of homeostasis at submaximal workloads • Headaches or stomachaches out of proportion to life events • Insomnia • Persistent low-grade stiffness and soreness of the muscles and joints; feeling of "heavy" legs • Frequent upper respiratory tract infections: sore throats, colds, or cold sores • Constipation or diarrhea • Loss of appetite; loss of body weight or muscle mass, or both, when no conscious attempt is being made to diet or when weight loss is undesirable • An elevation of ~10% in the morning resting heart rate taken immediately on awakening
Psychological/ behavioral	• Feelings of depression • General apathy, especially toward previously enjoyed activities • Decreased self-esteem • Emotional instability or mood changes • Difficulty concentrating • Loss of competitive drive or desire • Perceived insufficient recovery

Kindermann, 2000; Witlert, 2000). The sympathetic form is characterized by an increased sympathetic neural tone at rest and during exercise and down-regulation of beta (β) receptors. Restlessness and hyperexcitability dominate. For example, an elevated resting heart rate, slower heart rate recovery after exercise, decreased appetite and unintentional loss of body mass, excessive sweating, and disturbed sleep patterns are symptoms of the sympathetic form of overtraining (Fry et al., 1991; Lehmann et al., 1998b). The sympathetic form of overtraining is generally considered an early indication of overtraining. It appears to be most closely related to high-intensity anaerobic activities (Fry and Kraemer, 1997). The parasympathetic form of overtraining is characterized by sympathetic neural insufficiency, a decreased sensitivity to the pituitary and adrenal hormones, and increased parasympathetic tone at rest and during exercise. The symptoms of the parasympathetic form of overtraining are less obvious and in isolation may be difficult to distinguish from positive training adaptations (Fry et al., 1991; Lehmann et al., 1998b). For example, resting pulse rates may be lower, submaximal exercise heart rates and lactate responses lower, and heart rate recovery from exercise rapid, but these responses are typically associated with early fatigue and impaired

maximal work capacity markers, such as heart rate and lactate. Apathy, digestive disturbances, and altered immune and reproductive function are common. The parasympathetic form of the overtraining syndrome is the more advanced form. It appears most frequently associated with excessive volume training in both aerobic endurance activity and dynamic resistance exercise (Fry and Kraemer, 1997). Individual differences in the nervous system may predispose any given individual to either up-regulation (sympathetic form) or down-regulation (parasympathetic form) of the neuroendocrine homeostasis.

The signs and symptoms of OTS are outward manifestations of neuroendocrine imbalances, immune system activation and/or suppression, or a reversal of normal physiological adaptations. They provide a starting point for research investigating the physiological mechanisms behind OTS.

Hypothesized Causes and Mechanisms of Overtraining Syndrome (OTS)

The precise cause(s) and mechanism(s) of OTS are unknown. A high-volume training load performed at high intensity, applied in a monotonous manner, and without sufficient rest and recovery that alters metabolic processes

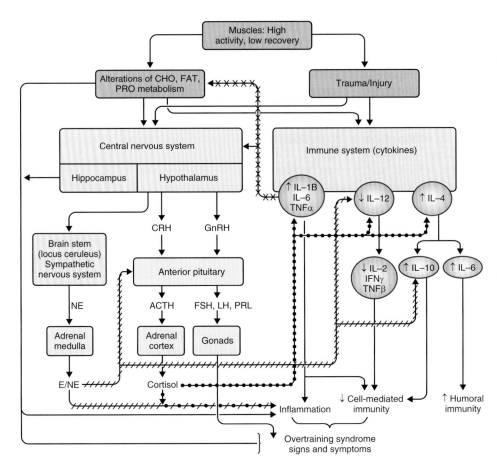

FIGURE 22.12 Hypothesized Mechanism of Overtraining Syndrome.
A high-volume training load performed at high intensity, applied in a monotonous manner, and without sufficient rest and recovery that alters metabolic processes and leads to an accumulation of muscle trauma appears to be the primary predisposing factor to the development of the overtraining syndrome. Alterations of carbohydrate (CHO), lipid (FAT), and/or protein (PRO) metabolism (represented on the left side of this flow chart) and microtrauma or tissue injury in muscles (presented on the right side of the flow chart) can individually or collectively impact both the central nervous system and the immune system. Full details describing this figure are included in the text. *Sources*: Budgett (1998); Chrousos and Gold (1992); Fry et al. (1992); Gastmann and Lehmann (1998); Keizer (1998); Kreider et al. (1998); Moldoveanu et al. (2001); Petibois et al. (2003); Robson (2003); Smith (2000, 2003a,b); Steinacker et al. (2004); Synder (1998).

and leads to an accumulation of muscle trauma appears to be the primary predisposing factor (**Figure 22.12**) (Armstrong and vanHeest, 2002; Budgett, 1998; Fry et al., 1991; Meussen et al., 2006; Petibois et al., 2002, 2003; Smith, 2000). Related stressors such as frequent competition, excessive travel, training and competing under inhospitable environmental conditions, and/or poor nutrition as well as unrelated stressors such as family, school, or work commitments accumulate and are likely peripheral causes. Thus OTS may represent the sum of multiple life stressors and can be understood, at least partially with the context of Selye's General Adaptation Syndrome (see Chapter 1) (Meeusen et al., 2006).

Several hypotheses have been developed to explain the physiological mechanisms by which probable causative factors actually bring about OTS. Remember that a hypothesis by definition is "an assumption not proved by experiment or observation. It is assumed for the sake of testing its soundness or to facilitate investigation of a class of phenomena" (Thomas, 1985). Thus, while research data can account for some observed symptoms of OTS, these data are generally insufficient to justify calling any hypothesis a theory. In short, the underlying mechanism(s) remain(s) unproven at this time (Armstrong and vanHeest, 2002).

These hypotheses may be categorized in three major areas: biochemical/metabolic, neuroendocrine, and immunological. **Figure 22.12** indicates how these areas may interact in producing OTS. Refer to this figure throughout the following discussion.

Alterations of Carbohydrate, Lipid, and Protein Metabolism

Muscles obviously use fuel for contractions in exercise training. Indeed, a major objective of exercise training, especially endurance training, is to increase metabolism to support competition. OTS in endurance athletes thus may be mediated primarily through dysfunctions of carbohydrate (CHO), lipid (FAT), and/or protein (PRO) metabolism (Kreider et al., 1998; Petibois et al., 2002, 2003; Synder, 1998). Glycogen depletion may become a reality with insufficient CHO ingestion after successive training bouts. Low glycogen can in itself lead to the defining signs of OTS, early fatigue, and poor performance (Synder, 1998).

The predominant backup fuel to CHO for exercise is, of course, FAT in the form of triglyceride derived free fatty acids (FFA). While the utilization of higher amounts of FFA and the sparing of glycogen is a beneficial adaptation of training, this typically occurs in the presence of adequate glycogen stores. Without sufficient CHO stores and in the presence of the oxidative stress that accompanies endurance activity, alterations occur in the triglyceride/fatty acid cycle, and polyunsaturated fatty acids (PUFAs) increase. These changes have been linked to the pathogenesis of inflammation and immunosuppression (Petibois et al., 2002, 2003; Steinacker et al., 2004). Additionally, leptin is released from adipose cells. Leptin provides feedback for satiety, may act as a metabolic hormone, and helps regulate hypothalamic-pituitary function. Movement of fatty acid from adipocytes may inhibit leptin secretion. Low plasma leptin levels activate the hypothalamus-pituitary-adrenal axis (HPAA) as well as sympathetic activity, and, as a cytokine, leptin is closely linked to immune function (Saris, 2001; Steinacker et al., 2004).

These alterations in CHO (insufficient) and FAT metabolism (increased FFA utilization) also lead to shifts in PRO metabolism. Protein is not normally utilized extensively as fuel. However, under conditions of high-intensity, long-duration training or competition, especially when CHO stores are inadequate, PRO (particularly the branched chain amino acids [BCAA]) is utilized as fuel. Furthermore, the increased circulating FFA, which must be transported in blood by albumin, leads to release of another amino acid (AA), tryptophan (TRY). TRY also normally binds to albumin. In addition to competing for albumin, BCAA and TRY normally compete for the same carrier to enter the brain. The decreased BCAAs (when utilized to supply fuel) and increased TRY favor the entry of TRY into the brain. In the brain, TRY is converted into serotonin. Increased levels of serotonin are responsible for decreased motor excitability, decreased appetite, increased sleep, and altered neuroendocrine function—among the signs and symptoms often seen in OTS (Budgett, 1998; Gastmann and Lehmann, 1998; Kreider et al., 1998).

Glutamine is the most abundant AA in human muscle and plasma. Glutamine is an energy source essential for kidney function, used by the liver during exercise for the production and release of the antioxidant glutathione, important at the neural level in the perception of exertion, lethargy, and energy levels, and a precursor of substances essential for immune cell replication. Specifically, macrophages cannot synthesize certain cytokines (such as interleukin-1 [IL-1]) if glutamine is in short supply. Cytokines are essential for communication between immune cells and other body cells. Muscles are the main source of glutamine. Psychological, environmental, and exercise stresses, especially with insufficient rest periods between bouts, may decrease glutamine flux from muscle during recovery. Immune function may consequently be depressed after exercise due to the decreased availability of glutamine. This in turn may be linked to the high incidence of upper respiratory tract infections (URTI) common in athletes after excessive exercise (such as a marathon) or in an overreached/overtrained state (Budgett, 1998; Fry et al., 1991; Gotovtseva et al., 1998; Papacosta and Nassis, 2011; Petibois et al., 2002, 2003; Robson, 2003;

Rowbottom et al., 1996). Note that only cell-mediated immunity seems adversely affected (**Figure 22.12**).

Altered neuroendocrine function is predominantly mediated through the hypothalamus in Selye's classic stress response. The primary neural component is the brainstem (locus ceruleus)-sympathetic nervous system pathway. The primarily hormonal component is the hypothalamus-pituitary-adrenal axis (HPAA). The hypothalamus, as both a neural structure and an endocrine gland, can orchestrate the body's response by stimulating both the sympathetic nervous system and the endocrine glands.

Muscle Trauma and Injury/Cytokine Theory

Microtrauma or tissue injury in muscles can impact both the central nervous system (CNS) and the immune system. Activation of the CNS by cytokines explains many of the signs and symptoms of OTS. Anti-inflammatory cytokines define the role of T cells. T cells divide into two distinct functional subsets: TH1, associated with cell-mediated immunity, and TH2, associated with humoral immunity. The up-regulation of TH1 cells primarily depends on IL-12; the up-regulation of TH2 cells primarily depends on IL-4. In addition, IL-4 and IL-10 coordinate to inhibit TH1 development. Thus 1L-10 suppresses cell-mediated immunity and macrophage function. The response to trauma/injury is a shift to a TH2 lymphocyte response, resulting in an up-regulation of humoral immunity and down-regulation of cell-mediated immunity. The individual is thus more susceptible to URTI (Moldoveanu et al., 2001; Smith, 2003a). The binding of cytokines (particularly IL-6) in the hypothalamus activates the hypothalamic-pituitary-adrenal axis (HPAA) and the sympathetic nervous system, resulting in the release of E/NE and cortisol (Moldoveanu et al., 2001; Steinacker et al., 2004). These stress hormones bring about physical changes and are associated with mood changes such as depression and anxiety. The activation of the hippocampus may explain loss of attention and the return of previously corrected errors (Armstrong and vanHeest, 2002; Keizer, 1998; Smith, 2000, 2003b; Steinacker et al., 2004). Experimental evidence in support of this cytokine hypothesis is growing (Main et al., 2010).

Markers and Monitoring of Training to Predict Overtraining Syndrome (OTS)

Research is ongoing to determine the mechanisms of OTS and identify a marker such as a level of some hormone or specific change that could help detect early on whether an athlete is on the brink of overtraining. Once known, this could lead to intervention or, ideally, prevention (Budgett, 1998; Urhausen and Kindermann, 2000).

Despite numerous attempts to identify such a marker, the overwhelming consensus remains that no reliable and valid variable or index is available to predict OTS or even to distinguish among well-trained, overreached, or overtrained athletes. Making matters still more difficult, there is no clear demarcation for when overload becomes overtraining load. The margin between adaptation/super-compensation and the functional impairment of OTS is fluid both among athletes and within individual athletes. Nonetheless, there is consensus that monitoring athletes is extremely important. The difficulty is how and what to monitor (Achten and Jeukendrup, 2003; Duclos, 2008; Flynn, 1998; Gabriel et al., 1998; Hartmann and Mester, 2000; Hooper and Mackinnon, 1995; Kuipers, 1998; Lac and Maso, 2004; Meeusen et al., 2006; Urhausen and Kindermann, 2002). Training, performance, and mood state appear to be reasonable and practical places to begin.

Monitor Training

All athletes should be encouraged to keep a daily training log. This should include body weight (with periodic evaluation of body composition), morning resting heart rate (often difficult because many athletes do not like doing this), training goal, training achieved, subjective ratings of perceived exertion during training, any noticeable muscle/tendon/joint aches or pains, and any symptoms of URTI (Calder, 2004).

Athletes should be aware of and report (before beginning the day's workout) any meaningful changes (a rise ≥20%) in resting heart rate, any muscle/tendon/joint soreness, or URTI symptoms persisting from the day before. These could be indications that it is necessary to cut back the volume and intensity of the workout on this day to possibly avoid longer setbacks in the future (Hooper and Mackinnon, 1995).

At the end of each macrocycle (see Chapter 1), the training log should be carefully evaluated to determine the athlete's response to the training load. The training plan for the next cycle should be based on this evaluation (Smith, 2003a).

Monitor Performance

The most obvious item to monitor is, of course, the specific sport performance, including not only the outcome but also the effort involved and apparent recovery. Performance in training workouts should also be monitored. In some events, individualized ergometric tests can reproduce specific levels of performance in the exercise physiology laboratory or training room (Meeusen et al., 2006; Urhausen and Kindermann, 2002). Because athletes suffering from OTS often start a normal training workout, race, or other event but do not complete the performance as expected, the analysis should include splits in relation to a predetermined strategy. A two-bout exercise test protocol might be best for detecting differences in training status.

Meeusen et al. (2004) detected subtle differences in HPAA hormonal responses to two bouts of maximal exercise 4 hours apart between cyclists in a well-trained (N = 7) state and in an intentionally overreached state (same seven athletes), and in one diagnosed OTS motocross athlete that would have been missed had only one exercise bout been used. Performance itself was also sensitive to the training status. Time to exhaustion in bout 2 decreased only 3% from bout 1 in the well-trained state, doubled to –6% in the overreached condition, and almost doubled again to –11% in the OTS athlete. Follow-up studies (Meeusen et al., 2010; Nederhof et al., 2008) have supported the sensitivity of the hormonal response (particularly ACTH and prolactin) to a two-bout exercise test in being able to distinguish between NFOR and OTS athletes and NFOR, NFOR recovering, and normal athletes. Performance of an interval shuttle run test (alternately running for 30 seconds and walking for 15 seconds starting at speeds of 10 km·hr^{-1}) has also been shown to be sensitive to detecting NFOR (Schmikli et al., 2011).

Although some individual studies have reported changes in performance (submaximal and maximal), exercise heart rate, or heart rate variability as a convenient method for monitoring overreaching, a meta-analysis (Bosquet et al., 2008) has determined that while such changes are statistically valid they have very limited practical value for athletes, coaches, and physicians as they typically fall within the day-to-day variability of heart rate.

Performance tests must be conducted after a recovery or regeneration cycle (see Chapter 1) when adaptation or maladaptation can accurately be evaluated and not confused with the normal fatigue of training (Fry et al., 1992; Rowbottom et al., 1998). This analysis requires, of course, baseline data previously established for the athlete. The Focus on Application box describes a study that suggests that the 20-meter shuttle test (20 MST or PACER) may be an easy way to monitor for OTS in team sport athletes.

Monitor Mood State

Subjective ratings of mood, fatigue, athletic and nonathletic stress, and muscle soreness have been suggested as the most cost-effective strategy for early detection of OTS and thus for monitoring training (Hooper and Mackinnon, 1995; Lehmann et al., 1993; Meeusen et al., 2006; Meyers and Whelan, 1998; Urhausen and Kindermann, 2002). The Profile of Mood States (POMS) (McNair et al., 1971) has been most extensively studied. This 65-item test provides subjective ratings of tension-anxiety, depression, anger, vigor, fatigue, confusion, and total mood. A shorter 24-item version is also available but is sometimes called the BRUMS, Brunel Mood Scale (Rohlfs et al., 2008; Terry et al., 2003). Although Profile of Mood States cannot diagnose OTS, it can document mood changes consistent with the condition (such as increased depression and tension-anxiety and decreased vigor and total mood score) in some athletes (Hawley and Schoene, 2003; Hooper and Mackinnon, 1995). The deterioration in mood states often coincides with an increased training load and usually precedes a decrement in performance (Urhausen and

FOCUS ON APPLICATION
Monitoring Overreaching/Overtraining

The authors were concerned about the lack of clear practical tests for the overtraining syndrome (which they called nonfunctional overreaching), which is problematic both for scientists studying the issue and for coaches trying to prevent it. They designed their study to investigate changes in a variety of biochemical, immunological, physiological, and psychological markers for monitoring fatigue and recovery.

Eighteen Australian male rugby league players in a semiprofessional club volunteered and were divided into two matched groups. All players completed 6 weeks of five to seven training sessions per week of progressive endurance development, resistance training, speed and agility training, and rugby drills. The intensive training (IT) group was intentionally overtrained, while the other group was normally trained (NT). (The training load for each individual was set using the method of Foster outlined in the Focus on Application—Clinically Relevant box presented later in this chapter.) The average training load for the two groups is presented in the graph below, which shows the IT group did approximately 21% more training than the NT group.

Following 6 weeks of training, all players completed the same taper. This was a step-reduction taper consisting primarily of a reduction in training session duration while maintaining training intensity. The activities included three field sessions and two resistance training sessions.

All players were tested before the training protocol, after the 6 weeks of training (except for the 20 MST run each week), and at the completion of the 7-day taper. All measures were taken after 24 hours of rest after the last training session and at the same time of day. The only significantly different variables between the IT and NT groups after the 6-week overload period were the 20 MST, $\dot{V}O_2$max, and glutamine/glutamate ratio. Because of its ease of administration, only the 20 MST results are discussed here. The NT group incrementally

improved their 20 MST performance by approximately 1% per week through the first 5 weeks and then decreased slightly, for an overall improvement of $+3.3 \pm 7.7\%$ at week 6. In contrast, the IT group showed basically no change through week 3, approximately 1% decrease at week 4, and a decrease of $-9.2 \pm 3.8\%$ by week 6. After the taper, both groups showed an equal improvement of approximately +6% from the start of the training program, with no difference between groups. These results suggest that the 20 MST may be a useful measure for monitoring response to training and that a short taper is useful even for team sports players.

Source: Coutts et al. (2007).

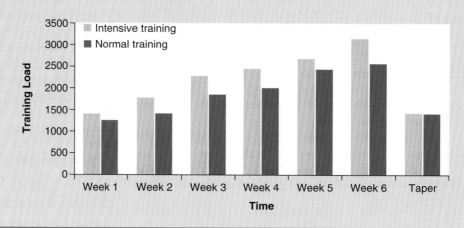

Kindermann, 2002). Self-analysis questionnaires using well-being ratings can prove useful, including ratings of fatigue, stress level, muscle soreness (especially "heavy" legs), training enjoyment, health concerns, irritability, self-confidence/self-esteem, attitude toward work/study/teammates, communication with teammates and coaches, and sleep quality/disorders. Although verbal reports are very important, all of these items should be recorded in a written training log. Subjective portions of this log require candor and complete honesty by the athlete and must be evaluated in light of training and performance. The usefulness of the log depends heavily on the coach's or athletic trainer's interpretation. A new 22-item questionnaire that includes six distinct symptom clusters (depression, vigor, physical symptoms, sleep disturbance, stress, and fatigue) covering three domains (mood, stress, and behavioral/physical symptoms) is informative for coaches and

user-friendly for athletes but requires further validation (Main and Grove, 2009).

Prevention and Treatment of Overtraining Syndrome (OTS)

Prevention

Attempts to prevent the Overtraining Syndrome center on periodization of the exercise training with an emphasis on adequate recovery for adaptation and proper nutrition.

PERIODIZATION The key to preventing the OTS is careful periodization of training (see Chapter 1). It is difficult to attain the delicate balance between overload/progression (avoiding large immediate increases in overload) and sufficient rest/recovery, but this balance is essential for each individual (Meeusen et al., 2006; Smith, 2003a).

Periodization allows the athlete to peak for specific competitions. Peak performance cannot be maintained indefinitely, so competitions must be prioritized and periodization phases matched to these priorities. The more frequently peaks are attempted, the more vulnerable the athlete is to overtraining (Bompa, 2004; Smith, 2003a). Few studies have actually compared the effectiveness of periodization. However, Rhea and Alderman (2004) and Steinacker et al. (1998) have shown positive results for strength/power (weight lifting) and aerobic/anaerobic (rowing) programs using periodization.

The main protection against OTS is the inclusion of sufficient recovery after heavy physical training, including each daily training session and each competition. Athletes and coaches indoctrinated with the philosophy of "if some is good, more is better" often find it difficult to accept that "less can actually be more." Possible components of daily recovery include hydration and refueling as soon as possible to deal with metabolic fatigue; light activity, stretching, and hydrotherapy (showering or pool/spa activities) to deal with neural fatigue; and unwinding with activities such as debriefing or listening to music to deal with psychological fatigue (Calder, 2004). This recovery should be monitored. The monitoring system proposed by Kenttä and Hassmén (1998) is described in the Focus on Application box. Restful sleep of 8–9 hours is essential. Sufficient recovery should also be included within the training progression itself through the inclusion of easy days, days of active cross-training, rest days emphasizing stretching and relaxation techniques, or days of compete rest (Kenttä and Hassmén, 1998). The Focus on Application: Clinically Relevant box also describes a technique for evaluating the adequacy of the variation of training.

NUTRITION Adequate nutrition, with the possible periodization of carbohydrate intake to match glycogen needs, is also critical. A key goal is to ensure sufficient glycogen stores to support high-intensity training or competition. Maintaining blood glucose is also important for attenuating increases in stress hormones (especially cortisol), diminishing the changes in immunity mediated through cytokines. Ingestion of carbohydrate during prolonged high-intensity exercise has been shown to blunt the inflammatory response (Coyle, 2004; Kreider et al., 1998; Venkatraman and Pendergast, 2002).

One to two hours of high-intensity exercise or as little as 20–30 minutes of heavy interval training can result in glycogen depletion. Full replenishment of glycogen under optimal dietary conditions takes 20–24 hours. Optimal conditions include ingestion of 50–100 g of high-glycemic carbohydrate within 15–20 minutes of stopping exercise, and continuing each hour for the first 4 hours of recovery at a rate of 1–1.2 g CHO per kg of body weight. If the next day's workout is scheduled to be moderate- or heavy-endurance activity, the 24-hour recovery diet should consist of 7–12 g CHO per kg; if moderate duration but low intensity, the 24-hour recovery diet can be 5–7 g CHO per kg. Extreme-duration training or competition necessitates 10–12 g CHO per kg. From these numbers it should be obvious that "two-a-days" will not allow for full glycogen replenishment between sessions. This represents a form of metabolic underrecovery (Coyle, 2004).

Adequate nutrition involves more than just carbohydrate ingestion, however. The most basic consideration is that, unless the athlete is trying to lose weight during the general preparatory cycle, caloric intake must balance caloric output. Days of lower carbohydrate intake (if carbohydrate is periodized as suggested) allow for increases in fat and protein while still maintaining caloric balance.

Fat and protein ingestion are critical. Low-fat diets (<20%) compromise endurance performance and lead to possible deficiencies in micronutrients. Both the quantity and type of fats alter immune functioning. Diets very low (<20%) or very high (>60%) in protein have negative effects on immune function as well. Diets unbalanced in fat and protein may be a factor in overtraining. In addition, the inclusion of protein in the food consumed immediately after exercise may aid in glycogen storage (Coyle, 2004).

Hydration, the last critical component, should include both water and sports drinks. Thirst is not a reliable indication of the amount of fluid needed. Chapter 6 discusses fluid needs for adequate hydration and rehydration.

The quest to find the foods or nutritional supplements to support the immune system during strenuous training has motivated scientists, athletes, and commercial entities for many years. The accompanying Focus on Application box reviews the current recommendations regarding nutritional supplements to lessen immune disruption with strenuous training.

Treatment

If training adjustments are insufficient and OTS develops, treatment is needed. The first step in treatment is a medical examination to rule out possible illnesses or injuries as the underlying cause of a performance decrement. Once these possible causes have been ruled out, the individual must be guided through a recovery program. This must be done carefully, because active—and especially competitive—individuals often resist recommendations to cut down or cease training. Rest may be a four-letter word to an athlete, but rest is the only established treatment (Meeusen et al., 2006; Mujika and Padilla, 2000). As with recovery, rest need not mean total inactivity, however.

Armstrong and Van Heest (2002) point out that OTS and clinical (major) depression involve very similar signs and symptoms, brain structures, neurotransmitters, endocrine pathways, and immune responses and thus probably have similar causes. Given these communalities they and others (American College of Sports Medicine, 2000) suggest treating overtrained athletes with antidepressant

Ratings of Perceived Exertion and Recovery

Researchers have begun to promote monitoring the adequacy of recovery from training using rating scales. One system (Kenttä and Hassmén, 1998) proposes assessing recovery from training using two total quality recovery (TQR) scales. The TQR perceived (TQR$_{per}$) scale is a subjective rating by the individual to the query "How do you rate your overall recovery for the previous 24 hours?" The TQR action scale (TQR$_{act}$) allows the athlete to accumulate "recovery points" based on his/her activities in the previous 24 hours. Up to 10 points can be awarded for nutrition and hydration, up to 4 for sleep and rest, up to 3 for relaxation and emotional support, and up to 3 for stretching and active rest. Because the point values for the action items are not set in stone but are determined by the athlete and his/her coach or trainer, specific point values should be established before implementing this scale. Based on this system, recovery is adequate if both the TQR$_{per}$ and TQR$_{act}$ are at or above the training stress value as measured by the Borg Rating of Perceived Exertion Scale

(Borg, 1998) for the workout preceding the recovery.

Foster (1998) bases his technique on Borg's category ratio scale (CR-10) (Borg, 1998) and the duration of each day's workout, multiplying the two together to obtain a training session load. Each

week the mean and standard deviation of the training load is computed as an index of training variability. The monotony of the weekly training load is calculated by dividing the daily mean load by the standard deviation (SD). A small SD and a high quotient indicate little day-to-day

Borg's RPE Scale	TQR per Scale	Borg's CR-10 Scale
6	6	0.0
7 very, very light	7 very, very poor	0.0
8	8	0.5
9 very light	9 very poor	1.0
10	10	1.5
11 fairly light	11 poor	2.0
12	12	3.0
13 somewhat hard	13 reasonable	3.5
14	14	4.5
15 hard	15 good	5.5
16	16	6.5
17 very hard	17	7.5
18	18	9.0
19 very, very hard	19	10.0
20	20	10.0+

medications and professional psychological counseling. Research supporting the use of specific antidepressants is needed.

Just as there is no definitive marker for overtraining, so too is there no definitive marker to indicate recovery. Resumption of training must be gradual. The best "treatment," of course, is prevention (American College of Sports Medicine, 2000; Flynn, 1998; Meeusen et al., 2006).

Selected Interactions of Exercise and Immune Function

Exercise, the Immune System, and Upper Respiratory Tract Infection

Many people believe that individuals who exercise regularly are less likely to acquire a cold or the flu, whereas others believe that highly trained, competitive athletes are more susceptible to upper respiratory tract infections (URTI). This section considers scientific evidence that both positions may be correct. The relationship between exercise and URTI is apparently mediated by

the exercise intensity and overall training load (Gleeson, 2007: Mackinnon, 1999; Mathews et al., 2002; Nieman, 2000; Nieman et al., 1990, 1993a).

Figure 22.6 shows a schematic model explaining the relationship between exercise and incidence of infection. This model suggests that exercise is a stressor that can lead to immunomodulation (either immunoenhancement or immunosuppression) via various mechanisms and that immune enhancement or suppression can lead to a decreased or increased risk of infections, respectively.

As discussed earlier, an acute bout of exercise leads to changes in immune cell number and cell function. **Figure 22.13** presents the "open window" hypothesis, which suggests that the suppression of immune function is greater and more prolonged after severe exercise than after moderate exercise (Pedersen and Ullum, 1994). Notice the similarities between the theoretical curve in Figures 22.7 and 22.13, which depicts NK cell activity. The suppression of the T cells and NK cells during recovery from strenuous exercise may provide a period of increased susceptibility (the "open window" represented by the rectangular shaded area) for infection. This hypothesis is not universally accepted. Changes in variation, that is, high monotony. The strain of the weekly load is determined by multiplying the daily load by 7 d·wk⁻¹ and the monotony factor. Both consistent high training monotony and high training strain appear related to training maladaptation.

The example below shows how simply substituting one rest day for a long cycling ride reduces the training monotony and strain. Many elite athletes work at a training load of 4000 U·wk⁻¹; thus the 7-day-a-week program would be considered excessive even for an elite athlete. This biathlete could substitute the long bike ride for the long run on alternate weeks.

Day	Training Session	Duration (min)	Perceived Exertion CR-10	Load (units)
Monday	Weight lifting	90	4	360
Tuesday	Running (8 km)	45	3	135
Wednesday	Cycling (48 km)	120	4	480
Thursday	Weight lifting	90	4	360
Friday	Cycling (80 km)	200	6	1200
Saturday	Track intervals	75	7	525
Sunday	Long run (29 km)	180	6	1080

A. Daily Mean Load 591
Standard Deviation of Daily Load 396
Monotony (daily load ÷SD) 1.49
Weekly Load (daily load × 7) 4140
Strain (weekly load × monotony) 6169

B. Daily Mean Load 420
Standard Deviation of Daily Load 345
Monotony (daily load ÷SD) 1.21
Weekly Load (daily load × 7) 2940
Strain (weekly load × monotony) 3557

Day	Training Session	Duration (min)	Perceived Exertion CR-10	Load (units)
Monday	Weight lifting	90	4	360
Tuesday	Running (8 km)	45	3	135
Wednesday	Cycling (48 km)	120	4	480
Thursday	Rest day	0	0	0
Friday	Weight lifting	90	4	360
Saturday	Track intervals	75	7	525
Sunday	Long run (29 km)	180	6	1080

immune cell number and function measured in recovery may have little or no effect on health outcomes, such as infections (Rowbottom and Green, 2000). Or the decrease in immune cells in the blood may reflect their movement into tissue where they can provide increased immune surveillance and even immunoenhancement (Edwards et al., 2007). However, there is a consensus that immune cell number and function, as well as other measures of immune function, are suppressed for at least several hours during recovery from prolonged, intense endurance exercise (Walsh et al., 2011).

Exercise Training and Incidence of Upper Respiratory Tract Infection (URTI)

Initial epidemiological studies supported the theory that prolonged, strenuous exercise, such as marathon running, led to a higher incidence of URTI (Nieman, 1997b). On the other hand, moderate exercise training has been associated with a lower self-reported incidence of URTI (Mathews et al., 2002). Based on these findings, a J-shaped model of the relationship between exercise workload and risk of URTI (see **Figure 22.14**) has been proposed (Nieman et al., 1990; Woods et al., 1999). This model suggests that a moderate level of exercise is beneficial but that very high levels of training may be detrimental. However, not all studies have found intense training associated with

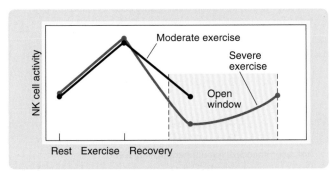

FIGURE 22.13 The "Open Window" Hypothesis.
The open window (shaded rectangular area) is a period after severe exercise when NK cell activity decreases. It is proposed that during this period, microbial agents can establish an infection.
Source: Adapted from Pedersen, B. K. & H. Ullum: NK cell response to physical activity: Possible mechanisms of action. *Medicine and Science in Sports and Exercise*. 26(2):140–146 (1994). Reprinted by permission of Lippincott Williams & Wilkins.

The Role of Nutritional Supplements in Lessening Immune Disruption with Strenuous Training

Walk into any nutritional supplement store (or even your local grocery store or drug store) and you will see numerous supplements claiming to boost immune function. Nutritional supplements to bolster immunity have long been used during periods of physiological stress, such as during surgery or during recovery from trauma. This has led many to speculate that nutritional agents may be useful in attenuating immune changes and inflammation following strenuous exercise, and thus may lower the risk of upper respiratory tract infection. While there are theoretical reasons to believe that different supplements may be useful and some evidence in animal models to suggest the utility of supplementation, the majority of studies conducted with human athletes have been disappointing.

The International Society of Exercise and Immunology recently published a Position Statement on Immune Function and Exercise. In that statement they reviewed many of the proposed nutritional supplements and their rationale for use, and provided a recommendation based on current research literature (see accompanying table).

The results of this systematic analysis suggest that there are few nutritional supplements that are effective in dampening immune disruption with exercise or in reducing risk of upper respiratory tract infection in well-fed healthy athletes. An exception appears to be carbohydrate supplementation. Carbohydrate ingestion before and/or during prolonged exercise attenuates the increase in blood neutrophil and monocyte counts, stress hormones, and anti-inflammatory cytokines, but has little or no effect on decrements in salivary IgA output and T cell and NKC activity. Thus, carbohydrate ingestion during heavy exercise may provide a partial countermeasure to immune dysfunction exercise.

There is also some encouraging research findings regarding quercetin, a dietary polyphenol found in tea, apples, some fruits (e.g., apples, grapes, citrus fruits, raspberries, cranberries), and green leafy vegetables. Most of the research on the effectiveness of this supplement has been done in animal models and more work is required in humans; however, initial results are encouraging. Importantly, quercetin is found in many foods that are recommended as part of a healthy diet.

While the idea of a nutritional supplement to boast immune function is attractive, the available evidence suggests that athletes should eat a sound health diet, ensure they have sufficient carbohydrates immediately before or after exercise, and perhaps recover with a cup of green tea.

Source: Walsh et al. (2011).

Immunonutritional Supplement	Proposed Rationale	Recommendation Based on Current Evidence
Macronutrients		
Carbohydrate	Maintains blood glucose during exercise, lowers stress hormones, and thus counters immune dysfunction	Recommended; up to 60 g·hr^{-1} of heavy exertion helps dampen immune inflammatory responses, but not immune dysfunction
Branched chain amino acids (BCAAs)	BCAAs (valine, isoleucine, and leucine) are the major nitrogen source for glutamine synthesis in muscle	Not recommended; data inconclusive, and rationale based on glutamine is faulty
Vitamins/Minerals		
Vitamin E	Quenches exercise-induced reactive oxygen species (ROS) and augments immunity	Not recommended; may be pro-oxidative with heavy exertion
Vitamin C	Quenches ROS and augments immunity	Not recommended; not consistently different from placebo
Multiple vitamins and minerals	Work together to quench ROS and reduce inflammation	Not recommended; not different from placebo; balanced diet is sufficient
Advanced Supplements		
Glutamine	Important immune cell energy substrate that is lowered with prolonged exercise	Not recommended; body stores exceed exercise-lowering effects
Bovine colostrums	Mix of immune, growth, and hormonal factors improve immune function and the neuroendocrine system, and lower illness risk	Data are inconclusive, mixed research results
Probiotics	Improve intestinal microbial flora, and thereby enhance gut and systemic immune function	Data are inconclusive, mixed research results
N-3 PUFAs (fish oil)	Exerts anti-inflammatory effects postexercise	Not recommended; not different from placebo
β-Glucan	Receptors found on immune cells, and animal data show supplementation improves innate immunity and reduces infection rates	Not recommended; human study with athletes showed no benefits
Herbal supplements (e.g., ginseng, Echinacea)	Contain bioactive molecules that augment immunity and counter infection	Not recommended; humans studies do not show consistent support within an athletic context
Quercetin	In vitro studies show strong anti-inflammatory, antioxidative, and antipathogenic effects. Animal data indicate increase in mitochondrial biogenesis and endurance performance, reduction in illness	Recommended, especially when mixed with other flavonoids and nutrients; human studies show reduction in illness rates during heavy training, mild stimulations of mitochondrial biogenesis, and improved endurance performance in untrained subjects; anti-inflammatory and antioxidative effects when mixed with green tea extract and fish oil

FOCUS ON RESEARCH: *Clinically Relevant*

Effect of Football Training on Upper Respiratory Tract Infection and Salivary IgA

Coaches and athletes are concerned about URTI infections because they impair performance and may limit the ability to train. Given the detrimental effects, many are interested in finding immune markers to predict who is at risk for a URTI. Salivary immunoglobin A (s-IgA) is a potential marker to predict URTI because the oral mucosa is the first line of defense against pathogens that may enter the body through this route.

Researchers investigated s-IgA and incidence of URTI in collegiate football players and normally active controls over 12 months. Data collected at eight specific times representing different training phases included both s-IgA data and self-reported data about symptoms of URTI.

As seen in the graph below, the incidence of URTI increased dramatically following the first 6 weeks of training in both the fall and spring season (times 2 and 6, respectively) and during the fall and spring season (times 3 and 7). Analysis of the s-IgA data revealed that both the concentration of s-IgA and the secretion rate of s-IgA decreased in the football players during the same period. A regression analysis of this data revealed that the rate of s-IgA secretion was the most predictive of URTI.

These results have several important implications for those who work with athletes. Following intensive preseason training and during the in-season training phase, the incidence of URTI may be very high (>50%) among athletes—much higher than among normally active controls. The increased incidence of URTI is associated with suppression of s-IgA. The exact cause for this higher incidence of URTI is not certain but likely includes the stress of intensive training and competition along with more frequent exposure to the infections of other players because football players spend so much time in close contact. One interesting finding was that s-IgA secretion rates below 40 µg·min⁻¹ were predictive of URTI, suggesting that in the future coaches and trainers may be able to measure this variable to predict who is at greatest risk for developing a URTI and who would therefore benefit from reduced training.

Source: Fahlman and Engels (2005).

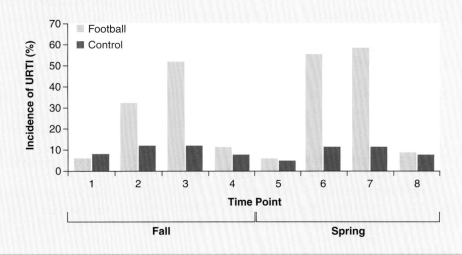

an increased risk of URTI (Gleeson et al., 1996; Hemilä et al., 2003; Pyne et al., 1995). Thus, although the theory that intense training may lead to an increase incidence of URTI has some support, the research findings are not unequivocal. Furthermore, some researchers have questioned whether reported sore throats following intense training periods are due to URTI or rather an inflammation caused by dry mucosal lining in the throat. A recent study investigated both self-reported symptoms and incidence of pathogenic infection in sedentary controls, recreationally competitive athletes, and elite athletes. In this study the distribution of symptoms mimicked the J-shaped curve. However, in only 30% of cases were pathogens identified as causing an URTI (Spence et al., 2005).

On balance, research suggests that moderate exercise enhances immune function and may play an important role in reducing an individual's susceptibility to infection. Exercise is immunomodulatory; whether exercise is immunosuppressive or immunopotentiating likely depends on the overall magnitude of the stress, including

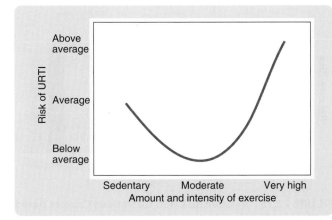

FIGURE 22.14 J-Shaped Model of Relationship between Exercise Intensity and URTI.
Source: Nieman, D. C., L. M. Johanssen, J. W. Lee, & K. Arabatzis: Infectious episodes in runners before and after the Los Angeles Marathon. *Journal of Sports Medicine and Physical Fitness*. 30:316–328 (1990). Reprinted by permission of Lippincott Williams & Wilkins.

not only the physiological stress of exercise but also environmental, psychological, and nutritional stress. The immune response to exercise is mediated largely through the neuroendocrine system. Currently, evidence is insufficient to recommend any given laboratory test of immune function to ascertain whether an individual is at high risk for an infectious episode linked with overtraining or psychological stress. See the Focus on Research box for a look at how investigators are exploring this possibility.

Precautions to Lessen Risk of Upper Respiratory Tract Infection (URTI)

Because competitive endurance athletes often do not have the option of training moderately, the precautions listed below can help lessen their risk of URTI (Brenner et al., 1994; Heath et al., 1992; Nieman, 1994; Walsh et al., 2011):

1. Eat a well-balanced diet. Improper nutrition can compound the negative influence of heavy exertion on the immune system.
2. Minimize other life stresses. Psychological stress may be additive.
3. Avoid overtraining and chronic fatigue. Get plenty of rest, and space vigorous workout and race events as far apart as possible.
4. Consume plenty of carbohydrates before and/or during prolonged exercise.
5. Get a flu shot. Flu shots are especially important for athletes competing in the winter.
6. Avoid excessive muscular soreness. Soreness may activate immune system involvement, and interfere with its ability to ward off viruses.
7. Try to avoid being around sick people.

Guidelines for Postponing Training Due to Upper Respiratory Tract Infection (URTI)

One of the challenges facing exercise enthusiasts, athletes, and occupational workers is knowing when exercise can be safely and effectively performed during an illness. The following guidelines suggest when exercise training is and is not appropriate.

1. Maintain training if the URTI is only minor and a systemic infection is lacking (no fever, aching muscles, extreme fatigue, or swollen glands); or just stop for a couple of days. Consider using decongestants during the day and antihistamines at night.
2. If the URTI causes positive signs of systemic infection (fever, aching muscles, extreme fatigue, swollen glands), stop training for 2–4 weeks. If training is not stopped, viral cardiomyopathy or severe viral infection may result.
3. If symptoms occur above the neck (runny or stuffy nose, scratchy throat), begin sessions with a short or light activity. If symptoms worsen, stop; if symptoms

lessen, continue. If symptoms are below the neck (muscle ache, vomiting, diarrhea, fever), stop training until the symptoms go away.

Exercise, the Immune System, and Cancer

The NK cells and macrophages are important cells in the innate immune system defense against the development and spread of malignancies (Woods and Davis, 1994). Acute dynamic aerobic exercise causes an increase in these cells. Therefore, there is a theoretical link between physical activity and cancer. Furthermore, epidemiological studies have found a negative relationship between physical activity and certain cancers (Blair and Minocha, 1989; Lee, 2003; Sternfeld, 1992;). **Figure 22.15** presents the median relative risk (RR) for developing certain site-specific cancers for the most active individuals versus the least active (Lee, 2003). Higher levels of physical activity are associated with a lower relative risk of colon cancer (in both males and females), breast cancer in women, and prostate cancer in men. Although some evidence suggests that physically active individuals may have less risk for lung cancer, this is a difficult relationship to demonstrate due to the confounding influence of smoking. In almost all large-scale studies demonstrating a reduced risk (RR < 1.0), a dose-response curve suggests that higher levels of physical activity are associated with greater risk reduction.

Although many studies have found an association between physical activity and cancer risk (site specific and overall risk), the shape of the dose-response curve and the specific exercise and intensity associated with the decreased risk is not clearly established (Thune and Furberg, 2001). Furthermore, the mechanisms responsible for the effects of exercise on cancer are unknown. Although scientists have noted that higher levels of physical activity are associated with a better overall life-

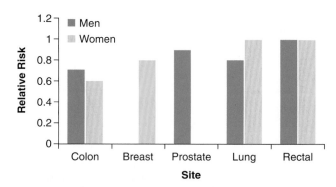

FIGURE 22.15   Relative Risk (RR) for Various Cancers Based on Physical Activity Level.
Values indicate median RR for the most active versus the least active. A RR of 1.0 represents the risk for inactive individuals. A RR of less than 1.0 is associated with a reduced risk.
Source: Based on data in Lee, I. M.: Physical activity and cancer prevention—Data from epidemiological studies. *Medicine & Science in Sports & Exercise.* 35(11):1823–1827 (2003).

style, lower body fat, decreased stool transit time, and enhancement of antioxidant enzyme systems (Woods and Davis, 1994), these healthy outcomes are unlikely the reason for the inverse relationship between physical activity and colon cancer, because the relationship between colon cancer and physical activity persists even after adjusting for these confounding variables (Lee, 2003).

Exercise, the Immune System, and AIDS

Acquired immune deficiency syndrome (AIDS) is a disease caused by the human immunodeficiency virus (HIV) and characterized by severe CD4 cell depletion. This virus infects the CD4-bearing T cells (helper T cells), which orchestrate much of the immune response of the body. As the infection progresses, there is greater depletion of the CD4 cells, leading ultimately to immunodysregulation (Brenner et al., 1994). HIV infection is considered a chronic disease involving three stages (Phair, 1990):

1. *Healthy carrier*: During this stage the virus infects relatively few CD4-bearing cells and is not clinically detectable except by blood testing. An individual may remain in this stage up to 10 years. These individuals are viral carriers and potentially infectious despite the absence of outward signs of infection.
2. *Symptomatic infections*: Mild symptoms of HIV infection such as fatigue, intermittent fever, and weight loss become evident during this phase. The CD4 count is further diminished.
3. *AIDS*: Severe CD4 cell depletion occurs along with major complications resulting from opportunistic infection or malignancy. At this stage of the disease, the individual's entire health is compromised.

In the early stage of the disease, when individuals are asymptomatic, moderate aerobic exercise training appears to be a useful strategy; some evidence suggests that exercise training may delay the progression of the disease (Brenner et al., 1994). These data may reflect the immune benefits of exercise training (increased number of CD4 cells) and/or psychological benefits of exercise training (Brenner et al., 1994; Mackinnon, 1992). Furthermore, evidence suggests that exercise may be a safe activity throughout the course of the disease.

The use of highly active antiretroviral therapy (HAART) has dramatically changed the treatment of HIV and AIDS, significantly lessoning the mortality and opportunistic infections. As a result of this new treatment, HIV infection is now treated as a chronic illness, though it remains a life-threatening disease (Ciccolo et al., 2004; O'Brien et al., 2004). The downside is that HAART treatment results in serious adverse effects, including, headache, fatigue, nausea, vomiting, and altered metabolic processes. Exercise is a possible management strategy for these problems, but it is often difficult to maintain an exercise

program in face of these challenges. Although a systematic review has suggested that aerobic and resistance training confers benefit to individuals with HIV and AIDS, the need for additional research is recognized (O'Brien et al., 2004). Available studies were performed before the development of HAART treatment, involved small numbers of patients, and had high dropout rates. Currently, it appears that exercise is safe and may confer health benefits, but much more research is required to clarify the benefits of exercise in individuals with HIV or AIDS.

SUMMARY

1. The immune system can be functionally divided into the innate and the adaptive branches. The innate branch protects against foreign substances or cells without having to recognize them. In the adaptive branch of the immune system, immune cells recognize a foreign material and react specifically and selectively to destroy it.
2. Moderate aerobic exercise leads to an increase in the number and activity of neutrophils; an increase in the number, percentage, and activity of NK cells; an increase in phagocytic activity and secretion of cytokines from macrophages; an increase in the number of acute phase proteins; and an increase in the number of B and T cells.
3. Exhaustive aerobic exercise is associated with a reduction in NK cell number and activity and a decrease in lymphocytes and neutrophils.
4. The depressed levels of NK cells following strenuous exercise is a likely explanation of the vulnerability to acute infection associated with high-level competition and chronic overtraining.
5. The neuroendocrine system and the immune system overlap considerably. Hormonal control of the immune response is mediated primarily by the action of epinephrine and cortisol.
6. A sustained mismatch between exercise training stress and inadequate recovery can lead to training maladaptation. Maladaptation occurs over a continuum. The least serious is functional overreaching (FOR). FOR refers to short-term performance decrement (days to weeks) and is often done intentionally during a shock microcycle of periodization. Non-functional overreaching (NFOR) is more severe with a performance decrement that lasts from weeks to months and usually is accompanied by severe signs and symptoms. The overtraining syndrome (OTS) is the most serious stage of the continuum with the greatest disruption and a performance recovery that takes months to years.
7. Although no single marker has been identified to predict NFOR or OTS, it is important to monitor training load, performance, mood state and ensure adequate recovery and nutrition in an attempt to

prevent maladaptation. The primary treatment is rest.

8. Severe exercise training is associated with immuno-suppression and an increased risk of URTI.

9. Physical activity is associated with lower prevalence and mortality rates for cancers involving the colon, breast, prostate, and lung.

10. Exercise training appears to be beneficial to individuals infected with HIV.

REVIEW QUESTIONS

1. Graphically present the two branches of the immune system, emphasizing how they work together.

2. Identify the primary cells of the innate and adaptive branches of the immune system, and indicate the mechanisms by which each leads to antigen destruction.

3. Describe the sequence of events in inflammation.

4. Describe the immune response to moderate aerobic exercise and to a severe exercise bout.

5. Differentiate between the training adaptations of the immune system to a moderate training program and to overtraining.

6. Describe the continuum for training maladaptation. Discuss the current hypotheses that explain overtraining. What factors should be monitored to attempt to prevent non-functional overreaching and the overtraining syndrome?

7. Describe the relationship between exercise and the incidence of upper respiratory tract infection (URTI).

8. Describe the relationship between physical activity levels and the risk of various cancers.

9. Describe the role of physical activity for an individual infected with HIV.

For further review and additional study tools, visit the website at http://thePoint.lww.com/Plowman4e ✳ ▶

REFERENCES

Achten, J. & A. E. Jeukendrup: Heart rate monitoring: Applications and limitations. *Sports Medicine*. 33:517–538 (2003).

American College of Sports Medicine, American Dietetic Association, Dietitians of Canada: Nutrition and athletic performance joint position statement. *Medicine & Science in Sports & Exercise*. 32:2130–2145 (2000).

Armstrong, L. E. & J. L. vanHeest: The unknown mechanism of the overtraining syndrome: Clues from depression and psychoneuroimmunology. *Sports Medicine*. 32:185–209 (2002).

Blair, S. N. & H. C. Minocha: Physical fitness and all-cause mortality: A prospective study of healthy men and women. *The Journal of the American Medical Association*. 262:2395–2401 (1989).

Bompa, T. O.: Primer on periodization, US Olympic Coach E-Magazine. http://coaching.usolympicteam.com/coaching/kpub.nsf/v/0504b (2004).

Borg, G.: *Borg's Perceived Exertion and Pain Scales*. Champaign, IL: Human Kinetics (1998).

Bosquet, L., S. Merkari, D. Arvisais, & A. E. Aubert: Is heart rate a convenient tool to monitor over-reaching? A systematic review of the literature. *British Journal of Sports Medicine*. 42:709–714 (2008).

Brenner, I. K. M., P. N. Shek, & R. J. Shephard: Infection in athletes. *Sports Medicine*. 17(2):86–107 (1994).

Brolinson, P. G. & D. Elliott: Exercise and the immune system. *Clinical Sports Medicine*. 26:311–319 (2007).

Budgett, R.: Fatigue and underperformance in athletes: The overtraining syndrome. *British Journal of Sports Medicine*. 32:107–110 (1998).

Calder, A.: Recovery strategies for sports performance. US Olympic Coach E-Magazine. http://coaching.usolympicteam.com/coaching/kpub.nsf/v/3Sept03 (2004).

Chrousos, G. P. & P. W. Gold: The concepts of stress and stress system disorders: Overview of physical and behavioral homeostasis. *Journal of the American Medical Association*. 267:1244–1252 (1992).

Ciccolo, J. T., E. M. Jowers, & J. B. Bartholomew: The benefits of exercise training for quality of life in HIV/AIDS in the post-HAART era. *Sports Medicine*. 34(8):487–499 (2004).

Coutts, A. J., P. Reaburn, T. J. Piva, & G. J. Rowsell: Monitoring for overreaching in rugby league players. *European Journal of Applied Physiology*. 99(3):313–324 (2007).

Coyle, E. F.: Highs and lows of carbohydrate diets. Gatorade Sports Science Institute. *Sports Science Exchange* 17:1–6 (2004).

Duclos, M.: A critical assessment of hormonal methods used in monitoring training status in athletes. *International SportMed Journal*. 9(2):56–66 (2008).

Edwards, K. M., V. E. Burns, D. Carroll, M. Drayson, & C. Ring: The acute stress-induced immunoenhancement hypothesis. *Exercise and Sport Sciences Reviews*. 35(3):150–155 (2007).

Fahlman, M. M. & H.-J. Engles: Mucosal IgA and URTI in American college football players: A year longitudinal study. *Medicine & Science in Sports & Exercise*. 37(3):374–380 (2005).

Febraio, M. A. & B. K. Pedersen: Muscle-derived interleukin-6: Mechanisms for activation and possible biological roles. *The Federation of American Societies for Experimental Biology*. 16:1335–1347 (2002).

Fleshner, M.: Physical activity and stress resistance: Sympathetic nervous system adaptations prevent stress-induced immunosuppression. *Exercise and Sport Sciences Reviews*. 33(3):120–126 (2005).

Flynn, M. G.: Future research needs and directions. In Kreider, R. B., A. C. Fry, & M. L. O'Toole (eds.): *Overtraining in Sport*. Champaign, IL: Human Kinetics, 373–383 (1998).

Foster, C.: Monitoring training in athletes with reference to overtraining syndrome. *Medicine & Science in Sports & Exercise*. 30:1164–1168 (1998).

Fragala, M. S., W. J. Kramer, C. R. Denegar, C. M. Maresh, A. M. Mastro, & J. S. Volek: Neuroendocrine-immune interactions and response to exercise. *Sports Medicine*. 41(8):621–639 (2011).

Fry, A. C. & W. J. Kraemer: Resistance exercise overtraining and overreaching: Neuroendocrine responses. *Sports Medicine*. 23:106–129 (1997).

Fry, R. W., A. R. Morton, & D. Keast: Periodization and the prevention of overtraining. *Canadian Journal of Sports Sciences.* 17:241–248 (1992).

Fry, R. W., A. R. Morton, & D. Keast: Overtraining in athletes: An update. *Sports Medicine.* 12:32–65 (1991).

Gabriel, H. H. W., A. Urhausen, G. Valet, U. Heidelbach, & W. Kindermann: Overtraining and immune system: A prospective longitudinal study in endurance athletes. *Medicine & Science in Sports & Exercise.* 30:1151–1157 (1998).

Gastmann, U. A. L. & M. J. Lehmann: Overtraining and the BCAA hypothesis. *Medicine & Science in Sports & Exercise.* 30:1173–1178 (1998).

Gleeson, M.: Immune function in sport and exercise. *Journal of Applied Physiology.* 103:693–699 (2007).

Gleeson, M., N. Bishop, M. Oliverira, & P. Tauler: Influence of training load on upper respiratory tract infection incidence and antigen-stimulated cytokine production. *Scandinavian Journal of Medicine and Science in Sports.* (2011). DOI: 10.1111/j.1600–0838.2011.01422.x

Gokhale, R., S. Chandrashekara, & K. C. Vasanthakumar: Cytokine response to strenuous exercise in athletes and non-athletes—An adaptive response. *Cytokine.* 40:123–127 (2007).

Gotovtseva, E. P., I. D. Surkina, & P. N. Uchakin: Potential interventions to prevent immunosuppression during training. In Kreider, R. B., A. C. Fry, & M. L. O'Toole (eds.): *Overtraining in Sport.* Champaign, IL: Human Kinetics, 243–272 (1998).

Halson, S. L. & A. E. Jeukendrup: Does overtraining exist? An analysis of overreaching and overtraining research. *Sports Medicine.* 34:967–981 (2004).

Hartmann, U. & J. Mester: Training and overtraining markers in selected sports events. *Medicine & Science in Sports & Exercise.* 32:209–215 (2000).

Hawley, C. J. & R. B. Schoene: Overtraining syndrome: A guide to diagnosis, treatment, and prevention. *The Physician and Sports Medicine.* 31:25–31 (2003).

Heath, G. W., C. A. Macera, & D. C. Nieman: Exercise and upper respiratory tract infections: Is there a relationship? *Sports Medicine.* 14(6):353–365 (1992).

Hemilä, H., J. Virtamo, D. Albanes, & J. Kaprio: Physical activity and the common cold in men administered vitamin and β-Carotene. *Medicine & Science in Sports & Exercise.* 35(11):1815–1820 (2003).

Hooper, S. L. & L. T. Mackinnon: Monitoring overtraining in athletes: Recommendations. *Sports Medicine.* 20:321–327 (1995).

Keizer, H. A.: Neuroendocrine aspects of overtraining. In Kreider, R. B., A. C. Fry, & M. L. O'Toole (eds.): *Overtraining in Sport.* Champaign, IL: Human Kinetics, 145–167 (1998).

Kenttä, G. & P. Hassmén: Overtraining and recovery: A conceptual model. *Sports Medicine.* 26:1–16 (1998).

Kohut, M. L., J. M. Davis, D. A. Jackson, et al.: Exercise effects on IFN-b expression and viral replication in lung macrophages following HSV-1 infection. *American Journal of Physiology.* 275:L1089–L1094 (1998).

Kreider, R. B., A. C. Fry, & M. L. O'Toole: Overtraining in sport: Terms, definitions, and prevalence. In Kreider, R. B., A. C. Fry, & M. L. O'Toole (eds.): *Overtraining in Sport.* Champaign, IL: Human Kinetics, vii–ix (1998).

Kuipers, H.: Training and overtraining: An introduction. *Medicine & Science in Sports & Exercise.* 30:1137–1139 (1998).

Lac, G. & F. Maso: Biological markers for the follow-up of athletes throughout the training season. *Pathologie-biologie (Paris).* 52:43–49 (2004).

Lee, I. M.: Physical activity and cancer prevention—dData from epidemiological studies. *Medicine & Science in Sports & Exercise.* 35(11):1823–1827 (2003).

Lehmann, M., C. Foster, H. H. Dickhuth, & U. Gastmann: Autonomic imbalance hypothesis and overtraining syndrome. *Medicine & Science in Sports & Exercise.* 30:1140–1145 (1998a).

Lehmann, M., C. Foster, & J. Keul: Overtraining in endurance athletes: A brief review. *Medicine and Science in Sports and Exercise.* 25:854–862 (1993).

Lehmann, M., C. Foster, N. Netzer, W. Lormes, J. M. Steinacker, Y. Liu, A. Opitz-Gress, & U. Gastmann: Physiological responses to short- and long-term overtraining in endurance athletes. In Kreider, R. B., A. C. Fry, & M. L. O'Toole (eds.): *Overtraining in Sport.* Champaign, IL: Human Kinetics, 19–46 (1998b).

Mackinnon, L. T.: *Advances in Exercise Immunology.* Champaign, IL: Human Kinetics (1999).

Mackinnon, L. T.: Chronic exercise training effects on immune function. *Medicine & Science in Sports & Exercise.* 32(7):S369–S376 (2000).

Mackinnon, L. T.: *Exercise and Immunology.* Champaign, IL: Human Kinetics (1992).

Mackinnon, L. T., T. W. Chick, A. Van As, & T. B. Tomasi: The effect of exercise on secretory and natural immunity. *Advances in Experimental Medicine and Biology.* 216:869–876 (1987).

Main, L. C., B. Dawson, K. Heel, J. R. Grove, G. J. Landers, & C. Goodman: Relationship between inflammatory cytokines and self-report measures of training overload. *Research in Sports Medicine.* 18:127–139 (2010).

Main, L. C., & J. R. Grove: A multi-component assessment model for monitoring training distress among athletes. *European Journal of Sport Science.* 9(4):195–202 (2009).

Marieb, E. N. & K. Hoehn: *Anatomy and Physiology* (4th edition). Redwood City, CA: Benjamin Cummings (2010).

Mastro A. M., & R. H. Bonneau: Exercise and immunity. In W. J. Kraemer, & A. D. Rogol (eds.), *The Endocrine System in Sports and Exercise (IOC Encyclopedia).* Oxford, UK: Blackwell Publishing, 368–390 (2005).

Matthews, C. E., I. S. Ockene, P. S. Freedson, M. C. Rosal, P. A. Merriam, & J. R. Herbert: Moderate to vigorous physical activity and risk of upper-respiratory tract infection. *Medicine & Science in Sports & Exercise.* 34(8):1242–1248 (2002).

McNair, D. M., M. Lorr, & L. F. Droppleman: *EDITS Manual for the Profile of Mood States.* San Diego, CA: Educational and Industrial Testing Service, 1–29 (1971).

Meeusen, R., M. Duclos, M. Gleeson, G. Rietjens, J. Steinacker, & A. Urhausen: Prevention, diagnosis and treatment of the overtraining syndrome. *European Journal of Sport Science.* 6(1):1–14 (2006).

Meeusen, R., E. Nederhof, L. Buyse, G. DeShutter, & M. F. Piacetini: Diagnosing overtraining in athletes using the two-bout exercise protocol. *British Journal of Sports Medicine.* 44:642–648 (2010).

Meeusen, R., M. F. Piacentini, B. Busscharert, L. Buyse, G. DeSchutter, & J. Stray-Gundersen: Hormonal responses in athletes: The use of a two bout exercise protocol to detect subtle differences in (over)training status. *European Journal of Applied Physiology.* 91:140–146 (2004).

Meyers, A. W. & J. P. Whelan: A systematic model for understanding psychosocial influences in overtraining. In Kreider, R. B., A. C. Fry, & M. L. O'Toole (eds.): *Overtraining in Sport.* Champaign, IL: Human Kinetics, 335–369 (1998).

Miles, M. P.: Neuroendocrine modulation of the immune system with exercise and muscle damage. In Kramer, W. J., & A. D. Rogol (eds.): *The Endocrine System in Sports and Exercise.* Malden, MA: Blackwell Publishing (2005).

Moldoveanu, A. I., R. J. Shephard, & P. N. Shek: The cytokine response to physical activity and training. *Sports Medicine.* 31(2):115–144 (2001).

Mujika, I., & S. Padilla: Detraining: Loss of training-induced physiological and performance adaptations. Part I: Short term insufficient training stimulus. *Sports Medicine.* 30(2): 79–87 (2000).

Nash, M. S.: Exercise and immunology. *Medicine and Science in Sports and Exercise.* 26(2):125–127 (1994).

Nederhof, E., J. Zwerver, M. Brink, R. Meeusen, & K. Lemmink: Different diagnostic tools in nonfunctional overreaching. *International Journal of Sports Medicine.* 29:590–597 (2008).

Nieman, D. C.: Is infection risk linked to exercise workload? *Medicine & Science in Sports & Exercise.* 32:S406–S411 (2000).

Nieman, D. C.: Exercise, upper respiratory tract and the immune system. *Medicine and Science in Sports and Exercise.* 26(2):128–139 (1994).

Nieman, D. C.: Immune response to heavy exertion. *Journal of Applied Physiology.* 82(5):1385–1394 (1997a).

Nieman, D. C.: Risk of upper respiratory tract infection in athletes: An epidemiologic and immunologic perspective. *Journal of Athletic Training.* 32(4):344–349 (1997b).

Nieman, D. C., A. R. Miller, D. A. Henson, B. J. Warren, G. Gusewitch, B. J. Johnson, J. M. Davis, D. E. Butterworth, & S. L. Nehlsen-Cannarella: Effects of high- vs moderate-intensity exercise on natural killer activity. *Medicine and Science in Sports and Exercise.* 25(10):1126–1134 (1993).

Nieman, D. C., J. C. Ahle, D. A. Henson, B. J. Warren, J. Suttles, J. M. Davis, K. S. Buckley, S. Simandle, D. E. Butterworth, O. R. Fagoaga, & S. L. Nehlsen-Cannarella: Indomethacin does not alter natural killer cell response to 2.5 h of running. *Journal of Applied Physiology.* 79:748–755 (1995a).

Nieman, D. C., K. S. Buckley, D. A. Henson, B. J. Warren, J. Suttles, J. C. Ahle, S. Simandle, O. R. Fagoaga, & S. L. Nehlsen-Cannarella: Immune function in marathon runners versus sedentary controls. *Medicine and Science in Sports and Exercise.* 27:5986–5992 (1995b).

Nieman, D. C., L. M. Johanssen, J. W. Lee, & K. Arabatzis: Infectious episodes in runners before and after the Los Angeles Marathon. *Journal of Sports Medicine and Physical Fitness.* 30:316–328 (1990).

Novas, A. M. P., D. G. Rowbottom, & D. G. Jenkins: Tennis, Incidence of URTI and Salivary IgA. *International Journal of Sports Medicine.* 24:223–229 (2003).

O'Brien, K., S. Nixon, A. M. Tynan, & R. H. Glazier: Effectiveness of aerobic exercise in adults living with HIV/AIDS: Systematic review. *Medicine & Science in Sports & Exercise.* 36(10):1659–1666 (2004).

Pedersen, B. K. & L. Hoffman-Goetz: Exercise and the immune system: Regulation, integration, and adaption. *Physiological Reviews.* 80(3):1055–1081 (2000).

Papacosta, E., & G. P. Nassis: Saliva as a tool for monitoring steroid, peptide and immune markers in sport and exercise science. *Journal of Science and Medicine in Sport.* 14:424–434 (2011).

Pedersen, B. K., & H. Ullum: NK cell response to physical activity: Possible mechanisms of action. *Medicine and Science in Sports and Exercise.* 26(2):140–146 (1994).

Pedersen, B. K., T. C. A. Åkerström, A. R. Nielsen, & C. P. Fischer: Role of myokines in exercise and metabolism. *Journal of Applied Physiology.* 103:1093–1098 (2007).

Peters, E. M. & E. D. Bateman: Ultramarathon running and URTI: An epidemiological survey. *South Africa Medical Journal.* 64:582–584 (1983).

Petersen, A. M. W. & B. K. Pedersen: The anti-inflammatory effect of exercise. *Journal of Applied Physiology.* 98:1154–1162 (2005).

Petibois, C., G. Cazorla, J. R. Poortmans, & G. Déléris: Biochemical aspects of overtraining in endurance sports: A review. *Sports Medicine.* 32:867–878 (2002).

Petibois, C., G. Cazorla, J. R. Poortmans, & G. Déléris: Biochemical aspects of overtraining in endurance sports: The metabolism alteration process syndrome. *Sports Medicine.* 33:83–94 (2003).

Phair, J. D.: The natural history of HIV infection. In Sande, M. A., & P. A. Volberding (eds.): *The Medical Management of AIDS.* Philadelphia, PA: Saunders (1990).

Pyne, D. B., M. S. Baker, P. A. Fricker, W. A. McDonald, R. D. Telford, & M. J. Wwidemann: The effects of an intensive 12-wk training program by elite swimmers on neutrophil oxidative activity. *Medicine and Science in Sports and Exercise.* 27:536–542 (1995).

Rhea, M. R. & B. L. Alderman: A meta-analysis of periodized versus non-periodized strength and power training programs. *Research Quarterly for Exercise and Sport.* 75:413–422 (2004).

Rhind, S. G., G. A. Gannon, P. N. Shek, I. K. M. Brenner, Y. Severs, J. Zamecnik, A. Buguet, V. M. Natale, R. J. Shephard, & M. W. Radomski: Contribution of exertional hyperthermia to sympathoadrenal-mediated lymphocyte subset redistribution. *Journal of Applied Physiology.* 87(3):1178–1185 (1999).

Robson, P. J.: Elucidating the unexplained underperformance syndrome in endurance athletes: The interleukin-6 hypothesis. *Sports Medicine.* 33:771–781 (2003).

Rohlfs, I. C. P. D., T. M. Rotta, C. D. Luft, A. Andrade, R. J. Krebs, & T. deCarvalho: Brunel Mood Scale (BRUMS): An instrument for early detection of overtraining syndrome. *Revista Brasileira de Medicina do Esporte.* 14(3):176–181 (2008).

Roitt, I., J. Brostoff, & D. Male: *Immunology* (4th edition). Baltimore, MD: Mosby (1998).

Rowbottom, D. G., D. Keast, & A. R. Morton: Monitoring and preventing of overreaching and overtraining in endurance athletes. In Kreider, R. B., A. C. Fry, & M. L. O'Toole (eds.): *Overtraining in Sport.* Champaign, IL: Human Kinetics, 47–66 (1998).

Rowbottom, D. G., D. Keast, & A. R. Morton: The emerging role of glutamine as an indicator of exercise stress and overtraining. *Sports Medicine.* 21:80–97 (1996).

Rowbottom, D. G. & K. J. Green: Acute exercise effects on the immune system. *Medicine & Science in Sports & Exercise.* 32(7):S396–S405 (2000).

Saris, W.H.: The concept of energy homeostasis for optimal health during training. *Canadian Journal of Applied Physiology.* 26(Suppl):S167–S175 (2001).

Schmikli, S. L., M. S. Brink, W. R. deVries, & F. J. G. Backx: Can we detect non-functional overreaching in young elite soccer players and middle-long distance runners using field performance tests? *British Journal of Sports Medicine.* 45:631–636 (2011).

Selye, H.: *The Stress of Life.* New York, NY: McGraw-Hill (1956).

Shephard, R. J., S. Rhind, & P. N. Shek: The impact of exercise on the immune system: NK cells, interleukins 1 and 2, and related responses. In Holloszy, J. O., (ed.): *Exercise and Sport Sciences Reviews.* Baltimore, MD: Williams & Wilkins (1995).

Smith, D. J.: A framework for understanding the training process leading to elite performance. *Sports Medicine.* 33:1103–1126 (2003a).

Smith, J. A.: Guidelines, standards, and perspectives in exercise immunology. *Medicine and Science in Sports and Exercise.* 27(4):497–506 (1995).

Smith, L. L.: Cytokine hypothesis of overtraining: A physiological adaptation to excessive stress. *Medicine & Science in Sports & Exercise.* 32(2):317–331 (2000).

Smith, L. L.: Overtraining, excessive exercise, and altered immunity: Is this a T helper-1 versus T helper-2 lymphocyte response? *Sports Medicine.* 33:347–364 (2003b).

Snyder, A.C.: Overtraining and glycogen depletion hypothesis. *Medicine & Science in Sports & Exercise.* 30:1146–1150 (1998).

Spence, L., M. D. Nissen, T. P. Sloots, J. G. McCormack, A. S. Locke, D. B. Pyne, P. A. Fricker, & W. J. Brown. Upper respiratory illness aetiology and symptomatology in elite and recreationally-competitive athletes. *Brian and Behavioral Immunology.* 19:469–470 (2005).

Steensberg, A., G. van Hall, T. Osada, M. Sacchetti, B. Saltin, & B. K. Pedersen: Production of interleukin-6 in contracting human skeletal muscles can account for the exercise-induced increase in plasma interleukin-6. *Journal of Physiology.* 529(1):237–242 (2000).

Steinacker, J. M. & W. Lormes: New aspects of the hormone and cytokine response to training. *European Journal of Applied Physiology.* 91:382–391 (2004).

Steinacker, J. M., W. Lormes, M. Lehman, & D. Altenburg: Training of rowers before world championships. *Medicine & Science in Sports & Exercise.* 30:1158–1163 (1998).

Sternfeld, B.: Cancer and the protective effect of physical activity: the epidemiological evidence. *Medicine and Science in Sports and Exercise.* 24(11):1195–1209 (1992).

Steinacker, J. M., W. Lormes, S. Reissnecker, & Y. Liu: New aspects of the hormone and cytokine response to training. *European Journal of Applied Physiology.* 91:382–391 (2004).

Terry, P. C., A. M. Lane, & G. L. Fogarty: Construct validity of the profile of mood states—Adolescents for use with adults. *Psychology of Sport and Exercise.* 4(2):125–139 (2003).

Thomas, C. L. (ed): *Taber's Cyclodedic Medical Dictionary* (16th edition). Philadelphia, PA: FA Davis (1985).

Thune, I. & A. S. Furberg: Physical activity and cancer risk: Dose-response and cancer, all sites and site-specific. *Medicine & Science in Sports & Exercise.* 33(6):S530–S550 (2001).

Tomasi, T. B., F. B. Trudeau, D. Czerwinski, & S. Erredge: Immune parameters in athletes before and after strenuous exercise. *Journal of Clinical Immunology.* 2:173–178 (1982).

Urhausen, A. & W. Kindermann: Diagnosis of overtraining: What tools do we have? *Sports Medicine.* 32(2):95–102 (2002).

Urhausen, A. & W. Kindermann: The endocrine system in overtraining. In Warren, M. P. & N. W. Constantini (eds.): *Sports Endocrinology.* Totowa, NJ: Humana Press, 347–370 (2000).

Venkatraman, J. T. & D. R. Pendergast: Effect of dietary intake on immune function in athletes. *Sports Medicine.* 32:323–337 (2002).

Walsh, N. P., M. Gleeson, R. J. Shephard, M. Gleeson, J. A. Woods, N. C. Bishop, M. Fleshner, C. Green, B. K. Pedersen, L. Hoffman-Goetz, C. J. Rogers, H. Northoff, A. Abbasi, & P. Simon: Position statement part one: Immune function and exercise. *Exercise Immunology Review.* 17:6–63 (2011).

Walsh, N. P., M. Gleeson, D. B. Pyne, D. C. Nieman, F. S. Dhabhar, R. J. Shephard, S. J. Oliver, S. Bermon, & A. Kajeniene: Position statement part II: Maintaining immune health. *Exercise Immunology Review.* 17:64–103 (2011).

Walsh, N. P. & M. Whitham: Exercising in environmental extremes: A greater threat to immune function? *Sports Medicine.* 36(11):941–976 (2006).

Witlert, G.: The effects of exercise on the hypothalamo-pituitary-adrenal axis. In Warren, M. P. & N. W. Constantini (eds.): *Sports Endocrinology.* Totowa, NJ: Humana Press, 43–56 (2000).

Woods, J. A., M. A. Ceddia, C. Kozak, & B. Wolters: Effect of exercise on the macrophage MHC II response to inflammation. *International Journal of Sports Medicine.* 18:483–488 (1997).

Woods, J. A., & J. M. Davis: Exercise, monocyte/macrophage function, and cancer. *Medicine and Science in Sports and Exercise.* 26(2):147–157 (1994).

Woods, J. A., J. M. Davis, E. P. Mayer, A. Ghaffar, & R. R. Pate: Exercise increases inflammatory macrophage anti-tumor cytotoxicity. *Journal of Applied Physiology.* 75:879–886 (1993).

Woods, J. A., J. M. Davis, J. A. Smith, & D. C. Nieman: Exercise and cellular innate immune function. *Medicine & Science in Sports & Exercise.* 31(1):57–66 (1999).

Appendix A

Units of Measure, the Metric System, and Conversions between the English and Metric Systems of Measurement

TABLE A.1 SI Units (Système International) (Metric)		
Physical Quantity	**Unit**	**Symbol**
Mass	kilogram	kg
Distance	meter	m
Volume (liquid or gas)	liter	L
Time	second	sec
Force	newton	N
Work	joule	J
Power	watt	W
Angle	radian	rad
Linear velocity	meters per second	$m \cdot sec^{-1}$
Angular velocity	radians per second	$rad \cdot sec^{-1}$
Temperature	degrees	°
Velocity	meters per second	$m \cdot sec^{-1}$
Torque	newton-meter	N-m
Acceleration	meters per second	$m \cdot sec^{-1}$
Amount of substance	mole	mol

TABLE A.2 SI Prefixes (Système International) (Metric)			
Prefix*	**Meaning**	**Scientific Notation**	**Symbol**
Makes Smaller			
deci-	one tenth of (0.1)	10^{-1}	d
centi-	one hundredth of (0.01)	10^{-2}	c
milli-	one thousandth of (0.001)	10^{-3}	m
micro-	one millionth of (0.000001)	10^{-6}	μ
Makes Larger			
kilo-	a thousand times (1000)	10^{3}	k

*Most commonly used in this text.

TABLE A.3 Conversions between the English and Metric Systems of Measurement

Measurement	Unit and Abbreviation	Metric Equivalent	English-to-Metric Conversion Factor	Metric-to-English Conversion Factor
Length	1 kilometer (km)	= 1000 meters	1 mile = 1.61 km	1 km = 0.62 mile
	1 meter (m)	= 100 centimeters	1 yard = 0.914 m	1 m = 1.09 yards
		= 1000 millimeters	1 foot = 0.305 m	1 m = 3.28 feet
	1 centimeter (cm)	= 0.01 meter	1 foot = 30.5 cm	1 m = 39.37 inches
	1 millimeter (mm)	= 0.001 meter	1 inch = 2.54 cm	1 cm = 0.394 inch
	1 micrometer (μm)	= 0.000001 meter		
Mass	1 kilogram (kg)	= 1000 grams	1 pound = 0.454 kg	1 kg = 2.205 pounds
	1 gram (g)	= 1000 milligrams	1 ounce = 28.35 g	1 g = 0.035 ounce
	1 milligram (mg)	= 0.001 gram		
Volume (liquids and gases)	1 liter (L)	= 1000 milliliters	1 quart = 0.946 L	1 L = 0.264 gallon
			1 quart = 946 mL	1 L = 1.057 quarts
			1 gallon = 3.785 L	
	1 milliliter (mL)	=0.001 liter		1 mL = 0.034 fluid ounce
		= 1 cubic centimeter	1 pint = 473 mL	
			1 fluid ounce = 29.57 mL	
	1 microliter (μL)	= 0.000001 liter		
Area	1 square meter (m^2)	= 10,000 square centimeters	1 square yard = 0.836 m^2	1 m^2 = 1.196 square yards
	1 square centimeter (cm^2)	= 100 square millimeters	1 square inch = 6.452 cm^2	1 cm^2 = 0.155 square inch
Temperature	Degrees Celsius (°C)		°C = 5/9 (°F − 32)	°F = (9/5°C) + 32
Force	1 Newton (N)	= 0.1019 kilopond	1 ft-lb·sec^{-1} = 0.138 N	
Linear velocity	1 (m·sec^{-1})		1 mi·hr^{-1} = 26 m·min^{-1}	
Angular velocity	1 radian per second (rad·s^{-1})			1 $radian^{-1}$ = 57.3°·s^{-1}
Work and energy	1 Joule (J)	= 1 N·m		1 J = 0.784 ft·lb
	1 kcal	= 426.85 kgm		1 J = 0.239 cal
		= 4.18 KJ		
	1 kgm	= 1 kpm		
		= 0.00234 kcal		
Power	1 watt (W)	1 W = 1 joule per sec (J·sec^{-1})	1 hp = 745.7 W	1 W = 0.0013 hp
		1 W = 6.12 kgm·min^{-1}		
Pressure	1 Newton per square meter (N·m^2)		1 mmHg = 133.32 N·m^2	760 mmHg = 29.02 inches
			1 atmosphere = 760 mmHg	

Appendix B

Metabolic Calculations

This appendix describes three methods used to calculate oxygen consumption ($\dot{V}O_2$cons). The first series of equations involves direct calculations using data obtained from open-circuit spirometry. This technique also allows for the calculation of carbon dioxide produced ($\dot{V}CO_2$prod), which the other two, because they are indirect techniques, do not. The second series of equations calculates submaximal oxygen consumption values for selected activities (walking, running, cycle ergometer riding, and stair stepping) using known rates of work. The third set of calculations estimates maximal oxygen consumption ($\dot{V}O_2$max) from selected field tests (the PACER, or 20-m shuttle test, and the Rockport Fitness Walking Test [RFWT]).

THE CALCULATION OF OXYGEN CONSUMED AND CARBON DIOXIDE PRODUCED FROM DATA OBTAINED BY OPEN-CIRCUIT SPIROMETRY

Basic Formulas

Theoretically, the amount of oxygen consumed is simply equal to the amount of oxygen in the inspired air minus the amount of oxygen in the expired air. All values are expressed in $mL \cdot min^{-1}$ or $L \cdot min^{-1}$.

B.1 oxygen consumption ($L \cdot min^{-1}$) = amount of oxygen inspired ($L \cdot min^{-1}$) − amount of oxygen expired ($L \cdot min^{-1}$)
$$\dot{V}O_2\text{cons} = \dot{V}_I O_2 - \dot{V}_E O_2$$

In practice, there is no way to obtain $\dot{V}_I O_2$ or $\dot{V}_E O_2$ directly, so a working formula is used. The working formula is based on the fact that the amount of a gas depends on the fraction (F) of the gas and the volume of the air containing that gas.

B.2 oxygen consumption ($L \cdot min^{-1}$) = [fraction of oxygen in inspired air × volume of inspired air ($L \cdot min^{-1}$)] − [fraction of oxygen in expired air × volume of expired air ($L \cdot min^{-1}$)]
$$\dot{V}O_2\text{cons} = (F_I O_2 \times \dot{V}_I) - (F_E O_2 \times \dot{V}_E)$$

Although the term *fraction* and the symbol F are always used in this equation, these values really represent the percentages of oxygen in inspired or expired air, and they are expressed mathematically as decimals. Thus, $F_I O_2$ is a constant 20.93%, or 0.2093. The inspired ventilation values either can be directly measured by a spirometer or pneumoscan, as described in Chapters 4 and 9, or can be calculated.

The $F_E O_2$ is measured by an oxygen analyzer, as described in Chapter 4. As with the inspired ventilation, expired ventilation can be either directly measured by a spirometer or pneumoscan or can be calculated. Either $\dot{V}_I$ or $\dot{V}_E$ must be directly measured. When the value of one of them is known, the other can be calculated.

Ventilation Conversions

As stated in Chapter 9, the volume of air (either inspired or expired) is collected under conditions known as ambient temperature and pressure saturated, or ATPS. To do metabolic calculations, air volumes must first be converted to standard temperature and pressure (STPD) values. This conversion is necessary so that the number of gas molecules in any given volume is equal. The equations vary slightly according to whether the measured volume is inspired or expired.

The conversion process is based on the impact of temperature, pressure, and water vapor molecules on volume. The effect of temperature on volume is described by Charles's law. *Charles's law* states that the volume of a gas is directly related to temperature assuming a constant pressure, that is,

$$\frac{T_1}{T_2} = \frac{V_1}{V_2}$$

Therefore, if the initial temperature (T_1) is increased (T_2), the initial volume (V_1) will also be increased (V_2). Conversely, if T_1 is decreased at T_2, then V_1 will also be decreased at V_2. In metabolic calculations, V_2 is the value that is unknown. Therefore, the working formula that takes into account the impact of temperature on volume becomes

$$V_2 \times T_1 = V_1 \times T_2 \quad or \quad V_2 = \frac{V_1 \times T_2}{T_1}$$

usually expressed as

$$V_2 = V_1\left(\frac{T_2}{T_1}\right)$$

The effect of pressure on volume is primarily described by Boyle's law. *Boyle's law* states that the volume of a gas is inversely related to pressure assuming a constant temperature, that is,

$$\frac{P_1}{P_2} = \frac{V_2}{V_1}$$

Therefore, if the initial pressure (P_1) is increased (P_2), the initial volume (V_1) will be decreased (V_2). Conversely, if P_1 is decreased at P_2, then V_1 will be increased at V_2. Because V_2 is again the value that is unknown, this formula rearranges to

$$V_2 \times P_2 = V_1 \times P_1 \quad or \quad V_2 = \frac{V_1 \times P_1}{P_2}$$

usually expressed as

$$V_2 = V_1\left(\frac{P_1}{P_2}\right)$$

Water vapor molecules evaporate into the air (or into other gases) and account for part of the pressure exerted by the gas. The amount of water vapor is related exponentially to temperature. If the temperature is constant and a gas goes from being saturated with water vapor (S) to dry (D), the volume of the gas decreases. Conversely, if a gas goes from D to S, the volume increases. Tables, such as the abbreviated version in **Table B.1**, are available to determine the water vapor pressure (PH_2O) at measured ambient temperatures.

In practice, the formulas just described are generally combined so that the effects of temperature and volume are calculated concurrently, as indicated in the following formula:

B.3
$$V_2 = V_1\left(\frac{T_2}{T_1}\right)\left(\frac{P_1}{P_2}\right)$$

TABLE B.1 Water Vapor Pressure (PH_2O) at Selected Ambient Temperatures

Ambient Temperature (°C)	Ambient Temperature (°F)	PH$_2$O (mmHg)
20	68	17.5
21	70	18.7
22	72	19.8
23	73	21.1
24	75	22.4
25	77	23.8

The order of the temperature and pressure components in this equation may be reversed. If necessary, pressure is adjusted for water vapor.

Table B.2 presents the factors that are used in converting ventilatory volumes from ATPS to BTPS or STPD using expired and inspired ventilation volumes. BTPS ventilations are not used in the calculation of $\dot{V}O_2$ consumed and $\dot{V}CO_2$ produced, but they are presented for completeness and because BTPS values are used in determining ventilatory thresholds (Chapter 10) and lung volumes (Chapter 9).

The Conversion of $\dot{V}_E$ from ATPS to BTPS

When any ventilation volume is converted, it is first important to identify P_1, P_2, T_1, and T_2. Thus, in converting from $\dot{V}_E$ATPS to $\dot{V}_E$BTPS, P_1 is the ambient pressure; P_2 is the body pressure, which equals barometric pressure; T_1 is the ambient temperature; and T_2 is the body temperature. Second, the factor representing each of these components should then be identified from **Table B.2**: that is, $P_1 = P_B - PH_2O$ at T°C; $P_2 = P_B - 47$; $T_1 = 273 + T°C$; and $T_2 = 273 + 37°C$. This 273 is 273°K, to which either

TABLE B.2 Ventilation Conversion Factors

Volume	Pressure	Temperature
$\dot{V}_E$ATPS	$P_B - PH_2O$ at T°C	273° + T°C
$\dot{V}_I$ATPS	$P_B - [RH \times PH_2O$ at T°C]	273° + T°C
$\dot{V}_E$STPD	760	273°
$\dot{V}_E$BTPS	$P_B - 47$	273° + 37°

P_B, measured barometric pressure in mmHg; PH$_2$O, water vapor pressure in mmHg; T°C, measured temperature in degrees Celsius; RH, relative humidity as a fraction; 273°K = 0°C, standard temperature; 37°C, normal body temperature; 47 mmHg, water vapor pressure at 37°C.

the measured temperature (T°C) or the normal body temperature (37°C) is added. Ambient pressure is the measured barometric pressure at the data collection site corrected for the water vapor pressure at the ambient temperature. **Table B.1** is used to determine the water vapor pressure. Body pressure is the measured barometric pressure corrected for water vapor pressure at body temperature. Normal body temperature is assumed to be 37°C. Water vapor pressure (PH_2O) at 37°C is 47 mmHg.

Based on Equation B.3, the conversion formula becomes

B.4 minute ventilation (L·min⁻¹) BTPS = minute ventilation (L·min⁻¹) ATPS × temperature correction (°Kelvin) × pressure correction (mmHg)

or

$$\dot{V}_E BTPS = \dot{V}_E ATPS \left(\frac{273° + 37°C}{273° + T°C} \right) \left(\frac{P_B - PH_2O \, at \, T°C}{P_B - 47} \right)$$

For example, given the following information, we can correct $\dot{V}_E$ from ATPS to BTPS conditions.

$$\dot{V}_E ATPS = 12 \, L \cdot min^{-1}$$
$$T \, ATPS = 22°C$$
$$P_B = 745 \, mmHg$$
$$\dot{V}_E BTPS =$$
$$12 \, L \cdot min^{-1} \left(\frac{273° + 37°C}{273° + 22°C} \right) \left(\frac{745 \, mmHg - 19.8 \, mmHg}{745 - 47 \, mmHg} \right)$$
$$\dot{V}_E BTPS = 10.6 \, L \cdot min^{-1}$$

Under typical ambient conditions (without extremely high heat or altitude), BTPS values will be larger numerically than ATPS values because body temperature is usually higher than ambient temperature (which increases volume). Also, the body pressure adjusted for water vapor pressure at body temperature is typically lower than the ambient pressure adjusted for water vapor pressure at ambient temperature (which also increases volume).

The Conversion of $\dot{V}_E$ from ATPS to STPD

In converting from $\dot{V}_E ATPS$ to $\dot{V}_E STPD$, we identify P_1 as ambient pressure, P_2 as standard pressure, T_1 as ambient temperature, and T_2 as standard temperature. Identifying each of these components from **Table B.2** results in the following: $P_1 = P_B - PH_2O$ at T°C, $P_2 = 760$, $T_1 = 273° + T°C$, and $T_2 = 273°$. The body (barometric) pressure must be adjusted for the water vapor pressure at the ambient temperature so that the conversion goes from saturated or wet air to unsaturated or dry conditions. The formula for converting $\dot{V}_E ATPS$ to

$\dot{V}_E STPD$ accounts for changes in temperature (T) and pressure (P) as follows:

B.5 minute ventilation (L·min⁻¹) STPD = minute ventilation (L·min⁻¹) ATPS × temperature correction (°Kelvin) × pressure correction (mmHg)

or

$$\dot{V}_E STPD = \dot{V}_E ATPS \left(\frac{273°}{273° + T°C} \right) \left(\frac{P_B - PH_2O \, at \, T°C}{760} \right)$$

In this equation, the 273 represents the standard temperature of 0°C, which equals 273°K. The T°C represents the ambient temperature in degrees Celsius. PH_2O represents the water vapor correction from **Table B.1** to the body or barometric pressure (P_B), and 760 mmHg is standard pressure. Thus, given the following information, we can correct $\dot{V}_E$ from ATPS to STPD conditions.

$$\dot{V}_E ATPS = 12 \, L \cdot min^{-1}$$
$$T \, ATPS = 22°C$$
$$P_B = 745 \, mmHg$$
$$\dot{V}_E STPD =$$
$$12 \, L \cdot min^{-1} \left(\frac{273°}{273° + 22°C} \right) \times \left(\frac{745 \, mmHg - 19.8 \, mmHg}{760 \, mmHg} \right)$$
$$\dot{V}_E STPD = 10.6 \, L \cdot min^{-1}$$

The Conversion of $\dot{V}_I$ from ATPS to STPD

The conversion of $\dot{V}_I$ from ATPS to $\dot{V}_I STPD$ is the same as from $\dot{V}_E ATPS$ to $\dot{V}_E STPD$, with one small addition: in most laboratory settings, the inspired air is not totally saturated; that is, the relative humidity is not 100%. The equation must therefore be modified to adjust for the measured relative humidity (RH), expressed as a decimal fraction at the ambient temperature. Thus, the conversion equation becomes

B.6 $$\dot{V}_I STPD =$$
$$\dot{V}_I ATPS \left(\frac{273°}{273° + T°C} \right) \left(\frac{P_B - [RH \times PH_2O \, at \, T°C]}{760} \right)$$

Again, **Table B.1** presents the water vapor pressures (PH_2O) at temperatures generally encountered in a laboratory (20–25°C or 67–77°F). Thus, under the conditions given in the previous example but with an RH of 46%, the calculations become

$$\dot{V}_I STPD = 12 \, L \cdot min^{-1}$$
$$\left(\frac{273°}{273° + 22°} \right) \left(\frac{745 \, mmHg - [0.46 \times 19.8 \, mmHg]}{760 \, mmHg} \right)$$
$$\dot{V}_I STPD = 10.8 \, L \cdot min^{-1}$$

Under typical ambient conditions (without extremely high heat or altitude), STPD values, whether derived from expired or inspired ventilation volumes, are smaller numerically than ATPS values. The reason is that standard temperature is usually lower than ambient temperature (which decreases volume), and standard pressure is usually higher than ambient pressure (which decreases volume). The number of gas molecules depends on the volume they occupy. Therefore, STPD volumes are used when it is important to know the number of gas molecules, as in the calculation of O_2 consumed and CO_2 produced. The number of gas molecules and the volume they occupy under STPD conditions are constant and independent of the particular gas involved.

The Conversion of $\dot{V}_I$ from BTPS to STPD and Vice Versa

Occasionally, it is necessary to convert between BTPS and STPD, often based on which values any particular software-driven printout is programmed to provide. When BTPS is converted to STPD, P_1 is body or barometric pressure, P_2 is standard pressure, T_1 is body temperature, and T_2 is standard temperature. From **Table B.2**, these factors are identified as $P_1 = P_B - 47$, $P_2 = 760$, $T_1 = 273° + 37°C$, and $T_2 = 273°$. Substituting these into the generic Equation B.3,

$$V_2 = V_1 \left(\frac{T_2}{T_1} \right) \left(\frac{P_1}{P_2} \right)$$

we get

B.7 $\quad \dot{V}_E STPD =$

$$\dot{V}_E BTPS \left(\frac{273°}{273° + 37°C} \right) \left(\frac{P_B - 47 \text{ mmHg}}{760 \text{ mmHg}} \right)$$

Using the values from our examples

$$\dot{V}_E BTPS = 13.1 \, L \cdot min^{-1}$$
$$P_B STPD = 745 \text{ mmHg}$$

we can calculate $\dot{V}_E STPD$ as

$$\dot{V}_E STPD =$$
$$13.1 \, L \cdot min^{-1} \left(\frac{273°}{273° + 37°} \right) \left(\frac{745 \text{ mmHg} - 47 \text{mmHg}}{760 \text{ mmHg}} \right)$$
$$\dot{V}_E STPD = 10.6 \, L \cdot min^{-1}$$

Conversely, when STPD is converted to BTPS, P_1 is standard pressure (760 mmHg), P_2 is body pressure ($P_B - 47$ mmHg), T_1 is standard temperature (0°C or 273°K), and T_2 is body temperature (assumed to be 273° + 37°C). Substituting these values into the generic equation, we get

B.8 $\quad \dot{V}_E BTPS =$

$$\dot{V}_E STPD \left(\frac{273° + 37°C}{273°} \right) \left(\frac{760 \text{ mmHg}}{P_B - 47 \text{ mmHg}} \right)$$

Again, using the values from our example:

$$\dot{V}_E STPD = 10.6 \, L \cdot min^{-1}$$
$$P_B = 745 \text{ mmHg}$$
$$\dot{V}_E BTPS =$$
$$10.6 \, L \cdot min^{-1} \left(\frac{273° + 37°}{273°} \right) \times \left(\frac{760 \text{ mmHg}}{745 \text{ mmHg} - 47 \text{ mmHg}} \right)$$
$$\dot{V}_E BTPS = 13.1 \, L \cdot min^{-1}$$

Calculation of the Unknown Ventilation Value

The Calculation of $\dot{V}_E$ from $\dot{V}_I$ and $\dot{V}_I$ from $\dot{V}_E$

Open-circuit metabolic systems measure either inspired or expired air, but not both. Typically, the volume of expired air does not equal the volume of inspired air. The reason is that the number of oxygen molecules used from the inspired air is not replaced by the same number of carbon dioxide molecules, except when an individual is burning pure carbohydrate and has an RER of exactly 1.0. When fewer CO_2 molecules replace the O_2 molecules, the RER value is less than 1.0, and $\dot{V}_E$ will be smaller than $\dot{V}_I$. If the RER value is greater than 1.0, $\dot{V}_E$ will be larger than $\dot{V}_I$. This occurs when both metabolic and nonmetabolic CO_2 molecules (primarily from the buffering of lactic acid) are produced.

In order to solve Equation B.2 (i.e., calculate $\dot{V}O_2$cons), we must have values for both $\dot{V}_E$ and $\dot{V}_I$. Fortunately, there is a way to convert $\dot{V}_E$ to $\dot{V}_I$ or $\dot{V}_I$ to $\dot{V}_E$ mathematically. This is called the *Haldane transformation* and is based on the fact that nitrogen (N_2) is an inert gas that does not participate in human metabolism nor does it easily combine with any blood constituents. The number of particles of nitrogen does not change, although the concentration or fraction of the nitrogen will change because the fractions of oxygen and carbon dioxide are changing. Thus, the amount (again defined as the fraction of the gas times the volume of air containing that gas) of gaseous nitrogen expired is exactly equal to the amount of gaseous nitrogen inspired. That is,

B.9 $\quad$ fraction of inspired nitrogen × the inspired minute ventilation = fraction of expired nitrogen × the expired minute ventilation

or

$$F_I N_2 \times \dot{V}_I = F_E N_2 \times \dot{V}_E$$

Rearranging the equation, it becomes

$$\dot{V}_I = \frac{F_E N_2 \times \dot{V}_E}{F_I N_2} \quad \text{or} \quad \dot{V}_E = \frac{F_I N_2 \times \dot{V}_I}{F_E N_2}$$

B.10
$$\dot{V}_I = \dot{V}_E \left(\frac{F_E N_2}{F_I N_2}\right) \quad \text{and} \quad \dot{V}_E = \dot{V}_I \left(\frac{F_I N_2}{F_E N_2}\right)$$

As usual in these formulas, the measurements are percentages, but they are expressed as decimal fractions. Both $F_I N_2$ and $F_E N_2$ are easily obtained from known and measured values. Air is composed of nitrogen, oxygen, and carbon dioxide, and the fractions of O_2 and CO_2 are known for room air (assumed to be the inspired air) and measured for expired air by the gas analyzers. Thus, N_2 can be calculated by simple subtraction:

$$F_I N_2 = 1 - [F_I O_2 + F_E CO_2] = 0.7904$$
$$0.2093 + 0.0003$$

and

$$F_E N_2 = 1 - [F_E O_2 + F_E CO_2] = \text{variables}$$
$$\text{measured by analyzers}$$

Therefore,

B.11
$$\dot{V}_I = \dot{V}_E \left(\frac{1 - [F_E O_2 + F_E CO_2]}{0.7904}\right)$$

B.12
$$\dot{V}_E = \dot{V}_I \left(\frac{0.7904}{1 - [F_E O_2 + F_E CO_2]}\right)$$

For example, given

$$\dot{V}_I \text{STPD} = 10.8 \text{ L} \cdot \text{min}^{-1}$$
$$O_2\% = 16.38$$
$$CO_2\% = 4.03$$

the computation becomes

$$\dot{V}_I \text{STPD} = 10.8 \text{ L} \cdot \text{min}^{-1} \left(\frac{0.7904}{1 - [0.1638 + 0.0403]}\right)$$
$$= 10.73 \text{ L} \cdot \text{min}^{-1}$$

Conversely, if we are given

$$\dot{V}_E \text{STPD} = 10.6 \text{ L} \cdot \text{min}^{-1}$$
$$O_2\% = 16.38$$
$$CO_2\% = 4.03$$

the computation becomes

$$\dot{V}_I \text{STPD} = 10.6 \text{ L} \cdot \text{min}^{-1} \left(\frac{1 - [0.1638 + 0.0403]}{0.7904}\right)$$
$$= 10.67 \text{ L} \cdot \text{min}^{-1}$$

Calculation of Oxygen Consumed

Now we are finally ready to go back to Equation B.2 and solve it.

$$\dot{V}O_2 \text{ L} \cdot \text{min}^{-1} = (F_I O_2 \times \dot{V}_I) - (F_E O_2 \times \dot{V}_E)$$

The available information is as follows:

$$F_I O_2 = 0.2093 \text{ (assumed constant)}$$
$$\dot{V}_I \text{STPD} = 10.8 \text{ L} \cdot \text{min}^{-1} \text{ (measured as } \dot{V}_I \text{ATPS by}$$
$$\text{pneumoscan and converted by Eq. B.6)}$$
$$F_E O_2 = 0.1638 \text{ (measured by oxygen analyzer)}$$
$$\dot{V}_E \text{STPD} = 10.73 \text{ L} \cdot \text{min}^{-1} \text{ (calculated by the Haldane}$$
$$\text{transformation in Eq. B.12)}$$

Substituting the given values into Equation B.2, we get

$$\dot{V}O_2 \text{ L} \cdot \text{min}^{-1} = (0.2093 \times 10.8 \text{ L} \cdot \text{min}^{-1})$$
$$- (0.1638 \times 10.73 \text{ L} \cdot \text{min}^{-1})$$
$$= 0.5 \text{ L} \cdot \text{min}^{-1} \text{ or } 500 \text{ mL} \cdot \text{min}^{-1}$$

Calculation of Carbon Dioxide Produced

Theoretically, the amount of carbon dioxide produced is simply equal to the amount of carbon dioxide in expired air minus the amount of carbon dioxide in inspired air.

B.13
$$\dot{V}_I CO_2 \text{prod} = \dot{V}_E CO_2 - \dot{V}_I CO_2$$

Because there is no way to obtain $\dot{V}_E CO_2$ or $\dot{V}_I CO_2$ directly, a working formula must again be used. Thus, the calculation of the amount of carbon dioxide produced is very similar to the calculation of oxygen consumed.

B.14 carbon dioxide produced (L · min^{-1}) = [fraction of carbon dioxide in expired air × volume of expired air (L · min^{-1})] − [fraction of inspired carbon dioxide × volume of inspired air (L × min^{-1})].
$$\dot{V}_I CO_2 \text{ L} \cdot \text{min}^{-1} = (F_E CO_2 \times \dot{V}_E) - (F_I CO_2 \times \dot{V}_I)$$

The $F_I CO_2$ is a constant 0.0003 because the percentage of carbon dioxide in room air is assumed to be 0.03%.

Because this number is so small and would have no meaningful effect on the calculation in Equation B.14, it is generally considered to be 0. As a result, only the expired portion of the equation needs to be computed. F_ECO_2 is measured by a carbon dioxide analyzer as described in Chapter 4. $\dot{V}_E$ either is directly measured by a spirometer or pneumoscan or is calculated as previously described.

Using the values of CO_2% and $\dot{V}_E$ given previously, the calculation becomes

$$\dot{V}_ICO_2 \ L \cdot min^{-1} = (0.0403 \times 10.73 \ L \cdot min^{-1})$$
$$= 0.43 \ L \cdot min^{-1} \ or \ 430 \ mL \cdot min^{-1}$$

Note that as mentioned in the section describing the calculation of $\dot{V}_E$ from $\dot{V}_I$, the oxygen consumed ($500 \ mL \cdot min^{-1}$) is not equaled by the amount of carbon dioxide produced ($430 \ mL \cdot min^{-1}$).

Complete the practice problems at the end of the appendix to determine your understanding of these concepts and calculations.

THE CALCULATION OF OXYGEN CONSUMED USING MECHANICAL WORK OR SPEED OF MOVEMENT

In exercise situations where an accurate assessment of mechanical work or speed of movement is possible but the actual measurement of oxygen consumed and carbon dioxide produced is not, the oxygen consumed can be estimated. These situations include walking, running, cycling on an ergometer, and bench stepping. Specific formulas recommended by the American College of Sports Medicine (2010) are available for each activity. The resulting oxygen consumption values will not be as accurate as the direct measurement of oxygen consumed, which was described in the last section. However, these estimated oxygen consumptions are much less difficult and much less expensive to obtain. They can be very useful in the practical field settings of health clubs, hospitals, and/or school gymnasia as the initial step in determining exercise prescriptions by MET level or determining the caloric cost of any activity. Because of differences in economy (Chapter 4), none of these equations should be used for children. Because no systematic differences in economy have been found between males and females, all of these equations can be used for both sexes.

The following computations show you how to determine the oxygen consumption values of the four activities specified earlier. Remember from Chapter 4 that converting to METs requires dividing the $O_2 \ mL \cdot kg^{-1} \cdot min^{-1}$ value by $3.5 \ mL \cdot kg^{-1} \cdot min^{-1}$. Caloric cost (also discussed in Chapter 4) can be estimated by multiplying the $O_2 \ L \cdot min^{-1}$ value by $5 \ kcal \cdot L \cdot min^{-1}$, because $5 \ kcal \cdot L \cdot min^{-1}$ is the estimated caloric equivalent if the RER is unknown.

Oxygen Consumed during Horizontal (Level) and Vertical (Graded) Walking

Level Walking

To determine the oxygen consumed while walking on level ground or on a treadmill at 0% elevation, it is necessary to determine the walking speed in meters per minute ($m \cdot min^{-1}$). It is known that for speeds between 1.9 and 3.7 $mi \cdot hr^{-1}$ (or 50–100 $m \cdot min^{-1}$; 26.8 $m \cdot min^{-1}$ = 1 $mi \cdot hr^{-1}$), the net oxygen cost of level walking is 0.1 $mL \cdot kg^{-1} \cdot min^{-1}$ per $m \cdot min^{-1}$. Because this oxygen consumption constant is a net value, the oxygen consumed during rest (1 MET or 3.5 $mL \cdot kg^{-1} \cdot min^{-1}$) is added to obtain the total amount of oxygen consumed. Therefore, the equation can be stated as follows:

B.15

oxygen consumed during horizontal walking

($mL \cdot kg^{-1} \cdot min^{-1}$) = horizontal

component ($mL \cdot kg^{-1} \cdot min^{-1}$) + resting

component ($mL \cdot kg^{-1} \cdot min^{-1}$)

or

$$\dot{V}O_2 cons \ (mL \cdot kg^{-1} \cdot min^{-1}) = \left[speed \ (m \cdot min^{-1}) \right.$$
$$\left. \times \frac{0.1 \ mL \cdot kg^{-1} \cdot min^{-1}}{m \cdot min^{-1}} \right] + 3.5 \ mL \cdot kg^{-1} \cdot min^{-1}$$

For example, if an individual were walking on a treadmill at 0% grade and 3 $mi \cdot hr^{-1}$, it would first be necessary to convert the speed to meters per minute (3 $mi \cdot hr^{-1} \times$ 26.8 $m \cdot min^{-1}/mi \cdot hr^{-1}$ = 80.4 $m \cdot min^{-1}$). Then, substituting this value into Equation B.15, we get

$$\dot{V}O_2 cons \ (mL \cdot kg^{-1} \cdot min^{-1}) = \left[80.4 \ (m \cdot min^{-1}) \right.$$
$$\left. \times \frac{0.1 \ mL \cdot kg^{-1} \cdot min^{-1}}{m \cdot min^{-1}} \right] + 3.5 \ mL \cdot kg^{-1} \cdot min^{-1}$$
$$\dot{V}O_2 cons = 11.54 \ mL \cdot kg^{-1} \cdot min^{-1}$$

Graded Walking

To determine the oxygen consumed during uphill walking or walking on a treadmill at a grade, a vertical component is added to Equation B.15. The vertical component is determined by the percent grade expressed as a decimal. Each $m \cdot min^{-1}$ of vertical rise consumes an additional 1.8 $mL \cdot kg^{-1} \cdot min^{-1}$ for each $m \cdot min^{-1}$ of speed.

The following formula incorporates the vertical component in Equation B.15:

B.16

oxygen consumed during vertical walking ($mL \cdot kg^{-1} \cdot min^{-1}$)

= horizontal component ($mL \cdot kg^{-1} \cdot min^{-1}$)

+ resting component ($mL \cdot kg^{-1} \cdot min^{-1}$)

+ vertical component ($mL \cdot kg^{-1} \cdot min^{-1}$)

or

$$\dot{V}O_2 cons\ (mL \cdot kg^{-1} \cdot min^{-1}) = \left[speed\ (m \cdot min^{-1}) \times \frac{0.1\ mL \times kg^{-1} \times min^{-1}}{m \times min^{-1}} \right] + 3.5\ mL \cdot kg^{-1} \cdot min^{-1} + \left[decimal\ grade \times speed\ (m \cdot min^{-1}) \times \frac{1.8\ mL \cdot kg^{-1} \cdot min^{-1}}{m \cdot min^{-1}} \right]$$

If we change the percent grade in the previous example from 0% to 5%, we now have only to calculate the vertical component.

$$vertical\ component = \left[0.05 \times 80.4\ m \cdot min^{-1} \times \frac{1.8\ mL \cdot kg^{-1} \cdot min^{-1}}{m \cdot min^{-1}} \right] = 7.24\ mL \cdot kg^{-1} \cdot min^{-1}$$

The vertical component is then added to the horizontal and resting components to get the total amount of oxygen consumed while walking at a speed of 3 $mi \cdot hr^{-1}$ with a 5% grade on a treadmill.

$$
\begin{aligned}
Horizontal\ component &= 8.04\ mL \cdot kg^{-1} \cdot min^{-1} \\
Resting\ component &= 3.50\ mL \cdot kg^{-1} \cdot min^{-1} \\
Vertical\ component &= \underline{7.24\ mL \cdot kg^{-1} \cdot min^{-1}} \\
Total\ \dot{V}O_2 cons &= 18.78\ mL \cdot kg^{-1} \cdot min^{-1}
\end{aligned}
$$

Oxygen Consumed during Horizontal (Level) and Vertical (Graded) Running

The formulas for estimating the amount of oxygen consumed during running differ from those for walking only in two factors. The first is that the net oxygen cost of level running is 0.2 $mL \cdot kg^{-1} \cdot min^{-1}$ per $m \cdot min^{-1}$, or double the same cost for walking. Conversely, the additional cost for the vertical components is only half as much as for walking, because of differences in the biomechanics of the two gaits, especially the greater forefoot pushoff in running. This difference necessitates multiplying the

vertical component by 0.5. Thus, 1.8 $mL \cdot kg^{-1} \cdot min^{-1}$ × 0.5 = 0.9 $mL \cdot kg^{-1} \cdot min^{-1}$.

Running is defined as speeds greater than 5 $mi \cdot hr^{-1}$ (134 $m \cdot min^{-1}$). This leaves a gap between the top walking speeds (3.7 $mi \cdot hr^{-1}$ or 100 $m \cdot min^{-1}$) and the lowest running speed. The best formula for these intermediate speeds depends on whether the individual is actually running or walking.

The formula for determining the oxygen consumed while running on level ground or a treadmill is as follows:

B.17

$$\dot{V}O_2 cons\ (mL \cdot kg^{-1} \cdot min^{-1}) = \left[speed\ (m \cdot min^{-1}) \times \frac{0.2\ mL \cdot kg^{-1} \cdot min^{-1}}{m \cdot min^{-1}} \right] + 3.5\ mL \cdot kg^{-1} \cdot min^{-1}$$

Graded running adds a vertical component to Equation B.17:

B.18

$$\dot{V}O_2 cons\ (mL \cdot kg^{-1} \cdot min^{-1}) = \left[speed\ (m \cdot min^{-1}) \times \frac{0.2\ mL \cdot kg^{-1} \cdot min^{-1}}{m \cdot min^{-1}} \right] + 3.5\ mL \cdot kg^{-1} \cdot min^{-1} + \left[decimal\ grade \times speed\ (m \cdot min^{-1}) \times \frac{0.9\ mL \cdot kg^{-1} \cdot min^{-1}}{m \cdot min^{-1}} \right]$$

If the individual in the previous example switches from walking at 3 $mi \cdot hr^{-1}$ up a 5% grade to running the same grade at 7 $mi \cdot hr^{-1}$ (188 $m \cdot min^{-1}$), this example works out as follows:

$$\dot{V}O_2\ cons\ (mL \cdot kg^{-1} \cdot min^{-1}) = \left[188\ m \cdot min^{-1} \times \frac{0.2\ mL \cdot kg^{-1} \cdot min^{-1}}{m \cdot min^{-1}} \right] + 3.5\ mL \cdot kg^{-1} \cdot min^{-1} + [0.05 \times 188\ m \cdot min^{-1}]$$

$$
\begin{aligned}
Horizontal\ component &= 37.60\ mL \cdot kg^{-1} \cdot min^{-1} \\
Resting\ component &= 3.50\ mL \cdot kg^{-1} \cdot min^{-1} \\
Vertical\ component &= \underline{8.46\ mL \cdot kg^{-1} \cdot min^{-1}} \\
Total\ \dot{V}O_2 cons &= 49.56\ mL \cdot kg^{-1} \cdot min^{-1}
\end{aligned}
$$

Oxygen Consumed during Cycling Using Either the Legs or the Arms

The formulas for calculating the amount of oxygen consumed during cycling are intended only for cycling on an ergometer, which permits the actual measurement of the workload. The mechanical work completed (as described in Chapter 4) is determined by multiplying the force exerted, in the form of the load or resistance overcome, in kilograms, by the distance traveled ($m \cdot min^{-1}$) using the following equation:

B.19 work rate ($kgm \cdot min^{-1}$) = kg of resistance $\times m \cdot rev^{-1} \times rev \cdot min^{-1}$

The distance traveled per revolution is the circumference off the flywheel. On many ergometers, including the often-used Monark Tunturi, and Bodyguard friction ergometers, this distance is 6 m. The pedaling rate, or revolutions per minute value, is typically displayed on the console of the ergometer and can vary from 30 to 110 $rev \cdot min^{-1}$, with 50 or 60 $rev \cdot min^{-1}$ being the most commonly used by fitness exercisers.

Leg Cycling

Oxygen consumed during leg cycling can be estimated using the following equation. This formula is most accurate when the work rate is between 300 and 1200 $kgm \cdot min^{-1}$ (50–200 W), but it may be used up to rates of 4200 $kgm \cdot min^{-1}$. The oxygen cost against the external load is equal to that of vertical walking, or 1.8 $mL \cdot kg^{-1} \cdot min^{-1}$ per $m \cdot min^{-1}$, and the oxygen associated with unloaded cycling is 3.5 $mL \cdot kg^{-1} \cdot min^{-1}$. In the example below, this latter value has been added to the resting component to equal 7.0 $mL \cdot kg^{-1} \cdot min^{-1}$.

B.20 oxygen consumed during leg cycling ($mL \cdot kg^{-1} \cdot min^{-1}$) = [oxygen consumed during the resistance component ($mL \cdot kg^{-1} \cdot min^{-1}$) divided by body weight (kg)] + oxygen consumed during the resting component ($mL \cdot kg^{-1} \cdot min^{-1}$) + oxygen associated with unloaded cycling

or

$$\dot{V}O_2 cons (mL \cdot kg^{-1} \cdot min^{-1})$$
$$= \left[\frac{1.8\ mL \cdot kg^{-1} \cdot min^{-1}}{m \cdot min^{-1}}\ \text{work rate}\ (kgm \cdot min^{-1}) \right.$$
$$\left. \div \text{body weight (kg)} \right] + 7\ mL \cdot kg^{-1} \cdot min^{-1}$$

For example, if a 50-kg individual pedals a Monark bike at 60 $rev \cdot min^{-1}$ at a load of 2 kg (denoted as 2 kp on the ergometer itself; 1 kg = 1 kp), he or she consumes 32.92 $mL \cdot kg^{-1} \cdot min^{-1}$, which is calculated as follows:

$$\dot{V}O_2\ (mL \cdot kg^{-1} \cdot min^{-1}) = \left[\frac{1.8\ mL \cdot kg^{-1} \cdot min^{-1}}{m \cdot min^{-1}} \right.$$
$$\left. (2\ kg \times 6\ m \cdot rev^{-1} \times 60\ rev \cdot min^{-1}) \div 50\ kg \right]$$
$$+ 7\ mL \cdot kg^{-1} \cdot min^{-1}$$

Resistance component = 25.92 $mL \cdot kg^{-1} \cdot min^{-1}$
Rest + unloaded component = 7.00 $mL \cdot kg^{-1} \cdot min^{-1}$
Total $\dot{V}O_2 cons$ = 32.92 $mL \cdot kg^{-1} \cdot min^{-1}$

Arm Cranking

Cycling with the arms is more properly referred to as arm cranking. The formula for arm cranking differs from leg cycling in the constant for oxygen use per kilogram of resistance. The arm musculature used in cranking is smaller than the leg musculature used in cycling; hence, there is no need for the addition of an unloaded cycling cost. However, additional muscles in the shoulders, back, and chest are recruited to stabilize the arms, elevating the oxygen cost. Thus, instead of a constant 1.8 $mL \cdot kg^{-1} \cdot min^{-1}$ per $m \cdot min^{-1}$, the value used is 3 $mL \cdot kg^{-1} \cdot min^{-1}$ per $m \cdot min^{-1}$. In addition, although some locations may modify a regular leg cycle ergometer for use with the arms, most places use a specialized arm crank ergometer. In this case, the flywheel size and thus distance is typically smaller. For the Monark arm ergometer, this value is 2.4 m. Hence, the workload and $\dot{V}O_2$ consumed will be lower at any given resistance and number of revolution per minute. This formula is appropriate for power outputs between 150 and 750 $kgm \cdot min^{-1}$ (25–125 W).

B.21 oxygen consumed during arm cranking ($mL \cdot kg^{-1} \cdot min^{-1}$) = [oxygen consumed during the resistance component ($mL \cdot kg^{-1} \cdot min^{-1}$ per $m \cdot min^{-1}$) divided by body weight] + oxygen consumed during rest

$$\dot{V}O_2 cons\ (mL \cdot kg^{-1} \cdot min^{-1}) = \left[\frac{3\ mL \cdot kg^{-1} \cdot min^{-1}}{m \cdot min^{-1}} \right.$$
$$\left. \text{work rate}\ (kgm \cdot min^{-1}) \div \text{body weight (kg)} \right]$$
$$3.5\ mL \cdot kg^{-1} \cdot min^{-1}$$

If the individual in the previous example switches from leg cycling to arm cranking and uses an arm ergometer, he or she now consumes 20.78 $mL \cdot kg^{-1} \cdot min^{-1}$ of oxygen, calculated as follows:

$$\dot{V}O_2 \text{cons (mL} \cdot \text{kg}^{-1} \cdot \text{min}^{-1}) = \left[\frac{3 \text{ mL} \cdot \text{kg}^{-1} \cdot \text{min}^{-1}}{\text{m} \cdot \text{min}^{-1}} \right.$$

$$\left. (2 \text{ kg} \times 2.4 \text{ m} \cdot \text{rev}^{-1} \times 60 \text{ rev} \cdot \text{min}^{-1}) \div 50 \text{ kg} \right]$$

$$+ 3.5 \text{ mL} \cdot \text{kg}^{-1} \cdot \text{min}^{-1}$$

Resistance component =	$17.28 \text{ mL} \cdot \text{kg}^{-1} \cdot \text{min}^{-1}$
Resting component =	$\underline{3.5 \text{ mL} \cdot \text{kg}^{-1} \cdot \text{min}^{-1}}$
Total $\dot{V}O_2$cons =	$20.78 \text{ mL} \cdot \text{kg}^{-1} \cdot \text{min}^{-1}$

The Oxygen Consumed during Bench Stepping

Like cycling, bench stepping allows for the exact computation of the work being done if the height of the step, the rate of stepping, and the body weight of the stepper are known.

B.22 oxygen consumed during bench stepping $(\text{mL} \cdot \text{kg}^{-1} \cdot \text{min}^{-1}) = $ [oxygen consumed during the horizontal component $(\text{mL} \cdot \text{kg}^{-1} \cdot \text{min}^{-1})$ + oxygen consumed during the vertical component $(\text{mL} \cdot \text{kg}^{-1} \cdot \text{min}^{-1})$ + oxygen consumed at rest

or

$$\dot{V}O_2 \text{cons (mL} \cdot \text{kg}^{-1} \cdot \text{min}^{-1}) =$$

$$\left[\frac{0.2 \text{ mL} \cdot \text{kg}^{-1} \cdot \text{min}^{-1}}{\text{steps} \cdot \text{min}^{-1}} \times (\text{stepping rate})(\text{steps} \cdot \text{min}^{-1}) \right]$$

$$+ \left[1.33 \times \frac{1.8 \text{ mL} \cdot \text{kg}^{-1} \cdot \text{min}^{-1}}{\text{m} \cdot \text{min}^{-1}} \times (\text{step height}) \right.$$

$$\left. \times (\text{m} \cdot \text{step}^{-1}) \times (\text{stepping rate})(\text{steps} \cdot \text{min}^{-1}) \right]$$

$$+ 3.5 \text{ mL} \cdot \text{kg}^{-1} \cdot \text{min}^{-1}$$

In the first component, $0.2 \text{ mL} \cdot \text{kg}^{-1} \cdot \text{min}^{-1}$ is the oxygen cost of stepping back and forth along the horizontal plane. In the second component, as with walking or running, each $\text{m} \cdot \text{min}^{-1}$ of vertical rise requires $1.8 \text{ mL} \cdot \text{kg}^{-1} \cdot \text{min}^{-1}$ of oxygen. The 0.33 in the constant 1.33 accounts for the fact that bench stepping has both a positive (up) and a negative (down) action. Negative work in this situation requires one third as much oxygen as positive work. The equation is most accurate for step heights between 1.6 and 15.7 in (0.04–0.40 m) and step rates of 12 and 30 steps·min⁻¹)

For an individual stepping up and down on a 10-in (0.254 m) bench at 24 steps·min⁻¹, oxygen consumption is calculated as follows:

$$\dot{V}O_2 \text{cons (mL} \cdot \text{kg}^{-1} \cdot \text{min}^{-1}) = \left[24 \text{ steps} \cdot \text{min}^{-1} \right.$$

$$\left. \times \frac{0.2 \text{ mL} \cdot \text{kg}^{-1} \cdot \text{min}^{-1}}{\text{steps} \cdot \text{min}^{-1}} \right] + 0.254 \text{ m} \cdot \text{step}^{-1}$$

$$\left. \times 24 \text{ steps} \cdot \text{min}^{-1} \times \frac{1.8 \text{ mL} \cdot \text{kg}^{-1} \text{min}^{-1}}{\text{m} \cdot \text{min}^{-1}} \times 1.33 \right]$$

$$+ 3.5 \text{ mL} \cdot \text{kg}^{-1} \cdot \text{min}^{-1}$$

Horizontal component =	$4.8 \text{ mL} \cdot \text{kg}^{-1} \cdot \text{min}^{-1}$
Vertical component =	$14.6 \text{ mL} \cdot \text{kg}^{-1} \cdot \text{min}^{-1}$
Resting component =	$\underline{3.5 \text{ mL} \cdot \text{kg}^{-1} \cdot \text{min}^{-1}}$
Total $\dot{V}O_2$cons =	$22.9 \text{ mL} \cdot \text{kg}^{-1} \cdot \text{min}^{-1}$

THE CALCULATION OF MAXIMAL OXYGEN CONSUMPTION FROM CARDIOVASCULAR ENDURANCE FIELD TESTS

The direct measurement of maximal oxygen consumption ($\dot{V}O_2$max) is the best indicator of cardiovascular respiratory fitness. However, the direct measurement of $\dot{V}O_2$max requires expensive equipment, trained technicians, and considerable time. This makes it unsuitable for mass testing. Therefore, as indicated in Chapter 12, field tests are often used to estimate $\dot{V}O_2$max. The calculation of $\dot{V}O_2$max from the 1-mi run/walk is explained in Chapter 12. This section details the calculation of $\dot{V}O_2$max from the PACER (originally known as the 20-m shuttle test) and from the Rockport Fitness Walking Test (RFWT).

PACER $\dot{V}O_2$max

Several different formulas are available to determine $\dot{V}O_2$max from the results of the PACER test. Two have been included here to cover as wide an age span as possible. The first equation should be used for both male and female children and adolescents (Léger et al., 1988). It requires knowing only the final speed at which the individual ran and the age of the individual.

B.23 $\dot{V}O_2$max $= 31.025 + 3.238$ (final speed in km·hr⁻¹) $- 3.248$ (age in yr) $+ 0.1536$ (final speed × age)

For example, if a 9-year-old boy had a final speed of 11 km·hr⁻¹, we would substitute into the equation as follows:

$$\dot{V}O_2 \text{max} = 31.025 + 3.238(11) - 3.248(9)$$

$$+ 0.1536 (11 \times 9) = 52.62 \text{ mL} \cdot \text{kg}^{-1} \cdot \text{min}^{-1}$$

The second equation should be used for young ≥18 years adult males and females (Leger et al., 1988; Plowman and

Liu, 1999). It requires knowing only the maximal speed the individual completed. Level 1 (minute 1) is run at a speed of 8.5 km·hr^{-1}. Each additional level (min) adds 0.5 km·hr^{-1}

B.24 $\quad \dot{V}O_2max = -23.4 + 5.8 \text{ (max speed in km·hr}^{-1})$

Thus, if a 20-year-old college student ran for 10 minutes, the calculation would be (13 km·hr^{-1})

$$\dot{V}O_2max = -23.4 + 5.8 \text{ (13 km·hr}^{-1}) = 52 \text{ mL·kg}^{-1}\cdot\text{min}^{-1}$$

Rockport Fitness Walking Test $\dot{V}O_2$max

The RFWT can be used to estimate $\dot{V}O_2$max in male and female adults from approximately age 30–70 years (Kline et al., 1987) and adolescents 14–18 years (McSwegin et al., 1998), but not young adults.

Five variables are needed to estimate $\dot{V}O_2$max: body weight in pounds, age in years, sex (females are coded as 0 and males are coded as 1), time for completion of the mile walk (in minutes, including a decimal), and heart rate in beats per minute (recorded by a heart rate monitor during the final quarter mile or manually in the 15 sec immediately postexercise).

B.25 $\quad \dot{V}O_2max = 132.853 - 0.0769 \text{ (body weight)}$
$\qquad - 0.3877 \text{ (age)} + 6.3150 \text{ (sex)}$
$\qquad - 3.2649 \text{ (walk time)} - 0.1565 \text{ (heart rate)}$

For example, if a 64-year-old, 195-lb male completed the mile walk in 19.01 minutes with a last quarter heart rate of 113 b·min^{-1}, the calculation would be as follows:

$$\dot{V}O_2max = 132.853 - 0.0769(195) - 0.3877(64)$$
$$+ 6.3150(1) - 3.2649(19.01) - 0.1565(113)$$
$$= 19.61 \text{ mL·kg}^{-1}\cdot\text{min}^{-1}$$

Standard Error of the Estimate

Because all of these formulas are estimates, knowing the accuracy of the estimate is helpful. Accuracy is determined during the development of the equations when the estimated values are compared to the actual values statistically and a standard error of the estimate (SEE) is obtained. The PACER equation for children and adolescents (Eq. B.23) has an SEE of 5.9 mL·kg^{-1}·min^{-1}. The PACER equation for young adults (Eq. B.24) has an SEE of 4.6–4.7 mL·kg^{-1}·min^{-1}. The RFWT equation (Eq. B.25) has an SEE of 5.0 mL·kg^{-1}·min^{-1}. Each SEE means that the calculated $\dot{V}O_2$max could differ from an actual measured value by one or two times the amount of the SEE. Most scores (68%) should vary only plus or minus one SEE from the calculated estimated value.

Thus, the $\dot{V}O_2$max 52 mL·kg^{-1}·min^{-1} calculated for the college student from Equation B.24 could actually be anywhere from 47.3 to 56.7 mL·kg^{-1}·min^{-1}. Obviously, the smaller the SEE, the greater the equation's accuracy (Jackson, 1989). All of these estimation equations are deemed to have acceptable accuracy.

PRACTICE PROBLEMS

Use the data in **Table B.3** to work the problems that follow. Answers are provided at the end of the section.

1. Correct the expired minute ventilations from ATPS to STPD.
2. Correct the inspired minute ventilations from ATPS to STPD
3. Calculate the inspired minute ventilations from the expired minute ventilations using the Haldane transformation.
4. Calculate the expired minute ventilations from the inspired minute ventilations using the Haldane transformation.
5. Calculate $\dot{V}O_2$cons substituting the information given and computed from the maximal treadmill results in Equation B.2. Present your answer in both relative (mL·kg^{-1}·min^{-1}) and absolute (L·min^{-1}) oxygen units.
6. Calculate the $\dot{V}CO_2$ produced using the information given and computed from the maximal treadmill results in L·min^{-1}.
7. Calculate the oxygen consumed during submaximal walking.
8. Calculate the oxygen consumed during submaximal running.
9. Calculate the oxygen consumed during submaximal cycling, assuming that subject 3 is doing leg work and subject 4 is doing arm cranking.
10. Calculate the oxygen consumed during bench stepping.
11. Calculate the estimated $\dot{V}O_2$max for each subject using the appropriate formula for the information presented.

SOLUTIONS AND ANSWERS

1. **Subject No. 1**

$\dot{V}_E$STPD =

$45 \text{ L·min}^{-1}\left(\dfrac{273°}{273° + 20°}\right) \times \left(\dfrac{740 - 17.5 \text{ mmHg}}{760}\right)$

$\qquad = 39.86 \text{ L·min}^{-1}$

Subject No. 3

$\dot{V}_E$STPD =

$130 \text{ L·min}^{-1}\left(\dfrac{273°}{273° + 21°}\right) \times \left(\dfrac{738 - 18.7 \text{ mmHg}}{760}\right)$

$\qquad = 114.25$

TABLE B.3	Practice Problem Data			
	Subjects			
Variables	**No. 1**	**No. 2**	**No. 3**	**No. 4**
Descriptive Information				
Sex	Female	Female	Male	Male
Age (yr)	15	24	32	58
Weight (lb)	108	132	175	201
Maximal Treadmill Data				
$\dot{V}_E$ATPS (L·min^{-1})	45		130	
P_B (mmHg)	740	742	738	739
T (°C)	20	23	21	24
F_EO_2(%)	16.08	16.2	16.04	16.75
F_ECO_2(%)	4.94	5.01	5.12	4.73
$\dot{V}_I$ATPS (L·min^{-1})		70		75
RH (%)		50		25
Submaximal Exercise Data				
Speed (m·min^{-1})	90	161		
Grade	11	0		
Ergometer load (kp)			4	3
Pedaling rate (rev·min^{-1})			80	50
Flywheel circumference (m)			6	2.4
Step height (m)		0.305		
Step rate (steps·min^{-1})		30		
Field Test Data				
PACER speed (km·hr^{-1})	10			
PACER time (min)	12.5	9	16	
1-mi walk time (min)				17.6
HR (b·min^{-1})				108

2. **Subject No. 2**

$\dot{V}_I$STPD =

$70 \text{ L} \cdot \text{min}^{-1} \left(\dfrac{273°}{273° + 23°} \right) \times \left(\dfrac{742 \, [0.5 \times 21.1] \text{ mmHg}}{760 \text{ mmHg}} \right)$

$= 62.13 \text{ L} \cdot \text{min}^{-1}$

Subject No. 4

$\dot{V}_I$STPD =

$75 \text{ L} \cdot \text{min}^{-1} \left(\dfrac{273°}{273° + 24°} \right) \times \left(\dfrac{739 \, [0.25 \times 22.4] \text{ mmHg}}{760} \right)$

$= 66.52 \text{ L} \cdot \text{min}^{-1}$

3. **Subject No. 1**

$\dot{V}_I$STPD =

$39.86 \text{ L} \cdot \text{min}^{-1} \left(\dfrac{1 - [0.1608 + 0.0494]}{0.7904} \right)$

$= 39.83$

Subject No. 3

$\dot{V}_I$STPD $= 114.25 \text{ L} \cdot \text{min}^{-1} \left(\dfrac{1 - [0.1604 + 0.0512]}{0.7904} \right)$

$= 113.96$

4. **Subject No. 2**

$\dot{V}_E$STPD $= 62.13 \text{ L} \cdot \text{min}^{-1} \left(\dfrac{0.7904}{1 - [0.1620 + 0.0510]} \right)$

$= 61.93$

Subject No. 4

$\dot{V}_E$ STPD $= 66.52 \text{ L} \cdot \text{min}^{-1} \left(\dfrac{0.7904}{1 - [0.1675 + 0.0473]} \right)$

$= 66.96 \text{ L} \cdot \text{min}^{-1}$

5. **Subject No. 1**

$\dot{V}O_2$cons $= (0.2093 \times 39.83 \text{ L} \cdot \text{min}^{-1})$

$- (0.1609 \times 39.86 \text{ L} \cdot \text{min}^{-1}) = 1.93 \text{ L} \cdot \text{min}^{-1}$

$= 1930 \text{ mL} \cdot \text{min}^{-1} \div 49.1 \text{ kg}$

$= 39.31 \text{ mL} \cdot \text{kg}^{-1} \cdot \text{min}^{-1}$

Subject No. 2

$\dot{V}O_2cons = (0.2093 \times 62.13 \text{ L} \cdot \text{min}^{-1})$

$- (0.1620 \times 61.93 \text{ L} \cdot \text{min}^{-1}) = 2.97 \text{ L} \cdot \text{min}^{-1}$

$= 2970 \text{ mL} \cdot \text{min}^{-1} \div 60 \text{ kg}$

$= 49.52 \text{ mL} \cdot \text{kg}^{-1} \cdot \text{min}^{-1}$

Subject No. 3

$\dot{V}O_2cons = (0.2093 \times 113.96 \text{ L} \cdot \text{min}^{-1})$

$- (0.1604 \times 114.25 \text{ L} \cdot \text{min}^{-1}) = 5.53 \text{ L} \cdot \text{min}^{-1}$

$= 5530 \text{ mL} \cdot \text{min}^{-1} \div 79.55 \text{ kg}$

$= 69.52 \text{ mL} \cdot \text{kg}^{-1} \cdot \text{min}^{-1}$

Subject No. 4

$\dot{V}O_2cons = (0.2093 \times 66.52 \text{ L} \cdot \text{min}^{-1})$

$- (0.1675 \times 66.96 \text{ L} \cdot \text{min}^{-1}) = 2.71 \text{ L} \cdot \text{min}^{-1}$

$= 2710 \text{ mL} \cdot \text{min}^{-1} \div 91.36 \text{ kg}$

$= 29.66 \text{ mL} \cdot \text{kg}^{-1} \cdot \text{min}^{-1}$

6. Subject No. 1

$\dot{V}CO_2prod = (0.0494 \times 39.86 \text{ L} \cdot \text{min}^{-1})$

$= 1.97 \text{ L} \cdot \text{min}^{-1}$

Subject No. 2

$\dot{V}CO_2prod = (0.0501 \times 61.93 \text{ L} \cdot \text{min}^{-1})$

$= 3.10 \text{ L} \cdot \text{min}^{-1}$

Subject No. 3

$\dot{V}CO_2prod = (0.0512 \times 114.25 \text{ L} \cdot \text{min}^{-1})$

$= 5.85 \text{ L} \cdot \text{min}^{-1}$

Subject No. 4

$\dot{V}CO_2prod = (0.0473 \times 66.96 \text{ L} \cdot \text{min}^{-1})$

$= 3.17 \text{ L} \cdot \text{min}^{-1}$

7. Subject No. 1

$\dot{V}O_2cons = 90 \text{ m} \cdot \text{min}^{-1} \times \dfrac{0.1 \text{ mL} \cdot \text{kg}^{-1} \cdot \text{min}^{-1}}{\text{m} \cdot \text{min}^{-1}}$

$+ 3.5 \text{ mL} \cdot \text{kg}^{-1} \cdot \text{min}^{-1} + 0.11 \times 90 \text{ m} \cdot \text{min}^{-1}$

$\times \dfrac{1.8 \text{ mL} \cdot \text{kg}^{-1} \cdot \text{min}^{-1}}{\text{m} \cdot \text{min}^{-1}} = 30.32 \text{ mL} \cdot \text{kg}^{-1} \cdot \text{min}^{-1}$

8. Subject No. 2

$\dot{V}O_2cons = 161 \text{ m} \cdot \text{min}^{-1} \times \dfrac{0.2 \text{ mL} \cdot \text{kg}^{-1} \cdot \text{min}^{-1}}{\text{m} \cdot \text{min}^{-1}}$

$+ 3.5 \text{ mL} \cdot \text{kg}^{-1} \cdot \text{min}^{-1} = 35.7 \text{ mL} \cdot \text{kg}^{-1} \cdot \text{min}^{-1}$

9. Subject No. 3

$\dot{V}O_2cons = \left[\dfrac{1.8 \text{ mL} \cdot \text{kg}^{-1} \cdot \text{min}^{-1}}{\text{m} \cdot \text{min}^{-1}} \times (4 \text{ kg} \times 6 \text{ m} \cdot \text{rev}^{-1} \right.$

$\left. \times 80 \text{ rev} \cdot \text{min}^{-1}) \div 79.55 \text{ kg} \right]$

$+ 7 \text{ mL} \cdot \text{kg}^{-1} \cdot \text{min}^{-1}$

$= 50.44 \text{ mL} \cdot \text{kg}^{-1} \cdot \text{min}^{-1}$

Subject No. 4

$\dot{V}O_2cons = \left[\dfrac{3 \text{ mL} \cdot \text{kg}^{-1} \cdot \text{min}^{-1}}{\text{m} \cdot \text{min}^{-1}} \times (3 \text{ kg} \times 2.4 \text{ m} \cdot \text{rev}^{-1} \right.$

$\left. \times 50 \text{ rev} \cdot \text{min}^{-1}) \div 91.4 \text{ kg} \right]$

$+ 3.5 \text{ mL} \cdot \text{kg}^{-1} \cdot \text{min}^{-1}$

$= 15.32 \text{ mL} \cdot \text{kg}^{-1} \cdot \text{min}^{-1}$

10. Subject No. 2

$\dot{V}O_2cons = \left[\dfrac{0.2 \text{ mL} \cdot \text{kg}^{-1} \cdot \text{min}^{-1}}{\text{m} \cdot \text{min}^{-1}} \times 30 \text{ steps} \cdot \text{min}^{-1} \right]$

$+ \left[1.33 \times \dfrac{1.8 \text{ mL} \cdot \text{kg}^{-1} \cdot \text{min}^{-1}}{\text{m} \cdot \text{min}^{-1}} \times 0.305 \text{ m} \cdot \text{step} \right.$

$\left. \times 30 \text{ steps} \cdot \text{min}^{-1} \right] + 3.5 \text{ mL} \cdot \text{kg}^{-1} \cdot \text{min}^{-1}$

$= 31.41 \text{ mL} \cdot \text{kg}^{-1} \cdot \text{min}^{-1}$

11. Subject No. 1 PACER $\dot{V}O_2$max (Eq. B.17)

$\dot{V}O_2max = 31.025 + 3.238 (10) - 3.248 (15)$

$+ 0.1536 (10 \times 15)$

$= 37.73 \text{ mL} \cdot \text{kg}^{-1} \cdot \text{min}^{-1}$

Subject No. 2 PACER $\dot{V}O_2$max (Eq. B.18)

$\dot{V}O_2max = -23.4 + 5.8(12.5) = 49.1 \text{ mL} \cdot \text{kg}^{-1} \cdot \text{min}^{-1}$

REFERENCES

American College of Sports Medicine: *Guidelines for Exercise Testing and Prescription* (8th edition). Philadelphia, PA: Lippincott Williams & Williams (2010).

Jackson, A. S.: Application of regression analysis to exercise science. In Safrit, M. J. & T. M. Wood (eds.): *Measurement Concepts in Physical Education and Exercise Science.* Champaign, IL: Human Kinetics (1989).

Kline, G. M., J. P. Porcari, R. Huntermeister, et al.: Estimation of $\dot{V}O_2$max from a one mile track walk, gender, age, and body weight. *Medicine and Science in Sports and Exercise.* 19:253–259 (1987).

Leger, L. A., D. Mercier, C. Gadoury, & J. Lambert: The multi-stage 20 metre shuttle run test for aerobic fitness. *Journal of Sport Sciences.* 6:93–101 (1988).

McSwegin, P. J., S. A. Plowman, G. M. Wolff, & G. L. Guttenburg: The validity of a one-mile walk test for high school age individuals. *Measurement in Physical Education and Exercise Science.* 2(1):47–63 (1998).

Plowman, S. A. & N. Y-S. Liu: Norm-reference and criterion-referenced validity of the one-mile run and PACER in college age individuals. *Measurement in Physical Education and Exercise Science.* 3:63–84 (1999).

Appendix C

Answers to Check Your Comprehension

CHAPTER 1

Check Your Comprehension 1

1. Static exercise
2. Static exercise
3. Short-term, light to moderate submaximal aerobic exercise
4. Incremental aerobic exercise to maximum
5. Long-term, moderate to heavy submaximal aerobic exercise
6. Very short-term, high-intensity anaerobic exercise
7. Dynamic resistance exercise
8. Long-term, moderate to heavy submaximal aerobic exercise
9. Incremental aerobic exercise to maximum
10. Short-term, light to moderate submaximal aerobic exercise
11. Dynamic resistance exercise
12. Very short-term, high-intensity anaerobic exercise

Check Your Comprehension 2

Pattern (c) is the best. This incorporates step loading with recovery/rejuvenation microcycles programmed into the overload progression. Pattern (b) remains for too long at one level and makes too large a jump between levels. Pattern (a) progresses in small increments but does not plan for any rest or recovery cycles. Overtraining is most likely to occur in individuals when large increases in training occur abruptly and when the rest and recovery periods included in the periodization program are insufficient.

Check Your Comprehension 3 (Case Study)

These responses may be discussed in any order.

1. Specificity—While cross-training can be good, Mark has insufficient specificity in his workouts to improve his 10-km time. His workouts are also too short as his race time shows.
   Suggestion: Mark needs to increase the number of days per week that he runs to at least 3; he also needs to gradually increase the distance he runs.

2. Overload—Mark's workouts are sufficient to maintain his fitness as indicated by his lack of change in his race time from the previous year. However, they are insufficient to improve his fitness and hence his time.
   Suggestion: Mark needs to prepare a miniperiodization steploading plan (remembering that he has only 3 months until the Turkey Trot) and follow it.
   Note: This may be stated in reverse as the maintenance principle with the suggestions being to overload.

3. Progression—There is no indication that Mark has any progression in either the intensity or the duration of his workouts.
   Suggestion: Mark needs to use steploading to progress to at least 10-km distance; he also needs to insert some high-intensity speed workouts.

4. Individualization—By letting Kristi set the pace, the training was individualized for her, but not for Mark.
   Suggestion: Mark and Kristi need to do at least some of their weekly workouts separately—perhaps in the same area but at individual paces.

CHAPTER 2

Check Your Comprehension 1

See **Table 2.1**.

Check Your Comprehension 2

The theoretical number of ATP produced from the 18-carbon fatty acid stearate.

1. $n/2 - 1 = 18/2 - 1 = 8$ cycles of beta-oxidation
2. $FADH2 = 8 \times 2$ ATP $= 16$ ATP
   $NADH2 = 8 \times 3$ ATP $= 24$ ATP
   8×5 ATP $= 40$ ATP
3. Acetyl CoA $= 9$:
   9×12 ATP $= 108$ ATP
4. Activation energy $= -2$ ATP
5. Total: 108 ATP
   $\underline{+ 40 \text{ ATP}}$
   148 ATP
   $\underline{-2 \text{ ATP}}$
   146 ATP

The actual number of ATP produced from the 18-carbon fatty acid stearate.

1. $n/2 - 1 = 18/2 - 1 = 8$ cycles of beta-oxidation
2. $FADH2 = 8 \times 1.5$ ATP $= 12$ ATP
   $NADH2 = 8 \times 2.5$ ATP $= 20$ ATP
   8×4 ATP $= 32$ ATP
3. Acetyl CoA $= 9$:
   9×10 ATP $= 90$ ATP
4. Activation energy $= -2$ ATP
5. Total: 90 ATP
   $\underline{+ 32}$ ATP
   122 ATP
   $\underline{-2}$ ATP
   120 ATP

CHAPTER 3

Recommend that this client do aerobic activity first, followed by resistance activity.

This sequence does cause a slightly larger EPOC, elevation in energy expenditure, for the first 10 min of recovery. This is unlikely to even be noticed by the exerciser. However, on the basis of the significantly higher HR and $\dot{V}O_2$ measures during the RE-RU sequence, it is easier physiologically to do the run first. If resistance work is done first, it could negatively impact the adherence of the beginning exerciser. Conversely, if a client were interested primarily in weight control and had been training consistently for some time, more calories would be burned doing the resistance activity before the aerobic activity.

CHAPTER 4

Check Your Comprehension 1

Yes, this is a true max. RER $= 1.34$ (>1.1 criterion level); HR $= 200$ b·min^{-1} (predicted $220 - 22 = 198 \pm 12 = 186 - 210$); $\dot{V}O_2$ mL·kg^{-1}·min^{-1} difference minutes $27 - 28 = 2.07$ (less than half the expected 5.8 mL·kg^{-1}·min^{-1}); $\dot{V}O_2$ reaches a plateau.

Check Your Comprehension 2

Minute 2:   RER $= 0.99$;   CHO $= 96.6\%$;   FAT $= 3.4\%$
Minute 14: RER $= 0.96$;   CHO $= 86.4\%$;   FAT $= 13.6\%$
Minute 28: RER $= 1.34$;   CHO $= 100\%$

Check Your Comprehension 3

RER $= 0.96$
$\dot{V}O_2$ L·min$^{-1} = 2.36$
kcal·L $O_2^{-1} = 4.998$ (from **Table 5.4**)
4.998 kcal·L $O_2^{-1} \times 2.36$ L O_2·min$^{-1} = 11.80$ kcal·min^{-1}
11.80 kcal·min$^{-1} \times 4.18$ kJ·kcal$^{-1} = 49.30$ kJ·min^{-1}

Check Your Comprehension 4

1200 mL·min^{-1} $O_2 = 1.2$ L·min^{-1} O_2
1.2 L·min$^{-1} \times 5$ kcal·L$^{-1} = 6$ kcal·min^{-1}
300 kcal/6 kcal·min$^{-1} = 50$ min

Check Your Comprehension 5

$$\frac{35.75 \text{ mL} \cdot \text{kg}^{-1} \cdot \text{min}^{-1}}{3.5 \text{ mL} \cdot \text{kg}^{-1} \cdot \text{min}^{-1}} = 10.21 \text{ METs}$$

Check Your Comprehension 6

Computing the $\%\dot{V}O_2$ values for the given oxygen costs of each individual at each speed, we get:

Oxygen Cost	Daughter	Son	Mother	Father	Grand-mother
10 min·mi^{-1}	77	78	60	62	83
9 min·mi^{-1}	83	86	64	65	90
8 min·mi^{-1}	94	98	76	79	100
7 min·mi^{-1}	100	100	86	88	—

Therefore, the family could probably stay together easily at a 10-min·mi^{-1} pace, a little less easily because of the grandmother's 9-min·mi^{-1} pace. Perhaps grandmother and the kids should run together somewhere between 9-min·mi^{-1} and 10-min·mi^{-1} and let mom and dad go faster.

CHAPTER 5

The shift to a higher amount and percentage of aerobic metabolism as a result of the warm-up is beneficial because when more oxygen is available sooner, less reliance is placed on anaerobic metabolism, and less lactate accumulates at any given heavy workload. The dancers should be able to perform longer before feeling the consequences of the H^+ from lactic acid.

CHAPTER 6

Rank order for the glycemic load (GL) (from lowest to highest):

1. Gatorade $= 16.7$; 2. Snickers bar $= 20.7$; 3. Banana $= 25.3$; 4. Bagel $= 36.1$; 5. Pizza (supreme) $= 37.4$; 6. Power Bar (chocolate) $= 39.0$

The calculation of glycemic load (GL) alters the impact of some foods, but not others. For example, Gatorade has the highest GI but the lowest GL; the pizza has the lowest GI but next to the highest GL. Both the banana and the Power Bar have moderate GI, but the banana has a moderate GL and the Power Bar the highest GL among the selected foods. Conversely, the bagel has both a high GI and GL, whereas the Snickers bar has both a low GI and GL. This occurs because of the higher number of grams of CHO in the typical portion of some foods than others.

CHAPTER 7

1. $M_A = 112 \text{ lb} \div 2.2 \text{ lb·kg}^{-1} = 50.91 \text{ kg}$
2. Selected weight from underwater trials
   8.35 kg (trial 4) is the highest weight, but it was only obtained once, not more than twice as specified in the selection criteria, so it cannot be used. 8.325 kg is the second-highest obtained weight, and it is observed more than once (trials 6 and 8), so it is the selected representative weight. 8.325 kg – 7.06 kg = 1.265 kg M_W.
3. $$D_B = \frac{50.91 \text{ kg}}{[(50.91 \text{ kg} - 1.265 \text{ kg}) \div 9941] - (1.2274\text{L} + 0.1 \text{ L})}$$

   $D_B = 1.0473 \text{ g·cc}^{-1}$
   %BF $= [4.570 \div 1.0473] - 4.142 \times 100 = 22.2\%$
4. FFW $= 112 \text{ lb} \times [100 - 22.2 \div 100] = 87.14 \text{ lb}$
   $WT_2 = [(100 \times 87.14) \div (100\% - 19\%)] = 107.58 \text{ lb}$
   $\Delta WT = 107.58 \text{ lb} - 112 \text{ lb} = -4.42 \text{ lb}$
5. Phyllis needs to lose approximately 4.5 lb to have 19% BF, assuming she maintains her muscle mass (FFW).

CHAPTER 8

Check Your Comprehension 1

Danladi: HT $= 6'2'' = 74 \text{ in} \times 2.54 \text{ cm·in}^{-1} = 187.96 \text{ cm}$
$\qquad = 188 \text{ cm}$
$\qquad$ WT $= 191 \text{ lb} \div 2.2 \text{ lb·kg}^{-1} = 86.8 \text{ kg}$
$\qquad$ RMR $= 88.362 + (4.799 \times \text{HT cm}) + (13.397 \times \text{WT kg})$
$\qquad\qquad - (5.677 \times \text{age yr})$
$\qquad = 88.362 + (4.799 \times 188) + (13.397 \times 86.8)$
$\qquad\qquad - (5.677 \times 48)$
$\qquad = 1881.2 \text{ kcal·d}^{-1}$

RMR PAL $= 1.4$; $1.6 - 1.4 = 0.2$; $0.2 \times 1881.2 \text{ kcal·d}^{-1} = 376.24 \text{ kcal·d}^{-1}$, more physical activity needed

Basketball $= 6$ METs
$\qquad$ 1 MET $= 1 \text{ kcal·kg}^{-1}\text{·hr}^{-1} \div 60 \text{ min·hr}^{-1} = \text{kcal·min}^{-1}$
$\qquad$ 6 MET $= 6 \text{ kcal·kg}^{-1}\text{·hr}^{-1} \times 86.8 \text{ kg} \div 60 \text{ min·hr}^{-1}$
$\qquad\qquad = 8.68 \text{ kcal·min}^{-1}$
376.24 kcal·d$^{-1} \div 8.68$ kcal·min$^{-1} = 43$ min·d^{-1}

Walking $= 3.3$ METs
$\qquad$ 1 MET $= 1 \text{ kcal·kg}^{-1}\text{·hr}^{-1} \div 60 \text{ min·hr}^{-1} = \text{kcal·min}^{-1}$
$\qquad$ 3.3 MET $= 3.3 \text{ kcal·kg}^{-1}\text{·hr}^{-1} \times 86.8 \text{ kg} \div 60 \text{ min·hr}^{-1}$
$\qquad\qquad = 4.77 \text{ kcal·min}^{-1}$
$\qquad$ 376.24 kcal·d$^{-1} \div 4.77$ kcal·min$^{-1} = 78.9$ min $= 79$ min
$\qquad$ 3.3 METs $= 3.0$ mi·hr^{-1}; 60 min·hr$^{-1} \div 3.0 = 20$ min·mi^{-1};
$\qquad$ 78 min $\div 20$ min·mi$^{-1} = 3.95$ mi

Most of the physical activities should come from sports or planned physical activity because the professor's job is primarily sedentary. Higher MET level activities will allow him to spend less time in activity.

Check Your Comprehension 2

Zachary's weight should be 132 lb. He needs to lose 6 lb. These results are computed as follows using Equation 8.2.

DB $= 1.0982 - [0.000815 (8 + 9 + 12) + 0.0000084$
$\qquad (8 + 9 + 12)^2]$
$\qquad = 1.0982 - [0.023635 + 0.0070644]$
$\qquad = 1.0982 - 0.0306994 = 1.0675 \text{ g·cc}^{-1}$

For a 14-year-old male, the %BF formula from **Table 7.1** is

$\qquad$ %BF $= ([5.07 \div 1.0675] - 4.64) \times 100 = 10.9$

Using Equation 7.4

$\qquad$ FFW $= 138 \text{ lb} \times ([100\% - 10.9\%] \div 100) = 123 \text{ lb}$

Zachary should wrestle at no less than 7%BF with a weight loss not exceeding 7% of body weight. Using Equation 7.5

$\qquad$ $WT_2 = ([100\% \times 123 \text{ lb}] \div [100\% - 7\%]) = 132.26 \text{ lb}$

Using Equation 7.6

$\qquad$ 132 lb $-$ 138 lb $= -6$ lb

CHAPTER 9

Check Your Comprehension 1

1. Pattern A: Alveolar ventilation

   $[(600 \text{ mL·br}^{-1}) - (150 \text{ mL·br}^{-1})] \times (10 \text{ br·min}^{-1})$
   $= (450 \text{ mL·br}^{-1}) \times (10 \text{ br·min}^{-1}) = 4500 \text{ mL·min}^{-1}$
   $\qquad \div 1000 \text{ mL·L}^{-1}$
   $= 4.5 \text{ L·min}^{-1}$

   Pattern B: Alveolar ventilation

   $[(200 \text{ mL·br}^{-1}) - (150 \text{ mL·br}^{-1})] \times (30 \text{ br·min}^{-1})$
   $= (50 \text{ mL·br}^{-1}) \times (30 \text{ br·min}^{-1}) = 1500 \text{ mL·min}^{-1}$
   $\qquad \div 1000 \text{ mL·L}^{-1}$
   $= 1.5 \text{ L·min}^{-1}$

   At identical minute ventilations, alveolar ventilation is greatly reduced as the depth (tidal volume) of the ventilation decreases. Increasing the frequency of breathing does not compensate for a small tidal volume at the alveolar level. Therefore, shallow, frequent breathing is not as effective as deep, infrequent breathing.

2. Both situations decrease alveolar ventilation. When tidal volume is low, as when trying to inhale without exhaling first or in taking short, quick gulps of air, the volume of the dead space has a negative impact on the amount of air available for exchange (the alveolar ventilation). This result is seen in the calculations in

problem 1. Inadequate alveolar ventilation can lead to dizziness or unconsciousness, which are dangerous situations, especially in water.

3. A snorkel extends the dead space. Thus, the tidal volume must be increased sufficiently to compensate for that volume as well as the anatomical dead space to maintain effective alveolar ventilation.

Check Your Comprehension 2

Site	PO_2	PCO_2
Alveoli	104 mmHg	
Pulmonary capillary	40 mmHg, arterial end; 104 mmHg, venous end	
Left side of heart	95 mmHg	
Systemic arteries	95 mmHg	40 mmHg
Tissue (resting)	40 mmHg	45 mmHg
Systemic capillary	95 mmHg, arterial end; 40 mmHg, venous end	40 mmHg, arterial end; 45 mmHg, venous end
Systemic veins	40 mmHg	45 mmHg
Right side of heart	40 mmHg	45 mmHg
Pulmonary artery	40 mmHg	45 mmHg
Alveoli		40 mmHg
Pulmonary capillary		45 mmHg, arterial end; 40 mmHg, venous end
Left side of heart		40 mmHg

Check Your Comprehension 3

HbO_2 $mLO_2 \cdot dL^{-1}$ = Hb $gm \cdot dL^{-1} \times 1.34$ $mLO_2 \cdot gmHb^{-1}$
$\times SbO_2\%$(as decimal)
Last year: $13.2 \times 1.34 \times 0.97 = 17.16$ $mLO_2 \cdot dL^{-1}$
This year: $11.9 \times 1.34 \times 0.97 = 15.47$ $mLO_2 \cdot dL^{-1}$

The difference in oxygen-carrying capacity between this year and last is 17.16 $mLO_2 \cdot dL^{-1}$ − 15.47 $mLO_2 \cdot dL^{-1}$ = 1.69 $mLO_2 \cdot dL^{-1}$ or a reduction of almost 10%.

CHAPTER 10

Check Your Comprehension 1

1. Marathon; 2. 10,000 m; 3. 400 m high hurdles; 4. 100 m sprint; 5. Shot put

The greatest impact will be seen in those events involving the largest dependence on oxygen transport and utilization over the longest period of time because of the decrease in $SaO_2\%$ and PaO_2 at altitude. The last three are basically anaerobic events. The last two may even show an improved performance at altitude as the air resistance is lowered.

Check Your Comprehension 2

Both exercise-induced arterial hypoxemia and altitude decrease maximal exercise performance. The common mechanism is a decrease in $SaO_2\%$ and PaO_2.

CHAPTER 11

Check Your Comprehension 1

1.

Normal	**Increased sympathetic nervous stimulation**
EDV = 150; SV ~ 80 $mL \cdot b^{-1}$	EDV = 150; SV ~ 90 $mL \cdot b^{-1}$
EDV = 200; SV~ 100 $mL \cdot b^{-1}$	EDV = 200; SV ~ 105 $mL \cdot b^{-1}$
EDV = 250; SV ~ 105 $mL \cdot b^{-1}$	EDV = 250; SV ~ 112 $mL \cdot b^{-1}$
EDV = 300; SV ~ 95 $mL \cdot b^{-1}$	EDV = 250; SV ~ 110 $mL \cdot b^{-1}$

2.

$EF = \dfrac{80}{150} = 53.3\%$ $EF = \dfrac{90}{150} = 60\%$

$EF = \dfrac{100}{200} = 50\%$ $EF = \dfrac{105}{200} = 52.5\%$

$EF = \dfrac{105}{250} = 42\%$ $EF = \dfrac{112}{250} = 44.8\%$

$EF = \dfrac{95}{300} = 31.7\%$ $EF = \dfrac{110}{250} = 44\%$

Check Your Comprehension 2

	HR (b·min⁻¹)	SV (mL·b⁻¹)	$\dot{Q}$(L·min⁻¹)
Mike	80	90	**7.20**
Keiko	60	120	**7.20**
Kirk	122	146.5	**17.87**
Don	72	**88.05**	6.34
Nora	**58**	98	5.68

Check Your Comprehension 3

PP = SBP − DBP = 150 − 90 = 60 mmHg

$MAP = \dfrac{PP}{3} + DBP = \dfrac{60}{3} + 90 = 110$ mmHg

$TPR = \dfrac{MAP}{\dot{Q}} = \dfrac{110 \text{ mmHg}}{5.1 \text{ L} \cdot \text{min}^{-1}} = 21.57$

CHAPTER 12

Check Your Comprehension 1

Condition	MAP (mmHg)	TPR (units)	RPP (units)
Rest	102*	17.0	107
Light aerobic	118†	11.8	195
Heavy aerobic	129†	9.9	263
Maximal aerobic	144†	9.6	360
Sustained static	155†	19.4	284
Dynamic resistance exercise	136†	13.6	227
*Use Equation 11.5a.			
†Use Equation 11.5b.			

Check Your Comprehension 2

No, exercise prescriptions should be adjusted when an individual is doing upper body exercise. Upper body exercise, particularly when it involves a static component, leads to greater sympathetic stimulation than occurs during lower body exercise and results in higher blood pressure and total peripheral resistance.

CHAPTER 13

Check Your Comprehension 1

%HRmax Method

Mei:
estimated HRmax = 220 − 50 = 170 b·min^{-1}
Training HR = 170 × 0.57 = 97 b·min^{-1}
Training HR = 170 × 0.63 = 107 b·min^{-1}
On the basis of the % HRmax method, a light exercise for Mei elicits a heart rate between 97 and 107 b·min^{-1}.

Serena:
estimated HRmax = 220 − 60 = 160 b·min^{-1}
Training HR = 160 × 0.57 = 91 b·min^{-1}
Training HR = 160 × 0.63 = 101 b·min^{-1}
Using the % HRmax method, a light exercise for Serena elicits a heart rate between 91 and 101 b·min^{-1}.

% HRR Method

Mei:
estimated HRmax = 220 − 50 = 170 b·min^{-1}
Training HHR = [(170 − 62) × 0.30] + 62 = 94 b·min^{-1}
Training HHR = [(170 − 62) × 0.39] + 62 = 104 b·min^{-1}
On the basis of the % HHR method, a light exercise for Mei elicits a heart rate between 94 and 104 b·min^{-1}.

Serena:
estimated HRmax = 220 − 60 = 160 b·min^{-1}
Training HHR = [(160 − 82) × 0.30] + 82 = 105 b·min^{-1}
Training HHR = [(160 − 82) × 0.39] + 82 = 112 b·min^{-1}
Using the % HHR method, a light exercise for Serena elicits a heart rate between 105 and 112 b·min^{-1}.

Check Your Comprehension 2

1. A moderate workout represents 40–59% $\dot{V}O_2R$ or HRR.

Individual	40%	59%
Janet	52 mL·kg^{-1}·min^{-1}	52 mL·kg^{-1}·min^{-1}
	−3.5 mL·kg^{-1}·min^{-1}	− 3.5 mL·kg^{-1}·min^{-1}
	48.5 mL·kg^{-1}·min^{-1}	48.5 mL·kg^{-1}·min^{-1}
	× 0.4	× 0.59
	19.4 mL·kg^{-1}·min^{-1}	28.6 mL·kg^{-1}·min^{-1}
	+3.5 mL·kg^{-1}·min^{-1}	± 3.5 mL·kg^{-1}·min^{-1}
	22.9 mL·kg^{-1}·min^{-1}	32.1 mL·kg^{-1}·min^{-1}
Juan	64 mL·kg^{-1}·min^{-1}	64 mL·kg^{-1}·min^{-1}
	−3.5 mL·kg^{-1}·min^{-1}	− 3.5 mL·kg^{-1}·min^{-1}
	60.5 mL·kg^{-1}·min^{-1}	60.5 mL·kg^{-1}·min^{-1}
	× 0.4	× 0.59
	24.2 mL·kg^{-1}·min^{-1}	35.7 mL·kg^{-1}·min^{-1}
	+3.5 mL·kg^{-1}·min^{-1}	± 3.5 mL·kg^{-1}·min^{-1}
	27.7 mL·kg^{-1}·min^{-1}	39.2 mL·kg^{-1}·min^{-1}
Mark	49 mL·kg^{-1}·min^{-1}	49 mL·kg^{-1}·min^{-1}
	−3.5 mL·kg^{-1}·min^{-1}	− 3.5 mL·kg^{-1}·min^{-1}
	45.5 mL·kg^{-1}·min^{-1}	45.5 mL·kg^{-1}·min^{-1}
	× 0.4	× 0.59
	18.2 mL·kg^{-1}·min^{-1}	26.9 mL·kg^{-1}·min^{-1}
	+3.5 mL·kg^{-1}·min^{-1}	± 3.5 mL·kg^{-1}·min^{-1}
	21.7 mL·kg^{-1}·min^{-1}	30.4 mL·kg^{-1}·min^{-1}
Gail	56 mL·kg^{-1}·min^{-1}	56 mL·kg^{-1}·min^{-1}
	−3.5 mL·kg^{-1}·min^{-1}	− 3.5 mL·kg^{-1}·min^{-1}
	52.5 mL·kg^{-1}·min^{-1}	52.5 mL·kg^{-1}·min^{-1}
	× 0.4	× 0.59
	21 mL·kg^{-1}·min^{-1}	31.0 mL·kg^{-1}·min^{-1}
	+3.5 mL·kg^{-1}·min^{-1}	± 3.5 mL·kg^{-1}·min^{-1}
	24.5 mL·kg^{-1}·min^{-1}	34.5 mL·kg^{-1}·min^{-1}

4 mph is too low for Juan. 7, 8, and 9 mph are too high for everyone. 6 mph is moderate only for Juan. 5 mph falls within the moderate range for all runners.

2. To determine the anticipated heart rate during the 5-mph run, first determine what percent $\dot{V}O_2$max (as a fraction) each individual is working at. Refer to the box in the chapter to find the $\dot{V}O_2$ for each individual and the oxygen cost of running 5 mph.

3. Rearrange the $TE\!\times\!\dot{V}O_2$ equation to solve for $\%\dot{V}O_2R$.

$$\%\dot{V}O_2R = \frac{Ex\dot{V}O_2 - \dot{V}O_2rest}{\dot{V}O_2R}$$

Janet:

$$\frac{30.3\ mL\cdot kg^{-1}\cdot min^{-1} - 3.5\ mL\cdot kg^{-1}\cdot min^{-1}}{52\ mL\cdot kg^{-1}\cdot min^{-1} - 3.5\ mL\cdot kg^{-1}\cdot min^{-1}} = \frac{26.8}{48.5} = 0.553$$

Juan:

$$\frac{30.3\ mL\cdot kg^{-1}\cdot min^{-1} - 3.5\ mL\cdot kg^{-1}\cdot min^{-1}}{64\ mL\cdot kg^{-1}\cdot min^{-1} - 3.5\ mL\cdot kg^{-1}\cdot min^{-1}} = \frac{26.8}{60.5} = 0.443$$

Mark:

$$\frac{30.3\ mL\cdot kg^{-1}\cdot min^{-1} - 3.5\ mL\cdot kg^{-1}\cdot min^{-1}}{49\ mL\cdot kg^{-1}\cdot min^{-1} - 3.5\ mL\cdot kg^{-1}\cdot min^{-1}} = \frac{26.8}{45.5} = 0.589$$

Gail:

$$\frac{30.3\ mL\cdot kg^{-1}\cdot min^{-1} - 3.5\ mL\cdot kg^{-1}\cdot min^{-1}}{56\ mL\cdot kg^{-1}\cdot min^{-1} - 3.5\ mL\cdot kg^{-1}\cdot min^{-1}} = \frac{26.8}{52.5} = 0.511$$

These percentages (as fractions) can then be used in the HRR equation.

Janet	Juan	
220	220	
− 23	− 35	Age (yr)
197	185	Predicted HRmax (b·min⁻¹)
− 60	− 48	RHR (b·min⁻¹)
137	137	
× 0.553	× 0.443	%$\dot{V}O_2$R = %HRR (b·min⁻¹)
76	61	
+ 60	+ 48	RHR (b·min⁻¹)
136	109	Exercise HR (b·min⁻¹)

Mark	Gail	
220	220	
− 22	− 28	Age (yr)
198	192	Predicted HRmax (b·min⁻¹)
− 64	− 58	RHR (b·min⁻¹)
134	134	
× 0.589	× 0.511	%$\dot{V}O_2$R = %HRR (b·min⁻¹)
79	69	
+ 64	± 58	RHR (b·min⁻¹)
143	127	Exercise HR (b·min⁻¹)

CHAPTER 14

Coach Brown should observe the temperature, humidity, degree of direct sunlight on the field, and degree to which the uniforms interfere with heat dissipation or increase absorption of radiant heat. He should assess environmental conditions (using WBGT or heat stress index) and adjust the practice appropriately. The coach should cancel practice or limit activity if conditions are extreme (see **Figure 14.1**). He can have some drills performed in the shade or devise drills that can be performed without full gear to lessen heat stress.

The coach should be mindful of the fitness level, degree of acclimatization, and hydration level of his players. He should develop a periodization plan for general conditioning for all potential players to follow during the summer and before reporting for formal practice. He should begin the season with limited practice/workouts including some that can be safely done without helmets until players become acclimatized to the heat. He must make sure that players are hydrated at the onset of practice by having players weigh in at the beginning of practice to ensure they do not have large fluctuations in daily weight attributable primarily to body water loss. Those whose weight loss appears to be hydration related need to be counseled about drinking throughout the day and possibly their NaCl intake checked. Water and sports drinks should be readily available during practice, and the coach should encourage drinking throughout practice and after practice. Coach Brown should also carefully monitor his player for signs and symptoms of heat stress and ensure that he has a way to cool and rehydrate any player he thinks may be suffering from early signs of heat illness. The culture of the team should encourage players to stop and seek shade and fluid if they feel any symptoms.

CHAPTER 15

The table below presents the CVD risk analysis for Vivian: How many total risk factors does Vivian have?
5

CHAPTER 16

1. Low-to-moderate impact-loading activities are recommended, including hiking, cross-country skiing, stair climbing activities on commercially available machines, and weight lifting. These are activities that promote bone health while minimizing the risk of injury.
2. High-impact-loading activities, such as sprinting, jumping, and soccer, would be recommended in order to promote the attainment of a high peak bone mass. High-impact activities increase the likelihood that an individual will attain her genetic potential for peak bone mass. She should also be careful to ensure adequate calcium intake in her diet.

CHAPTER 17

To determine the percentage of ST fibers, divide the number of ST fibers (~12) by the total number of fibers (~41) and multiply by 100. The percentage of FT fibers can also be determined by subtracting the percentage of ST fibers from 100. (Some staining techniques also permit the calculation of the percentage of the subcategories of FT [FOG and FG] using the same procedure as above, although this is not possible in this example.)

Total number of fibers = 41
Number of FT fibers = 12
Number of ST fibers = 29

$$\% \text{ of FT} = \frac{\text{Number of FT}}{\text{total fiber count}} \times 100$$

$$= \frac{12}{41} \times 100 = 29\%$$

$$\% \text{ of ST} = \frac{\text{Number of ST}}{\text{total fiber count}} \times 100$$

$$= \frac{29}{41} \times 100 = 71\%$$

CHAPTER 18

Check Your Comprehension 1

1. and 2.

Name	Absolute Strength MVC (kg)	Relative Strength (kg·kg⁻¹)	50% MVC
Jody	40.0	0.66	20.0
Jill	60.0	0.88	30.0
Pat	36.0	0.51	18.0
Scott	50.0	0.79	25.0
Tom	72.0	0.88	36.0
Mike	71.0	1.01	35.5

3. Tom; Mike
4. Tom

Name the Six Major Modifiable Risk Factors	Provide Cutoff Numerical Values Including Units for Each Risk Factor	Provide Values for Vivian from Her History and Determine Whether She Has This Risk Factor
Cigarette smoking	Currently or stopped <6 months	Stopped smoking only one month ago. Yes, has this risk factor
Hypertension	≥140/90 mmHg	124/82 mmHg. No, does not have this risk factor
Cholesterol-lipid fractions	≥240 mg·dL⁻¹ TC <40 mg·dL⁻¹ HDL	TC = 280 mg·dL⁻¹; HDL-C = 34 mg·dL⁻¹. Yes, has this risk factor
Impaired fasting glucose	≥100 mg·dL⁻¹ on two separate occasions	Fasting glucose = 116 and 118 mg·dL⁻¹. Yes, has this risk factor
Obesity	Waist/hip ratio >0.86 for female	95 cm/103 cm = 0.92. Yes, has this risk factor
Physically inactive/ sedentary lifestyle	No regular exercise program or less than SG recommendations	No regular exercise. Yes, has this risk factor

Check Your Comprehension 2

1. No, bending the knees (changing knee angle) does not eliminate the involvement of the thigh muscles. If the feet are supported (held down), the thigh muscles are more active than the rectus abdominis.
2. External obliques
3. Not held
4. From the available choices, you should have selected feet unsupported and knees bent at a 105° position in order to maximize the use of the abdominal muscles. These results indicate the best form of the sit-up from the standpoint of hip angle and foot support, but they do not take into account arm position. Also, they do not permit comparison with a curl-up or crunch (in which the head, shoulders, and trunk are lifted off the floor only about 30°). Other research has actually shown that the abdominal muscles are responsible for only the first 30–45° of the sit-up motion, and it is easier on the spinal discs if only a partial sit-up and not a full sit-up is performed. Combining this information, it must be concluded that on the basis of currently available information, a curl-up test with knees bent and feet unsupported is the exercise of choice for the abdominal muscles for most individuals.

CHAPTER 19

Check Your Comprehension 1

This player had indicated that her goal is to increase her strength during the preparation phase of her training. Since she is starting her fourth season as a forward, she should be considered intermediate or advanced in strength training. To maximize her strength gains she should perform multiple sets of 6–12 repetitions. For rest between sets, 1–2 minutes would be appropriate.

Check Your Comprehension 2

Lifts should be performed in the following order: power cleans, lat pull-downs, back squat, bench press, leg extension, shoulder press, calf raises, shrugs, sit-ups, and forearm curls

Check Your Comprehension 3

This woman has indicated that her goal is to gain muscle strength. Since she is just beginning a program, she should be considered a novice. You should therefore recommend that she becomes familiar with proper technique for each lift and then begin a program that includes all the major muscles of the body (probably 6–10 exercises). She should perform 1–3 sets of 8–12 reps at 60–70% of her 1-RM for each exercise. She should perform this exercise 2–3 d·wk^{-1}.

CHAPTER 20

1. A ballistic technique is to stand on a step and bounce on your toes so that your heal goes below step height and then above it. This exercise will not work on a level surface.
2. A static technique is the wall stretch. Extend one leg straight back and stretch it, with the other bent at the knee and forward. Hold the position.
3. A CR PNF technique is to assume the long sitting position, a jump rope (or a towel or sweats) around your foot in a neutral position. Resist a maximal isometric contraction of foot, attempting to plantarflex. Relax and pull your foot into dorsiflexion with the implement. Repeat.
4. A CRAC PNF technique is the same as the CR technique, except that you actively contract the shin muscles (dorsiflex). Repeat.

CHAPTER 21

Numerous hormones play a role in regulating metabolic responses to exercise, including insulin, glucagon, growth hormone, and cortisol. Collectively, these hormones maintain blood glucose, increase fuel (free fatty acids and glucose) availability, and enhance the oxidation of these fuels to provide energy to support increased muscular activity—in this case cycling.

CHAPTER 22

Check Your Comprehension 1

Nick's fall and the abrasion he received resulted in tissue damage and may have allowed a foreign antigen to enter the body. The swelling, redness, and pain were the result of the inflammatory process, a process mediated by several chemical factors (including cytokines, complement, histamines, and prostaglandins) that increase vasodilation and capillary permeability, and cause leukocytes to move to the site of injury. The inflammatory response helps to promote tissue repair by getting leukocytes to the damaged area so that they can ingest (and destroy) foreign invaders.

Check Your Comprehension 2

IL-6 is released primarily from skeletal muscle and thus is called *myo*kine. IL-6 plays a key regulatory role, helping to regulate pro- and anti-inflammatory responses to exercise and regulating glucose metabolism.

Glossary

Absolute Submaximal Workload A set exercise load performed at any intensity from just above resting to just below maximum.

Acclimatization The adaptive changes that occur when an individual undergoes prolonged or repeated exposure to a stressful environment; these changes reduce the physiological strain produced by such an environment.

Action Potential Reversal of polarity or change in electrical potential.

Adaptive Thermogenesis Either an increase or decrease in the efficiency of energy utilization.

Adenosine Triphosphate (ATP) Stored chemical energy that links the energy-yielding and energy-requiring functions within all cells.

Adequate Intake (AI) Used when an RDA cannot be determined. The AI is an estimate of intake by healthy individuals.

Aerobic In the presence of, requiring, or utilizing, oxygen.

Afterload Resistance presented to the contracting ventricle.

All-or-None Principle When a motor neuron is stimulated, all of the muscle fibers in that motor unit contract to their fullest extent or do not contract at all.

Alveolar Ventilation ($\dot{V}_A$) The volume of air available for gas exchange; calculated as tidal volume minus dead space volume times frequency.

Anaerobic In the absence of, not requiring, nor utilizing, oxygen.

Anorexia Athletica (AA) An eating disorder that is characterized by a food intake less than that required to support the training regimen and by a body weight less than 95% of normal.

Anorexia Nervosa (AN) An eating disorder characterized by marked self-induced weight loss accompanied by reproductive hormonal changes and an intense fear of fatness.

Apolipoprotein The protein portion of lipoproteins.

Archimedes' Principle The principle that a partially or fully submerged object will experience an upward bouyaut force equal to the weight on the volume of fluid displaced by the object.

Arteriosclerosis The natural aging changes that occur in blood vessels, including thickening of the walls, loss of elastic connective tissue, and hardening of the vessel wall.

Arteriovenous Oxygen Difference (a-vO$_2$diff) The difference between the amount of oxygen originally carried in arterial blood and the amount returned in venous blood.

Atherosclerosis A pathological process that results in the buildup of plaque inside blood vessels.

Ballistic Stretching A form of stretching, characterized by an action-reaction bouncing motion, in which the involved joints are placed into an extreme range of motion by fast, active contractions of agonistic muscle groups.

Basal Metabolic Rate (BMR) The level of energy required to sustain the body's vital functions in the waking state, when the individual is in a fasted condition, at normal body and room temperature, and without psychological stress.

Beta-Oxidation A cyclic series of steps that breaks off successive pairs of carbon atoms from FFA, which are then used to form acetyl CoA.

Body Composition The partitioning of body mass into FFM (weight or percentage) and fat mass (weight or percentage).

Body Mass Index (BMI) A ratio of the total body weight to height.

Bone Modeling The process of altering the shape of bone by bone resorption and bone deposition.

Bone Remodeling The continual process of bone breakdown (resorption) and formation (deposition of new bone).

Bulimia Nervosa (BN) An eating disorder marked by an unrealistic appraisal of body weight and/or shape that is manifested by alternating bingeing and purging behavior.

Caloric Balance Equation The mathematical summation of the caloric intake (+) and energy expenditure (−) from all sources.

Caloric Cost Energy expenditure of an activity performed for a specified period of time. It may be expressed as total calories (kcal) or calories or kilojoules per minute (kcal·min^{-1} or kJ·min^{-1}) or relative to body weight (kcal·kg^{-1}·min^{-1} or kJ·kg^{-1}·min^{-1}).

Caloric Equivalent The number of kilocalories produced per liter of oxygen consumed.

Calorimetry The measurement of heat energy liberated or absorbed in metabolic processes.

Capacitance Vessels Another name for veins because of their distensibility, which enables them to pool large volumes of blood and become reservoirs for blood.

Carbohydrate Loading (Glycogen Supercompensation) A process of nutritional modification that results in an additional storage of glycogen in muscle fiber up to two to three times the normal levels.

Carbon Dioxide Produced ($\dot{V}CO_2$) The amount or volume of carbon dioxide generated during metabolism.

Cardiac Cycle One complete sequence of contraction and relaxation of the heart.

Cardiac Output ($\dot{Q}$) The amount of blood pumped per unit of time, in liters per minute.

Cardiorespiratory Fitness The ability to deliver and use oxygen under the demands of intensive, prolonged exercise or work.

Cardiovascular Drift The changes in observed cardiovascular variables that occur during prolonged, heavy submaximal exercise without a change in workload.

Cellular Respiration The process by which cells transfer energy from food to ATP in a stepwise series of reactions. It relies heavily on the use of oxygen.

Central Cardiovascular Adaptations Adaptations that occur in the heart that increase the ability to deliver oxygen.

Central Cardiovascular Responses Responses directly related to the heart.

Cholesterol A derived fat that is essential for the body but may be detrimental in excessive amounts.

Coenzyme A nonprotein substance derived from a vitamin that activates an enzyme.

Concentric Contraction A dynamic muscle contraction that produces tension during shortening.

Concurrent Training The integration of endurance- and resistance-based training into a training program.

Contractility The ability of a muscle to respond to a stimulus by shortening; the force of contraction of the heart.

Contraction Tension-producing process of the contractile elements within muscle.

Coronary Heart Disease (CHD) Also called coronary artery disease or ischemic heart disease; results from damage to the coronary arteries supplying the heart muscle (myocardium).

Coupled Reactions Linked chemical processes in which a change in one substance is accompanied by a change in another.

Criterion Test The most accurate test for any given variable; the measurement standard against which other tests are judged.

Cross-Bridging Cycle The cyclic events necessary for the generation of force or tension within the myosin heads during muscle contraction.

Cross-Training The development or maintenance of cardiovascular fitness by alternating between or concurrently training in two or more modalities.

Cutting Decreasing body fat and body water content to very low levels in order to increase muscle definition.

Cytokines Proteins or peptides that are released from immune cells and other tissues (notably skeletal muscle and adipose tissue) and are involved in communication between immune cells (especially lymphocytes and phagocytes) and other cells of the body.

Delayed-Onset Muscle Soreness (DOMS) A condition characterized by muscle tenderness, pain on palpitation, and mechanical stiffness that appears approximately 8 hours after exercise, increases and peaks over the next 24–48 hours, and usually subsides within 96 hours.

Densitometry The measurement of mass per unit volume.

Detraining The partial or complete loss of training-induced adaptations as a result of a training reduction or cessation.

Diastole The relaxation phase of the cardiac cycle.

Diastolic Blood Pressure (DBP) The force exerted on the wall of blood vessels by blood during relaxation of the heart (diastole).

Diet (a) The food regularly consumed during the course of normal living; (b) a restriction of caloric intake.

Diffusion The tendency of gaseous, liquid, or solid molecules to move from an area of higher concentration to an area of lower concentration by constant random action.

Doppler Echocardiography A technique that calculates stroke volume from measurements of aortic cross-sectional area and time-velocity integrals in the ascending aorta.

Dose-Response relationship A description of how a change in one variable is associated with a corresponding change in another variable.

Dynamic Balance The ability to make necessary postural adjustments while the center of gravity and the base of support are in motion.

Dynamic Contraction A muscle contraction in which the force exerted varies as the muscle shortens to accommodate change in muscle length and/or joint angle throughout the range of motion while moving a constant external load.

Dyspnea Labored or difficult breathing.

Eating Disorders (ED) Disturbances of eating habits or weight-control behavior that can result in significant impairment of physical health or psychosocial functioning.

Eating Disorders Not Otherwise Specified (EDNOS) Conditions of disordered eating that do not meet the complete criteria for AN or BN.

Eccentric Contraction A dynamic muscle contraction that produces tension (force) while lengthening.

Economy The oxygen cost of any activity, but particularly walking or running at varying speeds.

Ejection Fraction (EF) The percentage of end diastolic volume (EDV) that is ejected from the heart.

Elasticity The ability of a muscle to return to resting length after being stretched.

Electrocardiogram (ECG) Tracing that provides a graphic illustration of the electrical current generated by excitation of the heart muscle.

Electromyography (EMG) The measurement of the neural or electrical activity that brings about muscle contraction.

Electron Transport System (ETS) The final metabolic pathway, which proceeds as a series of chemical reactions in the mitochondria that transfer electrons from the hydrogen atom carriers NAD and FAD to oxygen; water is formed as a by-product; the electrochemical energy released by the hydrogen ions is coupled to the formation of ATP from ADP and P_i.

End–Diastolic Volume (EDV) The volume of blood in the ventricle at the end of diastole.

Endothelium Single layer of epithelial tissue.

End–Systolic Volume (ESV) The volume of blood in the ventricle at the end of systole.

Energy Availability Dietary intake minus exercise energy expenditure.

Energy System Capacity The total amount of energy that can be produced by an energy system.

Energy System Power The maximal amount of energy that can be produced per unit of time.

Entrainment The synchronization of limb movement and breathing frequency that accompanies rhythmical exercise.

Enzyme A protein that accelerates the speed of a chemical reaction without itself being changed by the reaction.

Eupnea Normal respiration rate and rhythm.

Excess Postexercise Oxygen Consumption (EPOC) Oxygen consumption during recovery that is above normal resting values.

Exchange Vessels Another name for capillaries because this is the site of gas and nutrient exchange between the blood and tissues.

Excitation-Contraction Coupling The sequence of events by which an action potential in the sarcolemma initiates the sliding of the myofilaments, resulting in contraction.

Exercise A single acute bout of bodily exertion or muscular activity that requires an expenditure of energy above resting level and that in most, but not all, cases results in voluntary movement.

Exercise-Associated Hyponatremia (EAH) The occurrence of hyponatremia during or up to 24 hours after prolonged physical activity; it is diagnosed by a plasma sodium concentration below normal values (usually 135 mmol·L^{-1}).

Exercise-Induced Arterial Hypoxemia (EIAH) A condition in which the amount of oxygen carried in arterial blood is severely reduced by ≥4% consistently.

Exercise Modality or Mode The type of activity or sport; usually classified by energy demand or type of muscle action.

Exercise Physiology A basic and an applied science that describes, explains, and uses the body's response to exercise and adaptation to exercise training to maximize human physical potential.

Exercise Response The pattern of homeostatic disruption or change in physiological variables during a single acute bout of physical exertion.

Exertional Heat Exhaustion A moderate illness characterized by an inability to maintain adequate cardiac output at moderate (38.5°C/101.3°F) to high (>40°C/104°F) body temperatures.

Exertional Heat Illness (EHI) A range of multisystem illnesses related to elevated body core temperature and the cardiovascular and metabolic processes that result from exercise and the body's thermoregulatory response.

Exertional Heat Injury A moderate to severe progressive multisystem disorder, with hyperthermia accompanied by organ damage or severe dysfunction.

Exertional Heatstroke A life-threatening illness characterized by high body temperature and central nervous system dysfunction.

Extensibility The ability of a muscle to be stretched or lengthened.

External Respiration The exchange of gases between the lungs and the blood.

Fartlek Workout A type of training session, named from the Swedish word meaning "speed play," that combines the aerobic demands of a continuous run with the anaerobic demands of sporadic speed intervals.

Fast Glycolytic (FG, Type IIX or IIx) Fibers Fast-twitch muscle fibers that perform primarily under glycolytic conditions.

Fast Oxidative Glycolytic (FOG, Type IIA or IIa) Fibers Fast-twitch muscle fibers that can work under oxidative and glycolytic conditions.

Fat-Free Weight The weight of body tissue excluding extractable fat.

Fatigue Index (FI) Percentage of peak power drop-off during high-intensity, short-duration work.

Female Athlete Triad A syndrome of interrelated conditions including disordered eating, menstrual dysfunction, and skeletal demineralization.

Fick Equation An equation used to calculate cardiac output from oxygen consumption ($\dot{V}O_2$) and arteriovenous oxygen difference (a-vO_2diff).

Field Test A performance-based test that can be conducted anywhere and that estimates the values measured by the criterion test.

First Law of Thermodynamics or the Law of Conservation of Energy Energy can neither be created nor destroyed but only changed in form.

Flavin Adenine Dinucleotide (FAD) A hydrogen carrier in cellular respiration.

Flexibility The range of motion in a joint or series of joints that reflects the ability of the musculotendon structures to elongate within the physical limits of the joint.

Food Efficiency An index of the number of calories an individual needs to ingest to maintain a given weight or percent body fat.

Gluconeogenesis The creation of glucose in the liver from noncarbohydrate sources, particularly glycerol, lactate or pyruvate, and alanine.

Glycemic Index (GI) A measure that compares the elevation in blood glucose caused by the ingestion of 50 g of any carbohydrate food with the elevation caused by the ingestion of 50 g of white bread or glucose.

Glycogen Stored form of carbohydrate composed of chains of glucose molecules chemically linked together.

Glycogenolysis The process by which stored glycogen is broken down (hydrolyzed) to provide glucose.

Glycolysis The energy pathway responsible for the initial catabolism of glucose in a 10- or 11-step process that begins with glucose or glycogen and ends with the production of pyruvate (aerobic glycolysis) or lactate (anaerobic glycolysis).

Health-Related Physical Fitness That portion of physical fitness directed toward the prevention of or rehabilitation from disease, the development of a high level of functional capacity for the necessary and discretionary tasks of life, and the maintenance or enhancement of physiological functions in biological systems that are not involved in performance but are influenced by habitual activity.

Heart Rate (HR) The number of cardiac cycles per minute.

Heart Rate Variability The beat-to-beat variation in the time of the R to R intervals on a standard ECG.

Heat Strain The physiological responses and resulting thermoregulatory processes to combat heat stress.

Heat Stress The physical work and environmental components that combine to create heat load on an individual.

Heat Stress Index A scale used to determine the risk of heat stress from measures of ambient temperature and relative humidity.

Hematocrit The ratio of blood cells to total blood volume, expressed as a percentage.

Hemoglobin (Hb) The protein portion of the red blood cell that binds with oxygen, consisting of four iron-containing pigments called hemes and a protein called globin.

High-Density Lipoprotein (HDL-C) A lipoprotein in blood plasma composed primarily of protein and a minimum of cholesterol or triglyceride whose purpose is to transport cholesterol from the tissues to the liver.

Homeostasis The state of dynamic equilibrium (balance) of the internal environment of the body.

Hormones Chemical substances that originate in glandular tissue (or cells) and are transported through body fluids to a target cell to influence physiological activity.

Hydrolysis A chemical process in which a substance is split into simpler compounds by the addition of water.

Hydrostatic Weighing Criterion measure for determining body composition through the calculation of body density.

Hyperplasia Growth in a tissue or organ through an increase in the number of cells.

Hyperpnea Increased pulmonary ventilation that matches an increased metabolic demand, such as during exercise.

Hypertension High blood pressure, defined as adult values equal to or greater than 140/90 mmHg.

Hyperthermia The increase in body temperature with exercise.

Hyperventilation Increased pulmonary ventilation, especially ventilation that exceeds metabolic requirements; carbon dioxide is blown off, leading to a decrease in its partial pressure in arterial blood.

Hypokinetic Diseases Diseases caused by and/or associated with lack of physical activity.

Hypothermia A core temperature less than 35°C (95°F), resulting in the loss of normal function.

Immune System A precisely ordered system of cells, hormones, and chemicals that regulate susceptibility to, severity of, and recovery from infection and illness.

Impulse An electrical charge transmitted through certain tissue that results in the stimulation or inhibition of physiological activity.

Incidence The rate of new cases of a disease in a specific population.

Intercalated Discs The junction between adjacent cardiac muscle cells that forms a mechanical and electrical connection between cells.

Internal Respiration The exchange of gases between the blood and the tissues at the cellular level.

Interval Training An aerobic and/or anaerobic workout that consists of three elements: a selected work interval (usually a distance), a target time for that distance, and a predetermined recovery period before the next repetition of the work interval.

Irritability The ability of a muscle to receive and respond to stimuli.

Isokinematic Contraction A muscle contraction in which the rate of limb displacement or joint rotation is held constant with the use of specialized equipment.

Isokinetic Contraction A muscle fiber contraction in which the velocity of the contraction is kept constant.

Isometric Contraction A muscle fiber contraction that does not result in a length change in muscle fiber.

Isotonic Contraction A muscle fiber contraction in which the tension generated by the muscle fiber is constant through the range of motion.

Kilocalorie The amount of heat needed to raise the temperature of 1 kg of water by 1°C at 1 atmosphere.

Krebs Cycle A series of eight chemical reactions that begins and ends with the same substance; energy is liberated for direct substrate phosphorylation of ATP from ADP and P_i; carbon dioxide is formed and hydrogen atoms removed and carried by NAD and FAD to the electron transport system; does not directly utilize oxygen but requires its presence.

Laboratory Test Precise, direct measurement of physiological functions for the assessment of exercise responses or training adaptations; usually involves monitoring, collection, and analysis of expired air, blood, or electrical signals.

Lactate Thresholds Points on the linear-curvilinear continuum of lactate accumulation that appear to indicate sharp rises, often labeled as the first (LT1) and second (LT2) lactate threshold.

Leukocytosis An increase in circulating leukocytes (WBC).

Lipoprotein Water-soluble compound composed of apolipoprotein and lipid components that transport fat in the bloodstream.

Load Force exerted on the muscle.

Long Slow Distance (LSD) Workout A continuous aerobic training session performed at a steady-state pace for an extended time or distance.

Low-Density Lipoprotein (LDL-C) A lipoprotein in blood plasma composed of protein, a small portion of triglyceride, and a large portion of cholesterol whose purpose is to transport cholesterol to the cells.

Maximal (max) Exercise The highest intensity, greatest load, or longest duration exercise of which an individual is capable.

Maximal Lactate Steady State (MLSS) The highest workload that can be maintained over time without a continual rise in blood lactate; it indicates an exercise intensity above which lactate production exceeds clearance.

Maximal Oxygen Consumption ($\dot{V}O_2$max) The highest amount of oxygen an individual can take in, transport, and utilize to produce ATP aerobically while breathing air during heavy exercise.

Maximal Voluntary Contraction (MVC) The maximal force that the muscle can exert.

Mean Arterial Pressure (MAP) A weighted average of SBP and DBP, representing the mean driving force of blood throughout the arterial system.

Mean Power (MP) The average power (force times distance divided by time) exerted during short-duration (typically 30 sec) work.

Mechanical Efficiency The percentage of energy input that appears as useful external work.

Mechanotransduction The process by which a bone responds to a mechanical force on it.

MET A unit that represents the metabolic equivalent in multiples of the resting rate of oxygen consumption of any given activity.

Metabolic Pathway A sequence of enzyme-mediated chemical reactions resulting in a specified product.

Metabolism The total of all energy transformations that occur in the body.

Microcirculation Smallest vessels of the vascular system, including arterioles, true capillaries, arteriovenous anastomoses, metarterioles, and venules.

Minerals Elements, not of animal or plant origin, that are essential constituents of all cells and of many functions in the body.

Minute Ventilation or Minute Volume ($\dot{V}_I$ or $\dot{V}_E$) The amount of air inspired or expired each minute, or the pulmonary ventilation rate per minute; calculated as tidal volume times frequency of breathing.

Mitochondria Cell organelles in which the formation of acetyl CoA, Krebs cycle, electron transport, and oxidative phosphorylation take place.

Morbidity The number of people with a sickness or disease in a population.

Mortality The number of deaths in a population.

Motor Unit A motor neuron and the muscle fibers it innervates.

Muscle Tension Force developed when a contracting muscle acts on an object.

Muscle Tonus A state of low-level muscle contraction at rest.

Muscular Endurance The ability of a muscle or muscle group to repeatedly exert force against a resistance.

Myocardial Oxygen Consumption The amount of oxygen used by the heart muscle to produce energy for contraction.

Myocardium The heart muscle.

Myoclonus A twitching or spasm in a maximally stretched muscle group.

Myofibril Contractile organelles composed of myofilaments.

Myofilaments Contractile (thick and thin) proteins responsible for muscle contraction.

Neurotransmitters Chemical messengers with which neurons communicate with target cells of either other neurons or effector organs.

Nicotinamide Adenine Dinucleotide (NAD) A hydrogen carrier in cellular respiration.

Non–Weight-Bearing Exercise A movement performed in which the body weight is supported or suspended and thereby not working against the pull of gravity.

One Repetition Maximum (1 rep max; 1-RM) The most weight that can be lifted one time.

Osteoblasts Bone cells that cause the deposition of bone tissue (bone-forming cells).

Osteoclasts Bone cells that cause the resorption of bone tissue (bone-destroying cells).

Osteocytes Mature osteoblasts surrounded by calcified bone that help regulate the process of bone remodeling.

Osteopenia A condition of decreased bone mineral density (BMD), defined as a T-score of –1 to –2.5 which means a BMD value greater than one standard deviation (SD) below (but not more than 2.5 SD below) values for normal young adults.

Osteoporosis A condition of porosity and decreased bone mineral density, defined as a T-score below –2.5, which indicates a BMD greater than 2.5 SD below values for young, normal adults.

Overreaching (OR) A short-term decrement in performance capacity that generally lasts only a few days to 2 weeks and from which the individual easily recovers.

Overtraining Syndrome (OTS) A state of chronic decrement in performance and ability to train, in which restoration may take several weeks, months, or even years.

Oxidation A gain of oxygen, a loss of hydrogen, or the direct loss of electrons by an atom or substance.

Oxidative Phosphorylation (OP) The process in which NADH + H$^+$ and FADH$_2$ are oxidized in the electron transport system and the energy released is used to synthesize ATP from ADP and P$_i$.

Oxygen Consumption (V̇O$_2$) The amount or volume of oxygen taken up, transported, and used at the cellular level.

Oxygen Deficit The difference between the oxygen required during exercise and the oxygen supplied and utilized. Occurs at the onset of all activity.

Oxygen Dissociation The separation or release of oxygen from the RBCs to the tissues.

Oxygen Drift A situation that occurs in submaximal activity of long duration, or above 70% V̇O$_2$max, or in hot and humid conditions where the oxygen consumption increases, despite the fact that the oxygen requirement of the activity has not changed.

Partial Pressure of a Gas (P$_G$) The pressure exerted by an individual gas in a mixture; determined by multiplying the fraction of the gas by the total barometric pressure.

Peak Power (PP) The maximum power (force times distance divided by time) exerted during very short-duration (5 sec or less) work.

Percent Saturation of Hemoglobin (SbO$_2$%) The ratio of the amount of hemoglobin combined with oxygen to the total hemoglobin capacity for combining with oxygen, expressed as a percentage; indicated generally as SbO$_2$% or specifically as SaO$_2$% for arterial blood or as SvO$_2$% for venous blood.

Perfusion of the Lung Pulmonary circulation, especially capillary blood flow.

Periodization Plan for training based on a manipulation of the fitness components with the intent of peaking the athlete for the competitive season or varying health-related fitness training in cycles of harder or easier training.

Peripheral Cardiovascular Adaptations Adaptations that occur in the vasculature or muscles that increase the ability to extract oxygen.

Peripheral Cardiovascular Responses Responses directly related to the vessels.

Phosphorylation The addition of a phosphate (P$_i$).

Physical Activity Level (PAL) The ratio of total energy expenditure (TEE) to 24-hour resting or basal energy expenditure (RMR), that is, TEE/RMR.

Physical Fitness A physiological state of well-being that provides the foundation for the tasks of daily living, a degree of protection against hypokinetic disease, and a basis for participation in sport.

Power The amount of work done per unit of time; the product of force and velocity; the ability to exert force quickly.

Preload Volume of blood returned to the heart.

Pressor Response The rapid increase in both systolic pressure and diastolic pressure during static exercise.

Prevalence The number of cases of a disease in a specific population at a given time.

Proprioceptive Neuromuscular Facilitation (PNF) A stretching technique in which the muscle to be stretched is first contracted maximally. The muscle is then relaxed and either is actively stretched by contraction of the opposing muscle or is passively stretched.

Pulmonary Ventilation The process by which air is moved into and out of the lungs.

Rate Pressure Product (RPP) An estimate of the myocardial oxygen consumption, calculated as the product of heart rate (HR) and systolic blood pressure (SBP).

Rating of Perceived Exertion A subjective impression of overall physical effort, strain, and fatigue during acute exercise.

Reciprocal Inhibition The reflex relaxation of the antagonist muscle in response to the contraction of the agonist.

Recommended Daily Allowance (RDA) The average daily intake level that is sufficient to meet the nutrient requirement of 97–98% of healthy individuals by age and sex.

Reduction A loss of oxygen, a gain of electrons, or a gain of hydrogen by an atom or substance.

Reflex Rapid, involuntary response to stimuli in which a specific stimulus results in a specific motor response.

Relative Humidity The moisture in the air relative to how much moisture (water vapor) can be held by the air at any given ambient temperature.

Relative Submaximal Workload A workload above resting but below maximum that is prorated to each individual; typically set as some percentage of maximum.

Residual Volume (RV) The amount of air left in the lungs following a maximal exhalation.

Resistance Training A systematic program of exercises involving the exertion of force against a load, used to develop strength, endurance, and/or hypertrophy of the muscular system.

Resistance Vessels Another name for arterioles because this is the site of greatest resistance to blood flow in the vascular system.

Respiratory Cycle One inspiration and expiration.

Respiratory Exchange Ratio (RER) Ratio of the volume of CO_2 produced divided by the volume of O_2 consumed in the body as a whole.

Respiratory Quotient (RQ) Ratio of the amount of carbon dioxide produced divided by the amount of oxygen consumed at cellular level.

Resting Metabolic Rate (RMR) The energy expended while an individual is resting quietly in a supine position.

Risk Factor An aspect of personal behavior or lifestyle, an environmental exposure, or an inherited characteristic that has been shown by epidemiological evidence to predispose an individual to develop a specific disease.

Sarcomere The functional unit (contractile unit) of muscle fibers.

Sarcoplasmic Reticulum (SR) The specialized muscle cell organelle that stores and releases calcium.

Skinfolds The double thickness of skin plus the adipose tissue between the parallel layers of skin.

Sliding-Filament Theory of Muscle Contraction The theory that explains muscle contraction as the result of myofilaments sliding over each other.

Slow Oxidative (SO, Type I) Fibers Slow-twitch muscle fibers that rely primarily on oxidative metabolism to produce energy.

Spirometry An indirect calorimetry method for estimating heat production, in which expired air is analyzed for the amount of oxygen consumed and carbon dioxide produced.

Sports Anemia A transient decrease in red blood cells and hemoglobin level (grams per deciliter of blood).

Sport–Specific Physical Fitness That portion of physical fitness directed toward optimizing athletic performance.

Static Balance The ability to make adjustments to maintain posture while standing still.

Static Contraction A muscle contraction that produces an increase in muscle tension but does not cause meaningful limb displacement or joint displacement and therefore does not result in movement of the skeleton.

Static Stretching A form of stretching in which the muscle to be stretched is slowly put into a position of controlled maximal or near-maximal stretch by contraction of the opposing muscle group and held for 30–60 sec.

Steady-State A condition in which the energy provided during exercise is balanced with the energy required to perform that exercise, and factors responsible for the provision of this energy reach elevated levels of equilibrium.

Strength The ability of a muscle or muscle group to exert maximal force against a resistance in a single repetition.

Stress The state manifested by the specific syndrome that consists of all the nonspecifically induced changes within a biological system; a disruption in body homeostasis and all attempts by the body to regain homeostasis.

Stress Fracture A fine hairline break in bone that occurs without acute trauma, is clinically symptomatic, and is detectable by X-rays or bone scans.

Stress Reactions Maladaptive areas of bone hyperactivity where the balance between resorption and deposition is progressively lost such that resorption exceeds deposition.

Stroke Volume (SV) Amount of blood ejected from the ventricles with each beat of the heart.

Substrate Fuel substance acted on by an enzyme.

Substrate-Level Phosphorylation The transfer of P_i directly from a phosphorylated intermediate or substrates to ADP without any oxidation occurring.

Supramaximal Exercise An exercise bout in which the energy requirement is greater than what can be supplied aerobically at $\dot{V}O_2$max.

Synapse The gap, or junction, between terminal ends of the axon and other neurons, muscle cells, or glands.

Syncytium A group of cells of the myocardium that function collectively as a unit during depolarization.

Systole The contraction phase of the cardiac cycle.

Systolic Blood Pressure (SBP) The force exerted on the wall of blood vessels by the blood as a result of contraction of the heart (systole).

Thermic Effect of a Meal (TEM) The increased heat production as a result of food ingestion.

Thermogenesis The production of heat.

Thermoregulation The process whereby body temperature is maintained or controlled under a wide range of environmental conditions.

Tidal Volume (V_T) The amount of air that is inspired or expired in one breath.

Torque The capability of a force to produce rotation of a limb around a joint.

Total Lung Capacity (TLC) The greatest amount of air that the lungs can contain.

Total Peripheral Resistance (TPR) or Resistance (R) The factors that oppose blood flow.

Tracking A phenomenon in which a characteristic is maintained, in terms of relative rank, over a long time span or even a lifetime.

Training A consistent or chronic progression of exercise sessions designed to improve physiological function for better health or sport performance.

Training Adaptations Physiological changes or adjustments resulting from an exercise training program that promote optimal functioning.

Training Principles Fundamental guidelines that form the basis for the development of an exercise training program.

Training Taper A reduction in training load before an important competition that is intended to allow the athlete to recover from previous hard training, maintain physiological conditioning, and improve performance.

Training Volume The quantity of training overload calculated as frequency times duration for anaerobic or aerobic continuous exercise or number of sets times number of repetitions for resistance exercise).

Transamination The transfer of the NH_2 amino group from an amino acid to a keto acid.

Transverse Tubules (T Tubules) Organelles that carry the electrical signal from the sarcolemma into the interior of the cell.

Uncompensable Heat Stress A condition in which the evaporative cooling that is needed is greater than the evaporative cooling permitted by the environment.

Valsalva Maneuver Breath holding that involves closing of the glottis and contraction of the diaphragm and abdominal musculature.

Velocity at $\dot{V}O_2$max The speed at which an individual can run when working at his or her maximal oxygen consumption, based on both submaximal running economy and $\dot{V}O_2$max.

Ventilatory Equivalent The ratio of liters of air processed per liter of oxygen used ($\dot{V}_E/\dot{V}O_2$).

Ventilatory Thresholds Points where the rectilinear rise in minute ventilation breaks from linearity during an incremental exercise to maximum.

Vital Capacity (VC) The greatest amount of air that can be exhaled following a maximal inhalation.

Vitamins Organic substances of plant or animal origin that are essential for normal growth, development, metabolic processes, and energy transformations.

Voluntary Dehydration Exercise-induced dehydration that develops despite an individual's access to unlimited water.

Weight-Bearing Exercise A movement performed in which the body weight is supported by muscles and bones.

Weight Cycling Repeated bouts of weight loss and regain.

Wolff's Law Bone forms in areas of stress and is resorbed in areas of nonstress.

Index

Page numbers followed by "*fig*" indicate figures; those followed by "*t*" indicate tables; those followed by "*b*" indicate box.